CLINICAL

GYNECOLOGIC PATHOLOGY

CLINICAL GYNECOLOGIC PATHOLOGY

Enrique Hernandez, M.D.
Professor and Director, Division of
Gynecologic Oncology, and Vice-Chairman,
Department of Obstetrics and Gynecology
Medical College of Pennsylvania and
Hahnemann University School of Medicine
Philadelphia, Pennsylvania

Barbara F. Atkinson, M.D.
Professor and Chair, Department of
Pathology and Laboratory Medicine
Medical College of Pennsylvania and
Hahnemann University School of Medicine
Philadelphia, Pennsylvania

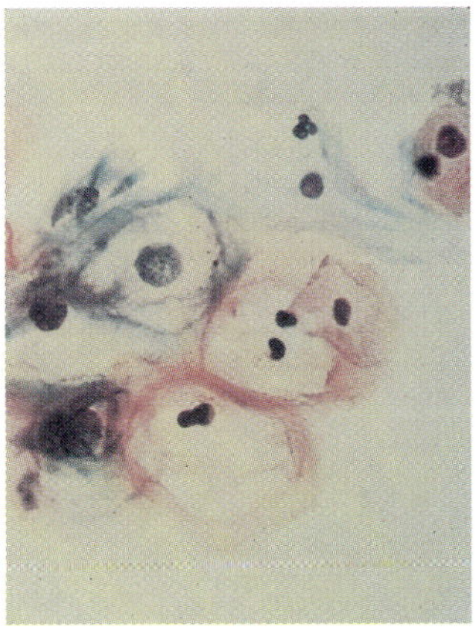

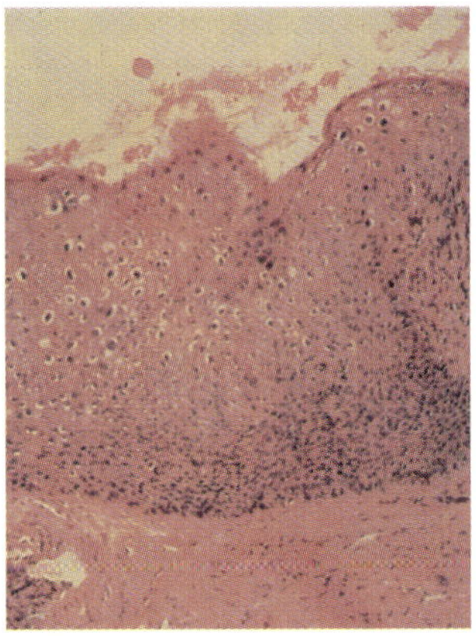

W.B. SAUNDERS COMPANY
A Division of Harcourt Brace & Company
Philadelphia London Toronto Montreal Sydney Tokyo

W.B. SAUNDERS COMPANY
A Division of
Harcourt Brace & Company

The Curtis Center
Independence Square West
Philadelphia, Pennsylvania 19106

Library of Congress Cataloging-in-Publication Data

Hernandez, Enrique.
Clinical gynecologic pathology/Enrique Hernandez, Barbara Atkinson.—1st ed.

p. cm.

ISBN 0–7216–5170–4

1. Pathology, Gynecological. I. Atkinson, Barbara F.
[DNLM: 1. Genital Diseases, Female—pathology. 2. Pathology, Clinical—methods. 3. Genitalia, Female—anatomy & histology. WP 141 H557c 1995]

RG77.H47 1995 618.1′07—dc20

DNLM/DLC 95-14246

Clinical Gynecologic Pathology ISBN 0–7216–5170–4

Printed in the United States of America

Last digit is the print number: 9 8 7 6 5 4 3 2 1

To Bill, Nancy and George, Mom and Dad

Barbara F. Atkinson, M.D.

To Dr. J. Donald Woodruff, friend and mentor,
who taught me the importance of understanding pathology
if you are to be a good gynecologist

Enrique Hernandez, M.D.

Contributors

Lisa L. Anderson, M.D.
Assistant Professor, Medical College of Pennsylvania and Hahnemann University School of Medicine, Department of Obstetrics and Gynecology, Division of Gynecologic Oncology, Philadelphia; Frankford Hospital, Philadelphia; Mercy Catholic Medical Center, Darby, Pennsylvania
Preinvasive Lesions of the Cervix and Vagina

Barbara F. Atkinson, M.D.
Professor and Chair, Department of Pathology and Laboratory Medicine, Medical College of Pennsylvania and Hahnemann University School of Medicine, Philadelphia, Pennsylvania
Preinvasive Lesions of the Cervix and Vagina / Malignant Neoplasms of the Cervix and Vagina

Gulnar Balsara, M.D.
Associate Professor, Department of Pathology and Laboratory Medicine, Medical College of Pennsylvania and Hahnemann University School of Medicine, Philadelphia, Pennsylvania
The Ovary: Normal, Physiologic Changes, Endometriosis, and Metastatic Tumors / Gestational Trophoblastic Disease

Paul B. Heller, M.D.
Associate Professor of Obstetrics and Gynecology, Division of Gynecologic Oncology, Medical College of Pennsylvania and Hahnemann University School of Medicine, Philadelphia, Pennsylvania
Malignant Neoplasms of the Cervix and Vagina

Enrique Hernandez, M.D.
Professor and Director, Division of Gynecologic Oncology, Medical College of Pennsylvania and Hahnemann University School of Medicine, Philadelphia, Pennsylvania
Benign Conditions of the Vagina and Cervix / Malignant Neoplasms of the Cervix and Vagina / The Ovary: Normal, Physiologic Changes, Endometriosis, and Metastatic Tumors / Tumors of the Ovarian Stroma / Gestational Trophoblastic Disease

Paul F. Kaminski, M.D.
Associate Professor, Department of Obstetrics and Gynecology, The Milton S. Hershey Medical Center, The Pennsylvania State University, Hershey, Pennsylvania
Benign Conditions of the Uterus / Premalignant and Malignant Conditions of the Uterus

Dennis M. O'Connor, M.D.
Associate Professor, Departments of Obstetrics and Gynecology and Pathology, University of Louisville School of Medicine, Louisville, Kentucky
Ovary–Germ Cell Tumors

Edward S. Podczaski, M.D.
Associate Professor, Department of Obstetrics and Gynecology, Division of Gynecologic Oncology, The Milton S. Hershey Medical Center, The Pennsylvania State University, Hershey, Pennsylvania
Benign Conditions of the Uterus / Premalignant and Malignant Conditions of the Uterus

Deborah E. Powell, M.D.
Professor and Chair, Department of Pathology and Laboratory Medicine, University of Kentucky College of Medicine and A.B. Chandler Medical Center, Lexington, Kentucky
Epithelial Tumors of the Ovary

Michael R. Spence, M.D., M.P.H.
Professor of Obstetrics and Gynecology and Medicine, Medical College of Pennsylvania and Hahnemann University School of Medicine, Philadelphia, Pennsylvania
Benign Conditions of the Vagina and Cervix

Richard J. Stock, M.D., M.P.H.
Captain, Medical Corps, United States Navy; Associate Professor of Clinical Obstetrics and Gynecology and Pathology, Eastern Virginia Medical School, Norfolk; Portsmouth General Hospital, Department of Obstetrics and Gynecology, Portsmouth Naval Hospital, Portsmouth, Virginia
The Fallopian Tubes

Cornelia Liu Trimble, M.D.
Clinical Fellow, Department of Gynecology and Obstetrics; Research Associate, Department of Pathology, The Johns Hopkins University School of Medicine, Baltimore, Maryland
Diseases of the Vulva / Tumors of the Ovarian Stroma

Edward L. Trimble, M.D., M.P.H.
Instructor, Department of Gynecology and Obstetrics, The Johns Hopkins University School of Medicine, Baltimore; Head, Surgery Section, Cancer Therapy Evaluation Program, National Cancer Institute, Bethesda, Maryland
Diseases of the Vulva / Tumors of the Ovarian Stroma

J. Donald Woodruff, M.D.
Richard W. Te Linde Professor Emeritus of Gynecologic Pathology, Professor Emeritus of Gynecology and Obstetrics, The Johns Hopkins University School of Medicine, Baltimore, Maryland
Diseases of the Vulva

Preface

My third year of residency in Gynecology and Obstetrics was the most formative of my professional career. During that year I had the opportunity to study gynecologic pathology under Professors J. Donald Woodruff and Tim H. Parmley at The Johns Hopkins Hospital. The experience in the pathology laboratory gave me a better understanding of the gross anatomy of the organs and structures that are removed in the operating suites. The clinical relevance of the pathologic diagnoses became clearer. The rationale behind the clinical approach to specific conditions was better defined. I also learned that arriving at a diagnosis is not any easier for the pathologist than it is for the clinician. Having a complete knowledge of the patient's medical history, physical examination, and laboratory and imaging studies, coupled with an understanding of the histopathology, would result in a more accurate diagnosis and treatment plan.

Gynecologic pathology in the United States started by accident when Dr. Thomas Cullen arrived from Canada at The Johns Hopkins Hospital, where there was no position for him. Dr. Howard Kelly, Gynecologist-in-Chief, sent him to Germany to study microscopy and bacteriology. Upon his return, Dr. Cullen became the Director of the newly established Gynecologic Pathology Laboratory. This laboratory gave gynecologists a better understanding of the diseases that they were treating and established the important relationship between pathology and gynecology. In 1900, Dr. Cullen described a typical case of carcinoma in situ of the cervix adjacent to invasive disease. The relationship between intraepithelial lesions of the cervix and invasive squamous cell carcinoma was better defined in 1944 by Dr. Cullen's successors, Drs. Galvin and Te Linde. At around the same time, Dr. George Papanicolaou introduced the study of cervical cytology. Although the field of pathology has expanded, histopathology and cytopathology continue to be the two techniques by which most gynecologic conditions are diagnosed and that are emphasized in this text. This textbook will allow the clinician to go through the diagnosis of a condition from the time the gross lesion is identified, examined with a colposcope (if applicable), biopsied or excised, and examined under the microscope. The clinicians will have a better understanding of the pathologic diagnosis and its implications for management. The pathologist, likewise, will gain a better understanding of the implications of his or her diagnosis with regard to management.

This textbook is composed of 12 chapters. Each chapter reviews the normal anatomy, cytology, and histology of the different genital structures. This is followed by the gross, cytologic, and histologic findings of benign and malignant conditions of the genital tract. Each condition is presented in a way that is familiar to clinicians. The gross findings are presented first, followed by cytology preparations, when applicable. The histopathologic findings are discussed in detail. Their clinical significance is presented, followed by a discussion on approaches to clinical management. The text is supported by over 500 color photographs of the gross, cytologic, and histopathologic findings that reflect what clinicians and pathologists see in actual practice. An extensive list of references is provided in each chapter.

We believe that this book will highlight the importance of pathology to the clinician. It is not enough to know whether a tumor is benign or malignant. An appreciation of the variety of pathologic diagnoses allows the clinician to better understand the prognosis and clinical approach to the disease. Likewise, the pathologist will realize the impact that the pathology diagnosis has on clinical management.

ENRIQUE HERNANDEZ, M.D.

I am convinced that the three most important factors in ensuring a correct pathology diagnosis in every case are the following: to have an adequate clinical history; to arrive at a differential diagnosis; and then to understand the entire context of the diagnostic entities being considered. This last factor means that it is necessary to understand the clinical features and presentation of the case as well as the gross and microscopic findings and the prognostic and treatment implications of a diagnosis. It should all fit together; if it doesn't, the diagnosis may be wrong or a new entity may be recognized.

In the same way the gynecologic surgeon must understand the cytopathology and histopathology and must communicate fully with the pathologist. Basic to all this is the correlation of the various types of pathology material, including biopsy, cytopathology, special stains, electron microscopy, immunocytochemistry, and molecular diagnostic techniques. In this book we have tried to incorporate all these aspects into a discussion of each of the gynecologic diseases. This will enable us all to more fully understand the significance and context of what we do.

As we edited this book our most important considerations were the correlation between clinical and pathology findings and the correlation of all kinds of pathology involved in a single entity. Another high priority was to provide color illustrations of the important aspects of each disease.

Anatomic pathology is predominantly a visual specialty. As in the cliché, "A picture is worth a thousand words," we have tried to provide a variety of illustrations, including those from the operating room, colposcopy, gross specimen examination, histopathology, cytopathology, and special stains. These were selected to show the most typical and diagnostic features of each case in an effort to tie together all the information.

BARBARA F. ATKINSON, M.D.

Contents

1

Diseases of the Vulva

Cornelia Liu Trimble / Edward L. Trimble / J. Donald Woodruff

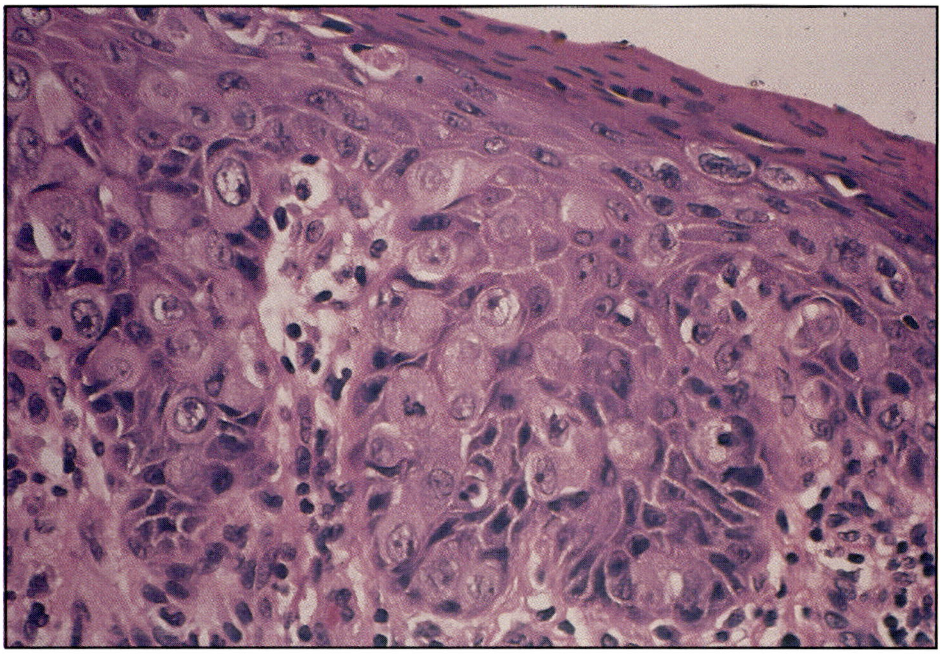

EMBRYOLOGY, NORMAL ANATOMY, AND HISTOLOGY

The vulva includes the labia majora, labia minora, mons pubis, clitoris, urinary meatus, vaginal orifice, hymen, vestibule, Bartholin's glands, Skene ducts, and vestibulovaginal bulbs. The vulvar epithelium is primarily of ectodermal origin. However, the shape of the vulva is the result of condensations of subepithelial mesoderm that appear during the third and fourth weeks of embryonic life. In the development of the external genitalia, the indifferent phase, which extends from the third to the eighth week of embryonic life, begins with the development of the genital tubercle (or eminence), which is anterior to the urogenital sinus (Fig. 1–1). This tubercle will become the clitoris. Both the urogenital folds (the future labia minora) and the labioscrotal folds (the future labia majora) develop between the fourth and sixth weeks of embryonic life. By the sixth week the cloacal membrane is divided into the urogenital membrane anteriorly and the anal membrane posteriorly. The urethra and the vestibule (or introitus) with its mucus-secreting glands are of endodermal (urogenital sinus) origin. The structures of the vulva have all been developed by the seventh to eighth week of embryonic life. Further differentiation involves the growth of these structures. Differentiation of the external genitalia into male-type structures begins to be recognizable by the tenth week of embryonic life.[1]

The anterior junction of the urogenital folds becomes the prepuce and the adjacent mons. The mons pubis (or mons veneris) is a cushion of fat covered by skin and its appendages. The labioscrotal folds (labia majora) are not fully developed until after puberty. These longitudinal folds of fat are covered by stratified squamous epithelium, which may have varying degrees of surface maturation and keratinization and an underlying layer of connective tissue that corresponds to the dartos of the male scrotum. The labia majora are virtually absent in a young child. Their development, which occurs primarily by the deposition of fat, is one of the secondary sex characteristics that herald puberty. The skin of the more prominent portions of the labia majora is pigmented and rich in hair follicles and sebaceous (holocrine) and sudoriferous glands (Figs. 1–2 and 1–3). The latter include the unique apocrine glands (Fig. 1–4), which are found only in specific areas (axilla, vulva, and perianal region). They are characterized by the presence of decapitation secretion, which means that the outer surface of the cell is shed as part of the secretory process. Because this secretion

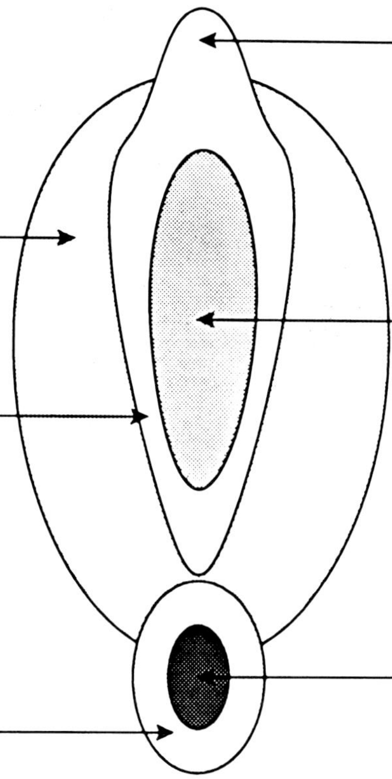

FIGURE 1-1
Schematic diagram of the external genitalia of the sixth- to eighth-week embryo. At this time sex differentiation has not occurred.

begins at puberty and because the cyclic nature of this activity follows that of the ovary, these apocrine glands may be designated accessory sex glands. An understanding of this cyclic activity is relevant to the diagnosis and treatment of certain vulvar diseases (e.g., Fox-Fordyce disease).

As previously described, the urogenital folds form the labia minora. However, in most women the labia minora do not join posteriorly. The fourchette of the vulva of the adult represents the posterior junction of the urogenital folds. The labia minora are composed primarily of vascular connective tissue. The surface stratified epithelium is characterized by a relative absence of the surface keratin and the underlying granular layer as well as hair follicles in the subcutaneous tissue. However, numerous sebaceous glands are present that, in the absence of hair follicles, secrete their contents directly onto the skin. Apocrine glands are rare in this area.

The corpora cavernosa in both sexes are formed by enlargement of vessels in the genital tubercle (penis or clitoris). The clitoris, like its male homologue the penis, is made up of vascular erectile tissue. However, the clitoris lacks the corpus spongiosum (Fig. 1–5). Nerve fibers are prominent in the clitoris, accounting for the response to tactile stimulation. The two vestibular bulbs, which are collections of veins situated beneath the anterior portion of the labial structures, are part of the corpus cavernosum.

The female urethra is mostly lined by transitional epithelium, but stratified squamous epithelium is present at or near the urethral meatus. It must be appreciated that the mesoderm of the wolffian (mesonephric) ducts contributes to the trigone and adjacent urethra and that the latter portion of epithelium responds to steroid hormone stimulation. The postmenopausal patient who has urinary tract irritation, manifested by symptoms such as urinary frequency and urgency, may achieve symptomatic relief when estrogen is used.

At each side of the dorsal border of the urethral meatus are the openings of the Skene (paraurethral) ducts, which are tiny, tortuous canals that course just beneath the urethra for a distance of about 1.5 cm. These are lined by squamous epithelium. These may be the seat of an infection that is inaccessible to treatment by local application of antibiotics. Also, it has been shown that the distal urethra is almost completely surrounded by a labyrinth of minor paraurethral glands. Occlusion of one or more of these glands produces a cyst. Subsequent infection may result in development of a suburethral abscess that occasionally causes urinary retention in women. In cases of recurrent urinary tract infection, the paraurethral canals should be suspected as a focus of infection, especially in the absence of other pathologic lesions. This is particularly true in patients whose urinary tract infections occur after coitus. Urethral

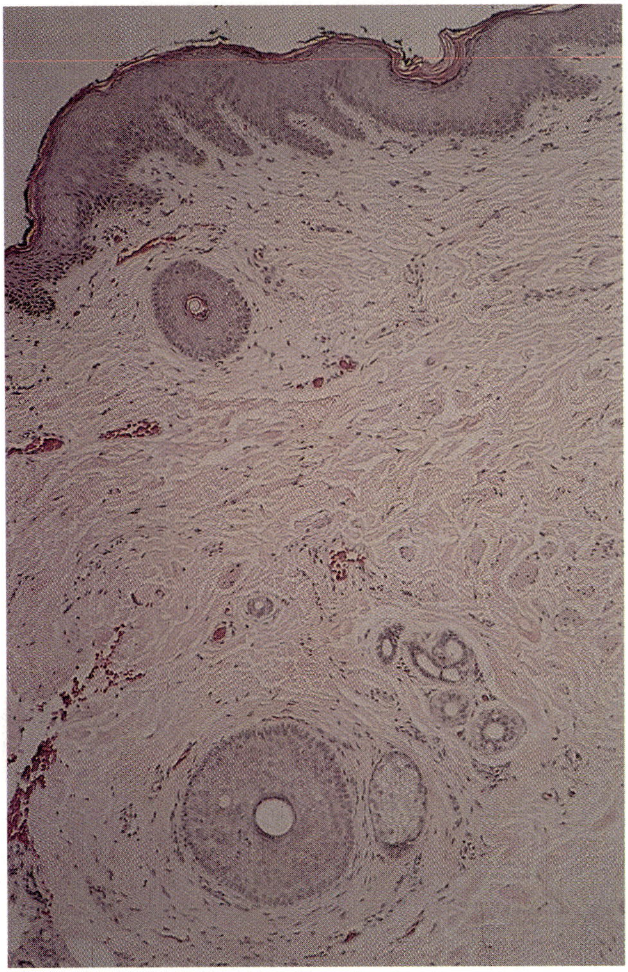

FIGURE 1-2
This section through the skin of the labium majus shows keratinized stratified squamous epithelium *(top)* and skin appendages in the underlying connective tissue. The keratinized stratified epithelium has several layers of acellular keratin on the surface that appears deep pink. The cells under the keratin layer have keratohyaline granules. This layer of cells is known as the granular zone or stratum granulosum. At the low magnification shown here, the granular zone appears as a bluish purple band immediately under the keratin layer (stratum corneum). The basal layer has a brownish color, which indicates the presence of melanin in the cells of the basal layer (stratum basale). Two hair follicles are seen cut on cross section. The hair shaft *(center)* is surrounded by multiple layers of squamous epithelium. Associated with the deeper hair follicle is a sebaceous gland immediately adjacent to it; lateral to that there are several sweat glands and ducts.

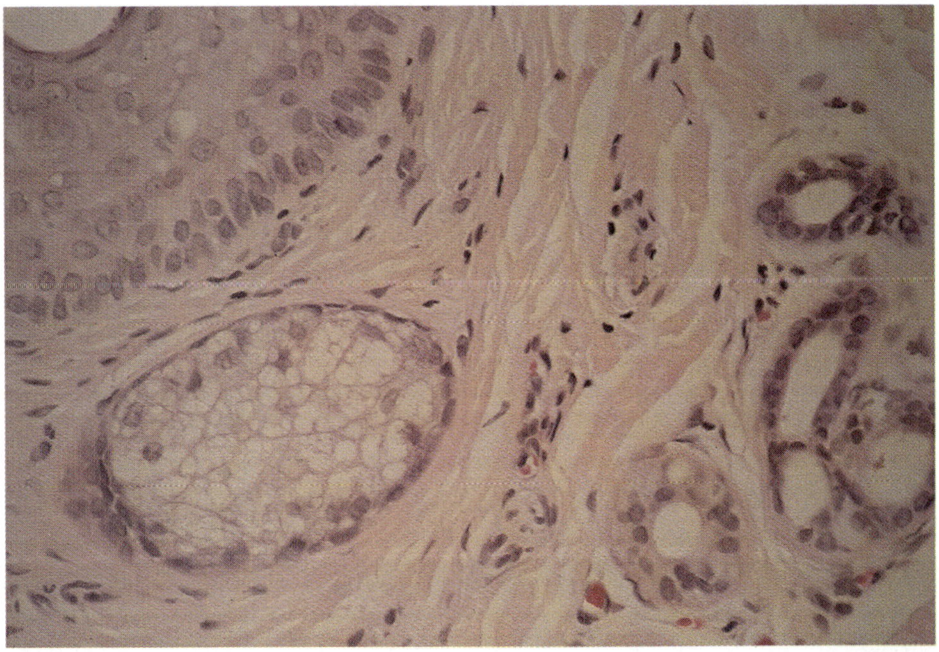

FIGURE 1-3
A portion of a hair follicle is seen *(left upper corner);* immediately under it is a sebaceous gland. A group of sweat glands and ducts is seen on the right. The ducts are lined by cuboidal to flattened cells with scant cytoplasm and a relatively hyperchromatic nuclear chromatin pattern. The cells of the glands are cuboidal but have more cytoplasm, which is lightly eosinophilic and has vacuoles.

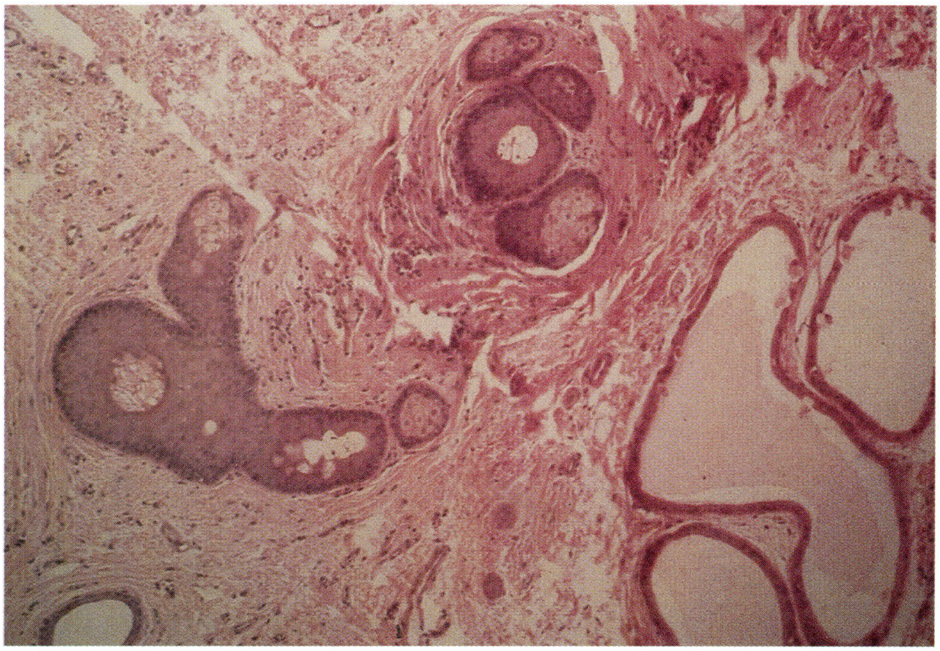

FIGURE 1-4
Various skin appendages are seen in this microphotograph. It can be appreciated that the sebaceous glands are incorporated within the stratified squamous epithelium of the hair follicle. Three dilated apocrine glands are seen *(bottom)*. They are lined by cells that contain abundant eosinophilic cytoplasm.

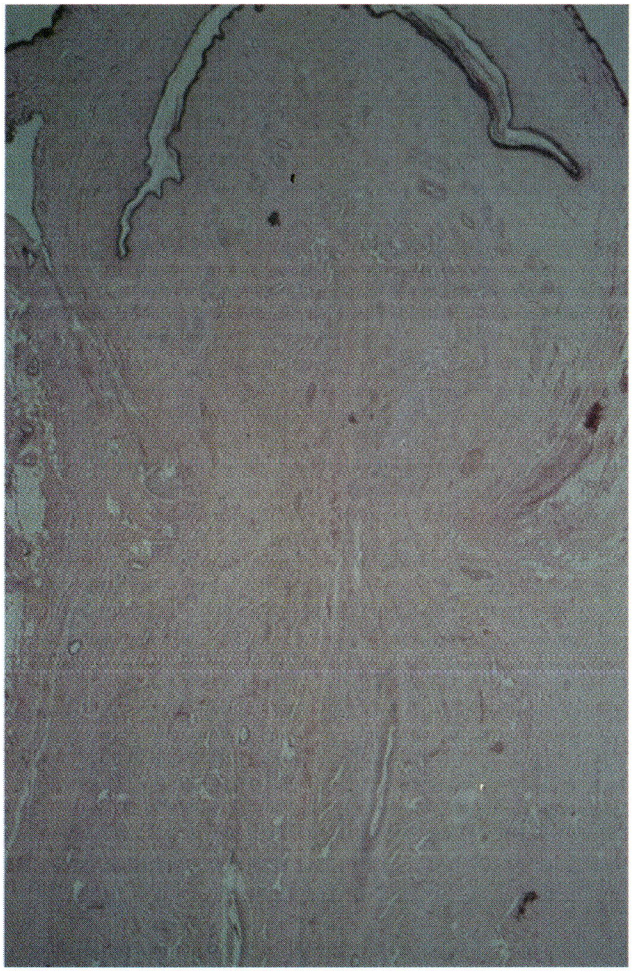

FIGURE 1-5
This is a cross section of the clitoris and its prepuce. The stratified squamous epithelium covering these structures is seen as a purple band. A prominent network of erectile tissue and vessels is seen through the middle of the connective tissue.

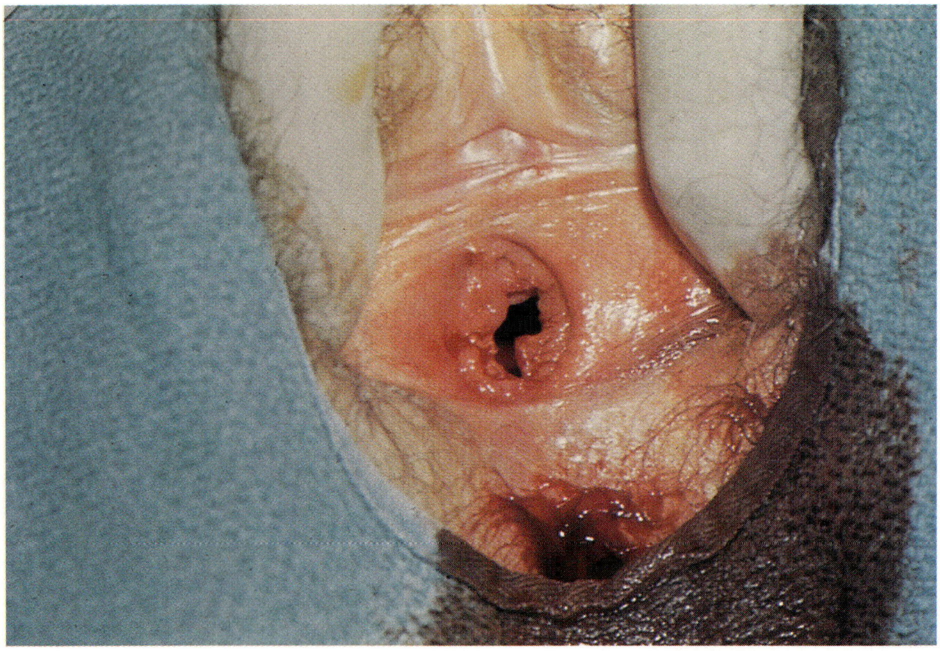

FIGURE 1-6
The vestibule seen here shows the hymen after it has been opened.

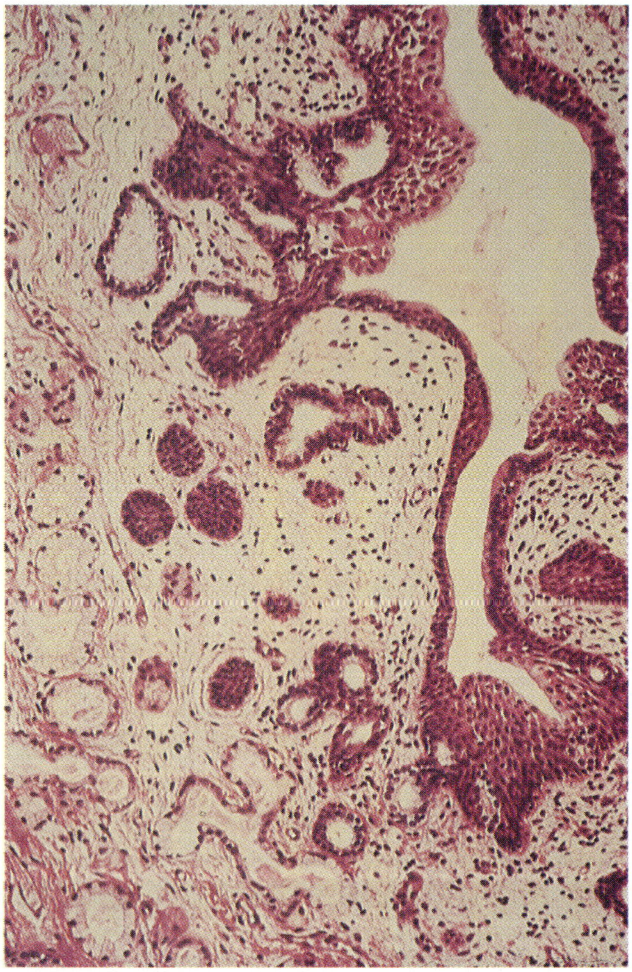

FIGURE 1-7
This is a cross section of Bartholin gland and duct. The duct is the large structure lined by squamous and transitional epithelium. The stratified squamous epithelium is seen best at the bottom of the duct, but even here the cells at the surface are cuboidal. At the top left border of the duct the epithelium is transitional. The mucus-secreting glands are seen *(left).*

diverticula may be the locus for these infections (see Chapter 2).

The hymen, which partially closes the orifice of the vagina in women who have not been sexually active, consists of a double plate of stratified squamous epithelium between which is a well-developed layer of dense but vascular connective tissue. Residual tags of the hymen (hymenal caruncles) are frequently noted at the introitus. "Hymenal polyps" have been reported in young girls and must be differentiated from sarcoma botryoides (see Chapter 3). An imperforated hymen causes no problems until menarche, when the patient develops cyclic pelvic pain and a hematocolpos. This can progress to hematometra, hematosalpinx, and hematoperitoneum. The last condition has been associated with pelvic endometriosis. A cruciate incision of the hymen will allow satisfactory drainage of the menstrual blood (Fig. 1–6).

The vestibule contains Bartholin's glands (vulvovaginal glands) situated on each side of the vulva beneath Colle's fascia within the depths of the perineum. These correspond histologically to Cowper glands, which empty into the membranous urethra of the male. The orifice of the gland occasionally may be seen at the introitus, approximately midway between the urethra and the fourchette and caudad to the hymenal ring. When the duct opening is quite conspicuous and surrounded by an erythematous areola it is known as the gonorrheal macule of Sanger. However, infection with organisms other than *Neisseria gonorrhoeae* may be responsible for this finding.

Bartholin's glands are racemose; their lobulation is significant when surgical excision is indicated. Care must be taken to remove the entire gland. Fortunately, such surgery is rarely necessary today because incision and marsupialization of the dilated duct usually results in adequate drainage and avoids an extensive dissection.[2] The incision for drainage should be placed in the region of the normal gland orifice at the introitus, not through the skin of the labia minora. Removal is indicated only when deep-seated infections recur or when the possibility of neoplasm exists.

The stratified epithelium at the orifice of Bartholin's gland changes to transitional epithelium in the main duct. As the duct divides, the epithelium has fewer and fewer layers, and the superficial layer of cells remains columnar or cuboidal. The acini are lined by a mucus-secreting epithelium, in which the nuclei are located near the basement membrane (Fig. 1–7).

It is important to appreciate that, as in the male, there are minor (Littre) as well as major vestibular glands. The introitus is ringed with these smaller glands, which are variants of Bartholin's gland. These superficial glands lie immediately external to the hymenal ring and may be the seat of chronic or recurrent infections that lead to irritation at the outlet, thus causing dyspareunia.

The blood supply to most of the vulva is derived from the internal pudendal artery, which is a branch of the internal iliac (hypogastric) artery. The veins follow a similar path but also communicate with the vesicovaginal plexus and the inferior hemorrhoidal veins. The dorsal vein of the clitoris runs beneath the symphysis pubis to reach the pelvic veins. The lymphatic drainage of lateral structures is to the ipsilateral inguinal nodes. However, contralateral node metastases in the absence of ipsilateral metastasis have been reported in 2.5 percent of unilateral squamous cell carcinomas of the vulva.[3] Rich lymphatic anastomoses occur in the perineum.[4] Therefore, malignancies in this area could drain to either groin. Direct metastasis to pelvic lymph nodes from a cancer located in the clitoris is rare.[5]

The innervation of the vulva has multiple sources. The pudendal nerve, which is derived from the second to the fourth sacral nerves, gives off the perineal nerve from which the posterior labial nerve arises. The latter innervates most of the vulva. Additional innervation is supplied by the perineal branch of the femoral cutaneous nerve and the anterior labial branch of the ilioinguinal nerve.[6]

MALFORMATIONS

Congenital anomalies of the vulva are rare. The most common relate to pseudohermaphroditism. A male pseudohermaphrodite has testes but also has some degree of incomplete masculinization of the genitalia (Fig. 1–8). A female pseudohermaphrodite has ovaries, but some degree of masculinization of the external genitalia is present as well. This is most often the result of congenital adrenal hyperplasia and frequently causes clitorimegaly (Fig. 1–9). The ingestion of androgenic steroids by the mother during pregnancy is an extremely rare cause of this problem.

On occasion, a cyst may be found at the introitus of the newborn. This disappears spontaneously in almost all cases and probably represents local edematous tissue enlargement rather than a true tumor.

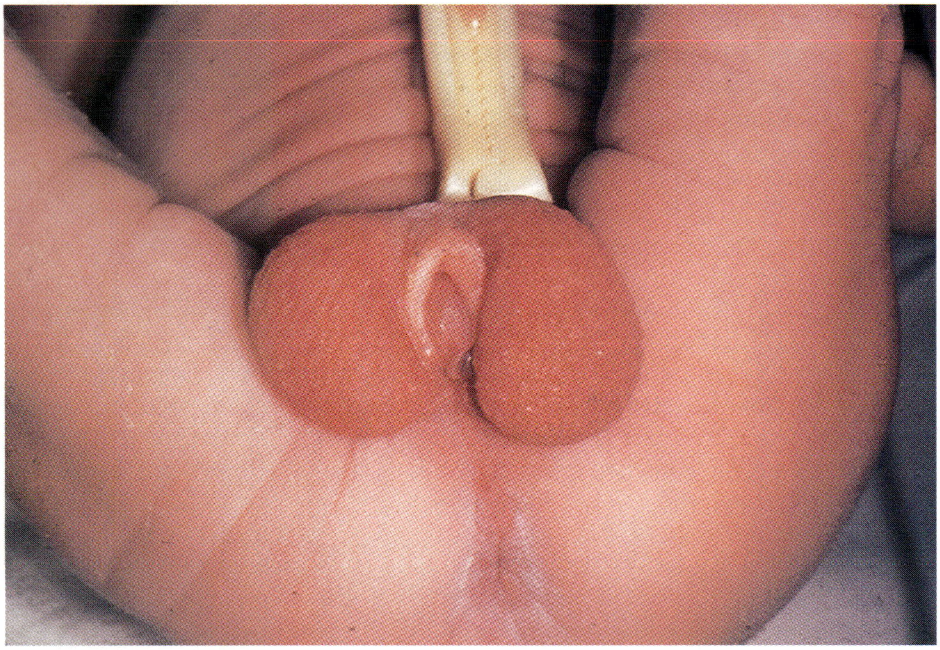

FIGURE 1-8
This baby was born with a congenital malformation that includes the presence of a scrotum but lack of development of a penis. This could be the result of either a female fetus exposed to androgens in utero or a male pseudohermaphrodite with incomplete development of the external genitalia.

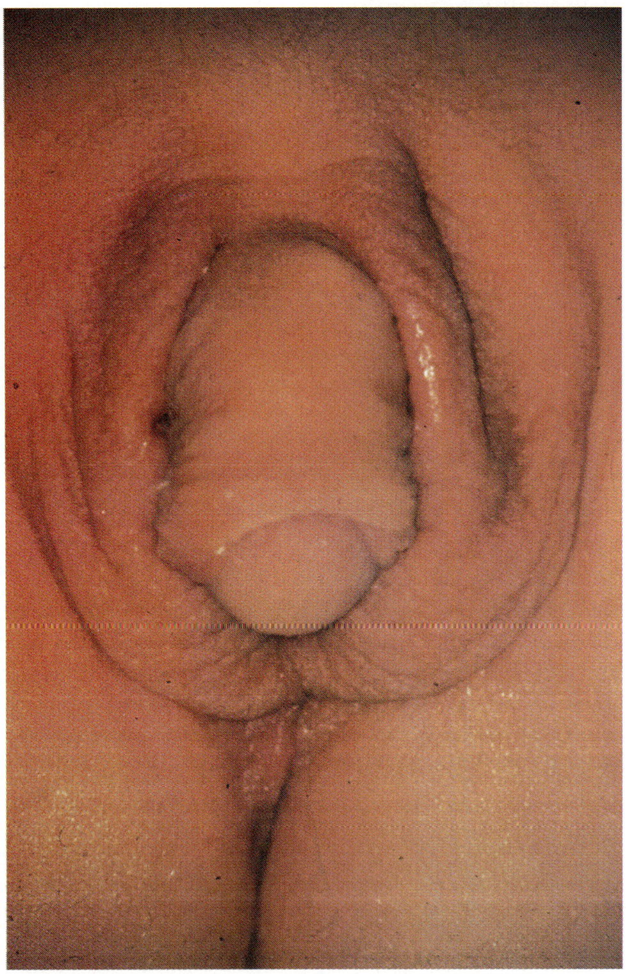

FIGURE 1-9
This female child has clitorimegaly. This was secondary to congenital adrenal hyperplasia.

INFLAMMATORY AND ULCERATIVE DISEASE

Reactive Vulvitis

Since the vulva is of ectodermal origin, the common inflammatory processes affecting it are similar to those found elsewhere on the skin. The most frequent type of dermatitis is irritative or reactive and results from an association of local moisture (retained by tight "nonbreathing" clothing) with local irritants (e.g., topical medications, colored or scented toilet paper, detergents, hygiene sprays). When vulvitis is present it is also important to examine the vagina because the vulvar inflammation may be caused by a reaction to a vaginal discharge. During the acute phase of the dermatitis, erythema and edema are the rule. This is often associated with superficial vulvar traumatic excoriation due to scratching (Fig. 1–10). If a biopsy is performed during the acute phase, a florid acute inflammatory cell infiltrate within the dermis is seen, and superficial epithelial ulcerations may be present. However, biopsy is recommended only when there are areas of hyperkeratosis, atypical pigmentation, or ulcerations that are thought to be possibly malignant. In the acute phase of dermatitis, the trauma of biopsy may accentuate the symptoms. In contrast, biopsy of chronic lesions is imperative if early neoplasia is to be diagnosed.

The pruritus of acute dermatitis is treated with a topical corticosteroid. The allergic or toxic agent must be eliminated. The use of loose-fitting clothing is recommended. A mixture of baby powder and cornstarch can be applied to the vulva to help keep it dry.

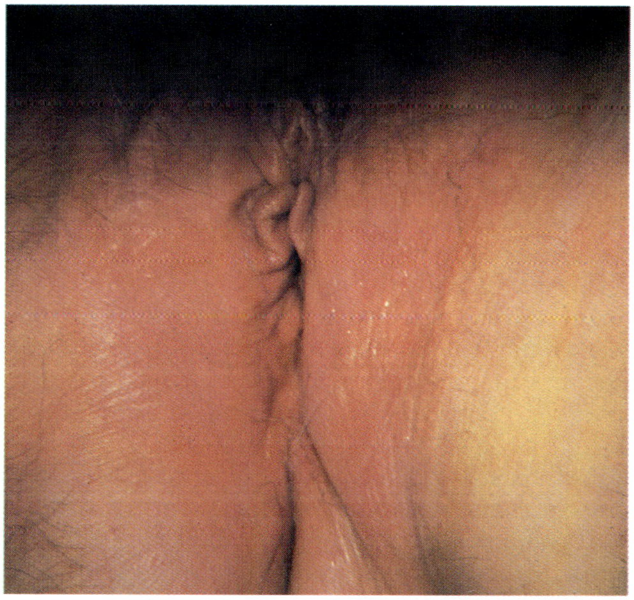

FIGURE 1–10
There is erythema and edema of the vulva in this patient who has acute dermatitis.

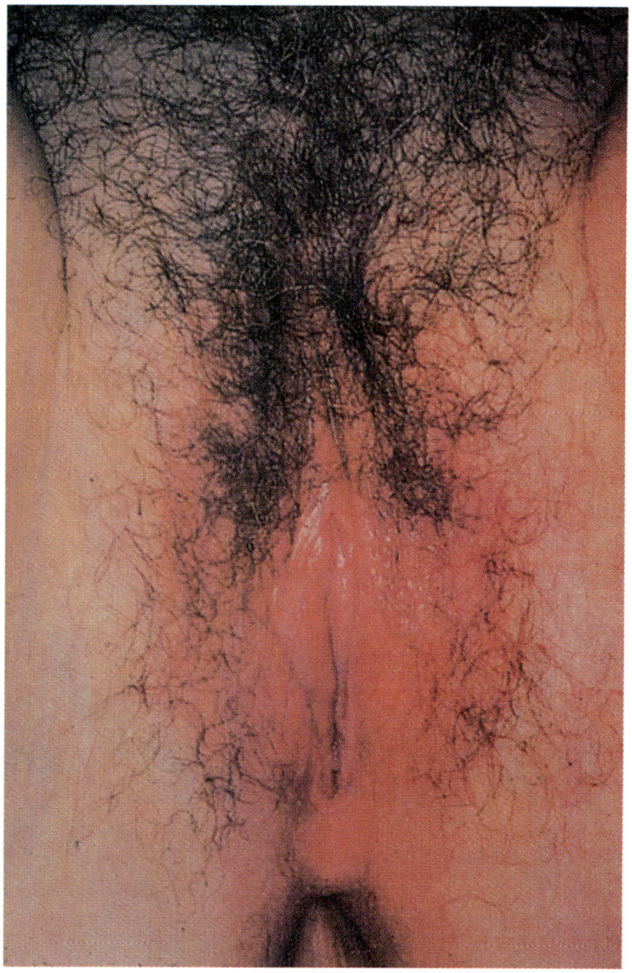

FIGURE 1–11
This case of acute seborrheic dermatitis shows generalized vulvar erythema. Scaly small white patches are seen on the left labium majus.

Seborrheic Dermatitis

Seborrheic dermatitis (dandruff) occurs on the vulva as in other areas of the skin (Fig. 1–11). These lesions are slightly elevated, scaly patches. In the acute phase they are erythematous. In the chronic phase the patches are grayish-white and become the site of intense pruritus. This is treated by topical fluorinated hydrocortisone (e.g., fluocinonide). It is now thought that seborrheic dermatitis is an inflammatory reaction to a commensal fungus, *Pityrosporum ovale.* The two widely used agents against dandruff, selenium sulfide and zinc pyrithione, are active against *Pityrosporum.* Another antifungal agent, ketoconazole, has recently been introduced as a shampoo for the treatment of dandruff.[6a] However, zinc pyrithione is effective, well tolerated, and costs one-tenth as much as ketoconazole. Seborrheic dermatitis should not be confused clinically with psoriasis, which will be discussed later.

Intertrigo

Intertrigo or intertriginous dermatitis (eczema) is common in areas of the body where moist tissues are apposed, especially in obese patients. On the vulva during the acute phase there is fissuring of macerated, erythematous skin in the intercrural or interlabial folds (Fig. 1–12). In the chronic phase there are thickened and grayish-white skin features that are just as typical of any long-standing dermatitis characterized by hyperkeratosis. Weight loss and elimination of moisture at the site is the best therapy, but this may be difficult for many patients. The application of a mixture of baby powder and cornstarch helps to absorb moisture. Loose-fitting cotton clothes should be worn. The lesions are frequently intensely pruritic. This pruritus can be controlled by using a potent topical corticosteroid that is thoroughly rubbed into the area. Eurax is a nonsteroidal agent that is a good topical antipruritic agent and can also be used. Its mechanism of action is not well defined.

Chronic Dermatitis

The gross appearance of lesions of chronic dermatitis is caused by hyperkeratosis, which produces a whitish or grayish-white discoloration of the skin (Fig. 1–13) or a white plaque. This white plaque has been called leukoplakia. The idea that "leukoplakia" is premalignant has led to confusion. The term leukoplakia should be avoided because it encompasses many different clinical lesions that have different causes. The microscopic appearance of chronic dermatitis is characterized by hyperkeratosis, acanthosis (elongation of the rete pegs), and a chronic inflammatory cell infiltrate in the dermis. There is no mitotic activity or abnormal maturation (Fig. 1–14).

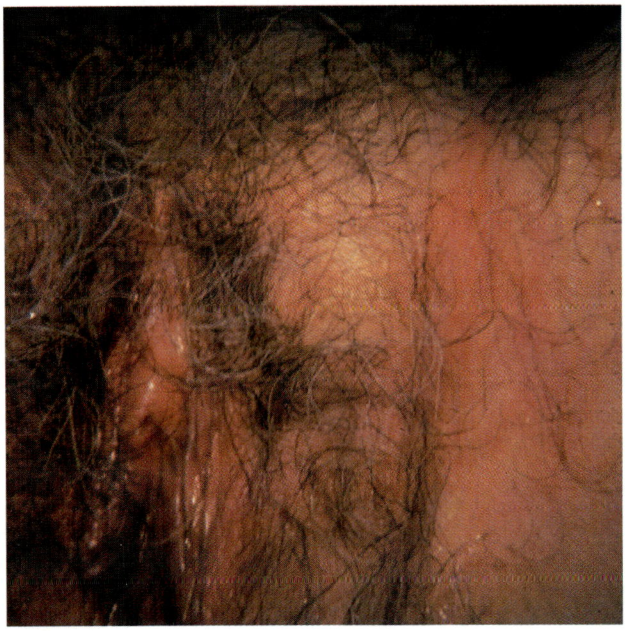

FIGURE 1–12
This intercrural area shows moist, erythematous, macerated skin. This is known as intertrigo.

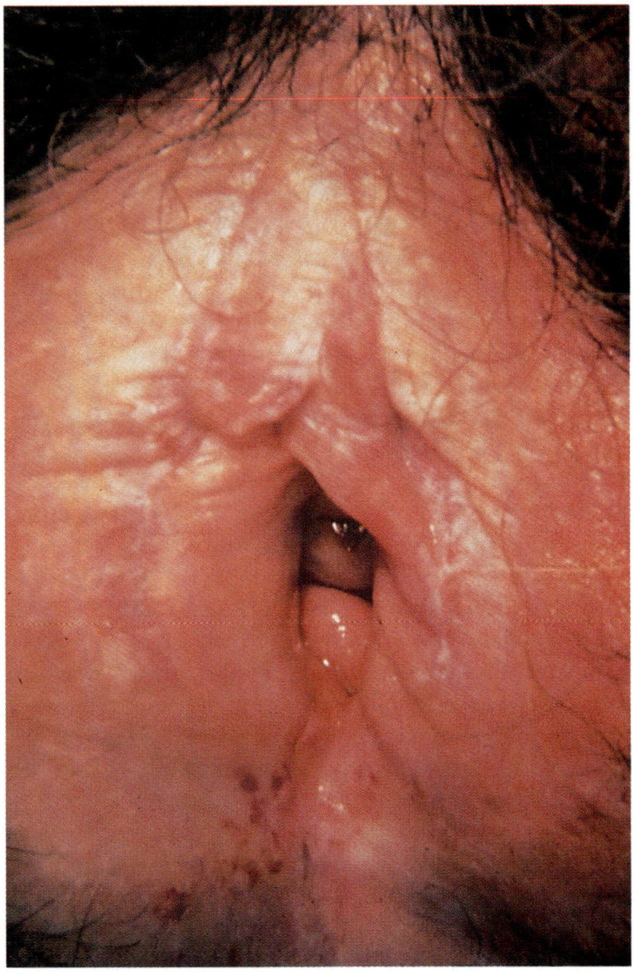

FIGURE 1–13
The skin of this vulva, which shows chronic dermatitis, appears dry, constricted, and whitish. Excoriation marks are seen in the perineum. The chronic changes distort the normal appearance of the vulva.

Chronic dermatitis causes severe pruritus. It has been suggested that chronic irritation from scratching could initiate a neoplastic transformation in the vulvar skin that may lead to malignancy.[7, 8] Biopsy with microscopic examination should be used to classify appropriately a "white lesion" on the vulva as chronic dermatitis, vulvar intraepithelial neoplasia, or cancer.

A potent topical corticosteroid such as fluorinated hydrocortisone can be used initially to treat a patient who has chronic vulvitis. However, a thick keratin layer may prevent penetration of the

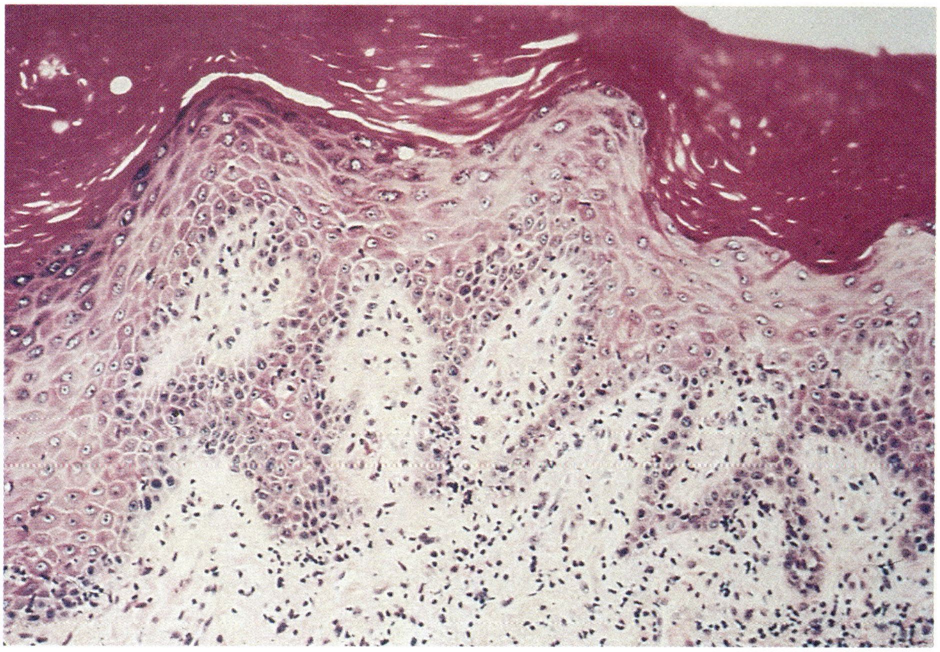

FIGURE 1–14
This is a biopsy from a patient who had chronic dermatitis. There is marked hyperkeratosis and acanthosis. A round cell infiltrate is present in the dermis.

steroid into the dermis. Subcutaneous corticosteroid (e.g., triamcinolone acetonide suspension 10 mg/ml) injections have been used successfully.[9] Hydroxyzine hydrochloride can also be used at bedtime to break the "itch-scratch" cycle. In recalcitrant cases, subcutaneous alcohol injection performed under general anesthesia interferes with the nerve endings and achieves relief for up to 6 months to a year.[10] The Mering procedure, which denervates the vulva, can be considered when all other approaches fail.[11]

In some patients with chronic dermatitis a diagnosis of neurodermatitis is made.[12] This suggests a psychological component in the cause of the condition. The use of psychotropic drugs may be a helpful adjunct to local therapy in these cases.

Lichen Planus

Lichen planus is an uncommon cutaneous disease that is probably of autoimmune origin and may rarely affect the vulva. A patient who has lichen planus of the vulva typically complains of vulvar burning and sometimes of pruritus. The labia minora and the vestibule are typically involved; the vagina can also be affected. Erythema and atrophy are present. Ulceration can occur and may lead to coaptation of the labia with obliteration of the introitus (Fig. 1–15). Lichen planus of the vulva is frequently misdiagnosed as atrophic or infectious vulvovaginitis. When treatment is unsuccessful a biopsy may be helpful. This leads to a correct diagnosis. The biopsy shows acanthosis, basal cell degeneration with formation of necrotic keratinocytes, and a heavy, bandlike, lymphocytic and histiocytic infiltrate in the adjacent dermis (Fig. 1–16). If an area of ulceration or erosion is taken as a sample for biopsy, the epithelium will be absent, and the correct diagnosis will be missed. Instead, a diagnosis of chronic ulcerative vulvitis is made.

Patients who have lichen planus on the vulva may have lesions at other sites as well, including the mouth and limbs. The oral lesions are characterized by interlacing white lines on an erythematous mucosa. On the skin, the lesions are very small, polygonal, glistening papules that frequently have central umbilication.

Corticosteroids or tretinoin used topically have had limited success.[13] We have recently treated a patient successfully with subcutaneous injections of triamcinolone acetonide suspension, 10 mg/ml. This approach deserves further consideration.

Vulvitis circumscripta plasmacellularis is considered by some to be an erosive variant of lichen planus.[13a] A well-circumscribed, glistening, erythematous lesion that has an orange hue is seen at the introitus or lateral aspect of the labium minus (Fig. 1–17). The histopathologic findings are marked epithelial edema, hemosiderin deposition, and a bandlike infiltrate containing many plasma cells that is found in the underlying connective tissue. Prominent small vessels are also seen. Degeneration of the basal layer of epithelium, which is characteristic of lichen planus, may not be present in vulvitis circumscripta plasmacellularis.

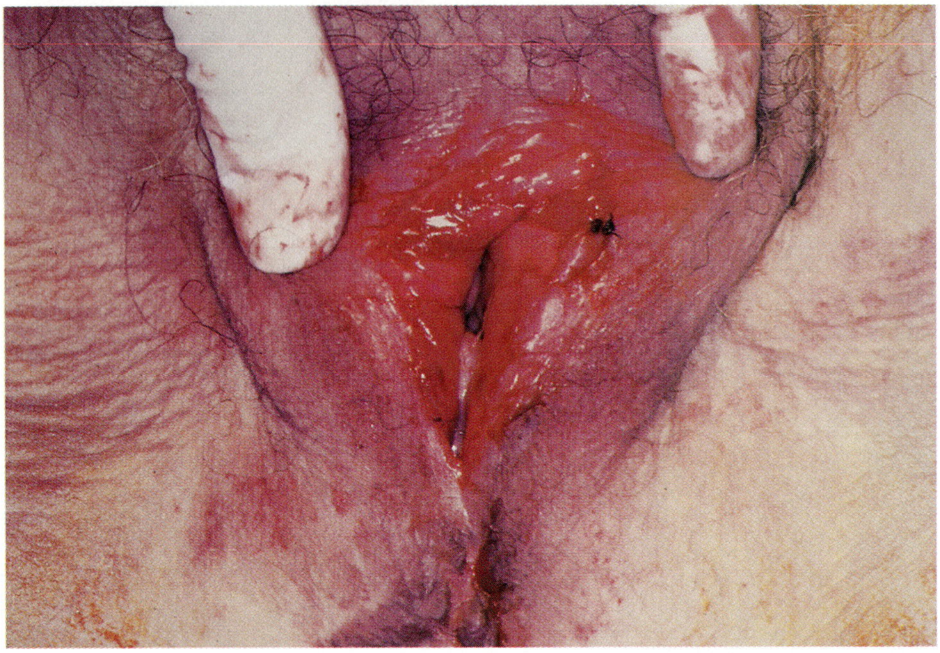

FIGURE 1-15
In this patient who has lichen planus the lower labia minora have been fused and have just been separated. They show marked erythema and atrophy. A suture is present at a biopsy site on the left labium.

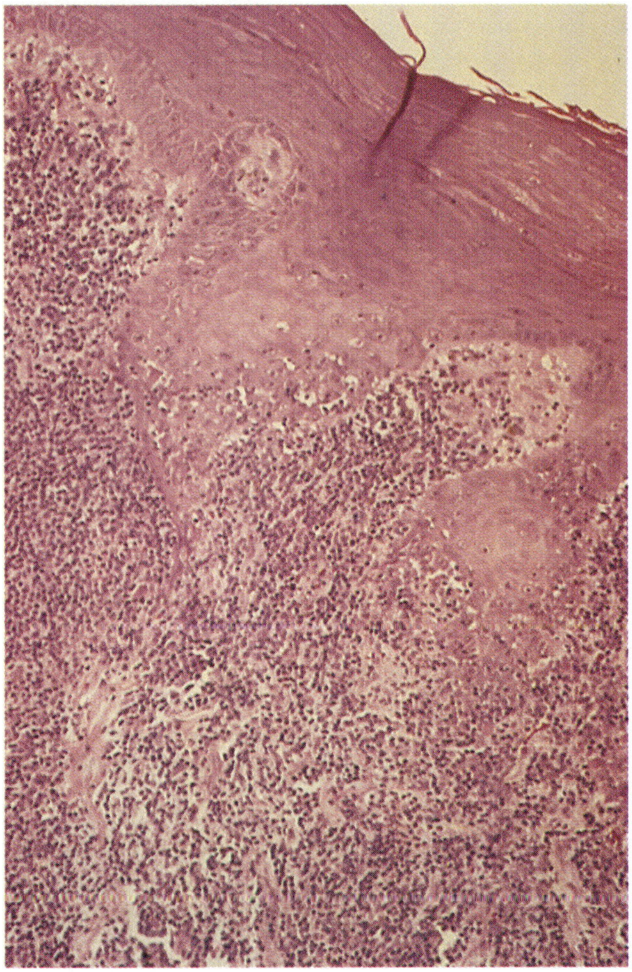

FIGURE 1-16
This biopsy of lichen planus shows a marked round cell infiltrate filling the dermis. The basal layers of the epithelium are disrupted by the infiltrate. The rete pegs are wide, and there is parakeratosis.

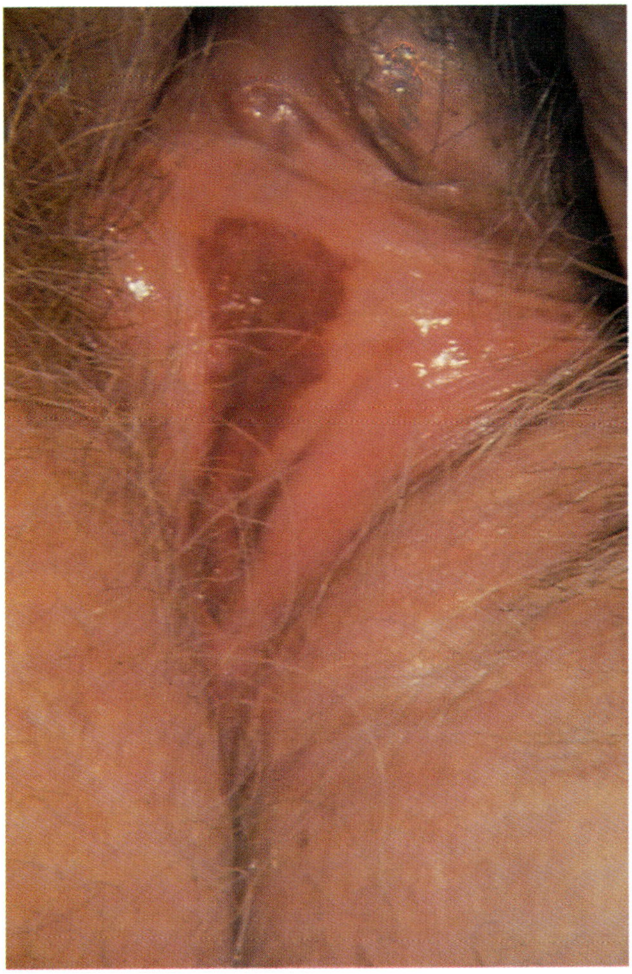

FIGURE 1-17
A well-circumscribed, shiny, red lesion occupies the introitus. This finding is typical of vulvitis circumscripta plasmacellularis.

Vulvar Vestibulitis

A relatively common disorder, vulvar vestibulitis is characterized by vulvar pain and severe, acquired entry dyspareunia. Slightly erythematous, tender macules are found in the mucosa of the vestibule (Fig. 1–18). These commonly involve the fourchette. Biopsy shows a nonspecific chronic inflammatory infiltrate in the subepithelial stroma surrounding the minor vestibular glands (Fig. 1–19). The etiology of this condition is not known. Perineoplasty (Fig. 1–20) offers the best treatment results. Symptomatic improvement occurs in approximately one-third of patients.[13b, 13c]

Psoriasis

The mons and crural folds are relatively common sites of psoriasis; however, the vulva is rarely the sole site of involvement on the body. The gross appearance of psoriasis on the vulva is often atypical and frequently does not resemble psoriasis elsewhere (Fig. 1–21). The characteristic "silver scales" are often absent owing to the moisture in the area. Nevertheless, the classic features are usually apparent on lesions elsewhere on the body. The lesions are irregular, multifocal patches that have an erythematous background. Elevated silver scales may be prominent (Fig. 1–22). The adjacent skin may demonstrate excoriations, accentuation of the skin markings, or lichenification.

Fox-Fordyce Disease

Fox-Fordyce disease is caused by obstruction of the apocrine gland. The labia majora and mons are dotted with tiny, slightly elevated, firm, intensely pruritic papules (Fig. 1–23). The labia minora, prepuce, and clitoris, which do not contain apocrine glands, are spared in this disease, but these areas may be edematous. On microscopic examination focal nests of dilated apocrine glands are found that show little, if any, evidence of inflammatory reaction (Fig. 1–24). The process is usually cyclic and is related to the secretory activity of the apocrine glands. Oral contraceptives

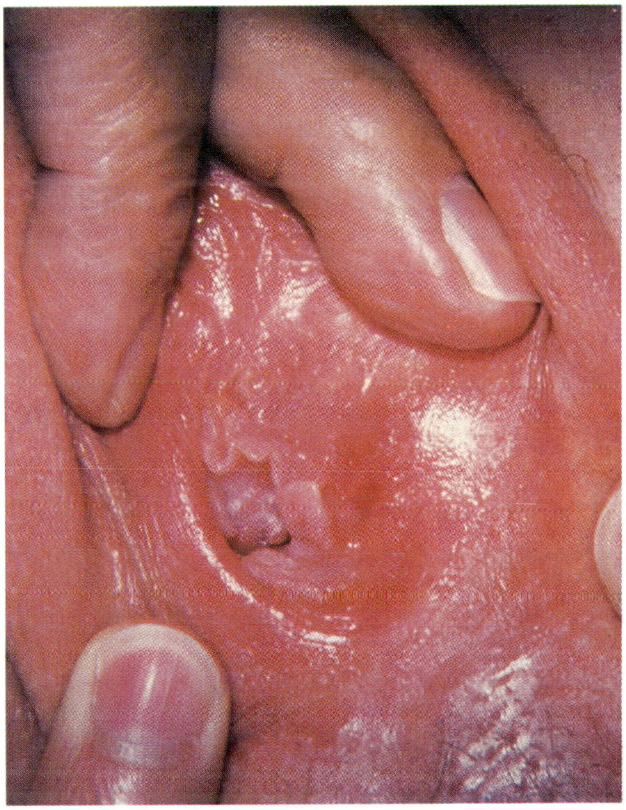

FIGURE 1-18
An erythematous macule is seen on the left vulva just beside the hymenal ring. This is characteristic of vulvar vestibulitis.

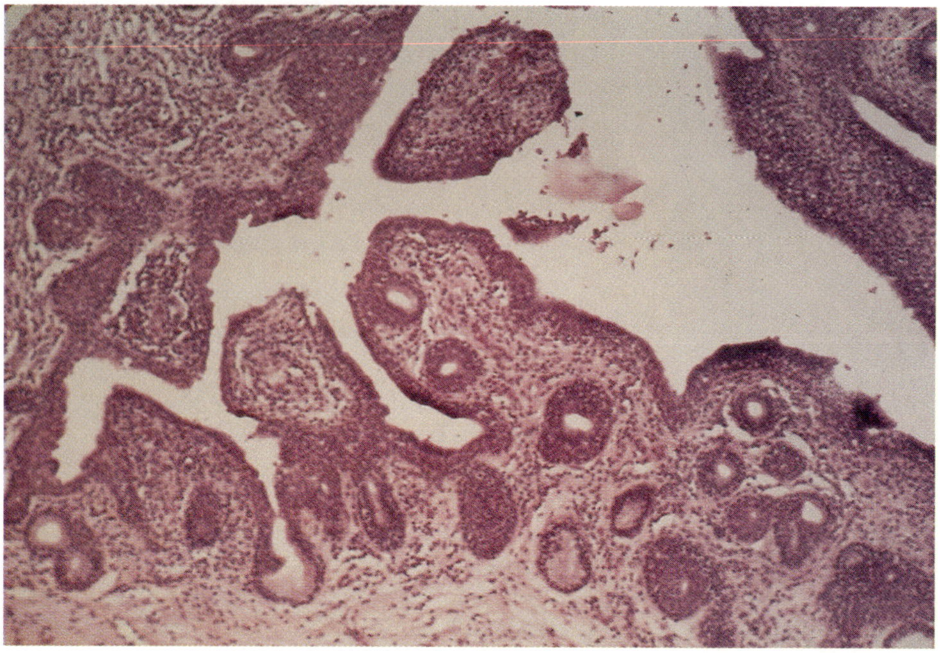

FIGURE 1-19
This cross section of the vestibule shows squamous epithelium and minor vestibular glands. There is a round cell infiltrate in the subepithelial stroma.

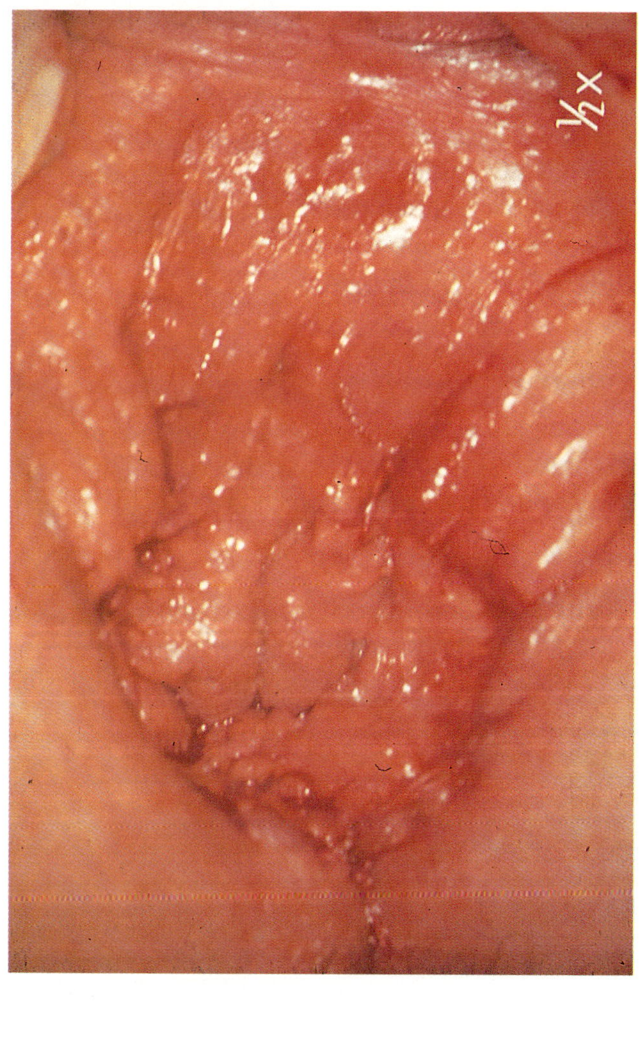

FIGURE 1-20
This patient has had a perineoplasty for vulvar vestibulitis. The vestibule has been excised. The mucosa of the posterior vaginal wall has been mobilized and sutured to the perineum at the bottom. The vaginal tube is in the center, and just above it is the urethral opening.

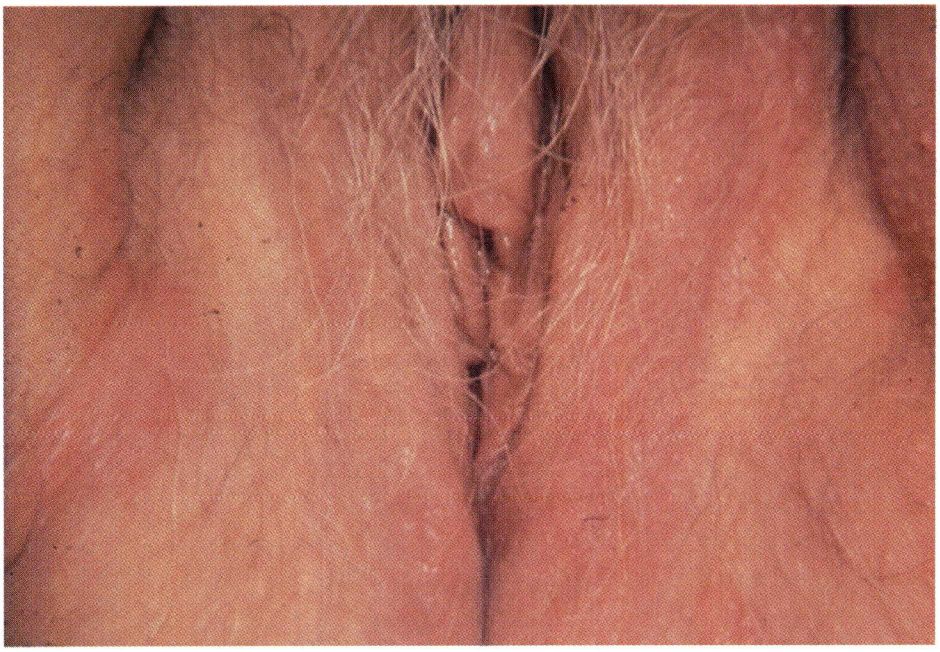

FIGURE 1-21
This patient has psoriasis on the vulva. Several well-demarcated, raised, erythematous patches are seen. Some lesions have grayish white scales.

(which reduce apocrine gland secretions) and local antipruritic medications are usually effective. In unusual cases treatment similar to that described for chronic dermatitis may be necessary.

Crohn Disease

Crohn disease (regional enteritis) may involve the lower genital tract (Fig. 1–25). Draining sinuses and rectoperineal or rectovaginal fistulae develop in approximately 20 to 25 percent of patients with documented intestinal disease.[14, 15] These may drain into the posterior fourchette. The adjacent vulva may show linear excoriations and edema. The diagnosis is difficult unless the clinician is aware of the patient's disease and this association. On rare occasions, there may be little or no definite evidence of intestinal Crohn disease. Biopsy of the intestines or fistulae shows a chronic inflammatory infiltrate, and occasionally noncaseating granulomas may be present (Fig. 1–26). Treatment includes systemic steroids and metronidazole.[16] Surgery to remove or repair the affected area without the use of these medications perioperatively is doomed to fail.

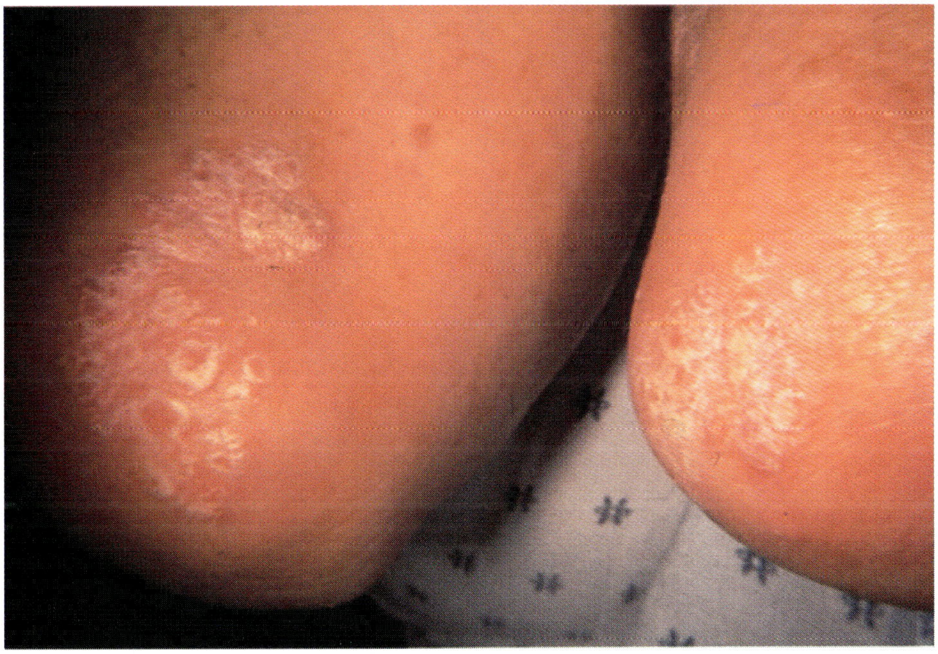

FIGURE 1-22
This is the same patient shown in Figure 1–21 who also has lesions on the elbows. Here the raised, irregular patches have prominent silvery scales.

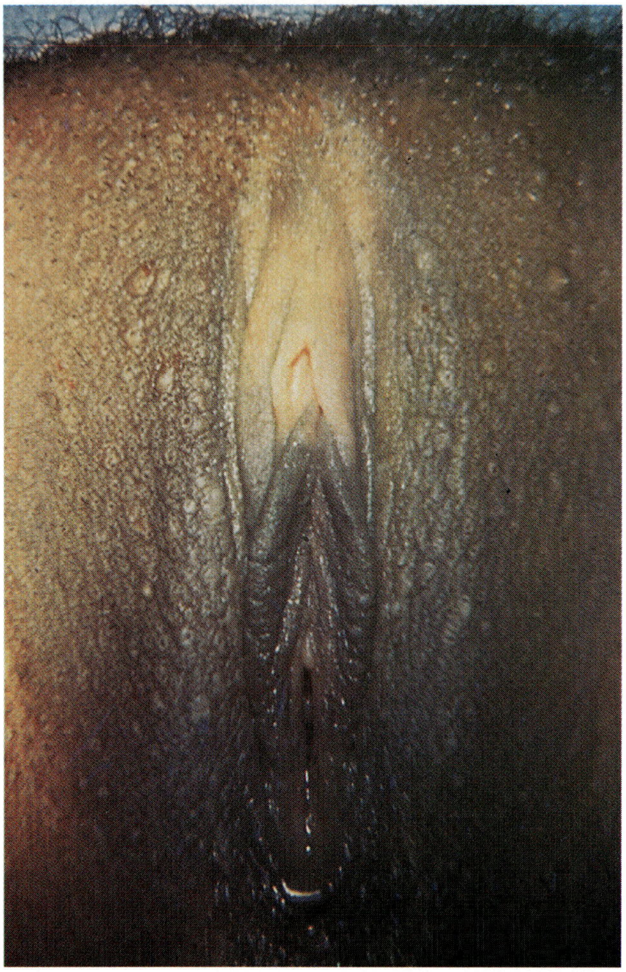

FIGURE 1-23
Multiple small papules are seen on the labia majora and mons of this patient who has Fox-Fordyce disease.

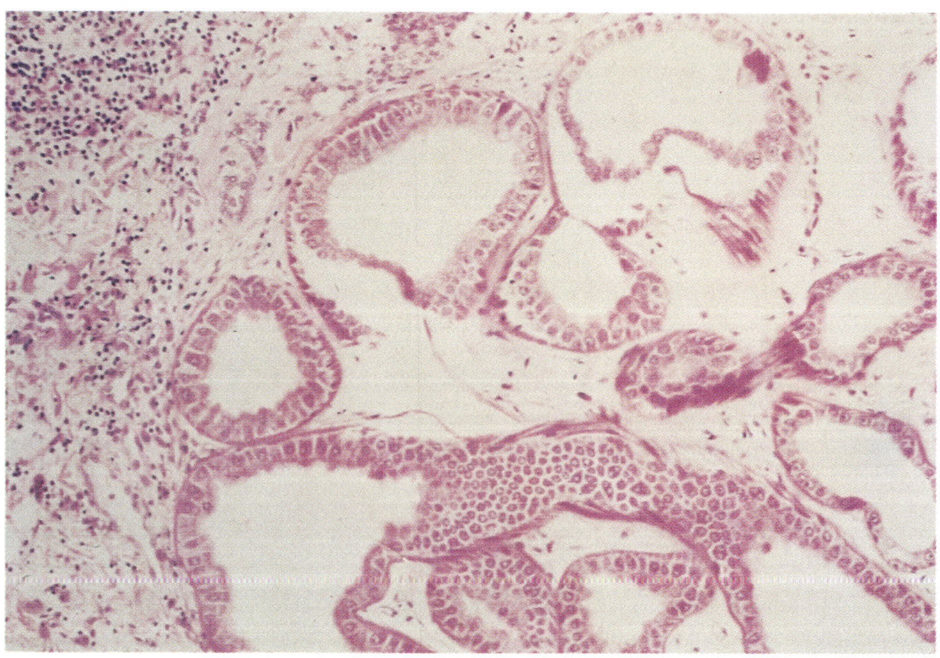

FIGURE 1-24
A group of dilated apocrine glands is seen. A chronic inflammatory infiltrate is present. This is a biopsy from a patient who has Fox-Fordyce disease.

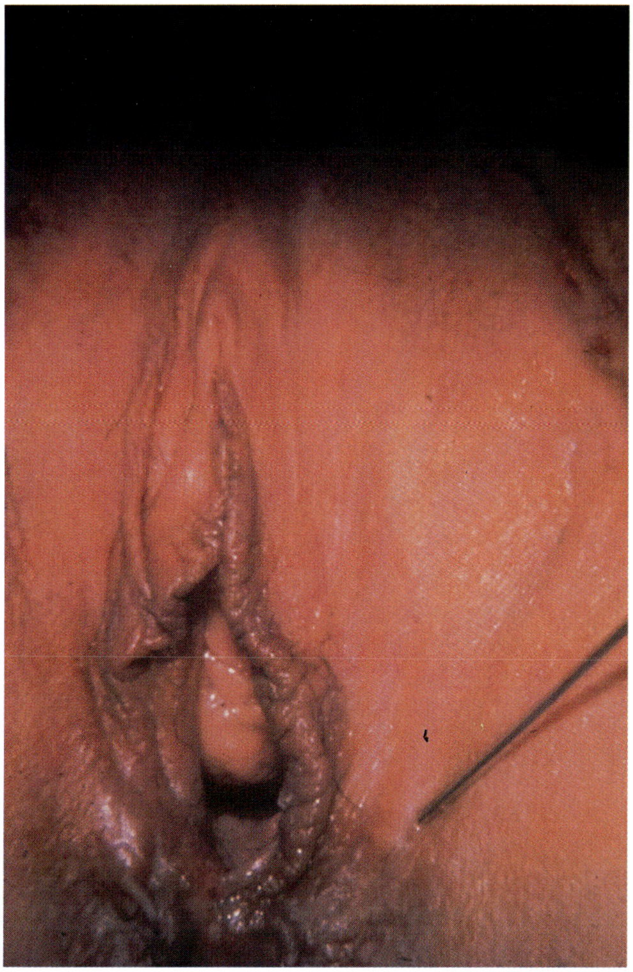

FIGURE 1-25
A metal probe has been inserted into a draining sinus of a patient who has Crohn disease affecting the vulva. Scars from other draining sinuses are seen in the intercrural areas.

Behçet Syndrome

Behçet disease or syndrome is characterized by a triad of recurrent aphthous ulcerations in the mouth (Fig. 1–27) and on the vulva that are associated with inflammatory vasculitis of the eye. Any one or all three of these components may be present, but uveitis is less frequent than vulvar and oral ulcerations. The patient with Behçet disease may also experience meningoencephalitis, recurrent synovitis, cutaneous pustules or nodules resembling erythema nodosum, phlebitis of large and small veins, arterial aneurysms in the systemic and pulmonary circulation, and discrete gastrointestinal ulcers that can bleed or perforate.

An acute ulcer of Behçet disease is sharply marginated and has a grayish-white necrotic center when it occurs in the mouth. On the vulva it may be reddish-yellow (Fig. 1–28). Surprisingly, these ulcers may produce no symptoms. In the chronic phase distortion of the labia with tissue fenestrations may develop. Biopsy in the chronic phase shows an intense mucosal and submucosal chronic inflammatory infiltrate with accompanying florid vasculitis, which culminates in occlusion of the submucosal vessels (Fig. 1–29).

The cause of the disease is unknown, but vasculitis is the key factor in the pathogenesis. An autoimmune process has been suggested.[17] The clinical diagnosis is frequently one of exclusion after other destructive lesions affecting the vulva, such as Crohn disease, pemphigus, herpes, and syphilis, have been excluded. The lesions are usually self-limiting and thus the effectiveness of various therapies is difficult to assess. Fatal cases are almost always associated with eye lesions and involvement of the central nervous system. Of interest is the reported association of exacerbations with the menstrual cycle. Improvement with the use of oral contraceptives has been noted. This may be coincidental and may be related to the frequent sponta-

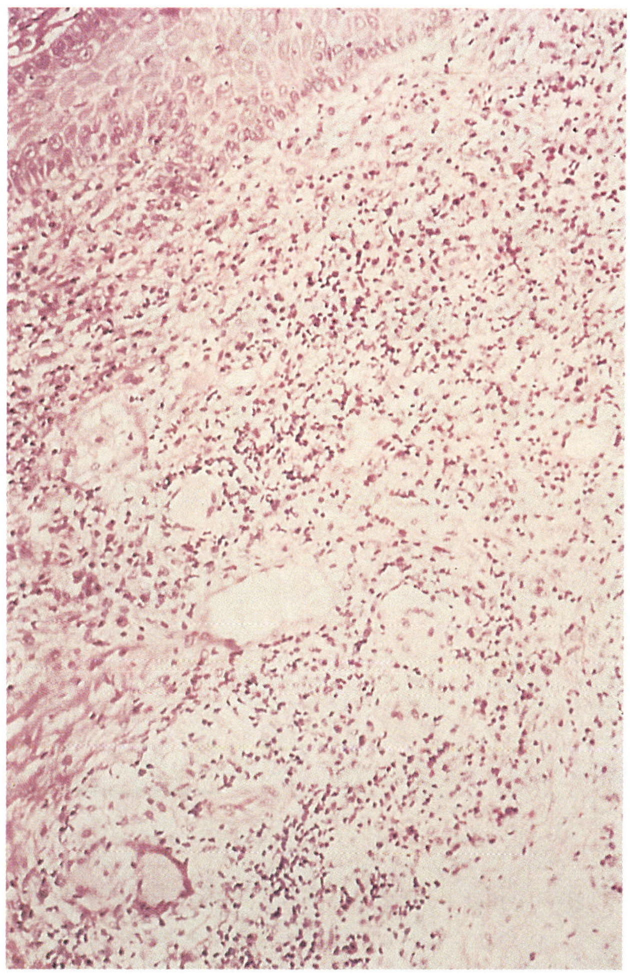

FIGURE 1-26
This biopsy specimen from a vulvar draining sinus of a patient who has Crohn disease shows squamous epithelium *(top)*, chronic inflammatory infiltrate, and giant cells.

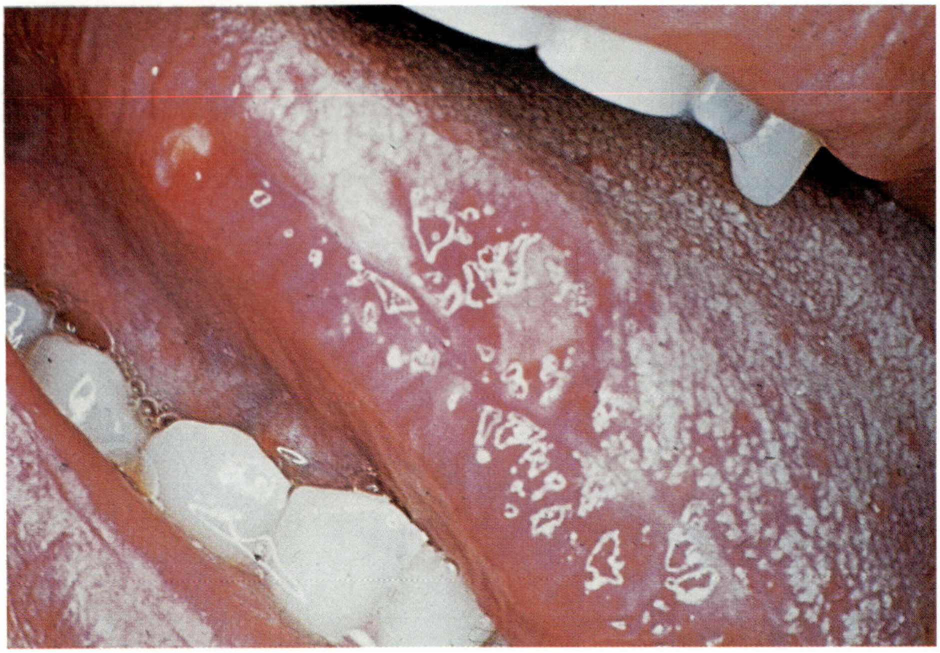

FIGURE 1-27
Two aphthous ulcers are seen on the edge of this tongue of a patient who has Behçet syndrome. The center of the ulcers is grayish white.

neous exacerbations and regressions for which this disease is noted. Systemic corticosteroid treatment is the most widely used and effective therapy.[18]

Aphthous Ulcers

Aphthous ulcers occur in the vulvar area where they are usually asymptomatic. These are shallow ulcers that are probably caused by trauma. No treatment is necessary because spontaneous healing is rapid. A topical anesthetic can be used if the lesion is painful. If the lesion does not heal, biopsy is mandatory to exclude a malignant disease.

Other Ulcers

Pemphigus vulgaris, Darier disease (keratosis follicularis), and Hailey-Hailey disease (familial benign chronic pemphigus) can also involve the vulva (Fig. 1–30). Biopsy, which is mandatory for all ulcerative lesions of the vulva, demonstrates acantholysis in patients with pemphigus (Fig.

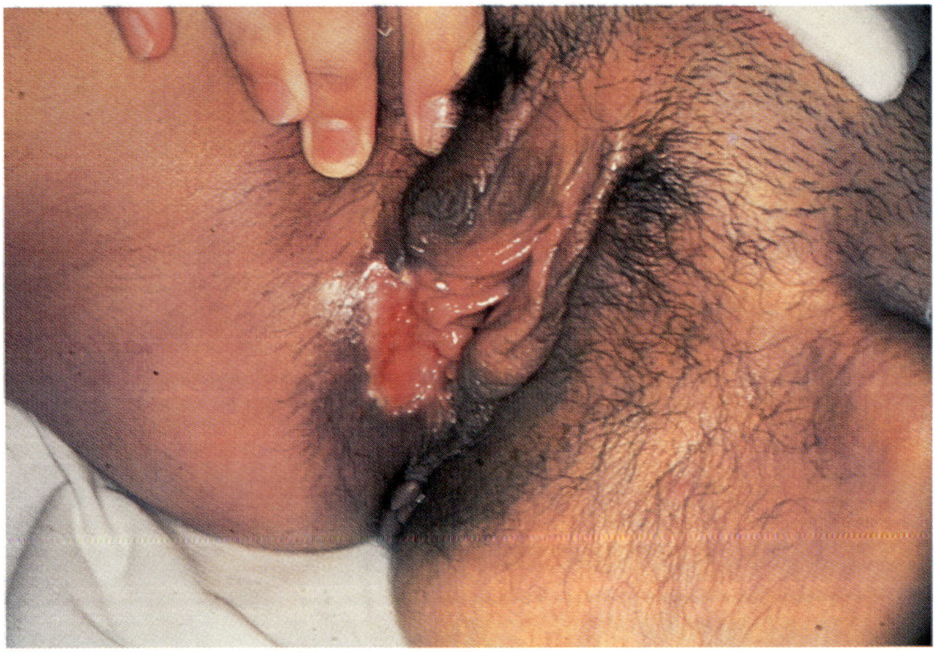

FIGURE 1-28
A vulvar ulcer is also present in the patient shown in Figure 1–27. The vulvar ulcer is large and well demarcated and has a reddish yellow center.

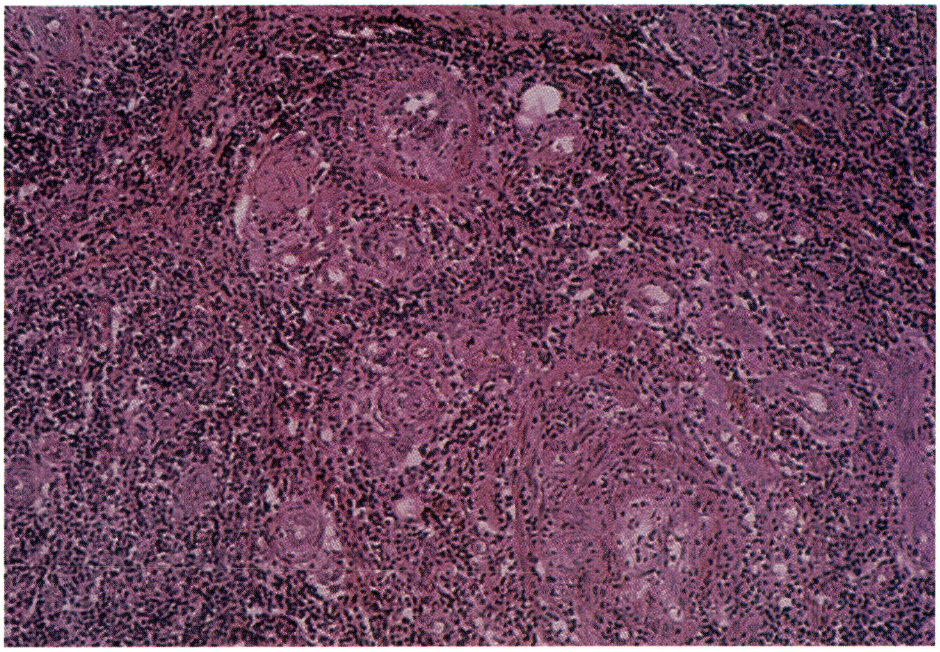

FIGURE 1-29
This biopsy from an ulcer of a patient who has Behçet syndrome shows an intense chronic inflammatory infiltrate with prominent vasculitis. The inflammatory cells are present within the vessel walls. This has led to occlusion of the large vessel *(lower right)*.

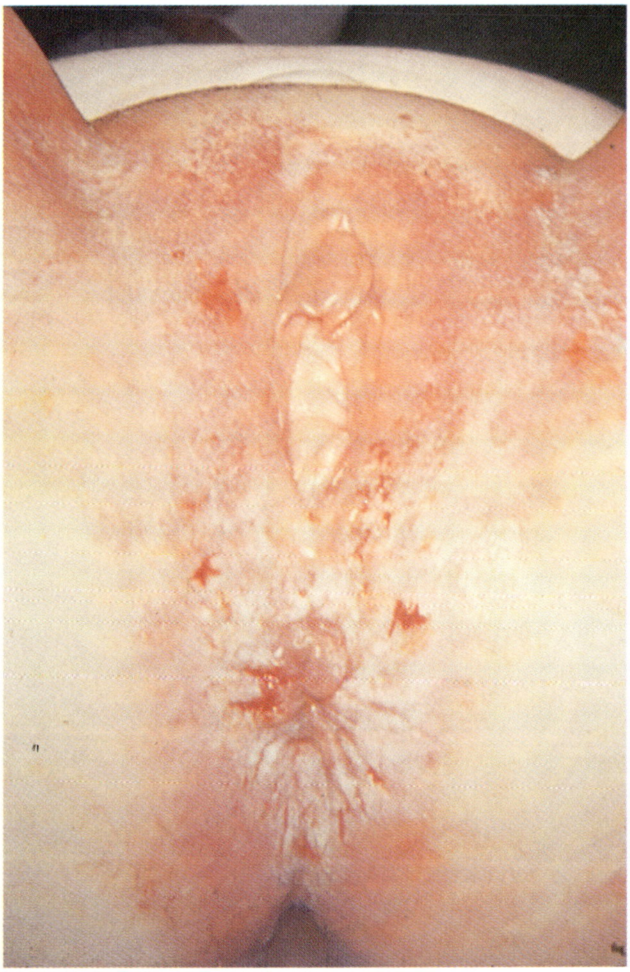

FIGURE 1-30
Darier disease starts as greasy, gray-white papules seen on the upper vulva. These eventually coalesce, as is seen in the perianal region. Fissures and superficial ulcerations are seen as reddish areas. Biopsy of this lesion revealed findings similar to those of pemphigus except that suprabasal clefts are present instead of bullae.

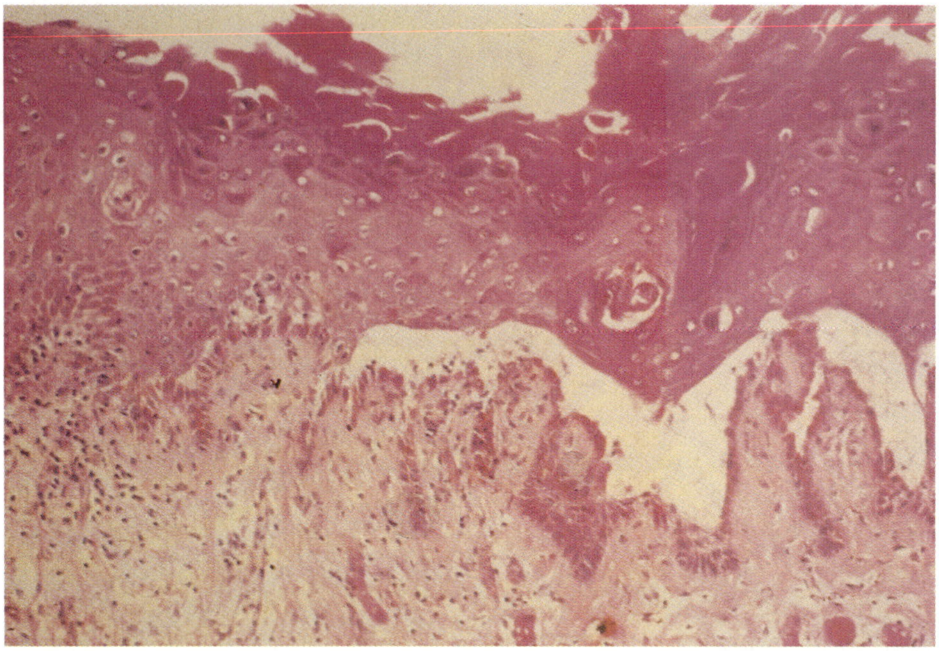

FIGURE 1-31
This is a biopsy specimen of a vulvar lesion of pemphigus. A bulla is formed by the separation of the surface epithelium from the basal layer of cells. Hyperkeratosis is present. A scattered lymphoid infiltrate is seen.

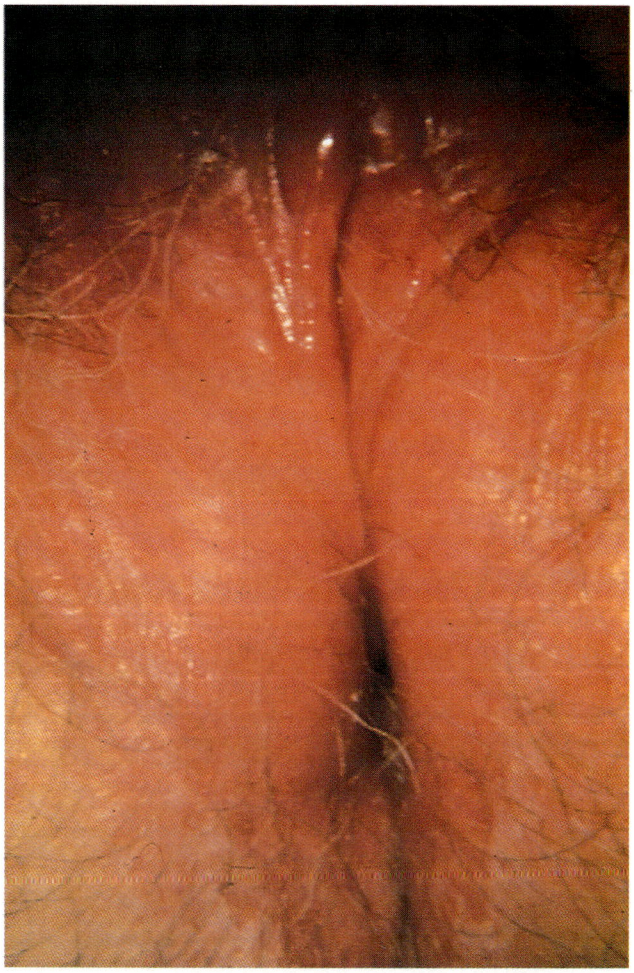

FIGURE 1-32
This vulva has marked erythema and edema secondary to *Candida albicans* infection. Satellite lesions are seen on the right inner thigh.

1–31). This is the process of disintegration of the intercellular bridges between the keratinocytes, which leads to an intraepidermal cleft or bulla. The superficial epithelium is separated from the first two to three cell layers of the basal zone. Acantholytic cells line the bulla and also lie free within the cavity of the bulla. These cells have a large basophilic nucleus that may be surrounded by a clear halo. Nucleoli are prominent and may be bullet shaped. Moderate lymphocytic infiltration is found in the dermis. Hyperkeratosis is seen over the bulla.

Finally, it should be noted that both decubitus and factitious (self-induced) ulcerations may be present on the vulva as in other locations on the body. The former are usually self-evident and occur most frequently in patients with poor circulation. Factitious ulcers present a clinical rather than a histopathologic challenge because the psychologic aspects of the problem may be bizarre and difficult to characterize.

SYSTEMIC DISEASE

The vulva, like the skin elsewhere, may reflect the presence of systemic disease. A patient who has poorly controlled diabetes mellitus may complain of vulvar pruritus. This is usually due to an infection with *Candida albicans.* In the acute phase there is intense erythema of the labia minora and majora and satellite erythematous lesions that involve the intracrural folds and inner thighs (Fig. 1–32). In the chronic phase of candidal infection hyperkeratosis is present. On physical examination thickened and grayish epithelium is found, interspersed by small superficial reddish areas (Fig. 1–33). Excoriations from scratching are usually present. A dramatic response to topical antifungal agents and control of the diabetes is seen.

Chronic anemia is occasionally accompanied by vulvar ulceration. Uremic frost may be appreciated as brownish-yellow patches on the vulva. Systemic sarcoidosis may present on the vulva as grayish-white thickened skin. This is due to hyperkeratosis, which is characteristic of most chronic inflammatory conditions of the vulva. Biopsy reveals noncaseating granulomas with multiple giant cells seen in the dermis. These may be seen in many other conditions, and the diagnosis of sarcoidosis depends on their presence at other more typical sites including the lung, lymph nodes, and liver and the lack of infectious agents or other diseases such as Crohn disease.

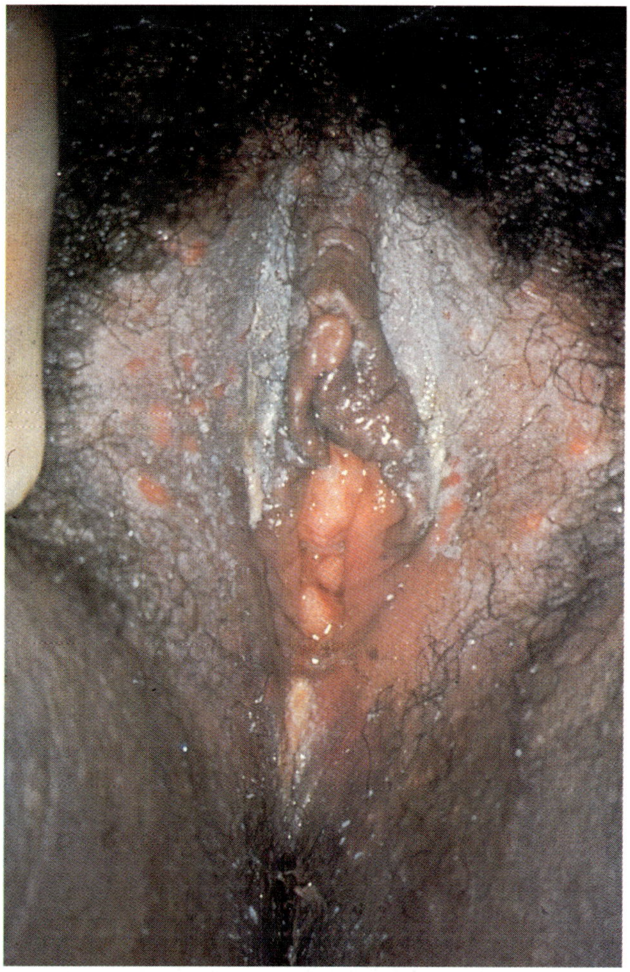

FIGURE 1–33
This patient has chronic *Candida* vulvitis. The vulvar skin is thickened and grayish white, and it is interspersed by erythematous patches.

VIRAL DISEASE

Herpes Simplex Virus

Herpes simplex virus (HSV) infection in the lower genital tract is a sexually transmitted disease. The great majority of lesions are caused by HSV type 2. A small percentage of cases (10 to 15 percent) are caused by HSV type 1, which is most typically associated with cold sores in the oropharyngeal mucosa.

Although HSV infection of the vulva is common, the initial symptoms often pass unnoticed. The symptoms of the primary infection occur within 2 to 7 days of exposure. These vary from a local tingling sensation to a constellation of symptoms which include general malaise, fever, headache, myalgia, and inguinal adenopathy. Small, painful vesicles scattered over the surface of the vulva are present (Fig. 1–34). This stage is rarely seen by the clinician. More commonly, the clinician sees the patient when the lesions have progressed to the stage of superficial serpiginous ulcerations formed by the confluence of ruptured vesicles (Fig. 1–35). These lesions may become superinfected. Urethral involvement may cause dysuria, which may result in urinary retention.

Biopsy or a cytologic smear of an intradermal or subepithelial vesicle or an ulcer should be diagnostic. There is marked inflammation at the base of the lesion, but the diagnostic cells are found at the edge. These cells are enlarged and multinucleated. The nuclei have a ground-glass chromatin appearance. The nuclei may contain a basophilic or eosinophilic inclusion if the lesion is older. A scraping taken from the edge of the base of the ulcer can be prepared with Papanicolaou stain or Wright stain for cytologic examination. The best diagnostic material is obtained when a vesicle is unroofed and the base and lateral borders of the lesion are scraped. If the lesion is dry, a better cytologic sample will be obtained if a gauze pad saturated with normal saline solution is placed on the lesion before obtaining the specimen. The multinucleated cells with the characteristic chromatin pattern are then seen (Fig. 1–36).

The primary lesions persist for 2 to 3 weeks. The virus has been recovered from asymptomatic patients as long as 180 days after a clinical infection, and the potential for infectivity may persist long after the lesions appear to be healed. It is also important to note that vulvar herpetic lesions are undoubtedly only a local manifestation of an infection that is present throughout the lower genital tract. Careful examination often reveals lesions on the cervix, urethra, and anal mucosa. HSV infection is of serious significance when the patient is pregnant and near term. If there is evidence of viral shedding during the third trimester or of active lesions within 2 weeks of predicted delivery, cesarean section has been recommended as the optimum approach to delivery. Cesarean section should be undertaken before rupture of the membranes has occurred to minimize the chances of neonatal herpetic encephalitis. It must be appreciated, however, that cesarean section may not totally prevent infection of the fetus, but it will reduce the incidence of serious neonatal complications.[19]

Oral acyclovir has been found to be effective in shortening the healing time for ulcers and in decreasing the time of active viral shedding.[20, 21] There is no evidence that the agent is teratogenic, but it should be used with caution during pregnancy.

The virus remains latent in the dorsal root ganglia (S2–S4). Latent or recurrent infections are common and are usually less symptomatic than the primary infection. Approximately half of patients who have primary infections develop a symptomatic recurrence within 6 months of the primary infection. Chronic oral acyclovir has been recommended for patients who experience multiple recurrences every year.

Herpes Zoster

Herpes zoster in the vulvar area is rare but causes marked distress owing to severe burning pain along the distribution of a nerve. The varicella-zoster virus causes herpes zoster. Unilateral lesions are traced along the course of the pudendal nerve and its branches. This nerve radiates toward the adjacent buttock or into the inguinal region and lower abdomen (Fig. 1–37). High doses of acyclovir have been used to shorten the acute process.[21] Recurrences are rare.

Molluscum Contagiosum

The vulva is a common site of involvement with molluscum contagiosum. The lesions can be asymptomatic or pruritic. They are single or multiple, rounded, dome-shaped, waxy papules 2 to 5 mm in diameter (Fig. 1–38). A central depression and umbilication may be present, which contains a "waxen kernel" that may be evacuated by a tiny dermatologic curette or even with the tip of a 25-gauge needle. Biopsy of a solitary lesion may be performed to confirm the diagnosis, but this is seldom necessary. The microscopic appearance is characteristic. The central area contains cells harboring large inclusion bodies. At the base of a lesion the molluscum bodies are eosinophilic, but they become basophilic as they move closer to the surface (Fig. 1–39). There is little to no inflammatory reaction. Since this disease is sexually transmitted, the patient should be evaluated for other sexually transmitted diseases. Treatment consists of evacuation of the central core. This is achieved with the tip of a 25-gauge needle after an antiseptic has been applied. Recurrence is rare.

Human Papillomavirus

Human papillomavirus as well as other benign papillomas are discussed later under Benign Tumors.

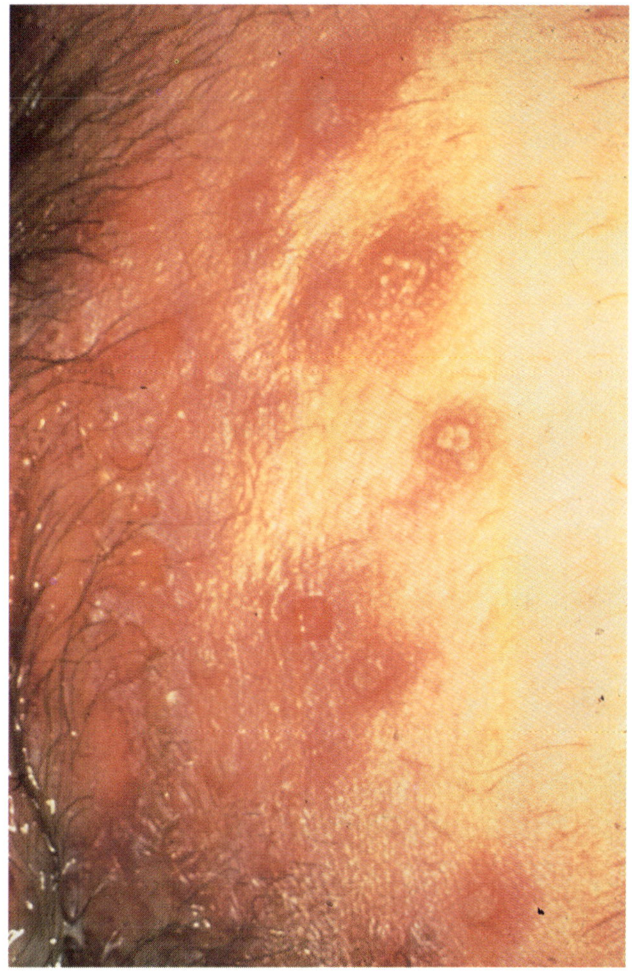

FIGURE 1-34
This patient has early vesicular lesions of herpes simplex virus. The vesicles are small and surrounded by intense erythema.

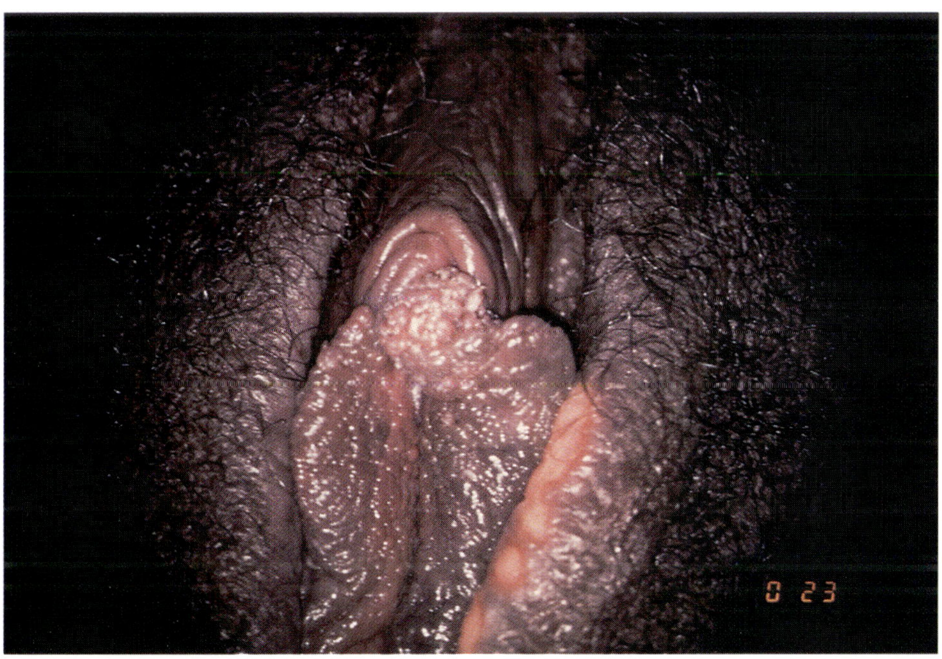

FIGURE 1-35
Superficial, yellow-pink, serpiginous ulcerations are seen on the left labium majus. These are caused by herpes simplex virus infection. A condylomatous lesion is also seen near the clitoris. This is caused by human papillomavirus infection.

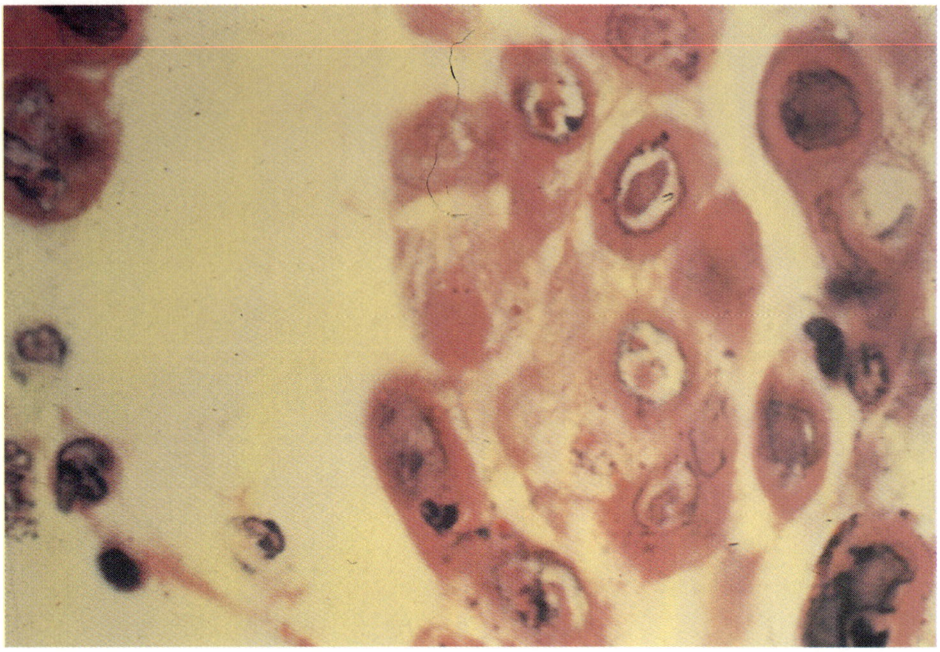

FIGURE 1-36
This is a hematoxylin and eosin stain of a vulvar biopsy specimen from a patient who has late-stage lesions of herpes simplex virus infection. A group of cells *(center)* have very large, reddish intranuclear inclusions surrounded by a clear halo. The nuclear chromatin is pushed to the periphery, making a dense nuclear rim.

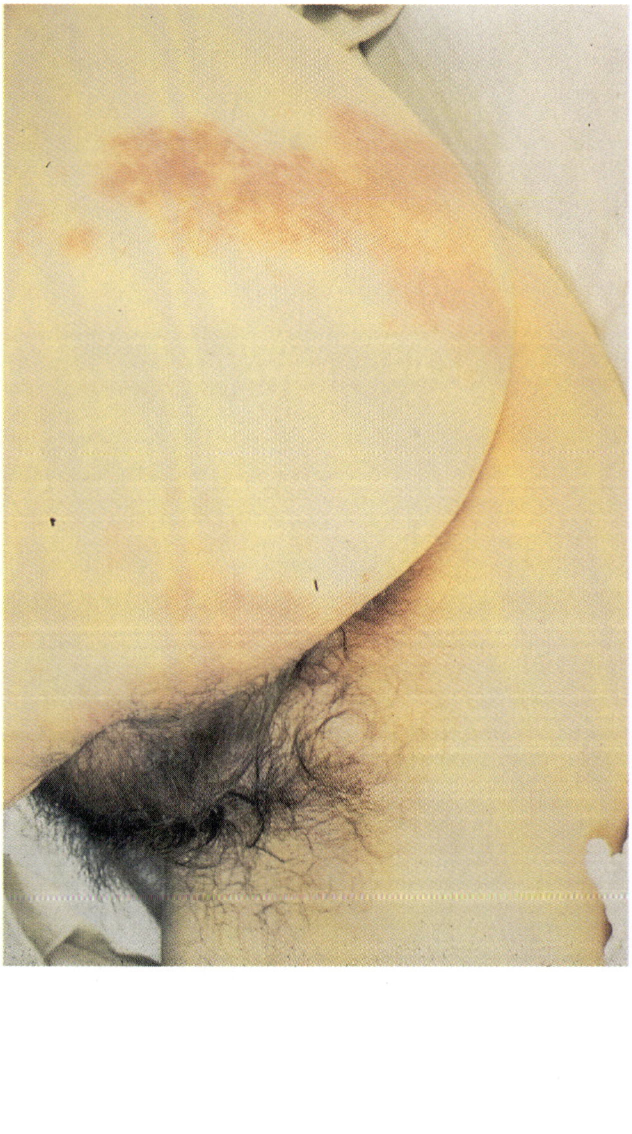

FIGURE 1-37
Crops of vesicles are seen on the left buttock and inner thigh following the nerve distribution. This patient has herpes zoster.

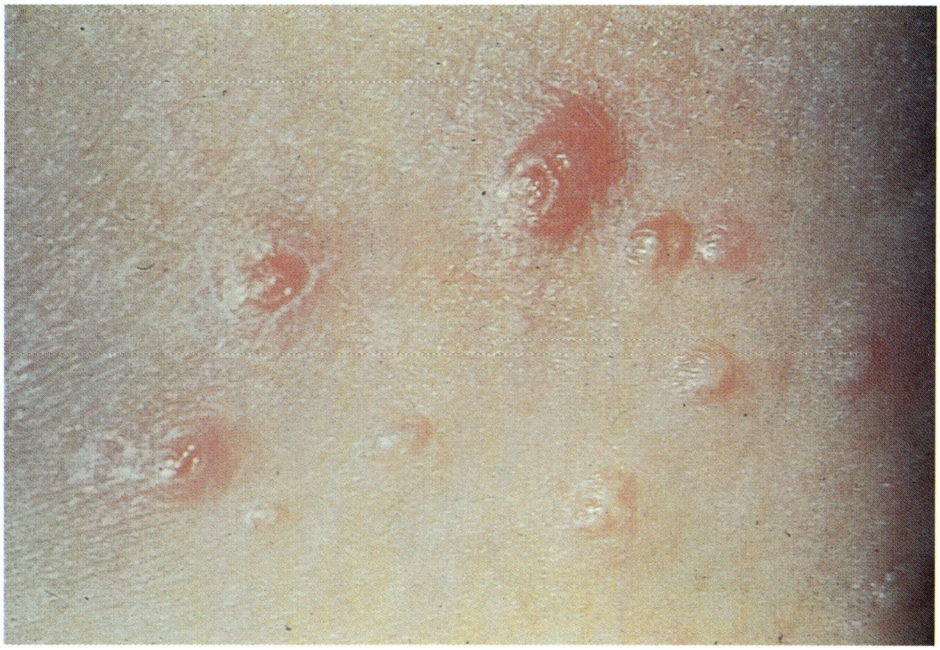

FIGURE 1-38
Multiple small rounded papules of molluscum contagiosum are seen. Some have central umbilication and erythema.

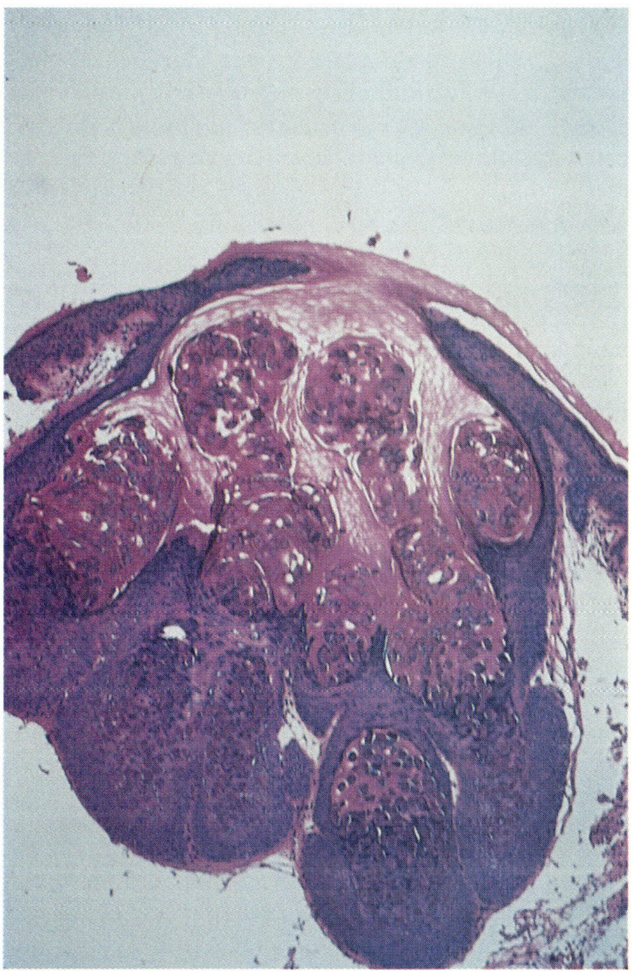

FIGURE 1-39
This is a biopsy specimen of a molluscum contagiosum lesion. The squamous cells at the base contain large intracytoplasmic viral inclusions. The inclusions are also found in a central area under the surface epithelium, which is umbilicated.

BACTERIAL DISEASE

Nonspecific

Folliculitis

Pustular disease or folliculitis is not uncommon in the external genitalia. The hair follicle and its associated sebaceous gland are ideal sites for the entrapment of secretions after the shaft has been occluded and subsequent focal infection has occurred (Fig. 1–40). These conditions are usually self-limiting and require no intervention. If necessary, local heat and oral antibiotics can be used to hasten the resolution. Aggressive management is recommended in diabetic patients to avoid the development of necrotizing fasciitis.[22]

Ecthyma

A more diffuse and dramatic form of folliculitis is known as ecthyma (Fig. 1–41). These lesions need to be distinguished from condyloma latum. Ecthyma is characterized by pustule formation with central umbilication. There is no more extensive surrounding induration than is found with typical condyloma lata, but if the condyloma lata lesion is secondarily infected it may be similar. Examination of secretions from the lesions under the darkfield microscope and serologic studies for syphilis assist in the differential diagnosis. The lesions may progress to abscess formation, which necessitates drainage. The infection is not deep seated and does not produce interconnecting sinuses such as those seen with suppurative hidradenitis. Local heat and oral antibiotics produce a relatively rapid response.

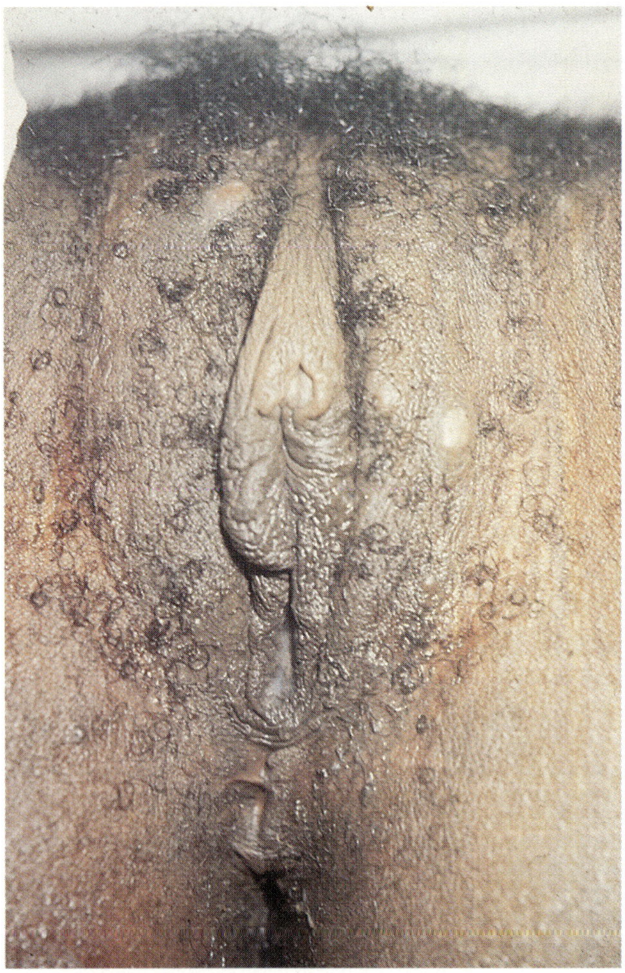

FIGURE 1–40
An infected hair follicle is present on the left labium majus and is seen as a pinkish white papule. Another one is present on the right mons.

Hidradenitis

Hidradenitis is an infectious or inflammatory process of the apocrine glands. These glands are located in the labia majora, mons, and perianal area. The infections are usually cyclic, and the patient complains of painful swellings on the mons and labia majora during the secretory phase of the menstrual cycle. The process may also involve the axillae, which also have apocrine glands. The cyclic nature of hidradenitis in its early and minor stages suggests a therapeutic approach to the problem, namely, modification of secretory activity of the glands by the use of oral contraceptives or antiandrogens.[23, 24] Antibiotics and local heat are used to treat the acute phase.

The cyclic nature of the infection disappears as the infection becomes deep seated and changes to suppurative hidradenitis. In this suppurative phase, draining sinuses communicate with each other subcutaneously (Fig. 1–42). The labia minora, clitoris, and prepuce are not involved by the infection because they do not have apocrine glands, but they may become edematous. Oral contraceptives are ineffective in the suppurative stage. Extensive “unroofing” incisions may be necessary to treat deep-seated infection. In performing this procedure, the incisions are carried down to Colles' fascia and then are left open. The base of the incisions is curetted. These incisions heal remarkably well within 2 to 3 weeks. Laser ablation of the infected sinuses has also been used, and satisfactory results have been reported.[25] Preoperative and postoperative antibiotics and warm whirlpool baths are useful adjuncts to treatment. Oral isotretinoin can be tried in patients who have severe disease. It is imperative that pregnancy be avoided while the patient is taking this medication because it is a potent teratogen. One patient with suppurative hidradenitis that responded to a

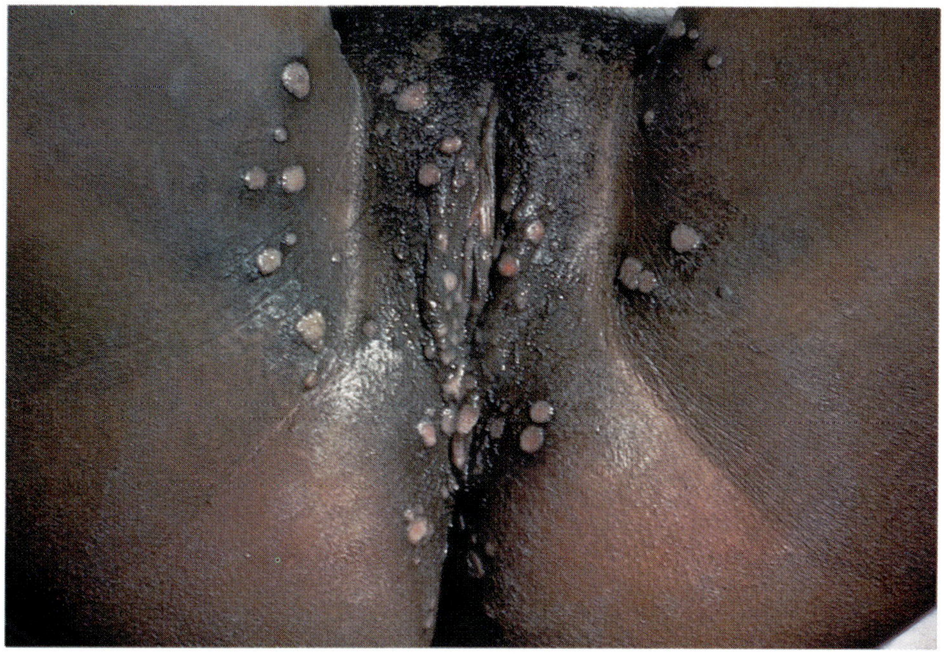

FIGURE 1-41
Multiple papules, some of which have central erythema, are seen in this patient who has ecthyma. This can be confused with condyloma latum. Darkfield microscopic examination of secretions and serologic studies for syphilis are needed to exclude condyloma latum.

gonadotropin-releasing hormone agonist and estrogen replacement has been reported.[26] She subsequently underwent a total abdominal hysterectomy and bilateral salpingo-oophorectomy followed by estrogen replacement. No recurrences were observed during the 6 months of follow-up after castration. Antiprogesterone agents (e.g., RU-486) now being introduced in the United States may play a role in controlling this disease in the future.

Hidradenitis can be confused with diffuse folliculitis (i.e., ecthyma). The latter involves the hair follicles and sebaceous glands and is not cyclic in nature. The labia minora, which have an abundance of sebaceous glands without hair follicles, may be involved in ecthyma. Suppurative hidradenitis may simulate the chronic phase of lymphogranuloma venereum; however, in lymphogranuloma there is more distortion of the anatomy, and lymphedema and tissue destruction involve both the labia minora and the labia majora.

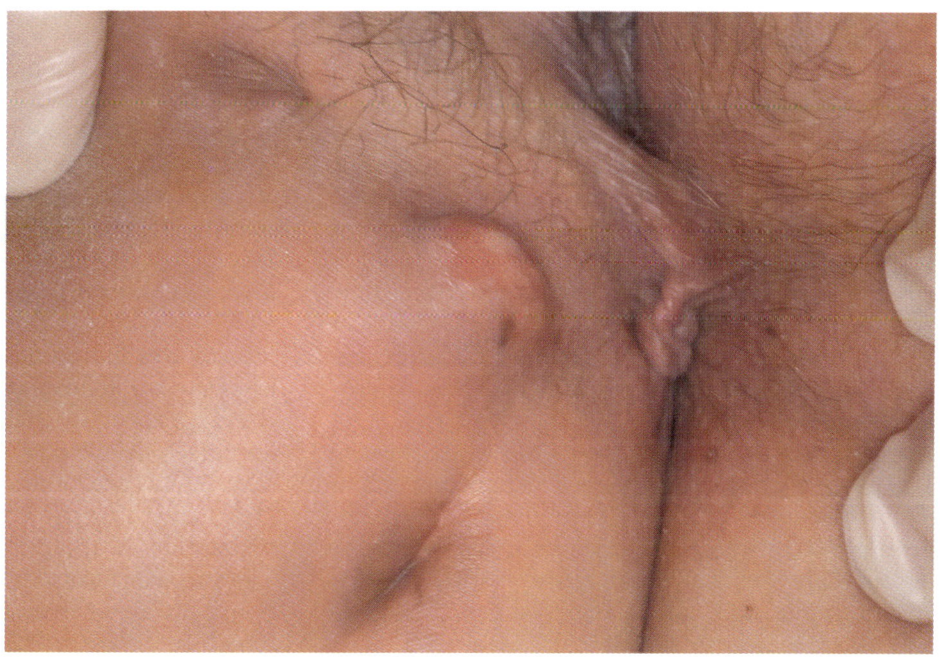

FIGURE 1-42
This patient who has suppurative hidradenitis presents with sinuses on the perineum, buttock, and inner thigh. (Courtesy of Dr. Gordon Davis, Phoenix, AZ.)

Gonorrhea

The vulvar mucosa, with its many layers of stratified squamous epithelium, is relatively resistant to gonorrheal infection. The vulnerable structures in the vulva are the vulvovaginal glands, the urethra, and the associated Skene glands. However, because of the thinness of the vulvovaginal mucous membrane before menarche, gonorrheal vulvovaginitis may occur in a young child who has been sexually molested. At present, intramuscular ceftriaxone is the treatment of choice. Spectinomycin is used when a patient is allergic to ceftriaxone.

Bartholin Adenitis

Inflammation of Bartholin's gland may be the result of a gonorrheal infection. However, in most cases culture of a Bartholin abscess reveals a mixed bacterial flora. In the acute stage, infection of Bartholin's gland results in edema, and the area becomes turgid and painful. The overlying skin is erythematous. Pressure over the gland may result in the expression of pus from the duct orifice. However, exquisite tenderness usually precludes attempting this.

Microscopic examination of the gland during this stage shows the usual evidence of acute suppurative inflammation which includes extensive infiltration with polymorphonuclear leukocytes, hyperemia, edema, epithelial degeneration, and sometimes desquamation.

The process may progress in one of two directions. Most often, abscess formation occurs, and the swelling and pain become more pronounced. There is focal fluctuation in the mass (Fig. 1–43). Incision and evacuation of the purulent contents result in immediate relief. This is usually done under anesthesia for patient comfort. The procedure includes breaking up of loculations and complete drainage of the abscess cavity. Marsupialization can be performed to provide a large enough opening for continuous drainage. Word has advocated the introduction of a small catheter into the incision instead of marsupialization.[27] Sometimes this may serve only to occlude the drainage site, and in many instances the catheter falls out prematurely instead of staying in for the recommended 3 to 4 weeks.

Spontaneous rupture of the abscess may occur. The resultant small perforation provides inadequate drainage and thus can prolong the acute process. Recurrences are common unless the opening is enlarged and premature closure is prevented. Again, this can be achieved using a variety of techniques: the Word catheter, surgical marsupialization of the abscess, or laser incision with vaporization of the cyst wall.[28]

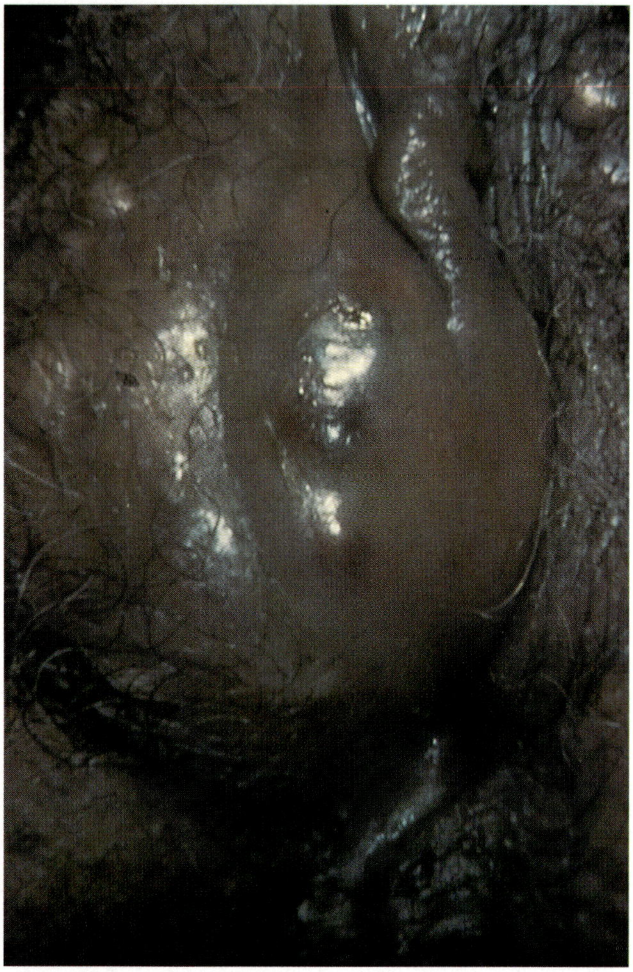

FIGURE 1–43
Marked swelling of the lower right labium minus distorts the introitus. This is secondary to an abscess of the Bartholin gland.

In less virulent infections, the process may subside without abscess formation if the gland duct is not occluded. This allows for spontaneous drainage of the exudate. Resolution of the process is occasionally incomplete, and chronic inflammation of the gland persists. Chronic Bartholin adenitis presents clinically as an induration of the gland, which is palpable deep in the perineum and lateral to the fourchette. This chronic inflammatory process usually remains asymptomatic for years. Rarely, exacerbations occur and lead to recurrent abscesses. More commonly, cysts of varying sizes (Fig. 1–44) are produced owing to occlusion of the gland duct by the chronic inflammation. Marsupialization of the cyst is the treatment of choice. The incision is made on the labial mucosa close to the vestibule to avoid labial fenestrations. Chronic

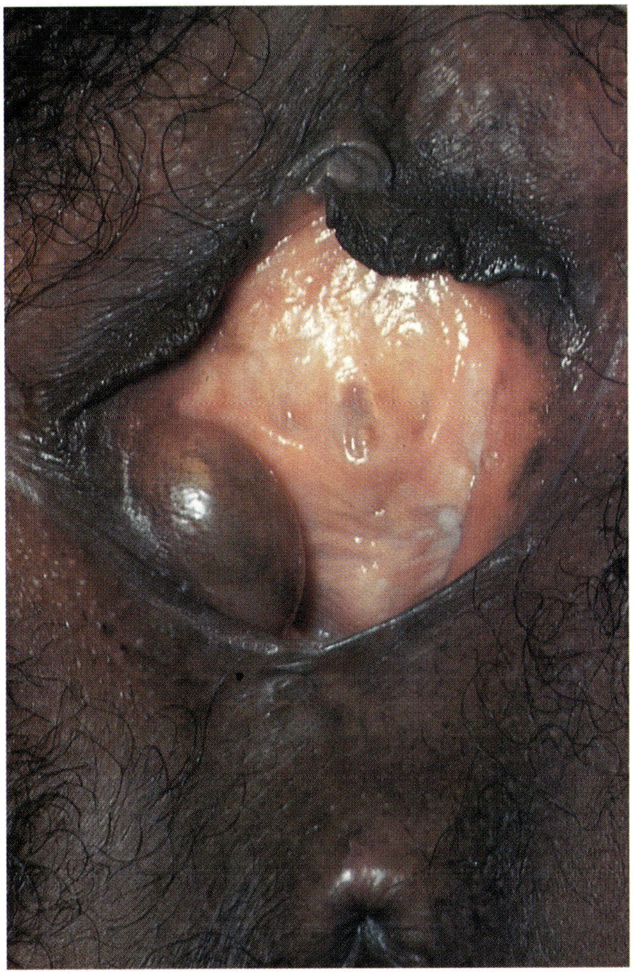

FIGURE 1-44
A Bartholin cyst is seen at the right side of the introitus. The surface is smooth and rounded. The cyst was not tender.

recurrent cysts may necessitate removal of the entire gland.

The lining of Bartholin duct cysts varies greatly from the classic transitional epithelium of the normal duct to a flattened single cell layer. The latter is due to the intracystic pressure on the epithelium and the destruction produced by the inflammatory process. In the absence of a transitional epithelial lining, difficulty may be encountered in making an accurate histopathologic diagnosis. However, in most instances, mucus-secreting acini (see Fig. 1–7), similar in many aspects to those of the salivary gland, are found in the chronically infected underlying tissue.

Chancroid

Chancroid is a sexually transmitted disease caused by the gram-negative bacillus *Haemophilus ducreyi.* A macule or pustule develops 1 to 3 days after exposure. The pustule ruptures a few days later. One or more ulcers may develop. The ulceration of chancroid is typically ragged and irregular, especially in its later stages. It has an excavated appearance or undermined edges. The base is covered by a purulent exudate. There is little or no surrounding induration, leading to what has been called "soft" chancre. In contrast to the nontender syphilitic chancre, the chancroid ulcer is very tender. It also bleeds easily. Often the ulcer arises in the region of the clitoris or in the vestibule, and frequently there is edema of the adjacent vulvar structures. Inguinal adenitis may be present, and in half of all cases a bubo (i.e., inflammatory swelling of lymph nodes) develops. Pain is a more common clinical feature of chancroid than of the other ulcerative lesions of the vulva.

This lesion cannot be distinguished from other chronic ulcerative lesions by microscopic examination, and the organism may not grow in culture. Gram stain of material recovered from the undermined border of the lesion may demonstrate short, plump, gram-negative bacilli, which are commonly found in clusters oriented in one direction, the so-called school of fish arrangement that is characteristic. Because the organism is not identified by culture or Gram stain in almost half the cases, the diagnosis is usually based on the clinical findings.[29] Syphilis and granuloma inguinale must be excluded (see following section). HSV infection and traumatic ulcers are also part of the differential diagnosis.

Effective treatment includes oral trimethoprim-sulfamethoxazole, oral erythromycin, or intramuscular ceftriaxone. Since the 1970s, reports have noted increasing resistance of this organism to tetracycline, so this agent is not recommended.[30]

Granuloma Inguinale

Granuloma inguinale is a contagious, chronic sexually transmitted disease of tropical countries, but a few cases are seen in the United States. The causative organism is the gram-negative bacillus *Calymmatobacterium (Donovania) granulomatis.* The lesions are granulomatous and locally destructive. The disease usually begins as a small papular lesion or nodule on the labia minora or majora or on the mons pubis. It can also occur perianally. This soon develops into several superficial painless ulcers that tend to coalesce and spread along the inguinal and pubic regions. Initially, the ulcers have a clean base of granulation tissue and slightly raised edges (Fig. 1–45). Pro-

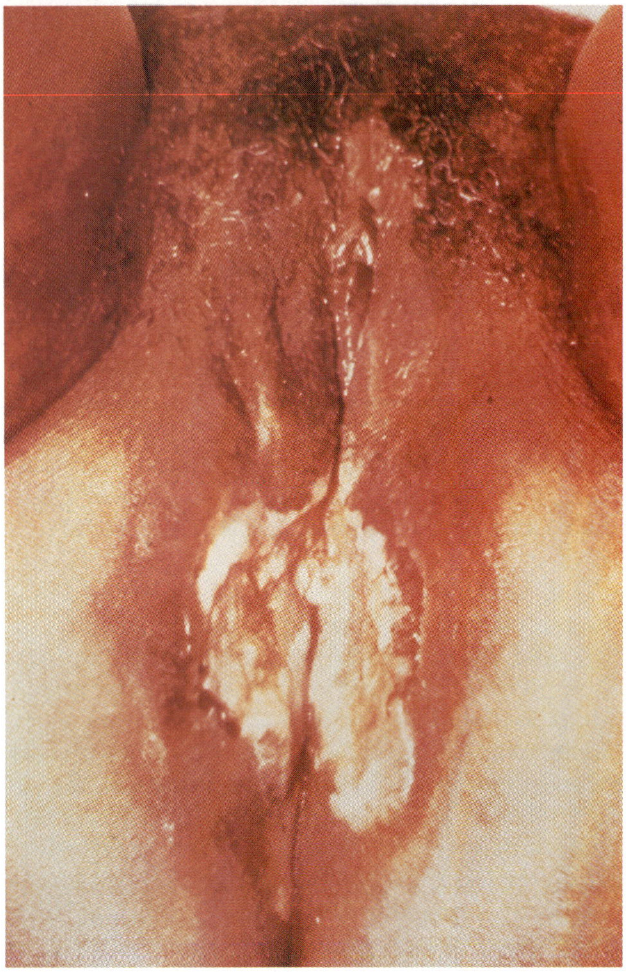

FIGURE 1–45
This is a vulvar ulcer of granuloma inguinale involving the perineum. The ulcer edges are sharp and raised. The base of the ulcer is white and clean.

gression of the granulomatous process may result in papillomatous-like tumors. The lesions cause irritation but are rarely painful. In the later stages of the disease, the infection may be deep, and extensive cicatrization may result. Hematogenous or lymphatic spread of the infection may occur. Granuloma inguinale of the cervix, uterus, fallopian tubes, and ovaries as well as some instances of extragenital infection have been reported.

The diagnosis can be made by obtaining scrapings with a scalpel from the periphery of the skin lesions. These are stained with Wright, Giemsa, or hematoxylin and eosin stain. The causative organism is usually found in the large mononuclear cells as a small, bilobed, encapsulated body that appears red with Giemsa stain (Donovan body). Chronic granulomatous diseases such as granuloma inguinale have been associated with squamous cell carcinoma.[31] Therefore, although the scrapings are adequate in most cases for making the diagnosis of the acute infection, biopsy is necessary in the chronic distorting lesions to eliminate the presence of malignancy. The histopathologic features include a transitory phase of subcutaneous infiltration with plasma cells, polymorphonuclear leukocytes, and histiocytes that have phagocytized cellular debris (foam cells). Later stages show formed granuloma in the subcutaneous tissue. Marked pseudocarcinomatous (pseudoepitheliomatous) epithelial hyperplasia is seen in the chronic stage, and differentiation from a neoplastic change may be difficult. The presence of abnormal maturation in the tips of the rete pegs, like cellular keratinization or keratin pearl formation, must be regarded with suspicion, and a more adequate tissue specimen may show definite malignancy.

The acute lesions of granuloma inguinale usually respond to orally administered tetracycline. In the chronic stages, surgery may be indicated to remove the areas of chronic infection and distortion.

Lymphogranuloma Venereum

Lymphogranuloma venereum (LGV, lymphogranuloma inguinale, lymphopathia venereum) is another granulomatous disease that is rare in temperate climates. The organism responsible for the lesions of LGV are the L_1, L_2, and L_3 subtypes of *Chlamydia trachomatis.* Confirmation of the diagnosis is based on culture of the organism or its identification with nucleic acid probes.

In women the disease is first recognized as small superficial ulcers on the vulva followed by development of pronounced inguinal adenitis (Fig. 1–46). Systemic symptoms such as malaise, fever, loss of appetite, loss of weight, and arthralgias may accompany the lymphadenitis. Further progress of the disease is characterized by extensive ulceration and marked lymphedema, which may lead to elephantiasis. On occasion, large indolent ulcers destroy the vulvar structures and extend to the perineum and rectum (Fig. 1–47). The combination of lymphatic obstruction and tissue damage may lead to either rectal or urethral stricture, or the destruction in these areas may result in incontinence. Fenestration of the labia is not uncommon. Marked lymphedema and draining sinuses are the hallmarks of chronic LGV of the vulva, which is confused only with extensive suppurative hidradenitis. In the differential diagnosis it must be reemphasized that suppurative hidradenitis rarely involves the labia minora except with minimal degrees of edema in contrast to the widespread tissue destruction associated with LGV.

The microscopic appearance of the skin lesions

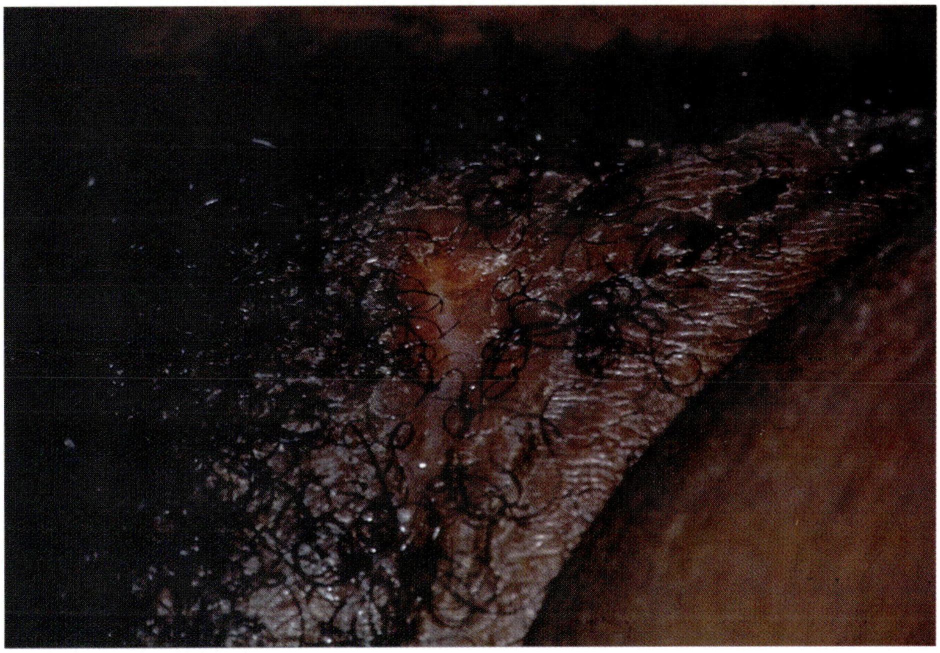

FIGURE 1-46
This patient has LGV. The mons is on the left and the thigh at the right of the picture. An infected inguinal node is seen draining in the groin.

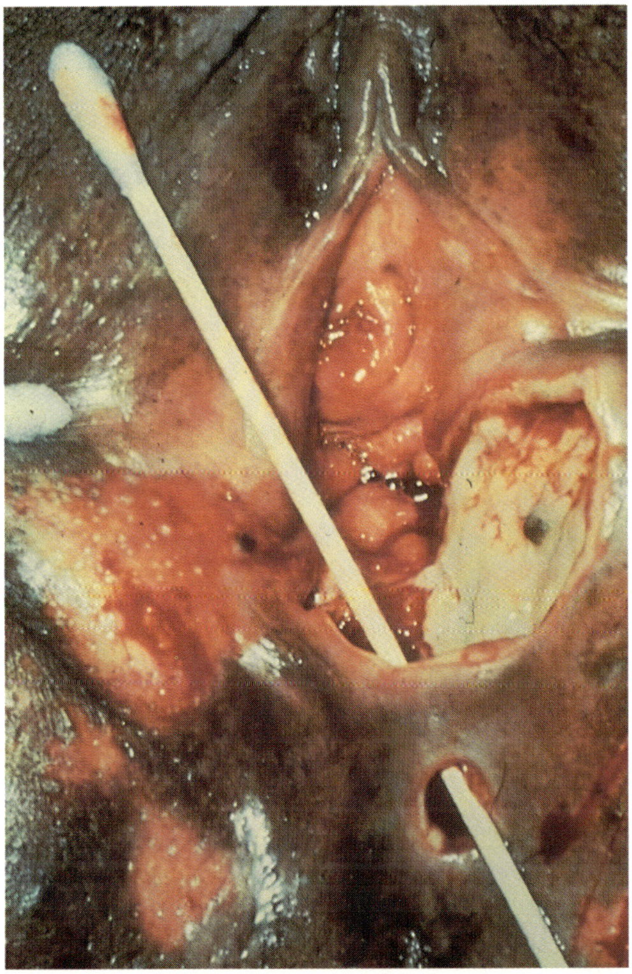

FIGURE 1-47
This patient who has LGV has a large ulcer in the left labium minus that has extended to and destroyed an area of the perineum.

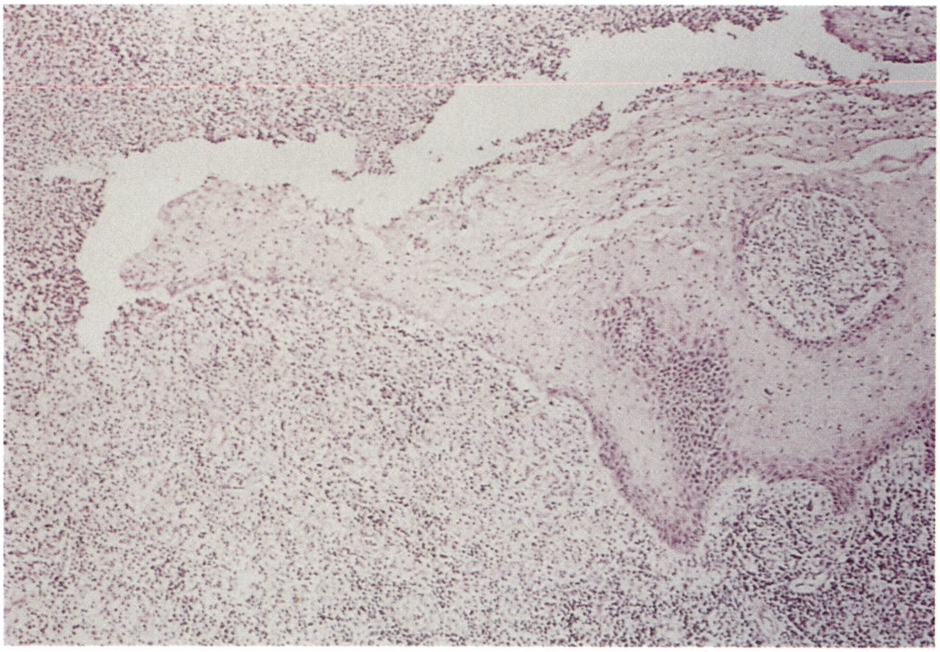

FIGURE 1–48
This is a biopsy specimen of a draining sinus of a patient with LGV. There is marked acute and chronic inflammation disrupting the squamous epithelium.

is characterized by extensive infiltration with plasma cells and lymphocytes. There is dilation of the lymphatic vessels, endothelial cell proliferation, and, in the later stages, marked fibrosis and scarring. Microabscesses and giant cells with pseudotubercle formation are noted in the subacute phase. The microabscesses are found at the site of the draining sinuses (Fig. 1–48). Pseudocarcinomatous hyperplasia of the overlying squamous epithelium with marked elongation and distortion of the rete pegs may simulate a malignancy. Conversely, carcinoma may develop in the background of chronic lymphogranulomatous lesions and may be clinically overlooked because of the tissue distortion.

Extragenital manifestations of LGV are well known. Extensive intestinal disease with cicatricial constrictions, particularly of the large bowel, have been reported. Cases of meningitis have also been reported. The preferred antibiotics against *Chlamydia* include doxycycline, tetracycline, and azithromycin.

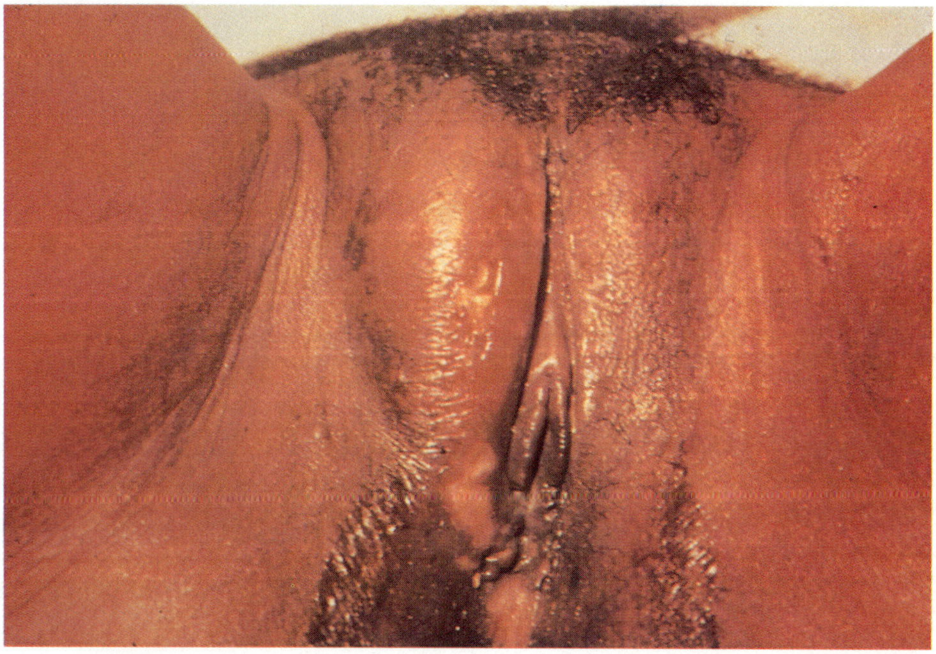

FIGURE 1–49
This patient who has primary syphilis has several chancres. The ulcers have sharp and raised edges. The center of the ulcers is clean and yellowish. In this case there is edema of the right labium majus.

Syphilis

Syphilis is caused by the spirochete *Treponema pallidum*. Primary, secondary, or tertiary syphilitic lesions may occur on the vulva. In women, the primary lesion (a chancre) heals spontaneously in 2 to 6 weeks and may be unnoticed. In some patients it may remain for 3 to 6 months. The "hard" chancre of syphilis is a painless, firm ulcer that has raised borders (i.e., a "punched out" appearance) and a non-necrotic base. In contrast to primary syphilis in men, in women the primary lesion is more apt to be multiple and there is less induration (Fig. 1–49). The chancre is commonly located on the labia minora or at the introitus. Inguinal lymphadenitis is routinely present, although it is not as striking as that associated with LGV. Although the appearance of the primary chancre is characteristic, it must be appreciated that primary syphilis may masquerade in many guises, and thus syphilis must be considered in all patients with ulcerated lesions (Table 1–1).

The characteristic secondary lesion of syphilis on the vulva is the condyloma latum. This appears 1 to 6 months after the primary lesion. It is a grayish-pink, moist papule that is usually multiple. They are often confluent and involve not only the vulva but also the adjacent perineum, perianal region, and the inner sides of the thighs (Fig. 1–50).

Tertiary lesions on the vulva are rarely seen. They occur either as gummatous tumors or ulcerations. They are often found in visceral sites; however, if on the vulva the ulcers may extend widely and may destroy the vulvar structures as well as the surrounding tissues.

TABLE 1–1.
Differential Diagnosis of Vulvar Ulcers

Trauma (aphthous or factitious ulcers)
Behçet syndrome
Herpes simplex
Chancroid
Granuloma inguinale
Lymphogranuloma venereum
Syphilis
Tuberculosis
Histiocytosis X
Cancer

The primary chancre is characterized by dense infiltration with lymphocytes, plasma cells, and fibroblasts. Giant cells may be present. Arteritis of the deep cutaneous vessels is seen. A Warthin-Starry silver impregnation stain or fluorescent techniques may demonstrate presence of the spirochete. The condyloma latum is a granulomatous lesion that may show superficial epithelial necrosis. Both superficial and deep vessels are involved. The vessel wall shows edema and a marked perivascular inflammatory infiltrate.

The gummatous tertiary skin lesion is a granulomatous nodule composed of plasma cells, lymphocytes, epithelioid cells, and fibroblasts. A variable number of giant cells are present. The nodule extends from the epidermis deep into the subcuta-

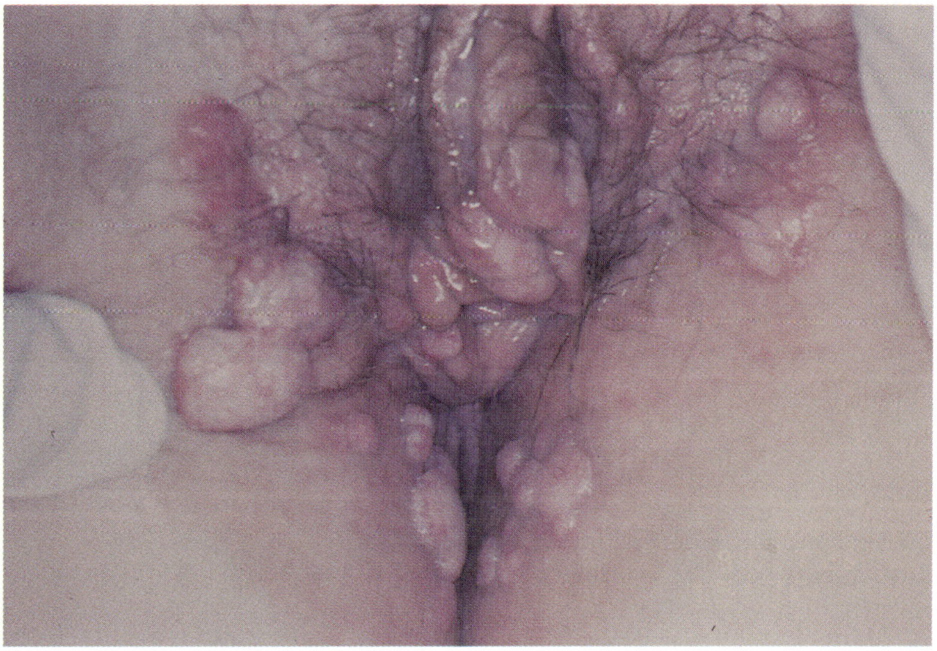

FIGURE 1–50
Multiple condylomata lata of secondary syphilis are shown. The lesions are grayish pink, moist papules. Some are confluent. The surface of the papules is slightly convoluted but smoother than that of the typical condyloma acuminatum.

neous tissue. There is obliterative endarteritis within the gumma. The overlying skin may be thinned or eroded, and this causes the ulcer.

The most specific method of making a diagnosis of syphilis is to identify the *T. pallidum* organism. The spirochete is readily identifiable by darkfield microscopic examination of serum from both primary and secondary lesions but not from tertiary lesions. To obtain a specimen for darkfield examination the chancre or condylomatous lesion is first cleaned with saline solution. After drying, the lesion is abraded with dry gauze until minimal bleeding occurs. Then, by applying pressure, a clear serum is expressed from the lesion and applied to a clean glass slide. A coverslip is placed over the serum and sealed by applying petroleum jelly around its periphery.

Most cases of syphilis are diagnosed in the latent stage. Serologic tests in the latent stage, as in other stages of the disease, are of diagnostic importance. Serologic tests are divided into those based on nonspecific reagin-type antibodies and those based on antitreponemal antibodies. Nonspecific tests include the VDRL and the rapid plasma reagin (RPR) tests. Specific tests include the *T. pallidum* immobilization (TPI) test, the fluorescent treponemal antibody absorption (FTA-ABS) test, and the micro hemagglutination assay (MHA). One of the specific tests should be performed in patients with a reactive VDRL or RPR test to confirm the diagnosis. Sometimes no spirochetes are identified in material from primary or secondary lesions or in patients who have latent or tertiary syphilis. Again, a specific test is indicated. In patients with very early disease serologic tests may be negative even though the chancre is present and it is possible to identify the spirochetes by darkfield examination. It takes several weeks for the serology to convert to positive.

Penicillin is the drug of choice for treating syphilis. Erythromycin and tetracycline are alternatives that can be used if a patient is allergic to penicillin. The dose and duration of therapy vary according to the stage of the disease. The treatment schedules recommended by the United States Centers for Disease Control are found in many infectious diseases textbooks and manuals.[32]

Tuberculosis

Tuberculous ulceration of the vulva is extremely rare. It may occur as a primary lesion due to exogenous infection generally caused by direct inoculation from an infected sexual partner. The lesion is usually found in the vestibule where it begins as a nodule that later ulcerates. The characteristic-appearance is that of an irregular, ragged ulcer of granulomatous or even caseous appearance (Fig. 1–51).

The microscopic diagnosis is based on the demonstration of tubercles similar to those seen elsewhere. There are large or small granulomas that have classic Langhans-type giant cells surrounded by epithelioid cells (Fig. 1–52). Necrosis may be present in the granulomatous center. Differentiation from other granulomatous diseases and confirmation of the diagnosis requires special techniques (acid-fast or fluorescent stain) to identify the presence of the organism. The use of skin tests (e.g., Tine test, purified protein derivative) may help in establishing the diagnosis.

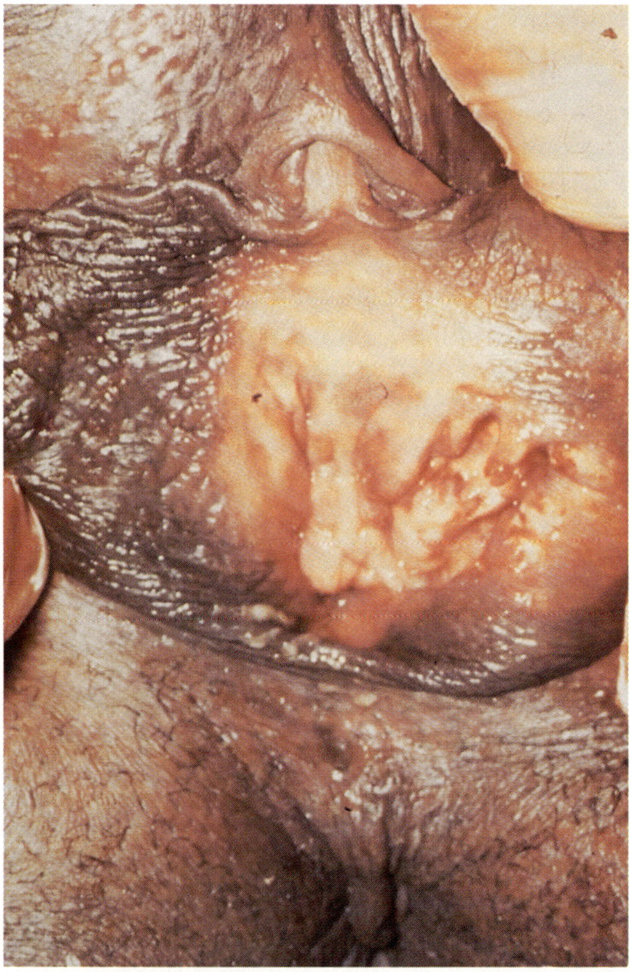

FIGURE 1–51
This is an example of tuberculosis involving the vulva. An irregular, ragged ulcer destroys the left labium minus. The raised whitish areas in the center of the ulcer contain caseating granulomas.

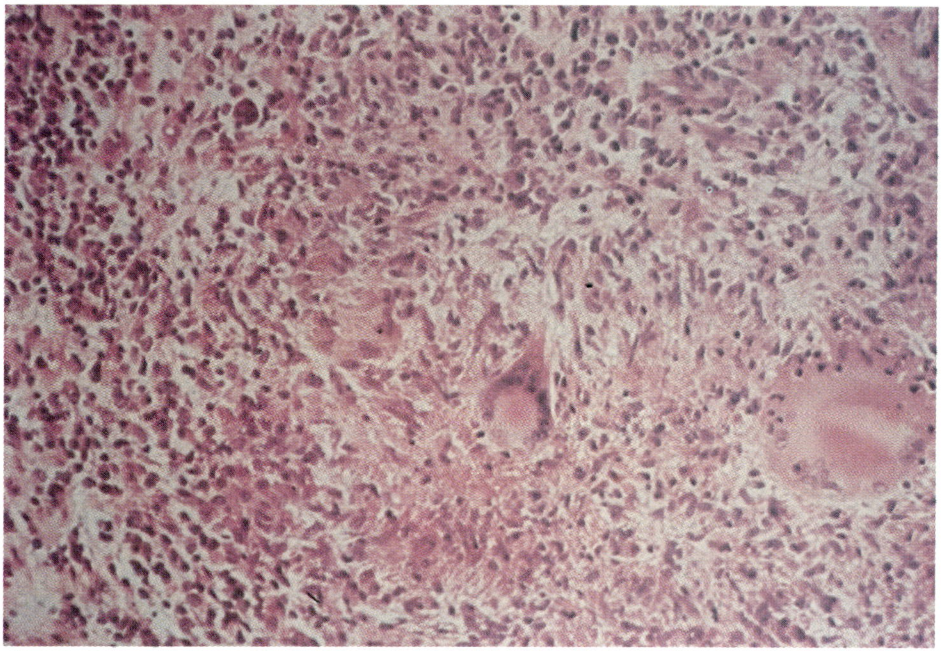

FIGURE 1-52
A granuloma of tuberculosis is shown. A Langhans-type cell is seen in the center. Its nuclei are arranged around the periphery of the cell. Epithelioid cells surround the giant cell. A chronic inflammatory infiltrate surrounds the granuloma and is seen best at the left.

OTHER INFECTIOUS DISEASES

Tinea

Tinea versicolor is occasionally seen in the vulvar area and typically involves the mons, the labia majora, and the inner thighs. This condition is caused by the fungus *Malassezia (Pityrosporum) furfur*. A product of the fungus interferes with the oxidation of melanin, resulting in hypopigmented or depigmented patches that are fine and scaly. The patient may experience mild pruritus.

Tinea cruris is caused by the fungus *Epidermophyton floccosum*. Heat and humidity are necessary for the development of tinea cruris. The lesion begins as a small erythematous, scaly patch on the upper inner thigh and intercrural area. The lesion spreads from the edges while the center clears partially. The border of the lesion is well demarcated. It may extend toward the labia majora or perianally. Tinea cruris produces intense pruritus.

Both tinea versicolor and tinea cruris respond well to clotrimazole and to many other topical antifungal agents.

Pediculosis

Pediculosis is caused by the louse *Phthirus pubis*. Infestation with the pubic louse can cause intense pruritus. The diagnosis is made by identification of the lice or their nits on the hair shaft using a hand-held magnifying glass. Microscopic examination reveals the typical crablike morphology of the louse. The lice can be eradicated by the use of topical 0.5% malathion (e.g., Ovide) or 1% permethrin (e.g., Nix, Elimite).[33] Lindane (e.g., Kwell) and pyrethrins with piperonyl butoxide (e.g., Rid) are alternative preparations. Underclothing, linens, and towels must be thoroughly washed to prevent reinfection.

Scabies

Scabies is caused by the mite *Sarcoptes scabiei*.[34] In the United States infestation with this mite appears to occur in intervals of 30 years, and the cycle lasts about 15 years. The last cycle ended between 1979 and 1980. Therefore we should now be seeing the beginning of a new cycle. The female mite burrows a tunnel in the skin where it lays its eggs. This causes a marked inflammatory response and intense pruritus. The skin lesions are characterized by the burrows, a papular erythematous rash, and the presence of pruritic nodules. The mite can be identified under the microscope by examining material obtained from a fresh lesion. The scrapings are placed in potassium hydroxide or mineral oil. However, identification of the mite is not always possible and the diagnosis must be based on the history of insidious onset, the presence of nocturnal pruritus and the characteristic skin lesions, and involvement of typical areas, including the wrists, finger webs, elbows, axillae, external genitalia, and buttocks. The treatment of choice is topical 5% permethrin (e.g., Nix, Elimite). Lindane (e.g., Kwell) lotion and 10% crotamiton (e.g., Eurax) are also effective. As with pediculosis, all underclothing, linens, and towels must be thoroughly washed to prevent reinfection.

HYPERPLASTIC AND ATROPHIC CHANGES

The identification of leukoplakia of the tongue as a precancerous lesion was first described by Schwimmer[35] in 1877. Of the 20 patients reported, one also had patchy whitening of the vulva. Bonney[36] was impressed with the inflammatory origin of such lesions and recognized a relationship between the atrophic and hypertrophic stages. He suggested that the hypertrophic stage preceded the atrophic stage and that a malignant potential was associated only with the hypertrophic alterations. Taussig[37] believed that malignant potential was high in both stages and definitive therapy was necessary in both situations. The gross appearance of hyperplastic and atrophic changes of the vulva was described by Taussig as follows: (1) erythema, edema, excoriation, and dryness, (2) thickening and whitening of the vulvar skin with flattening of vulvar folds, and (3) cracking and superficial ulcerations with a parchment-like appearance of white or bluish-white skin. The microscopic stages were described as (1) minimal hyperkeratosis and acanthosis with inflammatory infiltrate, (2) hyperkeratosis and acanthosis with epithelial hypertrophy and round cell infiltration, and (3) hyperkeratosis, flattened rete pegs, and a frayed basement layer with dermal collagen and inflammatory infiltrate.

The confusion that exists in descriptions of the gross appearance of the white lesions of the vulva is reflected in the microscopic interpretation of such lesions. Sometimes the presence of mild hyperkeratosis, acanthosis, and inflammatory infiltrate has led to a diagnosis of leukoplakia when the lesion was actually chronic dermatitis with lichenification. Furthermore, quite commonly the atrophic conditions have been diagnosed as leukoplakia simply on the basis of the presence of hyperkeratosis. The result of an erroneous diagnosis and the presumed malignant potential of leukoplakia has led to unnecessary surgery for chronic dermatitis or lichen sclerosus. Thus, it is important to convey to the clinician the degree of epithelial atypicality and the potential for malignant transformation. Ideally, this will lead to an appropriate clinical management plan.

The term dystrophy was first applied to vulvar lesions (usually to white lesions) by Jeffcoate in 1966.[38] The International Society for the Study of Vulvar Disease (ISSVD) has adopted and publicized a classification (Table 1–2) of the vulvar "dystrophies" in an effort to standardize the nomenclature applied to the classic histopathologic features of the many lesions previously diagnosed as leukoplakia (e.g., hypertrophic and atrophic lesions, lichen sclerosus et atrophicus, kraurosis, primary senile atrophy, and others).[39] This system will be used here.

TABLE 1–2.
Current Classification of Vulvar Dystrophies

Squamous hyperplasia
Without atypia (e.g., chronic dermatitis with hyperkeratosis)
With atypia (mild, moderate, or marked atypia or VIN 1, VIN 2, and VIN 3)
Lichen sclerosus*
Without atypia
With atypia? (no cases identified)
Mixed
Focal lichen sclerosus with areas of hyperplasia, with or without atypia

* The term "et atrophicus" is no longer used because cellular overactivity rather than atrophy has been identified in these lesions.

Squamous Hyperplasia Without Atypia

The term squamous hyperplasia, with or without atypia, has been applied to proliferating epithelial lesions of the vulva. Such a term seems more meaningful to the clinician because it provides a point of reference compared to other proliferations in the cervix and endometrium. Typical hyperplastic dystrophy (squamous hyperplasia without atypia) corresponds to the classic picture of chronic dermatitis with hyperkeratosis previously described (Fig. 1–14). The epithelium has proliferated and there is acanthosis but no cellular atypia and no abnormal maturation. There is no malignant potential of this lesion.

Vulvar Intraepithelial Neoplasia

It is suggested that atypical hyperplasia (squamous hyperplasia with atypia) be diagnosed as vulvar intraepithelial neoplasia (VIN).[39] These lesions are characterized by squamous cellular atypia and disorganization, an increased nuclear to cytoplasmic ratio, nuclear pleomorphism, and abnormal maturation of the epithelium. The hyperkeratosis that is usually present in these lesions gives them their white color (Fig. 1–53). In some cases parakeratosis is also seen, and this

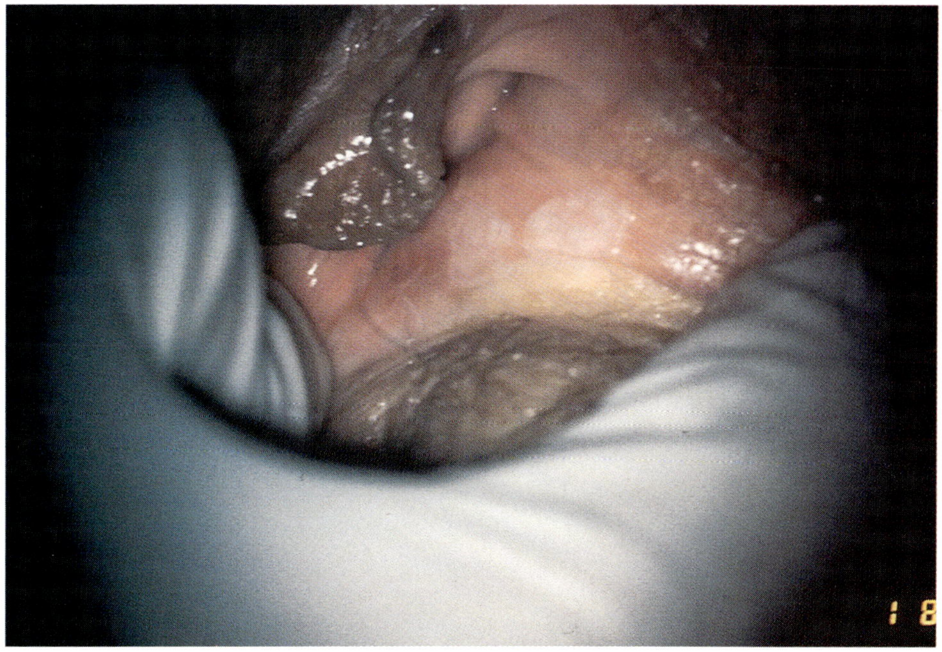

FIGURE 1-53
There is a slightly raised white patch on the left labium minus. Biopsy showed VIN 3.

may lead to a more reddish color of the lesion (Fig. 1–54). Increased mitotic activity, mitoses higher in the epithelium, and abnormal mitotic figures are present. Proliferation of the basal and parabasal cell layers leads to acanthosis, and in some cases there is distortion of the rete pegs (Fig. 1–55). Cellular atypia and mitotic activity confined to the lower third of the epithelium is classified as VIN 1. If these changes extend to the middle third or the upper third of the epithelium the lesion is classified as VIN 2 or VIN 3, respectively.[40] If the full thickness of the epithelium demonstrates cellular atypia the diagnosis is carcinoma in situ or VIN 3 (Fig. 1–56). VIN 3 now replaces other terms such as Bowen disease, erythroplasia of Queyrat, carcinoma in situ, and bowenoid papulosis.

There is controversy about whether bowenoid papulosis should be maintained as a separate diagnosis. The typical patient with bowenoid papulosis is in the fourth decade of life and presents with multiple gray-brown papules on the vulva (Fig. 1–57). Sometimes the papules have a verrucous appearance. Spontaneous regression of the

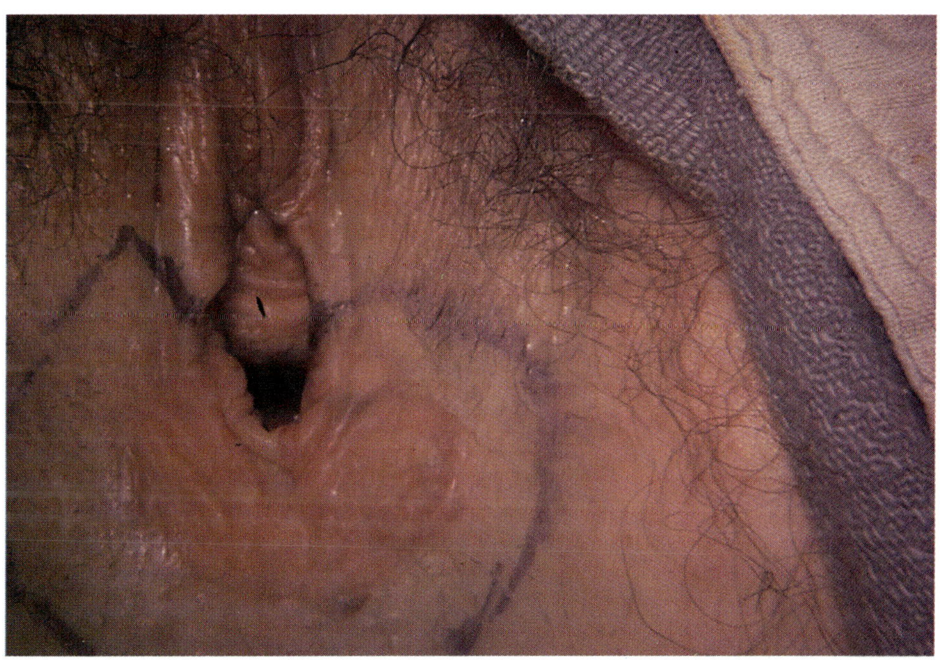

FIGURE 1-54
This reddish lesion on the perineum is VIN 3. The purple mark represents the planned excision line. VIN 3 is treated by wide local excision.

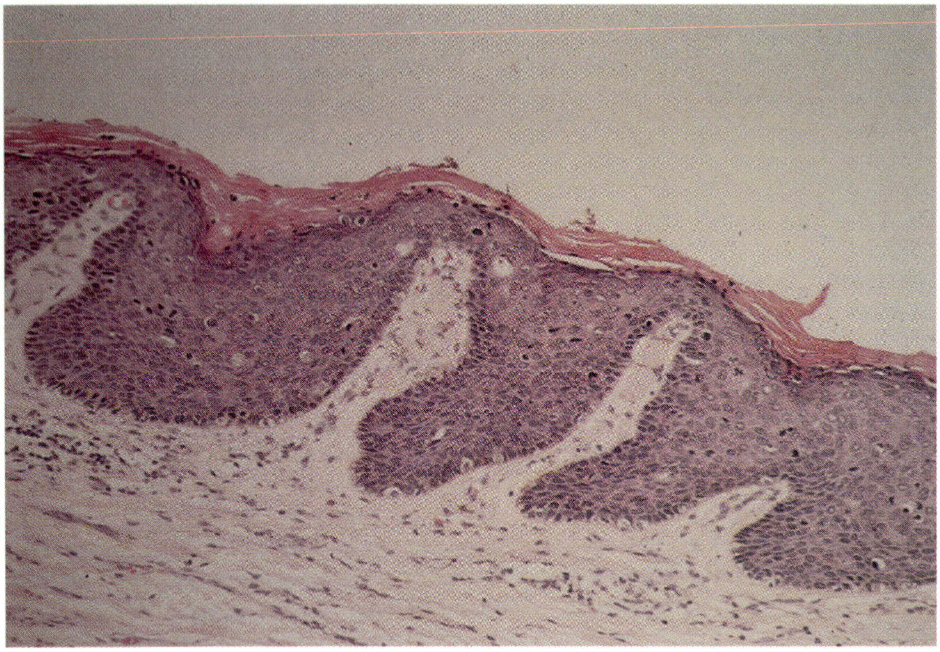

FIGURE 1-55
This biopsy specimen shows VIN 3. Abnormal nuclei are present throughout the full thickness of the epithelium. Numerous mitotic figures are present, some of which are close to the surface. There are hyperkeratosis, parakeratosis, and acanthosis.

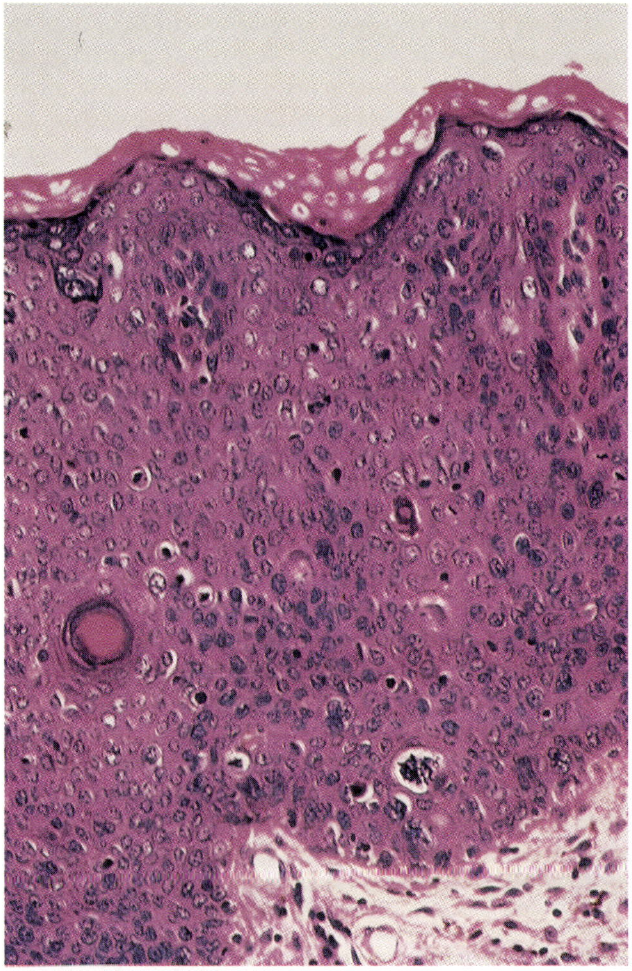

FIGURE 1-56
A high-power view of VIN 3. There is marked atypia throughout the full thickness of the epithelium. The cytoplasm is scant in all the cells. There is a pearl formation *(left)*. An abnormal mitotic figure is seen in a cell a few layers above the basement membrane.

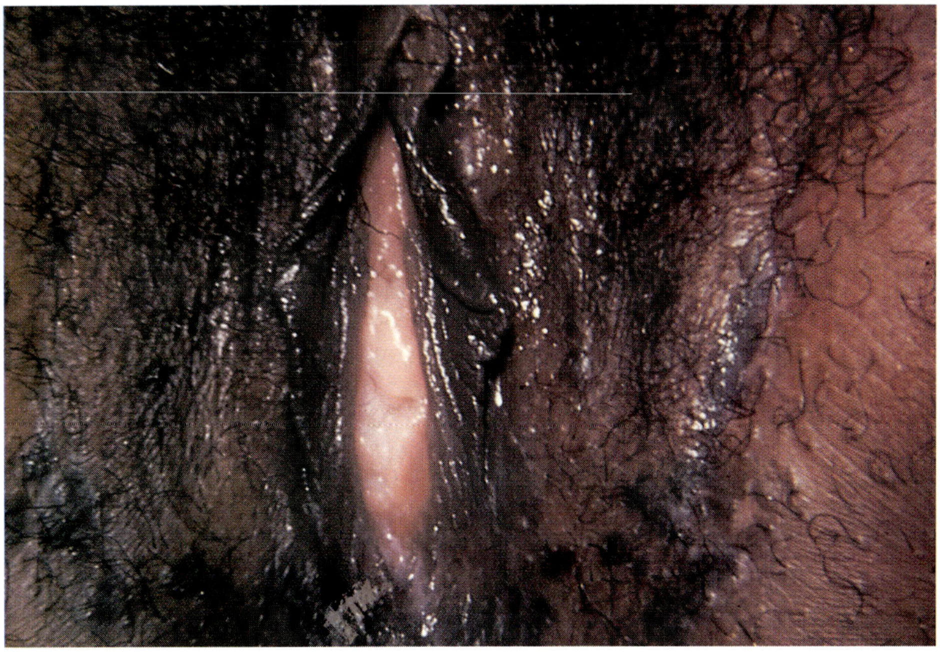

FIGURE 1-57
Multiple grayish papules are seen on the labia majora of this patient who has bowenoid papulosis.

lesions has been reported.[41] On microscopic examination, bowenoid papulosis may be indistinguishable from VIN 3. It has been suggested that cellular uniformity and absence of hair follicle involvement distinguishes bowenoid papulosis from VIN 3.[42]

It is important to appreciate that in the vulva invasive carcinoma may occur without full-thickness cellular atypia and disorganization (Fig. 1–58). Abnormal cell maturation may be observed in the form of individual cell keratinization in the lower half of the epithelium. Marked atypicality is characterized by "keratin pearl" formation at the tips of the rete pegs (Fig. 1–59). This finding is of concern because this abnormal maturation of deeper areas may be a harbinger of invasion. These cases should be diagnosed as markedly atypical squamous hyperplasia.

The average age range of patients with VIN 3 is the third to fourth decades of life.[43–45] Koilocytotic atypia, characteristic of human papillomavirus (HPV) infection, and HPV DNA is found in over 80 percent of VIN 3 lesions.[46] Progression of VIN 3 to invasive squamous cell carcinoma rarely occurs.

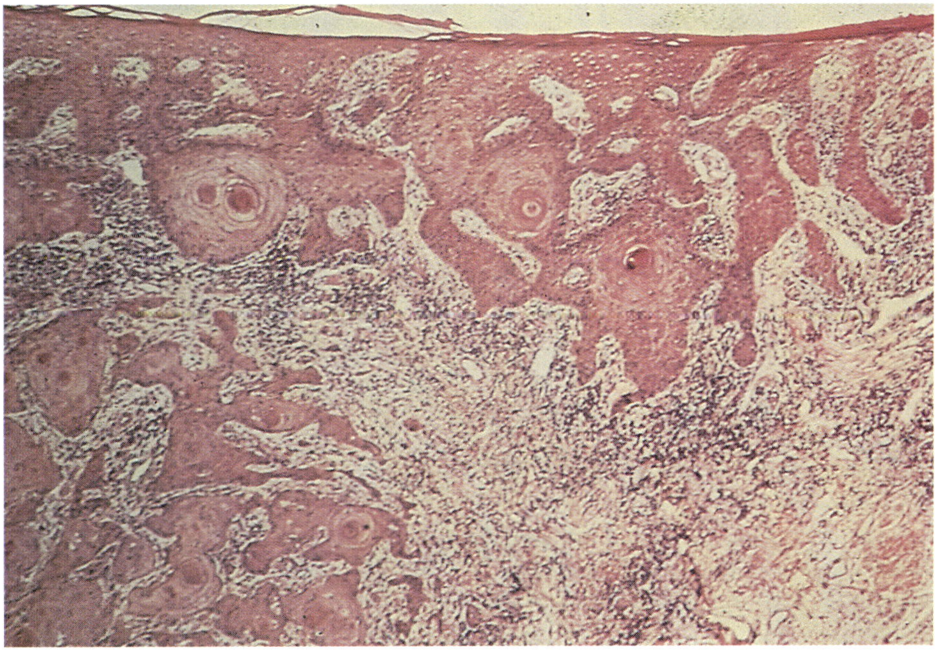

FIGURE 1-58
The maturation of the squamous epithelium at the surface of this lesion is relatively normal. However, pearl formation is present within the tips of the rete pegs. This has given rise to the well-differentiated squamous cell carcinoma seen here.

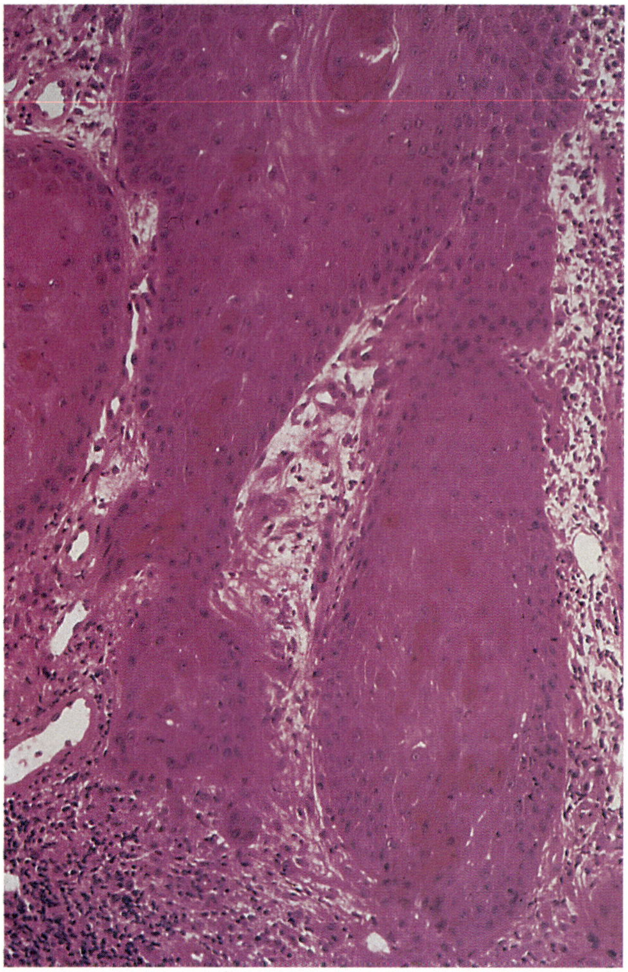

FIGURE 1-59
This is a biopsy specimen of markedly atypical squamous hyperplasia, which is characterized by abnormal keratinization of the cells at the tip of the rete pegs. A squamous pearl is seen *(top)*.

However, patients who have immunosuppression and women over the age of 60 years seem to have a greater risk of progression to cancer than other women.[47, 48] In contrast, the average age range of patients with invasive squamous cell carcinoma of the vulva is the seventh to eighth decades of life. HPV DNA is found in only 20 to 30 percent of these cases.[49, 50]

The role of HPV infection in the development of VIN is highlighted by the presence of multifocal (multiple sites on the vulva) as well as multicentric (involvement of vulva, cervix, or vagina) disease. Numerous instances of carcinoma in situ occurring simultaneously on the perineum, vulva, and cervix have been reported.[51, 52] Therefore, in a patient who has VIN all these sites should be carefully examined, and biopsies should be obtained if a lesion is identified. The vulva can be examined with a colposcope (see Chapter 3) or a magnifying glass.

The treatment of VIN is wide local excision. This allows for the identification of the presence of occult invasion. In one series such invasion was found to be present in 19 percent of the specimens.[53] In some patients a wide geographic distribution of multiple lesions requires a simple vulvectomy and skin graft. However, thorough evaluation of the vulva by colposcopy and multiple biopsies to exclude invasion may spare a vulvectomy. If there is no invasion the lesions on the hair-bearing areas are excised, and those on the labia minora, fourchette, and around the clitoris can be vaporized with laser treatment.[54]

Lichen Sclerosus

Lichen sclerosus is a genetically inherited disease, but a specific gene has not yet been identified.[55] It may occur in various areas of the body and in any age group but is more common in postmenopausal women. When it occurs in children, resolution

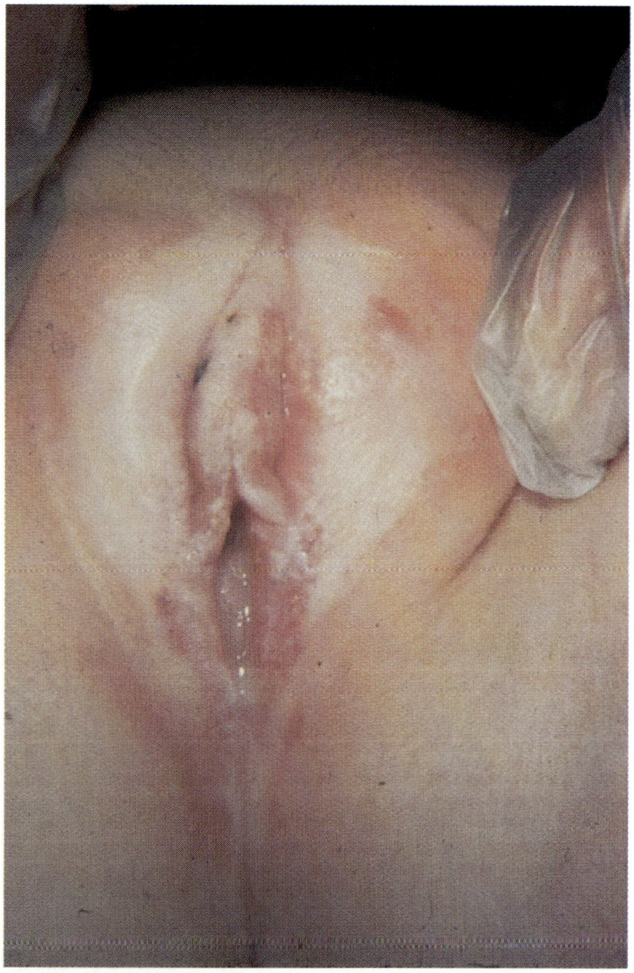

FIGURE 1-60
This young girl has extensive changes of lichen sclerosus. The skin of the labia, prepuce, and perineum is shiny white, dry, and thin. Excoriation marks are seen.

usually occurs before or after puberty.[56] Lichen sclerosus is more common and more extensive on the vulva than in any other area of the body. In the earliest phase the lesion appears as a yellowish-blue papule. With coalescence of multiple lesions, an entire area becomes grayish-white, thin, and often parchment-like (Fig. 1–60). The lesion may involve any area of the vulva and may extend to the inner thighs and to the perianal region. As the condition progresses, the labia minora may shrink to the point of disappearance. This may result in constriction of the introitus. The shrinking of the prepuce may constrict the clitoris. Generally, there are no early symptoms; however, the thinned tissue is easily irritated, and this results in pruritus. This happens most commonly in postmenopausal women. On the vulva the chronic pruritus results in excoriations. Symptoms do not exist when lichen sclerosus occurs in other areas of the body.

The histopathologic characteristics of lichen sclerosus are hyperkeratosis, thinning of the epithelium with loss of rete pegs, a subepithelial zone of collagen, and a chronic inflammatory cell infiltrate beneath the collagen (Fig. 1–61). Often the layer of keratin is thicker than the epithelium. The homogeneous collagen band is often strikingly edematous when the process is acute or has been recently irritated. The underlying infiltrate is made up of a variable number of lymphocytes and plasma cells, and there are occasional melanophages (pigment-laden macrophages). These are seen in many other chronic lesions as well. Keratin plugging of the follicles is commonly seen. The basal cells are vacuolated and subepidermal bullae are occasionally present. Melanocytes and melanin pigment in the epithelium are absent. The chronic trauma caused by scratching can result in epithelial hyperplasia next to the lichen sclerosus lesions. This is known as a mixed dystrophy. Although the term "et atrophicus" has usually been appended to lichen sclerosus, studies have demonstrated that the epithelium is more metabolically active than normal tissues.[57] Thus, the appellation is not justified and is no longer used.

The histologic changes occurring in lichen sclerosus are similar to those described by Taussig[58] for chronic atrophic vulvitis, later known as atrophic leukoplakia, kraurosis, and primary senile atrophy. Kraurosis is a clinical term (not a histopathologic diagnosis) that describes shrinkage of the vulvar structures with a decrease in or complete absence of the subcutaneous fat. This results in loss of the normal architecture that reduces the normal appearance of the vulva to a flattened, smooth, grayish-white area, often superficially excoriated or fissured, especially at the fourchette. The introitus is constricted so that coitus is painful or impossible. Although a diagnosis of kraurosis has often been made on the basis of the microscopic findings, one cannot determine the degree of shrinkage of the vulvar structures by microscopic examination of a small fragment of tissue. Therefore, lichen sclerosus is the diagnosis used when the histopathologic findings correspond to those noted earlier, whereas kraurosis is used to describe the gross appearance of the vulva.

Because lichen sclerosus is more common in

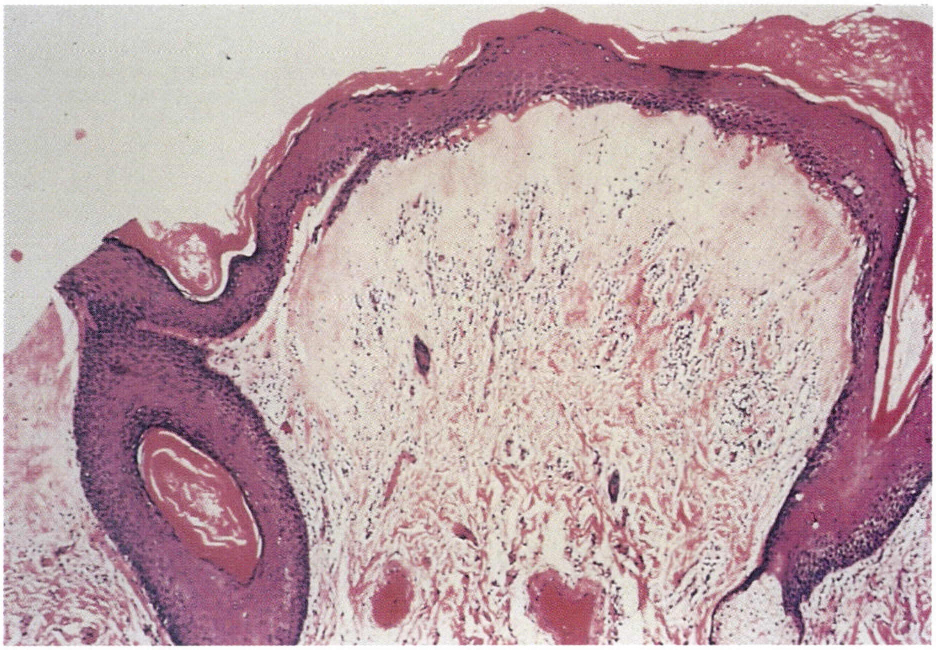

FIGURE 1–61
This is a biopsy of an area of lichen sclerosus. There is hyperkeratosis, particularly prominent on the right. The epithelium is thin, with loss of rete pegs. A subepithelial band of dense collagen is present, under which there is an inflammatory infiltrate. A hair follicle *(left)* contains a keratin plug.

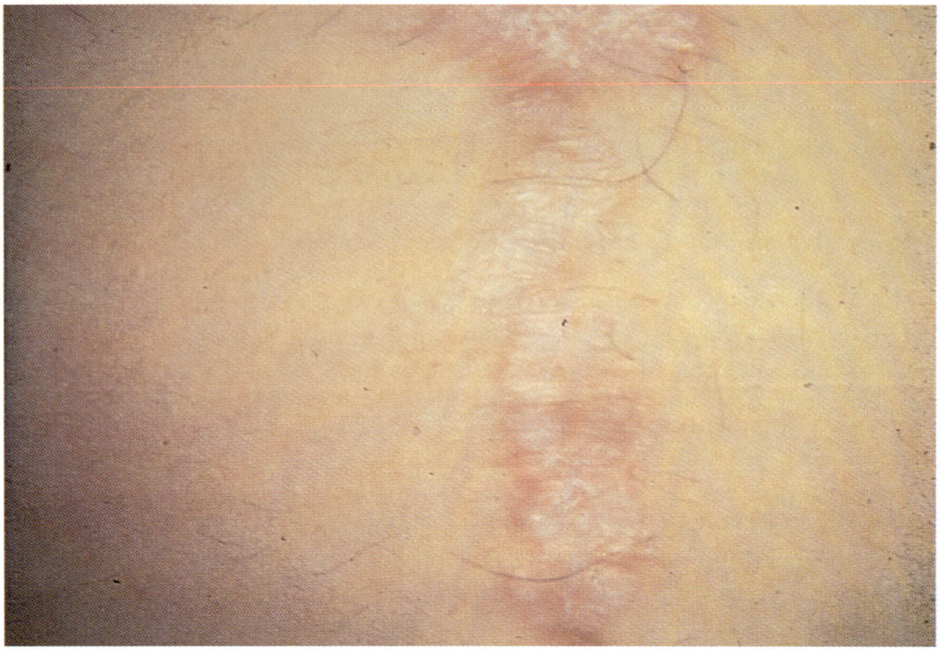

FIGURE 1-62
This abdominal scar shows changes characteristic of lichen sclerosus. The skin is shiny white, dry, and thin.

postmenopausal women the obvious explanation for its pathogenesis is the lack of sex hormones. However, this does not explain the occurrence of lichen sclerosus in women who are younger and have normal ovarian function. One can only assume that for some unknown reason the vulvar tissues lose their responsiveness to the ovarian hormones. Because similar changes occur in "nonsexual skin" (Fig. 1–62), other causes such as local vascular alterations and trauma must be considered.

Lichen sclerosus rarely if ever progresses to invasive squamous cell carcinoma and is not considered a premalignant condition.[59] However, hyperplastic and atrophic changes are frequently found in the skin next to vulvar cancer.[60] This may be coincidental. Conversely, the chronic irritation of the skin caused by the "itch-scratch" cycle of the vulvar dystrophies may lay the foundation for neoplastic transformation. Therefore, it is important to control the pruritus and not to hesitate in performing a biopsy of ulcerations or areas of skin

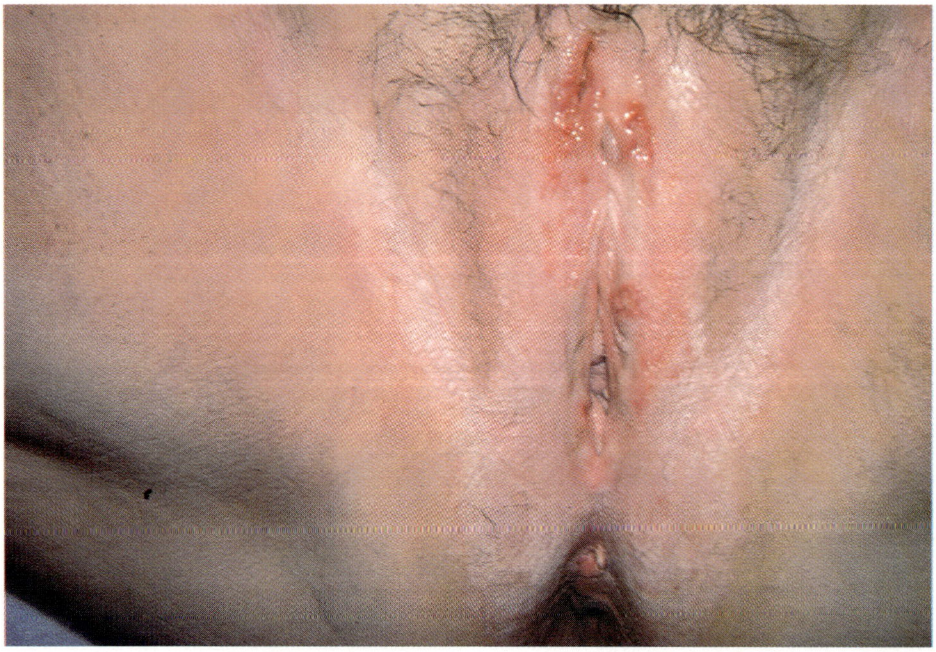

FIGURE 1-63
This patient has extensive lichen sclerosus of the vulva and multiple excoriation marks. Two ulcers are present on either side of the clitoris. Biopsy showed squamous cell carcinoma.

thickening when identified (Fig. 1–63). Wide local excision is necessary if cellular atypicality or abnormal maturation is seen. Lichen sclerosus has been successfully treated with topical testosterone (2%) or with progesterone (2%) and corticosteroids. Recently, good results have been reported using only the potent topical steroid 0.05% clobetasol propionate (e.g., Temovate).[61, 62]

VULVAR EDEMA

Generalized vulvar edema is caused by blockage or stasis of either lymphatic or vascular channels, or both. Probably the most common situation in which such stasis exists is pregnancy (Fig. 1–64). The best illustration of lymphatic blockage leading to vulvar edema is tropical elephantiasis in which the parasitic worm *Filaria sanguinis hominis* is responsible for the lymphatic blockage. Other conditions associated with generalized vulvar edema include lymphogranuloma venereum, chronic suppurative hidradenitis, Crohn's disease, debilitating neurologic disease, and extensive metastases to the inguinal lymph nodes. In a patient with long-term lymphatic obstruction, the skin covering the enlarged edematous labia is greatly thickened and resembles elephant hide. The subcutaneous tissues are edematous and focally infiltrated with lymphocytes and plasma cells. The lymphatics are dilated, and endothelial proliferation may be striking. Occasional giant cells may be recognized, but a classic granuloma with epithelioid cells is missing.

BENIGN TUMORS

Cystic Tumors

Bartholin Duct Cyst

The Bartholin duct cyst or vulvovaginal cyst was described earlier in the section on vestibular adenitis.

Sebaceous and Epidermal Inclusion Cysts

Sebaceous and epidermal inclusion cysts are relatively common on the vulva and usually produce no symptoms. Sebaceous cysts arise as a result of blockage of the ducts of the sebaceous glands. These are abundant in both the labia majora and minora. The gross appearance of the contents of a sebaceous cyst are characteristically cheesy. Like sebaceous cysts elsewhere, they are prone to infection and abscess formation. The lining of the sebaceous cyst is characterized by the presence of irregular clumps of cells that have small, dark nuclei and clear cytoplasm. An inflammatory cell infiltrate and giant cells are seen. The giant cells are part of the tissue reaction to the foreign sebaceous material. Carcinoma arising in these cysts is rare.

The residual of the obstructed pilosebaceous

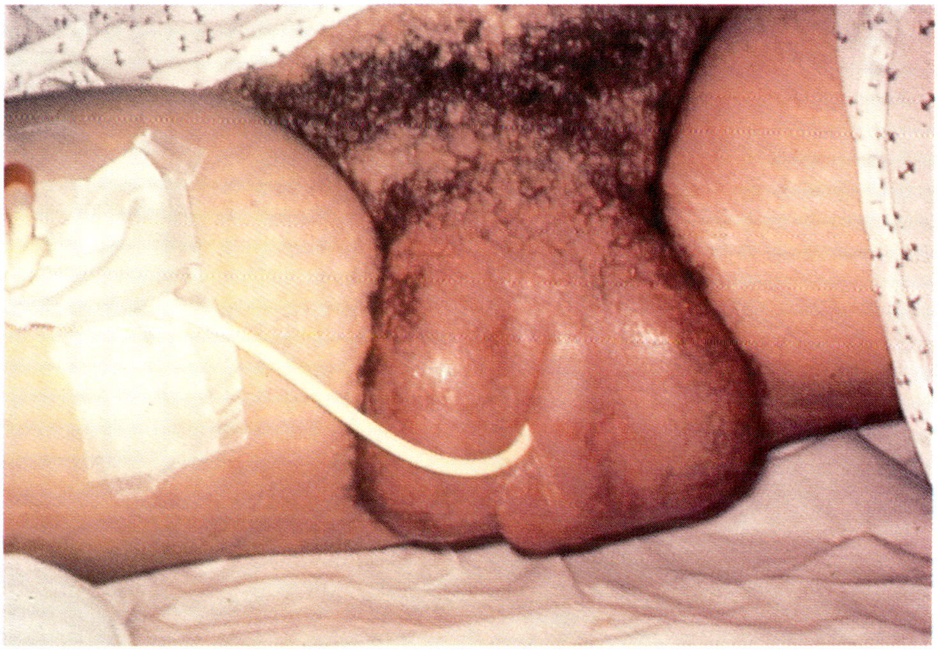

FIGURE 1–64
This patient has massive vulvar edema. She is pregnant and has preeclampsia and nephrotic syndrome.

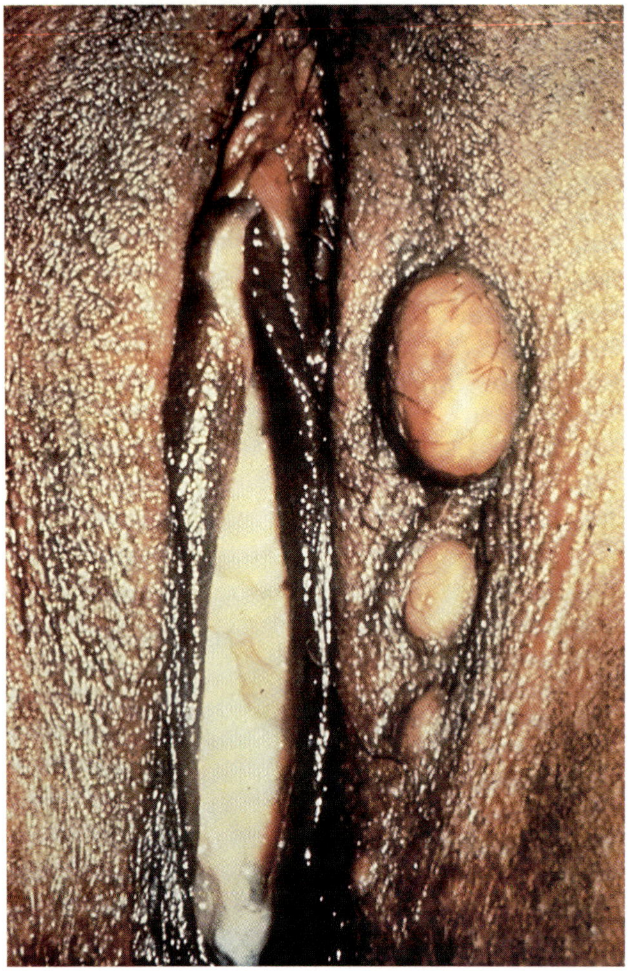

FIGURE 1-65
Three smooth, rounded nodules are seen on the left labium majus. These are epithelial inclusion cysts.

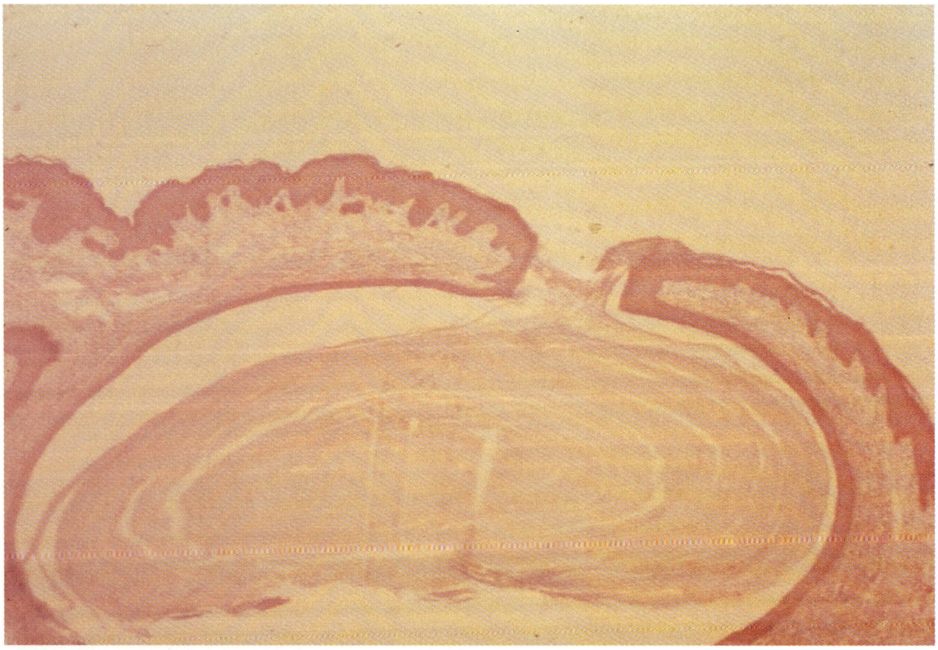

FIGURE 1-66
This is the microscopic appearance of an epithelial inclusion cyst. The cyst is lined by squamous epithelium, which in this case is continuous with the surface epithelium.

unit is the more common epithelial inclusion cyst. These cysts may be single or multiple, and they are small, round to oval, firm subcutaneous nodules that produce no symptoms. They are found on the labia majora (Fig. 1–65). Desquamated superficial epithelial cells make up the contents of these cysts. This material also looks cheesy. The cyst is lined by stratified squamous epithelium as in a hair follicle (Fig. 1–66).

Because sebaceous and epidermal inclusion cysts are rarely associated with symptoms, excision is seldom necessary. Frequently after excision more cysts appear at the incision line. If infected, incision and drainage with cauterization of the cyst cavity is performed. Broad spectrum oral antibiotics are prescribed. If the diagnosis is not clear by gross examination and excision is necessary, care must be taken if the lesion is located in the labium minus. The paucity of subcutaneous tissue in this structure and the possibility of wound breakdown may result in fenestrations. Alternatively, a portion of the labium may be removed with the cyst. Whatever approach is used, the patient must understand that there may be distortion of the normal anatomy after the procedure.

Mucinous Cyst

Mucinous or mucous cysts of the vulva are rare and occur lateral to the clitoris or in the inner aspect of the labium minus (Fig. 1–67). These cysts are commonly pedunculated and may represent aberrant mucinous epithelium, misplaced at the time of division of the cloaca by the anal fold (also known as the urorectal fold). Another possible origin of such a cyst is the minor vestibular glands. These structures, like Bartholin's gland, have mucus-secreting acini. These may undergo the same occlusive processes that affect the major vestibular glands.

Mucinous cysts of the vulva are usually unilocular and contain abundant mucoid material. The cyst wall is lined by a single layer of tall columnar, mucin-secreting cells that have a basally placed nucleus (Fig. 1–68). Squamous metaplasia, ciliated cells, reserve cell hyperplasia, and papillary groups of cells may also be seen. The cyst lining is surrounded by a fibrovascular stroma. Muscle is not seen.

Excision of the mucinous cyst is necessary only when other diagnoses must be excluded. Because a mucinous cyst may be slightly raised above the skin surface and blue in color, sometimes it must be differentiated from a pigmented lesion.

Skene Duct Cyst

A Skene duct cyst (paraurethral cyst) is a small cyst that on occasion may be enlarged to up to 2 cm in diameter and may cause urethral obstruction. The cyst is usually lined by transitional epithelium, but either squamous or ciliated metaplasia may also be seen.

Cyst of the Canal of Nuck

Cysts may arise from the peritoneal covering that has been carried down with the round ligament to

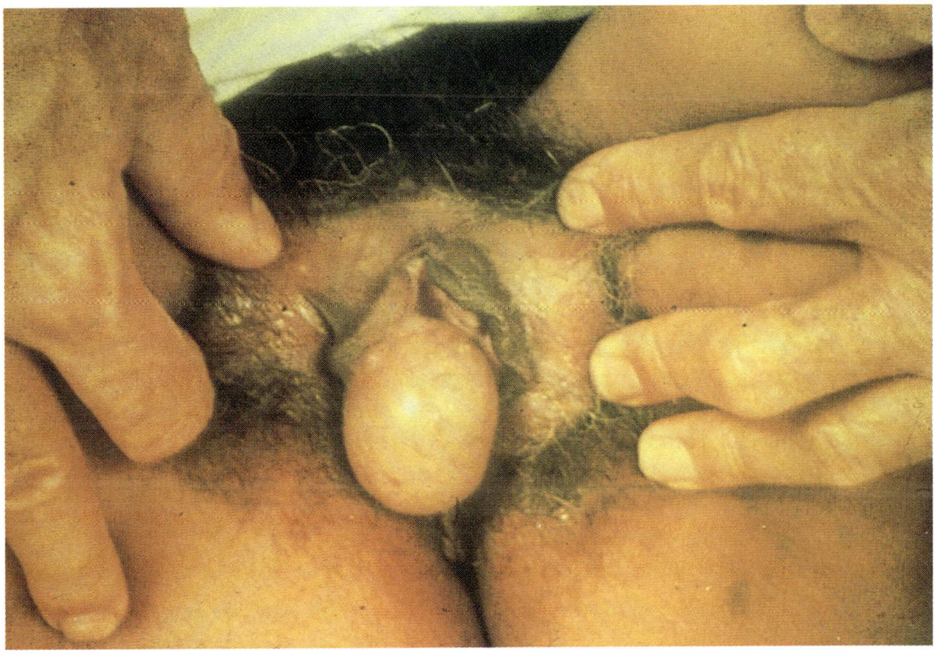

FIGURE 1–67
A mucinous cyst is seen on the inner aspect of the right labium minus.

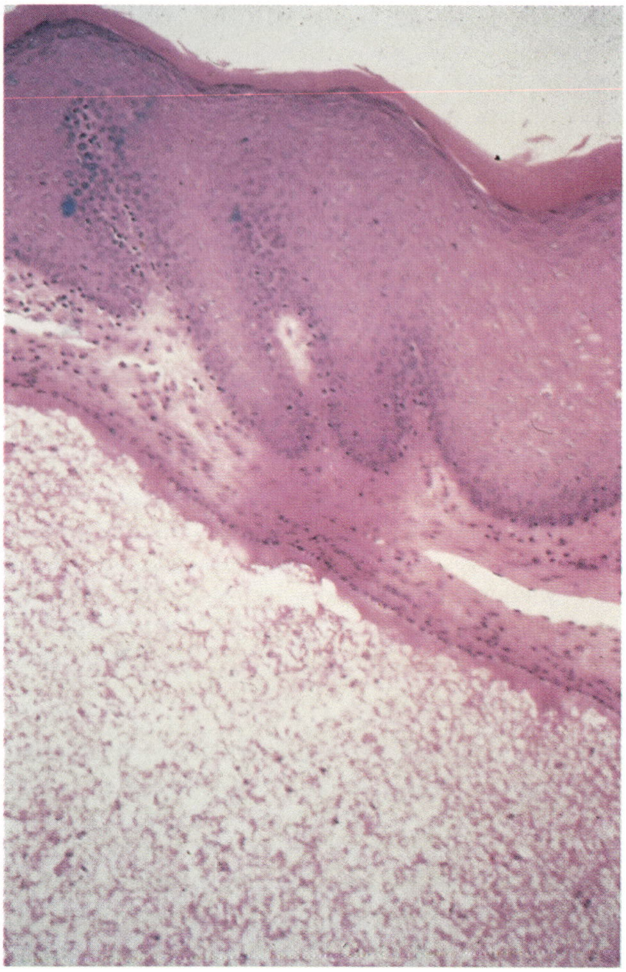

FIGURE 1-68
This is the microscopic appearance of the mucinous cyst shown in Figure 1-67. The outside surface is covered by squamous epithelium. The cyst cavity is seen at the bottom. The cyst is lined by a single layer of mucinous columnar epithelium with basally oriented nuclei. There is edema in the connective tissue between the cyst and the surface epithelium.

its insertion in the labium majus. The cyst of the canal of Nuck, which corresponds to the hydrocele in the male, is therefore found in the labium majus (Fig. 1-69). Direct and persistent communication with the peritoneal reflection along the inguinal canal and its associated round ligament may result in development of an indirect inguinal hernia. Excision of the cyst or sac, without ligation of the sac's neck and closure of the associated fascial defect (herniorrhaphy), will only lead to recurrence because the communication with the peritoneal lining persists.

The cyst of the canal of Nuck contains clear peritoneal fluid. The cyst wall is lined by a single layer of mesothelial cells that are cuboidal to flattened in shape. Mesothelial proliferation (see Chapter 9) may be present and may be erroneously diagnosed as cancer.

The cyst of the canal of Nuck may be mistaken for a Bartholin duct cyst on physical examination. The Bartholin duct cyst is found in the inferior aspect of the vulva whereas the cyst of the canal of Nuck is located on its superior aspect.

Solid Tumors

A number of solid growths can occur in the vulvar area. These include the verrucous lesions (e.g., condyloma acuminatum), acrochordon, fibroma, myoma, lipoma, sebaceous adenoma, vestibular adenoma, granular cell tumor (myoblastoma), hidradenoma, syringoma, ectopic breast tissue, endometriosis, and angioma. Isolated cases of lymphangioma and neurofibroma have also been reported.

Papillomas

Verrucous lesions of the vulva occur in one of two forms, the relatively rare true papilloma and the

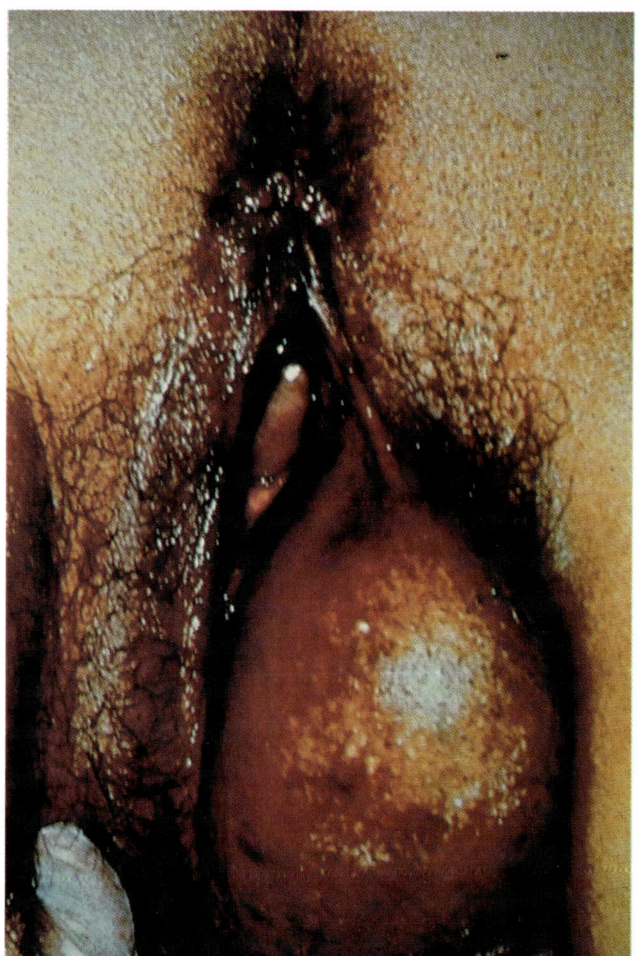

FIGURE 1-69
A cyst of the canal of Nuck is seen in the left labium majus, pushing toward the labium minus.

common condyloma acuminatum. A squamous papilloma is a warty growth which is usually found on the labia majora of a peri- or postmenopausal woman. It is characterized by a tree-like fibrovascular structure lined by stratified, keratinizing squamous epithelium which does not have evidence of HPV infection (e.g., koilocytosis).

Condyloma Acuminatum

Condyloma acuminatum is known as a venereal wart because it is sexually transmitted in almost all cases. It is caused by an HPV infection that causes squamous proliferation of the skin and mucous membranes. Over 60 genotypes of HPV have been identified. Those that affect the lower genital tract most commonly include types 6, 11, 16, 18, 31, 32, and 33. Types 6 and 11 are the ones most frequently found in vulvar condyloma acuminatum. HPV infection is epidemic in Western societies. The incubation period from contact until the appearance of the lesion is approximately 3 to 6 months.

Condyloma acuminatum is a verrucous lesion that is different in appearance from the condyloma latum of syphilis, which was discussed previously. By definition, the lesion is a "pointed excrescence." The warts may be solitary; however, most frequently they are multiple, involving the labia, the perineal and perianal regions, the upper inner thigh, and often the vagina and cervix (Fig. 1–70). The lesions may be grayish pink, reddish gray, or grayish tan. They may produce no symptoms or may cause itching and irritation. They may bleed when traumatized.

Condyloma acuminatum is a warty growth in which a heavy covering mantle of stratified squamous epithelium shows marked acanthosis (elongation of rete pegs) and parakeratosis (Fig. 1–71). Papillomatosis may be present to a minor degree and hyperkeratosis is noted, particularly in the older lesions. A sharp line of demarcation between the epithelium and the edematous vascularized underlying connective tissue is seen. The latter always shows some amount of infiltration by inflammatory cells.

Hyperkeratosis is a dense layer of noncellular keratin over the surface of the epithelium. This is superimposed on a well-defined granular layer (stratum granulosum). The keratin is composed of eosinophilic (acidophilic) material, which is cellular cytoplasm with no nuclei or just the shadowy outlines of nuclei. When parakeratosis (which looks like miniature nucleated squamous cells by cytology) is present, the granular zone is absent and the layer below the hyperkeratosis is composed of cells that have eosinophilic cytoplasm but retain a small, dark nucleus. Typically, hyperkeratosis appears to be white or grayish on physical examination whereas parakeratosis appears brown or reddish-brown.

The parabasal layer of condyloma acuminatum is thickened. The nuclei may be enlarged and pleomorphic, but cellular maturation and orientation progress normally as the cells move toward the surface. Normal mitotic figures may be seen in the basal layer of the epithelium. Koilocytosis, which is the diagnostic cytopathic effect of HPV infection, is seen (Fig. 1–72). Koilocytotic cells are found in the intermediate and superficial layers of

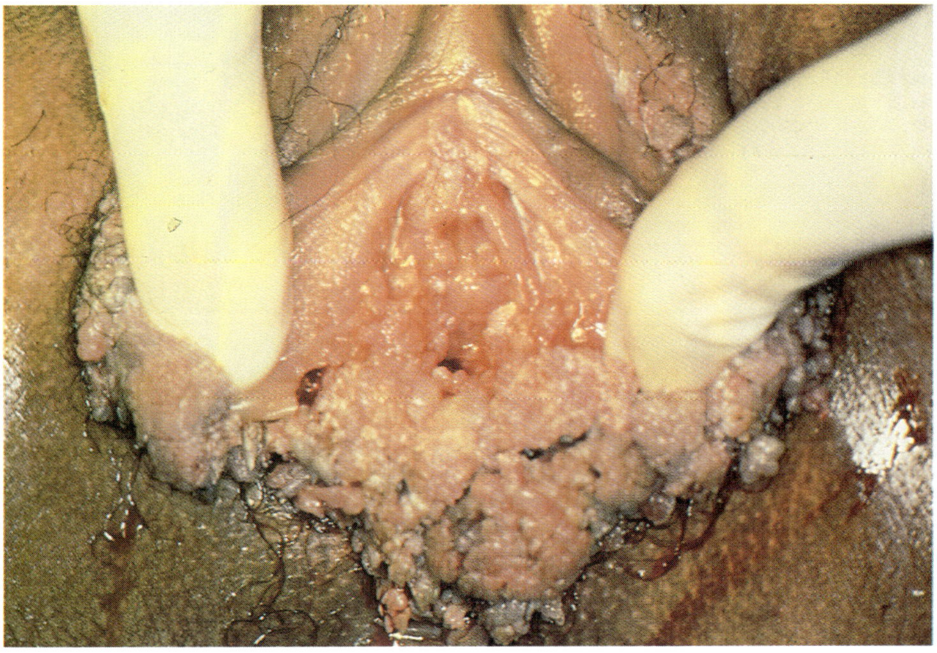

FIGURE 1–70
Extensive involvement of the vulva with condyloma acuminatum is seen here. The warty lesions are present on the labia, clitoris, vestibule, and perineum.

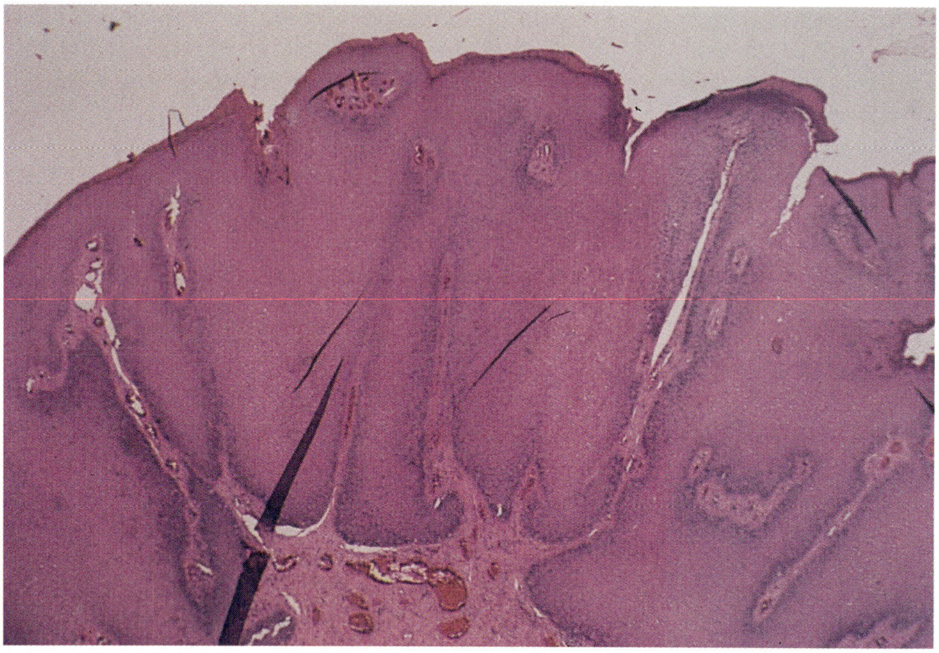

FIGURE 1-71
This is a biopsy of vulvar condyloma acuminatum. The epithelium is thickened, and the rete pegs are elongated and widened. The surface is slightly papillary. There is hyperkeratosis. Vascular engorgement is present in the connective tissue.

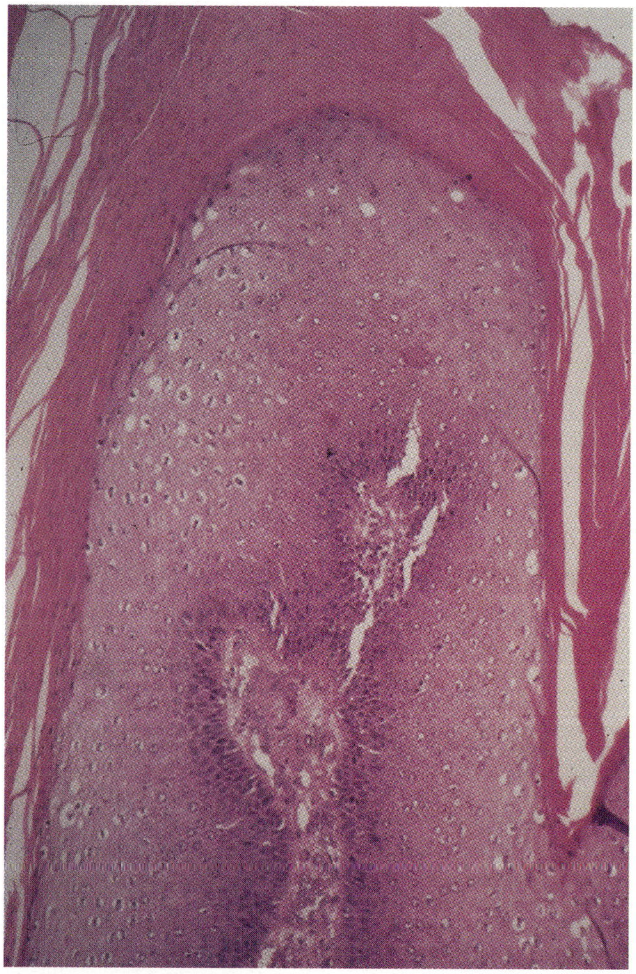

FIGURE 1-72
This is a high-power view of a papillary frond of vulvar condyloma acuminatum. There is hyperkeratosis. Ghost nuclei are seen in the lower layers of the stratum corneum. This represents atypical parakeratosis. Just under this area, koilocytes are seen. These cells are characterized by enlarged nuclei surrounded by a large clear cavity.

the epithelium. The koilocytes are frequently binucleated or multinucleated. The nuclei are enlarged, wrinkled, and sometimes hyperchromatic. The nucleus is surrounded by a large clear halo that gives the cell its name. However, the presence of this halo alone is not enough to classify the cell as a koilocyte. Nuclear atypia must be present.

Condyloma acuminatum may be misdiagnosed as carcinoma in situ or even invasive squamous cell carcinoma if tangential cutting of the specimen is misinterpreted as invasion. Condyloma acuminatum does not have the abnormal maturation, disorderly cellular orientation, and abnormal mitotic figures characteristic of VIN or invasive carcinoma.

Malignant alteration may occur in either condyloma acuminatum or true papilloma. Its incidence is difficult to establish, but it is probably rare. It may be difficult to differentiate the appearance of the benign from the malignant lesion by simple inspection. Therefore, verrucous lesions that do not respond to treatment, recur, change color, or become ulcerated should undergo biopsy.

At present, there is no treatment that will eradicate the chronic viral infection. Recurrences following local ablative therapy (e.g., podophyllin, tri- or bichloroacetic acid, 5-fluorouracil, electrocoagulation, cryosurgery, laser, or wide local excision) or systemic therapy (e.g., interferon) are common. Recalcitrant and recurrent lesions are frequent in diabetics and immunosuppressed patients and during pregnancy. Following termination of the pregnancy, the lesions may disappear spontaneously. Cesarean section should be considered as the optimal mode of delivery if the lower genital tract is extensively involved with condylomata. The elasticity of the vagina appears to be decreased when it is involved with condylomata, and this may lead to lacerations at the time of vaginal delivery. Suturing of tissue studded by condylomata is difficult. Furthermore, laryngeal papillomas have been reported in infants delivered vaginally to mothers who have condyloma acuminatum.[63, 64] This may also occur by transplacental transmission.

For 1 week after treatment with podophyllin resin cytologic changes mimicking those characteristic of intraepithelial neoplasia may be seen. There is intercellular edema, necrosis of the lower half of the epidermis, edema of the underlying dermis, and an inflammatory infiltrate. Mitotic activity is markedly increased, and a few abnormal mitotic figures may be seen. However, unlike the situation in VIN, the maturation and orientation of the cells remains orderly.

In general, simple condylomata acuminata are associated with HPV genotypes 6 and 11 whereas HPV types 16 and 18 are more closely associated with vulvar intraepithelial and malignant neoplasia. Infection with several HPV genotypes may occur. Patients who have HPV infection should be followed closely with regular gynecologic examinations, cervical or vaginal cytology evaluation, and biopsy of suspicious lesions.[65]

Micropapillomatosis Labialis (Physiologic Papillomatosis)

Micropapillomatosis labialis comprises diffuse, generally symmetrical, finger-like fibroepithelial projections found in the introitus and lower vagina of young women (Fig. 1–73). Although superficially they may resemble condyloma acuminatum, they do not seem to be caused by an HPV infection.[65a] Spontaneous resolution of these lesions may occur. No therapy is necessary.

Acrochordons

Acrochordons (skin tags) are small, skin-colored, teardrop-shaped tags that occur predominantly on the neck but are also seen on the vulva, axillae, eyelids, and occasionally on the trunk. They are frequently pedunculated but can be sessile. They may appear white if hyperkeratosis is present. Conversely, they may appear dark as a result of melanosis and the accumulation of subcutaneous melanophages such as is frequently seen with any chronic irritation. They usually produce no symptoms but can become irritated or gangrenous if twisting of the pedicle occurs. Acrochordons do not need to be removed unless they are irritated or unless their color raises concern about whether they could be a melanoma. Microscopic examination reveals an edematous core of connective tissue covered by keratinized squamous epithelium (Fig. 1–74).

Fibromas

Fibromas of the vulva are uncommon. They often contain smooth muscle or fibroadipose tissue; if so, the accurate diagnosis is fibromyoma or fibrolipoma. If the tumor is composed primarily of adipose tissue, it should be diagnosed as a lipoma. These tumors do not always arise from the vulvar tissues but may merely present in the external genitalia. The sites of origin are occasionally the round ligament or the intrapelvic fibromuscular tissue. Those arising from the round ligament or deeper pelvic structures may present as a firm, often nodular, indistinct mass. Lesions arising in

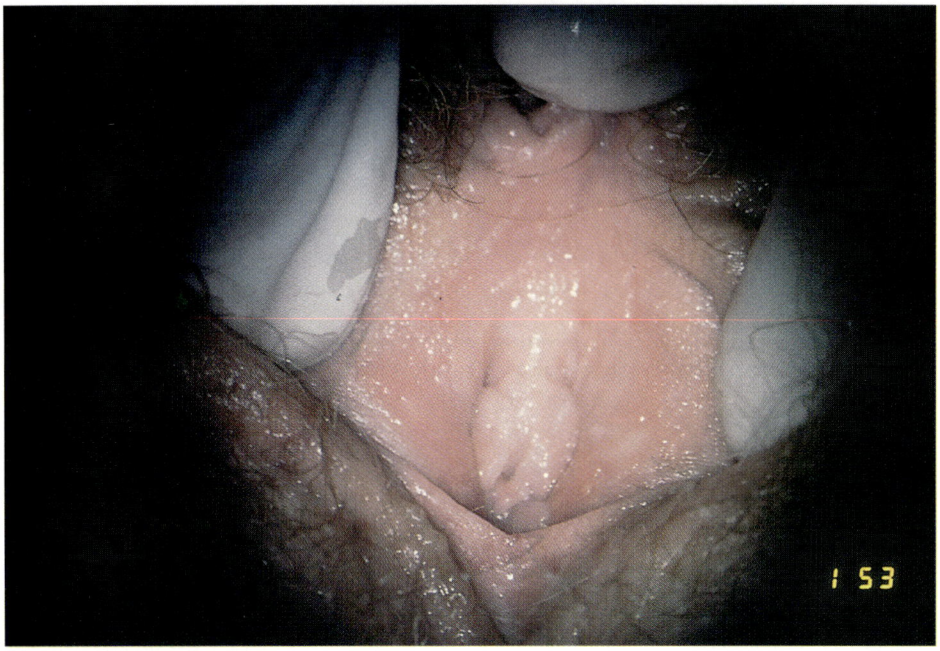

FIGURE 1-73
Symmetric, minute, papillary-like lesions are seen on the inner surface of both labia minora. This is micropapillomatosis labialis.

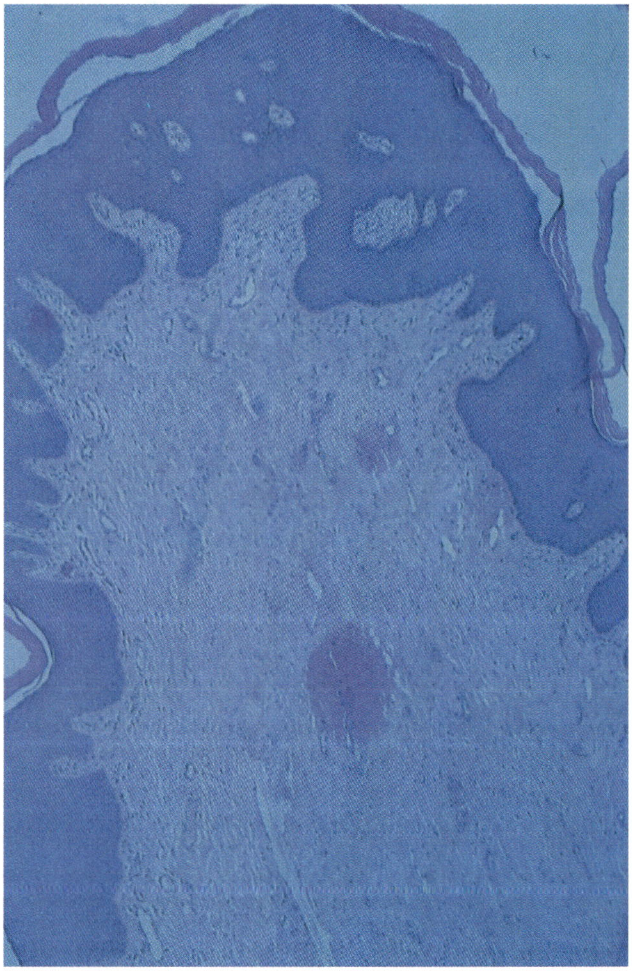

FIGURE 1-74
This is the microscopic appearance of a skin tag that shows a core of connective tissue covered by squamous epithelium.

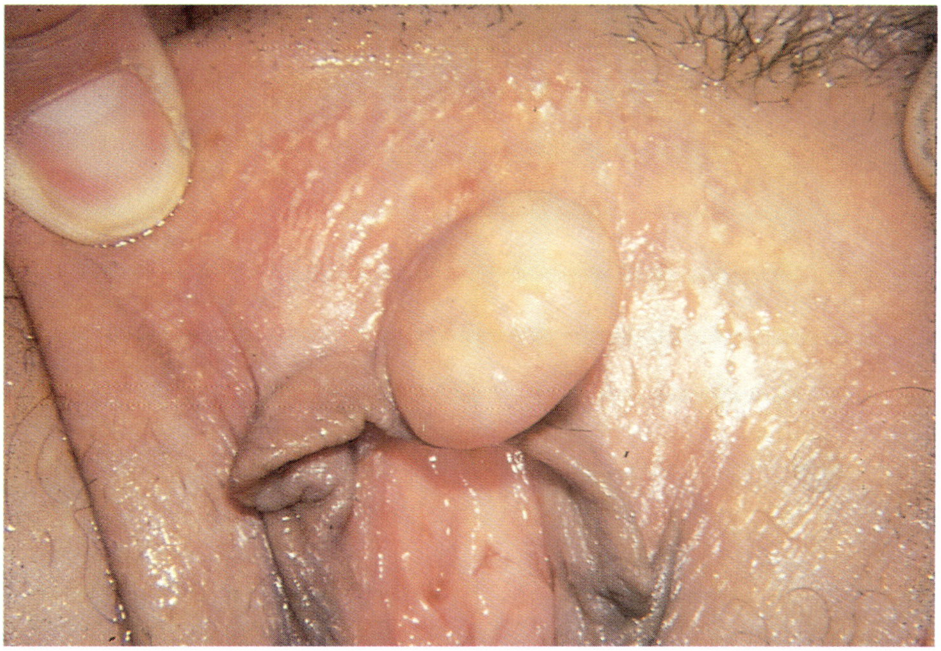

FIGURE 1-75
This is a fibroma of the clitoris which felt firm to palpation.

the vulva may rarely involve the clitoris and then present a diagnostic and therapeutic problem (Fig. 1–75). Others arising in the labia tend to become pedunculated (Fig. 1–76). Excision is necessary for the comfort of the patient and for accurate diagnosis.

The microscopic features are similar to those described for similar tumors at extrapelvic sites. A fibroma is characterized by parallel bundles of fibrocytes associated with variable amounts of collagen. In larger tumors, extensive hyaline or cystic degeneration may occur. Malignancy arising in these lesions is rare.

Dermatofibroma presents as a small vascular subcutaneous nodule and is included in this group of tumors because of the fibromatous component. It is characterized by fibroblast proliferation and disrupted collagen fibers within which is found an abundance of small capillaries that have a prominent endothelial lining. The prominent vascularity has led to the alternate diagnosis of sclerosing hemangioma. The overlying epidermis shows acanthosis (Fig. 1–77).

Sebaceous Gland Hyperplasia or Sebaceous Adenoma

Sebaceous hyperplasia occurs on the labia minora more commonly than on the labia majora. Multiple small, reddish-yellow, soft papules that produce no symptoms are present (Fig. 1–78). The lesions are composed of multiple sebaceous glands that show a proliferation of basal cells from which the gland arises. It is composed of an abnormal proliferation

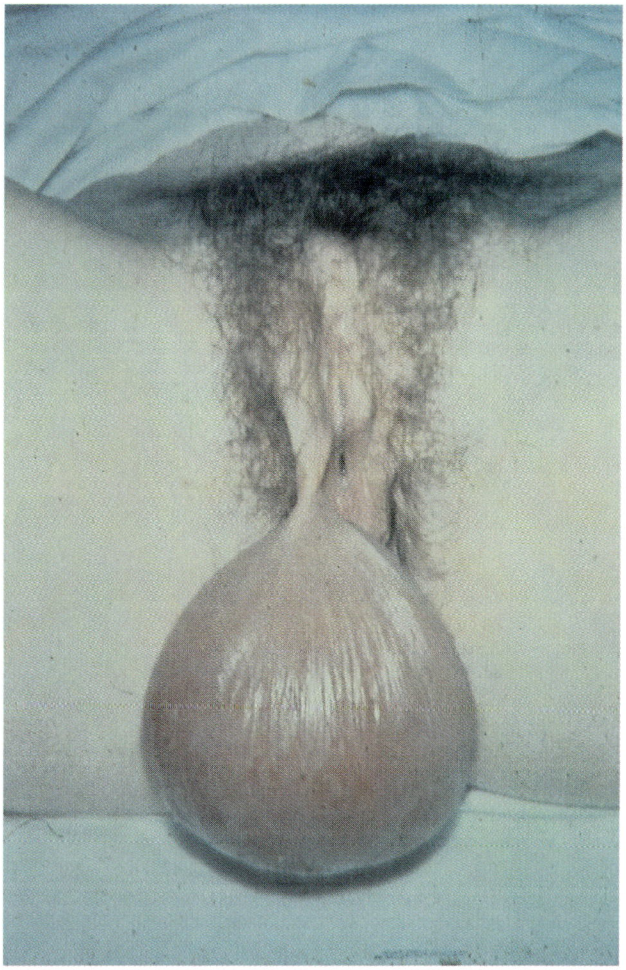

FIGURE 1-76
A pedunculated fibroma of the right labium majus is seen here.

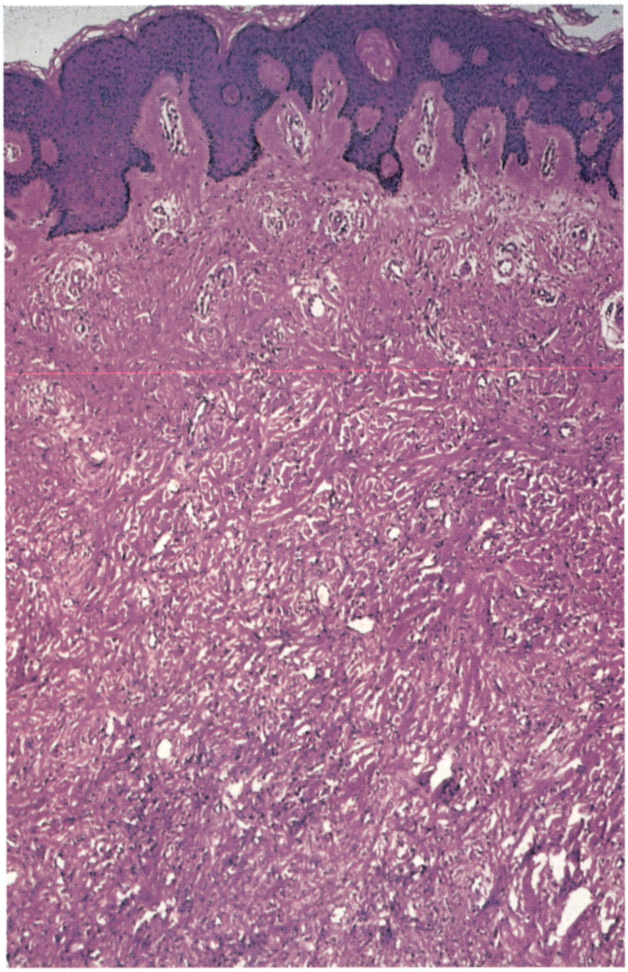

FIGURE 1-77
This is a biopsy specimen of dermatofibroma, which shows interdigitating collagen bundles interspersed by capillaries. The overlying squamous epithelium shows acanthosis.

of well-differentiated glands (Fig. 1–79). There is no cellular atypia. These lesions need no treatment.

Minor Vestibular Gland Adenoma

This is a rare lesion that presents as a firm, small nodule in the vestibule.[66] It is never larger than 2 cm in diameter. Microscopic examination reveals proliferation of mucus-secreting glands (Fig. 1–80). The adenoma is surrounded by dense fibrous tissue, and dense fibrous bands may traverse the nodule, resulting in a nestlike arrangement of the acini. The interstitial tissue within and adjacent to the adenoma may be filled with mucin and macrophages.

Granular Cell Tumor (Myoblastoma)

Granular cell tumor is a rare tumor of the vulva but is found more commonly in other areas of the body; the most frequent site is the tongue.[67–70] Although the older name, granular cell myoblastoma, suggests an origin from smooth muscle, the lesion is now known to arise from the nerve sheath and would be more accurately described as a type of schwannoma. The majority of vulvar lesions have been found on the labia majora. They may present as subcutaneous nodules that rarely exceed 2 to 3 cm in diameter. The surface may become superficially ulcerated. The base of the ulcer is clean and yellow in color. The border of the lesion is well demarcated, and the edge appears to be rolled up (Fig. 1–81). The cells forming the tumor are large and contain abundant cytoplasm filled with eosinophilic granules of various sizes. The nucleus is relatively small and has basophilic chromatin (Fig. 1–82). The overlying epithelium frequently shows pseudocarcinomatous hyperplasia. This is an epithelial reaction to the subepithelial tumor and should not be confused with VIN or squamous cell carcinoma. Because the

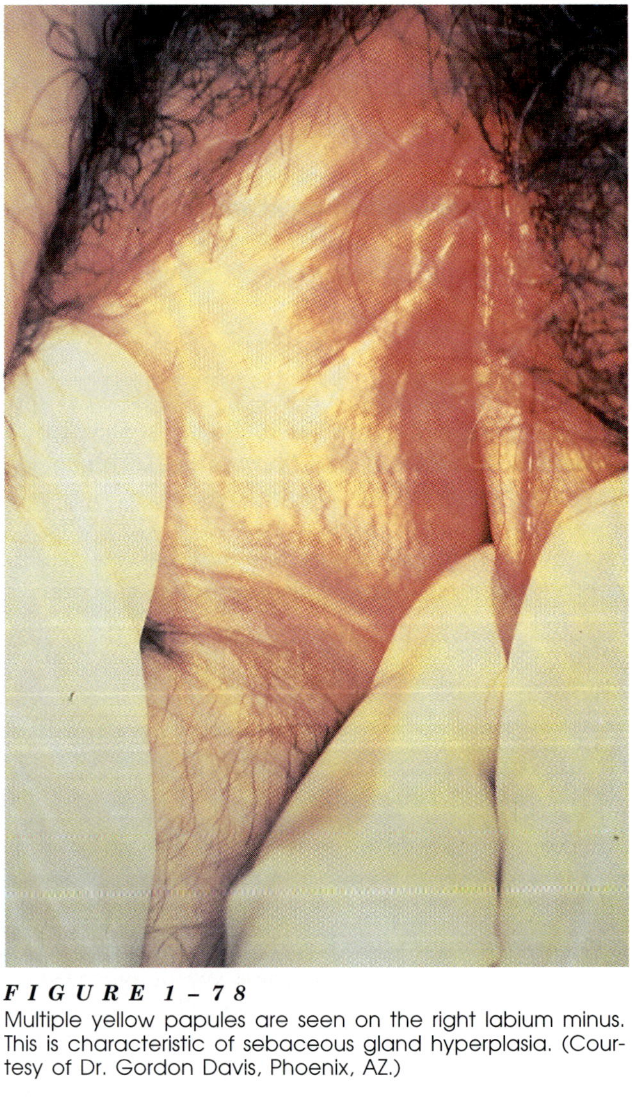

FIGURE 1-78
Multiple yellow papules are seen on the right labium minus. This is characteristic of sebaceous gland hyperplasia. (Courtesy of Dr. Gordon Davis, Phoenix, AZ.)

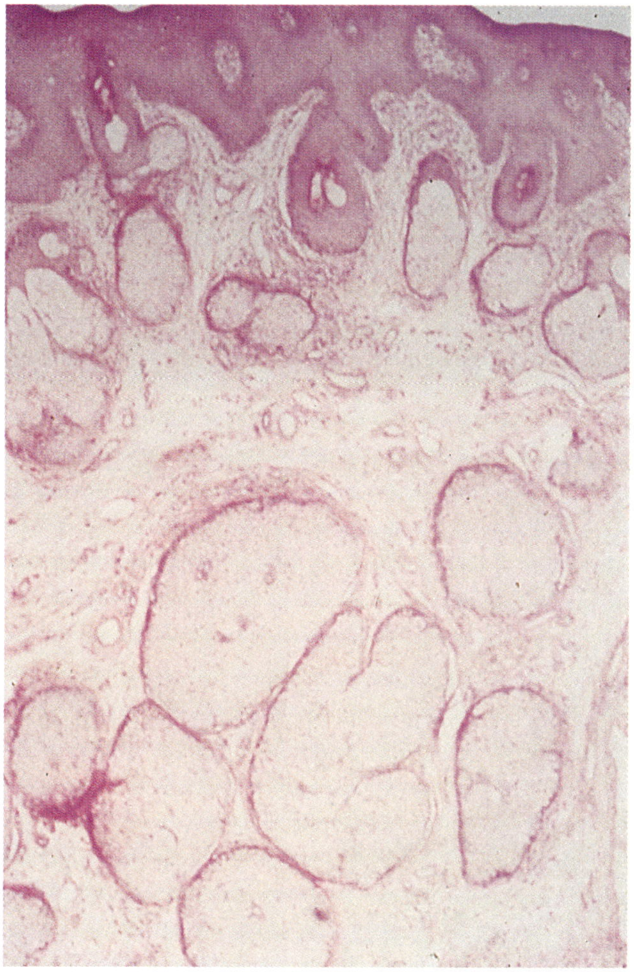

FIGURE 1-79
Marked proliferation of sebaceous glands is seen in this case of sebaceous gland hyperplasia.

locally infiltrative nature of the lesion makes complete excision difficult, the margins of resection are frequently involved. Although local recurrences and rare cases of malignant changes have been reported, most cases of "metastases" are, in reality, instances of multiple primary tumors.[70a]

Hidradenoma

Hidradenoma of the vulva is a rare tumor but one that deserves special consideration because this benign lesion has been mistaken for adenocarcinoma. This tumor arises from the apocrine sweat glands. In some cases a direct continuity from tumor to the normal sweat gland can be demonstrated.

Hidradenomas occur in postpubertal, predominantly white women. The lesion presents as a sharply circumscribed, slightly elevated lesion, rarely more than 1 cm in diameter (Fig. 1–83), although Kaufmann et al[71] have reported an 8-cm hidradenoma. The skin overlying the nodule may be reddened or slightly ulcerated and granular. Slight bleeding may at times be a clinical symptom. Most commonly, however, the lesions are asymptomatic and are found on routine examination of the genitalia. The most frequent location is on the labia majora or in the interlabial folds. These lesions are generally solitary, although a rare case of multiple hidradenomas has been described.

The histopathologic appearance is quite characteristic. The architectural growth pattern is papillary-adenomatous. It is this complex branching nature of the lesion which has on occasion led to an erroneous diagnosis of carcinoma. The epithelial lining is characteristically composed of a double layer of nonciliated columnar cells that have clear cytoplasm and hyperchromatic nuclei (Fig. 1–84). Large cells with abundant pale eosinophilic cytoplasm are also seen. These are the mature superficial glandular cells that are the actively se-

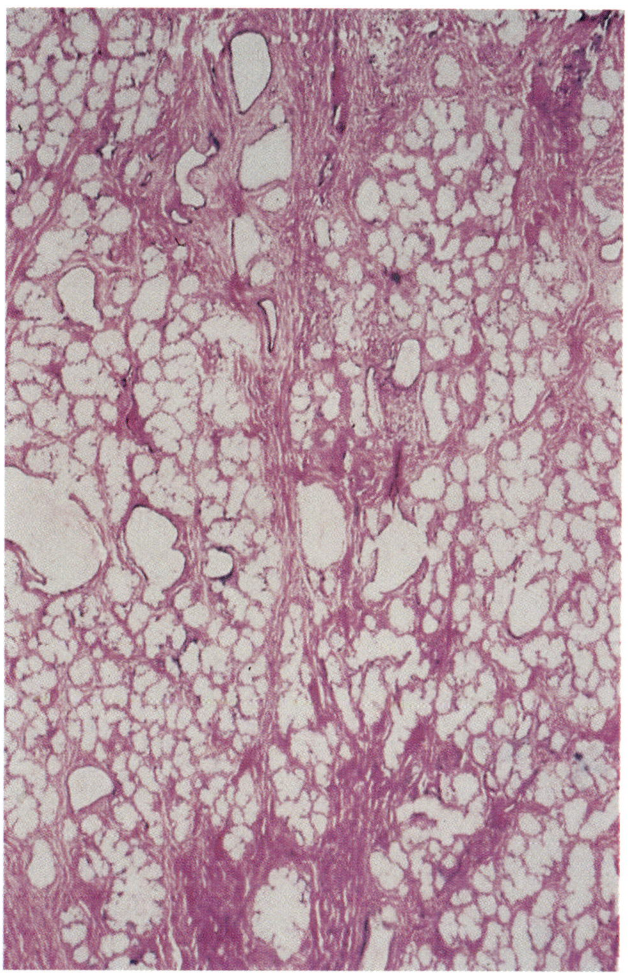

FIGURE 1-80
A minor vestibular gland adenoma shows marked proliferation of mucin-secreting glands in the vestibule. The glands are lined by a single layer of cells.

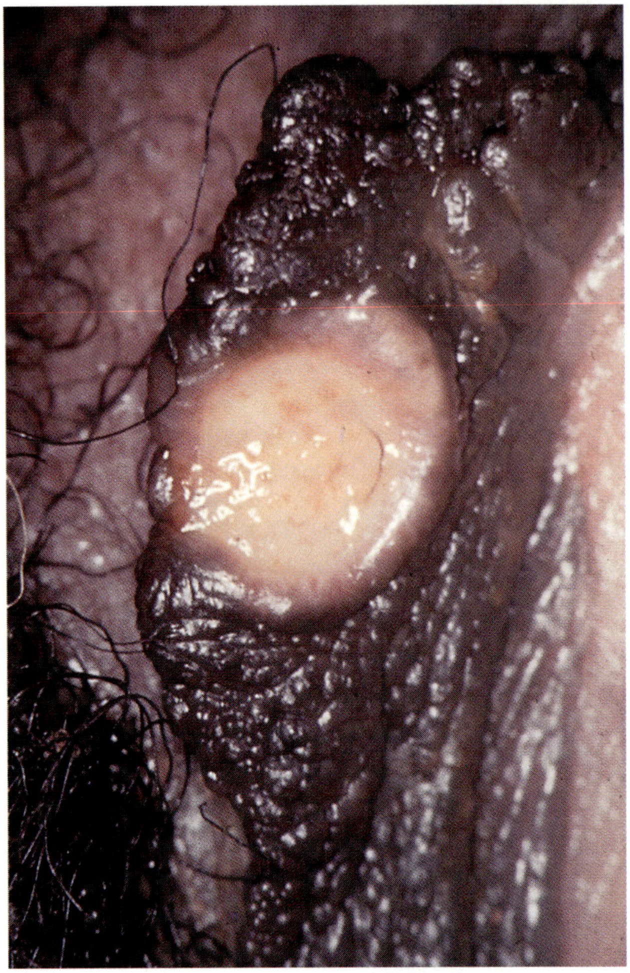

FIGURE 1-81
This ulcer has a shiny, clean, yellow base. The edge of the ulcer is raised and well demarcated. This is the typical appearance of granular cell tumor.

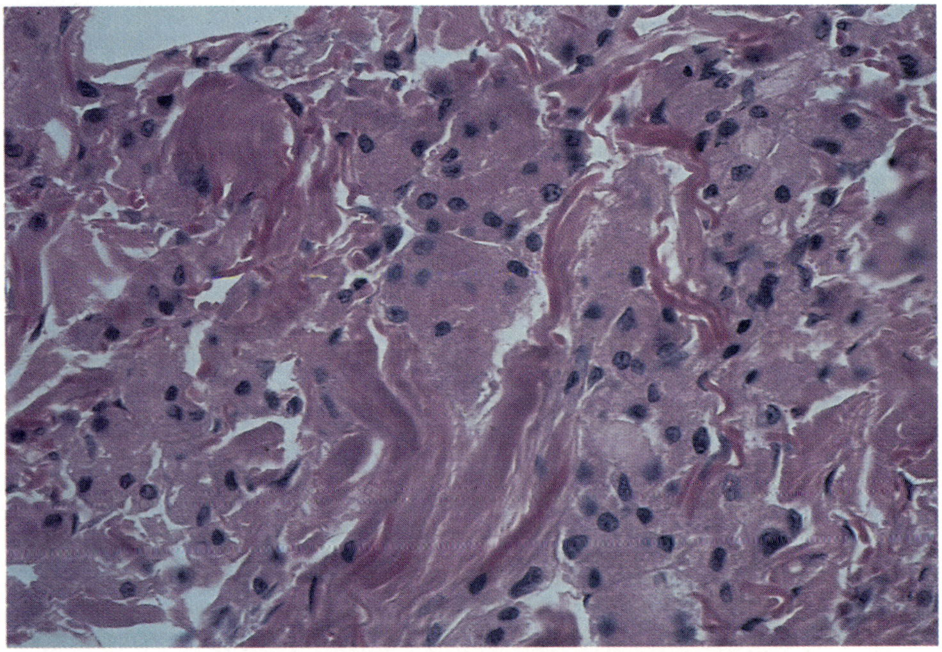

FIGURE 1-82
This granular cell tumor is composed of large cells with small nuclei. The cytoplasm is granular and eosinophilic. The nuclei are slightly hyperchromatic.

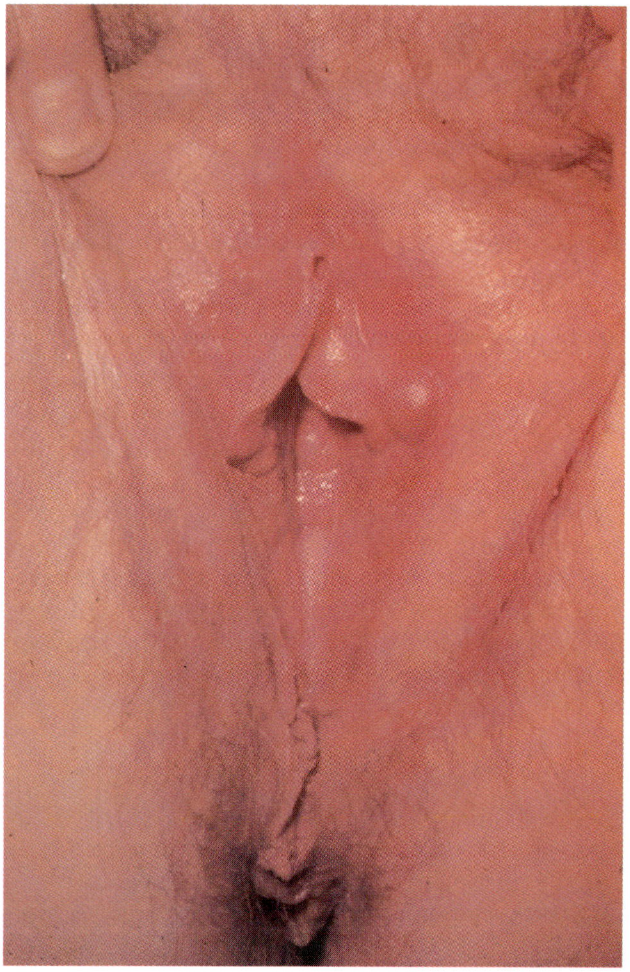

FIGURE 1-83
A solitary nodule is seen in the left interlabial fold. On biopsy this proved to be a hidradenoma.

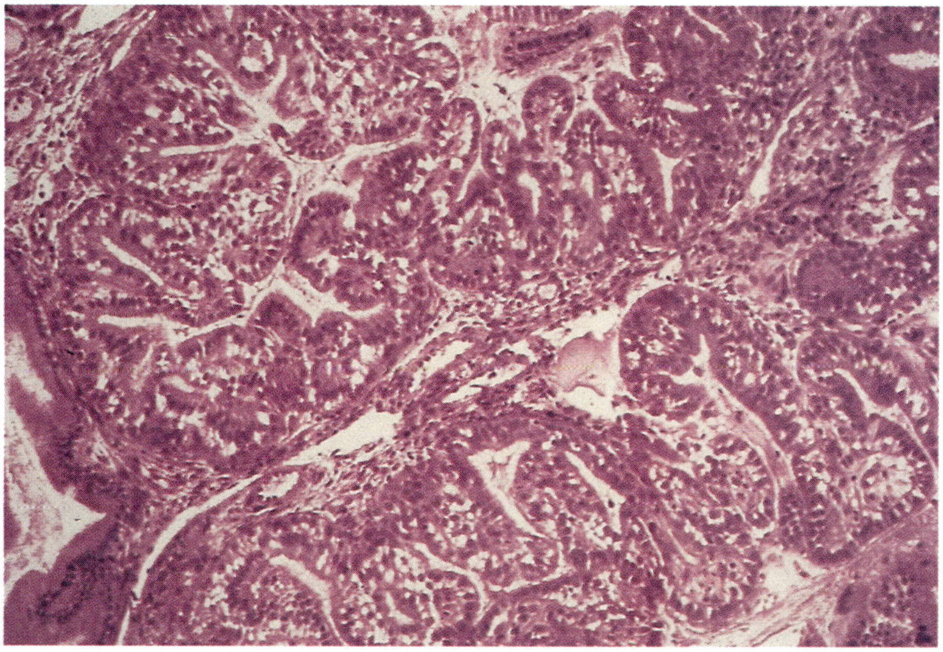

FIGURE 1-84
This hidradenoma is composed of glandular epithelium that forms a complex papillary pattern. The glands are lined by columnar cells with basally oriented nuclei. Clear cells are also present.

creting elements of the acinus. Near the basement membrane, especially in the smaller acini, rounded or cuboidal cells simulating the reserve or indifferent cells of the cervix are found. Flattened myoepithelial cells are also seen at the basement membrane. Simple excision of the lesion results in permanent cure in nearly all cases. Rare cases of hidradenocarcinoma have been reported.[72, 73]

Syringocystadenoma papilliferum is a lesion that occurs in the ducts of the apocrine glands. It is characterized by papillary invaginations into the dilated ducts. These lesions simulate and may actually represent ectopic breast tissue.

Syringoma

Syringoma is a common skin lesion. It is rarely diagnosed because most tumors are small and asymptomatic. They are usually multiple, tiny, elevated, nontender nodules. The lesion is characterized by slightly dilated eccrine glands with terminal comma-like tails. The glands are lined by flattened epithelium (Fig. 1–85).[74, 75]

Ectopic Breast Tissue

Aberrant breast tissue is probably relatively common in the vulva but is rarely diagnosed. It is usually recognized during pregnancy because the glands at the ectopic site proliferate just as normal breast tissue does under hormonal stimulation. Biopsy at this time is fraught with the hazard of excessive bleeding. Milk production may sometimes be recognized; it was present in a small tumor removed from the vulva at the time of delivery (Fig. 1–86). A few cases of breast carcinoma have been reported as arising in the vulva or the adjacent mons pubis.[76–78]

Endometriosis

Endometriosis is an uncommon lesion in the vulvar area. It may occur in the area of Bartholin's gland (especially in the scar from previous surgery on this gland) and in the fourchette at the site of a previous episiotomy. This presumably is the result of implantation of endometrium at the time of the surgical procedure. The lesion may appear as a bluish or bluish-red nodule that may be cyclically enlarged, bleed into itself, and become painful. The cyclic nature of the symptoms usually suggests the correct diagnosis. Examination of the excised tissue confirms the clinical diagnosis when both normal endometrial glands and stroma are identified (Fig. 1–87). Sometimes the diagnosis is suggested by old or new hemorrhage associated with either glands or a stromal component. On occasion endometriosis has been found in the upper labium majus along the peritoneal investment of the round ligament. This may be the result of metaplasia of the mesothelial lining. Excision of the lesion is the treatment of choice. Medical therapy (discussed in Chapter 8 under Endometriosis) can be used if there is a recurrence.

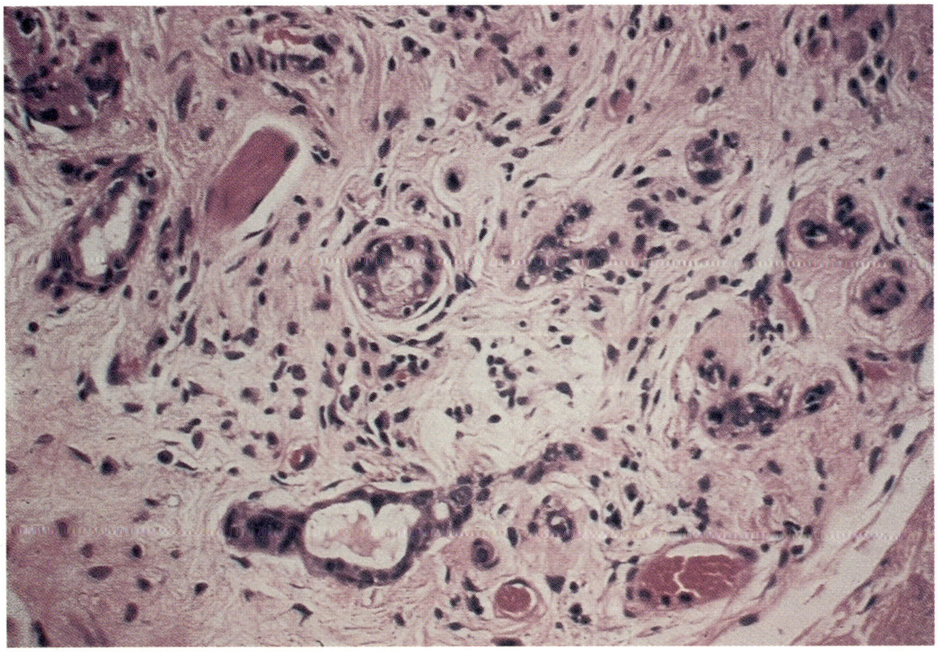

FIGURE 1–85
This biopsy specimen of a syringoma shows eccrine glands with dense connective tissue. Some of the glands seem to have a tail.

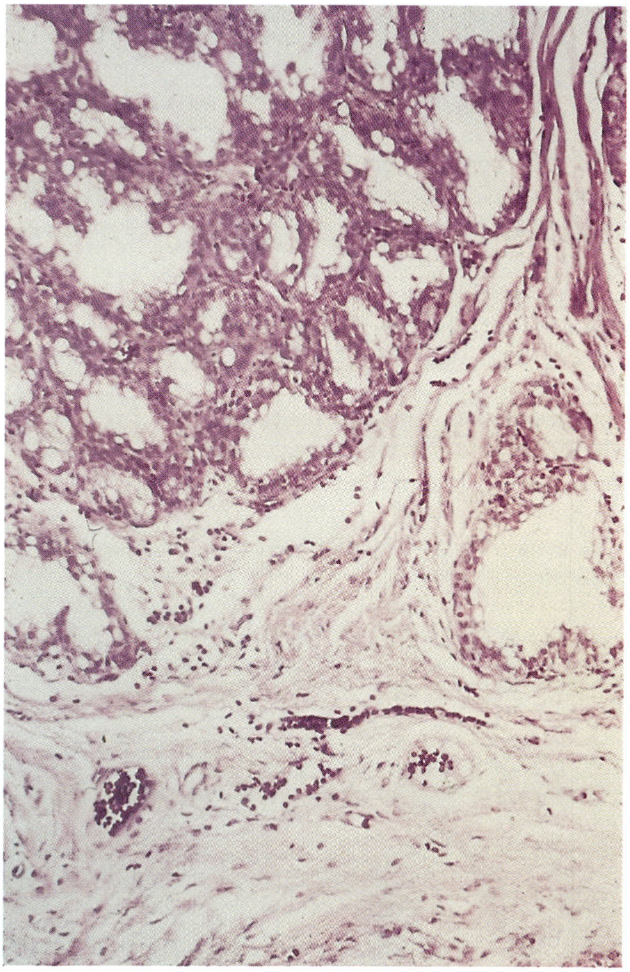

FIGURE 1-86
Proliferating glandular epithelium is seen. Multiple large vacuoles are present within the epithelial cells. This represents lactational changes in ectopic breast tissue on the vulva. The patient was post partum.

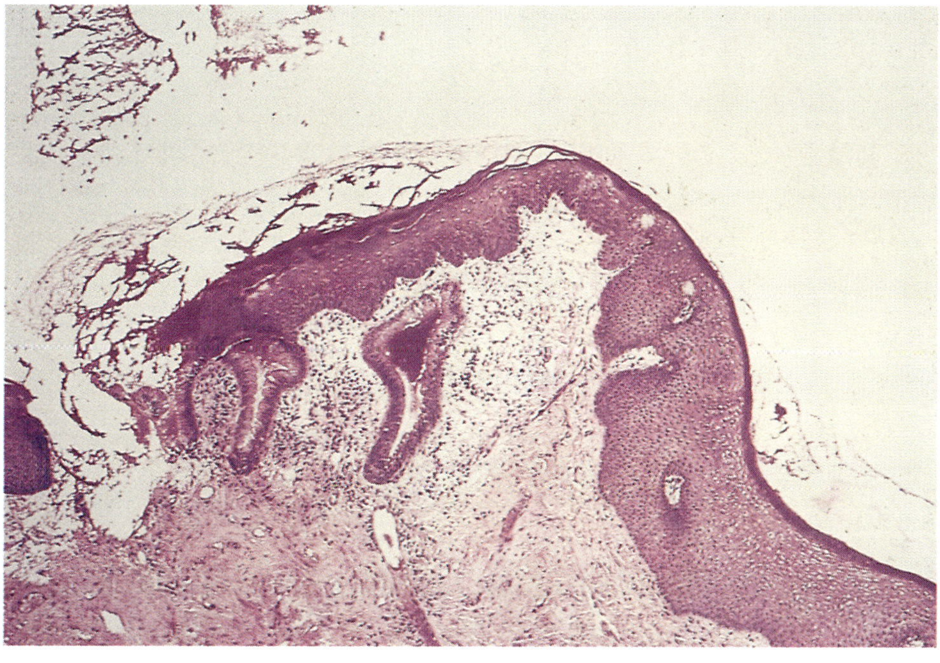

FIGURE 1-87
Glands and edematous stroma are seen under the squamous epithelium *(left)* in this vulvar biopsy. The glands are lined by columnar epithelium. Some of the cells resemble those of the endocervix. This is endometriosis with endocervical metaplasia.

Vascular Lesions (Hemangioma, Angiokeratoma, Varices)

Hemangioma of the vulva may occur as a congenital lesion and usually involves other sites in addition to the vulva. Hemangioma cavernosum is a purplish-red, rounded, and spongy lesion (Fig. 1–88). It is readily compressible. These lesions typically regress spontaneously and rarely need active treatment. Surgery is reserved for the management of excessive bleeding.

Small hemangiomas may appear at any time during life. They look like small, reddish papules (Fig. 1–89) that do not need to be excised unless there is a question about whether they are a pigmented neoplasm (e.g., melanoma). If they bleed, they can be easily cauterized. Hyperkeratosis may occur over the surface of a hemangioma. Then the surface appears to be white or grayish white on a red background. These are known as angiokeratomas (Fig. 1–90).

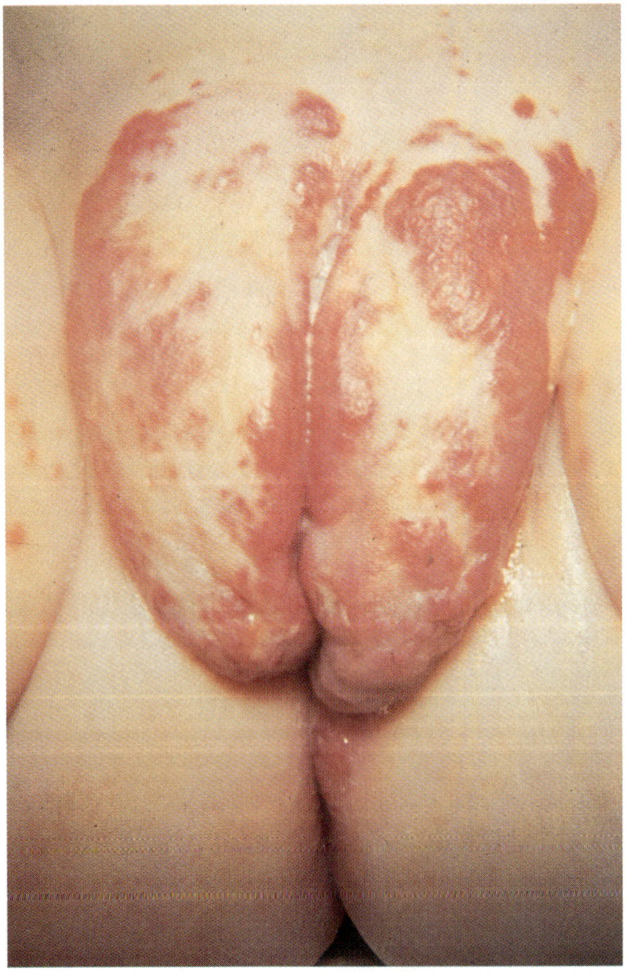

FIGURE 1–88
This child has a reddish purple, raised, irregular hemangioma of the vulva.

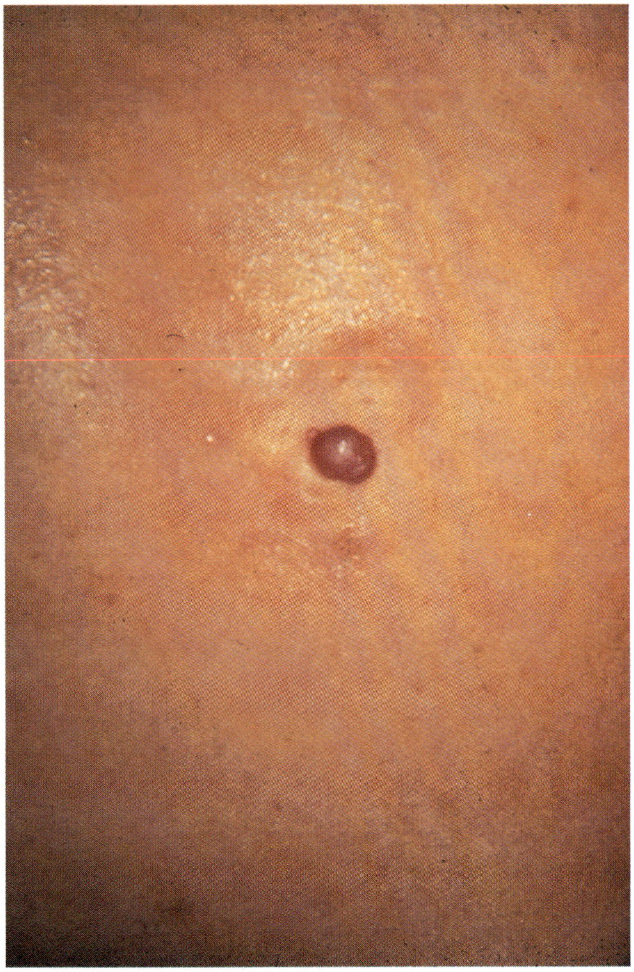

FIGURE 1–89
This solitary, reddish purple nodule is a hemangioma. A depigmented zone surrounds it. This appearance can be difficult to differentiate from melanoma, and biopsy may be necessary.

Small, elevated hemorrhagic lesions are common on the vulva of postmenopausal patients. Although confused with hemangioma, they usually represent multiple tiny varicosities (Fig. 1–91). They may cause bleeding if rubbed too vigorously or scratched. Even when these varicosities are identified in patients with postmenopausal bleeding, a thorough evaluation of the entire genital tract is necessary to exclude other lesions, especially endometrial carcinoma.

The microscopic appearance of a true hemangioma is the same as that in such lesions elsewhere. They are focal nests of dilated vessels that show varying degrees of endothelial proliferation (Fig. 1–92).

Dramatic varicosities of the vulva may occur, usually in older parous women. They are almost always unilateral. The classic type of varicocele that occurs in men is unusual in women. When it

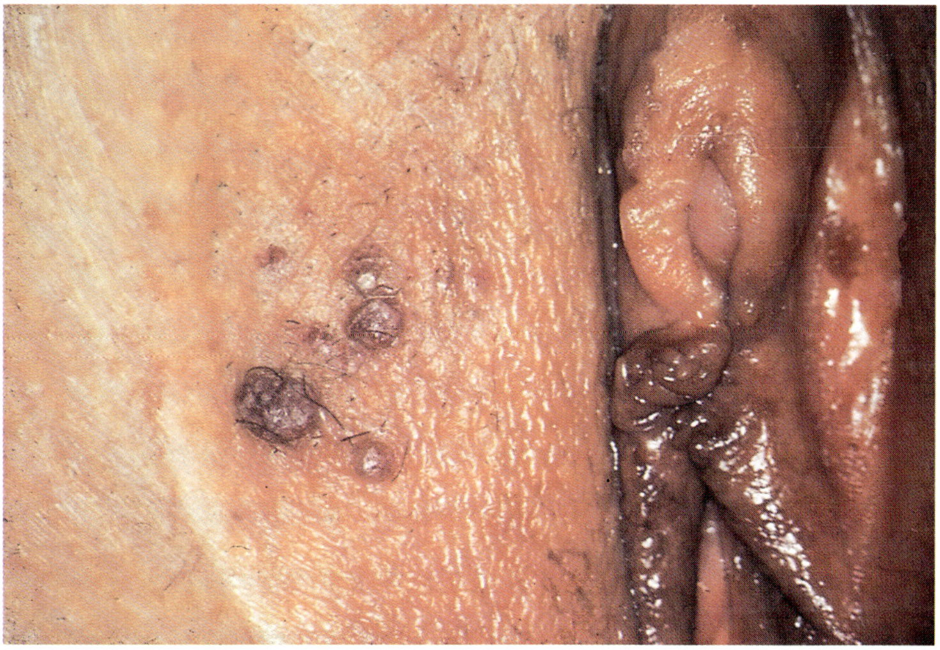

FIGURE 1-90
The surface of these hemangiomas is grayish white. This color is caused by hyperkeratosis of the epithelium overlying the hemangioma. These lesions are known as angiokeratomas.

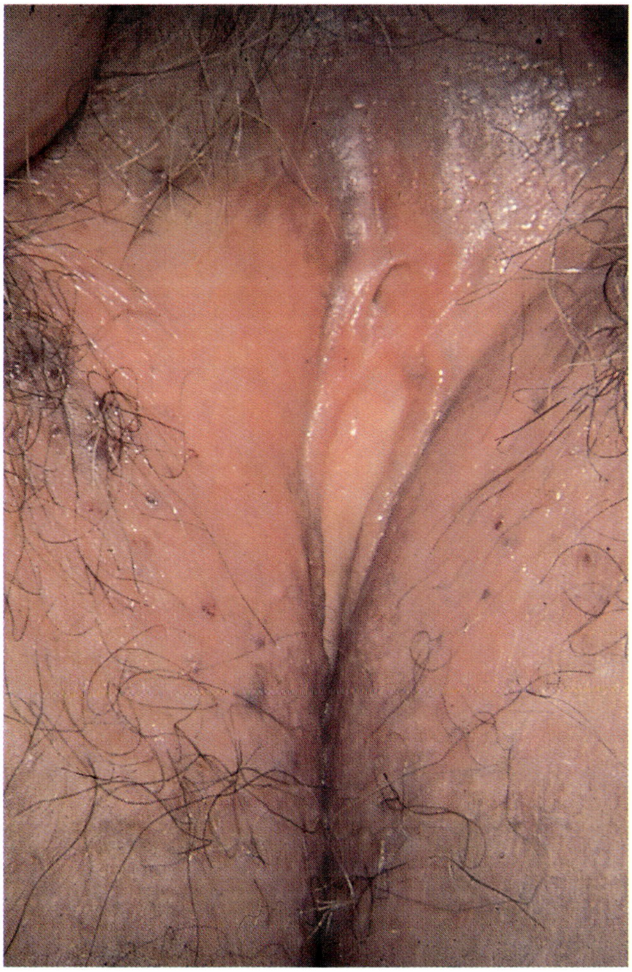

FIGURE 1-91
This vulva has multiple small varicosities (purple-black) that could be confused with hemangiomas.

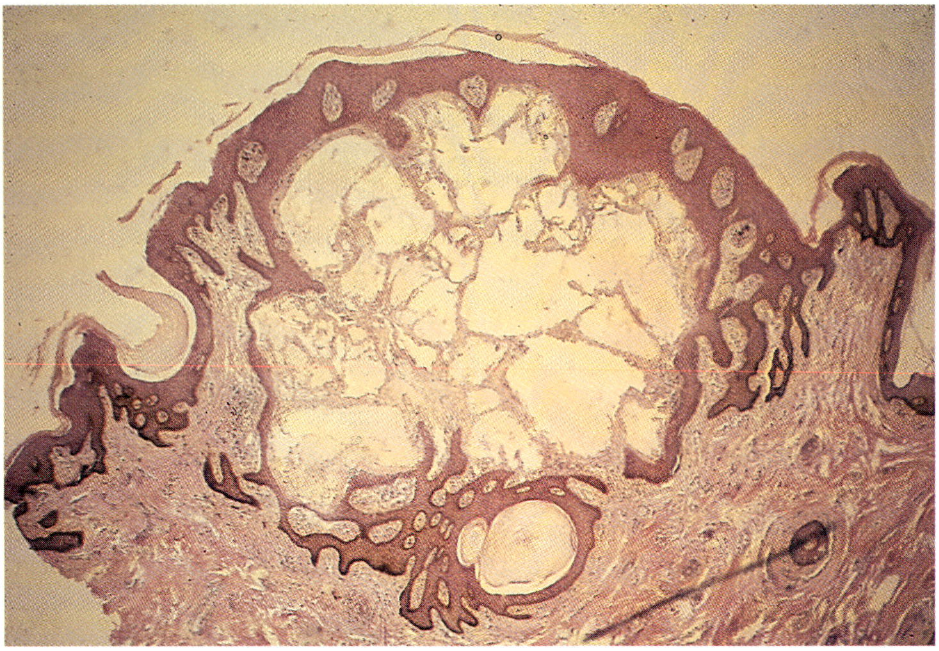

FIGURE 1-92
In this biopsy specimen of a superficial hemangioma multiple, dilated, vascular spaces are present under the squamous epithelium in the papillary dermis.

does occur, therapy involves excision of the entire lesion with careful ligation of the major vessels. Although in men the varicocele originates from occlusion of the pampiniform plexus, in women it usually results from occlusion of the pudendal vessels.

Traumatic hematomas are sometimes confused with melanoma based on appearance alone (Fig. 1–93). However, the clinical history and physical examination usually allow one to reach the correct diagnosis. A traumatic hematoma may present as a tense, tender mass with edema of the surrounding tissues. It should be managed conservatively unless it continues to enlarge. The application of ice may limit the continued expansion of the hematoma.

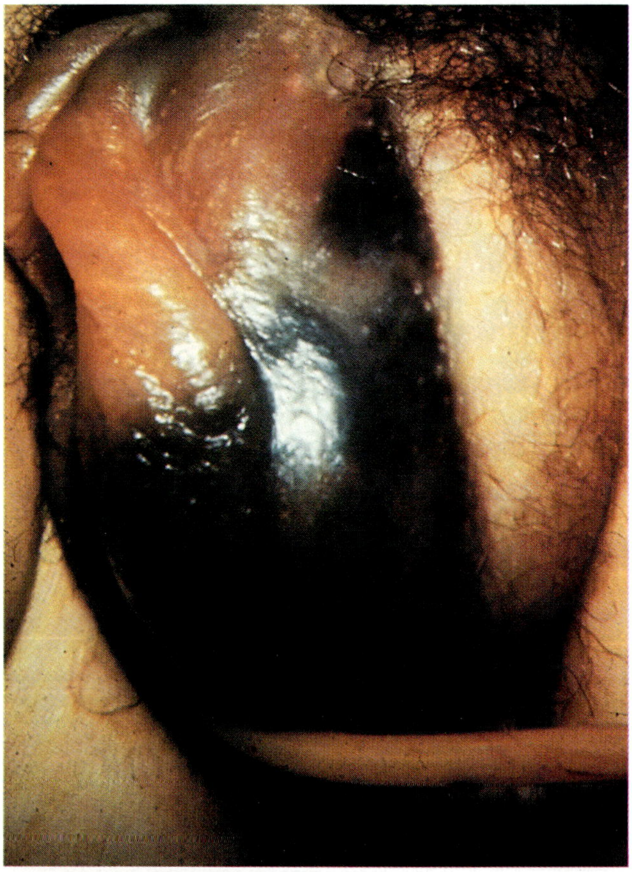

FIGURE 1-93
A large vulvar hematoma causing blue-black discoloration of the vulva is shown.

Pyogenic Granuloma

Pyogenic granuloma or granuloma pyogenicum appears as a slighted elevated, painless, yellow-white lesion that is usually situated on the inner surface of the labia near the introitus (Fig. 1–94). These lesions have also been described as pedunculated and dull red in color; they look similar to granulation tissue. The surface epithelium is ulcerated, and the epithelium at the edges of the ulcer shows pseudoepitheliomatous hyperplasia. This hyperplasia may form an "epidermal collarette" around the lesion. These changes represent a benign epithelial reaction to inflammation and are not indicative of malignant alteration. The lesion itself is a nodule of granulation-like tissue composed of multiple

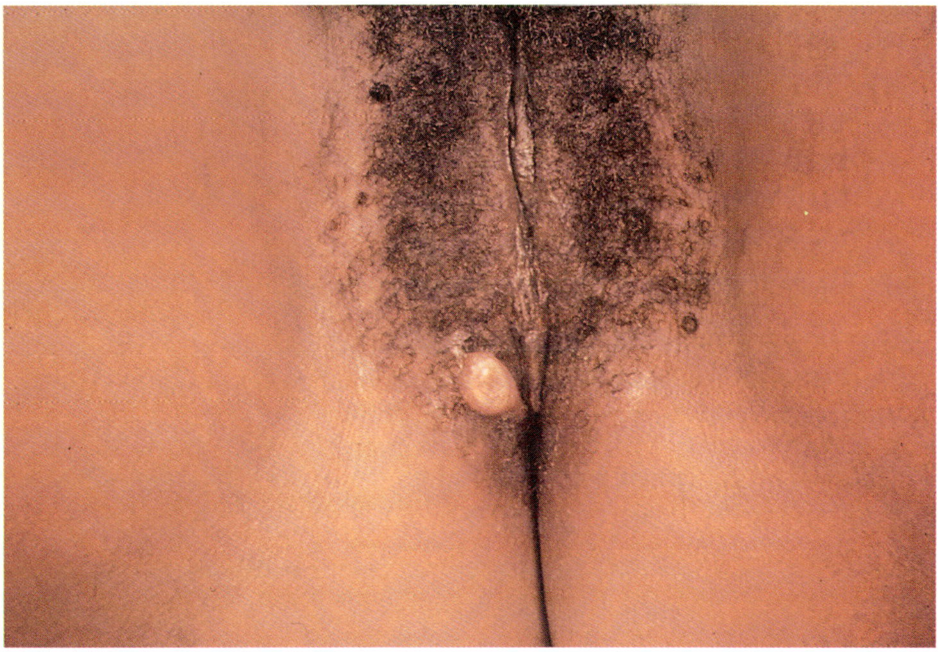

FIGURE 1-94
This raised, shiny, pinkish white nodule was found to be a pyogenic granuloma.

small vessels in the dermis surrounded by lymphocytes. The angiomatous pattern suggests that the lesion is actually a hemangioma (Fig. 1–95). Simple excision is curative.

Neurofibroma (Schwannoma)

Neurofibromas are most often small polypoid nodules and are found in children and young adults. They may occur as isolated lesions or as part of von Recklinghausen disease.[79, 80] Neurofibromas are found on the vulva of almost 50 percent of patients who have von Recklinghausen disease. These tumors are composed of spindle-shaped cells that form wavy bundles and whorls. Antibodies to neural antigens stain these long, thin nerve fibers.

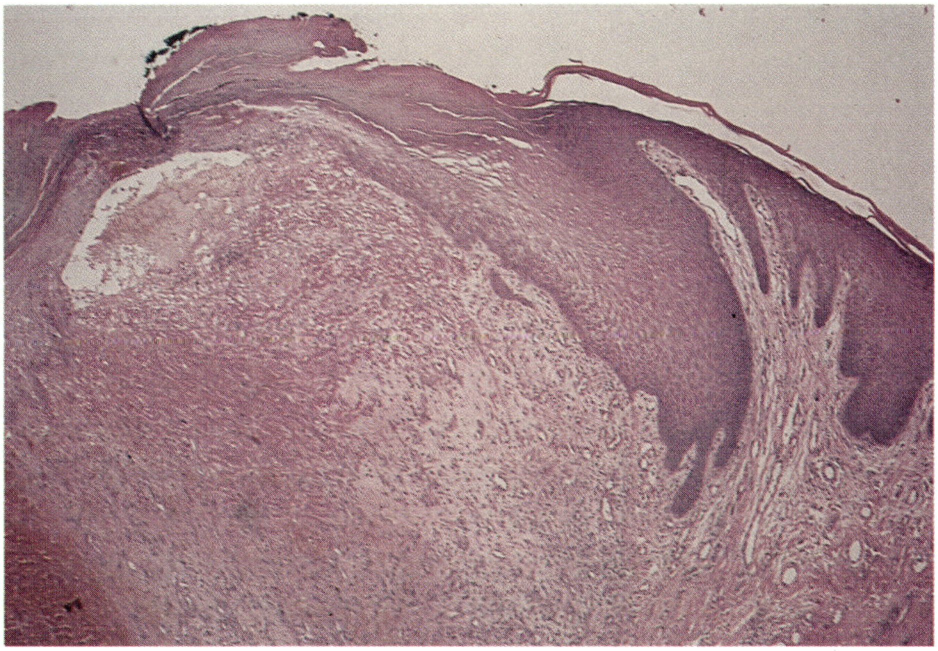

FIGURE 1-95
This biopsy of a pyogenic granuloma shows a superficial ulceration *(top left)*. There is hyperkeratosis and elongation of the rete pegs flanking the lesion. This epithelial change is known as pseudoepitheliomatous hyperplasia. The lesion *(center)* is formed by proliferation of capillaries.

PIGMENTED LESIONS

Lentigo

Pigmented vulvar lesions are common. The one most frequently encountered is the simple lentigo or lentiginous spot. It resembles a freckle. Lentigines are generally multiple and flat (Fig. 1–96). If a biopsy is taken, the histologic findings include slight acanthosis with increased melanin deposition in the basal layer of the epithelium, which may be confused with chronic dermatitis in black patients. However, hyperkeratosis and a dermal inflammatory infiltrate are seen in chronic dermatitis, and inflammation is not present in lentigo. Lentigo has no malignant potential, and no treatment is necessary. Biopsy is necessary only if a more serious pigmented lesion is suspected.

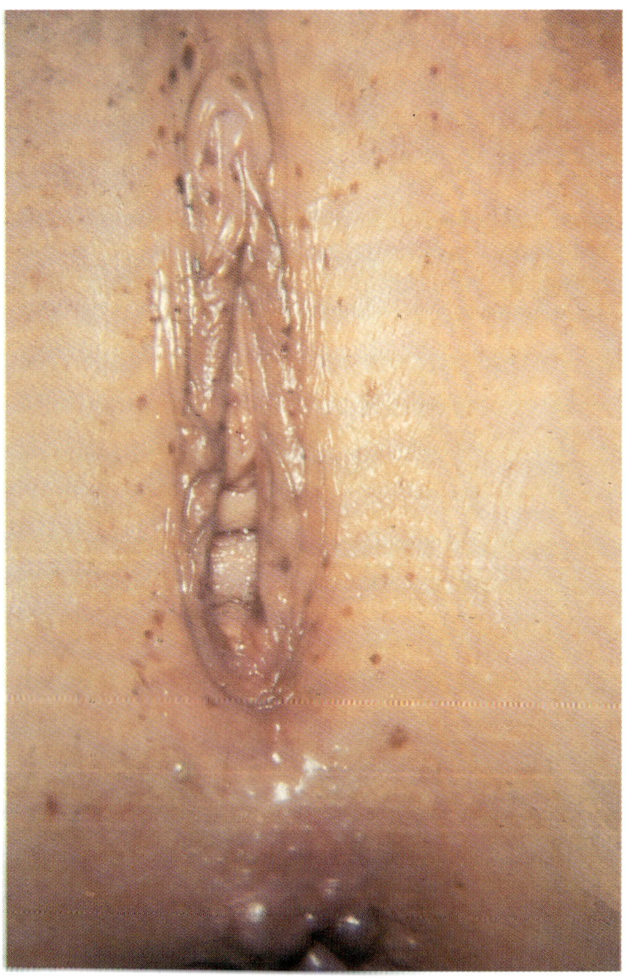

FIGURE 1–96
Multiple small, flat, freckle-like spots are seen on this vulva. This is simple lentigo.

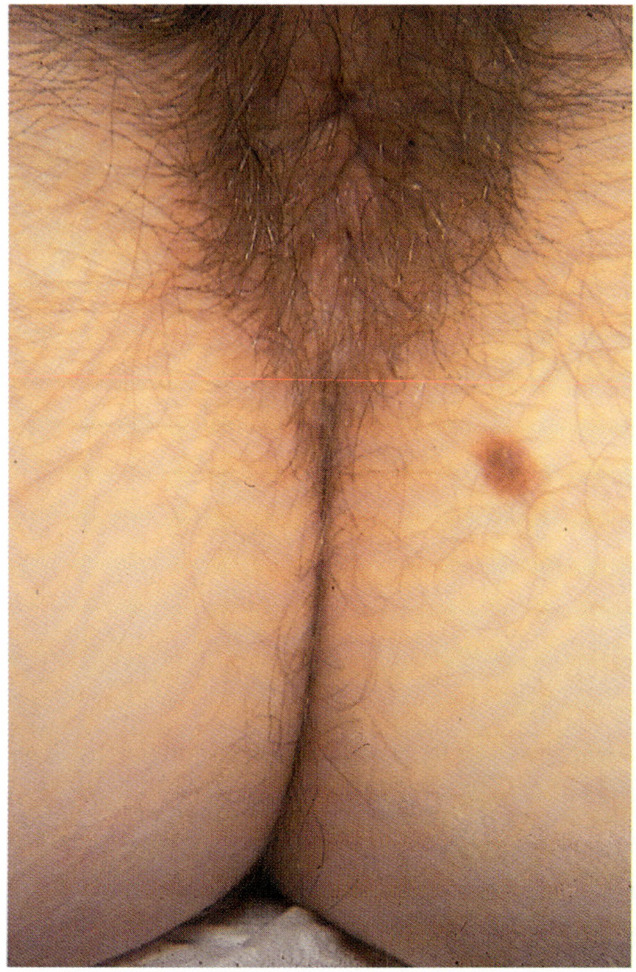

FIGURE 1–97
A brown nevus is seen on the left buttock. This should be removed for histopathologic examination to confirm that it is a nevus and not a melanoma.

Nevi

Nevi of the intradermal, junctional, and compound varieties are frequent on the external genitalia.[81] They may be melanotic or amelanotic. They are usually single. Most are dark brown, but red and skin-colored nevi are also seen (Fig. 1–97). They may be flat or raised. The diagnosis of type of nevus can be made only by biopsy.

Melanocytes, which are of neural crest origin, can be found in the basal layer of the epidermis (also known as the junction), in the dermis, or in both areas. An intradermal nevus has normal squamous epithelium overlying nests of nevus cells. These are uniform small cells that have a hyperchromatic nucleus (Fig. 1–98). Pigment is usually absent. These lesions have no malignant potential. In a junctional nevus, nests of cells that

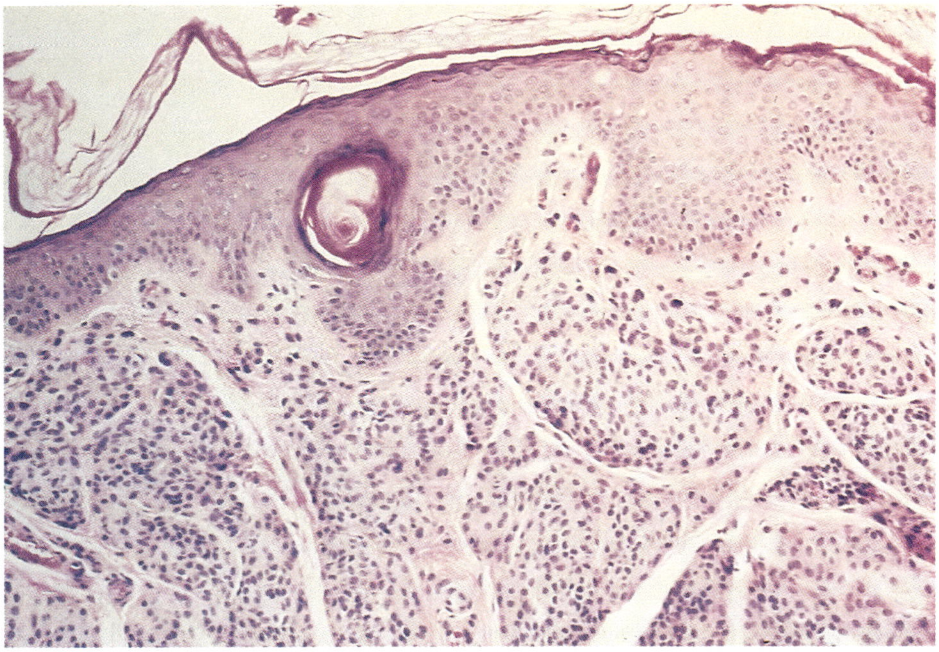

FIGURE 1–98
Nests of proliferating nevus cells are seen in the dermis. A band of collagen separates the proliferating nevus cells from the normal squamous epithelium.

often contain pigment are present within the basal layer of the epithelium. These cells may seem to drop off into the dermis because the basement membrane is difficult to identify. Mitotic activity is absent, and there is no pleomorphism. Junctional nevus activity was formerly considered an ominous feature and suggested a risk of invasion. However, these lesions are benign and require only wide local excision. A compound nevus is a combination of both junctional and intradermal nevi (Fig. 1–99). The intradermal component should not be interpreted as invasion into the underlying dermis. Differentiation of this nevus from melanoma is based on the uniformity of the cells and the lack of nuclear atypia and mitotic activity. Again, local excision of the lesion with clear margins is the only treatment necessary. Atypical melanocytic proliferation (atypical melanocytic hyperplasia) at the epidermal-dermal junction associated with an inflammatory infiltrate and free

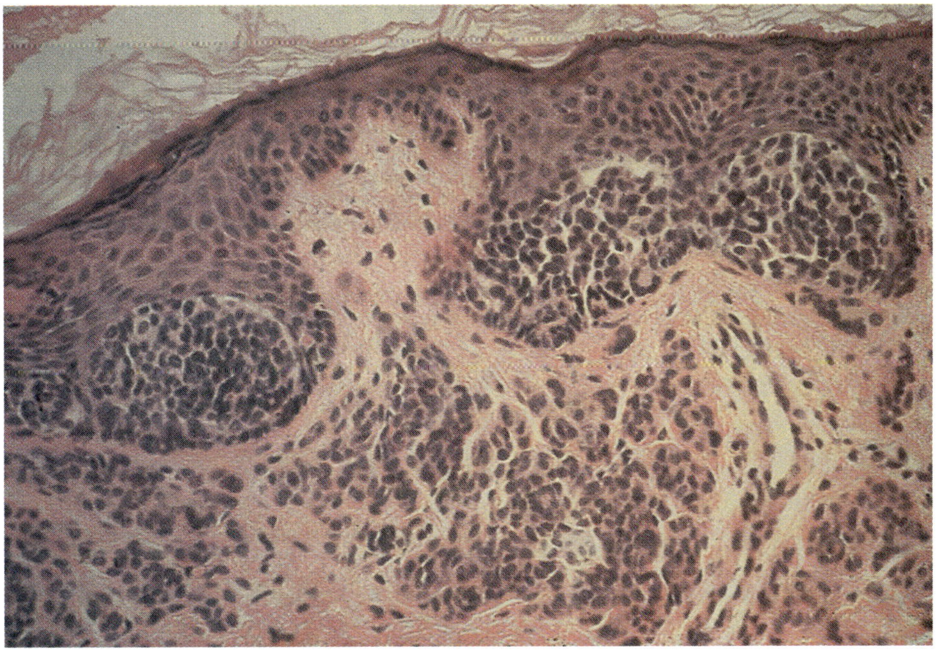

FIGURE 1–99
This compound nevus has proliferating nevus cells in the dermis and in nests in the lower layer of the squamous epithelium. The cells are very uniform in both the junctional and the dermal areas.

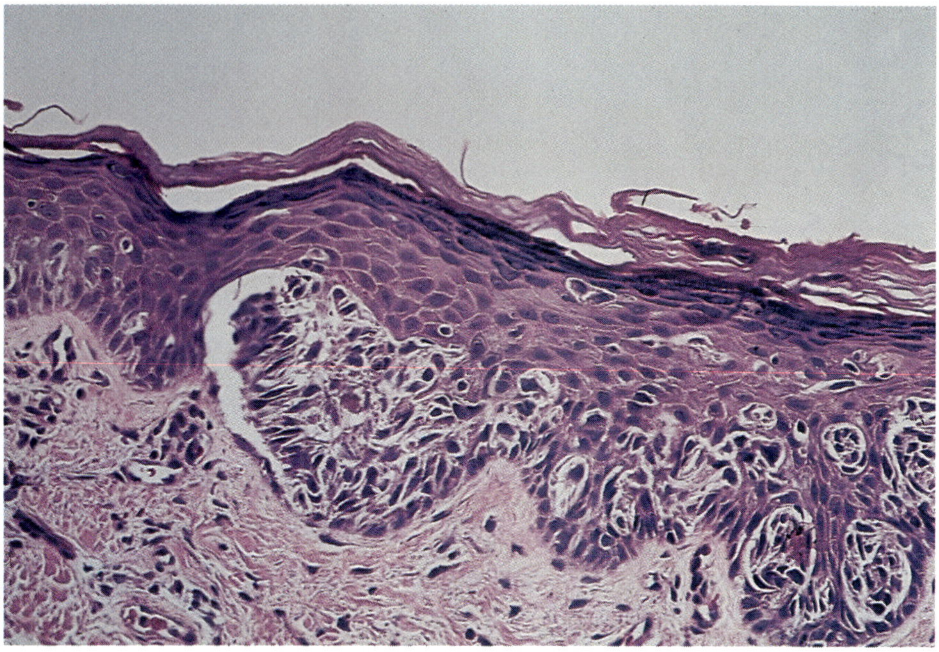

FIGURE 1-100
There is proliferation of atypical melanocytes at the base of the epithelium. A few melanocytes (round cells with clear cytoplasm and a hyperchromatic nucleus) are seen on the upper layers of the squamous epithelium. The melanocytes are confined within the epithelium. This lesion is known as melanoma in situ.

pigment in the dermis has been called by some melanoma in situ (Fig. 1-100). Wide local excision with clear margins of resection is also the treatment of choice for this.

The juvenile nevus, often called a giant or spindle cell nevus, is a benign lesion. It may be misinterpreted, however, as malignant melanoma. The juvenile nevus appears as a slightly scaly, pink, round, firm, hairless nodule that has a smooth surface. It may also be purplish red in color. It most frequently occurs during the first two decades of life. The juvenile nevus is a variant of a compound nevus. Usually it is associated with thinning of the epithelium, irregular acanthosis, and pseudoepitheliomatous hyperplasia of the squamous surface. The dermis is edematous and contains dilated vessles. The nevus cells are pleomorphic, which may raise a question of melanoma. The cells are spindle shaped or, less frequently, epithelioid (polygonal). Giant cells with eosinophilic cytoplasm and a large nucleus may also be seen. Multinucleated giant cells are seen less frequently. It is important to recognize that this nevus is benign because complete excision of the lesion is adequate treatment.

Seborrheic Keratoses

Seborrheic keratoses are as common on the vulva as they are on the skin elsewhere. Grossly, the pigmented lesion may occasionally be confused with carcinoma in situ or melanoma (Fig. 1-101). A biopsy, which is clearly indicated in these cases, will confirm the histopathologic diagnosis. Thickened squamous epithelium with keratin inclusions is pathognomonic of seborrheic lesions (Fig. 1-102).

Other Lesions

As previously mentioned, VIN 3 may appear as a pigmented lesion. Only microscopic examination of a biopsy specimen can identify the true nature of this lesion. Chronically irritated skin becomes thickened and may show an increase in pigmentation, especially in black patients. Mucosal pigmentation in the vulva and elsewhere has been reported secondary to lead exposure, irradiation, and ingestion of bismuth or quinacrine hydrochloride and in patients with the Peutz-Jeghers syndrome.[82-84]

Benign vulvar melanosis may grossly resemble malignant melanoma.[85] Melanosis is usually found on the labia minora and may be single or multiple. Melanosis is an irregular hyperpigmented area that has brown to brown-black streaks (Fig. 1-103). The size of the lesion varies and ranges from 1 to 4 cm in maximum diameter. Lesions are flat and have no evidence of induration and no ulceration. Microscopic examination reveals increased melanin in the basal layer of the epithelium, normal rete pegs, and an absence of nevus cells. No therapy is needed once a biopsy has been obtained to exclude melanoma and establish the correct diagnosis.

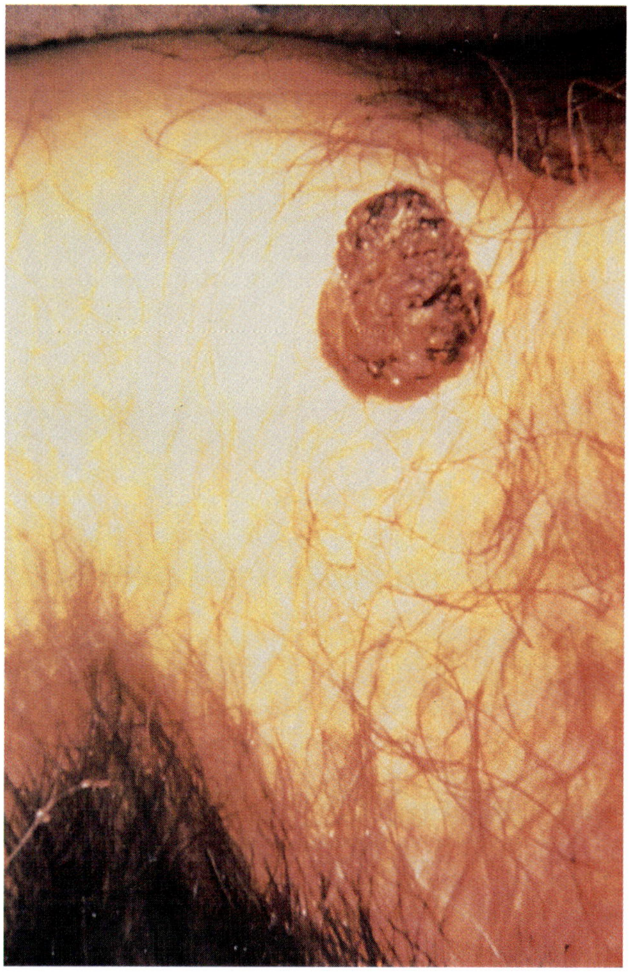

FIGURE 1-101
A solitary, verrucous pigmented lesion is present on the mons. This is seborrheic keratosis but may require biopsy for accurate diagnosis.

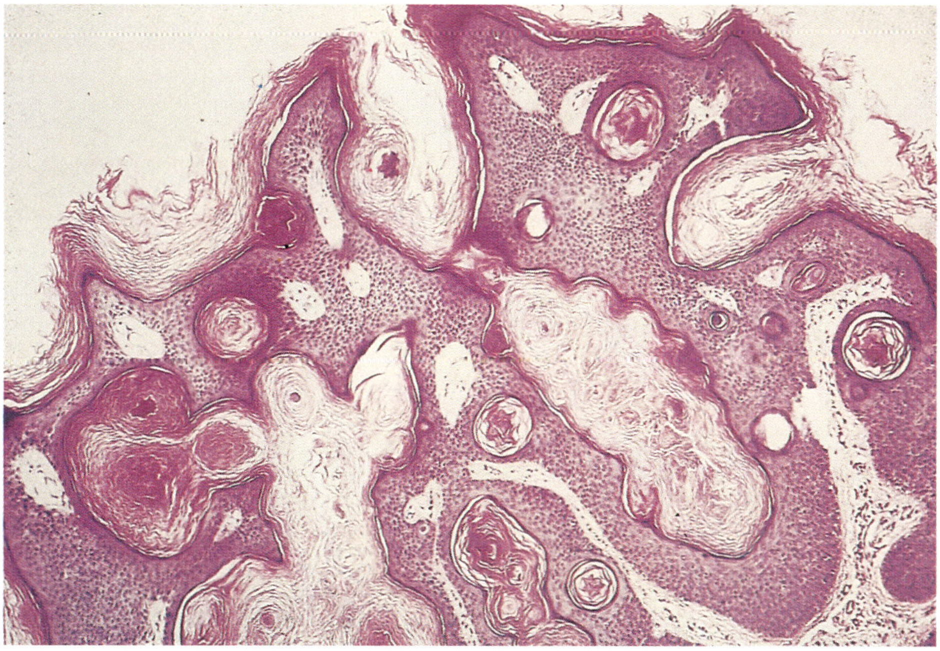

FIGURE 1-102
Convoluted (warty) squamous epithelium with hyperkeratosis and keratin inclusions is characteristic of seborrheic keratosis.

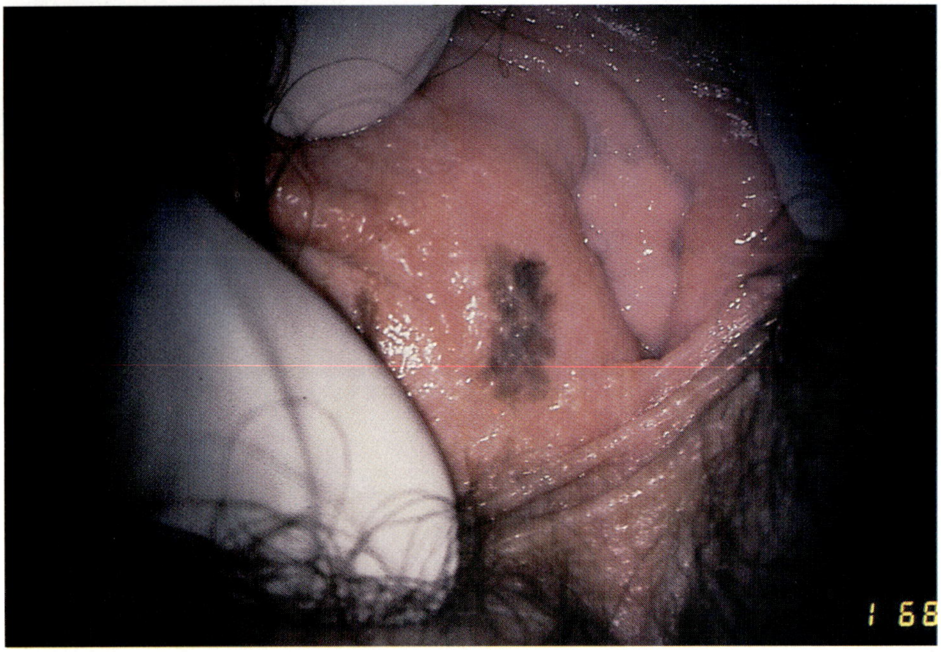

FIGURE 1–103
This is benign vulvar melanosis. The lesion is flat, with irregular borders and variable coloration. Biopsy must be done to exclude melanoma.

Malignant melanoma is discussed in the subsequent section on malignant tumors.

DEPIGMENTATION

Focal lack of pigmentation can be seen on the vulva as in other areas of the body (Fig. 1–104). Congenital absence of pigment is called leukoderma. Pigment may also be lost as a result of scarring or trauma (e.g., after laser ablation of vulvar lesions). This acquired loss of pigment is termed vitiligo.

MALIGNANT TUMORS

Paget Disease

Paget disease of the vulva is rare. Most patients with Paget disease of the vulva are in their seventh or eighth decade of life. The patient usually complains of pruritus or irritation. Paget disease of the vulva is similar in appearance to Paget disease of the breast. The lesion has slightly raised edges and a brick-red background. Within this background there are a variable number of islands of white epithelium (Fig. 1–105). Breast lesions of Paget disease are often associated with an underlying intraductal adenocarcinoma. Invasive ductal carcinoma may also be present. In contrast, in the majority of cases of vulvar Paget disease no origin in a gland is found, and there is no associated invasive disease.

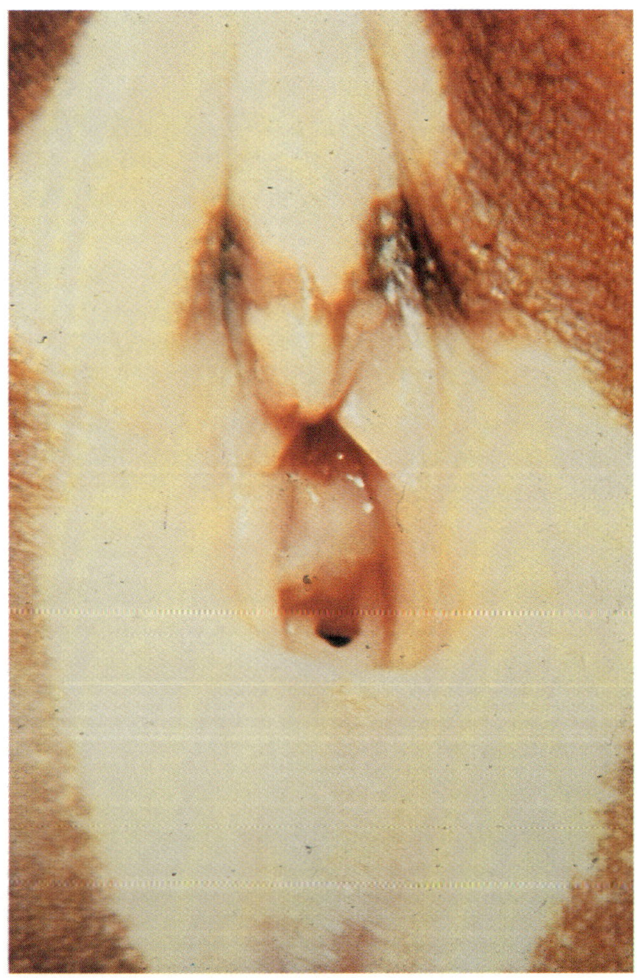

FIGURE 1–104
This congenital absence of pigment is known as leukoderma.

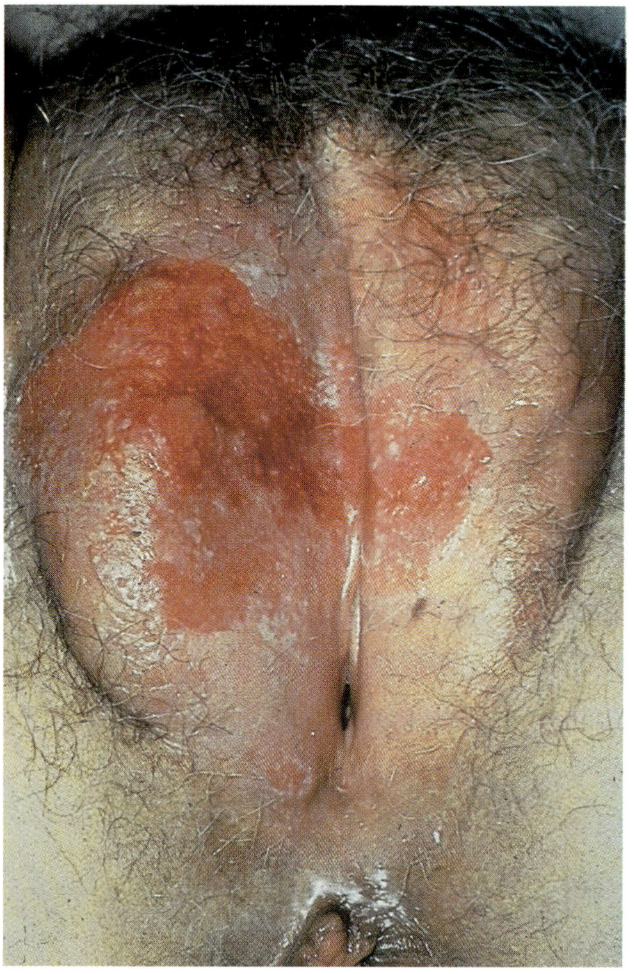

FIGURE 1-105
This deep red lesion is surrounded by shiny white epithelium. The surface of the lesion is irregular. Biopsy showed Paget disease associated with hyperkeratosis.

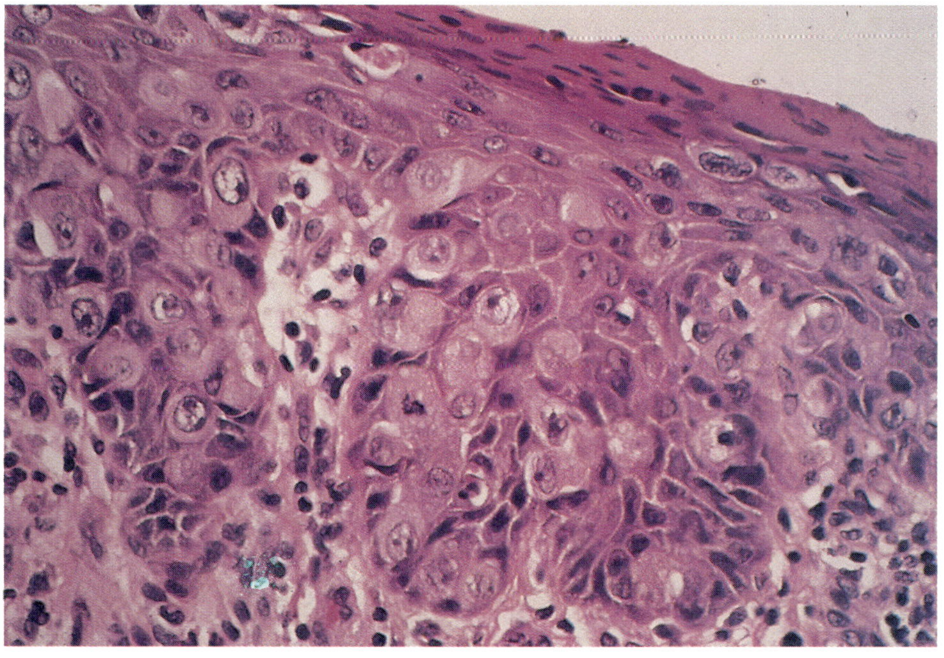

FIGURE 1-106
This is the microscopic appearance of Paget disease. The Paget cells are large and have abundant cytoplasm and a large nucleus with a prominent nucleolus. Most of the Paget cells are in the basal layer of the epithelium. However, two Paget cells are seen near the surface *(upper right)*. Parakeratosis is seen above these cells.

The histopathologic appearance of Paget disease is characteristic. The Paget cell is large and contains abundant, finely granular cytoplasm, which is amphophilic to clear. The nucleus is large, round to oval, and often eccentric in location. The chromatin pattern is vesicular, and nucleoli are prominent. Mitotic figures are frequently seen. These cells are seen primarily in the basal layer of the epithelium in groups or singly (Fig. 1–106). Scattered Paget cells may also be present throughout the various epithelial layers as well as in the underlying appendages. Parakeratosis, which is responsible for the lesion's reddish appearance, is present. Focal areas of hyperkeratosis are also seen.

The Paget cell may stain positive for mucin with mucicarmine stain. Periodic acid–Schiff stain (PAS) after diastase pretreatment can also be used to demonstrate mucin production. Paget cells are also immunoreactive for carcinoembryonic antigen (CEA), cytokeratin, and epithelial membrane antigen. Immunoreactivity for CEA is seen in normal eccrine and apocrine glands but not in squamous epithelium, hair follicles, and sebaceous glands.[86] Paget disease needs to be differentiated from the "pagetoid" growth seen in some melanoma cases. Paget lesions may contain cells with a few coarse melanin granules. Melanoma cells are immunoreactive for S-100, HMB-45, and other specific melanoma-associated antigens, whereas Paget cells are not.[87] Melanoma cells do not have mucin and are not immunoreactive for CEA.

The origin of the Paget cell remains controversial. It has been suggested that it arises from a totipotential cell of the embryonal stratum germinativum that was destined to be part of the apocrine system.[88] This idea is supported by electron microscopic studies and the immunocytochemistry findings mentioned earlier that suggest that the Paget cell is similar to the cells lining the apocrine glands. The local dermal milieu may play a role in causing the differentiation of basal epithelial cells into Paget cells. This concept is supported by the recurrence of Paget disease on a skin graft after a simple vulvectomy.[89]

There may be two varieties of vulvar Paget disease. The most common lesion begins and remains an intraepithelial disease. It is characterized by a series of lesions that are excised but recur over a period of years. This recurrence is not accompanied by metastasis. However, the second variety, which is more rare, comprises those cases of intraepithelial Paget disease that progress to invasive disease[90] or that present de novo as invasive lesions originating from the surface epithelium or from the skin appendages. Intraepithelial involvement of skin appendages should not be misinterpreted as invasion. The cells of invasive Paget disease infiltrate the dermis as cords, nests, and sheets (Fig. 1–107). Neoplasms that begin in the skin appendages and invade early, often develop metastases before the surface epithelium is involved. The metastases may simulate a squamous carcinoma with "pagetoid cells."

An adenocarcinoma of the underlying sweat glands is found in 15 to 20 percent of patients who have intraepithelial Paget disease (Fig. 1–108).[91] In addition, approximately 30 percent of patients with vulvar Paget disease have a noncontiguous carcinoma such as breast, rectal, bladder, urethral,

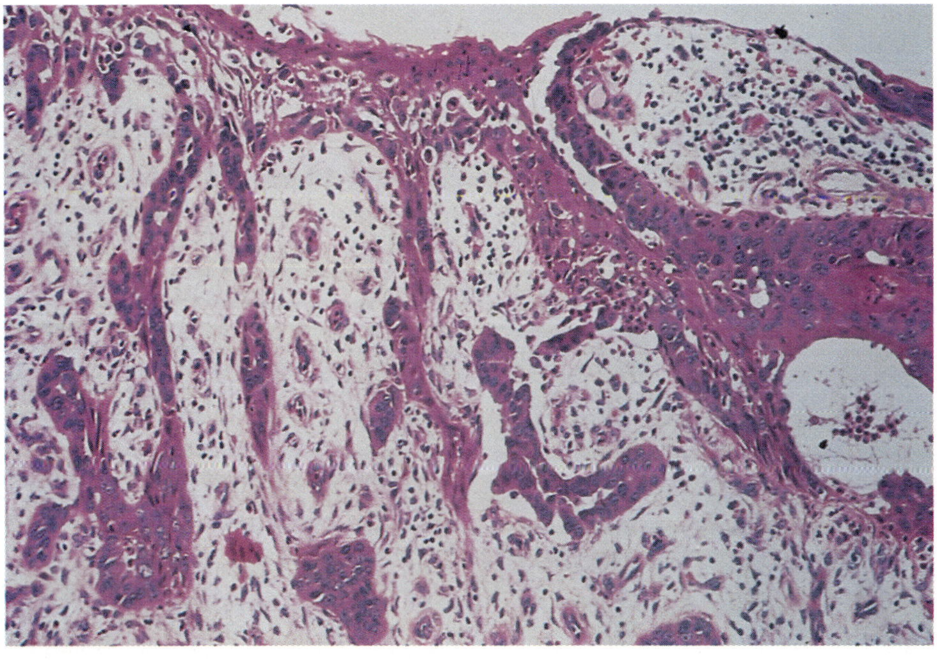

FIGURE 1–107
The cells of this invasive Paget disease invade the dermis in cords and nests. The surface epithelium is almost completely replaced by Paget cells. There is marked dermal edema.

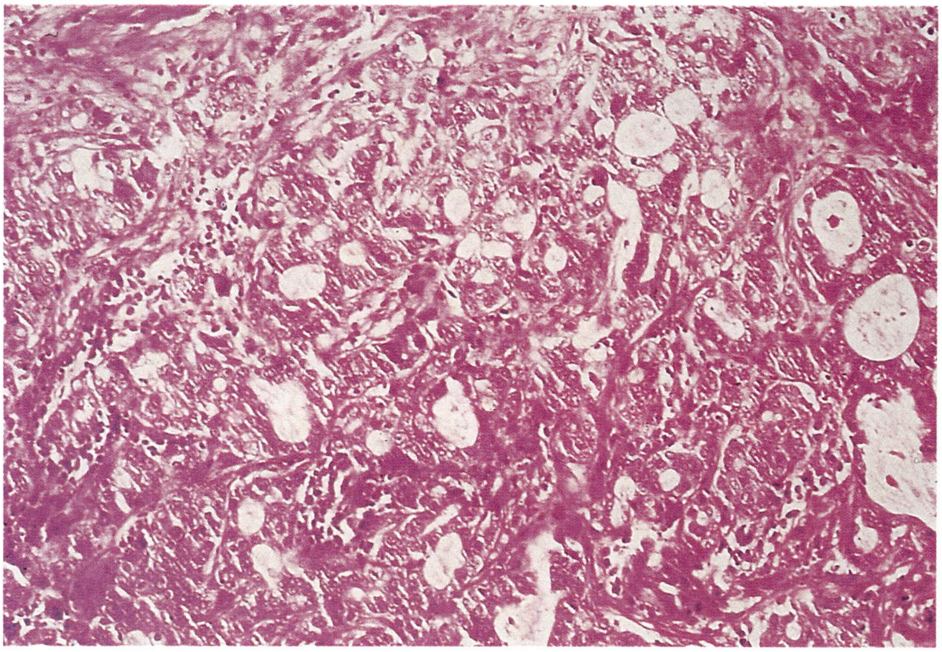

FIGURE 1-108
This is a poorly differentiated adenocarcinoma that arose in the sweat glands of the vulva of a patient who had intraepithelial Paget disease.

cervical, or ovarian carcinoma. Therefore, a patient who has Paget disease of the vulva should be evaluated for the possibility of synchronous neoplasms.

Standard treatment for intraepithelial Paget disease is simple excision. This excision should be at least 0.5 cm deep and have a 1-cm margin. In patients with extensive disease, a skinning vulvectomy with split-thickness skin grafts may be necessary. It is important to attempt to achieve negative margins because patients who have positive margins are at high risk for recurrence. Because Paget disease is typically more extensive on microscopic examination than on clinical examination, some have recommended frozen sections for evaluation of the margins.[92] This is not always practical because it may result in unacceptable prolongation of the operative time and may make definitive evaluation of the margin difficult. On occasion, a clear margin is not obtained despite extensive excision. Recurrences of intraepithelial Paget disease can be treated by laser vaporization.[93] Invasive Paget disease is treated by radical vulvectomy and bilateral inguinal lymphadenectomy. The presence of lymph node metastasis is an ominous sign.

Classification and Staging of Vulvar Malignancies

Malignancies of the vulva other than those associated with Paget disease may be classified as shown in Table 1–3. Staging of carcinoma of the vulva according to the International Federation of

TABLE 1–3.

Classification of Malignant Tumors Occurring in the Vulva

- I. Epithelial
  - A. Squamous
    1. Typical
    2. Basaloid
    3. Warty
  - B. Basal cell
  - C. Verrucous
  - D. Adenocarcinoma
    1. Bartholin gland
    2. Other
  - E. Paget disease
- II. Melanoma
- III. Sarcomas
  - A. Leiomyosarcoma
  - B. Rhabdomyosarcoma
  - C. Alveolar soft part
  - D. Kaposi
  - E. Dermatofibrosarcoma protuberans
  - F. Malignant fibrous histiocytoma
- IV. Other
  - A. Lymphoma
  - B. Endodermal sinus tumor
  - C. Neuroendocrine carcinoma
  - D. Primitive neuroectodermal tumor
  - E. Histiocytosis X
  - F. Desmoid tumor
  - G. Metastasis to vulva

Gynecology and Obstetrics (FIGO)[94] is shown in Table 1–4. Two recent retrospective analyses suggest that this surgical staging system places patients in more accurate risk categories than does the clinical staging system previously used.[95,96]

Squamous Cell Carcinoma

Approximately 3 to 4 percent of all primary malignancies of the genital tract in women arise in the vulva. Squamous cell carcinoma is the most frequent histopathologic type, comprising over 85 percent of cases, and this is followed by melanoma. Pruritus is the most frequent complaint among patients who have squamous cell carcinoma of the vulva.[97] The patient may also complain of irritation, pain, bleeding, discharge, or urinary or rectal symptoms, or she may be asymptomatic and seek medical attention after discovering a vulvar lesion. As discussed under hyperplastic and atrophic lesions of the vulva, vulvar dystrophies are frequently found in the skin adjacent to vulvar squamous cell carcinoma. However, vulvar dystrophy is relatively common among postmenopausal women (the group most frequently affected with vulvar cancer), whereas vulvar cancer is rare. Therefore, vulvar dystrophy is probably not a premalignant lesion, but the chronic skin damage caused by the "itch-scratch" cycle associated with it may prepare the ground for malignant transformation.

TABLE 1–4.
Staging of Vulvar Carcinoma According to TNM Classification of the International Federation of Gynecology and Obstetrics (FIGO)

Stage 0:	Carcinoma in situ
	T_{is}
Stage I:	Tumor confined to the vulva or perineum; more than 2 cm in greatest dimension. No nodal metastasis
	$T_1N_0M_0$
Stage II:	Tumor confined to the vulva or perineum; more than 2 cm in greatest dimension. No nodal metastasis
	$T_2N_0M_0$
Stage III:	Tumor of any size with adjacent spread to the lower urethra, vagina, or anus and/or unilateral regional lymph node metastasis
	$T_3N_0M_0$
	$T_3N_1M_0$
	$T_1N_1M_0$
	$T_2N_1M_0$
Stage IVA:	Tumor invasion of any of the following: upper urethra, bladder mucosa, rectal mucosa, pelvic bone, and/or bilateral regional lymph node metastasis
	$T_1N_2M_0$
	$T_2N_2M_0$
	$T_3N_2M_0$
	T_4, any N, M_0
Stage IVB:	Any distant metastasis (including metastasis to pelvic lymph nodes)
	any T, any N, M_1

TNM Classification

T (primary tumor)
- T_1: Tumor confined to the vulva and/or perineum; 2 cm or less in greatest dimension
- T_2: Tumor confined to the vulva and/or perineum; >2 cm in greatest dimension
- T_3: Tumor of any size with adjacent spread to the lower urethra, vagina, or anus
- T_4: Tumor invasion of any of the following: upper urethra, bladder mucosa, rectal mucosa, pelvic bone

N (regional lymph nodes)
- N_0: No nodal metastasis (surgically proven)
- N_1: Unilateral inguinal lymph node metastasis
- N_2: Bilateral inguinal lymph node metastasis

M (distant metastasis)
- M_0 : No distant metastasis
- M_{1a}: Pelvic lymph node metastasis
- M_{1b}: Other distant metastasis

Squamous cell carcinoma of the vulva may present as a fungating mass (Fig. 1–109), a nodule (Fig. 1–110), or a plaque that may or may not be ulcerated (Fig. 1–111). The color of the lesion may be white (Fig. 1–112), pink, or red. Some lesions may have increased pigmentation or no pigmentation. Almost all are unifocal, and most are located on the labia. Labial lesions are fairly evenly distributed between the labia minora and majora. Some are located in the perineum, fourchette, or mons, and a few are found on the clitoris.

There appear to be two subtypes of vulvar squamous cell carcinoma. One type is associated with HPV infection (predominantly of genotypes 16 and 18) and is found in relatively younger women (mean age 58.9 years). Epidemiologic risk factors associated with this type of vulvar squamous cell carcinoma include early age at first intercourse, multiple lifetime sexual partners, and cigarette smoking. The other type of carcinoma does not appear to be associated with HPV infection, sexual history, or smoking. It occurs in older women (mean age 66.8 years).[98–100] This is the most frequent type of vulvar squamous cell carcinoma. Most of these lesions are well-differentiated squamous carcinomas and show keratin pearl formation (see Fig. 1–58).

HPV-associated vulvar squamous cell carcinoma has two characteristic histopathologic appearances, basaloid and warty. Basaloid lesions are composed of sheets and nests of relatively uniform populations of small ovoid cells with a high nuclear to cytoplasmic ratio. There is little evidence of maturation. The cells resemble the most basal layer of cells in the squamous epithelium, and

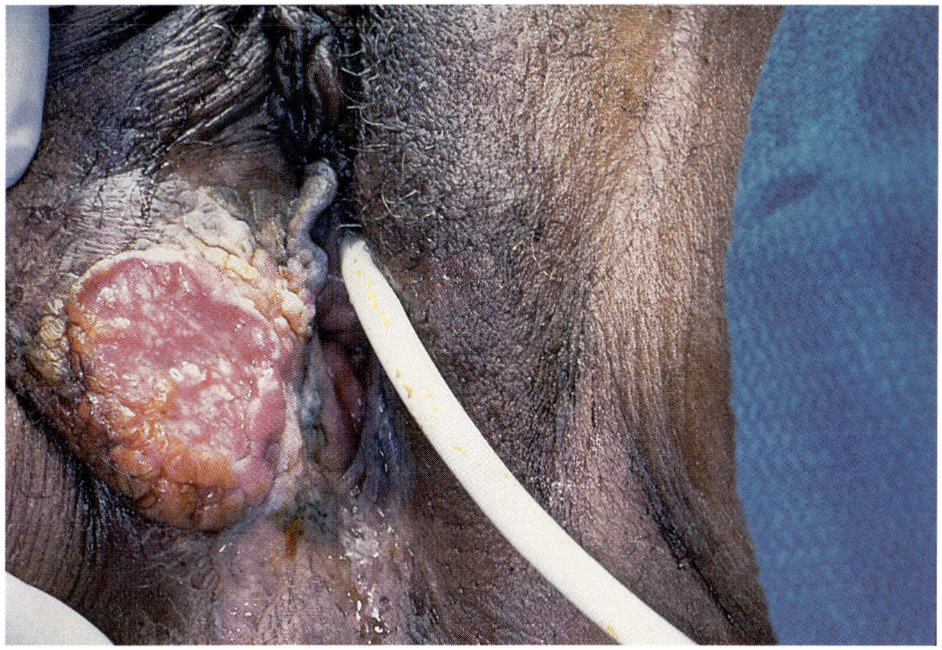

FIGURE 1-109
A fungating squamous cell carcinoma is seen on the right labium majus.

keratinization is absent or minimal. Occasionally, the cells in the center of the nests have more cytoplasm, and keratinization is seen (Fig. 1–113). The invasive front of basaloid squamous cell carcinoma tends to be rounded rather than spiky or wispy, with the tumor arranged in variably sized nests and cords. Often the centers of larger nests display necrosis. Keratin pearls are occasionally seen. Basaloid carcinoma must be differentiated from basal cell carcinoma (see later discussion). Basaloid carcinoma does not have the characteristic palisading of the outermost layer of cells that is seen in the nests of basal cell carcinoma. Warty carcinoma demonstrates marked koilocytotic changes (Fig. 1–114). This lesion is exophytic and displays spiky "church-spire" extensions in a manner similar to, but not as exuberant as, those seen in condyloma acuminatum. Some degree of maturation is often seen. Hyperkeratosis, parakeratosis, and marked cytologic atypia are present. Central keratinization may be quite prominent in invasive nests of warty squamous cell carcinoma. The non-

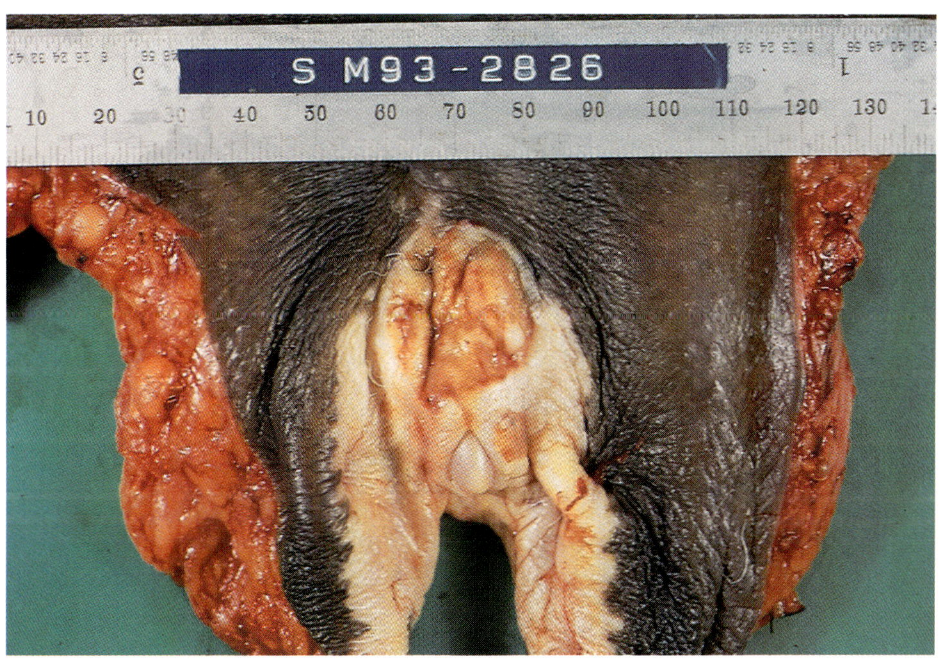

FIGURE 1-110
A nodular squamous cell carcinoma is seen on the prepuce. Vitiligo surrounds the introitus. This patient had chronic vulvar pruritus and over the years had multiple biopsies that showed squamous hyperplasia without atypia.

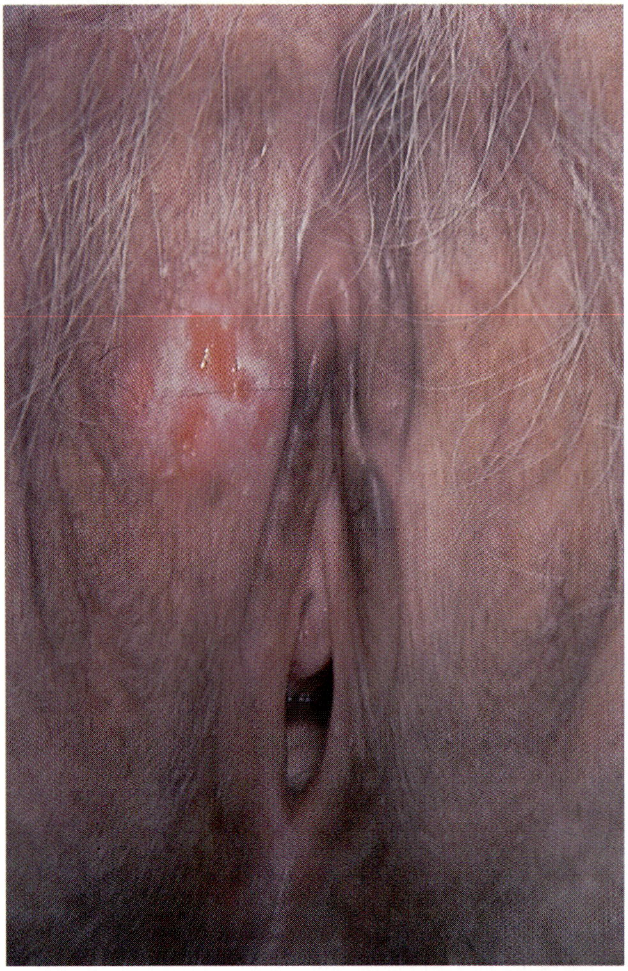

FIGURE 1-111
This ulcerated white lesion proved on biopsy to be squamous cell carcinoma.

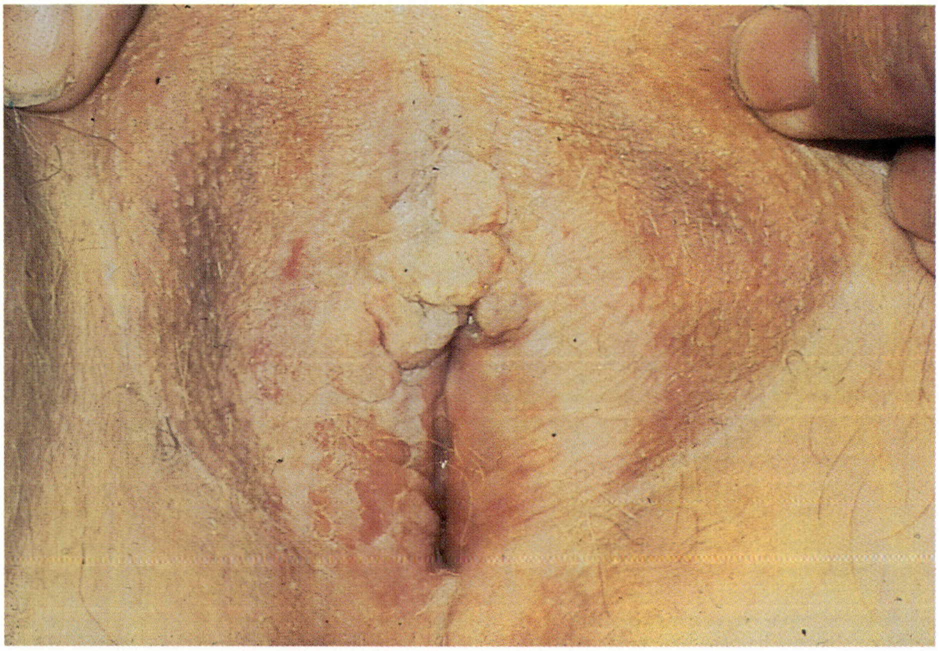

FIGURE 1-112
This hyperkeratotic, warty lesion in the area of the clitoris is squamous cell carcinoma.

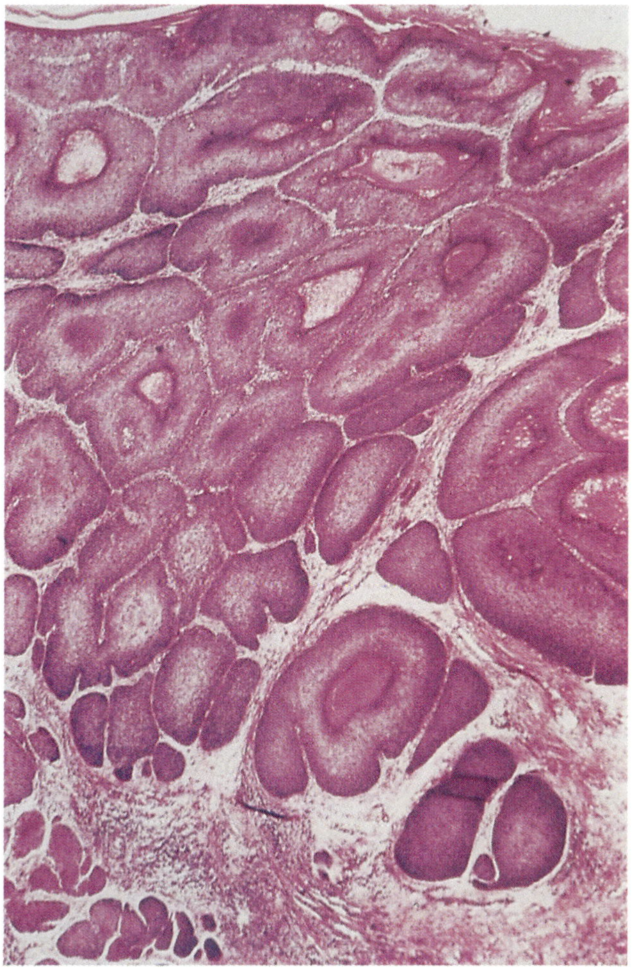

FIGURE 1-113
This is a basaloid squamous cell carcinoma of the vulva. Multiple nests of tumor infiltrate the stroma. The nests have rounded borders. The tumor nests appear dark purple because the cells are small and the nuclei are relatively large and hyperchromatic. In this example there is some maturation of the cells in the center of the nests; there are also keratinization and necrosis.

HPV-associated vulvar squamous cell carcinoma does not have the warty architecture but does have the other cellular features of keratinization just described.

Multiple factors have been found to be associated with tumor recurrence or metastasis to inguinal lymph nodes from vulvar squamous cell carcinoma. These include tumor size and location, tumor thickness or depth of invasion, tumor differentiation, tumor growth pattern, invasion of lymphovascular spaces, and the status of the surgical margins. An almost linear relationship exists between the depth of invasion and lymph node metastasis. In one study the incidence of inguinal lymph node metastasis was 2.6 percent when the tumor thickness (depth of invasion) was equal to or less than 1 mm, whereas it was 48 percent when tumor thickness was over 5 mm.[3] Depth of invasion is particularly important when one is defining the prognosis of patients who have superficially invasive tumors.[101, 102] To compare the different reports, the method used to determine the extent of invasion needs to be clear. Tumor thickness is defined as the distance from the surface of the tumor to the deepest point of invasion (Fig. 1-115). This method is thought by many to be the easiest and most accurate and reproducible.[3, 103] The depth of invasion can be measured from the tip of the adjacent deepest non-neoplastic rete peg to the deepest point of invasion or from the epidermal-dermal junction of the most superficial adjacent papilla. The latter is considered most accurate in determining the risk of lymph node

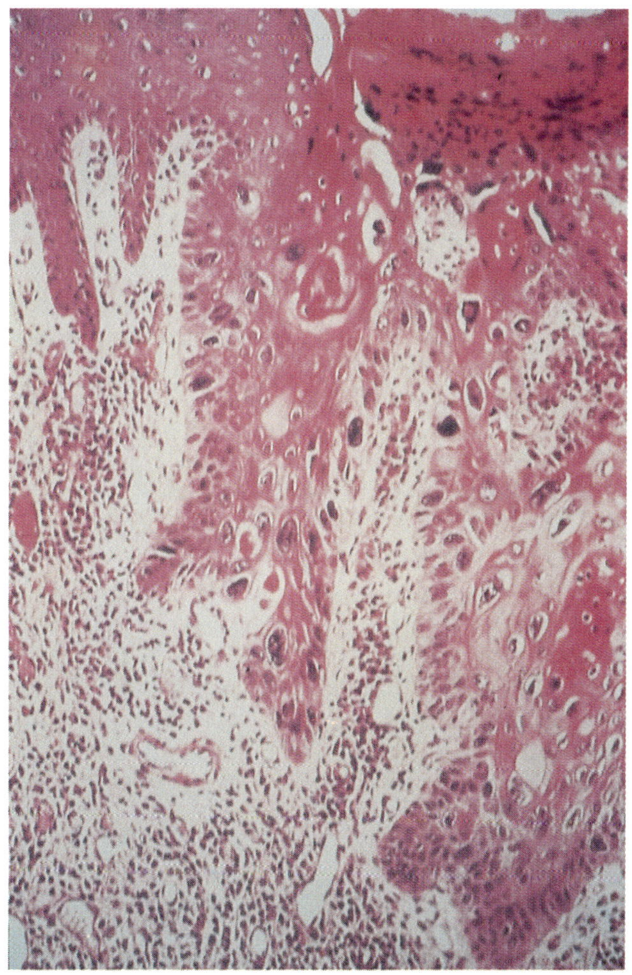

FIGURE 1-114
This vulvar biopsy specimen shows a warty squamous cell carcinoma arising from epithelium demonstrating koilocytotic atypia *(left)*. Irregular tongues of carcinoma invade the underlying stroma. A lymphocytic infiltrate is seen in the stroma. There is parakeratosis. Koilocytotic change is prominent in the invasive tumor. Some of the tumor cells have large, bizarre nuclei. Koilocytotic cavities surround many of the atypical nuclei. Keratinization is present in the invasive tongues.

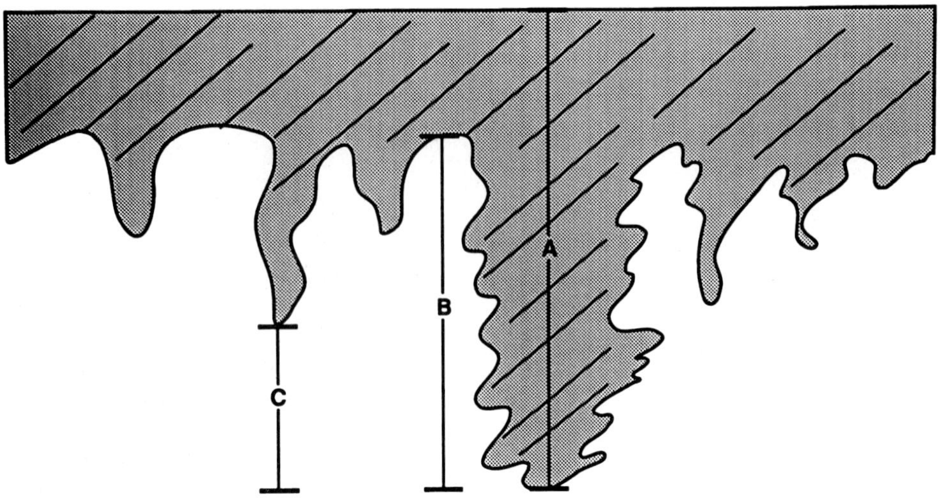

FIGURE 1-115
Various proposed methods for measuring depth of invasion in vulvar squamous cell carcinoma are compared. Method A measures tumor thickness from the surface of the tumor to the deepest point of invasion. Method B measures depth of invasion from the basement membrane of the most superficial adjacent dermal papilla. Method C measures depth of invasion from the tip of the deepest adjacent normal rete peg.

metastasis and recurrence in patients with very early superficial tumors. The International Society for the Study of Vulvar Diseases (ISSVD) recommends that vulvar cancer that is less than 2 cm in diameter and has a depth of invasion of less than 1 mm measured from the adjacent dermal papilla be classified as stage IA.[104] The risk of lymph node metastasis or recurrence in patients who have this early lesion is nil. These patients may be treated by wide local excision of the lesion.

Tumor differentiation is also a strong predictor of inguinal lymph node metastasis in both superficial and deeply invasive tumors.[3] This is true regardless of whether the traditional histopathologic grading classification of well, moderately, and poorly differentiated carcinoma or that proposed by the Gynecologic Oncology Group (GOG), which will be described subsequently, is used.[105] Well-differentiated vulvar squamous cell carcinoma is characterized by cells with prominent intercellular bridges, intracytoplasmic keratin, mild nuclear atypia, and low mitotic count. Squamous pearls and necrosis with keratin debris may also be present. Moderately differentiated tumors have less keratin, increased nuclear atypia, and mitotic activity, whereas poorly differentiated tumors have marked nuclear pleomorphism, brisk mitotic activity, and focal cytoplasmic keratin and no intercellular bridges. The GOG classification consists of four grades and is based on the proportion of the tumor comprising a poorly differentiated pattern. The poorly differentiated pattern is usually present at the epidermal-dermal junction. It consists of small cells with scant cytoplasm and little to no differentiation. These cells infiltrate the stroma either in elongated streaks or small clusters. A GOG grade 1 vulvar squamous cell carcinoma has no undifferentiated component. A grade 2 lesion has 1 to 30 percent, a grade 3 has 31 to 50 percent, and a grade 4 lesion has more than 50 percent of an undifferentiated component. In one large study, only 3 percent of patients who had a GOG grade 1 squamous cell carcinoma had inguinal lymph node metastasis, whereas 60 percent of those with grade 4 tumors had metastasis.[3] In the same study, using the traditional grading classification, 27 percent of patients with well-differentiated tumors had lymph node metastasis, whereas 55 percent of those with poorly differentiated tumors had lymph node metastasis. In both cases this difference was statistically significant.

The tumor growth pattern also seems to be associated with the frequency of nodal metastasis and recurrence, especially in patients with superficially invasive lesions. Three growth patterns have been identified: isolated foci originating from VIN-3, pushing pattern, and an infiltrative pattern. The first pattern consists of one or more isolated foci of single cords or narrow tongues of cells that arise directly from VIN-3 lesions and penetrate the stroma without coalescence. The tongues may be of any length. The depth of invasion (measured from the epidermal-dermal junction of the most superficial adjacent papilla) in this pattern is virtually always less than 2 mm. This pattern is reportedly associated with no risk of lymph node metastasis.[106]

The pushing growth pattern is characterized by an invasive front composed of well-defined and circumscribed tumor masses that have few or no tumor cords or nests arising from them (Fig. 1–116). Tumors exhibiting this pattern typically are less than 5 mm thick. They are generally well differentiated and rarely invade lymphovascular spaces. Stromal desmoplasia is often not seen. In a large series of patients with stage I through stage IV vulvar squamous cell carcinoma, none of those with a pushing growth pattern developed local re-

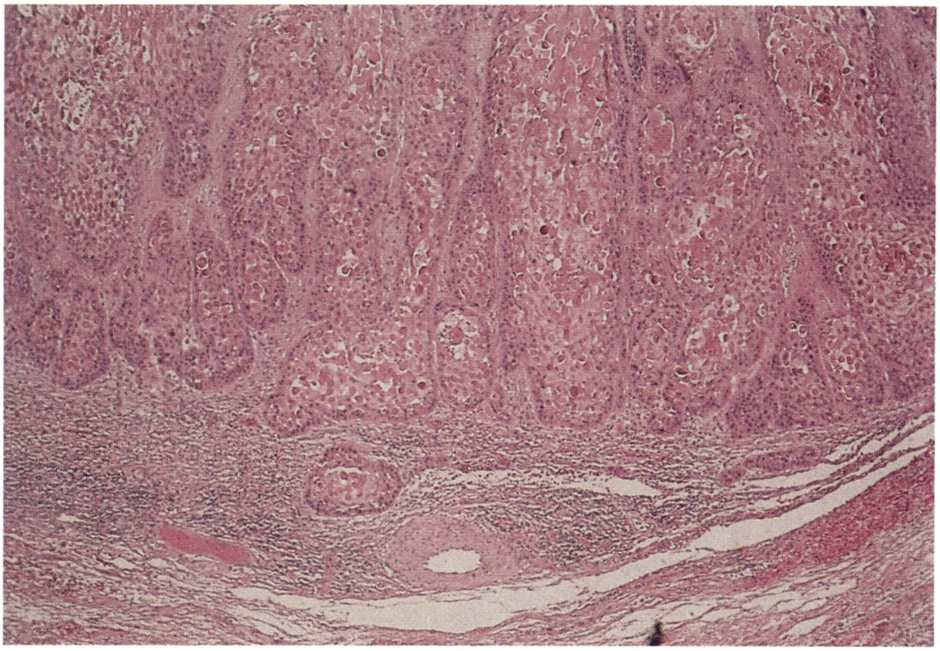

FIGURE 1-116
This well-differentiated squamous cell carcinoma of the vulva has a pushing growth pattern. There is a prominent band of lymphoid cells under the pushing front of the tumor.

currence.[107] This better prognosis associated with the pushing growth pattern has also been reported by others.[106]

The infiltrative growth pattern is also known as "spray," "diffuse," or "stellate" growth. This growth pattern consists predominantly of infiltrating, dissociated tumor nests, cords, ribbons, or single cells that often originate from a central tumor mass (see Fig. 1–58). Both a desmoplastic stromal response and lymphocytic inflammatory infiltrate are frequently seen. Vascular space involvement is more common with this pattern of growth than with compact tumors.[105] Local recurrences are common (26 percent in one series) when this tumor growth pattern is present.[107]

The pushing and infiltrative growth patterns may or may not show confluence, and the significance of confluence is controversial.[106] Confluence is defined as the presence of a compact mass of invading tumor that completely fills a 1-mm or greater field. In one series of cases of superficially invasive vulvar squamous cell carcinoma 27 of 47 patients (36 percent) whose tumors exhibited confluence had lymph node metastasis, whereas none of 31 patients whose tumor did not have confluence had lymph node metastasis.[108] However, others have reported lymph node metastasis in patients with superficially invasive tumors with no confluence.[106]

Lymphovascular space invasion is also associated with an increased frequency of lymph node metastasis and recurrence.[109–111] Such invasion should be diagnosed only if islands of tumor cells are found within spaces that are clearly lined by endothelium. In the GOG experience, lymph node metastasis was present in 75 percent of patients who had tumors with lymphovascular space invasion compared to 27 percent in whom no lymphovascular space invasion was present.[3]

In one study, the amount of acellular keratin was correlated with local recurrence.[107] Seventy-five percent of the outcomes could have been predicted using only the amount of keratin present. Recurrences were reported in 11 of 102 patients (11 percent) whose tumors were composed of less than 25 percent keratin and in 10 of 33 (33 percent) with greater than 25 percent keratin.

The status of the surgical margin is an important predictor of local recurrence. None of 91 patients in whom vulvar squamous cell carcinoma was excised with a tumor-free margin of 8 mm or larger developed recurrence, whereas 21 of 44 (48 percent) who had margins of less than 8 mm did have local recurrence.[107] Tumor-free margins and depth of invasion, when combined, are the best predictors of local recurrence.

The status of the inguinal nodes as determined by histopathology is the most important independent prognostic factor.[95] The corrected actuarial 5-year survival for patients who have vulvar squamous cell carcinoma and negative lymph nodes is 96 percent.[112] It is 94 percent in the presence of one inguinal lymph node with metastasis, 80 percent with two positive nodes, and 12 percent with three or more positive nodes. Similar data have been reported by the GOG. They report a relative 5-year survival of 75 percent when one to two nodes are involved with tumor, 36 percent when three to four nodes are positive, 24 percent when five to six nodes are involved, and none when seven or more nodes are involved by metastases from vulvar squamous cell carcinoma.[95]

Although tumor size is a predictor of inguinal lymph node status in most series, tumor size and tumor location have not been found to be independent prognostic factors in the GOG experience. The strong correlation between histopathologically proven lymph node status and tumor grade, depth of invasion, and the presence or absence of lymphovascular space invasion overshadows the significance of tumor size. The patient's age is also a strong predictor of the presence of inguinal lymph node metastasis. In the GOG experience, 25 percent of patients younger than 55 years had lymph node metastasis, whereas 46 percent of patients 75 years of age or older had metastasis.[3]

Squamous cell carcinoma of the vulva spreads locally and through the lymphatics. The vulvar lymphatics drain laterally to the superficial inguinal and femoral groin nodes and then to the pelvic wall lymphatics. It has been established that in the absence of inguinal lymph node metastasis, pelvic lymph node involvement is insignificant.[113, 114] Approximately 15 to 20 percent of patients with inguinal lymph node metastasis have metastasis in the pelvic lymph nodes as well.

Treatment should include management of the primary lesion and the regional lymph nodes based on the factors previously discussed. There has been increasing interest in conservative, less radical surgery designed to minimize the postoperative anatomic changes and sexual dysfunction while maintaining the potential for cure.[115] Patients who have minimally invasive disease (stage IA) may be treated by wide local excision only. The lateral margins should be clear of the tumor by at least 1 cm. Patients with small lesions that invade deeper than 1 mm may be treated with radical excision or radical hemivulvectomy (Fig. 1–117).[116] The incision is carried down to the inferior fascia of the urogenital diaphragm, and the lateral margins should be clear of the tumor by at least 1 cm. An ipsilateral inguinal node dissection should be done when the lesion is unilateral and the tumor thickness is 2 mm or less (but more than 1 mm).[3] Contralateral lymph node metastasis in this situation does not occur. However, more than 3 percent of patients who have a tumor 3 to 5 mm in thickness have metastases to the contralateral nodes. Therefore, bilateral inguinal node dissection should be considered for patients who have unilateral vulvar squamous cell carcinoma when the tumor thickness increases. Midline lesions require a modified radical vulvectomy (anterior or posterior radical vulvectomy) or a complete radical vulvectomy if there are multiple areas of abnormal skin (Fig. 1–118). Bilateral inguinal node dissection is performed when there is a midline lesion. If the inguinal nodes are positive for metastasis, adjuvant whole pelvis and inguinal irradiation is administered.[117] Neoadjuvant radiation or chemotherapy (or both) has been advocated for patients with locally advanced disease because this therapy can lead to less radical surgery and increase the success rate of resection.[118] Due to complicating medical conditions and the debilitated status of

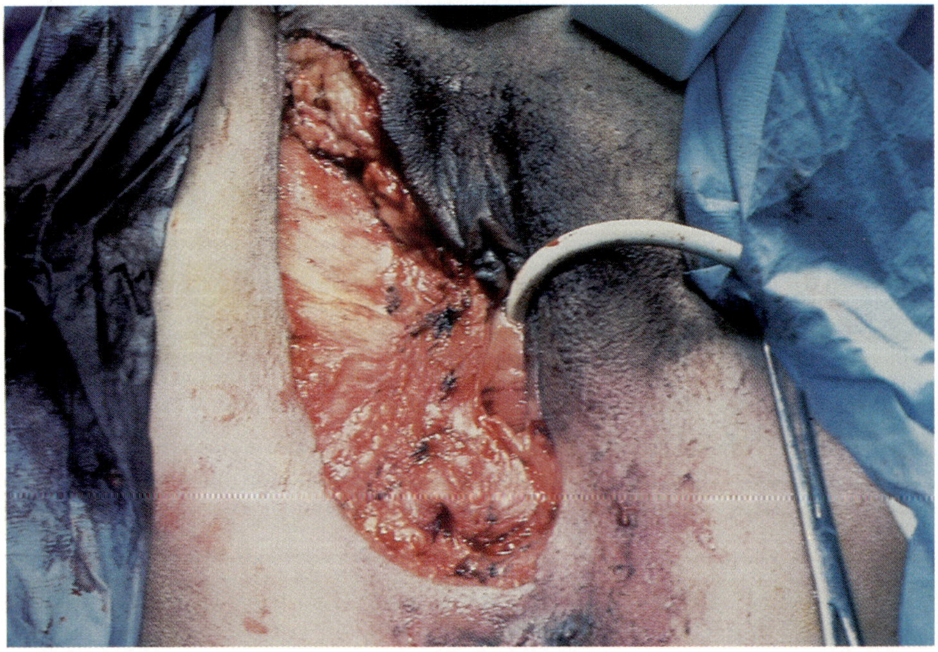

FIGURE 1–117
This is a patient who has had a radical right hemivulvectomy for stage I squamous cell carcinoma of the vulva. The exposed fascia lata is seen *(upper right)*.

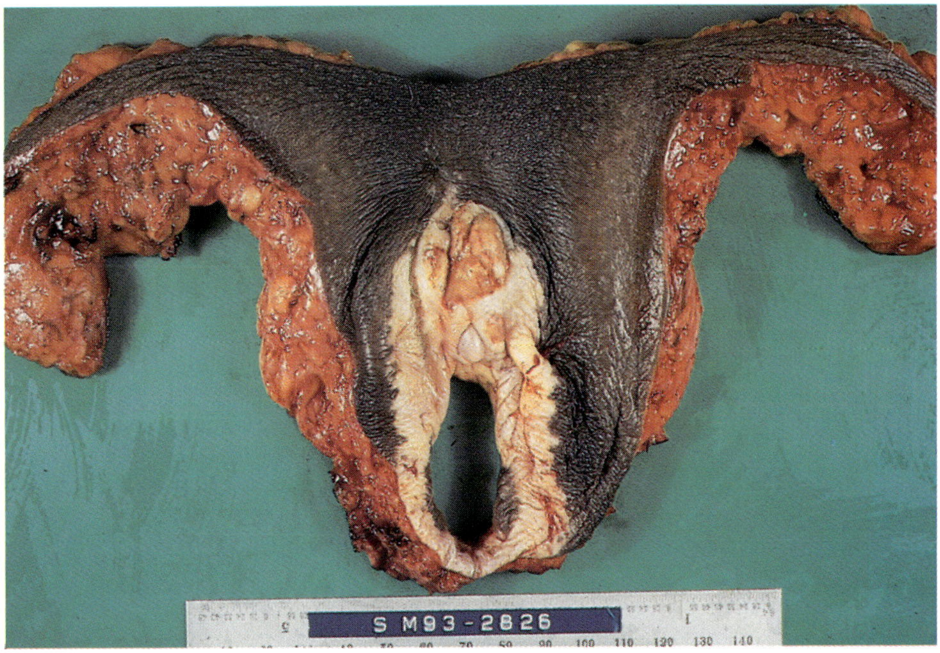

FIGURE 1-118
The same patient as in Figure 1-110 had a central lesion above the clitoris. She had a modified complete radical vulvectomy and en bloc inguinal lymph node dissection. The fat and lymphatic tissue are still attached to the skin of the groins.

some patients radiation therapy alone may be used.[119] Radiation vulvitis and radiation necrosis are among the possible complications (Fig. 1-119). Modern radiation therapy techniques should result in a decrease in the incidence of these complications.

Morrow and colleagues[120] suggest that the design of therapy for vulvar squamous cell carcinoma should take into account: (1) lesion size and location, (2) depth of invasion, (3) lymphovascular space involvement, (4) degree of histopathologic differentiation, (5) clinical status of the inguinal nodes, (6) the health and wishes of the patient, (7) condition of the vulvar skin not involved by cancer, (8) presence of associated problems such as genital prolapse, and (9) other sites of lower genital tract squamous neoplasia. The frequent association of vulvar squamous cell carcinoma with other premalignant and malignant neoplasms, especially of the cervix and vagina, is well known.[101,106]

Basal Cell Carcinoma

Basal cell carcinoma of the vulva is a rare tumor constituting only 2 to 3 percent of all vulvar cancers. It occurs primarily in postmenopausal white women. The mean age is 65 years. The most common complaints at presentation are pruritus and the presence of a mass. Most basal cell carcinomas of the vulva occur on the labia majora, but some occur on the labia minora, urethral meatus, prepuce, and clitoris. The gross appearance may be that of a nodule or plaque, with or without ulceration. The reported lesions have ranged in size from 0.2 to 10 cm. Some are multifocal. The typical microscopic appearance of basal cell carcinoma is similar to that of this tumor on other skin. There are masses or nests of small cells that have a uniform appearance (Fig. 1-120). These cells have round to oval nuclei, a high nuclear to cytoplasmic ratio, infrequent mitoses, and indistinct cell borders. The tumor masses may be solid or may show an adenoid pattern, which is characterized by the formation of glandlike spaces of various sizes with peripheral palisading of the cells. This pattern must be differentiated from the more aggressive adenoid cystic carcinoma, which more commonly arises from Bartholin's gland.[121] Squamous cell metaplasia may be seen in vulvar basal cell carcinoma but does not alter the prognosis.[122] Basal cell carcinoma must be distinguished from the even rarer basosquamous carcinoma, which contains a malignant squamous component and has a poorer prognosis. The long-term prognosis of patients with vulvar basal cell carcinoma is good despite a 20 percent risk of local recurrence.[123] Metastases to the inguinal nodes are rare, and wide local excision is considered standard treatment unless involvement of the inguinal lymph nodes is suspected.[124] If suspicious lymph nodes are present, a lymphadenectomy should be considered.

Verrucous Carcinoma

Verrucous carcinoma is a variant of squamous cell carcinoma that occurs most commonly in the naso-

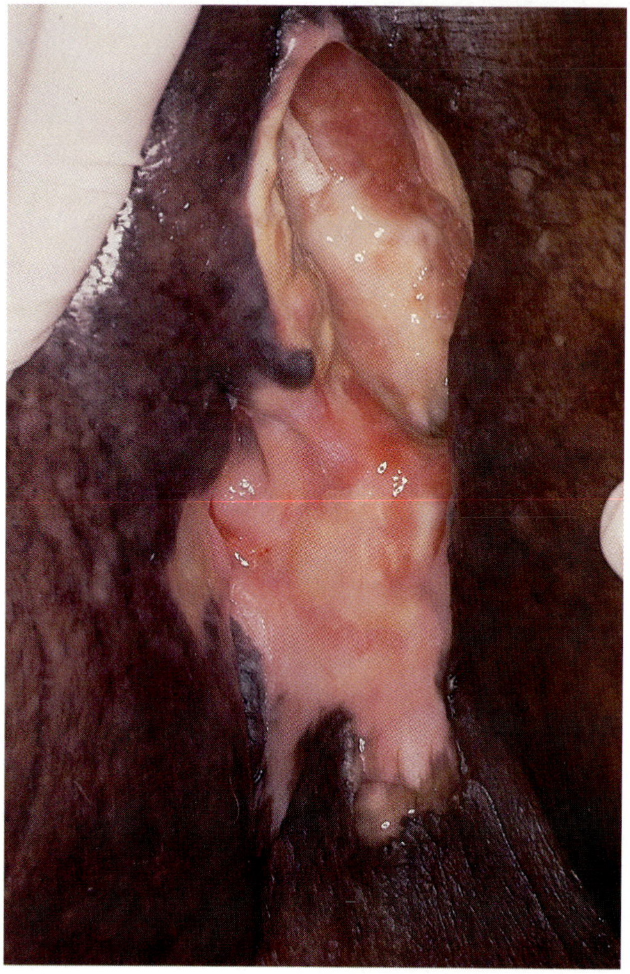

FIGURE 1-119
This necrotic ulcer is seen in a patient who received radiation therapy for treatment of squamous cell carcinoma of the vulva. This ulcer was aggressively debrided, and multiple biopsies were obtained to exclude recurrence. Biopsies showed only necrosis and radiation effect.

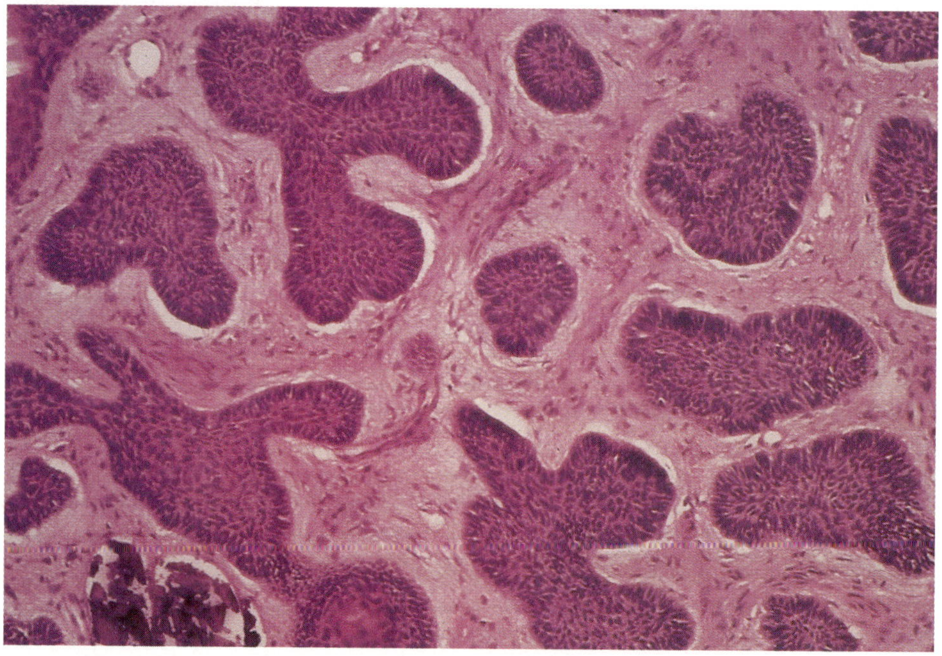

FIGURE 1-120
This vulvar biopsy specimen shows multiple nests of basal cell carcinoma. The nests are composed of a relatively uniform population of small cells that have large, elongated, hyperchromatic nuclei. There is palisading of the nuclei at the periphery of the nests. There is artificial separation ("cracking") of the stroma from the tumor nests. This is a frequent finding in this lesion.

pharyngeal region. A handful of cases of vulvar verrucous carcinomas have been reported.[125, 126] This carcinoma tends to occur in postmenopausal women, and almost all patients are older than 40 years of age at the time of diagnosis. In half of the cases there is a past history of vulvar condyloma acuminatum. Another squamous cancer, usually of the cervix or vagina, is simultaneously or subsequently discovered in 25 percent of cases. As in other squamous cancers of the vulva, patients complain of pruritus, pain, bleeding, or discharge. Large, fungating cauliflower-like masses that resemble condyloma acuminatum may be found, usually on the labia majora (Fig. 1–121). The appearance of this tumor may lead to a mistaken diagnosis of a condyloma acuminatum that is recalcitrant to treatment. Even the microscopic diagnosis may be missed unless a sufficiently deep and well-oriented biopsy is obtained. The tumor is composed of papillary fronds of mature squamous epithelium that infiltrate the underlying stroma with a pushing border (Fig. 1–122). There is lack of individual cell anaplasia. Keratin pearl formation may be seen but not at the tip of the rete pegs. There is marked hyperkeratosis and acanthosis. A chronic inflammatory cell infiltrate is seen in the dermal papillae. Verrucous carcinoma can be differentiated from condyloma acuminatum by the presence of bulbous, voluminous rete pegs and keratin pearls in verrucous carcinoma and the presence of slender fibrovascular stalks in condyloma. Verrucous carcinoma must also be distinguished from warty squamous cell carcinoma. Warty squamous cell carcinoma has individual cell anaplasia and keratin pearls within the underlying stroma, features that are absent in verrucous carcinoma.

Lymph node metastasis does not occur in patients with verrucous carcinoma despite deep local invasion. Wide local excision is generally adequate therapy. The depth of the incision should reach the inferior fascia of the urogenital diaphragm. Recurrences are common despite aggressive surgical therapy. However, in one series the corrected 5-year survival was 94 percent.[127]

Bartholin Gland Carcinoma

Bartholin gland carcinoma is another rare tumor of the vulva. It is associated with a high frequency of lymph node metastasis because this deep gland has a rich lymphatic supply.[128, 129] The mean and median age of patients with cancer of Bartholin gland is 50 years. By far the most common presenting complaint in patients with this tumor is the presence of a mass; however, pain and drainage may also occur (Fig. 1–123). It is generally accepted that three criteria must be met to make the diagnosis of Bartholin gland cancer: (1) a histologically documented transition from a normal gland to a malignant gland, (2) clinical location of the tumor in the anatomic position of Bartholin gland, and (3) absence of another primary tumor. The histopathologic types of Bartholin gland carcinoma include squamous cell carcinoma (40 percent), adenocarcinoma (40 percent), and adenoid cystic carcinoma (15 percent) (Fig. 1–124).[130, 131] Standard treatment is radical vul-

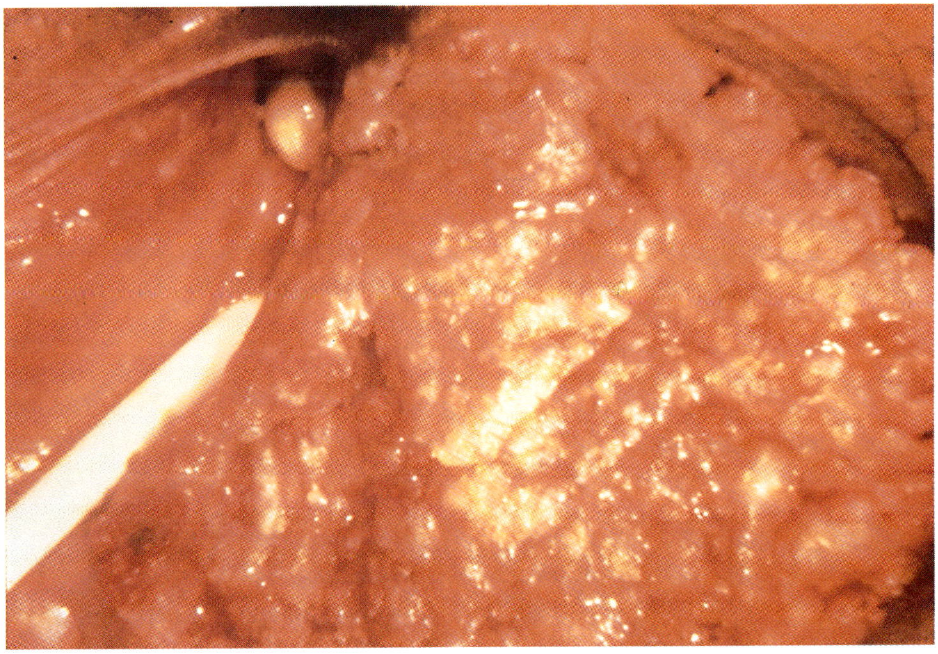

FIGURE 1–121
This is a large fungating verrucous carcinoma on the left vulva.

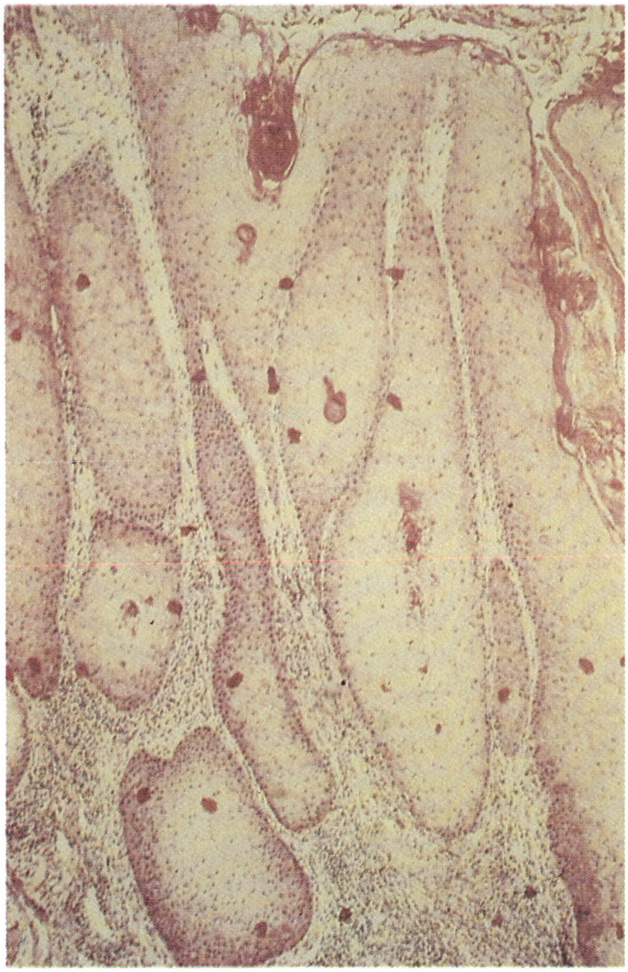

FIGURE 1-122
This biopsy specimen was taken from a patient who had verrucous carcinoma of the vulva. Bulbous tongues of tumor extend deep into the stroma. The tips of the tongues are rounded. Within the tumor tongues there is normal maturation of the epithelium that progresses from the periphery toward the center. There is no cellular anaplasia. There is an inflammatory infiltrate in the stroma. Marked hyperkeratosis is seen *(top)*. The surface has a convoluted appearance. (Courtesy of Dr. Tung Van Dinh, University of Texas Medical Branch at Galveston, TX.)

vectomy and bilateral inguinal lymph node dissection. Lymph node metastasis is found in half of the cases and is sometimes bilateral.

Recently, radical wide excision with ipsilateral inguinal lymphadenectomy and adjunctive irradiation has been advocated as treatment for this carcinoma. The cumulative 5-year survival was 84 percent in one series of 36 cases treated this way in one institution.[132] In general, an enlarged Bartholin gland in women over the age of 50 years who do not have a history of Bartholin adenitis should be removed to rule out the possibility of cancer. Alternatively, multiple needle biopsies can be obtained, and it may be possible to make the diagnosis this way.

Other Adenocarcinomas

Besides adenocarcinoma of Bartholin gland and Paget disease, primary adenocarcinoma of the vulva may originate in the skin appendages, minor vestibular glands, periurethral glands, and ectopic breast tissue.[132a]

Melanoma

Melanoma is the second most common histopathologic type of cancer found in the vulva, comprising approximately 5 percent of vulvar malignancies. Melanoma occurs predominantly in white women. The peak frequency occurs in the sixth and seventh decades of life. At the time of diagnosis the patient may complain of a lump or a new or changing pigmented lesion that may be associated with bleeding, itching, burning, or pruritus. The lesions are typically raised, irregular, and multi-

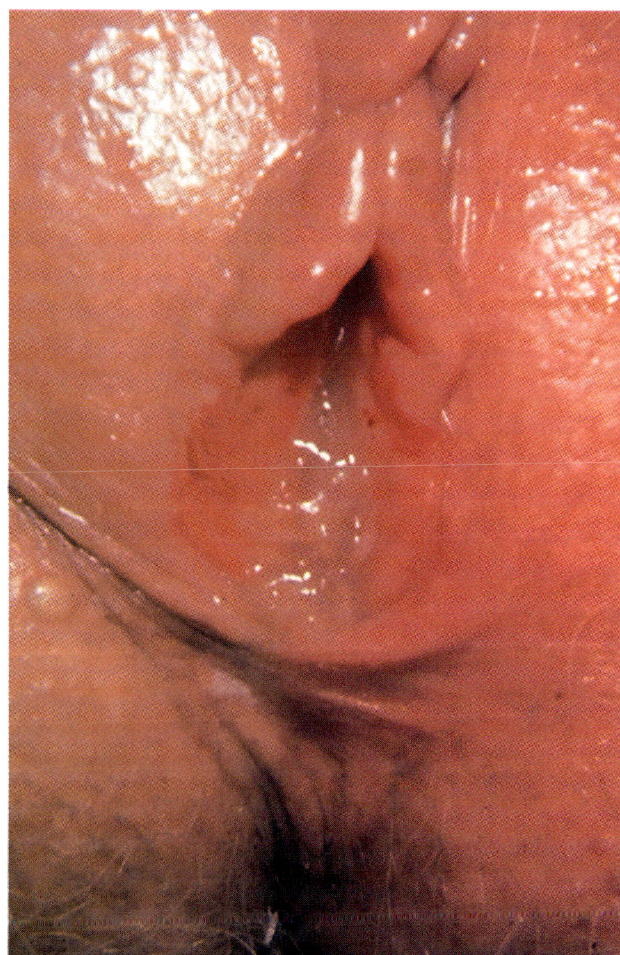

FIGURE 1-123
There is mucus secretion at the introitus as well as erythema and edema. A firm mass was palpated deep and lateral to the perineum in this case of Bartholin gland carcinoma.

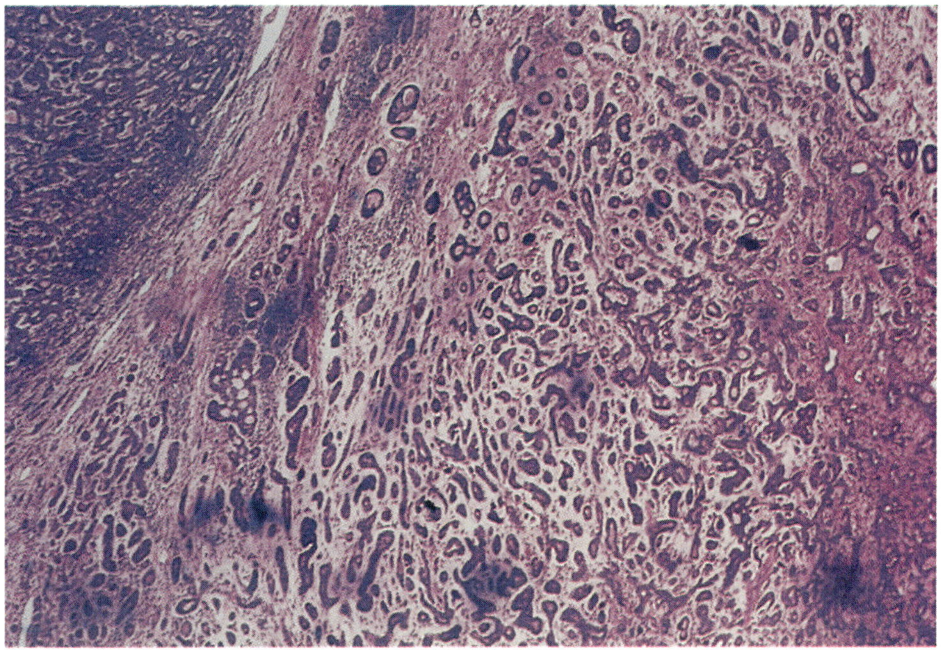

FIGURE 1-124
This is a low-power view of an adenoid cystic carcinoma of the Bartholin gland. Dense pink material is surrounded by small cells with dark nuclei.

colored (Fig. 1–125). They are found with almost equal frequency on the labia majora and on mucosal surfaces such as the labia minora, clitoris, and urethra. The clinical and pathologic characteristics of vulvar melanoma parallel those of melanomas elsewhere in the body. Three growth patterns occur in the vulva: nodular (Fig. 1–126), superficial spreading, and mucocutaneous.[133] The growth pattern and the histopathologic type (e.g., epithelioid, spindle, nevoid, mixed) do not appear to influence the prognosis. Immunocytochemical techniques may be necessary to distinguish "pagetoid" vulvar melanoma from Paget disease (see earlier discussion of Paget disease). Prognosis is largely influenced by tumor thickness as measured from the surface of the epithelium (Breslow microstaging) or by specific histologic levels (Clark microstaging), and the presence or absence of lymph node metastasis.[134–137] A modification of the Clark levels was proposed by Chung et al[133] in 1975 (Table 1–5). This microstaging classification is more applicable to the microanatomy of the vulvar skin than to skin elsewhere in the body. The surface of the vulvar skin and the epithelial-stroma

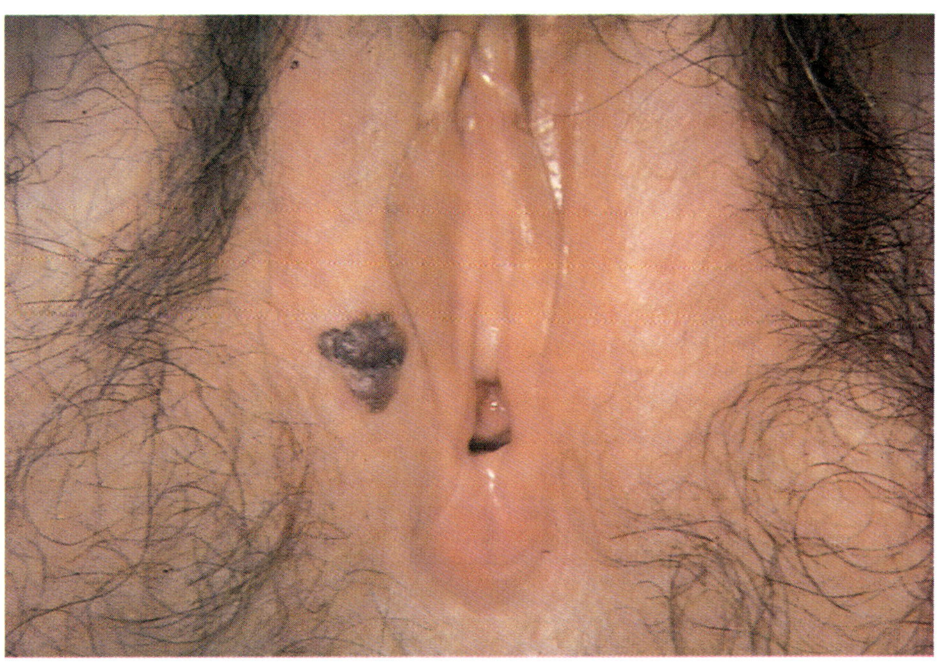

FIGURE 1-125
A raised, irregular nodule that varies from purplish to reddish pink is seen. Excisional biopsy showed it to be an invasive melanoma.

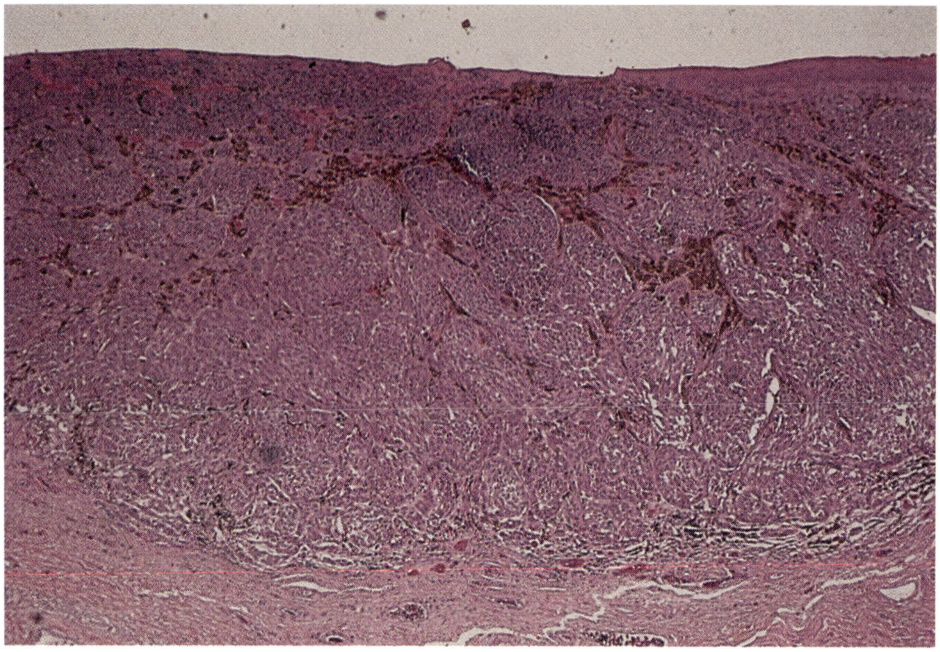

FIGURE 1-126
This is a nodular melanoma. The surface epithelium is intact on the right, but it is ulcerated over the lesion on the left. Although most of the tumor cells are not pigmented, pigment is present in the connective tissue between tumor nests. The lesion has a pushing border. At this power the fusiform shape of the cells is barely visible.

junction are more irregular than they are in other areas of the body. The amount of fat is variable.

By tradition most patients with vulvar melanoma have been treated by radical vulvectomy and regional lymphadenectomy. However, experience with cutaneous melanoma elsewhere in the body has led to a reconsideration of this traditional approach, resulting in more conservative surgery for this disease.[138] Radical local excision is recommended for the primary lesion. The role of regional lymphadenectomy is not well defined.[139–141] Regional lymphadenectomy may be reasonable in patients who have Chung level III to V lesions. Half of patients with level III to V vulvar melanomas have inguinal lymph node metastasis, and removal of the involved nodes has resulted in some unusual cases of long-term survival.[142] There is not yet an effective chemotherapy for malignant melanoma.

TABLE 1-5.

Microstaging of Vulvar Melanoma According to Breslow and Chung et al and Its Relationship to Survival[142]

	Definition	10-Year Survival (%)
Chung Level		
I	Intraepithelial	100
II	Invasion* 1 mm or less	81
III	Invasion 1 to 2 mm	87
IV	Invasion greater than 2 mm	11
IV	Invasion to subcutaneous fat	33
Breslow Level (Tumor Thickness)		
<0.75 mm		48
0.75 to 1.5 mm		68
1.51 to 3.0 mm		44
>3.0 mm		22

* Measured from the stratum granulosum of the surface epithelium

Sarcomas

Leiomyosarcoma

Sarcomas of the vulva are rare, but leiomyosarcoma is the most common of these tumors. It arises most often in the labium majus or the Bartholin's gland area.[143] It is usually greater than 5 cm in diameter at the time of diagnosis. On microscopic examination spindle-shaped cells, occasionally with an epithelioid appearance, are seen. An infiltrating border, nuclear atypia, and pleomorphism are present. In a bland-appearing tumor, a mitotic count of 10 or more per 10 high power microscopic fields is necessary to make a diagnosis of leiomyosarcoma; otherwise the tumor is a leiomyoma. Abnormal mitoses may be seen. Immunocytochemical studies show a positive reaction using antibodies to desmin. Leiomyosarcoma should not be confused with nodular fasciitis (pseudosarcomatous fasciitis), a benign condition of which a handful of cases have occurred in the vulva.[144] Standard treatment of vulvar leiomyosarcoma is radical local excision.[145–146] Distant metastases are common, but there is no effective chemotherapy for this. The prognosis is poor.

Rhabdomyosarcoma

Rhabdomyosarcoma is the most common soft tissue tumor of childhood. In 20 percent of cases the pelvis or genitourinary system is involved. When the genital tract is involved, the lesion is found more frequently in the vagina than in the cervix. It is extremely rare in the vulva. This tumor is discussed in more detail in Chapter 4.

Alveolar Soft Part Sarcoma

Alveolar soft part sarcoma in general occurs in the soft tissue of the extremities in young adults. It can arise in the vulva.[147] On microscopic examination one sees polygonal cells with granular cytoplasm that are arrayed on fibrovascular stalks. They can form alveolar-like structures. Mitoses are infrequent. Standard therapy is radical local excision.

Kaposi Sarcoma

Kaposi sarcoma is a malignant tumor of endothelial origin that is associated with the acquired immunodeficiency syndrome (AIDS). Clinically, it progresses from a patch to a plaque and then to a nodule. At the earliest stage, increased vascularity associated with a mononuclear cell infiltrate is seen in the dermis. As the lesion progresses, there is a further increase in vascularity associated with atypical spindle cells.[148]

Dermatofibrosarcoma Protuberans

Dermatofibrosarcoma protuberans is a rare tumor that has a marked propensity for local recurrence but not for systemic metastasis.[149] It can occur on any skin surface except the palms and soles. It is densely cellular, but there is little cytologic atypia, few mitoses, and no giant cells. It commonly grows intradermally. At the tumor base there is an infiltrative growth pattern. Radical local excision is standard treatment.

Malignant Fibrous Histiocytoma

Malignant fibrous histiocytoma arises from undifferentiated mesenchymal cells. This tumor is associated with deep soft tissue and skeletal muscle. It affects men more often than women.[150] Malignant fibrous histiocytoma of the vulva is extremely rare.[151] It presents as a solitary mass that grows relatively rapidly. On cut section the tumor is gray-white in color; it may have areas of hemorrhage and necrosis and there may be grossly visible whorled bundles. There are plump and spindle-shaped cells arranged in a cartwheel pattern. Large epithelioid cells and giant malignant cells can be seen. The nuclei are ovoid to round and pleomorphic. Nucleoli are easily identified. Other areas may be myxoid. In these areas the tumor cells have abundant cytoplasm and a more rounded nucleus. The cytoplasm stains slightly bluish and contains both small and large vacuoles. The standard therapy of malignant fibrous histiocytoma is radical local excision.[152] Radiation therapy has been reported to decrease the rate of local recurrence.[153]

Other Sarcomas

Other sarcomas that rarely occur in the vulva include angiosarcoma, neurofibrosarcoma, and reticulosarcoma.[147]

Other Rare Tumors of the Vulva

Lymphoma most often involves the genital tract as part of a systemic disease (Fig. 1–127), although primary genital lymphomas have been reported.[154–157] The cervix (see Chapter 4) is involved by primary or secondary lymphoma more frequently than the vulva or vagina. Seventy to 80 percent of primary genital lymphomas are diffuse large cell type (working formulation) or diffuse histiocytic type (Rappaport classification) of non-Hodgkin's lymphomas; the rest are nodular types or Burkitt lymphomas. Multidisciplinary therapy, including chemotherapy, radiation therapy, and surgery, has been used to treat primary genital lymphomas.[158, 159] When the vulvar lesion is associated with systemic disease chemotherapy is the treatment of choice.

A few cases of primary vulvar *endodermal sinus tumor* have been reported.[160] Its pathologic characteristics and clinical behavior are similar to those of tumor occurring in the ovary (see Chapter 10). Aggressive surgery followed by chemotherapy consisting of bleomycin, ctoposide, and cisplatin is recommended.

Neuroendocrine (small cell) carcinoma has also been reported in the vulva.[161] It is associated with a poor prognosis as when it occurs at other sites. There are two case reports of *peripheral primitive neuroectodermal tumor* of the vulva.[162]

Histicytosis X (eosinophilic granuloma) is a rare systemic disease that may affect the vulva.[162] In this disease there is diffuse proliferation of atypical histiocytes. These cells have cytoplasm like a typical macrophage but an enlarged and atypical nucleus. On electron microscopic examination

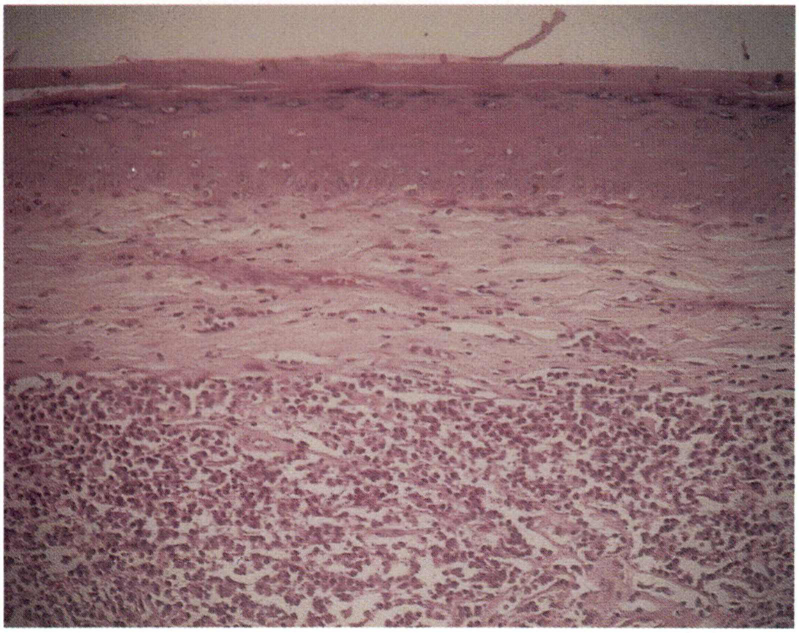

FIGURE 1-127
This is a biopsy specimen of a vulvar nodule found in a patient who had generalized lymphadenopathy. The surface epithelium is intact. There is dense infiltration of the underlying connective tissue by lymphoid cells that extended to the deep margin of the biopsy specimen. At higher magnification the lymphoid cells appeared to be highly atypical. Immunocytochemistry and flow cytometry confirmed that this is a malignant non-Hodgkin's lymphoma.

Langerhans granules seen in the cytoplasm of the cells are diagnostic. The etiology of histiocytosis X is unknown. Aggressive treatment that includes systemic chemotherapy has improved the 5-year survival of patients with disseminated disease from 30 percent to 90 percent.[164]

A *desmoid tumor* is a locally invasive fibrous tumor that occurs in muscle or fascia and frequently recurs after excision. One case of a desmoid tumor occurring in the vulva has been reported.[165] Wide excision followed by treatment with tamoxifen can be used in the treatment of these tumors.

The vulva is sometimes the site of metastatic disease. This usually originates from other genital tract cancers, most commonly those of the cervix and endometrium (Fig. 1–128). Involvement of the vulva by lymphoma and histiocytosis X has already been discussed. We have seen recurrent rectal adenocarcinoma present with multiple vulvar subcutaneous nodules. Some of these lesions were ulcerated and had associated edema. Metastases to the vulva from ovary, breast, kidney, stomach, and lung cancer as well as from invasive melanoma, choriocarcinoma, and neuroblastoma have also been reported.[166]

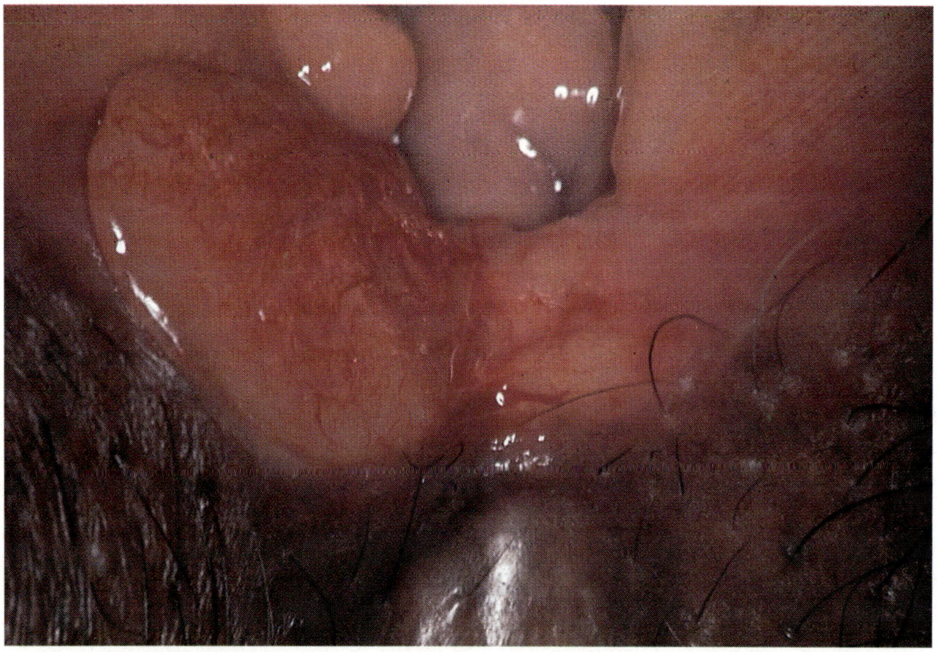

FIGURE 1-128
This raised nodule with a vascular pattern on its surface is located at the posterior fourchette. Biopsy proved that it was metastatic endometrial adenocarcinoma.

URETHRA

Prolapse of the urethra may occur in premenarchal girls and postmenopausal women. Most commonly, prolapse involves the posterior urethra. This prolapse is seen at the meatus as deep red irregular mucosa. Biopsy is not necessary but if performed it shows an inflammatory infiltrate in the underlying connective tissue, and the mucosa may demonstrate ulceration. In its embryologic development the posterior wall of the urethra is partially formed by mesoderm. This mesoderm is responsive to sex hormones. Lack of estrogen stimulation is responsible for the urethral mucosal eversion. Postmenopausal women also may develop caruncles, which are polypoid or sessile masses arising from the urethral meatus. These probably are areas of prolapsed, chronically inflamed urethral mucosa. They can be tender and may bleed. On microscopic examination the submucosa may be found to contain large venous channels. In the connective tissue there are chronic inflammatory cells, and occasionally a myxomatous or granulomatous stroma is seen. Condyloma acuminatum frequently involves the urethra, and this area should be carefully evaluated in the patient who is undergoing treatment of vulvar condylomata.

Urethral carcinoma is rare. It accounts for less than 1 percent of malignancies of the female genital tract. The great majority of these are squamous carcinomas that arise in the distal urethra. Transitional cell (urothelial) carcinoma and adenocarcinoma may be seen in the proximal and distal urethra.[167] Patients with tumors limited to the meatus (Fig. 1–129) and clinically negative lymph node may be treated with interstitial radiation and local excision.[168] Radical surgery or radiation therapy may be necessary for patients with more advanced disease.[169]

SURGICAL PATHOLOGY CONSIDERATIONS

The true nature of many vulvar lesions is difficult to determine without obtaining a biopsy. Before performing a vulvar biopsy a careful medical history and physical examination should be performed because the vulvar lesion may be a manifestation of systemic disease. The groins, mons pubis, perineum, and entire vulva should be carefully inspected so that multifocal disease is not missed. In addition, the vagina and cervix should be inspected because multicentric disease (e.g., condyloma acuminatum, squamous intraepithelial neoplasia, squamous carcinoma) may involve the vulva, vagina, and cervix. The proximity of the lesion to the urethra, vagina, and anus should be noted. The presence of symptomatic pelvic relaxation should be noted because it may influence the choice of subsequent surgery. A drawing of the vulva, including measurements of the lesion or lesions is critical in the pretreatment work-up. Photographs may also be useful.

Cytologic smears may be useful in diagnosis of infectious diseases such as herpes and molluscum contagiosum. Some tumors can also be diagnosed this way, but biopsy confirmation is necessary. It is often necessary to moisten the lesion by holding a saline-soaked gauze pad to it for a few minutes

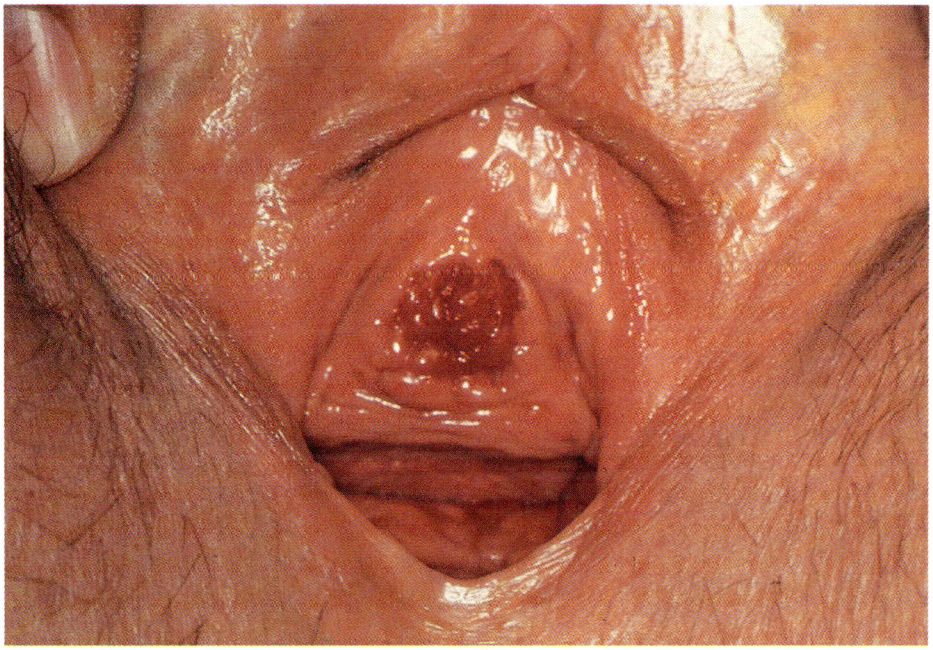

FIGURE 1–129
The urethral meatus is surrounded by a deep red polypoid lesion. Biopsy showed a urothelial carcinoma (transitional cell) that arose in the urethra.

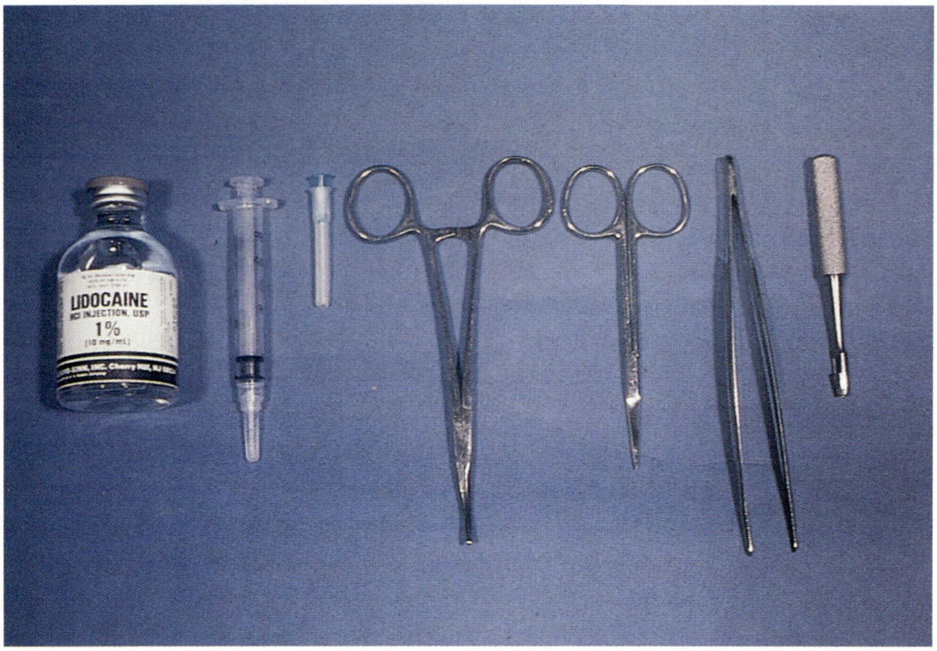

FIGURE 1–130
The equipment necessary for obtaining an adequate vulvar biopsy is shown. A Keyes punch biopsy instrument *(far right)* comes with different diameters to produce biopsy sizes of 2 mm, 3 mm, and 4 mm. We now use a disposable version of this instrument. We use a 25-gauge needle or smaller to infiltrate local anesthesia. A No. 15 or No. 10 blade scalpel (not shown) is used for excisional biopsy. Hemostasis is achieved by the use of silver nitrate sticks when a small punch biopsy is done. Excisional biopsies require suturing. We prefer 3-0 polyglactin suture (e.g., Vicryl) mounted on a small cutting needle.

before scraping. The optimal site to sample is the edge of the lesion or ulcer.

Biopsies should be full thickness. Lesions less than 1 cm in diameter may be removed in toto by excision biopsy using a scalpel. Larger lesions should be sampled by using a punch biopsy device (e.g., a Keyes punch) from the periphery of the lesion (Fig. 1–130). This punch biopsy should include the lesion as well as normal skin. Biopsy of lesions that have an ulcerated necrotic center may not be diagnostic if the biopsy is taken from the center of the lesion. In most situations the biopsy sample can be obtained in the office using local anesthesia.

At the time of definitive surgery it is essential to include drawings on the pathology consultation request form and in the patient's permanent medical record that show the lesion and the specimen resected. Photographs are also helpful. In some cases it is necessary to define the limits of resection intraoperatively. Biopsies performed at the beginning of the operation and sent immediately for frozen section analysis will facilitate this step. The sites of these biopsies should be recorded on

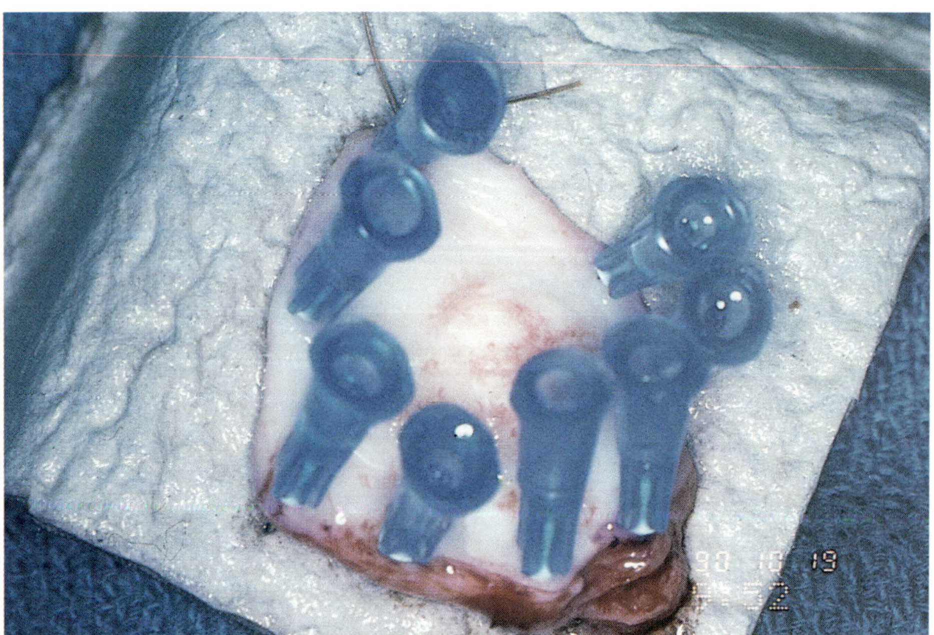

FIGURE 1–131
This was a wide local excision of VIN 3. The specimen has been pinned to corrugated cardboard. A suture has been used to indicate orientation. The next step will be to ink the margins. Subsequently, the prepared specimen is placed in formalin.

the drawings. The resection specimen should also be labeled or tagged to permit accurate orientation by the pathologist (Fig. 1–131). It is critical for the pathologist to be able to identify proximal, distal, medial, and lateral borders of the resection specimen. Such labeling may also include the proximity of the lesion to the urethra, vagina, and anus as appropriate. The specimen is stretched and pinned on corrugated cardboard or a wax block before fixation. This prevents curling and subsequent difficulties in orientation. The margins of the resection are inked with india ink for easy identification of the margins on the tissue sections. The tissue to be embedded in paraffin should be cut perpendicular to the skin surface and should include the full thickness of the epidermis, dermis, and subcutaneous fat. The tissue is laid flat on the cassette with the epidermis extending toward one side and the dermis or subcutaneous fat toward the other. This procedure results in full-thickness tissue sections and facilitates the diagnosis. The processing of lymph nodes is discussed in detail in Chapter 4.

REFERENCES

1. Kistner RW: Gynecology: Principles and Practice. Chicago, Year Book, 1979, pp 17–21.
2. Cohen SD, Wright F, Hernandez E, Dunton CJ: Management of the Bartholin abscess. Am J Gynecol Health 1990;4:99–102.
3. Homesley HD, Bundy BN, Sedlis A, Yordan E, Berek JS, Jahshan A, Mortel R: Prognostic factors for groin node metastasis in squamous cell carcinoma of the vulva (a Gynecologic Oncology Group study). Gynecol Oncol 1993;49:279–283.
4. Parry-Jones E: Lymphatics of the vulva. J Obstet Gynaecol Br Commonwlth 1963;70:751–765.
5. Eriksson E, Eldh J, Peterson L-E: Surgical treatment of carcinoma of the clitoris. Gynecol Oncol 1984;17:291–295.
6. Netter FH: The Ciba Collection of Medical Illustrations. Vol. 2: Reproductive System. Summit, NJ, Ciba Foundation, 1970, p 104.

6a. Anonymous: Ketoconazole shampoo for dandruff. Med Lett Drugs Ther 1994;36:68.

7. Zacur H, Genadry R, Woodruff JD: The patient at risk for development of vulvar cancer. Gynecol Oncol 1980;9:199–208.
8. Woodruff JD: Diagnosis and management of benign lesions of the vulva. Curr Prob Obstet Gynecol 1978; 1(11):43–50.
9. Kelly RA, Foster DC, Woodruff JD: Subcutaneous injection of triamcinolone acetonide in the treatment of chronic vulvar pruritus. Am J Obstet Gynecol 1993;169:568–570.
10. Wheeless CR Jr: Atlas of Pelvic Surgery, 2nd ed. Philadelphia, Lea & Febiger, 1988, pp 18–19.
11. Wheeless CR Jr: Atlas of Pelvic Surgery, 2nd ed. Philadelphia, Lea & Febiger, 1988, pp 22–23.
12. Woodruff JD: Diagnosis and management of benign lesions of the vulva. Curr Probl Obstet Gynecol 1978;1(11):7–8.
13. Soper DE, Patterson JW, Hurt WG, Fantl JA, Blaylock K: Lichen planus of the vulva. Obstet Gynecol 1988;72:74–76.

13a. Scurry J, Dennerstein G, Brenan J, Ostor A, Mason G, Dorevitch A: Vulvitis circumscripta plasmacellularis: A clinicopathologic entity? J Reprod Med 1993;38:14–18.

13b. Friedrich EG: Vulvar vestibulitis syndrome. J Reprod Med 1987;32:110–114.

13c. Mann MS, Kaufman RH, Brown D Jr, Adam E: Vulvar vestibulitis: Significant clinical variables and treatment outcomes. Obstet Gynecol 1992;79:122–125.

14. Donaldson LB: Crohn's disease: Its gynecologic aspect. Am J Obstet Gynecol 1978;131:196–202.
15. Kremer M, Nussenson E, Steinfeld M, Zuckerman P: Crohn's disease of the vulva. Am J Gastroenterol 1984;79:376–378.
16. Levine EM, Barton JJ, Grier EA: Metastatic Crohn's disease of the vulva. Obstet Gynecol 1982;60:395–397.
17. O'Duffy JD: Behçet's syndrome (editorial). N Engl J Med 1990;322:326–327.
18. Wong RC, Ellis CN, Diaz LA: Behcet's disease: A review. Int J Dermatol 1984;23:25–32.
19. American College of Obstetricians and Gynecologists: Perinatal herpes simplex virus infections. ACOG Tech Bull, No. 122, 1988.
20. Mertz GJ, Critchlow CW, Benedetti J, Reichman RC, Dolin R, Connor J, Redfield DC, Savoia MC, Richman DD, Tyrell DL, Miedzinski L, Portney J, Keeney RE, Corey L: Double-blind placebo-controlled trial of oral acyclovir in first-episode genital herpes simplex infection. JAMA 1984;252:1147–1151.
21. Whitley RJ, Gnann JW Jr: Acyclovir: A decade later. N Engl J Med 1992;327:782–789.
22. Stephenson H, Dotters DJ, Katz V, Droegemueller W: Necrotizing fasciitis of the vulva. Am J Obstet Gynecol 1992;166:1324–1327.
23. Mortimer PS, Dawber RPR, Gales MA, Moore RA, Fenoglio CM: Mediation of hidradenitis suppurativa by androgens. Br Med J 1986; 292:245–248.
24. Thomas R, Barnhill D, Bibro M, Hoskins W: Hidradenitis suppurativa: A case presentation and review of the literature. Obstet Gynecol 1985;66:592–595.
25. Sherman AI, Reid R: CO_2 laser for suppurative hidradenitis of the vulva. J Reprod Med 1991;36:113–117.
26. Bogers J-W, Minderhoud-Bassie W, Huikeshoven FJM: A case of hidradenitis suppurativa treated with gonadotropin-releasing hormone agonist and by total abdominal hysterectomy with bilateral salpingo-oophorectomy. Am J Obstet Gynecol 1992;167:517–518.
27. Word B: New instrument for office treatment of cysts and abscesses of Bartholin's gland. JAMA 1964;190:777–778.
28. Heah J: Methods of treatment for cysts and abscesses of Bartholin's gland. Br J Obstet Gynaecol 1988;95:321–322.
29. Sweet RL, Gibbs RS: Infectious Diseases of the Female Genital Tract. Baltimore, Williams & Wilkins, 1985, pp 31–34.
30. Marmar JL: The management of resistant chancroid in Vietnam. J Urol 1972;107:807–808.
31. Woodruff JD: The vulva. *In* Rosenwaks Z, Benjamin F, Stone ML (eds): Gynecology: Principles and Practice. New York, Macmillan, 1987, p 401.
32. Sweet RL, Gibbs RS: Infectious Diseases of the Female Genital Tract. Baltimore, Williams & Wilkins, 1985, pp 26–32.
33. Anonymous: Drugs for parasitic infections. Med Lett Drugs Ther, 1993;35:111–122.
34. Sweet RL, Gibbs RS: Infectious Diseases of the Female Genital Tract. Baltimore, Williams & Wilkins, 1985, pp 37–38.
35. Schwimmer E: Die idiopathischen Schleim haut Plaques der Mundhohle. Vrljschr Dermatol Syph 1877;9:510.
36. Bonney V: Leukoplakia vulvitia and the conditions liable to be confused with it. Proc R Soc Med 1938;31:1057.
37. Taussig FJ: Leukoplakia and cancer of the vulva. Arch Dermatol Syph 1930;21:413.
38. Jeffcoate TNA: Chronic vulvar dystrophies. Am J Obstet Gynecol 1966;95:61–74.

39. International Society for the Study of Vulvar Disease: New nomenclature for vulvar disease. Obstet Gynecol 1976;47:122–124.
40. Crum CP, Fu YS, Levine RU, et al: Intraepithelial squamous lesions of the vulva: Biologic and histologic criteria for the distinction of condylomas from vulvar intraepithelial neoplasia. Am J Obstet Gynecol 1982;144:77–83.
41. Patterson JW, Kao GF, Graham JH, Helwig EB: Bowenoid papulosis: A clinicopathologic study with ultrastructural observations. Cancer 1986;57:823–836.
42. Ulbright TM, Stehman FB, Roth LM, Ehrlich CE, Ransburg RC: Bowenoid dysplasia of the vulva. Cancer 1982;50:2910–2919.
43. Bernstein SG, Kovacs BR, Townsend DE, Morrow CP: Vulvar carcinoma in situ. Obstet Gynecol 1983;61:304–307.
44. Crum CP, Liskow A, Petras P, Keng WC, Frick HC: Vulvar intraepithelial neoplasia (severe atypia and carcinoma in situ). Cancer 1984;54:1429–1434.
45. Powell LC, Dinh TV, Rajaraman S, Hannigan EV, Dilland EA, Yandell RB, To T: Carcinoma in situ of the vulva: A clinicopathologic study of 50 cases. J Reprod Med 1986;31:808–814.
46. Kaufman RH, Bornstein J, Adam E, Burek J, Tessin B, Adler-Storthz K: Human papillomavirus and herpes simplex virus in vulvar squamous cell carcinoma in situ. Am J Obstet Gynecol 1988;158:862–871.
47. Carter J, Carlson J, Fowler J, Hartenbach E, Adcock L, Carson L, Twiggs L: Invasive vulvar tumors in young women: A disease of the immunosuppressed? Gynecol Oncol 1993;51:307–310.
48. Giorda G, Vaccher E, Volpe R, DePiero G, Tirelli U, Scarabelli C: An unusual presentation of vulvar carcinoma in a HIV patient: Case report. Gynecol Oncol 1992;44:191–194.
49. Toki T, Kurman RJ, Park JS, Kessis T, Daniel RW, Shah KV: Probable nonpapillomavirus etiology of squamous cell carcinoma of the vulva in older women: A clinicopathologic study using in situ hybridization and polymerase chain reaction. Int J Gynecol Pathol 1991;10:107–125.
50. Andersen WA, Franquemont W, Williams J, Taylor PT, Crum CP: Vulvar squamous cell carcinoma and papillomaviruses: Two separate entities? Am J Obstet Gynecol 1991;165:329–336.
51. Woodruff JD, Davis HJ, Jones HW, Recio RG, Salimi R, Park I-J: Correlated investigative techniques of multiple anaplasia in the lower genital canal. Obstet Gynecol 1969;33:609–616.
52. Bornstein J, Kaufman RH, Adam E, Adler-Storthz K: Multicentric intraepithelial neoplasia involving the vulva: Clinical features and association with human papillomavirus and herpes simplex virus. Cancer 1988;62:1601–1604.
53. Chaffe W, Richards A, Morgan L, Wilkinson E: Unrecognized invasive carcinoma in vulvar intraepithelial neoplasia (VIN). Gynecol Oncol 1988;31:154–162.
54. Wright CV, Davies E: Laser surgery for vulvar intraepithelial neoplasia: Principles and results. Am J Obstet Gynecol 1987;156:374–378.
55. Friedrich EG, MacLaren NK: Genetic aspects of vulvar lichen sclerosus. Am J Obstet Gynecol 1984;150:161–166.
56. Wallace HL: Lichen sclerosus et atrophicus. Trans St Johns Hosp Dermatol Soc 1971;57:9–30.
57. Kaufman RH, Gardner HL, Johnson PC: P-32 uptake in lichen sclerosus et atrophicus of the vulva. Am J Obstet Gynecol 1967;98:312–319.
58. Taussig F: Diseases of the Vulva. New York, Appleton Century Croft, 1921.
59. Hart WR, Norris HJ, Helwig EB: Relation of lichen sclerosus et atrophicus of the vulva to development of carcinoma. Obstet Gynecol 1975;45:369–377.
60. Rueda NG, Garcia A, Vighi S, Belardi MG, Cardinal L, di Paola G: Epithelial alterations adjacent to invasive squamous carcinoma of the vulva. J Reprod Med 1994;39:526–530.
61. Bracco GL, Carli P, Sonni L, Maestrini G, De Marco A, Taddei GL, Cattaneo A: Clinical and histologic effects of topical treatments of vulval lichen sclerosus: A critical evaluation. J Reprod Med 1993;38:37–40.
62. Carli P, Bracco, G, Taddei G, Sonni L, De Marco A, Maestrini G, Cattaneo A: Vulvar lichen sclerosus: Immunohistologic evaluation before and after therapy. J Reprod Med 1994;39:110–114.
63. Shah K, Kashima H, Polk BF, Shah F, Abbey H, Abramson A: Rarity of cesarean delivery in cases of juvenile onset respiratory papillomatosis. Obstet Gynecol 1986;68: 795–799.
64. Majimudar B, Hallden C: The relationship between juvenile laryngeal papillomatosis and maternal condylomata acuminata. J Reprod Med 1986;31:804–807.
65. Crum CP, Nuovo GJ: Genital Papillomaviruses and Related Neoplasms. New York, Raven Press, 1991.
65a. Bergeron C, Ferenczy A, Richart RM, Guralnick M: Micropapillomatosis labialis appears unrelated to human papillomavirus. Obstet Gynecol 1990;76:281–286.
66. Axe S, Parmley T, Woodruff JD: Adenomas in minor vestibular glands. Obstet Gynecol 1986;68:16–18.
67. Birch HC, Sondag DR: Granular cell myoblastoma of the vulva. Obstet Gynecol 1961;18:443–453.
68. King DF, Bustillo M, Broen EN, Hirose FM: Granular cell tumors of the vulva: A report of 3 cases. J Dermatol Surg Oncol 1979;5:794–798.
69. Leib SM, Gallousis S, Freedman H: Granular cell myoblastoma of the vulva. Gynecol Oncol 1979;8:12–20.
70. Majmudar B, Castellano PZ, Wilson KRW, Siegel RJ: Granular cell tumors of the vulva. J Reprod Med 1990;35:1008–1014.
70a. Khansur T, Balducci L, Tavassoli M: Granular cell tumor: Clinical spectrum of the benign and malignant entity. Cancer 1987;60:220–222.
71. Kaufmann T, Pawl NO, Soifer I, Grestar WM, Kleinen GJ: Cystic papillary hidradenoma of the vulva: Case report and review of the literature. Gynecol Oncol 1987;26:240–245.
72. Messing MJ, Richardson MS, Smith MT, King L, Gallup DG: Metastatic clear-cell hidradenocarcinoma of the vulva. Gynecol Oncol 1993;48:264–268.
73. Bannatyne P, Elliott P, Russell P: Vulvar adenosquamous carcinoma arising in a hidradenoma papilliferum, with rapidly fatal outcome: Case report. Gynecol Oncol 1989;35:395–398.
74. Isaacson D, Turner ML: Localized vulvar syringomas. J Am Acad Dermatol 1979;1:352–357.
75. Young AW, Herman EW, Tovel HMM: Syringoma of the vulva: Incidence, diagnosis, and cause of pruritus. Obstet Gynecol 1980;55:515–518.
76. Cho D, Buscema J, Rosenshein NB, Woodruff JD: Primary breast cancer of the vulva. Obstet Gynecol 1985;66:79S–81S.
77. Rose PG, Roman LD, Rale FR, Tak WK, Hunter REI: Primary adenocarcinoma of the breast arising in the vulva. Obstet Gynecol 1990;76:537–539.
78. Bailey CL, Sankey HZ, Donovan JT: Primary breast cancer of the vulva: Case report. Gynecol Oncol 1993;50:379–383.
79. Messina AM, Strauss RG: Pelvic neurofibromatosis. Obstet Gynecol 1976;47:63S–66S.
80. Schreiber MM: Vulvar von Recklinghausen's disease. Arch Dermatol 1963;88:320–321.
81. Friedrich EG, Burch K, Bahr JP: The vulvar clinic: An eight-year appraisal. Am J Obstet Gynecol 1979;135: 1030–1040.
82. Jones IS: An assessment of vulval pigmentation. N Z Med J 1979;89:348–350.
83. Weiner K: Vaginal melanosis caused by bismuth therapy and carcinoma of the cervix. Arch Dermatol 1940;42:23–29.

84. Lutterloh CH, Shellenberger PL: Unusual pigmentation developing after prolonged suppressive therapy with quinacrine hydrochloride. Arch Dermatol Syph 1946;53:349–354.
85. Estrada R, Kaufman R: Benign vulvar melanosis. J Reprod Med 1993;38:5–8.
86. Nadji M, Morales A, Girtanner RE, Ziegels-Weissman J, Penneys NS: Paget's disease of the skin: A unifying concept of histogenesis. Cancer 1982;50:2203–2206.
87. Bacchi CE, Goldfogel GA, Greer BE, Gown AM: Paget's disease and melanoma of the vulva: Use of a panel of monoclonal antibodies to identify cell type and to microscopically define adequacy of surgical margins. Gynecol Oncol 1992;46:216–221.
88. Parmley TH, Woodruff JD, Julian CG: Invasive vulvar Paget's disease. Obstet Gynecol 1975;46:341–346.
89. Misas JE, Larson JE, Podczaski E, Manetta A, Mortel R: Recurrent Paget disease of the vulva in a split-thickness graft. Obstet Gynecol 1990;76:543–544.
90. Feurer GA, Shevchuk M, Calanog A: Vulvar Paget's disease: The need to exclude an invasive lesion. Gynecol Oncol 1990;38:81–89.
91. Curtin JP, Rubin SC, Jones WB, Hoskins WJ, Lewis JL: Paget's disease of the vulva. Gynecol Oncol 1990;39:374–377.
92. Stacy D, Burrell MO, Franklin WE III: Extramammary Paget's disease of the vulva and anus: Use of intraoperative frozen-section margins. Am J Obstet Gynecol 1986;155:519–523.
93. Bergen S, DiSaia PJ, Liao SY, Berman ML: Conservative management of extramammary Paget's disease of the vulva. Gynecol Oncol 1989;33:151–156.
94. International Federation of Gynecology and Obstetrics (FIGO): Changes in gynecologic cancer staging by the International Federation of Gynecology and Obstetrics. Am J Obstet Gynecol 1990;162:610–611.
95. Homesley HD, Bundy BN, Sedlis A, Yordan E, Berek JS, Jahshan A, Mortel R: Assessment of current International Federation of Gynecology and Obstetrics staging of vulvar carcinoma relative to prognostic factors for survival (a Gynecology Oncology Group study). Am J Obstet Gynecol 1991;164:997–1004.
96. Shanbour KA, Mannel RS, Morris PC, Yadach A, Walker JL: Comparison of clinical versus surgical staging systems in vulvar cancer. Obstet Gynecol 1992;80:927–930.
97. Podratz KC, Symmonds RE, Taylor WF, Williams TJ: Carcinoma of the vulva: Analysis of treatment and survival. Obstet Gynecol 1983;61:63–74.
98. Brinton LA, Nasca PC, Mallin K, Baptiste MS, Wilbanks Gd, Richart RM: Case control study of cancer of the vulva. Obstet Gynecol 1990;75:859–866.
99. Parazzini F, La Vecchia C, Garsia S, Nagri E, Sideri M, Rogroni MT, Origoni M: Determinants of invasive vulvar cancer risk: An Italian case-control study. Gynecol Oncol 1993;48:50–55.
100. Trimble CL, Shah KV, Hildesheim A, Brinton LA, Kurman RJ: Two distinct types of squamous vulvar carcinoma. Obstet Gynecol (in press).
101. Buscema J, Stern JL, Woodruff JD: Early invasive carcinoma of the vulva. Am J Obstet Gynecol 1981;140:563–569.
102. Boice CR, Sera IM, Thrasher T, King A: Microinvasive squamous carcinoma of the vulva: Present status and reassessment. Gynecol Oncol 1984;18:71–76.
103. Kürzl R, Messerer D, Baltzer J, Lohe K, Zander J: Comparative morphometric study on the depth of invasion in vulvar carcinoma. Gynecol Oncol 1988;29:12–25.
104. Kneale BL, Cavanagh D, DiPaola GR, Frankman O, Girtanner RE, Gomez-Rueda N, Iversen T, Krupp PJ, Morley GW, Pichel H: Microinvasive cancer of the vulva: Report of the ISSVD task force. J Reprod Med 1984;29:454–456.
105. Sedlis A, Homesley H, Bundy BN, Marshall R, Yordan E, Hacker N, Lee JH, Whitney C: Positive groin lymph nodes in superficial squamous cell vulvar cancer: A Gynecologic Oncology Group study. Am J Obstet Gynecol 1987;156:1159–1164.
106. Ross MJ, Ehrmann RL: Histologic prognosticators in stage I squamous cell carcinoma of the vulva. Obstet Gynecol 1987;70:774–784.
107. Heaps JM, Fu YS, Montz FJ, Hacker NF, Berek JS: Surgical-pathologic variables predictive of local recurrence in squamous cell carcinoma of the vulva. Gynecol Oncol 1990;38:309–314.
108. Hoffman JS, Kumar NB, Morley GW: Microinvasive squamous carcinoma of the vulva: Search for a definition. Obstet Gynecol 1983;61:615–618.
109. Donaldson ES, Powell DE, Hanson MB, van Nagell J: Prognostic parameters in invasive vulvar cancer. Gynecol Oncol 1981;11:184–190.
110. Husseinzadeh N, Zaino R, Hahhas WA, Mortel R: The significance of histologic findings in predicting nodal metastases in invasive squamous cell carcinoma of the vulva. Gynecol Oncol 1983;16:105–111.
111. Boyce J, Fruchter RG, Kasambilides E, Nicastri AD, Sedlis A, Ramy JC: Prognostic factors in carcinoma of the vulva. Gynecol Oncol 1985;20:364–377.
112. Hacker NF, Berek JS, Lagasse LD, Leuchter RS, Moore JG: Management of regional lymph nodes and their prognostic influence in vulvar cancer. Obstet Gynecol 1983;61:408–412.
113. Hacker NF, Berek JS, Lagasse LD, Nieberg RA, Leuchter RS: Individualization of treatment for state I squamous cell vulvar carcinoma. Obstet Gynecol 1984;63:155–162.
114. Curry SL, Wharton JT, Rutledge F: Positive lymph nodes in vulvar squamous carcinoma. Gynecol Oncol 1980;9:63–67.
115. Thomas GM, Dembo AJ, Bryson SCP, Osborne R, DePetrillo AD: Changing concepts in the management of vulvar cancer. Gynecol Oncol 1991;42:9–21.
116. Farias-Eisner R, Cirisano FD, Grouse D, Leuchter RS, Karlan BY, Lagasse LD, Berek JS: Conservative and individualized surgery for early squamous carcinoma of the vulva: The treatment of choice for stage I and II (T_{1-2} N_{0-1} M_0) disease. Gynecol Oncol 1994;53:55–58.
117. Homesley HD, Bundy BN, Sedlis A, Adcock L: Radiation therapy versus node resection for carcinoma of the vulva with positive groin nodes. Obstet Gynecol 1986;68:733–740.
118. Berek JS, Heaps JM, Fu YS, Juillard GJF, Hacker NF: Concurrent cisplatin and 5-fluorouracil chemotherapy and radiation therapy for advanced-stage squamous carcinoma of the vulva. Gynecol Oncol 1991;42:197–201.
119. Perez CA, Grigsby PW, Galakatos A, Swanson R, Camel HM, Kao MS, Lockett MA: Radiation therapy in management of carcinoma of the vulva with emphasis on conservation therapy. Cancer 1993;71:3707–3716.
120. Morrow CP, Curtin JP, Townsend DE: Tumors of the vulva. *In* Morrow CP, Curtin JP, Townsend DE (eds): Synopsis of Gynecologic Oncology. New York, Churchill Livingstone, 1993, pp 65–92.
121. Merino MJ, LiVolsi VA, Schwartz PE, Rudnicki J: Adenoid basal cell carcinoma of the vulva. Int J Gynecol Pathol 1982;1:299–306.
122. Hoffman MS, Roberts WS, Ruffolo EH: Basal cell carcinoma of the vulva with inguinal lymph node metastases. Gynecol Oncol 1988;29:113–119.
123. Breen JL, Neubekcer RD, Greenwald E, Gregorio CA: Basal cell carcinoma of the vulva. Obstet Gynecol 1975;46:122–129.
124. Gleeson NC, Ruffolo EH, Hoffman MS, Cavanagh D: Basal cell carcinoma of the vulva with groin node metastasis. Gynecol Oncol 1994;53:366–368.
125. Andersen ES, Sorensen IM: Verrucous carcinoma of the female genital tract: Report of a case and review of the literature. Gynecol Oncol 1988;30:427–434.
126. Brisigotti M, Morena A, Murcia C, Matias-Guiu X, Prat J: Verrucous carcinoma of the vulva: A clinopathologic and

immunohistochemical study of five cases. Int J Gynecol Pathol 1989;8:1–7.

127. Japaze H, Dinh TV, Woodruff JD: Verrucous carcinoma of the vulva: Study of 24 cases. Obstet Gynecol 1982;60:462–466.
128. Leuchter RS, Hacker NF, Voet RL, Berek JS, Townsend DE, Lagasse LD: Primary carcinoma of the Bartholin gland: A report of 14 cases and review of the literature. Obstet Gynecol 1982;60:361–368.
129. Wheelock JB, Goplerud DR, Dunn LJ, Oates JF III: Primary carcinoma of the Bartholin gland: A report of ten cases. Obstet Gynecol 1984;63:820–824.
130. Zaino RJ: Carcinoma of the vulva, urethra and Bartholin's gland. *In* Wilkinson EJ (ed): Contemporary Issues in Surgical Pathology: Vol. 9. Pathology of the Vulva and Vagina. New York, Churchill Livingstone, 1987, p 119.
131. Rosenberg P, Simonsen E, Risberg B: Adenoid cystic carcinoma of Bartholin's gland: A report of five new cases treated with surgery and radiotherapy. Gynecol Oncol 1989;34:145–147.
132. Copeland LJ, Sneige N, Gershenson DM, McGuffee VB, Abdul-Karim F, Rutledge F: Bartholin gland carcinoma. Obstet Gynecol 1986;67:794–801.

132a. Simon KE, Dutcher JP, Runowicz CD, Wiernick P: Adenocarcinoma arising in vulvar breast tissue. Cancer 1988;62:2234–2238.

133. Chung AF, Woodruff JM, Lewis JL Jr: Malignant melanoma of the vulva: A report of 44 cases. Obstet Gynecol 1975;45:638–646.
134. Breslow A: Tumor thickness, level of invasion and node dissection in stage I cutaneous melanoma. Ann Surg 1975; 182:572–575.
135. Breslow A: Thickness, cross-sectional areas and depth of invasion in the prognosis of cutaneous melanoma. Ann Surg 1970;172:902–908.
136. Clark WH, From L, Bernadino EA, Mihm MC Jr.: The histogenesis and biologic behavior of primary human malignant melanoma of the skin. Cancer Res 1969;29:705–715.
137. Tasseron EWK, van der Esch EP, Hart AAM, de la Rivière GB, Aartsen EJ: A clinicopathological study of 30 melanomas of the vulva. Gynecol Oncol 1992;46:170–175.
138. Look KY, Roth LM, Sutton GP: Vulvar melanoma reconsidered. Cancer 1993;72:143–146.
139. Phillips KGL, Twiggs LB, Okagaki T: Vulvar melanoma: A microstaging study. Gynecol Oncol 1982;14:80–88.
140. Podratz KC, Gaffey TA, Symmonds RE, Johansen KL, O'Brien PC: Melanoma of the vulva: An update. Gynecol Oncol 1983;16:153–168.
141. Bailet JW, Figge DC, Tamimi HK: Malignant melanoma of the vulva: A case report of distal recurrence in a patient with a superficially invasive primary lesion. Obstet Gynecol 1987;70:515–517.
142. Trimble EL, Lewis JL Jr, Williams LL, Curtin JP, Chapman D, Woodruff JM, Rubin SC, Hoskins WJ: Management of vulvar melanoma. Gynecol Oncol 1992;45:254–258.
143. Tawfik O, Huntrakoon M, Collins J, Owiety T, Seoud MA-F, Weed J Jr: Leiomyosarcoma of the vulva: Report of a case. Gynecol Oncol 1994;54:242–249.
144. LiVolsi VA, Brooks JJ: Nodular fasciitis of the vulva: A report of two cases. Obstet Gynecol 1987;69:513–516.
145. Tavassoli FA, Norris HJ: Smooth muscle tumors of the vulva. Obstet Gynecol 1979;53:213–217.
146. Moller LB, Nielsen MN, Trolle C: Leiomyosarcoma vulvae: Case report. Acta Obstet Gynecol Scand 1990;69:187–189.
147. Shen JT, D'Ablaing G, Morrow CP: Alveolar soft part sarcoma of the vulva: Report of the first case and review of literature. Gynecol Oncol 1982;13:120–128.
148. LiVolsi VA, Brooks JJ: Soft tissue tumors of the vulva. *In* Wilkinson EJ (ed): Contemporary Issues in Surgical Pathology: Vol 9. Pathology of the Vulva and Vagina. New York, Churchill Livingstone, 1987, pp 209–231.
149. Bock JE, Andreasson B, Thorn A, Holck S: Dermatofibrosarcoma protuberans of the vulva. Gynecol Oncol 1985;20:129–135.
150. Stever MR, Hernandez E, Miyazawa K: Malignant fibrous histiocytoma of the pelvis. Gynecol Oncol 1988;30:285–290.
151. Taylor RN, Bottles K, Miller TR, Braga CA: Malignant fibrous histiocytoma of the vulva. Obstet Gynecol 1985;66:145–148.
152. Santala M, Suonio S, Syrjänen K, Uronen MT, Saarikoski S: Malignant fibrous histiocytoma of the vulva. Gynecol Oncol 1987;27:121–126.
153. Reagan MT, Clwry LJ, Cox JD, et al: Radiation therapy in the treatment of malignant fibrous histiocytoma. Int J Radiat Oncol 1981;7:311–315.
154. Plouffe L Jr, Tulandi T, Rosenberg A, Ferenczy A: Non-Hodgkin's lymphoma in Bartholin's gland: Case report and review of literature. Am J Obstet Gynecol 1984;148:608–609.
155. Labes J, Ring A: Ulcerating cutaneous Hodgkin's disease of the vulva. Am J Obstet Gynecol 1964;89:272–273.
156. Swanson S, Innes DJ Jr, Frierson HF Jr, Hess CE: T-immunoblastic lymphoma mimicking B-immunoblastic lymphoma. Arch Pathol Lab Med 1987;111:1077–1080.
157. Doss LL: Simultaneous extramedullary plasmacytomas of the vagina and vulva: A case report and review of the literature. Cancer 1978;141:2468–2474.
158. Harris NL, Scully RE: Malignant lymphoma and granulocytic sarcoma of the uterus and vagina. Cancer 1984;53:2530–2545.
159. Fu YS, Reagan JW: Nonepithelial and metastatic tumors of the lower genital tract. *In* Fu YS, Reagan JW (eds): Pathology of the Uterine Cervix, Vagina, and Vulva. Philadelphia, WB Saunders, 1989, pp 336–379.
160. Dudley Ag, Young RH, Lawrence WD, Scully RE: Endodermal sinus tumor of the vulva in an infant. Obstet Gynecol 1983;61:76S–79S.
161. Copeland LJ, Cleary K, Sneige N, Edwards CL: Neuroendocrine (Merkel cell) carcinoma of the vulva: A case report and review of the literature. Gynecol Oncol 1985;22:367–378.
162. Scerr GR, d'Ablaing G III, Ouzounian JG: Peripheral primitive neuroectodermal tumor of the vulva. Gynecol Oncol 1994;54:254–258.
163. Rose PG, Johnston GC, O'Toole RV: Pure cutaneous histiocytosis X of the vulva. Obstet Gynecol 1984;64:587–590.
164. Thomas R, Barnhill D, Bibro M, Hoskins W, Hambidge W: Histiocytosis-X in gynecology: A case presentation and review of the literature. Obstet Gynecol 1986;67:46S–49S.
165. Kfuri A, Rosenshein NB, Dorfman H, Goldstein P: Desmoid tumor of the vulva. J Reprod Med 1981;26:272–273.
166. Dehner LP: Metastatic and secondary tumors of the vulva. Obstet Gynecol 1973;42:47–57.
167. Grabstald H: Tumors of the urethra in men and women. Cancer 1973;32:1236–1255.
168. Antoniades J: Radiation therapy in carcinoma of the female urethra. Cancer 1969;24:70–76.
169. Ampil FL: Primary malignant neoplasm of the female urethra. Obstet Gynecol 1985;66:799–804.

2

Benign Conditions of the Vagina and Cervix

Michael R. Spence / Enrique Hernandez

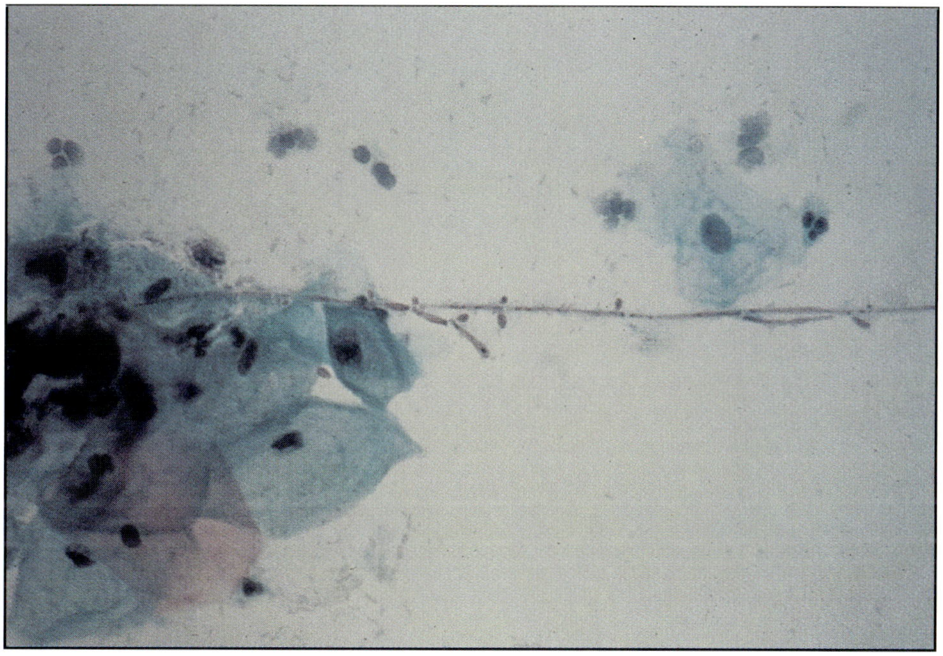

Many benign conditions affect the vagina and cervix, and most are found in both the cervix and the vagina; these will be discussed primarily in the section on the vagina. The benign conditions to be discussed here are mostly the result of alterations in development, inflammation, or infection.

THE VAGINA

Anatomy

The vagina is a tubular structure that is approximately 8 to 10 cm long in the normal woman. The anterior wall of the vagina is approximately 2 cm shorter than the posterior wall. Although the organ is normally collapsed anteroposteriorly, it is a potential cylinder. The boundaries of the vagina are the hymen inferiorly, the cervix uteri superiorly, the bladder and urethra anteriorly, and the rectum posteriorly.

The vagina is thought to be derived dually from the müllerian ducts, which are of mesodermal origin, and from the endoderm of the urogenital sinus. When the fused müllerian duct touches the urogenital sinus it causes the vaginal plate to develop. This is a hollow column of squamous epithelium that extends from the urogenital sinus to the tip of the fused müllerian duct. The vaginal plate and müllerian duct fuse to form the vagina. After this fusion, the columnar epithelium of the müllerian duct changes to squamous epithelium. This change occurs from the caudal to the cephalic direction. The mesonephric ducts (wolffian ducts) run parallel to the müllerian ducts, and their remnants can occasionally be seen in the lateral vaginal walls. The interactions of the urogenital sinus with the müllerian ducts and the wolffian ducts, and whether the vaginal plate is of mesodermal or endodermal origin, have been the subject of much controversy, and these issues have not been completely resolved.[1]

The vaginal mucosa is a nonkeratinized, stratified squamous epithelium. Figure 2–1 shows a schematic diagram of normal stratified squamous epithelium under various hormonal circumstances as would be seen in a histologic preparation. Figure 2–2 is a schematic of the cell types that would exfoliate from the surface epithelium as they would be seen on a cervicovaginal smear. The superficial layer of the vaginal mucosa under estrogen stimulation is composed of polygonal cells that have small pyknotic nuclei and abundant cytoplasm. When these superficial cells are seen in a Papanicolaou smear the cytoplasm may be either pink or blue (Fig. 2–3). At the top of the intermediate layer the cells are of the same size and shape as the superficial cells, but the nucleus is slightly larger and has an open chromatin pattern rather than the pyknotic one that is characteristic of a superficial cell (Fig. 2–3). Slightly deeper in the intermediate layer the cells are rounded and smaller and are about the size of squamous metaplastic cells (see Fig. 2–2). The basal layer contains small round cells that have a nuclear to cytoplasmic ratio of approximately 1 to 1. The long axis of the superficial cells aligns parallel to the surface, while that of the basal cells is perpendicular to the basement membrane, which lies directly below the basal cell layer. The vaginal epithelium responds to hormones. Estrogen causes an increase in the number of cell layers and maturation toward superficial cells (i.e., increase in cytoplasm and amount and type of intracytoplasmic keratin). The vaginal mucosa is nonkeratinized and the nuclei are preserved even in the superficial layers. However, the cells do contain intracytoplasmic keratin, which on Papanicolaou stain may appear pink, orange, or blue.

The vaginal submucosa lies under the basement membrane. The submucosa is composed of connective tissue with elastic fibers and numerous lymphatic and venous plexuses (Fig. 2–4). The sub-

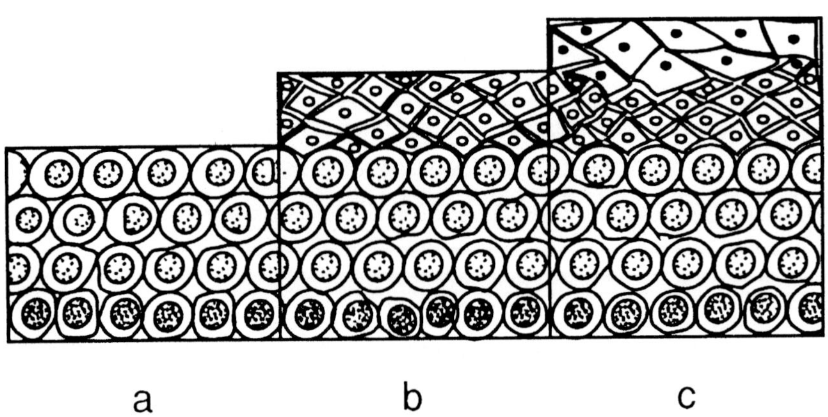

FIGURE 2–1
Schematic diagram of normal stratified squamous epithelium under various hormonal circumstances as seen in a histologic preparation: atrophic with parabasal cells at the surface *(a)*, intermediate pattern from progesterone *(b)*, superficial pattern from estrogen effect *(c)*. Note the increase in thickness of the epithelium, increased maturation of the cells, and larger size associated with increased keratin in the cytoplasm under the influence of sex hormones.

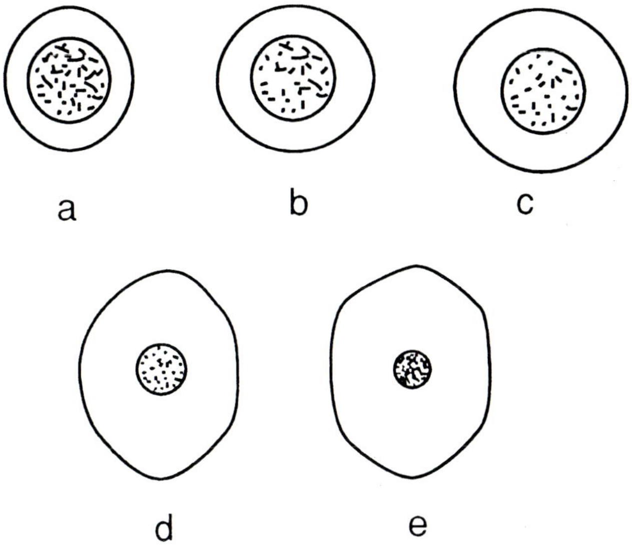

FIGURE 2-2

A schematic diagram of normal squamous epithelial cells that are exfoliated from cervix and vagina is shown. This allows for comparison of cell and nuclear sizes as well as nuclear to cytoplasmic ratio. The cells shown are basal *(a)*, parabasal *(b)*, squamous metaplastic *(c)*, intermediate *(d)*, and superficial *(e)*.

mucosa is surrounded by a muscularis (i.e., the tunica muscularis vaginae) composed of a circular layer of muscle overlaid by a longitudinal muscle layer. The muscularis, in turn, is covered by a layer of loose connective tissue.

The major arterial blood supply to the vagina is derived from the vaginal artery, which is a branch of the hypogastric artery. The vaginal artery may also originate from the uterine artery. Branches of the uterine, middle rectal, inferior vesical, and internal pudendal arteries also contribute to the blood supply of thc vagina. The venous drainage of the vagina is predominantly through a group of venous plexuses that anastomose with the parametrial uterine venous plexus. These anastomoses include the rectal, bladder, and pudendal plexuses as well as the vestibular bulb. These plexuses drain into the internal iliac (hypogastric) veins. The lymphatic drainage of the vagina is through a plexus of lymphatics that runs through the vaginal submucosa. The lymphatics of the upper two thirds connect to the lymphatics of the cervix, bladder, and rectum and drain to the internal iliac (hypogastric) and obturator lymph nodes. The lymphatics of the lower third of the vagina drain into the inguinal nodes. The parasympathetic innervation of the vagina is from L2, L3, and L4. The sympathetic innervation comes from the superior and inferior hypogastric (presacral) plexuses. The vagina does not have well-defined nerve endings. Painful stimuli to the vagina are usually not well perceived by the patient except when applied to the lower vagina close to the introitus. There are no distinct glands in the vagina. The lubrication that occurs during coitus is the result of a transudate from engorged pelvic vessels. Immunoglobulins A and E (IgA and IgE) are secreted locally. However, the mechanism for their production is not known.

The hormonal status of a patient can be judged from a Papanicolaou smear. If a complete hormonal status evaluation with a maturation index is needed, a scrape should be taken from the lateral vaginal wall so that squamous metaplastic

FIGURE 2-3

This vaginal smear shows several superficial cells (pink cytoplasm and pyknotic nuclei); one intermediate cell that has a larger nucleus, more open chromatin pattern, and blue cytoplasm *(top center)*; and a cluster of four metaplastic cells that have denser, blue-staining cytoplasm and larger nuclei. One macrophage is seen at the top, above the intermediate cell. Polymorphonuclear leukocytes are also present.

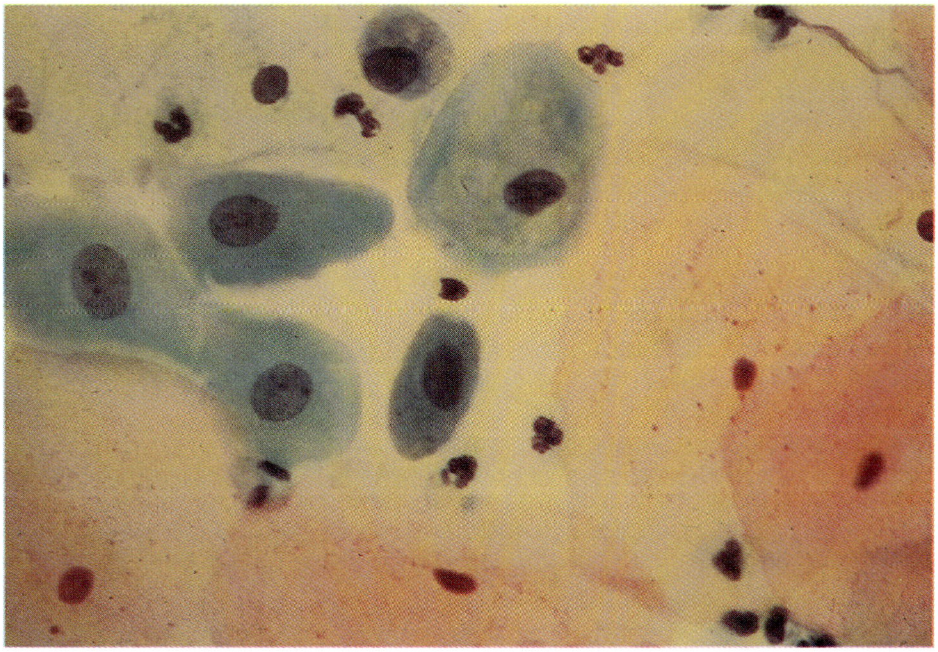

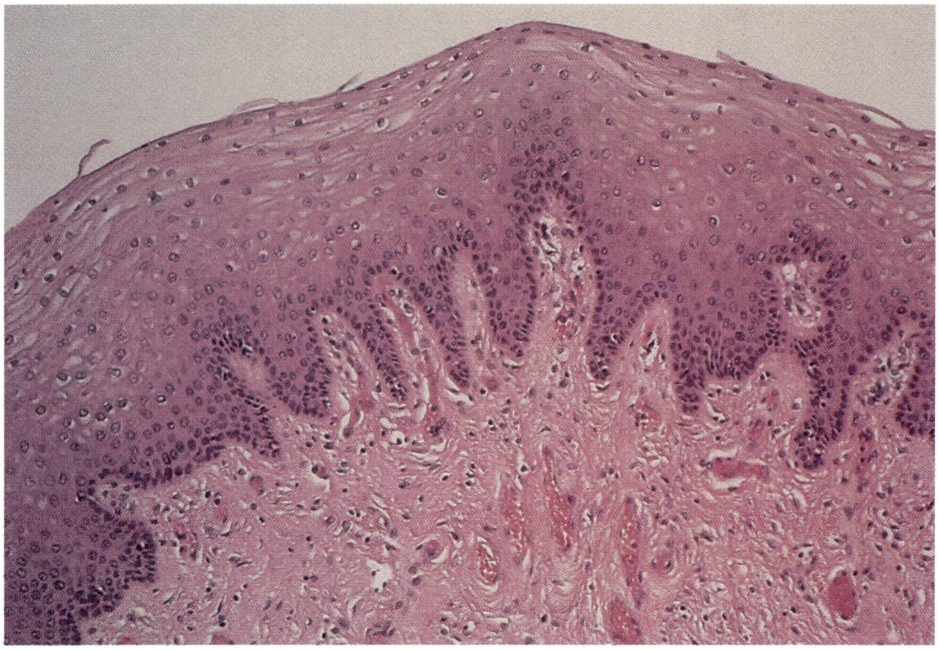

FIGURE 2-4
This vaginal biopsy specimen shows nonkeratinizing, stratified squamous epithelium. There is normal maturation and orientation of the cells. The submucosal stroma stains eosinophilic and contains lymphovascular spaces. The epithelial-stromal junction has a saw-toothed appearance. This is characteristic of the vaginal mucosa of a premenopausal woman. In postmenopausal women the epithelium may be thinner and the epithelial-stromal junction flat.

cells from the transformation zone do not interfere with the cell count. Maturation indexes are not used as often as in the past, since hormonal levels in serum can be easily measured. However, ordinary interpretation of a Papanicolaou smear requires a knowledge of the principles behind the cellular patterns seen in different hormonal milieus. To perform a maturation index the cytotechnologist counts and classifies a minimum of 200 cells and derives a ratio based on 100 cells. The comparison is the number of parabasal cells:intermediate cells:superficial cells. In the absence of inflammation or ulceration, all three cell types are never present on a smear; nor is there ever a combination of parabasal and superficial cells. A maturation index of 100:0:0 indicates that only parabasal cells are present; this pattern indicates atrophy as is seen during childhood and postmenopausally. If any progesterone is present the smear shows intermediate cells. Thus in a perimenopausal woman the maturation index may be 50:50:0. In a normally menstruating woman no parabasal cells are expected. The smear from most stages of the menstrual cycle shows a mixture of intermediate and superficial cells except just prior to ovulation, when the expected pattern is one of all superficial cells (0:0:100). In a woman receiving progesterone the pattern is one of intermediate cell predominance. Sometimes glycogenated intermediate cells are quite prominent, as they also may be during pregnancy (Fig. 2–5). If a woman is receiving estrogen, the pattern is one of superficial cell predominance. A significant population of superficial cells is evidence of exogenous or endogenous estrogen effect, since other hormones lead only to a predominance of intermediate cells. Some drugs such as digitalis and tamoxifen may lead to an inappropriate hormone effect in a postmenopausal woman.

Malformations

The malformations that occur in the vagina result from the lack of fusion of the paired müllerian ducts or from failure of the urogenital sinus and the fused müllerian duct to join. A failure to fuse or incomplete fusion of the müllerian ducts results in duplication of the vagina, cervix, or uterus. This lack of fusion is also responsible for a longitudinal vaginal septum (Fig. 2–6). Failure of the müllerian ducts and the urogenital sinus to join results either in complete vaginal agenesis or in a transverse vaginal septum that may be partial or complete. The transverse septum usually occurs in the middle third or the upper third of the vagina. The congenital changes associated with prenatal exposure to diethylstilbestrol (DES) are discussed later. A more complete description of the different congenital malformations of the genital tract can be found in several sources.[2]

Ecology

As described above, the maturation of the vaginal epithelium is dependent upon stimulation by estrogen and progesterone. The stimulation by progesterone results in the cells storing glycogen in their cytoplasm. This glycogen serves as an energy source for the microorganisms that reside in the

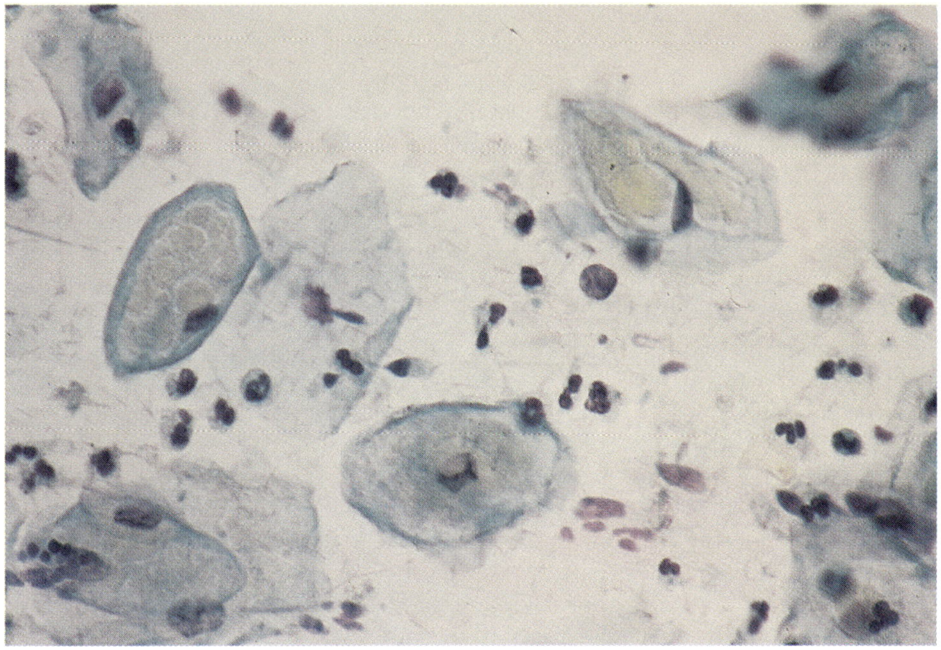

FIGURE 2-5
This cervical/vaginal smear from a pregnant woman shows several navicular cells. They contain yellow-staining glycogen. The cell borders are thick and sharp.

vagina. The vagina is colonized primarily by lactobacilli, and they are particularly prominent during the second half of the menstrual cycle. The proliferation and metabolism of the lactobacilli generate lactic acid. The production of lactic acid causes the pH of the vagina to be lowered to approximately 4.0, which is critical in the establishment of other organisms. The vagina of the normal woman is colonized by numerous microorganisms. It has been determined that approximately 10^5 to 10^{11} organisms are found in every gram of vaginal secretions.[3] Approximately 90 percent of these organisms are anaerobic in their growth requirements. The dominant species of the anaerobes are peptococci and peptostreptococci. However, *Bacteroides* species can also be found as part of the normal anaerobic flora. Other organisms that have been identified as commensal in the vagina include group B streptococci, which are found in 10 to 40 percent of normal women; *Escherichia coli,* which is present in 25 to 40 percent; and smaller numbers (1 to 5 percent) of other members of the En-

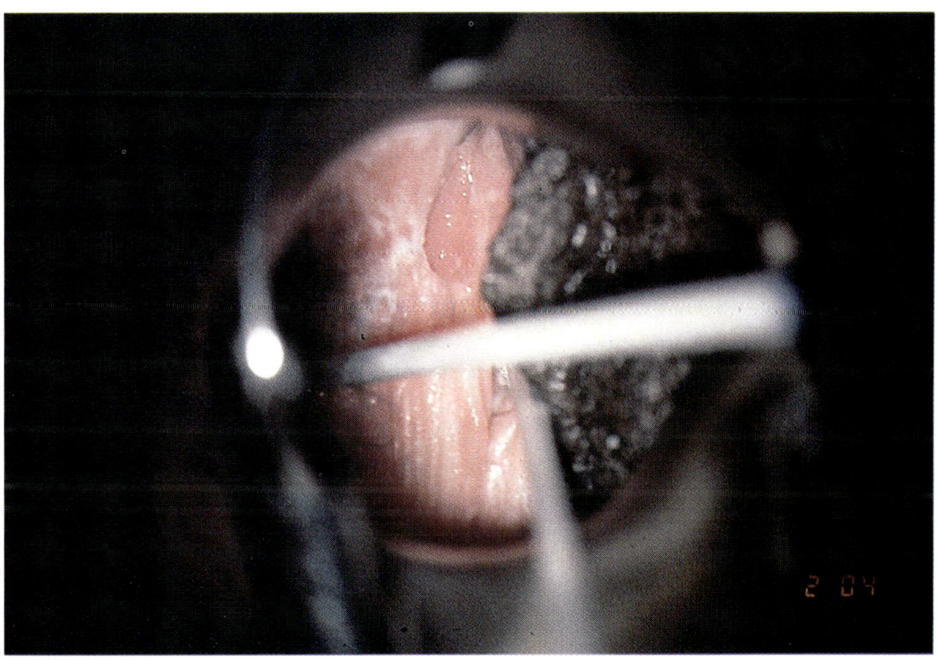

FIGURE 2-6
This patient has a longitudinal vaginal septum. The cotton-tipped applicators are in the vaginal cavities on either side. The septum is seen between them.

terobacteriaceae. In addition, up to 25 percent of normal women harbor *Candida* species without clinical evidence of infection. Although it has not been well defined, the proportions of the organisms normally found in the vagina vary with the phases of the menstrual cycle.

Infectious and Inflammatory Conditions

The majority of the infectious problems of the vagina are manifested by an abnormal vaginal discharge. All too often the inappropriate question "Do you have a vaginal discharge?" is asked of the patient. The response to this question is almost always yes, since most normal women produce vaginal secretions. These secretions are the result of desquamation of the vaginal epithelium admixed with the cervical mucus produced by the endocervical glands. In addition, there is a small contribution of transudate from the vaginal vasculature. Hence, the appropriate question is "Do you have a vaginal discharge that is abnormal for you?"

Although some of the vaginal secretions associated with inflammatory and infectious conditions have a characteristic presentation, these are not always diagnostic. In addition, there are situations in which infectious organisms are harbored in an asymptomatic patient who has no evidence of abnormality in the vaginal secretions. It is the poorly informed clinician who believes that inflammatory or infectious conditions of the vagina can be definitively diagnosed or excluded on the basis of their clinical presentation. The clinical findings need to be supported by laboratory data that include the microscopic examination of the vaginal secretions. This is best accomplished by utilizing nonbacteriostatic normal saline and 10 to 20 percent potassium hydroxide solution. A small amount of the vaginal secretions is mixed separately with 1 to 2 ml of each of these solutions, placed on clean microscope slides under a coverslip, and viewed at 100× and 400× magnification. This technique (wet preparation) helps confirm or refute the clinical impression. Other diagnostic methods that may be helpful include Gram stain and culture of the secretions. However, one must be very selective in the use of these techniques. In the identification of *Neisseria gonorrhoeae* the Gram stain of cervical secretions has a sensitivity of only 65% even if examined by well-trained observers. Culture is helpful for identification of pathogens such as *N. gonorrhoeae* and *Chlamydia trachomatis,* but nucleic acid probes may be best for these organisms. Culture is not of value in the management of other types of vaginitis.

Inflammatory Conditions

Foreign body vaginitis is relatively frequent. The patient with this problem usually complains of acute onset of a foul-smelling, watery, and sometimes bloody vaginal discharge. Although this condition commonly occurs in children, it is also encountered in adults. A retained tampon is the most common foreign body found in the vagina of the adult. Although one might think that this problem is seen predominantly in younger women just starting to use the device, it is actually more common in older women. The diagnosis is readily made by speculum examination. Upon removal of the object, erythema and denudation of the upper vaginal mucosa are seen. A wet preparation or culture could be done to exclude concomitant infections if this is clinically suspected. An antiseptic douche helps the patient get rid of the odor. Antimicrobial therapy is usually not necessary. The vaginal mucosa regenerates rapidly, and no abnormality is detected if the patient is examined 3 to 4 days after removal of the foreign body. If a culture has been obtained it usually reveals normal flora with increased anaerobes and decreased lactobacilli. The flora corrects itself within 4 to 7 days.

Another cause of noninfectious vaginitis is an allergic reaction or a contact inflammation and irritation. This can be secondary to perfumes and other chemicals that are added to tampons and sanitary napkins, or it may be a reaction to spermicide, intravaginal suppositories, and the latex of condoms, sponges, or diaphragms. The patient usually complains of severe burning and irritation of the vagina. There is often edema of the labia minora, and there can be a profuse, watery, often purulent vaginal discharge. Microscopic examination of this discharge shows polymorphonuclear leukocytes (PMNs), lymphocytes, and eosinophils. A careful history is required to identify the offending agent. Once it has been identified and removed there is a speedy recovery. This recovery can be hastened by the use of topical corticosteroids, although this is usually not necessary. There is a subset of patients in whom the allergic vaginitis is secondary to substances found in the seminal fluid. This can be resolved by the use of condoms.[4] One patient who had an allergic vaginitis that was thought to be secondary to atmospheric allergens was "cured" by the use of intravaginal cromolyn sodium. Cromolyn acts by stabilizing the mast cells and preventing the release of allergic reaction mediators.[5]

Desquamative inflammatory vaginitis (DIV) is a very distressing condition. The patient usually presents with an irritative, inflammatory vaginitis that is associated with a copious purulent discharge. The patient is frequently unable to engage in coitus owing to severe pain. The vaginal walls are erythematous; the labia minora are frequently edematous; and there is a copious, homogeneous, yellow discharge adherent to the vaginal walls and pooled in the posterior fornix. Microscopic examination of these secretions shows numerous PMNs, which may be in sheets (Fig. 2–7). Many of these PMNs are ameboid. They may have a long pseudopod extending from the cytoplasm, giving the cell somewhat the appearance of a tennis racket. Another hallmark of DIV is a large number of parabasal cells in the vaginal secretions. These cells have a rounded appearance, a moderate amount of cytoplasm, and a relatively large nucleus (see Fig. 2–2). Occasionally basal cells (which are smaller and have scanter cytoplasm) are also present. Autolysis of the cytoplasm of the parabasal and basal cells found in the vaginal secretions of the patient with DIV may also occur. This results in "bare nuclei." On a wet preparation these bare nuclei can be mistaken for parasite ova (vital stains can be useful in the identification of parasites).

The most common cause of DIV is lichen planus. Patients who have lichen planus of the vagina may have a white lacy pattern on the vaginal mucosa. This becomes evident once the discharge has been wiped off. This finding can be seen on other mucosal surfaces as well, including the buccal mucosa and the inner margins of the lower lip. It is interesting to note that in a subset of these individuals the diagnosis of interstitial cystitis or vulvar vestibulitis is made.[6, 7] Although the etiologic agents for these conditions have not been identified, the tissues affected have a common embryologic origin. This suggests an immune phenomenon or an epithelium-specific agent.

DIV has frequently been misdiagnosed as a severe trichomonal infection, since both cause a copious, yellow, foul-smelling discharge and marked vaginal erythema. The absence of motile trichomonads in a wet-mount specimen speaks against the diagnosis. Trichomonacidal therapy with metronidazole is of no benefit to the patient who has DIV. These patients often do respond to corticosteroids. These can be administered in the form of topical foams that contain 1 to 2 percent hydrocortisone. This is the same preparation (e.g., Proctofoam-HC) used for the treatment of anal and rectal conditions.

The treatment of DIV may require the intramuscular injection of long-acting corticosteroids or the administration of oral corticosteroids in high dosages. Even aggressive treatment may fail to control the condition. DIV is rarely "cured." A pattern of periodic remission and exacerbation is seen. Once remission is achieved, the time between exacerbations can be lengthened by having the patient use intravaginal boric acid capsules for the week prior to and during the week following menses. It is unclear why this works. One explanation is that it allows the reestablishment of the normal vaginal pH of approximately 4.0,

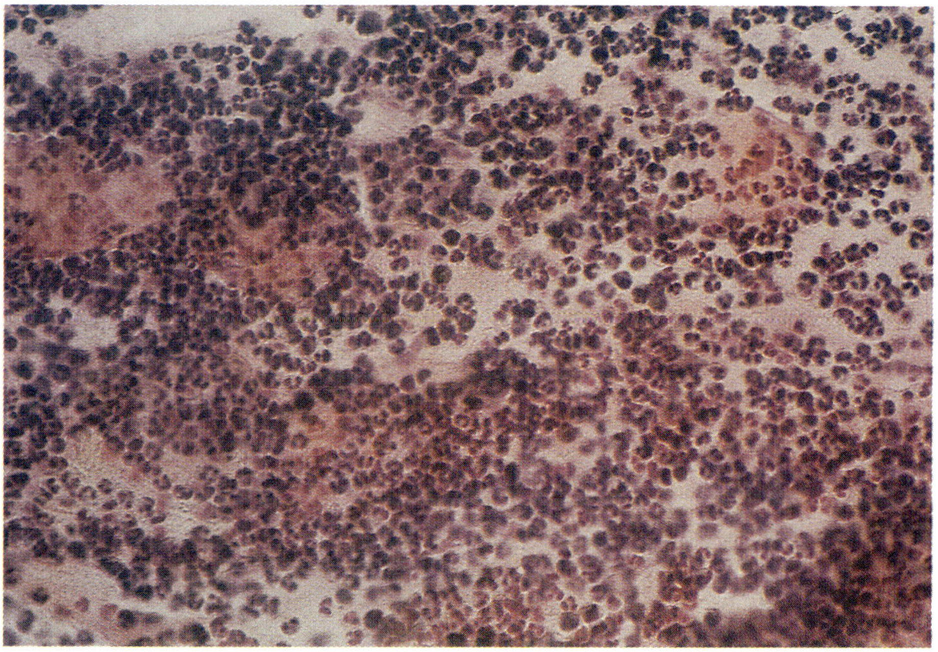

FIGURE 2–7
Sheets of polymorphonuclear leukocytes obscure the squamous cells in this vaginal smear.

leading to recolonization with the normal vaginal flora.

A subset of patients with DIV was recently described.[7a] The Gram stain of the vaginal secretions from these patients contained gram-positive cocci and no lactobacilli. A good therapeutic result was obtained with the use of topical 2 percent clindamycin.

A rare inflammatory condition of unknown origin that occurs in postpubertal women is emphysematous vaginitis. Multiple small gas-filled cysts are found in the vagina. The cystic spaces are lined by a syncytium of multinucleated giant cells. In some cysts there is a partial squamous epithelial lining. The cystic structures are in the submucosal stroma, and the overlying surface epithelium is normal. The stroma surrounding the cysts has an inflammatory infiltrate that includes lymphocytes. These lesions usually cause no symptoms and require no treatment.

Atrophic Vaginitis

Atrophic vaginitis occurs when there is a decrease in the proliferation and maturation of the vaginal squamous cells secondary to low levels of circulating estrogen. In women who have this condition, the vaginal mucosa is often pale, thin, and friable (Fig. 2–8). The patient often complains of a "dry vagina," painful intercourse, and a serous or serosanguineous vaginal discharge. Microscopic examination of the discharge reveals the presence of PMNs as well as a large number of parabasal and basal cells. A Papanicolaou smear obtained from a patient who has atrophic vaginitis shows parabasal cells, singly and in sheets (Fig. 2–9). When basal cells and degenerated parabasal cells are seen in association with the inflammation and necrosis of severe atrophy, an erroneous diagnosis of a high-grade squamous intraepithelial lesion may be made (Fig. 2–10). The treatment of atrophic vaginitis is estrogen administration in topical or oral form. If the Papanicolaou smear shows atypical squamous cells, the smear should be repeated after estrogen treatment. If the Papanicolaou smear shows changes consistent with a squamous intraepithelial lesion in a patient who has atrophic vaginitis and no identifiable lesions on colposcopy, intravaginal estrogen cream is prescribed. After a 4- to 6-week course of therapy the cytologic evaluation is repeated. However, only 5 days of topical estrogen suffices to cause a change in the vaginal epithelium.

Bacterial Infections

The normal ecology of the vagina includes many bacteria, and usually there is no inflammation. A true bacterial vaginitis is uncommon. When it occurs, it is often iatrogenic. The most common bacterial vaginitis is the result of alteration of the normal vaginal flora through the use of antimicrobial agents or topical spermicides. It is well established that the contraceptive sponge and spermicides containing nonoxynol 9 inhibit the growth of many microbes and are bactericidal for *Lactobacillus.* This results in a diminution of the total number of lactobacilli, which are replaced by members

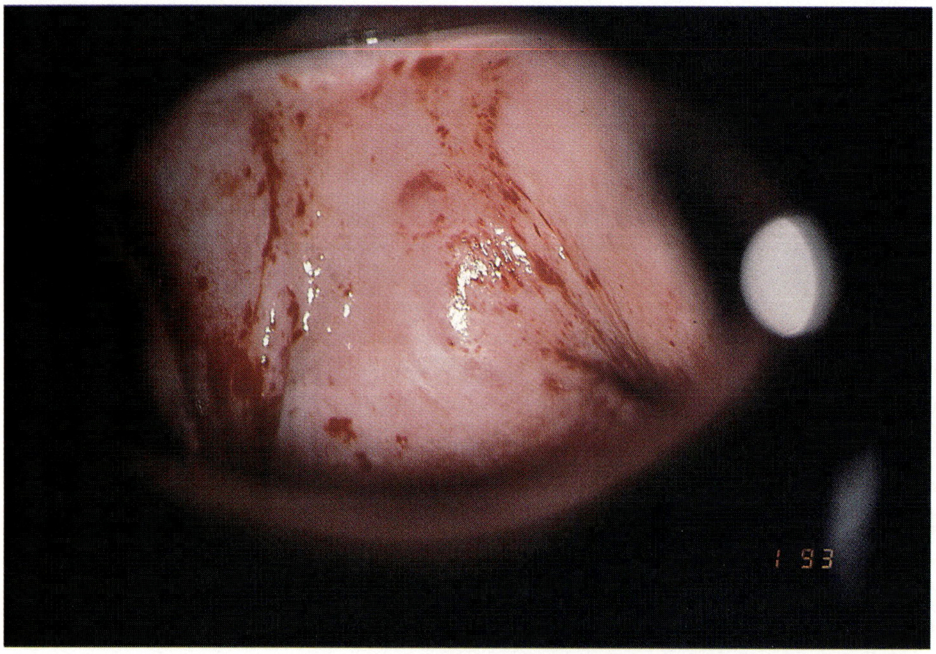

FIGURE 2–8
This is a colpophotograph of an atrophic vagina. The vaginal walls are smooth without the normal rugae. The mucosa is pale, and multiple petechiae are present.

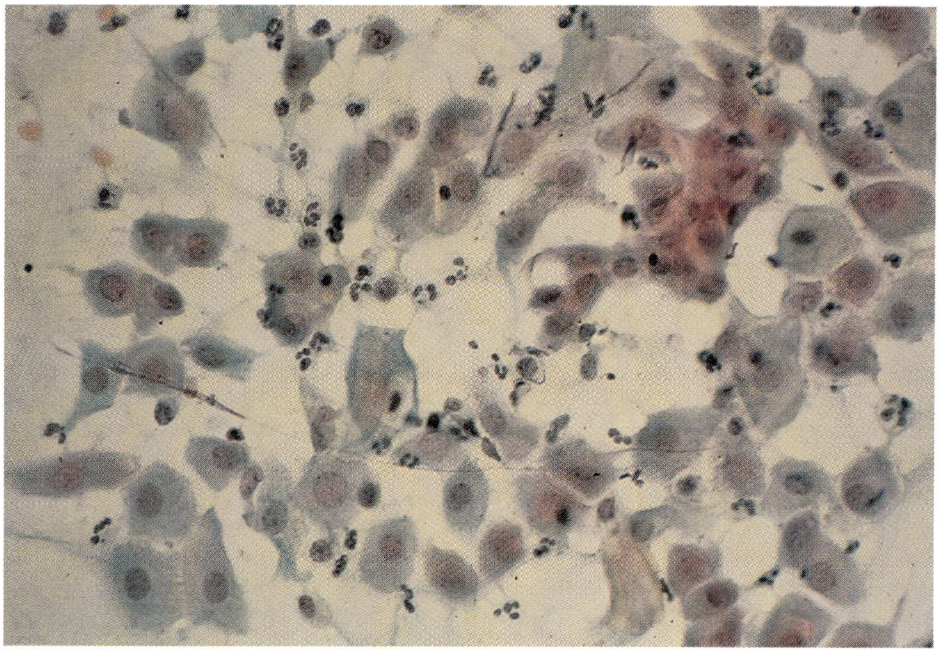

FIGURE 2-9
In this smear from a postmenopausal woman, a sheet of parabasal cells is seen in the upper right. The parabasal cells have a relatively high nuclear to cytoplasmic ratio. Polymorphonuclear leukocytes are present, as is common in vaginal atrophy.

of the Enterobacteriaceae and other pathogenic organisms. When this occurs, the patient often experiences an increased watery vaginal discharge and some degree of vulvar irritation. The diagnosis is usually made by the history and by microscopic inspection of the vaginal secretions. One sees large numbers of varied bacterial morphotypes rather than the long rods of *Lactobacillus.* Most frequently, a predominance of coccal chains or a mixed bacterial pattern that includes coccobacillary forms is seen. Numerous white blood cells are present. In cases of bacterial vaginitis the pH of the vaginal secretions is usually elevated above 4.5. This elevated pH enhances the ability of microorganisms to attach to epithelial cells, resulting in the formation of the so-called clue cells. This finding is usually associated with an overgrowth by *Haemophilus vaginalis* (see below) but may be seen in other bacterial overgrowths.

There is a temptation to obtain a culture of the vaginal secretions and then treat the patient with an antimicrobial agent chosen on the basis of culture results. Unfortunately, this is counterproductive and often worsens the condition. The goal

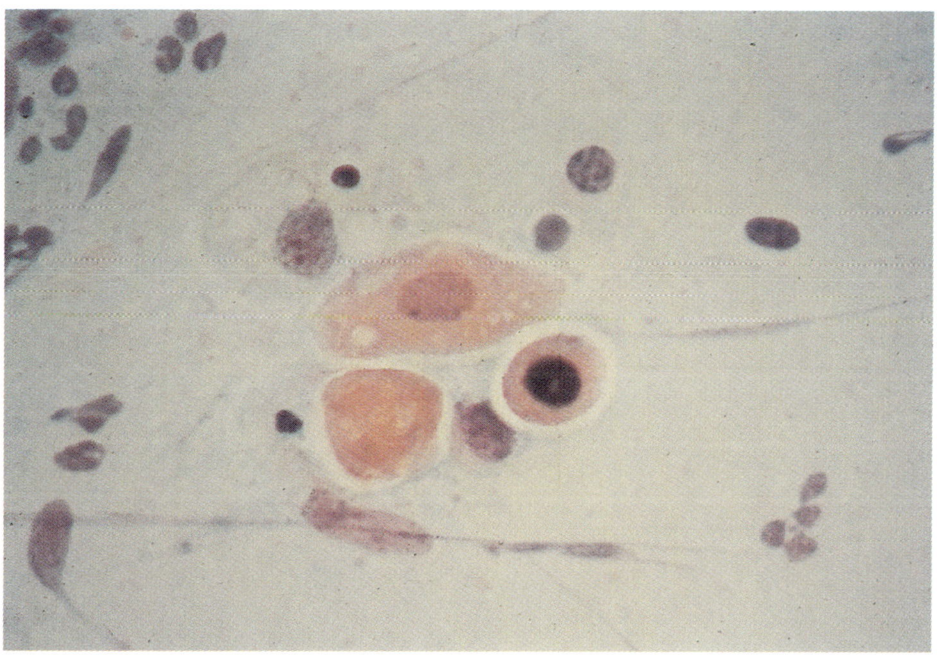

FIGURE 2-10
This smear was obtained from a woman with severe vaginal atrophy. There is an air-drying artifact. There is increase in the size of the cells, eosinophilia of the cytoplasm, and loss of cytoplasmic borders in a background of inflammatory cells. One of the cells has a very hyperchromatic nucleus and a high nuclear to cytoplasmic ratio. Such a finding may lead to an erroneous diagnosis of intraepithelial neoplasia.

should be to reestablish the normal vaginal ecology and restore *Lactobacillus* as the dominant genus. This can be easily accomplished by reacidifying the vagina to a pH that approximates 4.0 with the use of boric acid suppositories. These suppositories can be made up by the patient or her pharmacist by placing approximately 600 mg of boric acid powder into the small end of a size 0 gelatin capsule and then capping it. The patient inserts one of these capsules in the vagina at bedtime. The gelatin melts, and the boric acid is dispersed in the vagina. This lowers the vaginal pH to approximately 4.0, which enables reestablishment of the lactobacilli and also impedes the growth of pathogenic organisms. It may take up to 2 to 3 weeks before the results of this therapy are obtained.

One of the most common vaginal conditions is known as vaginal bacteriosis. It is estimated that up to one third of women who seek medical care for a complaint related to the vagina have vaginal bacteriosis.[8] The condition in the past was known as *Haemophilus vaginalis* vaginitis or by its older names *Corynebacterium vaginale* vaginitis and *Gardnerella* vaginitis. (A widely used but incorrect name for this entity is bacterial vaginosis.) This clinical condition is diagnosed by the presence of specific clinical findings and supporting laboratory data in a symptomatic patient. It does not appear to be sexually transmitted and is rarely, if ever, associated with an inflammatory response. The patient who has vaginal bacteriosis complains of an increase in the amount of vaginal discharge having an offensive odor. The patient may also complain of pruritus and irritation around the introitus as well as of dyspareunia. On physical examination, the patient is found to have a copious, gray-white vaginal discharge that is adherent to the inner aspect of the labia minora and the walls of the vagina. This discharge pools in the posterior vaginal fornix and is homogeneous in its consistency.

The diagnosis is confirmed by microscopic evaluation of the vaginal secretions mixed with saline, as described previously. Large numbers of coccobacilli and the so-called clue cells are seen. The clue cell is an epithelial cell that appears to be stippled owing to the bacteria that are densely adherent to it. The margins of the cell are obscured by the bacteria. Another important microscopic finding is the absence of, or a decrease in, the number of white blood cells. The pH of the secretions usually exceeds 4.5. For further confirmation some suggest mixing the vaginal discharge with potassium hydroxide solution. This results in the release of aromatic amines with an offensive fishy odor. This is known as the whiff test. If the patient complains of a vaginal discharge that has an offensive odor, this test is not necessary. Other diagnostic methods that have been employed in the diagnosis of vaginal bacteriosis include Papanicolaou smear recognition of clue cells (Fig. 2–11) and the Gram stain for coccobacilli.[9]

There have been numerous attempts to link the presence of vaginal bacteriosis with other conditions of the female reproductive tract, including endometritis, pelvic inflammatory disease, premature rupture of the fetal membranes, and preterm

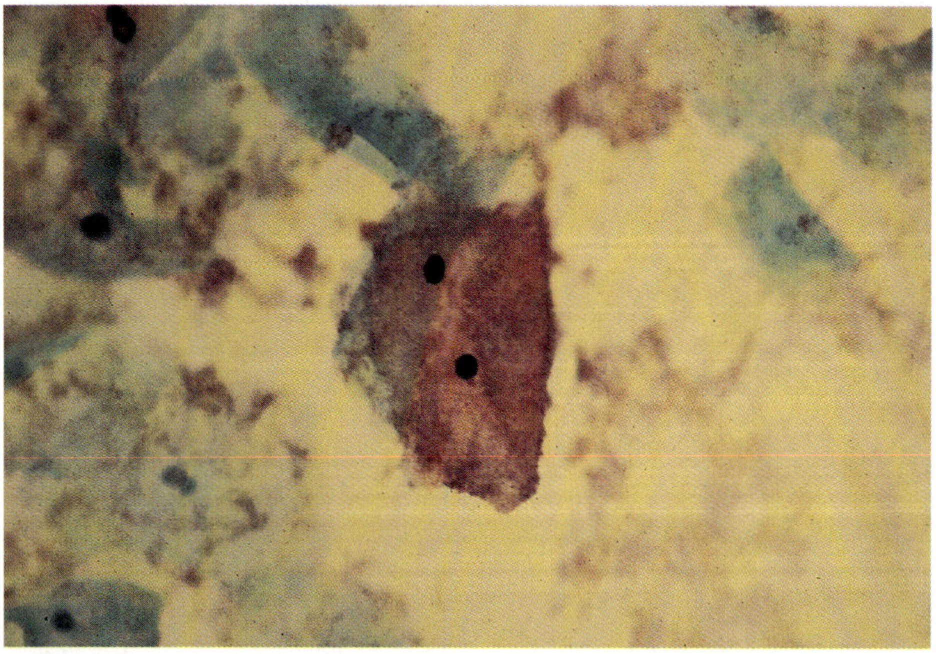

FIGURE 2–11
Two overlapping superficial squamous cells are seen in the center of this smear. The bluish purple coccobacilli cling to the epithelial cells and are also seen in the background. There is a clear zone around the epithelial cells.

labor.[10–16] The literature is controversial, and the role of vaginal bacteriosis in the foregoing conditions is still unclear. Another organism, *Mobiluncus curtisii,* a small, gram-negative, curved rod, is also thought by some to play a role in vaginal bacteriosis. However, this has not been confirmed by all observers. Patients who have vaginal bacteriosis can be treated either with topical (i.e., intravaginal) metronidazole or clindamycin or with oral metronidazole.[17] To minimize systemic effects the topical preparations are preferred. This therapy is aimed at eliminating the anaerobic bacteria that are associated with this condition.

Neisseria gonorrhoeae can cause abnormal vaginal bleeding. This is often caused by an inflammatory response of the cervix that results in a mucopurulent discharge. In prepubertal girls the vagina has not been influenced by estrogen, and the mucosa remains thin and vulnerable to infection by the gonococcus. *N. gonorrhoeae* vaginitis can occur in the young population. The isolation of *N. gonorrhoeae* from a prepubertal girl's vagina should alert the clinician to the possibility of sexual abuse. Gonorrheal vaginitis is characterized by an erythematous, tender vagina and an associated purulent, mucoid discharge. The wet preparation may demonstrate many acute inflammatory cells but is otherwise uninformative. The Gram stain may show intracellular gram-negative diplococci, but this infection can be only presumptively diagnosed using Gram stain of the vaginal secretions (Fig. 2–12). There are other nonpathogenic *Neisseria* species, such as *N. sicca* and *N. catarrhalis,* that reside in the vagina as normal flora and can resemble *N. gonorrhoeae* on Gram stain. For this reason, a culture or a specific fluorescent antibody, antigen probe, or nucleic acid probe must be utilized to make the diagnosis. Culture with sugar fermentation can also be used. Culture by itself, without sugar fermentation or other confirmatory test, is of no value, as the nonpathogenic *Neisseria* species also grow on the standard medium used for culture of *N. gonorrhoeae.* In the clinician's office, the vaginal secretions sample obtained with a sterile cotton-tipped applicator may be plated on Thayer-Martin, modified chocolate agar medium and placed in a 10% CO_2, oxygen-poor container (e.g., candle jar). Upon diagnosis of *N. gonorrhoeae* vaginitis, therapy is administered that assumes that the organism is β-lactam resistant. The current treatment of choice is ceftriaxone, 250 mg, as a single intramuscular dose.

Another intracellular organism implicated in "vaginitis" is *Chlamydia trachomatis.* However, *C. trachomatis,* unlike *N. gonorrhoeae,* has not been associated with vaginal discharge in females before puberty. If a vaginal discharge is found with *C. trachomatis* infection in an adult, it is secondary to a mucopurulent cervicitis. *C. trachomatis* is an intracellular pathogen that does not invade the vaginal epithelium. Thus far, there has not been a documented case of *C. trachomatis* vaginitis.

Treponema pallidum, the causative agent of syphilis, can infect the lower genital tract. However, the ulcers (i.e., chancre) of primary syphilis are usually found on the labia minora, labia majora, or cervix. They have been described in the posterior vaginal fornices, but this is an uncom-

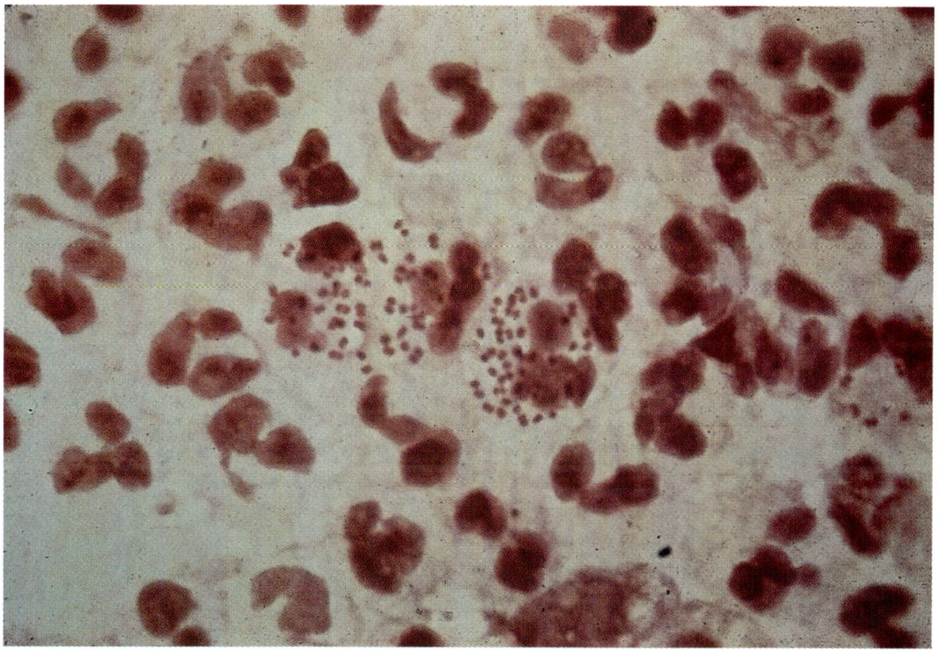

FIGURE 2–12
A Gram stain of vaginal discharge shows many polymorphonuclear leukocytes. Gram-negative diplococci are seen in the cytoplasm of some of the leukocytes; this suggests the presence of *Neisseria* species.

mon site. Secondary syphilis, manifested by the presence of mucous papules (i.e., condyloma latum), occurs on the labia minora and cervix. Involvement of the vagina is extremely rare.

A bacterium that is frequently found in women who have an abnormal vaginal discharge is *Leptothrix*. This long, filamentous, gram-positive rod is nonpathogenic. However, it grows well in an elevated pH (5.0 to 6.0) and is often found in patients who have *Trichomonas vaginalis* infection.

Mycobacterium tuberculosis can cause disease in the reproductive tract. The sites most commonly affected are the fallopian tubes and the endometrium. Vaginal infection probably does not occur.

Toxic shock syndrome is a systemic phenomenon that results from the release of a staphylococcal endotoxin. The clinical syndrome is diagnosed when the patient has a temperature above 39°C, a skin rash followed by desquamation, hypotension with a systolic blood pressure below 90 mmHg, and involvement of at least one organ system in addition to skin. Patients often have myalgia, vomiting, disorientation, and alteration in hepatic and/or renal function. The syndrome, when first described, occurred in menstruating women and was associated with prolonged use of a tampon. Subsequently, it was described in both genders and determined to be the result of infection with a coagulase-positive, penicillin-resistant *Staphylococcus aureus.*[18,19]

Parasitic Infections

The most common parasitic infection of the vagina is that caused by *Trichomonas vaginalis.* This motile protozoan is a unicellular parasite that has one recurrent and four anterior flagella, an undulating membrane, and an axostyle. It is frequently the cause of an abnormal vaginal discharge. Patients infected with *T. vaginalis* may be asymptomatic or may present with an array of complaints. These include vaginal discomfort, dyspareunia, dysuria, pruritus, and a copious, irritating, odoriferous vaginal discharge. The vaginal mucosa may appear normal in some cases, but in others there is marked erythema, edema, and scattered petechiae (Fig. 2–13). This is usually accompanied by a copious, frothy, salmon-colored (i.e., yellow-red), odoriferous discharge. In order to make the diagnosis of *Trichomonas* vaginitis, a wet-mount preparation is made as was described earlier. It is important not to use bacteriostatic saline, as this can immobilize the organisms, making their identification difficult. Motile organisms are seen as well as over ten white blood cells per high-power microscopic field. Although culture is the most sensitive technique to detect *T. vaginalis* infection, its cost is prohibitive.[20] Cytologic smears and wet preparations detect approximately 60 percent of the infections (Fig. 2–14).[21] However, the Papanicolaou smear may have a high false-positive rate.[22] In one study, 30 percent of patients would have been unnecessarily treated for trichomoniasis based on the Papanicolaou smear interpretation.[22] This can be avoided if the cytologic diagnosis is made only when well-preserved intact organisms are present. These should meet the following diagnostic criteria: The organism is oval to pear-shaped and has a small nucleus. There may be reddish cytoplasmic granules. In an inflammatory smear, degenerated

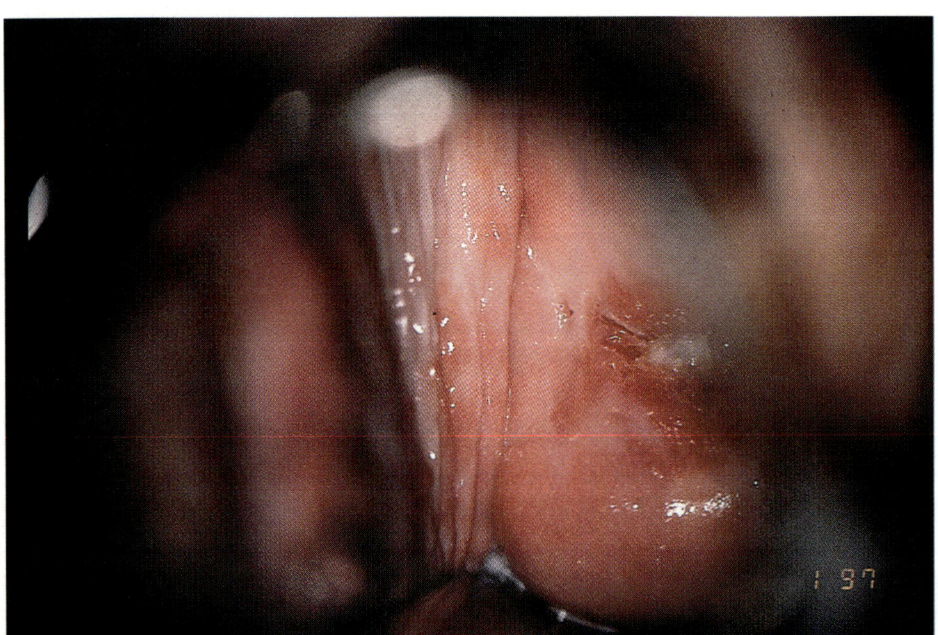

FIGURE 2–13
This colpophotograph shows the cervix on the right and the vaginal wall in the center and extending to the left. The vaginal wall has multiple erythematous macules typical of infection with *Trichomonas vaginalis.* The same macules are seen on the cervix. Normal mucus is seen in the cervical os. Columnar epithelium surrounds the cervical os and appears red.

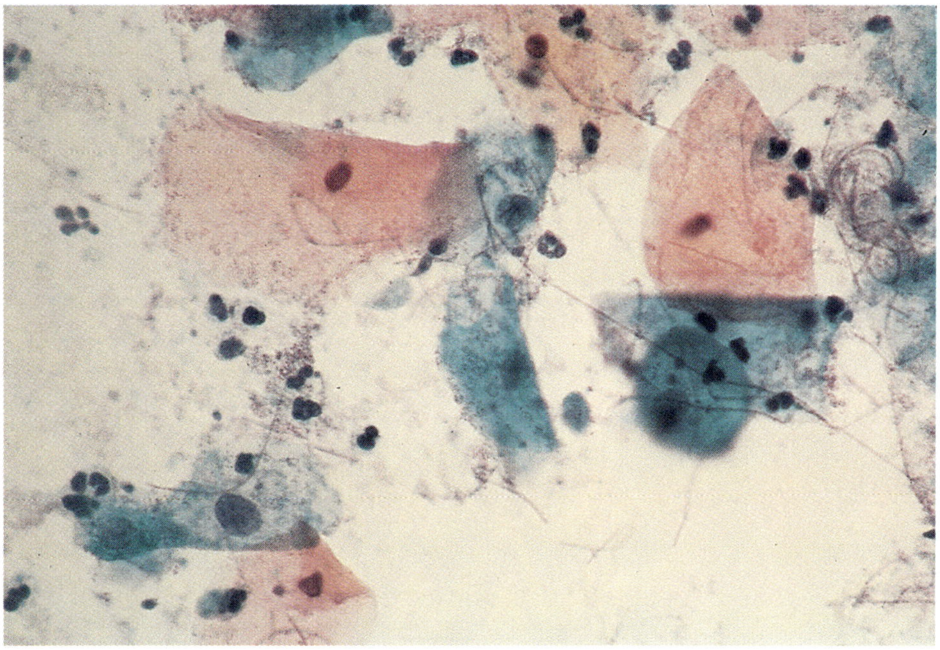

FIGURE 2-14
This cervical/vaginal smear shows superficial and intermediate squamous cells, leukocytes, *Leptothrix, Trichomonas,* and coccoid bacteria. Both an oval and a pear-shaped trichomonad are seen near the center. They stain blue and have a small, indistinct nucleus. The filamentous organisms are *Leptothrix.* When *Leptothrix* is present the cytopathologist should search for *Trichomonas,* since the two frequently coexist.

cells can mimic trichomonads, as can bare nuclei or degenerated parabasal cells in an atrophic smear. Direct immunofluorescence with monoclonal antibodies has been found to be both a sensitive and a specific technique for the rapid detection of *T. vaginalis* in vaginal discharge.[21]

Currently in the United States there is only one effective therapy for the treatment of trichomoniasis, and that is metronidazole. This can be administered as a single 2 gm oral dose or divided in two doses. An older regimen of 250 mg three to four times a day for 7 days is discouraged, since it may promote metronidazole resistance.

Another parasite that may be found in the vagina is the pinworm. This is most commonly found in children who have developed an infestation at the anus, which then can involve the vagina. Pinworm infestation is associated with intense perianal pruritus. Pinworm eggs are occasionally seen on Papanicolaou smears. *Entamoeba gingivalis* has also been reported to cause vaginitis.[23] Vaginal infestation with *Schistosoma haematobium* is extremely uncommon in North America but is endemic in Africa and Asia.[23] Infection with this organism results in a chronic inflammatory response and eosinophilia.

Viral Infections

The most common virus to infect the vagina is the human papillomavirus (HPV), the causative agent of condyloma acuminatum, or genital warts. Condyloma acuminatum of the vagina usually manifests as cauliflower-like lesions of varied size that project from the introitus and on the vaginal walls (Fig. 2–15). These lesions usually cause no symptoms. They can be denuded during the birthing process, and this results in significant bleeding. The diagnosis is usually made by clinical examination. Flat or slightly raised lesions (discussed under the section on the cervix) also can occur in the vagina. Biopsy is usually not performed, but the microscopic appearance is characteristic—finger-like projections of fibrovascular tissue which is lined by a thickened squamous epithelium. The epithelium retains its orderly maturation and orientation (i.e., polarity). Multiple koilocytotic cells, which represent the diagnostic cytopathic effect of HPV, are seen in the intermediate and superficial layers of the epithelium. The koilocytes are frequently bi- or multinucleate. The nuclei are enlarged, wrinkled, and sometimes hyperchromatic. The nucleus is surrounded by a clear space or halo (Fig. 2–16). A few normal mitotic figures may be present in the basal cell layer.[24]

The role of HPV in intraepithelial neoplasia (i.e., dysplasia) of the vagina and cervix has been extensively studied and is discussed in detail in Chapter 3. More than 60 HPV genotypes have been described. Although some HPV genotypes are more commonly associated with intraepithelial neoplasia, the management of condyloma acuminatum is not affected by the HPV genotype. Treatment may consist of removal or destruction of the warts or watchful waiting. Destruction of the lesions can be achieved with cryosurgery, cautery, laser, or surgical excision with a scalpel. Other therapeutic modalities include 5-fluorouracil ap-

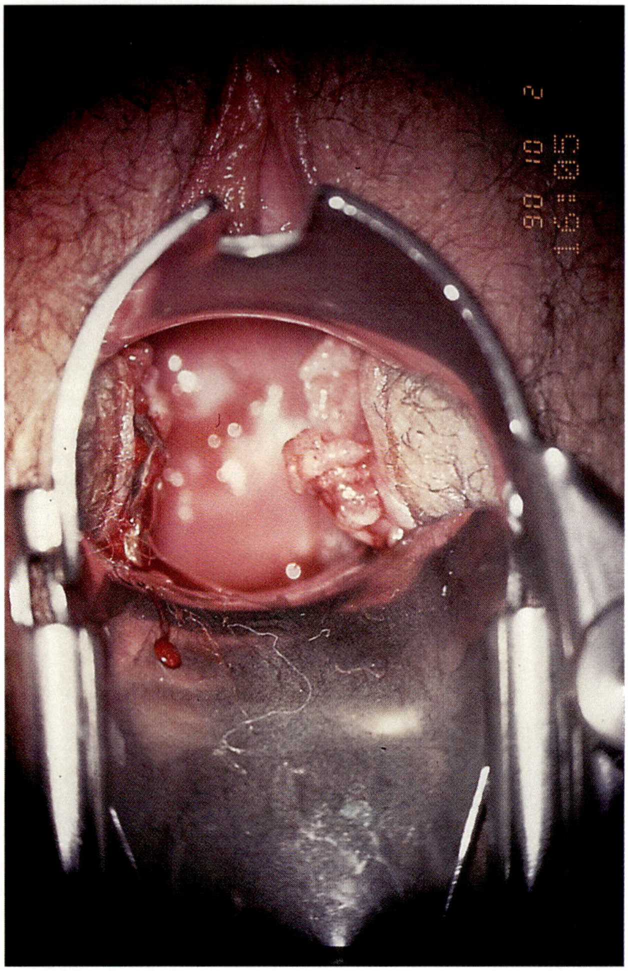

FIGURE 2-15
Cauliflower-like lesion of condyloma acuminatum is seen at the vaginal introitus on the right. A smaller lesion is present on the left. Denudation of the wart's epithelium by the speculum accounts for the bleeding.

plied topically and interferon injected either directly into the warts or intramuscularly.[25-28] Alternatively, trichloroacetic acid or a podophyllin preparation can be applied.[29] The clinician needs to be aware that most substances applied to the vagina are readily absorbed into the circulation. Hematologic toxicity may be seen with the prolonged use of podophyllins or 5-fluorouracil.

Since the vaginal warts are usually multiple and some may go unidentified, we favor topical 5-fluorouracil for the treatment of patients with these lesions. A generous amount of zinc oxide is applied to the vulva, perineum, and external urethral meatus to protect them from the burning effect of the fluorouracil. Approximately 2 gm (i.e., one half of a vaginal applicator) of 5-fluorouracil is inserted into the vagina every night for 5 to 7 days. The patient is reevaluated 3 to 4 weeks after treatment to ascertain whether there has been coaptation of the vaginal walls or formation of synechiae. Reexamination to confirm disappearance of the lesions is done a month later after the vagina has healed from the effects of the 5-fluorouracil.

Chronic epithelial ulcers occur in less than 6 percent of patients treated with this regimen.[30] These mucosal ulcerations are shallow and have sharp borders. The ulcer bed is flat and may bleed when touched. They occur in the vaginal fornices and/or the periphery of the ectocervix. They are usually single, and the median diameter is 2.5 cm. One quarter of patients with one of these ulcers have no symptoms. The others complain of serosanguineous or watery discharge, postcoital bleeding or spotting, irregular vaginal bleeding, and/or

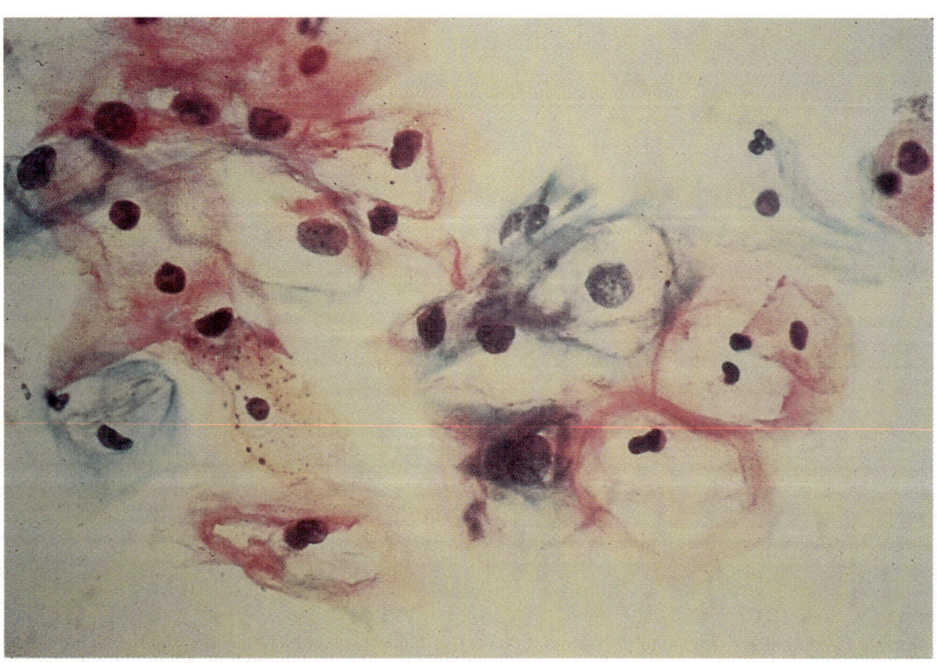

FIGURE 2-16
Multiple koilocytes are shown. A large clear space surrounds the nucleus. The peripheral cytoplasm is dense and folded at the edge of the cavity. Only the cells with an abnormal nucleus surrounded by a cavity are considered koilocytes.

pain. Surgical excision with primary closure is curative. Spontaneous healing occurs in 50 percent of cases.

All treatments for condyloma acuminatum should be considered only cosmetic, since the virus is resilient and recurrences are common.[31] Persistent or chronically recurrent warts should be submitted for biopsy to exclude a premalignant or malignant process. Patients who have florid and persistent warts should also be tested for human immunodeficiency virus (HIV) infection, since such lesions are the presenting complaint of many women with acquired immunodeficiency syndrome (AIDS).[32]

Herpes simplex virus (HSV) infections, both type 1 and type 2, occur in the cervix and the vulva. It is possible but unlikely that this virus causes vaginitis. The thickness of the vaginal epithelium and the lack of well-developed nerve endings in the vagina almost preclude infection with HSV. When HSV is associated with an abnormal vaginal discharge, the cause is usually superficial ulcerations of the cervix (Fig. 2–17). The cervical lesions produce a watery, serosanguineous discharge. The lesions begin as vesicles, and then the surface of the lesion breaks open and an ulcer base remains (Fig. 2–18). Pain is usually not a hallmark unless there is involvement at the level of the introitus or the rest of the vulva. The diagnosis of HSV infection is often confirmed by culture or by direct antigen or nucleic acid testing. HSV causes characteristic cellular changes that can be identified in cytologic preparations of the cervix and vagina (Fig. 2–19). The diagnostic cells on cervical/vaginal smears are enlarged and multinucleated. The nuclei mold to each other and have a characteristic ground-glass appearance. This is caused by the proliferation of viral particles pushing aside the nuclear chromatin so that it forms a rim against the nuclear membrane. A large red or blue viral inclusion surrounded by a ground-glass halo is sometimes seen in older lesions.

Currently the most widely used effective therapy for HSV infection is acyclovir.[33] This medication is usually administered orally, but on occasion it is given intravenously. Foscarnet, an agent used to treat cytomegalovirus (another virus in the herpes family) infection, is probably also effective against HSV. Its hematologic toxicity makes it a less desirable alternative, however.

In the past it was thought that HSV played an important role in the genesis of cervical intraepithelial neoplasia (CIN). It is now believed that HSV infection is a marker for individuals at risk for other sexually transmitted diseases such as HPV infection, which is associated with the development of CIN and cancer.

Fungal Infections

Fungal vaginitis is one of the most frequent problems encountered in the gynecologist's office. The most common causative agent is *Candida albicans*. This organism causes significant vaginal and vulvar pruritus and is often associated with a white, curdy discharge and white plaques on the vaginal walls. *C. albicans* and other *Candida* spe-

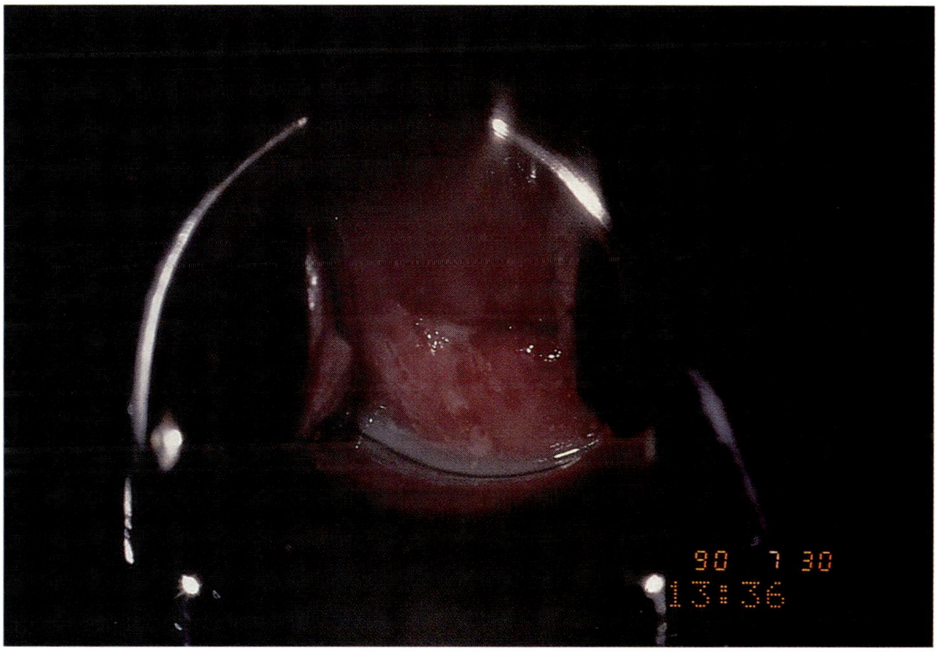

FIGURE 2-17
This cervix has lesions secondary to HSV infection. Multiple superficial small ulcers are present. Some coalesce, forming a serpiginous pattern.

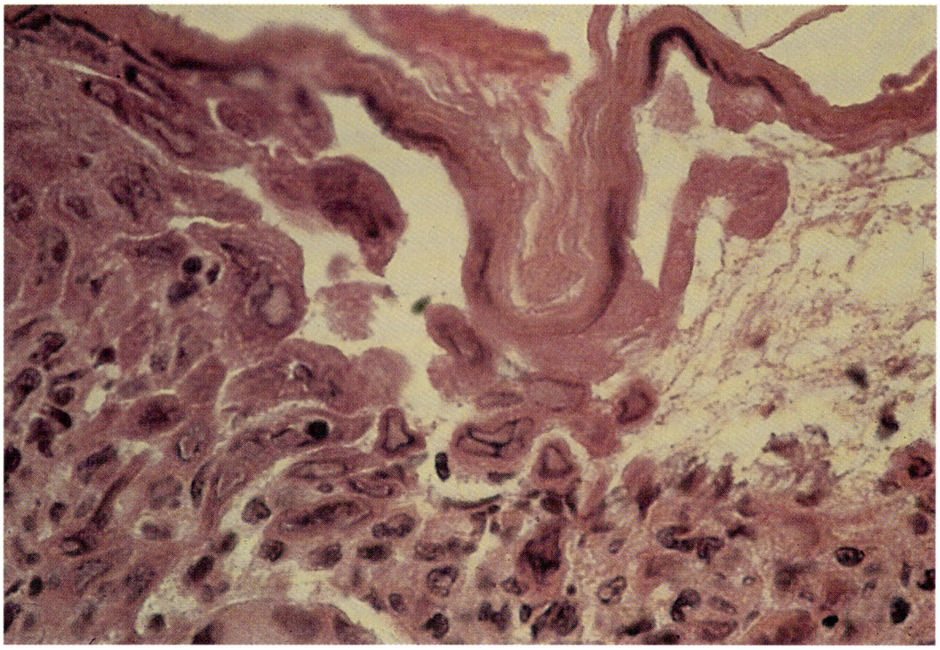

FIGURE 2-18
A histologic section of the edge of a herpetic lesion is shown. A vesicle is seen on the right, with the surface epithelium still intact but separated from the base. Some of the infected cells are multinucleated. The nuclei have an opaque, ground-glass appearance with a rim of dense chromatin.

cies are found in the vagina of up to 25 percent of women without causing symptoms. However, if the underlying bacterial flora is disturbed or if the intracellular glycogen stores increase, this fungus proliferates and may become the dominant species. This can lead to symptoms. Other *Candida* species that can become pathogenic include *C. tropicalis* and *C. parapsilosis. C. glabrata,* previously known as *Torulopsis glabrata,* is also frequently encountered in the vagina and can cause symptoms if it becomes dominant. *C. albicans, C. tropicalis,* and *C. parapsilosis* are all organisms that produce pseudohyphae and budding yeasts or blastospores. *C. glabrata* forms only blastospores, so it is more difficult to diagnose. The diagnosis of a vaginal fungal infection can be made only by microscopic examination of the secretions. This is usually accomplished by mixing a sample of the vaginal secretions with 10 to 20 percent potassium hydroxide and examining the specimen at 100× and 400× magnification. The presence of pseudohyphae or blastospores is diagnostic in the sympto-

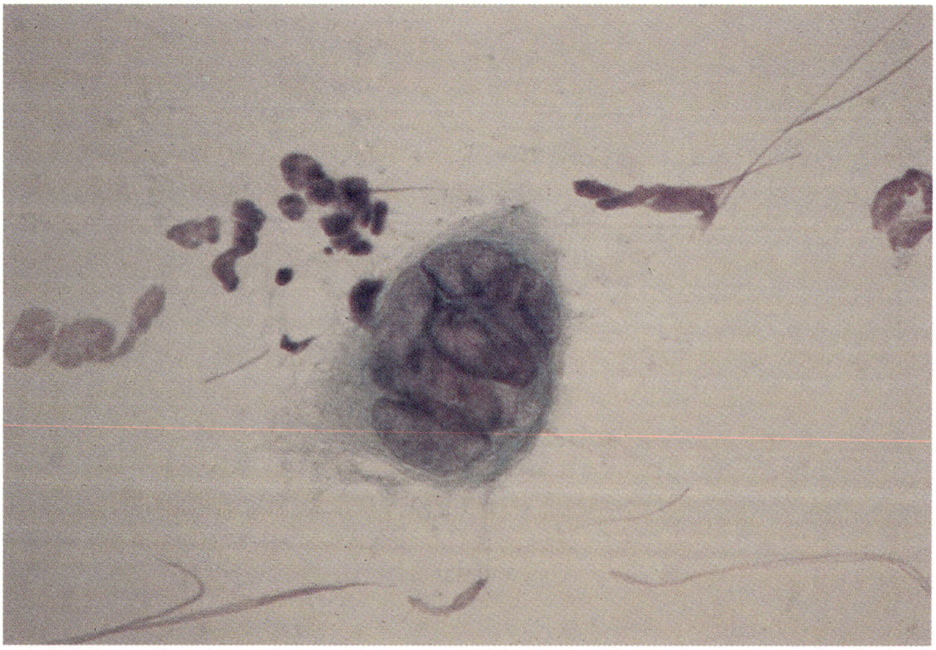

FIGURE 2-19
This smear shows a large multinucleated cell, diagnostic of HSV infection. The nuclei are molded. The centers of the nuclei have a ground-glass appearance surrounded by a dense rim of chromatin.

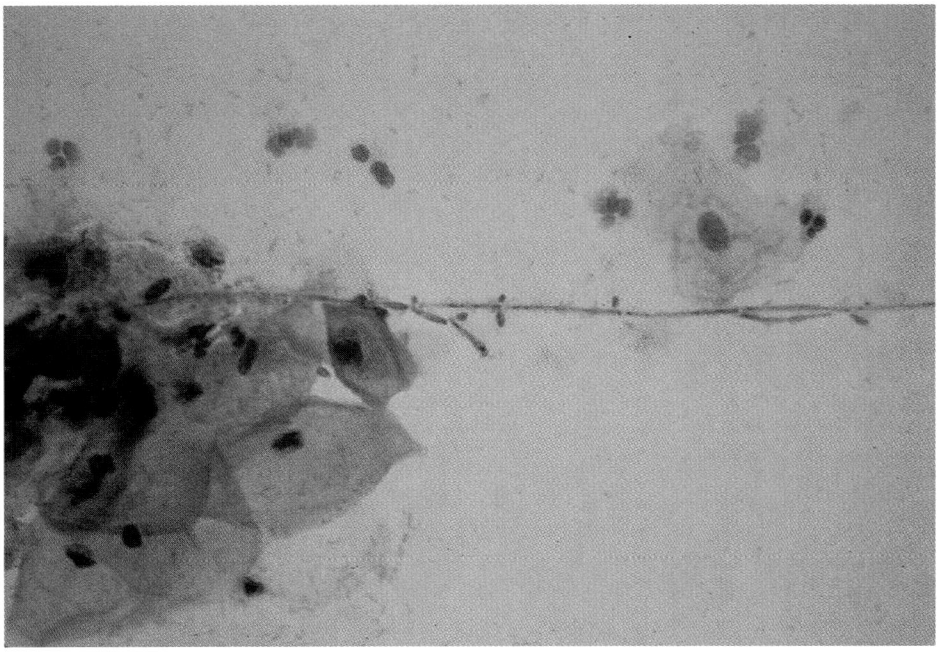

FIGURE 2-20
This vaginal smear shows pseudohyphae and blastospores, characteristic of *Candida* species. A sheet of squamous cells is also present.

matic patient. *Candida* infection can also be diagnosed by Papanicolaou smear (Fig. 2–20). It is common to see reactive and inflammatory changes in the squamous cells in the presence of candidal infection. It is important to note that patients who are asymptomatic and who harbor *C. albicans* as a commensal organism do not usually have the pseudohyphal morphotype but do have budding yeast forms. Obtaining a culture in an asymptomatic patient is counterproductive and may lead to unnecessary treatment.

The hallmark of a *Candida* infection is not the presence of a discharge but the presence of pruritus. One can mistake physiologic changes that occur in the middle of the menstrual cycle for evidence of fungal vaginitis. The increased production of cervical mucus and the desquamation of epithelial cells result in a thick, cottage cheese–like discharge that can be clinically misdiagnosed as a *Candida* infection. This results in the inappropriate treatment of a physiologic process with antifungal agents. Only the patient who has clinical signs and symptoms consistent with *Candida* infection and who has organisms confirmed by microscopy should be treated. Administration of one of the many topical imidazole formulations (e.g., miconazole, clotrimazole, terconazole) is usually effective. Patients with resistant infections can be treated with boric acid suppositories or with oral ketoconazole.[34, 35] Fluconazole and itraconazole, two recently introduced systemic antifungal agents that may be effective against vaginal fungal infections, are usually reserved for more serious systemic cases. Painting of the vulva and vaginal walls with gentian violet can be messy but is often successful.

Trauma

Traumatic vaginal injuries occur in both children and adults. In children, they are often related to sexual activity and usually associated with sexual assault. The most common site of traumatic vaginal injury in the child is in the introitus; this is due to forceful entry through its narrow caliber. When full penetration occurs the vaginal walls can also be damaged. These injuries can be severe and may result in significant blood loss that sometimes necessitates transfusion. Other vaginal injuries during childhood are those secondary to traumatic falls. These injuries usually involve the perineal body and may result in periurethral and hymenal tears. One of the adverse sequelae of these injuries is the scarring that may occur after the repair. To preclude scarring in prepubertal girls, the insertion of an intravaginal mold or the use of intravaginal estrogen has been suggested.[36]

Traumatic injury to the adult vagina can be due to coitus. Bleeding can occur from the hymenal ring at the time of the first intercourse; periurethral tears may also occur at this time. The majority of clinically significant nonobstetric vaginal tears in the adult occur in the vaginal vault and are most common in the posterior fornix. These usually appear as semilunar lacerations below the cervix at the vaginal reflection. They may extend to the parametrium and involve large pelvic vessels. Although these injuries are most commonly seen in premenopausal, sexually active women and are the result of vigorous sexual activity, they also occur in older patients. Traumatic vaginal injuries in adults have been associated with excessive alcohol intake. Surgical repair of the laceration is the only treatment. Although the vagina is colonized by a large number of bacteria, antibiotics are rarely needed. A thorough evaluation is necessary to exclude trauma to neighboring organs.

Traumatic ulcers are also seen in patients who have complete vaginal prolapse. Placement of the vagina back into its normal position, either by surgery or by use of a pessary, allows the ulcer to heal. Since this situation usually affects postmenopausal women, topical estrogen is used to assist in the healing process by stimulating the maturation of the vaginal epithelium.

Traumatic ulcerations of the vagina and cervix heal by the processes of reepithelialization and granulation. Cells scraped from the edge or base of a traumatic ulcer are seen on the cytologic preparation as sheets of proliferating epithelial cells that have been stimulated by the healing process (Fig. 2–21). The cells are large and form cohesive groups. These groups usually have a streaming appearance with all the cells oriented in the same direction. The nuclei are usually large, and the nucleoli are very prominent and often multiple. This cytologic appearance is termed repair and is a benign cellular change. Repair must be distinguished from carcinoma, particularly from adenocarcinoma, which may have similar nuclear features. This distinction is best done by recognizing the orientation of the groups of cells and the uniformity of the cell size and nuclear patterns.

Genital prolapse or some other process that causes recurring traumatic friction of the cervix or vagina leads to thickening of the epithelial layers by development of a surface maturation to parakeratosis and hyperkeratosis. Hyperkeratotic and parakeratotic cells are present on the surface of the normal skin, as is found in the vulva. Such epithelium is keratinized squamous, as opposed to the vaginal and cervical epithelium, which is normally nonkeratinized. If individual hyperkeratotic cells are seen on a cervical/vaginal smear, they may have come from the vulva. To make a cytologic diagnosis of vaginal or cervical hyperkeratosis or parakeratosis it is necessary to see groups, sheets, or plaques of cells that display those characteristics.

Hyperkeratotic plaques are composed of sheets of cells that do not have intact nuclei. The cytoplasm usually has increased keratinization. When the Papanicolaou stain is used, the cytoplasmic staining varies from pinkish to orange and yellow. Parakeratotic cells look like miniature squamous cells. They have a normal nuclear to cytoplasmic ratio, but the cell size is small and the nuclei are pyknotic and round to oval. Cytoplasmic keratinization in parakeratosis is similar to that seen in hyperkeratosis.

Almost all cases of hyperkeratosis and parakeratosis are due to a benign process. Of 170 women evaluated by colposcopy for a Papanicolaou smear with hyperkeratosis or parakeratosis, only six (3.5

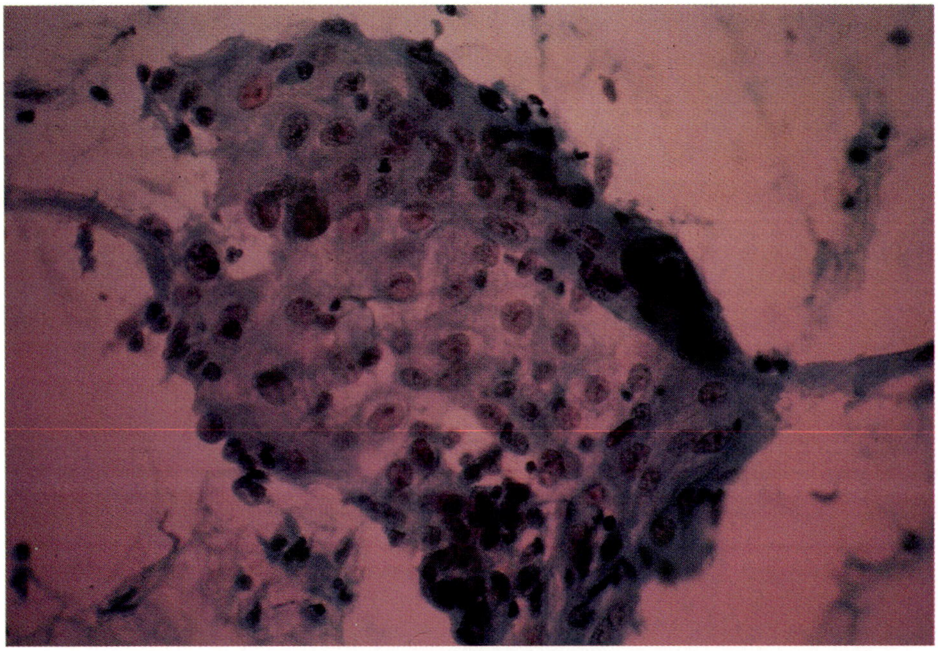

FIGURE 2–21
This vaginal smear shows changes consistent with repair. The patient from whom the smear was obtained had a vaginal ulcer caused by long-term use of a pessary. The sheet of squamous cells is cohesive. The cells at the bottom are orienting themselves in the same direction. The nuclei are enlarged, and the nucleoli are prominent.

percent) were found to have CIN, and in all six patients it was CIN 1.[36a] There are very rare cases of invasive keratinizing cervical cancer with a surface reaction that may shed hyperkeratotic or parakeratotic cells. Owing to this, in a patient who has had multiple smears that show hyperkeratosis or parakeratosis or if this finding is associated with any unusual sign or symptom, we suggest colposcopic examination of the cervix and vagina.

Cellular repair, hyperkeratosis, and parakeratosis in the absence of cellular atypia are classified under benign cellular changes by the Bethesda System for reporting cervical/vaginal cytologic diagnoses (see Chapter 3). If atypia is present, a cytopathologic diagnosis of atypical squamous cells of undetermined significance is made.

Benign Neoplasms

Benign neoplastic lesions of the vagina can be cystic or solid. The cystic lesions include Gartner cyst, epidermal inclusion cyst, endometriosis, and adenosis. These latter two conditions can also present as solid lesions.

A Gartner cyst usually occurs on the anterolateral wall of the vagina as a soft, nontender, thin-walled cystic structure. It is derived from wolffian (mesonephric) duct remnants. It is usually 2 to 4 cm in diameter and rarely presents a clinical problem. It is more commonly identified serendipitously at the time of routine pelvic examination. If it is small and asymptomatic it does not need to be removed. If it is associated with symptoms (e.g., dyspareunia) and its removal is technically difficult, marsupialization with biopsy of the cyst wall to confirm the clinical diagnosis is sufficient treatment. The cyst is filled with clear to light yellow fluid. Examination of the cyst wall shows that it is lined by a single layer of cuboidal or low columnar epithelium that may be ciliated. Occasionally the epithelium is flattened. Malignancy in a Gartner cyst has not been described.

The epithelial or epidermal inclusion cyst is common in the scalp and other areas of the skin but may also be found in the vagina, where it is usually the result of trauma or surgery. It is usually located in the posterior wall of the distal third of the vagina. An epithelial inclusion cyst is the result of infolding and incorporation of the vaginal epithelium into the submucosal stroma. A cystic space is filled by the continually proliferating epithelium with exfoliation of squamous cells and degenerated keratin. The cyst is lined by stratified squamous epithelium. The cyst content is yellow, thick, and caseous. Epithelial inclusion cysts are often misdiagnosed as granulomas. They can be associated with dyspareunia. These structures do not undergo malignant change and can be easily removed by surgical excision.

Vaginal endometriosis usually manifests as one or more red or blue-red, 2 to 5 mm cystic lesions in the posterior vaginal fornix. Clinically this condition may be confused with a hemangioma. The lesions, subject to cyclic hormonal change, may be completely excised and examined for diagnosis. The microscopic appearance is one of hemosiderin-laden macrophages associated with endometrial stroma with scanty or absent endometrial glands. These findings are no different from those in endometriosis found at other sites.

Vaginal adenosis occurs in the upper vagina and presents as a small cystic lesion (Fig. 2–22) or as solid, reddened epithelium that resembles a cervical ectropion. Owing to abnormal stromal development the epithelium can also be thrown onto firm, transverse ridges in the anterior vaginal fornix, including the upper ectocervix. The term "cockscomb cervix" is used to describe this finding (Fig. 2–23). This change is frequently associated with intrauterine exposure to DES before the 18th week of gestation but also occurs in patients who have no history of such exposure. Prenatal DES exposure prevents the transformation of the mucus-secreting columnar epithelium of the müllerian duct to squamous epithelium.[1] DES can also cause disorganization of the stromal proliferation that forms the cervix and other segments of the genital canal walls. This, in turn, causes the cockscomb cervix.

In adenosis the epithelium forms glandular structures lined by tall columnar, mucus-producing cells similar to those of the endocervix. The nuclei are uniformly located at the base of the epithelium and the vacuolated cytoplasm toward the lumen. When the adenosis glands are occluded by the transformation of the surface epithelium into squamous epithelium, a cyst develops from accumulation of mucus. This cyst resembles the nabothian cyst of the cervix and may look yellow or bluish (see Fig. 2–22). A single such cyst in the vagina is referred to as a mucinous cyst.

Benign solid neoplasms of the vagina include polyp, leiomyoma, papilloma, and hemangioma. Simple epithelial polyps are unusual but important to recognize, since they can be confused with sarcoma botryoides (see Chapter 4). This benign type of polyp is most often found in older women, while sarcoma botryoides is found in infants. Benign vaginal polyps are firm, irregular lesions measuring 1 to 2 cm in diameter. They have a central core of thick vessels embedded in a loose myxoid stroma that contains pleomorphic spindle-

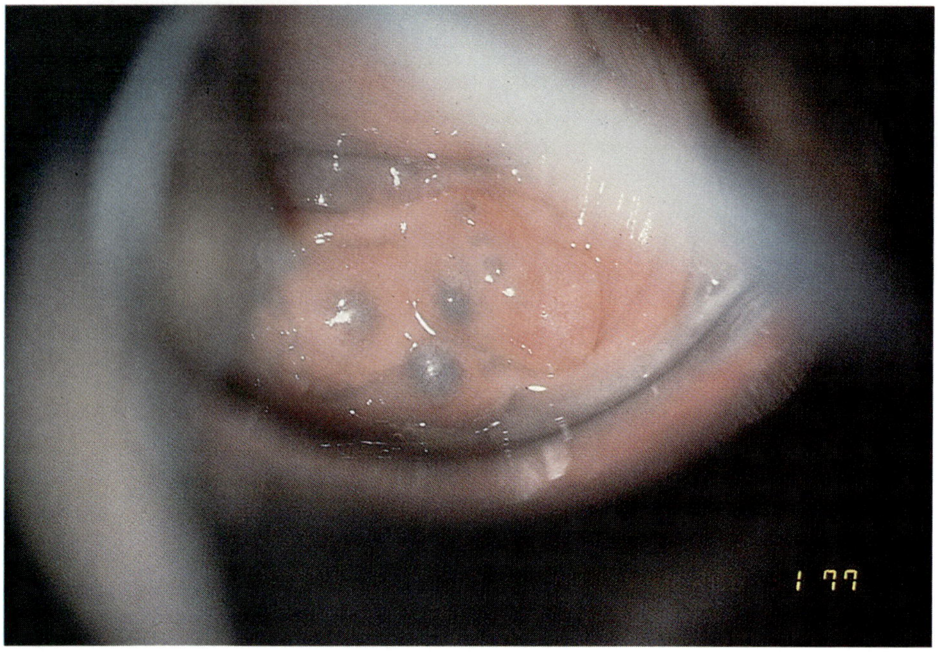

FIGURE 2-22
Several small blue cysts are seen in the superior aspect of this patient's posterior vaginal wall. She had a history of intrauterine exposure to diethylstilbestrol. Biopsy of one of the lesions showed changes consistent with adenosis (i.e., columnar, mucin-secreting cells lining glandular structures).

shaped cells. The surface is covered by normal vaginal mucosa. These polyps do not recur after excision.[37] Mucosal tags may look like a polyp. They are found in the lower vagina and are the result of healing following trauma. They are composed of epithelium and dense connective tissue, but they lack the central core of thick blood vessels that is the hallmark of a polyp.

Leiomyoma or vaginal fibroma is another seldom-seen vaginal tumor.[38] It is a firm nodule that is present beneath the mucosa of the lateral vaginal walls. Vaginal leiomyoma is usually a solitary lesion that, like its uterine counterpart, can attain large size. These lesions can be associated with dyspareunia or may cause dystocia during labor and delivery. Some women with a vaginal leiomyoma experience no symptoms. The leiomyoma is well circumscribed and on cut section appears off-white and dense. The tumor is composed of smooth muscle bundles arranged in whorls. It can undergo the same degenerative changes seen in a uterine leiomyoma (see Chapter 5). Other lesions that are rarely encountered in the vagina include hemangiomas,[39] pigmented lesions,[40–43] and tumors of

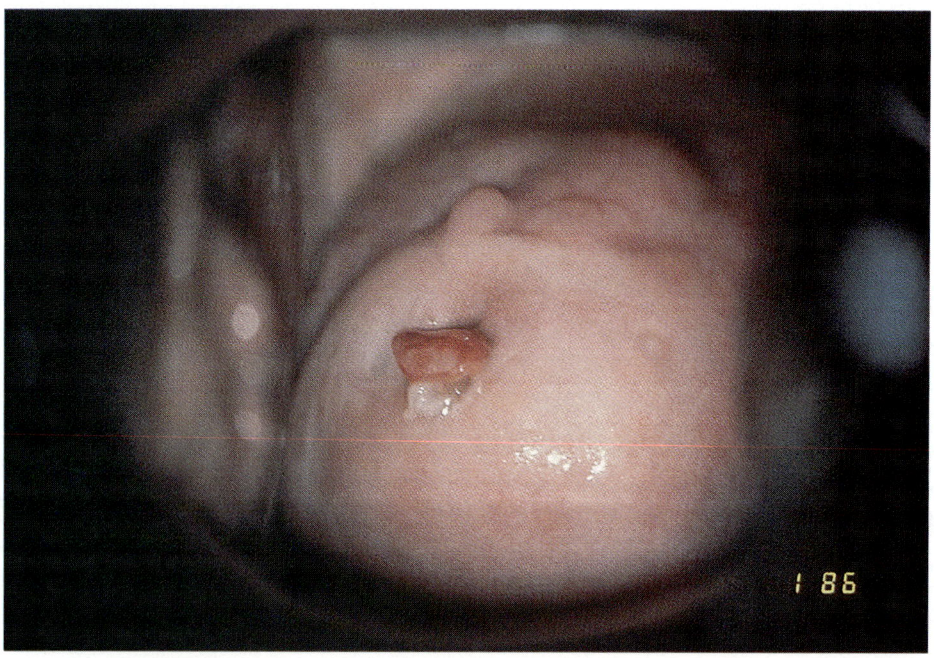

FIGURE 2-23
This cervix has a reddish endocervical polyp at the os. Several mucosal elevations are present on the anterior ectocervix of this patient, who was exposed in utero to diethylstilbestrol. These anterior cervical mucosal ridges are identified by the term "cockscomb cervix."

neural and perineural origin (e.g., neurofibroma, granular cell tumor, and paraganglioma).[44–48]

Miscellaneous Conditions

Fistulae

Vesicovaginal and rectovaginal fistulae usually are secondary to obstetric trauma or are a complication of surgery or radiation therapy.[49–51] Enterovaginal, colovaginal, and rectovaginal fistulae can occur after radiation or surgery or may be secondary to an inflammatory process (e.g., Crohn disease, diverticulitis, perirectal abscess).[52–55] Any of the above fistulae can also be secondary to cancer. Ureterovaginal fistulae are invariably a postsurgical complication. Examination of the fistula tract shows fibroconnective tissue associated with an inflammatory infiltrate. The tract may have become epithelialized by epithelium of the same type as that of one or both of the interconnecting organs (i.e., squamous, urothelial, columnar). Descriptions of the surgical management of fistulae can be found in a gynecologic surgery textbook.[56]

Suburethral Diverticulum

The suburethral diverticulum is an uncommon finding in the anterior vaginal wall. It is usually present in the middle or distal third as a mass or induration. Symptoms are usually urinary and include dysuria, frequency, and postmicturitional dribbling. Pus or urine may be expressed from the urethral meatus by pressing on the anterior vaginal wall mass. The diagnosis is confirmed by cystourethroscopy or radiographic studies utilizing a contrast agent (e.g., voiding cystourethrogram).[57] The origin of this lesion is not clear. It has been suggested that it is the result of obstruction and infection in paraurethral glands, with subsequent drainage into the urethral lumen.[57]

Suburethral diverticula may be single or multiple. They range in size between 0.5 and 6 cm but are usually between 2 and 3 cm. The opening of the diverticulum is into the posterior urethral wall. The ostium measures between 1 and 3 mm. The sac of the diverticulum may be lined by squamous, urothelial or columnar epithelium. In some cases the lining is not identifiable, and only granulation tissue is present. The wall of the diverticulum is thick and made up of fibromuscular tissue that has a dense inflammatory infiltrate of polymorphonuclear neutrophils and lymphocytes. Rare cases of adenocarcinoma, squamous cell carcinoma, and transitional cell carcinoma in such a diverticulum have been reported.[57] The diverticulum may contain urine, pus, or stones. Culture of the contents shows common urinary pathogens (e.g., *E. coli, Streptococcus faecalis, Proteus,* and *Pseudomonas*).

The treatment of choice is excision of the diverticulum through an anterior vaginal wall incision. The urethral and vaginal defects are closed in layers using a fine absorbable suture. In cases of very distal diverticula, a meatotomy that incises the urethral floor to the level of the diverticulum may be performed. The diverticular sac is marsupialized by suturing it to the vaginal mucosa.

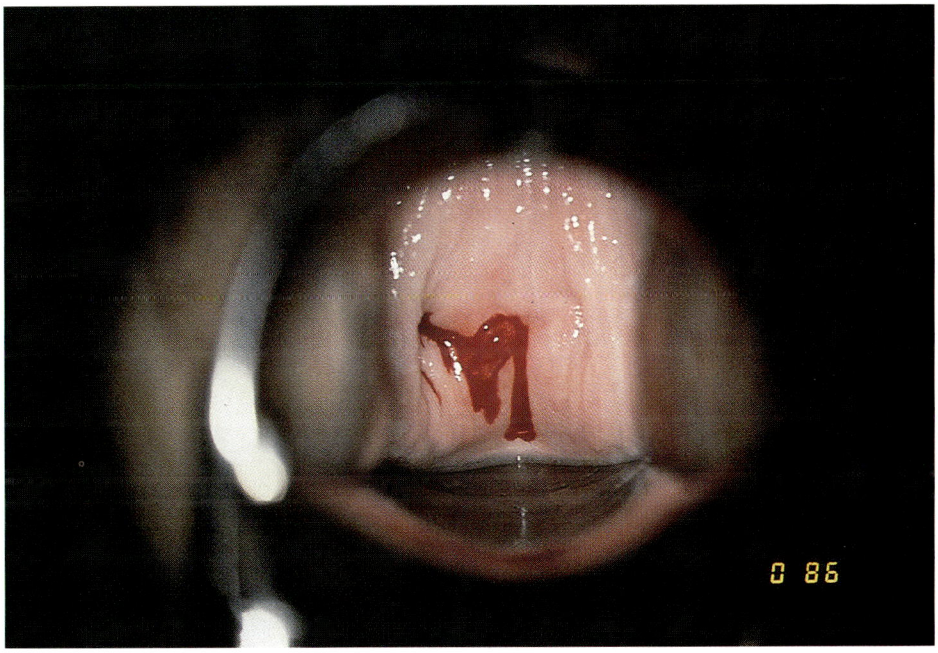

FIGURE 2-24
Red, friable granulation tissue is seen at the vaginal cuff in a patient who had recently undergone a vaginal hysterectomy. Manipulation of the lesion caused the patient no pain; in contrast, pain is invariably experienced when the lesion is a prolapsed fallopian tube. The patient's surgery was for a benign condition, and cancer is not a consideration in this case. The granulation tissue was cauterized using silver nitrate, which resulted in normal healing.

Granulation Tissue

Granulation tissue is often seen at the vaginal cuff following total hysterectomy. On examination it is an irregular, raised, red tissue nodule that bleeds easily on touch (Fig. 2–24). This can be confused with a prolapsed fallopian tube, which may occur as a complication following vaginal hysterectomy but is not usual after an abdominal hysterectomy. Manipulation of the prolapsed fallopian tube causes severe pain that is referred to the patient's flank. This does not occur with granulation tissue. A Papanicolaou smear from an area of granulation tissue shows reparative cellular changes (see Fig. 2–21). Granulation tissue must be differentiated from a neoplastic process, particularly recurrent carcinoma in the patient who has has been treated for uterine or cervical cancer.

THE CERVIX

Anatomy

The cervix is a solid, cylindrical structure approximately 2.5 to 3.0 cm in diameter and 3.0 to 5.0 cm in length. It is continuous with the body of the uterus, and it may constitute up to one third of the uterine length. Inferiorly the cervix projects into the vagina as the portio vaginalis, and the epithelium is continuous with that of the upper vagina (Fig. 2–25). The cervix is derived from the fused müllerian ducts, and its shape is the result of subepithelial stromal condensation.[1] Wolffian duct remnants are incorporated into the cervical stroma. The epithelium of the ectocervix is the result of transformation of the columnar epithelium that lines the müllerian ducts into stratified squamous epithelium.

The ectocervix projects into the upper vagina and is covered by nonkeratinized, stratified squamous epithelium that becomes continuous with the vaginal epithelium (Fig. 2–26). The endocervix extends from the cervical os to the lower uterine segment endometrium, and it is lined by a single layer of tall columnar, mucin-producing cells. The nucleus is located at the base of the cell. The cytoplasm may be clear, vacuolated, mucinous, or eosinophilic. Although these cells usually are nonciliated, ciliated cells may be present. Small reserve cells are seen between the columnar cells and the basement membrane. The endocervical epithelium also lines endocervical glands that penetrate the endocervical stroma and form an intricate system of interconnecting clefts. These glands have a lumen that allows the secretions to enter the endocervical canal. The cervical stroma is fibroconnective tissue that contains collagen and elastin.[58] Smooth muscle is also found in small amounts. The amount of smooth muscle in the cervix increases as the lower uterine segment is approached.

The epithelium of the ectocervix is similar to that of the vagina (see above). The junction of the columnar epithelium of the endocervix with the squamous epithelium of the ectocervix is the squamocolumnar junction. The anatomic location of this junction varies among patients and throughout a woman's life. While the squamocolumnar

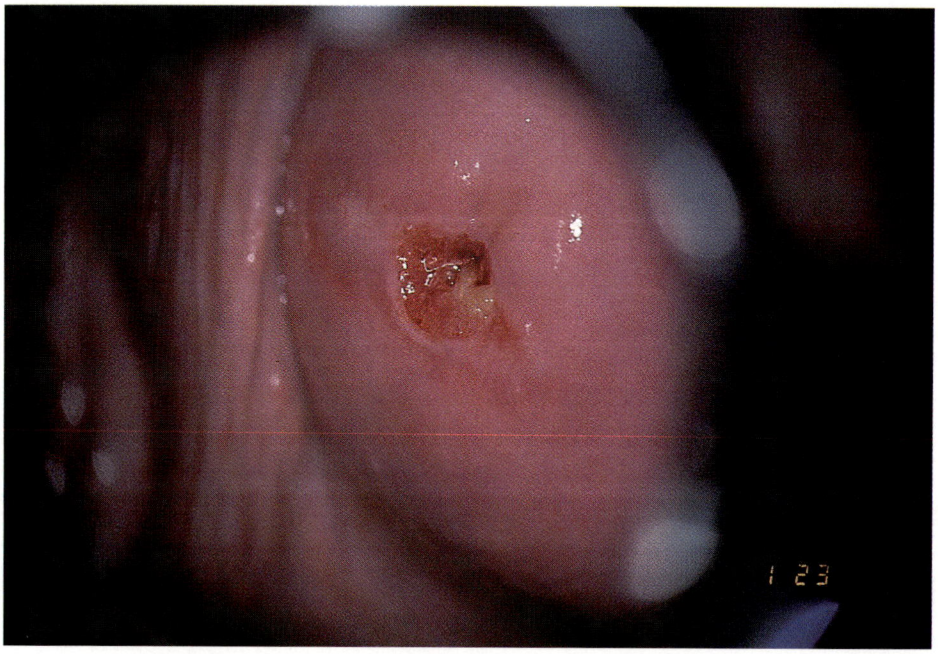

FIGURE 2–25
A normal cervix is shown in the center. The right vaginal wall is on the left and the posterior fornix at the bottom left. There is scant, thick mucus in the cervical os, consistent with progesterone effect. The cervical os is round, consistent with a history of no vaginal deliveries. The squamous epithelium of the cervix and vagina is pink. The columnar epithelium of the endocervix is seen at the os and is red. The pale area with slightly dilated overlying vessels at the 10 o'clock position on the cervix is a nabothian cyst.

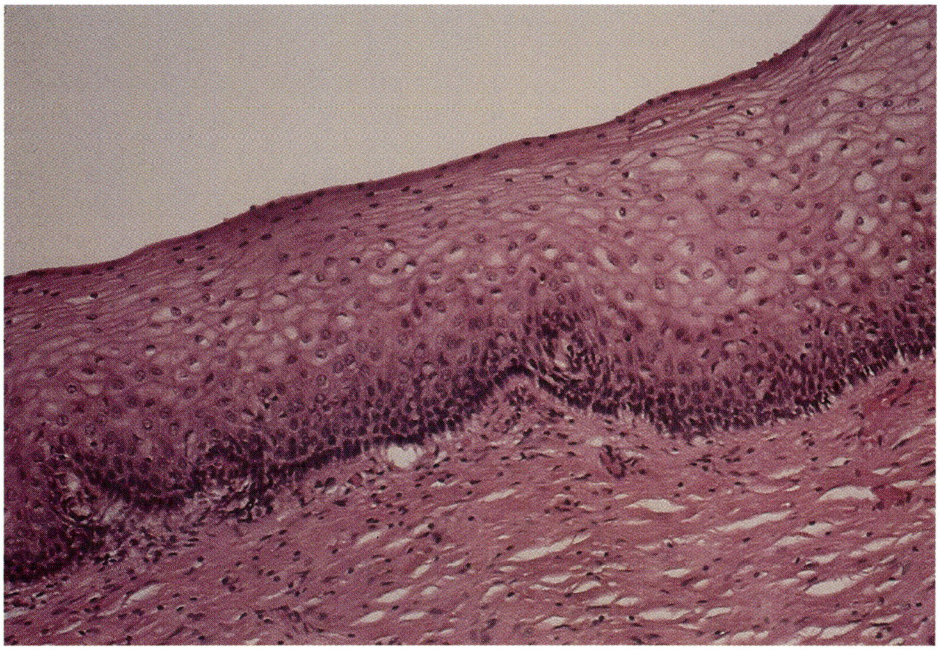

FIGURE 2-26
This cervical biopsy shows normal stratified nonkeratinizing squamous epithelium. The appearance and organization of the cells are similar to those seen in the vagina. The epithelial-stromal junction does not have the saw-toothed appearance that is seen in the vagina (see Fig. 2–4).

junction may be seen at the portio in a young woman, it is usually high in the endocervical canal in the postmenopausal woman. The columnar epithelium at the portio is converted to the more resistant squamous epithelium as the woman ages. This process is known as squamous metaplasia (Fig. 2–27). This transformation zone is particularly important in the development of CIN and is described in detail in Chapter 3.

The cervical epithelium responds to the cyclic ovarian hormones levels just as the vagina does. Under the influence of estrogen there is an increase in the layers of squamous cells. Estrogen stimulates the endocervical cells to produce more mucus. This increased mucus production peaks close to midcycle. The mucus produced as result of estrogen stimulation is thin, copious, and very elastic and aligns itself in parallel tubules of micelles made up of glycoproteins. This is seen as a fern pattern as the mucus is spread on a slide. This alignment of micelles is responsible for the elastic property of the mucus known as spinnbarkeit. The alignment of micelles facilitates the migration of spermatozoa into the upper genital

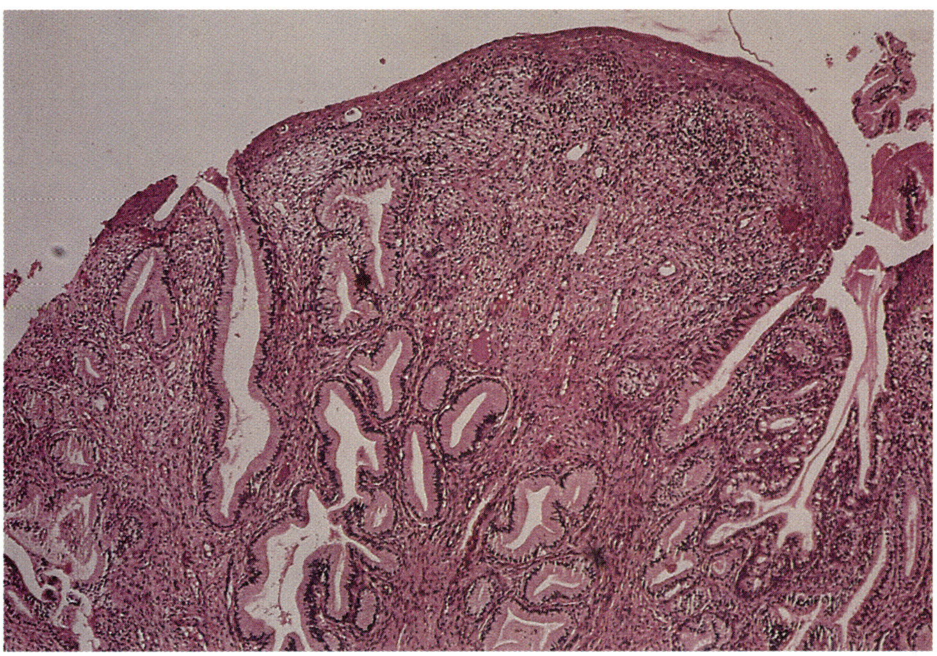

FIGURE 2-27
This biopsy specimen from the transformation zone shows normal endocervical glands in the cervical stroma and squamous metaplasia on the surface. The glands are lined by a single layer of tall columnar cells. The nuclei are at the base. Some of the glands are cut on cross section. The longitudinally cut glands show their lumens opening into the area of squamous metaplasia. The stroma has a lymphoid infiltrate seen best at the surface.

tract. After ovulation there is an increase in progesterone production; this results in the loss of the tubular alignment of the micelles, and the mucus becomes thick and tenacious (see Fig. 2–25). This cervical mucus phenomenon can best be observed by examining a cervical mucus specimen a day or two before ovulation and then after ovulation in the secretory (luteal) phase of the menstrual cycle. If ovulation does not occur there is no change in the mucus. In a postcoital specimen the movement of spermatozoa in the mucus obtained before ovulation is predominantly parallel, bidirectional, and progressive. The movement in mucus obtained during the luteal phase is disorganized. The qualities of the cervical mucus observed during the luteal phase are also seen in women taking the combined (estrogen and progestogen) oral contraceptives as well as in women taking a progestogen only. This includes medroxyprogesterone acetate, the progestogen-only (mini) pill, and the progestogen-containing Silastic implants (Norplant, Wyeth-Ayerst Laboratories). Through their effect on the cervical mucus these hormone formulations interfere with the ability of spermatozoa to reach the upper genital tract, although this is not the major mechanism of their contraceptive activity. An advantage of the tenacious, thick mucus is that it can block the ascent of microorganisms from the lower to the upper genital tract. Cervical mucus also contains significant quantities of IgE and IgA. These immunoglobulins are thought to play a role in decreasing the risk of acquiring sexually transmitted infections.

During pregnancy, changes occur in the cervical squamous epithelium, the columnar epithelium, and the stroma.[59] As pregnancy progresses there is a marked increase in the vascularity and edema of the stroma. An inflammatory infiltrate is usually present. The cervix becomes patulous. The squamous epithelium may show increased proliferation of the parabasal and intermediate cell layers. An increase in glycogenated intermediate cells may be seen on Papanicolaou smears (see Fig. 2–5). These cells have very distinct cell borders and shapes and are called navicular cells. The endocervical epithelium becomes hyperplastic, and this can even be confused with adenocarcinoma. Eversion of the endocervix occurs, and the columnar epithelium is evident at the portio (Fig. 2–28). Decidualization of the stroma is seen in a small proportion of cases. When this occurs the stromal cells become plump and have enlarged, eosinophilic, granular cytoplasm.

The major blood supply of the cervix is from the descending branches of the uterine arteries. These cervical branches are found in the lateral cervical stroma. Also contributing to the blood supply of the cervix are the vaginal arteries, which are branches of the internal iliac (hypogastric) arteries. The venous drainage is to veins that follow the course of the arteries (i.e., uterine and vaginal veins) as well as into the pampiniform plexuses. The primary lymphatic drainage is to the pelvic nodes, which include the parametrial, obturator, internal iliac, and external iliac nodes.[60, 61] The secondary drainage is to the presacral, common iliac, and para-aortic lymph nodes. The sensory innervation of the cervix is from the Franken-

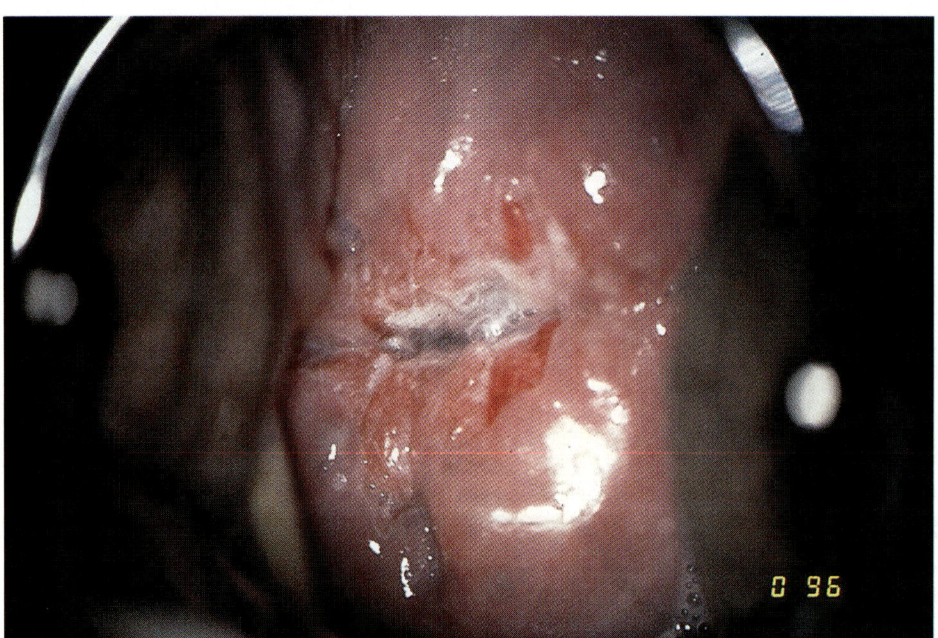

FIGURE 2–28
This cervix looks edematous, and the increased vascularity is suggested by the bluish pink color of the ectocervical epithelium. There is eversion of the endocervical epithelium, which is now present at the portio. This patient was in her last trimester of pregnancy. The cervical os is a transverse slit, which is consistent with this patient's history of previous vaginal deliveries.

häuser plexus, a terminal aspect of the superior and inferior hypogastric (presacral) plexuses. The nerves enter the lower uterine segment and upper cervix on either side at the back and form two lateral semicircular plexuses that are denser on the posterior cervix. Parasympathetic nerves from L4–S3 also innervate the cervix.

Congenital and Physiologic Changes

The major malformation of the cervix results from a lack of fusion of the paired müllerian ducts. This failure can result in duplication of the cervix and the uterus. In cases of incomplete distal fusion, the paired cervices connect to a single uterus. Cervical hypoplasia and aplasia can also occur. Another malformation is the so-called cockscomb cervix, described in the section on vaginal neoplasms. This anomaly as well as cervical rings and collars is found most commonly in females who were exposed to DES in utero. These women may also have a small uterus with a T-shaped endometrial cavity, which can be demonstrated by hysterosalpingography. This uterine anomaly has been associated with decreased fecundity and recurrent spontaneous abortions. Prenatal DES exposure has also been associated with vaginal adenosis (see above) and clear cell carcinoma of the vagina (see Chapter 4).

An anatomic variant that is frequently misdiagnosed as an epithelial erosion is the ectropion. This is the presence of columnar endocervical epithelium away from the cervical os on the portio vaginalis of the cervix (Fig. 2–29). Since the columnar epithelium is one cell thick and is more transparent than the stratified squamous epithelium, the underlying blood vessels are more apparent. This results in the area's having a beefy red, irregular appearance in contrast to the pink, smooth squamous epithelium. Since in columnar epithelium the blood vessels are found just below the surface, bleeding can occur with minimal trauma such as coitus or pelvic examination. The presence of columnar endocervical epithelium on the portio is most often seen in early puberty, when the cervical os opens and the endocervical epithelium is everted. The process of squamous metaplasia of the transformation zone is initiated by the changes in the vaginal pH that occur at menarche. This process is especially active during the second and third decades of life and during pregnancy (Fig. 2–30). This process is completed by the menopause, at which time the squamocolumnar junction is usually located within the endocervical canal.

The progressive transformation of columnar endocervical epithelium to squamous epithelium results in islands of columnar epithelium and gland openings being seen in the areas of squamous metaplasia (Fig. 2–31). The area of squamous metaplasia appears lighter in color than the native squamous epithelium, since the cells of squamous metaplasia have larger nuclei than the cells of a mature squamous epithelium and reflect light as the denser epithelium would. The gland openings in the areas of squamous metaplasia can become occluded. If there is still glandular epithelium producing mucin, this results in the

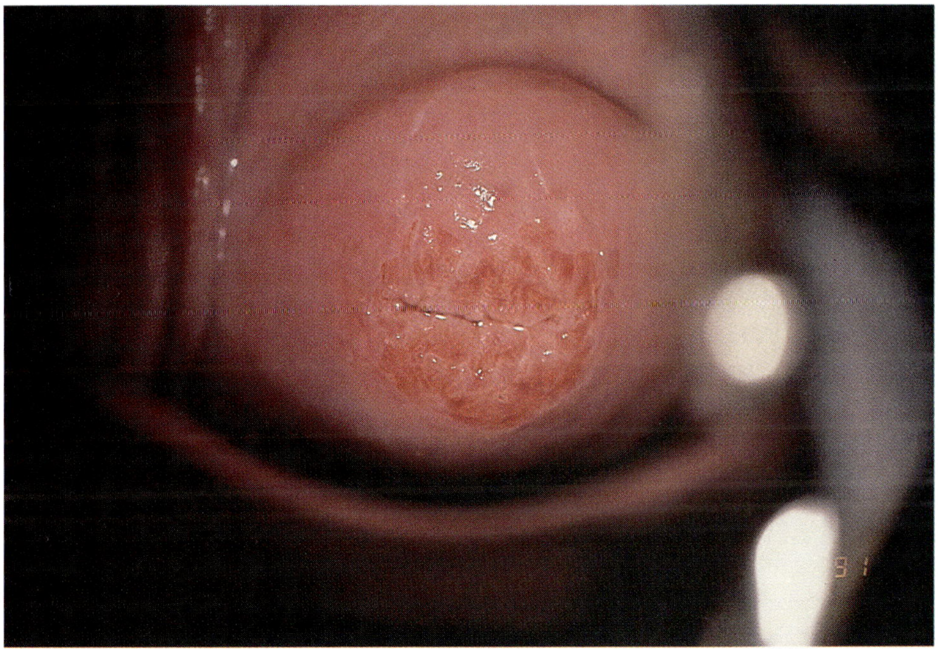

FIGURE 2–29
A normal cervix, which has an ectropion, in a nonpregnant woman is shown. The native ectocervical epithelium is shiny pink. The columnar endocervical epithelium is orange-red and extends to the portio. The cervical os is a transverse slit, which is characteristic of a parous woman. The anterior vaginal fornix is at the top of the photograph.

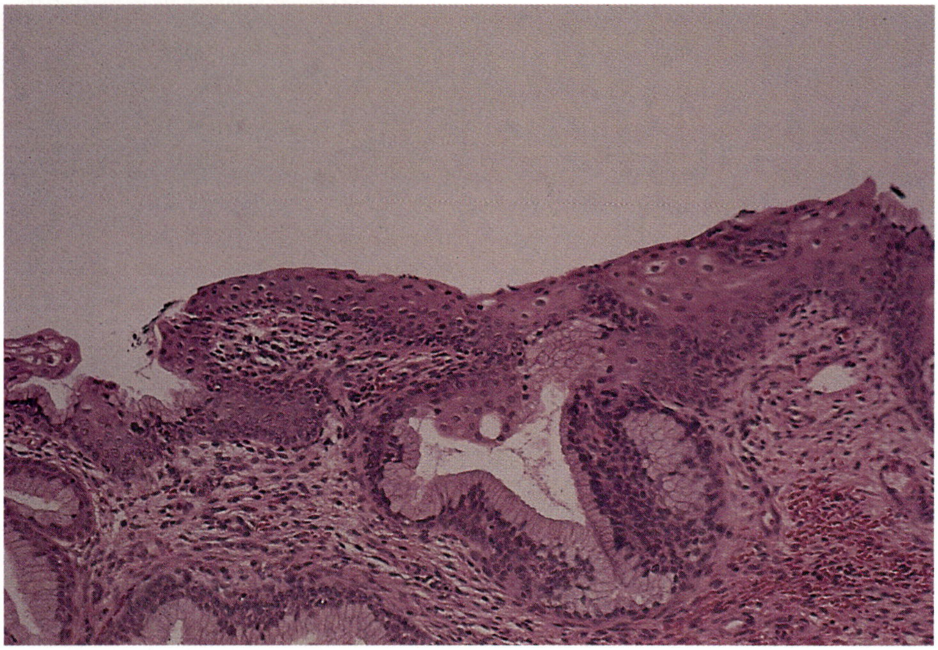

FIGURE 2-30
This biopsy specimen from the transformation zone shows squamous metaplasia and reserve cell hyperplasia. The squamous metaplasia is at the surface. It is immature (i.e., only a few layers thick) squamous epithelium. The endocervical glands show stratification of nuclei below the columnar cells. This is known as reserve cell hyperplasia. Ultimately these glands will also be replaced by squamous epithelium.

formation of a blue-domed or yellow-domed nabothian cyst. These cysts are 5 to 10 mm in diameter and frequently have overlying, normally branching, dilated blood vessels (Fig. 2–32). Nabothian cysts are benign and of no consequence. Opening the cyst with a sharp instrument, such as a needle or scalpel, results in the release of clear, odorless mucin (although this is not recommended). On microscopic examination the nabothian cyst reveals a lining of columnar, mucin-secreting cells with basally placed nuclei (Fig. 2–33). The cytoplasm of the cells is vacuolated and eosinophilic to pale. These cells empty their contents into the cyst cavity. Owing to compression the lining cells sometimes appear flattened.

Ecology

The ectocervix is bathed in the same milieu as the vaginal epithelium with which it is in continuity. Hence, the pH of the ectocervix and the organisms present on its surface is identical to that of the vagina. The mucus produced by the endocervical cells has a pH between 7.2 and 7.4. The majority

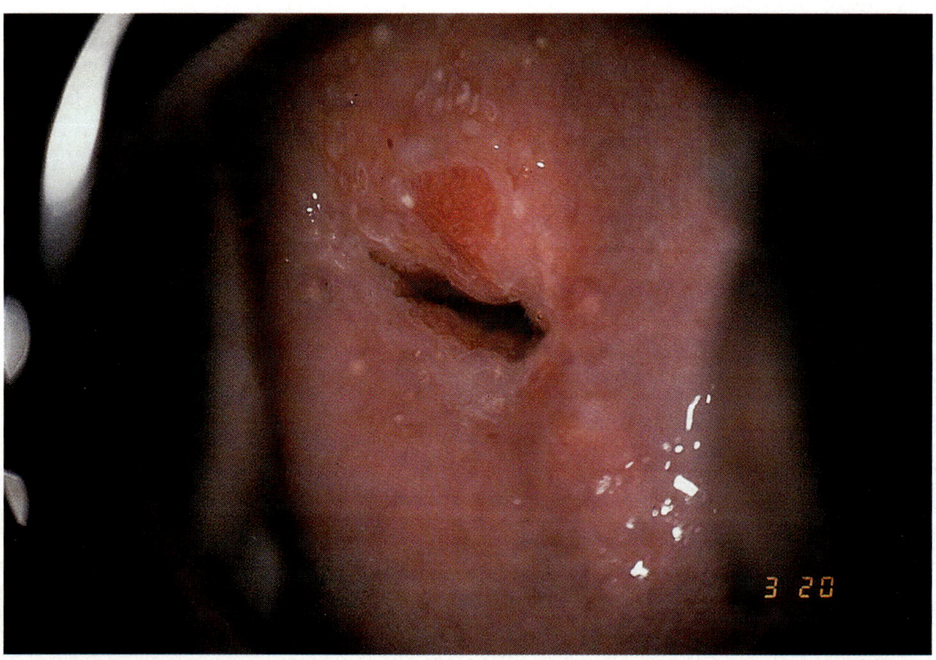

FIGURE 2-31
This cervix shows squamous metaplasia and multiple gland openings. The gland openings are the pink dots surrounded by white halos seen on the anterior ectocervix. The yellow papules are small nabothian cysts (see text). The cervical os is surrounded by faint, smooth white epithelium that blends with the pink ectocervical epithelium. This represents squamous metaplasia. An island of columnar epithelium that appears orange is seen within the squamous metaplasia on the anterior cervix at the 12 o'clock position.

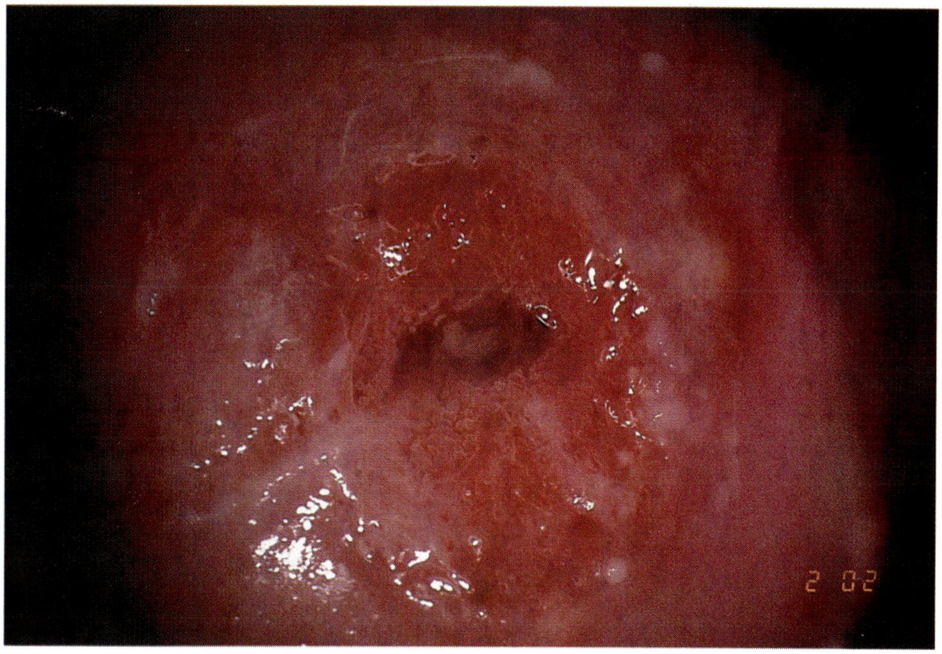

FIGURE 2-32
This cervix shows columnar epithelium surrounding the os at the portio. A yellow-domed nabothian cyst is seen at the 3 o'clock position of the ectocervix.

of commensal organisms do not tolerate this high pH, which results in little or no colonization of the endocervix. Some pathogenic species, which will be discussed, do flourish in this environment.

The cyclic change of the cervical mucus (described above), in concert with the exfoliation of the vaginal and cervical epithelial cells that proliferate under the influence of estrogen, can result in a curdy white discharge around midcycle. This may be confused with a fungal infection (see discussion of vaginal infections).

Inflammation and Infection

The cervix can be infected on the portio or in the endocervical canal. The site of infection is organism-specific, and this aids in the diagnosis and management.

Organisms infecting the portio can produce either exophytic or ulcerative lesions. These include HPV, HSV, *Treponema pallidum,* and *Haemophilus ducreyi.* Granuloma inguinale (donovanosis) rarely can infect the cervix and cause an exophytic lesion.[23]

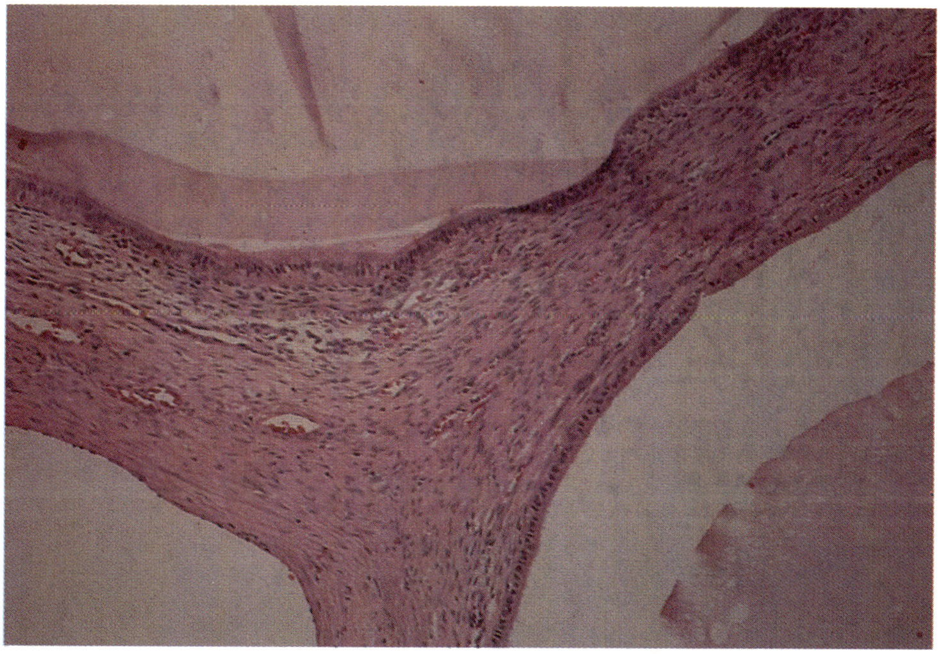

FIGURE 2-33
Three nabothian cysts are shown. The epithelial lining varies from tall columnar to flattened.

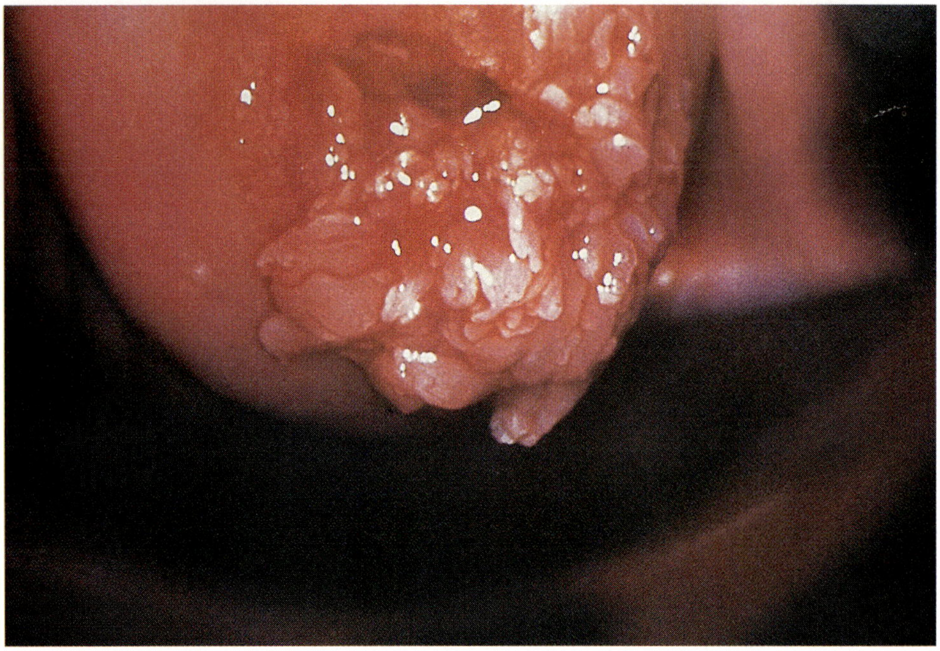

FIGURE 2-34
These finger-like projections on the posterior ectocervix are characteristic of condyloma acuminatum. The cervical os is seen above the lesion.

HPV can infect the ectocervix and cause warty lesions similar to those seen in the vagina or on the vulva (Fig. 2–34). However, cervical infection with this virus commonly results in papular or macular lesions (flat warts). Although the flat wart may not be readily seen, its visualization can be enhanced by swabbing the cervix with 3 to 5 percent acetic acid (white vinegar). This causes the area of involvement to become visible as a white plaque. The term aceto-white is used to describe this finding. This appearance may be confused with that of squamous metaplasia or of the more advanced lesions of CIN, which are discussed in Chapter 3. HPV lesions are flat and faint (Fig. 2–35). Their borders are indistinct and may be feathered. The lesion itself may appear "broken" or flocculated. Satellite lesions are frequently seen in the ectocervix, and reverse punctations (Fig. 2–36) may be present.[62] In some cases the lesion may be shiny and snow-white (Fig. 2–37) and may have fine-caliber vessels that do not form well-defined patterns. Micropapillae may also be seen. The clinical impression of HPV infection needs to be confirmed by biopsy. The cervical mu-

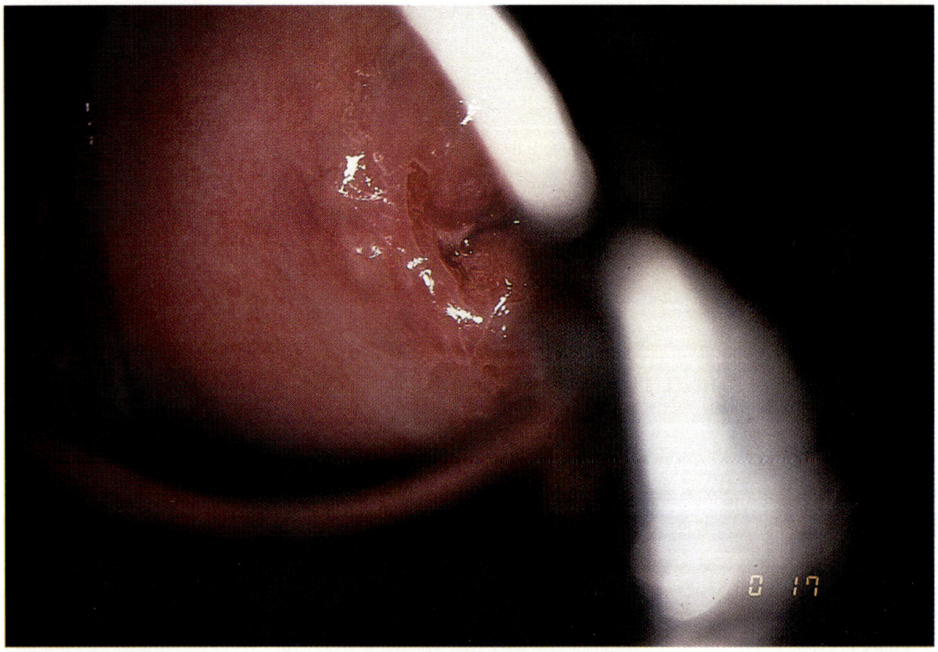

FIGURE 2-35
The cervical os is seen in the center of this colpophotograph. Very faint aceto-white epithelium is seen on the ectocervix at the 7 o'clock position. This subtle finding can be easily missed. This finding is consistent with HPV infection.

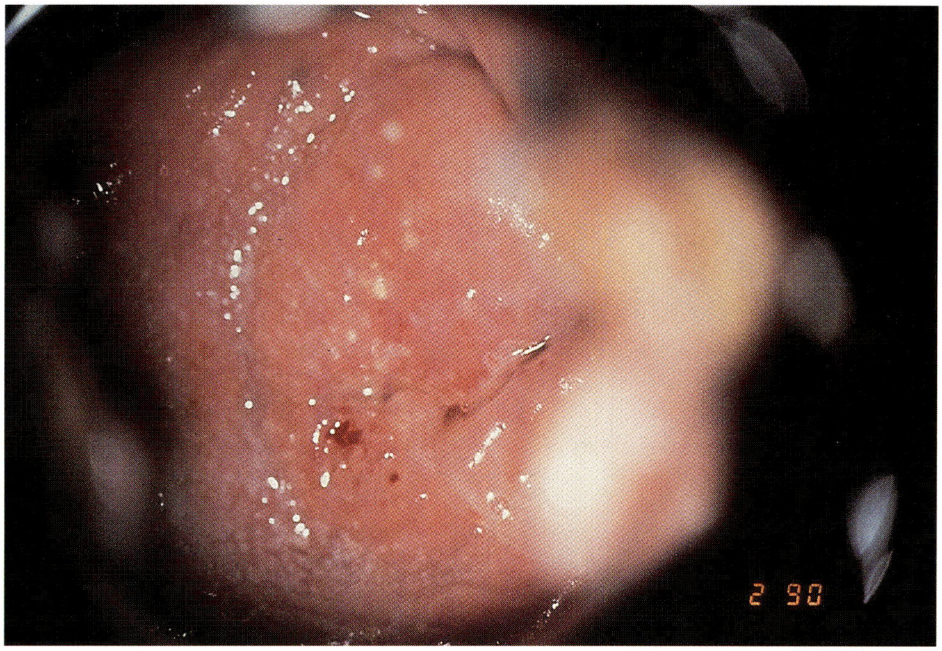

FIGURE 2-36
Multiple white dots are seen on the cervix and on the lateral vaginal fornix (left). These are known as reverse punctations and are caused by HPV infection. Small nabothian cysts, which are yellow, are also seen on the anterior ectocervix.

cosa infected with HPV shows basal cell hyperplasia and numerous koilocytes (Fig. 2–38).[63, 64] The koilocytes involve the intermediate and superficial cells. The nuclei are pleomorphic and hyperchromatic and have wrinkled nuclear membranes. There is bi- or multinucleation. The nuclei are surrounded by a clear halo, which gives the cell its name of koilocyte or hollow cell. The presence of a halo is not enough to identify a koilocyte or make the diagnosis of HPV infection; nuclear atypia must also be present. The nuclei rarely have basophilic inclusion bodies, which have been shown by electron microscopy to be arrays of viral particles. A few mitotic figures may be seen in the basal cell layer. In the absence of higher grades of CIN, the number of such figures is low, bizarre or abnormal figures are absent, and normal polarity of the cells is maintained. Both the histopathologic and the cytopathologic changes caused by HPV are discussed in Chapter 3.

Although there are currently over 60 genotypes of HPV and new ones are being discovered at a rapid rate, only a few cause genital tract lesions.[65] The dominant genotypes for external genital and

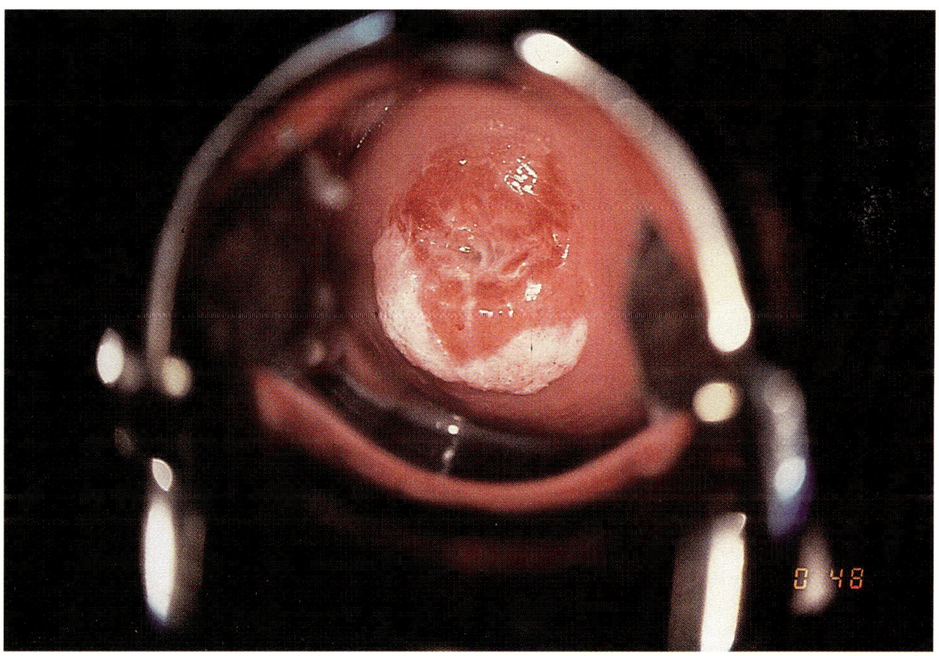

FIGURE 2-37
A raised, shiny, snow-white lesion is seen on the posterior ectocervix. This is condyloma acuminatum. Very faint acetowhite epithelium is seen on the ectocervix at the 12 o'clock position. This upper lesion is a subtle change also caused by the HPV.

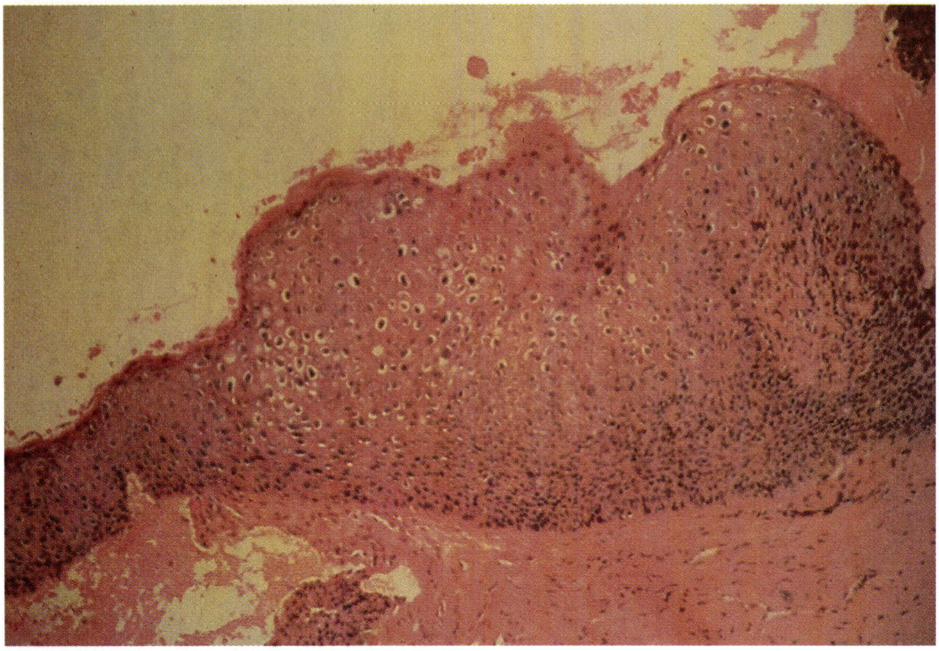

FIGURE 2-38
This microphotograph shows cervical epithelium infected with HPV. The lesion is raised and bulbous. The epithelium is thickened compared with the area seen on the left. Multiple koilocytes are seen from the intermediate cell layer up.

vaginal exophytic lesions are types 6 and 11. Types 16, 18, 31, 33, and 35 are more commonly associated with the flat warts that occur predominantly on the cervix. These latter five genotypes have been epidemiologically linked to CIN (see Chapter 3). HPV is encountered with such frequency that test kits are commercially available to identify the genotypes that usually infect the lower genital tract. Although typing may be of value for scientific investigation, the role (if any) of typing HPV lesions in clinical practice is not defined.

Since there is an association between genital warts, CIN, and cervical cancer, Papanicolaou smears and colposcopy should be performed when lesions are encountered. In addition, patients should be counseled regarding their need for continuing follow-up with annual or more frequent Papanicolaou smears. Therapy for venereal warts is not curative, since the virus is present in tissue that appears clinically normal.[66] In the absence of significant intraepithelial neoplasia, any medical intervention is for cosmetic reasons or to prevent bleeding from the warts should they be denuded during the birthing process. Common modalities of therapy include cryotherapy, cautery, laser, surgical excision, tri- or bichloroacetic acid, podophyllum resin, and 5-fluorouracil. These were discussed in the section on vaginal infections. Regardless of therapeutic modality, recurrence is commonplace.

Genital HSV infection, often referred to as herpes type 2, herpes genitalis, or herpes progenitalis, can occur in the ectocervix. Superficial small ulcers that produce a serosanguineous discharge are seen on the cervix (see Fig. 2–17). A patient who has cervical herpes infection usually also has vulvar lesions. It is more often the painful vulvar lesions that bring the patient to medical attention. Although the diagnosis is often determined presumptively by clinical examination, it can be readily confirmed by cytologic smear or by rapid diagnostic tests such as enzyme-linked immunosorbent assay or nucleic acid probes. A cervical Papanicolaou smear shows diagnostic cells as described earlier (see Fig. 2–19). Biopsy of the lesions is not necessary, but, if done, reveals either a vesicle or an ulcer with marked inflammation at the base. The diagnostic cells are found at the lateral edges of the base of the lesion. Therefore, when a sample is taken for cytologic examination of a suspected herpes infection lesion, a vesicle should be unroofed and the edges of the base of the ulcer scraped. Multinucleation, nuclear ground-glass appearance, and eosinophilic or basophilic intranuclear inclusions are seen. These inclusions are seen when the lesion is older and more advanced. Intraepithelial or subepithelial blebs may also be seen. Patients without symptoms may be given an antimicrobial (e.g., clindamycin) cream to use intravaginally to prevent secondary bacterial infection. Patients who have simultaneous vulvar lesions can be treated with acyclovir.[33]

Treponema pallidum, the causative agent of syphilis, can infect the cervix. Although a cervical chancre is uncommon, when present it is a nontender, well-circumscribed ulcer with an indurated, firm border. Secondary syphilis, in the form of mucosal papules known as condyloma latum, can also occur on the cervix. This lesion could be confused with a venereal wart (i.e., condyloma acuminatum). The surface of the condyloma latum is smooth, whereas that of condyloma acuminatum is irregular. If the cervical chancre or condyloma latum is scraped with a wooden spatula and the resultant exudate placed on a glass slide and examined by darkfield microscopy, hundreds of spirochetes are seen. Placing a drop of fluid from the cervical lesion on the slide without allowing it to dry may be technically difficult. Diagnosis sometimes requires serologic testing and/or biopsy. On tissue sections the typical small spiral organisms can be seen only if the tissue is stained with a specialized silver (Dieterle) stain. A chronic inflammatory infiltrate with lymphocytic perivascular cuffing is also noted. The primary and secondary lesions are self-limiting and heal without scarring. The treatment of choice for syphilis remains benzathine penicillin G.

Haemophilus ducreyi is the bacterium that causes chancroid. In the United States this sexually transmitted disease commonly occurs as miniepidemic outbreaks during the summer. The ulcerative lesions that result from this infection are usually multiple, are excavated in appearance, and have ragged, irregular borders. They are self-limiting and heal rapidly without scarring. The male partner may have a very painful penile ulcer. This identifies the woman as possibly infected and is what usually brings her to medical attention. Therapy for this condition currently consists of ceftriaxone, 250 mg intramuscularly.

Infections of the endocervical canal occur with *Neisseria gonorrhoeae* and *Chlamydia trachomatis*. These two sexually transmitted pathogens do not cause ulcerative lesions but are associated with an acute inflammatory response in the endocervix. The attendant cervicitis is associated with cervical erythema, friability, and a cervical mucopurulent discharge (Fig. 2–39). Identification of the causative organism can be accomplished with nucleic acid probes or cultures, as discussed in the section on bacterial vaginal infections. *N. gonorrhoeae* usually causes an acute endocervical infection, whereas *C. trachomatis* causes a chronic infection. Nests of lymphocytes are seen in the cervical stroma under the cervical epithelium with *C. trachomatis* infection.

In the past it was thought that there were characteristic cytologic features of cells infected with *C. trachomatis*. These are squamous intermediate cells with multiple vacuoles that may contain coccoid bodies. These cells are now recognized to be not diagnostic of *Chlamydia,* and there are no cytologic changes that are pathognomonic. Smears taken from patients who have this infection often show a repair reaction or the presence of germinal center lymphocytes, the so-called follicular cervicitis.

Both *N. gonorrhoeae* and *C. trachomatis* are readily amenable to eradication with antimicrobials. Since the treatment of these two infections

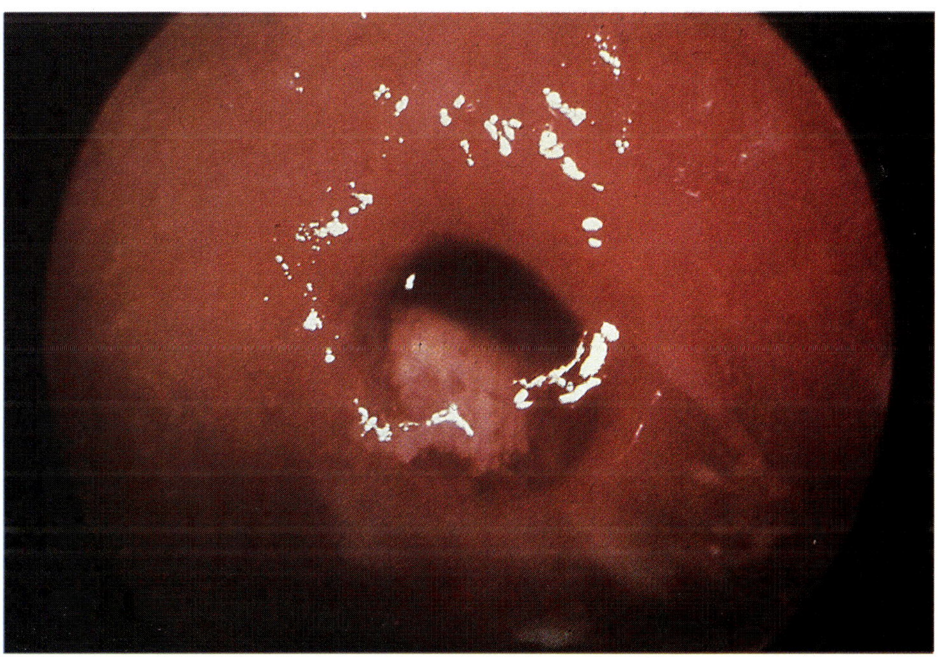

FIGURE 2–39
This colpophotograph shows mucopurulent cervicitis secondary to infection with *Chlamydia trachomatis*. A thick, yellow-white discharge is seen in the endocervix.

is a dynamic area of investigation, the current recommended therapy should be ascertained from the guidelines for the treatment of sexually transmitted diseases published by the United States Centers for Disease Control.[67]

Other uncommon infections of the uterine cervix include tuberculosis and schistosomiasis. Infection with *Schistosoma haematobium* has been associated with cervical cancer.[68]

Benign Neoplasms

The squamous papilloma is a benign solid tumor that is found on the ectocervix. It is a fibroepithelial polyp composed of squamous epithelium overlying a highly vascularized stroma. It is thought that the squamous papilloma most commonly arises as a result of inflammation or trauma. The squamous papilloma is usually no more than 2 to 5 mm in diameter. The surface epithelium may show acanthosis, parakeratosis, and hyperkeratosis. The stroma has increased vascularity and a round cell infiltrate. This lesion must be distinguished from condyloma acuminatum, which has similar histopathologic characteristics but in addition has koilocytotic cells as discussed above.

Leiomyoma, or fibroid tumor, is a benign neoplasm that is rarely encountered in the cervix. When it is, it is usually located under the cervical mucosa and is between 5 and 10 mm in diameter. It is difficult to differentiate a leiomyoma from a squamous papilloma by gross examination. However, microscopic examination of the leiomyoma shows the typical pattern of interlacing smooth muscle fibers identical to the leiomyoma that arises from the uterine body (see Chapter 5).

Adenomatous hyperplasia of the cervix may appear as a papule or cyst above the squamocolumnar junction. There is hyperplasia of the endocervical glands, forming a lacy pattern. Cystic dilatation of the glands is often present, their lining being composed of cuboidal and/or flattened epithelium (Fig. 2–40).

Another proliferation of the endocervical glands that is frequently misdiagnosed as a polyp, and occasionally as cancer, is microglandular hyperplasia. This cervical lesion may present as an inflamed ectropion or a reddish polypoid lesion. Microscopic examination reveals a proliferation of tightly packed glands, most of which are small and tubular. Occasionally the glands are separated by small amounts of bland fibrous stroma. The cytoplasm of the cells may contain subnuclear vacuoles (Fig. 2–41). Immature squamous metaplasia may be present (Fig. 2–42). The nuclei may be atypical. However, cellular stratification and mitotic activity, which distinguish this lesion from endocervical adenocarcinoma, are absent. On occasion a solid growth pattern is seen in association with microglandular hyperplasia.[69] In contrast to features observed in carcinoma, the nuclei are uniform and mitotic figures are absent. Microglandular hyperplasia used to be thought to only be a progestogen-dependent phenomenon that occurs in pregnant women and in those taking combination oral contraceptives. The lesion disappears after delivery or after stopping the oral contraceptive. However, microglandular hyperplasia is not a rea-

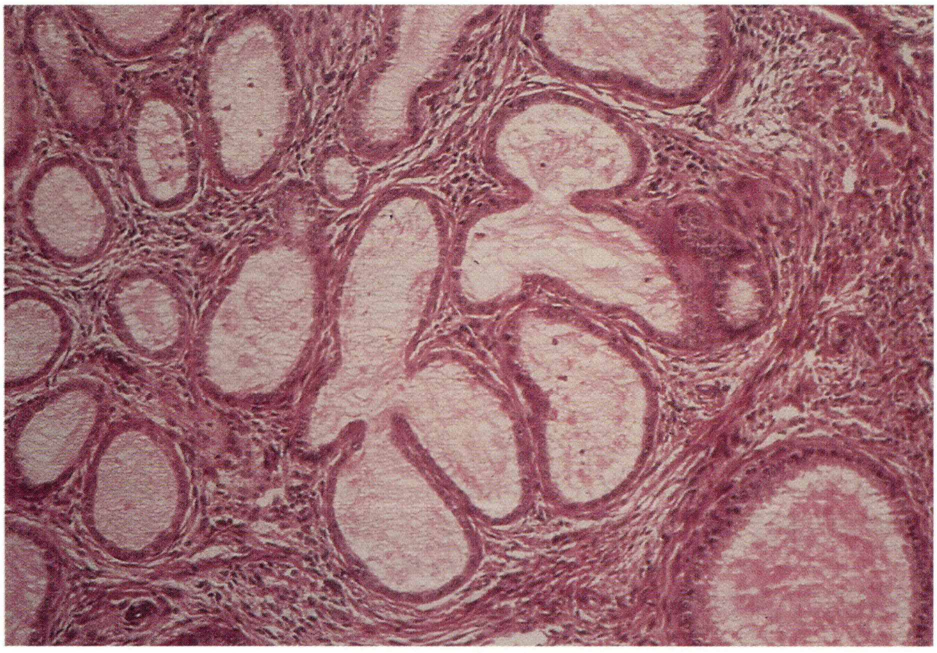

FIGURE 2–40
Endocervical gland proliferation is seen. There is cystic dilatation, and some of the glands are lined by a flattened epithelium. Secretions are seen in the gland's lumen.

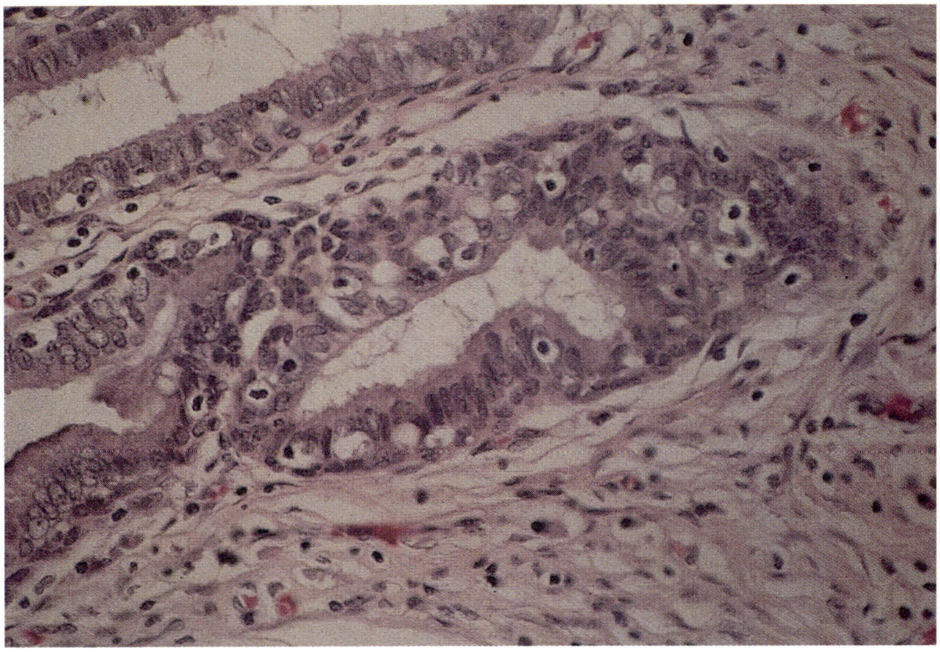

FIGURE 2-41
This is a high-power microscopic view of microglandular hyperplasia. Subnuclear vacuoles are seen. There is mild nuclear atypia, but there is no cellular stratification and no mitotic activity.

son to stop oral contraceptives unless there is significant cellular atypia. Cases of microglandular hyperplasia not associated with pregnancy or oral contraceptives are relatively common.[70]

Mesonephric duct remnants are found deep in the cervical stroma in approximately 10 percent of serially sectioned cervices. Hyperplasia and malignant proliferations of these remnants have been reported.[71] Mesonephric or wolffian duct remnant hyperplasia is usually an incidental histopathologic finding in a hysterectomy specimen. The lesion is found deep in the lateral cervical stroma and is usually no more than 3 mm in size. Diffuse involvement of the entire thickness of the cervix rarely occurs. There is proliferation of small round mesonephric tubules. The tubules are lined with cuboidal to columnar cells that contain clear to pale amphophilic cytoplasm. They have a bland, basally placed nucleus (Fig. 2–43). There is no cellular stratification and no mitotic activity. The lumina of the tubules may contain pink material that stains with periodic acid–Schiff (PAS), indicating that glycogen or mucin is present. Unlike in endocervical mucin-producing epithelium, the cyto-

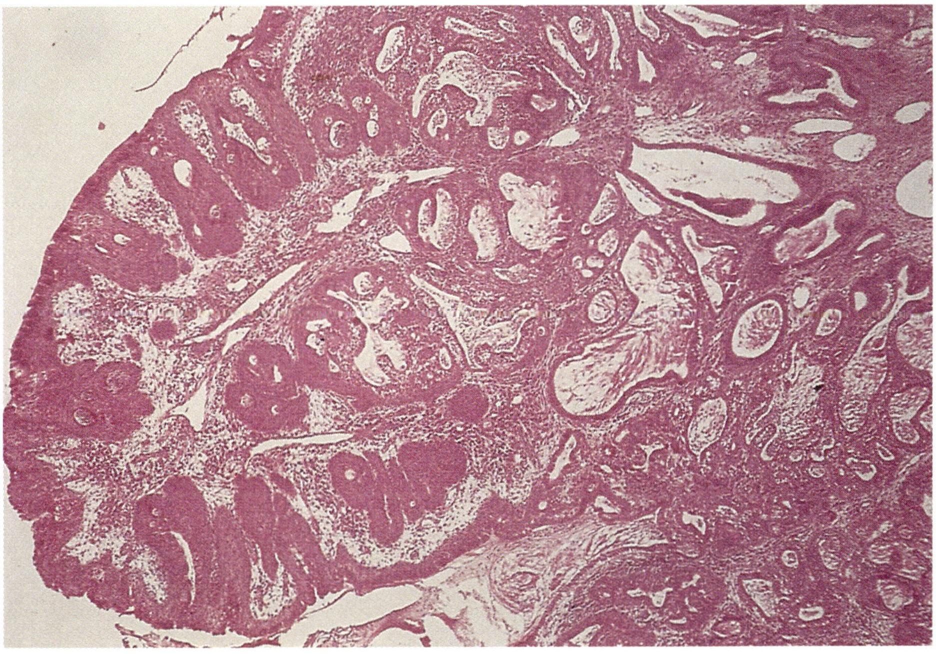

FIGURE 2-42
There is extensive squamous metaplasia of the endocervical mucin-secreting, columnar epithelium in this case of microglandular hyperplasia. The lesion protrudes toward the endocervical canal, which is on the left, and accounts for its polypoid appearance on gross examination.

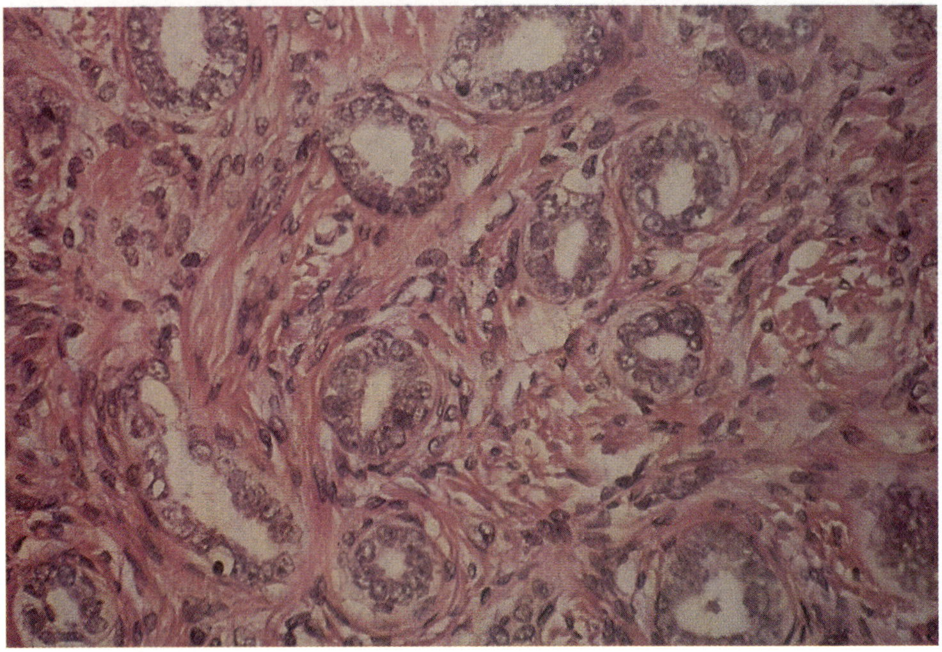

FIGURE 2-43
A high-power view of wolffian duct hyperplasia demonstrates that the tubules are lined by cuboidal cells. Their cytoplasm is pale and scant. The nuclei are round and occupy most of the cell. (Courtesy of Dr. Michael A. Jones, Maine Medical Center, Portland, ME.)

plasm does not stain with PAS. The intervening stroma is bland and lacks desmoplasia. This lesion should not be confused with adenoma malignum (minimal deviation adenocarcinoma), which exhibits proliferation of normal-appearing, mucin-secreting endocervical glands deep in the cervical stroma.[72]

Endometriosis can be found in the cervix. Frequently it is an incidental histopathologic finding on examination of a hysterectomy or cervical biopsy specimen. It may present as a bluish red or bluish black, 1 to 2 mm papule (Fig. 2–44). If the endometriosis implants are responsive to the cyclic hormonal changes of the menstrual cycle, they may bleed at the time of menstruation. Microscopic examination may show only scarring and hemosiderin-laden macrophages. Typical endometrial glands and stroma may also be seen (Fig. 2–45). Endometriosis is more commonly encountered in the cervix after it has been traumatized either by childbirth or by surgery. However, cervical endometriosis has also been reported in pa-

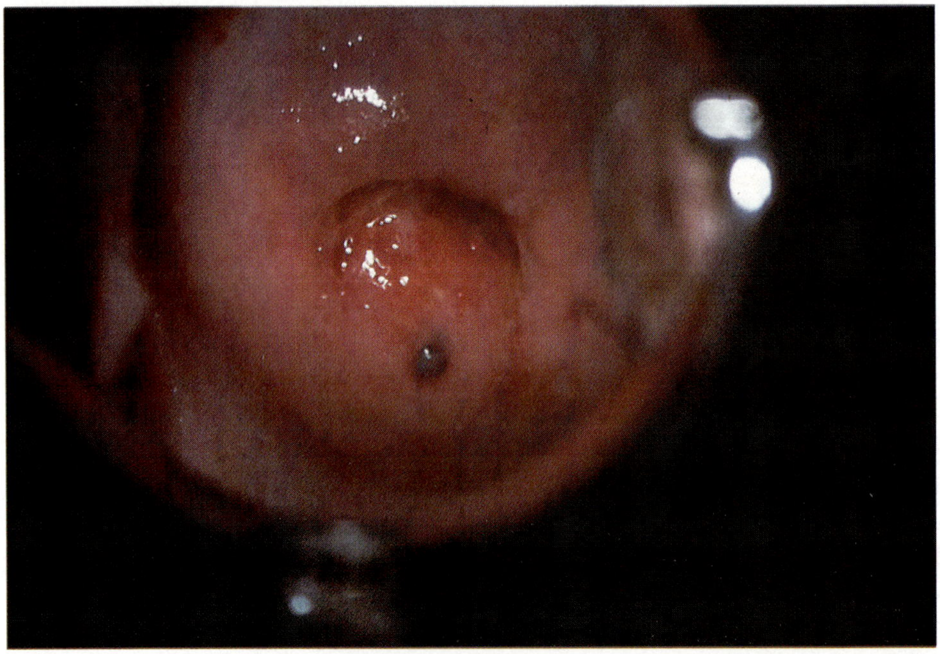

FIGURE 2-44
This blue-black cystic lesion at the 6 o'clock position on the ectocervix proved to be endometriosis.

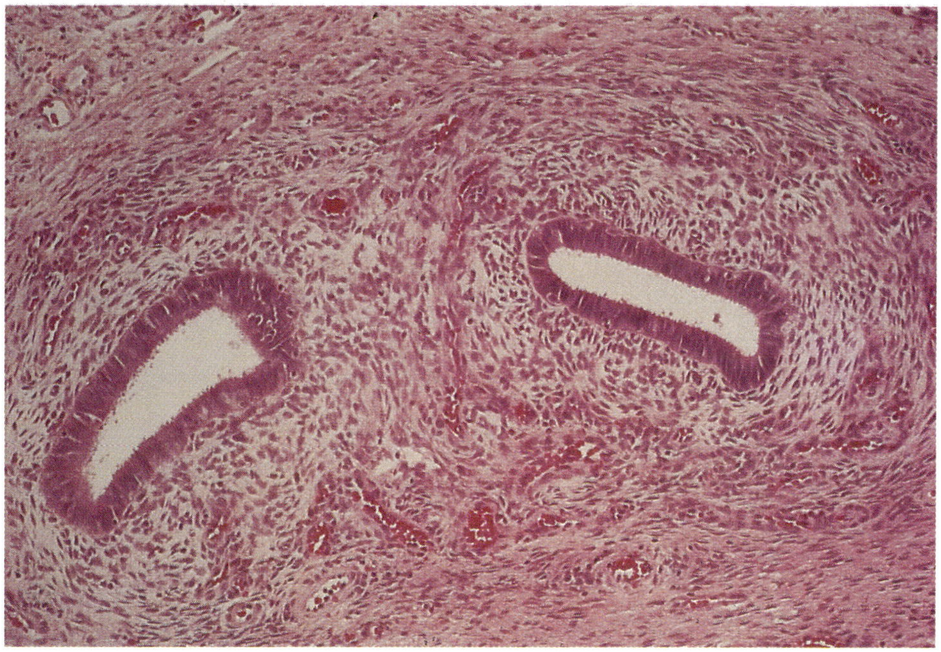

FIGURE 2-45
These two typical endometrial glands are surrounded by endometrial stroma that has cells with basophilic nuclei. The denser but less cellular cervical stroma surrounds the endometriosis. There is vascular engorgement.

tients who had no history of cervical trauma. These cases may be caused by direct implantation or may be the result of the capability of the müllerian-derived tissues to differentiate into any of the cell types found along the upper genital tract.

An endocervical polyp is a localized proliferation of endocervical glands and stroma. A patient with such a polyp may have postcoital bleeding or intermenstrual spotting. However, most patients who have an endocervical polyp are asymptomatic. Most endocervical polyps are found in women older than 40 years.[73] An endocervical polyp is usually a single, bright red, friable growth that arises from the endocervix and protrudes through the external cervical os. It rarely exceeds 5 to 10 mm in greatest diameter (Fig. 2–46). It is usually pedunculated but can also have a broad base. The base of the polyp is usually visualized only by using an endocervical speculum. If the pedicle is thin, the polyp can be twisted off in the clinician's office; otherwise, removal in the operating room is advised.

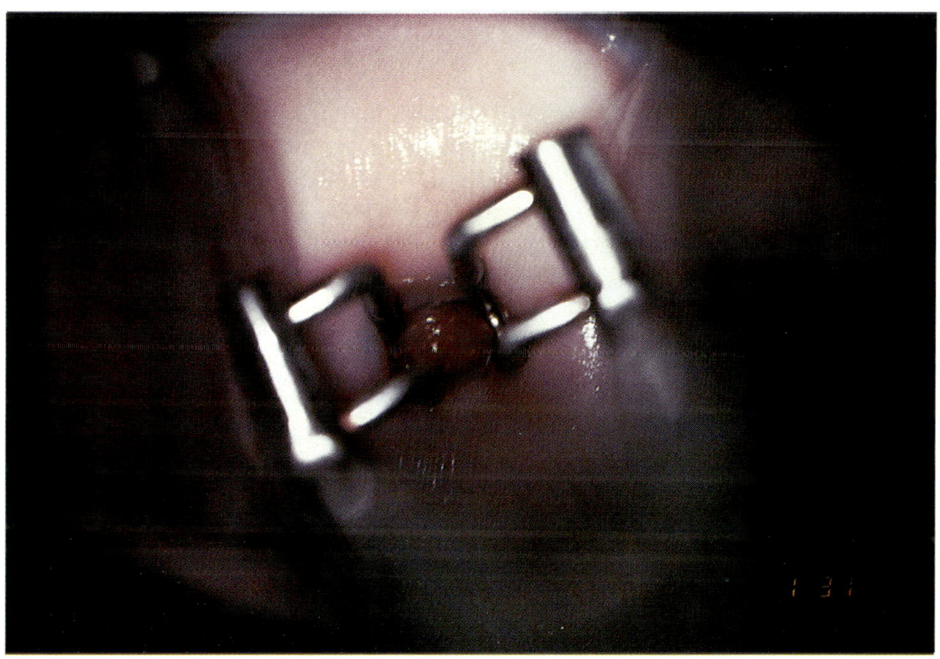

FIGURE 2-46
An endocervical polyp is seen in the endocervical canal. An endocervical speculum is used to enable better visualization. This polyp is bright red and approximately 5 mm in diameter.

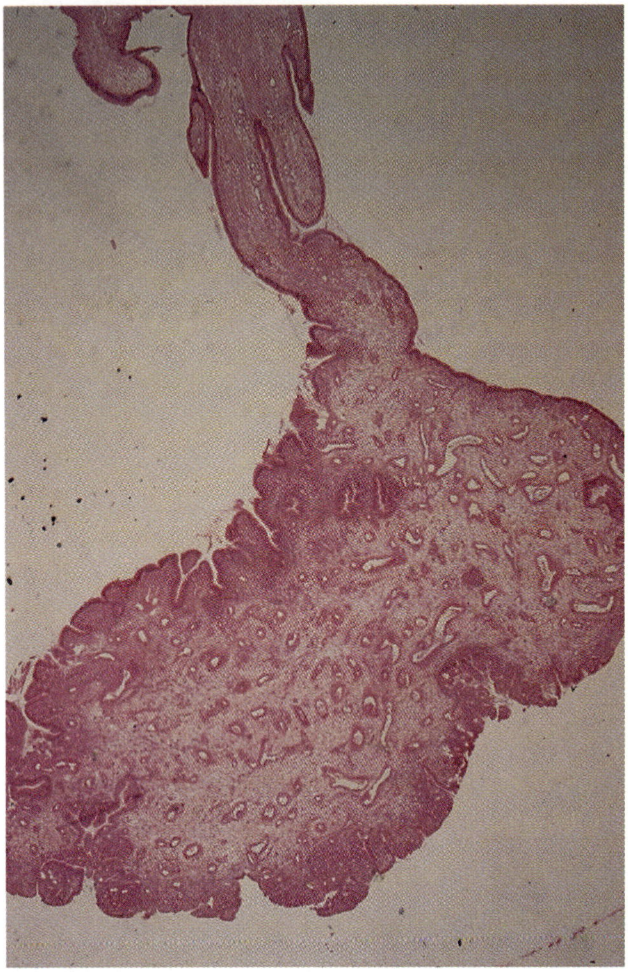

FIGURE 2-47
This endocervical polyp has a narrow stalk. The polyp is lined by a single layer of tall columnar, mucin-secreting cells. There is focal squamous metaplasia on the lower part of the polyp. The stroma is edematous, and dilated blood vessels are present.

The endocervical polyp consists of an inflamed, well-vascularized, and edematous stroma covered by tall columnar, mucin-secreting, endocervical type cells. The inflammatory infiltrate is composed predominantly of lymphocytes and macrophages. The blood vessels in the center of the polyp have thick walls. The endocervical epithelium of the polyp frequently shows squamous metaplasia (Fig. 2–47). Nabothian cysts within the polyp may also be seen. An endometrial polyp that protrudes through the external cervical os may have the same gross appearance as the endocervical polyp. The distinction can be made only by microscopic examination. Malignancy arising in a polyp is rare;[73] if malignancy is confined to the polyp, the prognosis is excellent.

Other lesions that rarely occur in the cervix include nevi,[74] hemangiomas,[75] lipomas,[76] gliomas,[77] and lymphangiomas.[78]

REFERENCES

1. Parmley TH: Clinical Review of the Embryology of the Female Genital Canal. Wichita, KS, Eagle Press, 1988.
2. Tjaden BL, Rock JA: Uterovaginal anomalies. *In* Carpenter SEK, Rock JA (eds): Pediatric and Adolescent Gynecology. New York, Raven Press, 1992, pp 313–330.
3. Barlett JG, Onderdonk AB, Drude C, et al: Quantitative bacteriology of the vaginal flora. J Infect Dis 1977;35:873–876.
4. Witkin SS, Jeremiah J, Ledger WJ: Recurrent vaginitis as a result of sexual transmission of IgE antibodies. Am J Obstet Gynecol 1988;159:32–36.
5. Dworetzky M: Allergic vaginitis (letter). Am J Obstet Gynecol 1989;161:1752–1753.
6. McCormack WM: Two urogenital sinus syndromes: interstitial cystitis and focal vulvitis. J Reprod Med 1990;35:873–876.
7. Fitzpatrick CC, DeLancey JO, Elkins TE, McGuine EJ: Vulvar vestibulitis and interstitial cystitis: a disorder of urogenital sinus–derived epithelium? Obstet Gynecol 1993;81:860–862.

7a. Sobel JD: Desquamative inflammatory vaginitis: a new subgroup of purulent vaginitis responsive to topical 2% clindamycin therapy. Am J Obstet Gynecol 1994;171:1215–1220.

8. Livengood CH III, Thomason JL, Hill GB: Bacterial vaginosis: treatment with topical intravaginal clindamycin phosphate. Obstet Gynecol 1990;76:118–123.
9. Nugent RP, Krohn MA, Hillier SL: Reliability of diagnosing bacterial vaginosis is improved by a standardized method of Gram stain interpretation. J Clin Microbiol 1991; 29:297–301.
10. Watts DH, Krohn MA, Hillier SL, Eschenbach DA: Bacterial vaginosis as a risk factor for post-cesarean endometritis. Obstet Gynecol 1990;75:52–58.
11. Soper DE: Bacterial vaginosis and postoperative infections. Am J Obstet Gynecol 1993;169:467–469.
12. McGregor JA, French JI, Seo K: Premature rupture of the membranes and bacterial vaginosis. Am J Obstet Gynecol 1993;169:463–466.
13. Gibbs RS: Chorioamnionitis and bacterial vaginosis. Am J Obstet Gynecol 1993;169:460–462.
14. Riluan JM, Hillier SI, Utomo B, et al: Bacterial vaginosis and prematurity in Indonesia: associations in early and late pregnancies. Am J Obstet Gynecol 1993;169:195–198.
15. Eschenbach DA: Bacterial vaginosis and anaerobes in obstetric-gynecologic infections. Clin Infect Dis 1993;4(Suppl 16):S282–S287.
16. Larson PG, Platz-Christensen JJ, Thejls H, et al: Incidence of pelvic inflammatory disease after first-trimester legal abortion in women with bacterial vaginosis after treatment with metronidazole: a double-blind, randomized study. Am J Obstet Gynecol 1992;166:100–103.
17. Greaves WL, Chungafung J, Morris B, et al: Clindamycin versus metronidazole in the treatment of bacterial vaginosis. Obstet Gynecol 1988;72:799–802.
18. Reingold AL: Epidemiology of toxic-shock syndrome, United States, 1960–1984. MMWR 1984;33(Suppl):SS-3.
19. Schlievert PM, MacDonald KL: Toxic shock syndrome. *In* Gorbach SL, Bartlett JG, Blacklow NR (eds): Infectious Diseases. Philadelphia, WB Saunders, 1992, pp 889–894.
20. Spence MR, Hollander DH, Smith J, et al: Clinical and laboratory diagnosis of *Trichomonas vaginalis* infection. Sex Transm Dis 1980;7:168–171.
21. Kreiger JN, Tam MR, Stevens CE, et al: Diagnosis of trichomoniasis: comparison of conventional wet-mount examination with cytologic studies, cultures, and monoclonal antibodies with staining of direct specimens. JAMA 1988;259:1223–1227
22. Weinberger MW, Harger JH: Accuracy of the Papanicolaou smear in the diagnosis of asymptomatic infection with *Trichomonas vaginalis.* Obstet Gynecol 1993;82:425–429.
23. Kauffman RH, Friedrich EG Jr, Gardner HL: Benign Dis-

eases of the Vulva and Vagina, 3rd ed. Chicago, Year Book, 1989, pp 441–444.
24. Nuovo GJ, Blanco JS, Silverstein SJ, Crum CP: Histologic correlates of papillomavirus infection of the vagina. Obstet Gynecol 1988;72:770–774.
25. Eron JL, Judson F, Tucker S, et al: Interferon therapy for condyloma acuminatum. N Engl J Med 1986;315:1059–1064.
26. Ferenczy A: Comparison of 5-fluorouracil and CO_2 laser for treatment of vaginal condylomata. Obstet Gynecol 1984;64:773–778.
27. Kreb H-B: Treatment of vaginal condylomata acuminata by weekly topical application of 5-fluorouracil. Obstet Gynecol 1987;70:68–71.
28. Krebs H-B: Prophylactic topical 5-fluorouracil following treatment of human papillomavirus associated lesions of the vulva and vagina. Obstet Gynecol 1986;68:837–841.
29. Malviya VK, Deppe G, Pluszczynski R, Boike G: Trichloroacetic acid in the treatment of human papillomavirus infection of the cervix without associated dysplasia. Obstet Gynecol 1987;70:72–74.
30. Krebs H-B, Helkamp BF: Chronic ulcerations following topical therapy with 5-fluorouracil for vaginal human papillomavirus associated lesions. Obstet Gynecol 1991;78:205–208.
31. Riva JM, Sedlacek TV, Cunnane MF, Mangan CE: Extended carbon dioxide laser vaporization in the treatment of subclinical papillomavirus infection of the lower genital tract. Obstet Gynecol 1989;73:25–30.
32. Matorras R, Ariceta JM, Rementeria A, et al: Human immune deficiency virus–induced immunosuppression: a risk factor for human papillomavirus infection. Am J Obstet Gynecol 1991;164:42–44.
33. Whitley RJ, Gnann JW Jr: Acyclovir: a decade later. N Engl J Med 1992;327:782–789.
34. Jovanovic R, Congema E, Nguyen HT: Antifungal agents vs boric acid for treating chronic mycotic vulvovaginitis. J Reprod Med 1991;36:593–597.
35. Sobel JD: Recurrent vulvovaginal candidiasis: a prospective study of the efficacy of maintenance ketoconazole therapy. N Engl J Med 1986;315:1455–1458.
36. Woodruff JD, Parmley TH: Nonobstetrical vaginal injuries. *In* Hafez ESE, Evans TN (eds): Human Reproductive Medicine–The Human Vagina. New York, North-Holland, 1978, pp 291–295.
36a. Andrews S, Miyazawa K: The significance of a negative Papanicolaou smear with hyperkeratosis or parakeratosis. Obstet Gynecol 1989;73:751–753.
37. Chirayil SJ, Tobon H: Polyps of the vagina: a clinicopathologic study of 18 cases. Cancer 1981;47:2904–2907.
38. Tavassoli FA, Norris HJ: Smooth muscle tumors of the vagina. Obstet Gynecol 1991;53:689–693.
39. Kaufman RH, Gardner HL: Benign mesodermal tumors. Clin Obstet Gynecol 1965;8:953–981.
40. Norris HJ, Taylor HB: Melanomas of the vagina. Am J Clin Pathol 1966;46:420–426.
41. Bottles K, Lacey CG, Miller TR: Atypical melanocytic hyperplasia of the vagina. Gynecol Oncol 1984;19:226–230.
42. Tobon H, Murphy AI: Benign blue nevus of the vagina. Cancer 1977;403:3174–3176.
43. Rodriguez HA, Ackerman LV: Cellular blue nevus: a clinicopathologic study of forty-five cases. Cancer 1968;21:393–405.
44. Gold BM: Neurofibromatosis of the bladder and vagina. Am J Obstet Gynecol 1972;113:1055–1056.
45. Azzopardi JG, Eusebi V, Tison V, Betts CM: Neurofibroma with rhabdomyomatous differentiation; benign "Triton" tumor of the vagina. Histopathology 1983;7:561–572.
46. Hertzig AT, Gore H: Tumors of the female organs. Atlas of Histopathology, Part 2, Section IX, Fascicle 33. Washington, DC, Armed Forces Institute of Pathology 1960; pp 66–67.
47. Pezershkpour G: Solitary paraganglioma of the vagina: report of a case. Am J Obstet Gynecol 1981;139:219–221.
48. Spitzer M, Molho L, Seltzer VL, Lipper S: Vaginal glomus tumor: case presentation and ultrastructural findings. Obstet Gynecol 1985;66(Suppl):86S–88S.
49. Elkins TE, Drescher C, Martey JO, Fort D: Vesicovaginal fistula revisited. Obstet Gynecol 1988;72:307–312.
50. Lee RA, Symmonds RE, Williams TJ: Current status of genitourinary fistula. Obstet Gynecol 1988;72:313–319.
51. Rosenshein NB, Genadry RR, Woodruff JD: An anatomic classification of rectovaginal septal defects. Am J Obstet Gynecol 1980;137:439–442.
52. Bandy LC, Addison A, Parker RT: Surgical management of rectovaginal fistulas in Crohn's disease. Am J Obstet Gynecol 1983;147:359–363.
53. Wiskind AK, Thompson JD: Transverse transperineal repair of rectovaginal fistulas in the lower vagina. Am J Obstet Gynecol 1992;167:694–699.
54. Curtin JP, Burt LL: Successful treatment of small intestine fistula with somatostatin analog. Gynecol Oncol 1990; 39:225–227.
55. Smith DH, Pierce VK, Lewis JL Jr: Enteric fistulas encountered on a gynecologic oncology service from 1969 through 1980. Surg Gynecol Obstet 1984;158:71–75.
56. Jelen I: Vaginal fistulas: operative management. *In* Gershenso DM, DeCherney AH, Curry SL (eds): Operative Gynecology, 1st ed. Philadelphia, WB Saunders, 1993, pp 213–229.
57. Ginsburg DS, Genadry R: Suburethral diverticulum. Obstet Gynecol Surv 1984;39:1–7.
58. Leppert PC, Cerreta JM, Mandl I: Orientation of elastic fibers in the human cervix. Am J Obstet Gynecol 1986;155:219–224.
59. Novak ER, Woodruff JD: Novak's Gynecologic and Obstetric Pathology, 8th ed. Philadelphia, WB Saunders, 1979, pp 82–92.
60. Holzaepfel JH, Ezell HE: Sites of metastases of uterine carcinoma. Am J Obstet Gynecol 1955;69:1027–1038.
61. Mangan CE, Rubin SE, Rabin DS, Mikuta JJ: Lymph node nomenclature in gynecologic oncology. Obstet Gynecol 1986;23:222–226.
62. Reid R, Scalzi P: Genital warts and cervical cancer: VII. an improved colposcopic index for differentiating benign papillomaviral infection from high-grade cervical intraepithelial neoplasia. Am J Obstet Gynecol 1985;153:611–618.
63. Reid R, Stanhope CR, Herschman BR, et al: Genital warts and cervical cancer: I. Evidence of an association between subclinical papillomavirus infection and cervical malignancy. Cancer 1982;50:377–387.
64. Reid R, Crum CP, Herschman BR, et al: Genital warts and cervical cancer: III. Subclinical papillomaviral infection and cervical neoplasia are linked by a spectrum of continuous morphologic and biologic change. Cancer 1984;53:943–953.
65. Wright TC Jr, Richart RM: Role of human papillomavirus in the pathogenesis of genital tract cancer. Gynecol Oncol 1990;37:151–164.
66. Ferenczy A, Mitow M, Nigai N, et al: Latent papillomavirus and recurring genital warts. N Engl J Med 1985;313:784–788.
67. Centers for Disease Control and Prevention: 1993 Sexually Transmitted Diseases Treatment Guidelines. MMWR 1993;42(RR14):1–102.
68. Schwartz DA: Carcinoma of the uterine cervix in West Africa. Gynecol Oncol 1984;19:365–370.
69. Young RH, Scully RE: Atypical forms of microglandular hyperplasia of the cervix simulating carcinoma: a report of five cases and review of the literature. Am J Surg Pathol 1989;13:50.
70. Chumas JC, Nelson B, Mann WJ, et al: Microglandular hyperplasia of the uterine cervix. Obstet Gynecol 1985;66:406–409.
71. Jones MA, Anrews J, Tarraza HM: Mesonephric remnant hyperplasia of the cervix: a clinicopathologic analysis of 14 cases. Gynecol Oncol 1993;49:41–47.
72. Giks CB, Young RH, Aguirre P, et al: Adenoma malignum (minimal deviation adenocarcinoma) of the cervix: a clinicopathologic and immunohistochemical analysis of 26 cases. Am J Surg Pathol 1989;13:717–729.

73. Aaro LA, Jacobson LJ, Soule EH: Endocervical polyps. Obstet Gynecol 1963;21:659–665.
74. Dundore W, Lamas C: Benign nevus (ephelis) of the uterine cervix. Am J Obstet Gynecol 1985;152:881–882.
75. Gusdon JT: Hemangioma of the cervix. Am J Obstet Gynecol 1965;91:204–209.
76. Rilke F, Cantaboni A: Lipomas of the uterus: presentation of 2 cases and review of the recent literature. Ann Obstet Gynecol 1964;86:645.
77. Luevano-Flores E, Sotelo J, Tena-Suck M: Glial polyp (glioma) of the uterine cervix: report of a case with demonstration of glial fibrillary acidic protein. Gynecol Oncol 1985;21:385–390.
78. Stout AP: Hemangioendothelioma: a tumor of blood vessels featuring vascular endothelial cells. Ann Surg 1943; 118:445–464.

3

Preinvasive Lesions of the Cervix and Vagina

Lisa L. Anderson/Barbara F. Atkinson

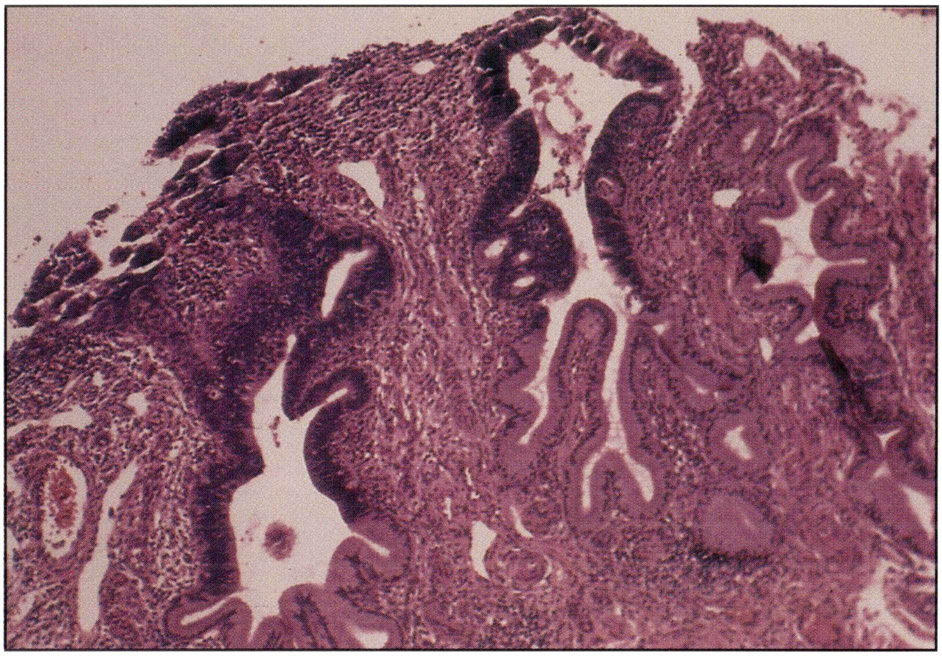

CLINICAL EMBRYOLOGY AND ANATOMY OF THE TRANSFORMATION ZONE

The uterus and upper vagina are formed by the fusion of the müllerian ducts.[1] During early embryogenesis the vagina and cervix are covered with columnar epithelium (see also Chapter 2). Through a process of squamous differentiation, the vagina and a variable portion of the ectocervix gradually become covered with squamous epithelium. Replacement of the müllerian-derived columnar epithelium by squamous epithelium ends around the fifth month postconception. The anatomic junction where the newly formed squamous epithelium of the ectocervix meets the mucin-secreting columnar epithelium of the endocervical canal is located in proximity to the external os and is referred to as the original squamocolumnar (SC) junction (Fig. 3–1). In women exposed to diethylstilbestrol (DES) in utero, the normal replacement of the columnar epithelium by squamous epithelium is prematurely halted, and the original SC junction may be located in the vagina rather than on the ectocervix, or it may be patchy and discontinuous.[2]

The transformation of endocervical columnar epithelium to squamous epithelium is a normal physiologic and dynamic process occurring throughout a woman's reproductive years. It occurs most prominently during fetal development, adolescence, and the first pregnancy. This process is influenced by changes in the local hormonal milieu and vaginal pH. At menarche, as a normal physiologic response to increasing levels of ovarian hormones, the cervix hypertrophies, with a subsequent "rolling out" or eversion of the most distal mucin-secreting endocervical tissue from inside the endocervical canal to an exposed position on the ectocervix. This endocervical epithelium is seen as a circumferential velvety red zone on the external os in contrast to the smooth pinkish appearance of the surrounding squamous epithelium of the ectocervix (see Fig. 3–1). This line of demarcation corresponds to the original SC junction. This exposure of the SC junction is an important anatomic event because it is in this zone that the physiologic transformation to a metaplastic squamous epithelium occurs and many neoplastic events originate.

The process of transformation begins after menarche when there is a drop in the vaginal pH.[3] Estrogen and progesterone levels lead to an increase in the cell layers of the vaginal squamous epithelium and intracytoplasmic glycogen storage. This allows establishment of the normal bacterial flora found in the adult, which was discussed in detail in the previous chapter. The byproducts of bacterial metabolism are responsible for the acidic vaginal pH. Other local irritants including trauma and infection may be involved as co-initiators in the normal process of squamous metaplasia. With exposure to the acidic environment of the vagina, the delicate mucin-secreting epithelium of the cervix becomes damaged and thus is stimulated to initiate a repair process. This transformation, whereby the everted columnar endocervical epithelium is converted to squamous epithelium, occurs by two separate histiogenetic mechanisms: squamous epithelialization and squamous metaplasia.

Squamous epithelialization is the direct ingrowth of the mature squamous epithelium of the adjacent ectocervix upward to the region of the everted columnar epithelium. The process of squamous metaplasia is one in which the delicate en-

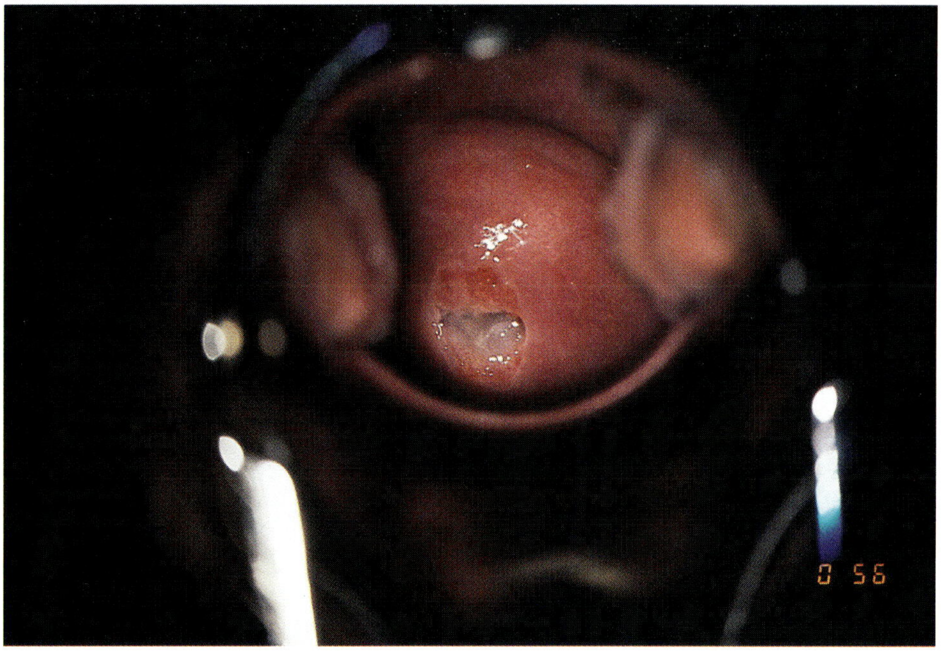

FIGURE 3-1
This colpophotograph of the cervix clearly shows the junction between the columnar epithelium, which appears irregular and red, and the squamous epithelium, which is smooth, shiny, and pink. A faint white line of squamous metaplasia is seen at the junction of the two epithelia. There is thick mucus in the endocervical canal. The diffuse prominent vascular pattern on the ectocervix and vaginal fornix suggests inflammation.

docervical cells are replaced by a more protective layer of mature squamous epithelium. Squamous metaplasia starts with the proliferation of the totipotential reserve cells, which lie just above the basement membrane of the endocervical columnar epithelium. Once stimulated, these cells stratify and differentiate, displacing the overlying columnar epithelium. At an early stage stratification of reserve cells occurs, but the columnar epithelium still forms a superficial layer. This is termed reserve cell hyperplasia. The next step is stratification with no residual glandular cells, known as immature metaplasia. Multiple foci or islands are produced that broaden, coalesce, and eventually join the squamous epithelium growing in from the periphery.[4] Eventually the immature squamous cells produced by this process differentiate into a mature squamous epithelium that can become glycogenated and is indistinguishable from the squamous epithelium that was native to the ectocervix.

In the majority of women during the reproductive years the transformation zone remains visible on the ectocervix and is clinically accessible for evaluation. However, with advancing age and the completion of metaplasia the transformation zone is usually found within the endocervical canal.

This transformation zone is important because it is the site of origin of almost all cervical intraepithelial neoplasia (CIN). This area must be sampled when obtaining cervical cytology. If a patient has an abnormal cervical cytologic result, this area must be visualized by colposcopy, which will be discussed in detail in this chapter. One of the criteria used to establish the adequacy of the colposcopic evaluation is the complete visualization of the transformation zone because the extent and limits of CIN usually coincide with the distribution of the transformation zone. Likewise, treatment of the patient with CIN involves destruction of the entire transformation zone.

EPIDEMIOLOGY OF CERVICAL INTRAEPITHELIAL NEOPLASIA AND CERVICAL CANCER

Age

The mean age of women with CIN is approximately 30 years, and that of patients with cervical squamous cell carcinoma is 50 years.[4a] The mode age of patients with CIN is 22 years, and that of patients with squamous cell carcinoma is 53 years. The age distribution of patients with cervical squamous cell carcinoma follows a normal curve, resulting in the small difference between the mean and mode ages of these patients. The age distribution of patients with CIN is skewed toward the younger age groups, resulting in an 8-year difference between the mean and mode ages of patients who have CIN.

Sexual Behavior

Cervical cancer and CIN are part of a spectrum of diseases that are now recognized to be sexually transmitted. This perspective is central in understanding the causal relationship between female sexual behavior and the pathogenesis of cervical

TABLE 3–1.
Risk Factors for Cervical Cancer

First coitus at a young age
Multiple sexual partners
"High-risk male"
Cigarette smoking
Immunosuppression
History of genital HPV infection
History of cervical intraepithelial neoplasia

neoplasia. It allows the identification of those risk factors (Table 3–1) linked with human sexuality and lifestyle that place women at risk for the development of cervical neoplasia. As a venereal disease, it implies that an infectious and transmissible agent is critically involved in the promotion of CIN and cervical cancer.

The results of extensive epidemiologic studies suggest that the risk of cervical neoplasia is associated with two independent variables: early sexual activity and multiple sexual partners.[5–9] The significance of an early age of first intercourse relates to the cause and effect of sexual activity on the adolescent cervix. As discussed previously, at menarche the process of squamous metaplasia and the formation of the transformation zone begin because this zone is present in the ectocervix in contact with the vaginal milieu. It is suggested that this process renders the cervix more susceptible to the incorporation of potential carcinogens[10, 11] and is a crucial event in the current model of cervical carcinogenesis. In addition, the risk of cervical cancer increases linearly as the number of male sexual partners increases, as seen in several case-control studies.[12, 13] It is theoretically possible that these two variables are not truly independent risk factors; instead, women who start sexual activity at an earlier age may have a longer lifetime exposure to coitus-related carcinogens.[14]

A woman's risk of cervical neoplasia may be independent of her own sexual activity and related to that of her male partner. Evidence favoring the high-risk male is suggested by the significantly higher incidence of cervical cancer among the wives of men who have penile cancer.[15–20] A case-control study analyzed the incidence of cervical cancer among the second wives of men whose first wife had had cervical cancer and found that these women had a 3.5 times higher risk of developing cervical cancer than a control population.[21] Additional evidence of a male factor predisposing to cervical neoplasia is found in several studies in which the sexual histories of husbands of women who had cervical cancer were compared to the sexual histories of a control group.[22–24] In these studies men in the case group reported significantly more female sexual partners than those in the control group. In one study, the husbands of affected women were also more likely to report prior venereal diseases, early sexual experiences, affairs during marriage, and visits to prostitutes.[23] A report from India, where the incidence of cervical cancer is among the highest in the world, examined the role of male behavior in the development of cervical cancer in a cohort of women who had only one lifetime sexual partner.[25] These authors found that the husbands' history of premarital or extramarital sexual relationships (especially an increasing number of these relationships) and a history of having had a sexually transmitted disease increase the risk of cervical cancer in their wives.

Cigarette Smoking

Winklestein in 1977 was the first to report on the association between cervical cancer and cigarette smoking.[26] Numerous reports since that time have confirmed the increased risk of cervical cancer and CIN in women who smoke.[27–30] Controlling for the number of sexual partners and the patient's age at the time of the first sexual intercourse, cigarette smoking emerges as an independent risk factor. Women who smoke are nearly twice as likely to develop cervical cancer as nonsmokers. The risk correlates with the number of cigarettes smoked daily, the number of cigarette pack years, the patient's age when she began smoking, and the use of nonfiltered cigarettes.[31] The association between cervical cancer and smoking is specific for squamous cell carcinoma; there is no association between smoking and the less common cervical adenocarcinoma or adenosquamous carcinoma.

Nicotine is known to be secreted in the cervical mucus, and although nicotine itself is not a carcinogen, its metabolic intermediates, the nitrosamines, are proven carcinogens.[32] Women who smoke shed higher levels of mutagens in their cervical mucus, and these may have a direct carcinogenic effect.[33] In addition, cigarette smoking has been shown to depress local immune defenses in the cervical epithelium. There is a reversal of the normal T4:T8 lymphocyte ratio and a diminution in the number of local Langerhans cells that are responsible for cell-mediated immunity.[34] Also, cervical human papillomavirus (HPV) infection and CIN have been associated with a local reduction in the number of Langerhans cells and decreased T-cell counts.[35] Several postulates have been made for the relationship of smoking to the induction of CIN and cervical carcinoma: the direct immunosuppressive effect of cigarette smoking may enhance the carcinogenic effect of infectious agents including HPV, and nitrosamines may have a direct cacinogenic effect on the cervical epithelium.[36]

Immunosuppression

The patient's immunologic status plays an important role in the clinical expression of genital HPV infection and CIN. An increased prevalence of HPV and CIN has been associated with the mild imunodeficiency that occurs during pregnancy[37] and is seen among immunosuppressed renal transplant patients.[38] The evidence for an association between human immunodeficiency virus (HIV), HPV, and cervical cancer is compelling. These are sexually transmitted diseases that share common behavioral risk factors. It is known that HIV-seropositive women have increased rates of genital HPV infection and CIN.[39–41] In one study, 70 percent of symptomatic HIV-positive women had genital HPV infection, and more than 50 percent of them had abnormal cervical cytologic results consistent with a squamous intraepithelial lesion (SIL).[42] CIN and cervical cancer appear to be more aggressive in HIV-positive women compared with HIV-negative women.

In women who are HIV-positive, recurrence rates for CIN after standard therapy are significantly higher than are the rates in controls, and this is related to the degree of immunosuppression.[42] Compared to uninfected women, HIV-positive women with cervical cancer have an overall poorer prognosis (i.e., higher recurrence and death rates).[43] The increased death rate in these patients is due to the cancer and not to other complications of the acquired immunodeficiency syndrome (AIDS). It is suggested that HIV infection impairs local cervical immunity, which allows the oncogenic progression of HPV-related lesions.[44] In addition, HPV may assume an important role in the sexual transmission of HIV infection either by disruption of the normal mucosal integrity or diminution of local immune surveillance.[42] As of January 1, 1993, the Centers for Disease Control (CDC) included invasive cervical cancer as one of four neoplastic and 23 AIDS-defining illnesses (i.e., a woman who has cervical cancer and who is HIV positive has AIDS).

Human Papillomavirus

HPV is probably the most common sexually transmitted disease in the United States. It is a highly infectious disease transmitted by genital–genital contact. Approximately 60 percent of sexual partners of persons who have condyloma acuminatum develop the infection themselves.[45] The incubation period can be from 3 weeks to 9 months.[46] Distribution of the virus is fairly ubiquitous, and it often involves the entire lower genital tract. Characteristically, some of these lesions regress spontaneously, whereas others persist or progress. A prolonged latent phase, up to 20 years prior to the appearance of clinical disease, has been recorded. This may be a function of age-related immune system changes.

Current epidemiologic, biologic, and molecular data support the idea that genital HPV infection plays an important and probably causal role in the etiology of CIN and cervical cancer. The compelling evidence in support of this hypothesis will be discussed. The epidemiology of HPV infection in women closely parallels that of CIN, and cervical cancer and risk factors such as early age of first intercourse, number of sexual partners, cigarette smoking, and immunosuppressive status are similar. Clinical evidence from one prospective study shows that women who have normal cervical cytologic results and who are infected with HPV have a significantly higher rate of subsequent development of CIN than HPV-negative women with normal cytologic findings.[47] A case-controlled study from Latin America examined risk factors for cervical cancer and found risk factors similar to those described previously but also found that the strongest independent risk factor was the presence of HPV DNA.[48]

The first evidence linking HPV infection with cervical cancer was the recognition that certain cytologic features interpreted in cervical smears as dysplasia were actually manifestations of HPV infection.[49] These HPV-infected cells were called koilocytes, meaning "hollow cell," because of their large perinuclear cytoplasmic clear zone or cavity. Such a cell must also have nuclear atypia to be considered a koilocyte.[50] Koilocytosis is now considered pathognomonic of HPV's cytopathic effect on the intermediate and superficial cell layers of squamous epithelium. The close association between HPV and cervical neoplasia is further substantiated by the detection of HPV in 80 to 90 percent of CIN and cervical cancer specimens.[51] In culture systems HPV has been shown to be capable of in vitro malignant human cell transformation and cell immortalization, although HPV infection alone does not lead to malignant transformation.[52, 53] It appears likely that HPV acts as a cellular promoter for proliferation, which may work together with an initiator to lead to malignant transformation.

Currently, more than 60 different genotypes of HPV have been identified. Research efforts have been directed toward analyzing the prevalence and distribution of genital HPV genotypes and their relationship to the natural history of CIN. HPV types 6 and 11 are often associated with condyloma acuminatum and low-grade squamous intraepithelial lesions (LSIL). These virus subtypes were considered to be low-risk because they are rarely associated with carcinoma and the lesions typically do not progress to high-grade squamous intraepithelial lesions (HSIL). HPV types 16, 18, and 33, on the other hand, appear to be the most oncogenic and have been associated with HSIL and cervical cancer. These "high-risk" types are thought to have a higher propensity for progression. It is important to recognize that HPV types 16 and 18 are the most common ones in both LSIL and HSIL, but many cases of LSIL do not progress.

The prognostic value of defining low- and high-risk HPV types and the role of HPV typing need to be clarified. In one recent study, the reverse of the findings described earlier was noted. HPV types 16, 18, and 33 were found more commonly in low-grade (CIN 1) lesions,[54] and HPV types 6 and 11 were identified in cervical cancers.[48] In contrast, prospective studies of women infected with high-risk HPV types have shown significant progression rates to HSIL compared to those without detectable HPV.[47, 55]

Infection with HPV types 16 and 18 does not consistently correlate with the geographic incidence of cervical cancer. A study from Greenland and Denmark compared the incidence of HPV and herpes simplex virus type 2 (HSV-2) in the normal population.[56] Although the incidence of cervical cancer is 5.6 times higher in Greenland, women in Denmark have a higher prevalence of HPV types 16 and 18 whereas that for HPV types 6 and 11 is the same in both countries. It is interesting to note that women in Greenland have a much higher incidence of HSV-2 antibodies and a significantly greater number of sexual partners than women in Denmark. This raises the possibility of a carcinogenic effect of HPV and HSV-2.

For HPV typing to be clinically useful it must serve a defined role in clinical management. Proponents of HPV typing see it as a useful adjunct to the standard approach of cytology screening followed by colposcopy. Women with latent HPV infection or LSIL caused by high-risk HPV types could be identified. However, given the uncertainty of the natural history of HPV infection and the fact that even those infected with HPV types 6 and 11 need close follow-up, this approach is not considered worthwhile.

At present, the natural history of low- and high-risk HPV types remains unknown and unpredictable. There are insufficient data regarding the appropriate evaluation, treatment, and follow-up of women infected with latent genital HPV. Currently, there is no effective treatment to eliminate the virus. Benign lesions are treated by local therapy if they produce symptoms. Women with SIL are managed according to the grade of the neoplasia. Standard treatment of women who have CIN or cervical cancer is based strictly on the histopathologic diagnosis regardless of the HPV genotype.[56a]

The actual prevalence of genital HPV is unknown because only clinically evident disease is reported and the majority of HPV infections remain subclinical or latent. More important, population studies using the polymerase chain reaction (PCR) method estimate that as many as 40 to 70 percent of sexually active, "disease-free" women who have normal cervical cytologic findings, normal colposcopy results, and normal cervical biopsies are infected with HPV.[57, 58] HPV infection alone does not result in CIN or cervical cancer because only about 5 percent of sexually active women develop HPV-associated lesions. Because of this discrepancy, progression from latent HPV infection to CIN appears to be dependent on the cumulative effect of other cofactors such as smoking, immune status, or other sexually transmitted diseases.

NOMENCLATURE AND HISTOPATHOLOGIC GRADING OF PREINVASIVE LESIONS OF THE CERVIX AND VAGINA

The nomenclature used to describe the preinvasive lesions of the cervix and vagina has changed several times during the last 20 years. It is important to understand each of the nomenclature systems to compare the literature in this area. Traditionally, preinvasive lesions were divided into mild, moderate, or severe dysplasia and carcinoma in situ (CIS).[59] A schematic representation comparing the patterns of intraepithelial neoplasia from normal epithelium to microinvasive squamous carcinoma of the cervix is shown in Figure 3–2. In this representation, segment *A* represents normal epithelium, *B* a very mild dysplasia, *C* mild dysplasia, *D* moderate dysplasia, *E* severe dysplasia, *F* carcinoma in situ, and *G* microinvasive carcinoma. In the CIN nomenclature panels *A* and *B* are classified as normal or benign changes, *C* as CIN 1, *D* as CIN 2, and both *E* and *F* as CIN 3. Under the Bethesda system (TBS), which was designed to standardize the nomenclature for cytologic diagnoses, cells retrieved from the surface of *B* would

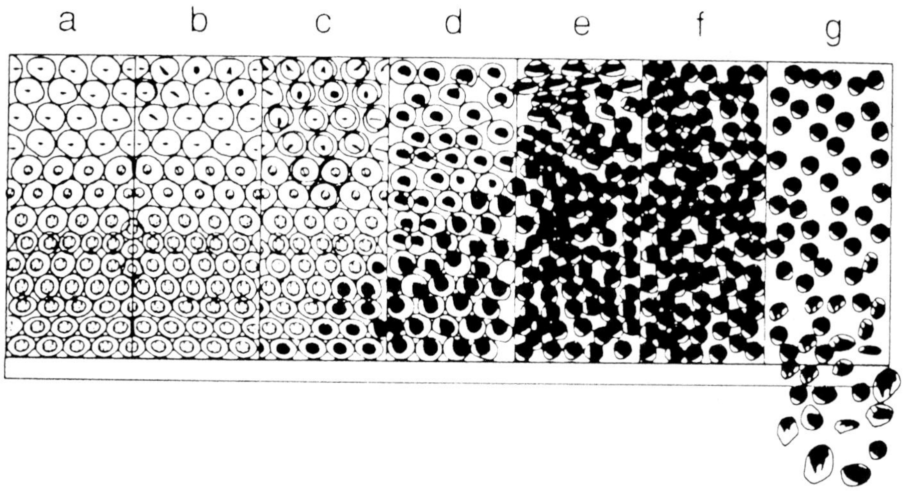

FIGURE 3-2
A schematic representation of the spectrum of intraepithelial neoplasia and microinvasive squamous carcinoma of the cervix is compared with the normal cervical epithelium. Normal epithelium (*a*), very mild dysplasia (*b*), mild dysplasia (*c*), moderate dysplasia (*d*), severe dysplasia (*e*), carcinoma in situ (*f*), microinvasive carcinoma (*g*). The cervical intraepithelial neoplasia (CIN) nomenclature would classify *a* and *b* as normal or benign changes, *c* as CIN 1, *d* as CIN 2, and *e* and *f* as CIN 3. Under the Bethesda system, which was designed to standardize the nomenclature of cytologic diagnoses, cells retrieved from the surface of *b* would be diagnosed as atypical squamous cells of undetermined significance (ASCUS), *c* as low-grade squamous intraepithelial lesion (LSIL), and *d*, *e*, and *f* as high-grade squamous intraepithelial lesion (HSIL).

be diagnosed as atypical squamous cells of undetermined significance (ASCUS), *C* would be diagnosed as LSIL, and *D*, *E*, and *F* would be classified as HSIL.

As can be seen from this comparison, the dysplasia/CIS nomenclature is a system with four tiers of diagnostic choice (mild, moderate, or severe dysplasia and CIS), whereas the CIN system has three tiers (CIN 1, 2, and 3), and TBS has two tiers (LSIL and HSIL). TBS does allow for an ASCUS category to diagnose a more minimal change than occurs in the LSIL category. ASCUS is further qualified as to whether a benign or premalignant process is favored (see subsequent discussion).

At the current time the standard of practice for cytopathologic diagnosis is to use the TBS.[60] For histopathologic diagnosis the dysplasia/CIS nomenclature has been generally replaced by the CIN nomenclature. A Papanicolaou smear diagnosed using TBS can be easily correlated with a histopathologic diagnosis made using the CIN nomenclature. It is possible for histopathologists to use TBS when rendering a diagnosis on a tissue specimen. However, more information is transmitted using the CIN nomenclature. The major advantages of the CIN nomenclature are the recognition that minimal lesions should not be called CIN and that because the significance of severe dysplasia versus carcinoma in situ is similar, both are called CIN 3. Lesions may progress directly from either severe dysplasia or CIS to invasive carcinoma.

In considering a comparison of the cytologic diagnosis to the histopathologic one, it is important to recognize that a cervical-vaginal cytologic smear retrieves cells that either have been exfoliated or are within the top one or two layers of the surface epithelium. The cytopathologist uses the appearance of these cells to make a diagnosis that is used to predict the severity of the changes seen in a full-thickness biopsy of the epithelium. Obviously, there are many variables in this analysis. The cytologic smear samples cells from a broad surface of the cervical and endocervical epithelium, whereas a biopsy samples one or more small localized areas that are selected based on abnormalities identified by visual inspection, usually by colposcopy (see later discussion). This difference may also lead to difficulty in correlation between the specimens. The surface cells may not reflect the lesions at the bottom of the epithelium. Invasion, for instance, may be covered by a surface that is only minimally abnormal or by necrosis and nonviable cells. If there is disagreement by more than one level or grade and the cytologic findings show a higher grade than the biopsy, then additional studies such as conization should be considered. Prior to this the cytology should be reviewed, however, to be sure that a correct diagnosis was made originally.

To arrive at the histopathologic grade in a biopsy specimen the portion of the total thickness of the epithelium that is filled with premalignant transformed cells is estimated. As shown in Figure 3–2, the transformed cells are smaller and have a

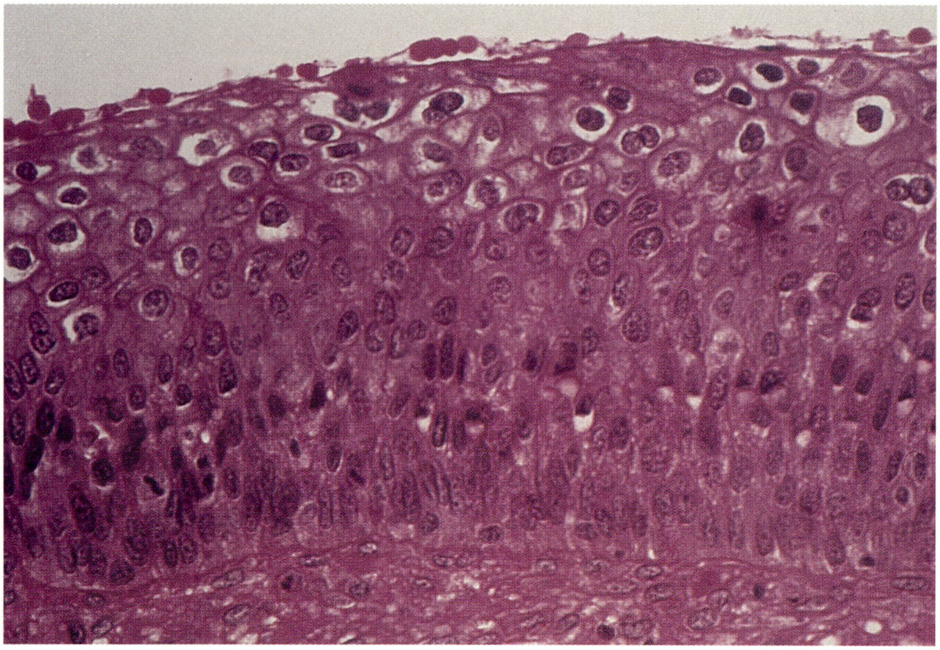

FIGURE 3-3
This cervical biopsy demonstrates CIN 1. The cells in the bottom one third of the epithelium are smaller and have scant cytoplasm. Some have lost their normal orientation. There is nuclear pleomorphism. Mitoses are seen above the basal layer; the cells above have more cytoplasm but still have abnormal nuclei. A clear cavity surrounds the abnormal nuclei of the cells, which are known as koilocytes.

darker nucleus than the normal basal cells (basaloid appearance). This change begins at the basal cell layer, and the cells proliferate to expand throughout the epithelium. In a CIN 1 lesion the basaloid cells are confined to the lower third of the epithelium (Fig. 3–3). These cells have an irregular nuclear membrane and scant cytoplasm. The orientation of the cells in the lower third of the epithelium is random. In CIN 1 lesions the cells in the upper two-thirds of the epithelium gain cytoplasm and orient themselves in a uniform pattern with their long axis parallel to the surface. The nuclei however, continue to be atypical. In CIN 2 lesions the basaloid cells occupy up to two-thirds of the epithelium (Fig. 3–4), and in CIN 3 lesions the abnormality involves almost all (severe dysplasia) or all (CIS) of the epithelial thickness (Fig. 3–5). With the passage of time some cells gain the

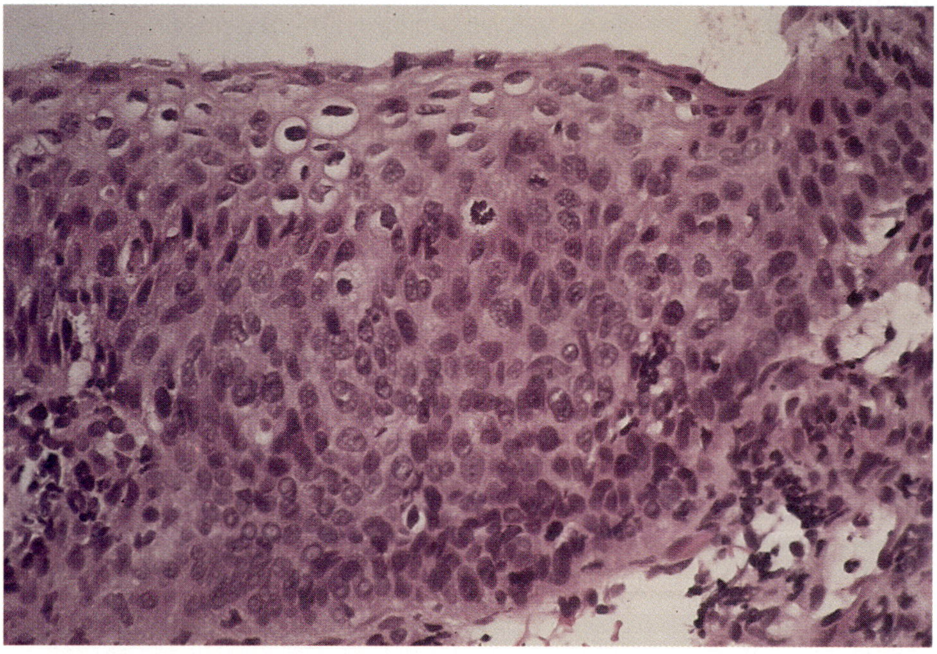

FIGURE 3-4
This cervical biopsy demonstrates CIN 2. Basaloid cells occupy two thirds of the epithelium. Mitoses are seen high in the epithelium. Koilocytes are present near the surface.

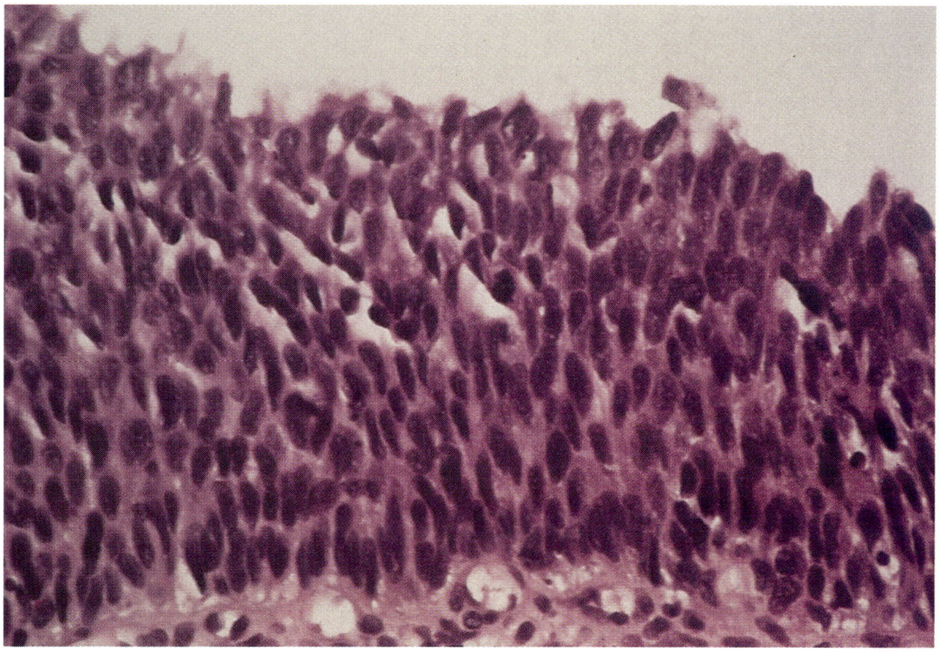

FIGURE 3–5
This cervical biopsy demonstrates CIN 3. The basaloid cells occupy the full thickness of the epithelium. The orientation of the cells is somewhat disorganized, but many of the nuclei have their long axis perpendicular to the basement membrane. There is prominent hyperchromasia.

potential to break through the basement membrane. At this time the appearance of the cells becomes more pleomorphic. Often there is an increased amount of cytoplasm.

In estimating the degree of CIN that is present, it is important to have a full-thickness biopsy section that demonstrates the epithelium from the basement membrane to the surface. In a small colposcopic biopsy specimen it may be easy to misorient the specimen, resulting in a tangential or horizontal cut. These specimens must not be graded because it is easy to overestimate the degree of intraepithelial neoplasia. If the histopathologic section exhibits a tangential cut, the biopsy specimen can sometimes be rotated in the block and recut. It is also important to recognize that neoplastic transformation begins at the transformation zone in most cases and often occurs in an immature squamous metaplasia. This immature epithelium may not have as many cell layers as the one shown in the schematic diagram (Fig. 3–2). There may be as few as five or six layers of cells present. These cases may be more difficult to classify but the degree of intraepithelial neoplasia should not be underestimated. CIN also occurs in metaplasia within endocervical glands (Fig. 3–6). The degree of CIN in endocervical glands can be very difficult to judge and should not be attempted at all unless there is a distinct glandular lumen connecting with the surface. When this occurs, the same criteria are used as when evaluating the lesion in surface epithelium. It is also important to recognize the difference in appearance between CIN within glands and invasive carcinoma. Endocervical glands have a basement membrane. If there is a question of invasion, deeper cuts may help to recognize the difference between an attachment of a gland to the surface and the presence of definite invasion. In determining whether there is invasion, the presence of an inflammatory infiltrate may be helpful, although this is not a diagnostic criterion by itself, since benign cervicitis also has a marked inflammatory infiltrate. The best criterion for invasion is the presence of larger and more pleomorphic cells below a basement membrane. These cells have more pleomorphic nuclei than is seen in CIN 3 lesions and may have nucleoli. Their cytoplasm is often abundant and eosinophilic.

The diagnosis of HPV in histologic sections is made by the recognition of koilocytic cells, which indicates an HPV infection. These cells have a large cavity or hole surrounding an abnormal nucleus. There is usually condensation of the cytoplasmic border around the cavity. The nucleus is often wrinkled or raisin-shaped and may be slightly hyperchromatic. The appearance of rows of cells that have koilocytic cavities leads to an irregular cellular arrangement resembling chicken wire. This appearance must be distinguished from that of the normal glycogenated epithelium. Glycogenated cells may sometimes have clear spaces around the nuclei, but glycogenation is very uniform and the cells form regular rows, whereas the

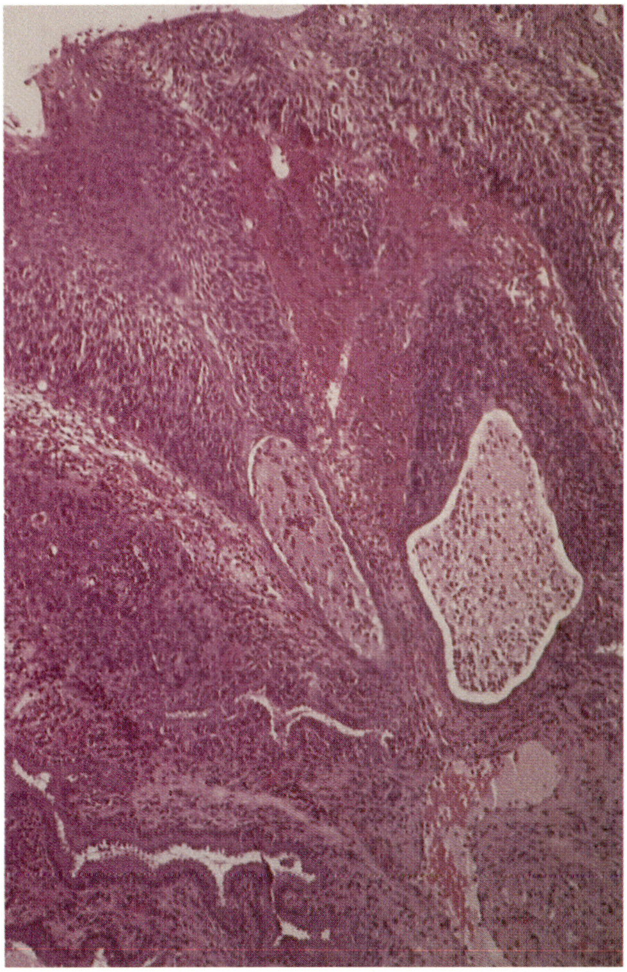

FIGURE 3-6
This cervical biopsy demonstrates squamous intraepithelial neoplasia (SIL) in glands. Normal endocervical glands are seen *(bottom left)*. A transition from normal endocervical epithelium to neoplastic squamous epithelium is seen in three other glands. SIL in glands should not be graded.

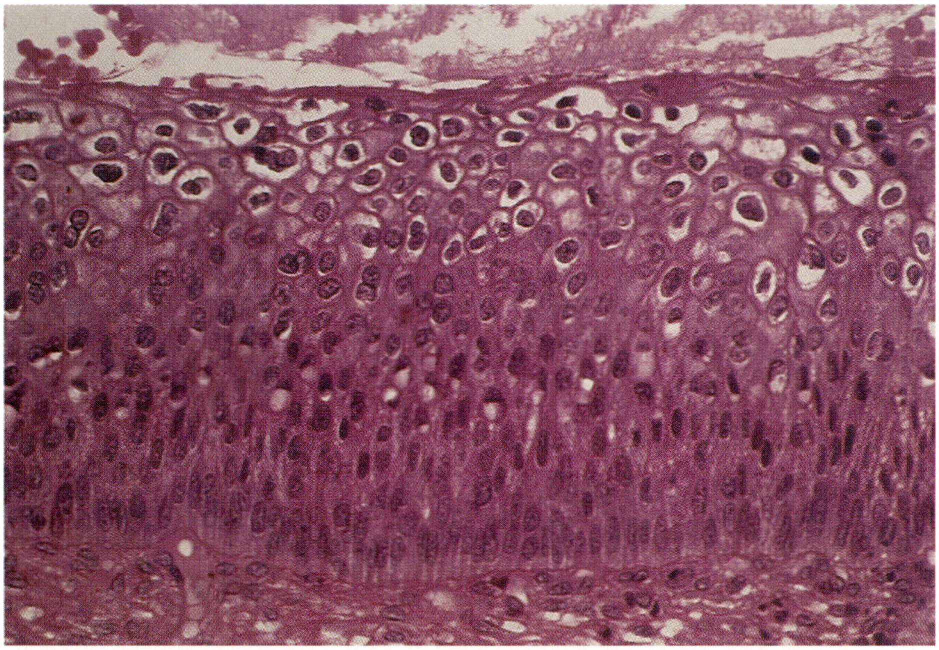

FIGURE 3-7
This cervical biopsy demonstrates koilocytotic changes extending to the epithelial surface, which is flat. Basaloid cells occupy the lower one-third of the epithelium. This is consistent with CIN 1.

koilocytes of an HPV infection are irregularly spaced and have a haphazard arrangement.

Cervical epithelial changes caused by HPV infection are considered the equivalent of LSIL in TBS and usually warrant a diagnosis of CIN 1. The surface of an HPV-infected cervical lesion is most commonly flat (Fig. 3–7). Koilocytes often extend to the surface, so they are present on a Papanicolaou smear. HPV-associated changes, however, may be apparent as a raised, bulbous, peaky, or warty surface (Fig. 3–8). When one of these raised lesions is present the surface epithelium often shows an abnormal keratinized plaque covering the underlying koilocytes. The surface cells and plaque have been called dyskeratosis when seen on cytologic examination. This terminology is used to indicate that there is an abnormal degree of cytoplasmic keratinization (yellow, orange, or fuchsia-colored cytoplasm rather than the normal blue or pink color of a superficial cell that has been stained using the Papanicolaou technique), and this abnormal keratinization is associated with a dyssynchronous and irregular nuclear maturation. Sometimes the surface of HPV-related lesions shows parakeratosis or hyperkeratosis, which represent a normal type of hyperkeratinization. Such changes are normally found in the skin but are abnormal in mucosa like that of the cervix and vagina. The presence of parakeratosis or hyperkeratosis in the cervix and vagina may be a surface change typical of HPV-associated lesions, or it may be a traumatically induced epithelial reaction as seen in patients who have uterine prolapse or who use a pessary or have used tampons or a diaphragm for a long time.

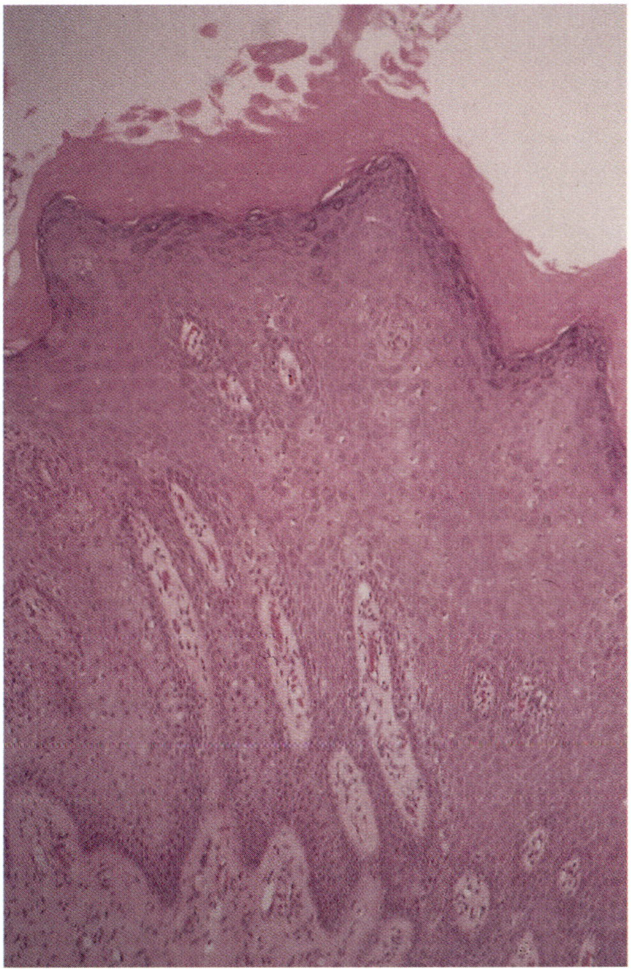

FIGURE 3–8
This cervical lesion has a peaky or warty hyperkeratinized surface. In this lesion, koilocytes are present but they are not on the surface.

CERVICAL AND VAGINAL SMEAR COLLECTION TECHNIQUE

Two factors that will help to ensure a correct cytopathologic diagnosis are provision of the necessary and appropriate clinical information with the cytopathologic consultation request and use of the correct technique to collect the cytologic specimen. In an effort to standardize techniques the National Committee for Clinical Laboratory Standards[61] has proposed guidelines for correct cervical sampling, and the Candadian Laboratory Testing Program has circulated similar guidelines.[62] A smear is taken preferably during the last 2 weeks of the menstrual cycle. However, if the woman is menstruating at the time of the visit the smear can still be taken. This specimen is usually adequate for evaluation unless excessive blood obscures the epithelial cells. Women should be advised not to use vaginal medications, contraceptives, or douches during the 48 hours prior to the office visit to avoid destroying or obscuring abnormal cells.

For a sample to be considered adequate it is necessary to obtain a specimen from both the ectocervix and the transformation zone. The adequacy of the sample is recognized by the cytopathologist by the presence of squamous metaplasia or endocervical cells on the smear. If a hormonal evaluation is required, a scrape from the lateral vaginal wall is necessary.[63, 64] If the clinician identifies any lesions on the vagina or cervix these should be individually scraped. Likewise, any vulvar lesions should be scraped. HPV and herpes lesions may be more obvious on the vulva than on the cervix. Because the vulvar lesions are often dry, resulting in an "air-dried" specimen, it is suggested that a saline-soaked gauze pad be held to the lesion for a few minutes to moisten the area before performing the scrape. A vaginal pool specimen is not recommended unless there is a specific suspicion that endometrial cancer or hyperplasia might be present.[65] If that is the case, then a vaginal pool specimen should be obtained in addition to the usual ectocervical or endocervical sample.

A variety of devices for obtaining cervical or vaginal cytologic samples are available (Fig. 3–9). Data are available comparing the efficacy of different sampling devices in obtaining proof of sampling of the transformation zone (i.e., an endocervical component).[66] The most commonly employed device for taking an ectocervical sample is a wooden or plastic spatula (e.g., Ayre spatula). Both are available in a variety of shapes. The spatula is placed firmly but gently against the cervix and rotated slightly past 360 degrees. In the past an endocervical specimen was usually obtained using a saline-moistened cotton-tipped applicator. The endocervical brush (e.g., Cytobrush) appears to be much more satisfactory in obtaining endocervical cells and is now used by many clinics to obtain the endocervical sample in nonpregnant women.[67] Other devices that have a brush (e.g., Cervex-Brush, Bayne Pap Brush, and others) obtain both the ectocervical and endocervical samples at the same time.[68] The sample obtained with the brush can be either put into a liquid fixative or smeared directly on a glass slide.

When using any of these endocervical sampling devices it is important to be gentle and not overly aggressive or bleeding may occur. The endocervical brush should not be forced too high into the endocervical canal. Because the brush is longer than the endocervical canal of some women, lower uterine segment endometrial sampling is obtained when sampling is too vigorous. The endocervical sample is taken by gently inserting the brush into the endocervical canal and turning it slightly past 360 degrees.

Currently, most cytopathologists prefer to have both the cervical and endocervical samples placed on only one glass slide. There are now federal regulations (CLIA 1988)[69] restricting the number of slides that a cytotechnologist can screen in one day (100 is the maximum). Because there is currently a significant shortage of cytotechnologists in the United States, it is important for each cytotechnologist to be able to screen as many individual cases as possible.

The sample should be spread quickly and uniformly across a slide that has a frosted end on which the patient's name has been written. The goal is to smear the material as quickly and evenly as possible and to fix the specimen immediately. After the specimen has been spread the slide is generally fixed with spray fixative. Ninety-five percent ethanol is widely accepted as the ideal fixative for cells. When this is used the slides must remain in the alcohol until they reach the laboratory. This is seldom practical, and spray fixative is routinely used by most clinicians. Commercial cytofixative should be used according to the directions of the manufacturer. When coating or spray fixatives are used, the nozzle of the spraying apparatus should be held approximately 12 inches from the slide. Holding the spray fixative container too close to the slide can result in cel-

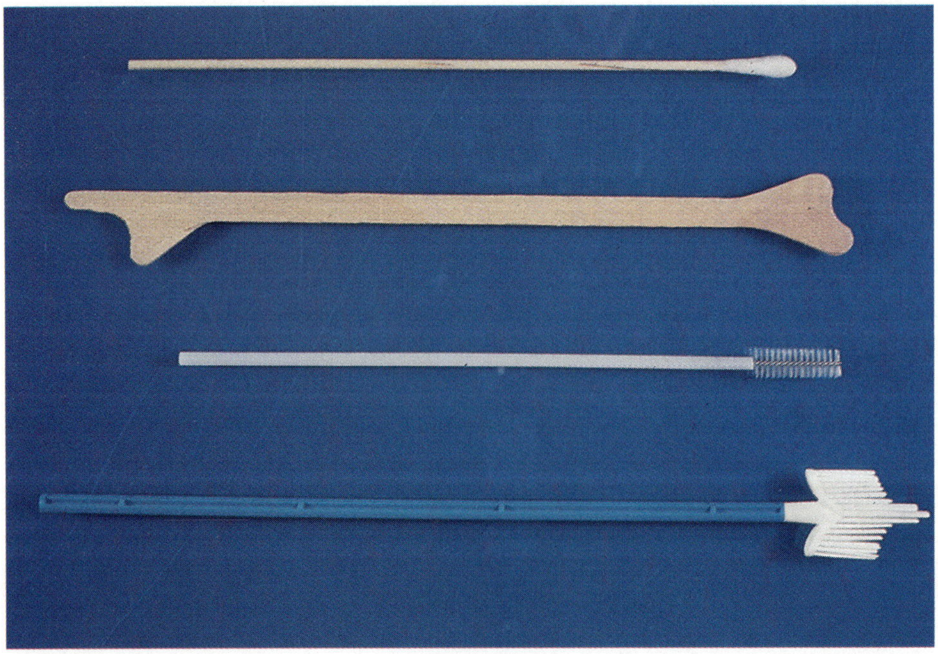

FIGURE 3–9
Commonly used cervical cytology sampling devices are shown. *From top to bottom;* Cotton-tipped applicator, wooden Ayre spatula, endocervical brush, Cervex-Brush.

lular artifacts, whereas holding the container too far away from the slide may result in drying artifacts or uneven fixation. Hair spray should not be used as a cell fixative because there is variability in its composition that may lead to poor fixation.

We routinely place the ectocervical sample on the slide first; then we mix it with the endocervical sample and then smear the mixed sample evenly. If separate ectocervical and endocervical samples are desired, the ectocervical sample is obtained first and placed longitudinally on one-half of the slide, and the endocervical specimen is then placed longitudinally on the opposite half of the slide. The smear is then fixed immediately because the endocervical sample dries very quickly when exposed to air. Alternatively, the ectocervical sample can be placed first on one side of the slide and spray fixative applied while a piece of cardboard protects the empty half of the slide. When the endocervical sample is placed on the other side of the slide it is also fixed. This method is more time consuming and impractical.

It is essential to label the slide with the patient's name and to fill out the cytopathology consultation request form completely and accurately. This form should show the patient's identification, the date of collection, the source of material, and other pertinent information. The latter includes the patient's age, last menstrual period, hormonal status, exogenous hormonal therapy, the presence or absence of an intrauterine contraceptive device (IUD), a history of in utero exposure to DES, a history of CIN, cervical cancer, or any other cancer, and any other pertinent information. The number of slides submitted and the submitting physician's name and phone number are also important information. The laboratory will consider any slides not accompanied by a requisition form as unacceptable for processing or interpretation. If pertinent clinical information is missing, the specimen should be classified as unsatisfactory for evaluation or satisfactory but limited depending on which information is missing. According to TBS criteria, a specimen should be considered unsatisfactory for evaluation if there is a lack of patient identification on the slide or requisition form or if the slide is broken and cannot be repaired. A case is satisfactory for evaluation but limited if pertinent clinical information is lacking (age and last menstrual period are the minimum).

THE BETHESDA SYSTEM AND CYTOLOGIC DIAGNOSES OF PREINVASIVE LESIONS

TBS for reporting cervical or vaginal cytologic diagnoses was originally devised in 1988 and modified in 1991.[70] It was designed to standardize the nomenclature used in describing the cytopathology of lesions of the cervix and vagina. By the time of the 1991 Bethesda workshop the use of TBS had become widespread nationally, and it is now the standard of practice in the United States for cytologic diagnoses on gynecologic specimens. TBS as modified in 1991 is shown in Table 3–2. After the revisions to TBS were made, specific criteria were developed for the diagnosis of each of these categories. A monograph has recently been published listing the criteria and showing pictures of each of these diagnoses and the important difficult diagnoses.[60]

The first diagnostic decision that is made upon review of a cytologic specimen is whether the specimen is adequate. If the specimen is adequate, the terminology used is satisfactory for evaluation. If the specimen is unsatisfactory for evaluation, the reason is specified. Four elements determine the adequacy of the specimen: (1) patient and specimen identification, (2) pertinent clinical information, (3) technical interpretability, and (4) cellular composition and sampling of the transformation zone. The first two have already been discussed. Technical interpretability has to do with whether the cells on the smear are obscured by blood, inflammation, thick areas, poor fixation, air drying artifact, contaminants, and so on. The smear is considered unsatisfactory for evaluation if approximately 75 percent or more of the epithelial cells are obscured by any of these elements. If 50 to 75 percent of the epithelial cells are obscured, the smear is considered satisfactory for interpretation but limited owing to that fact. If less than 10 percent of the surface of the slide is covered by well-preserved and well-visualized squamous epithelial cells this also makes the smear unsatisfactory for interpretation because of the scant squamous component. A specimen is also classified as satisfactory for evaluation but limited when an endocervical or transformation zone component is absent in a specimen from a patient who still has a cervix. An endocervical or transformation zone component consists at a minimum of two clusters of well-preserved endocervical glandular or squamous metaplastic cells with each cluster composed of at least five cells. This definition applies to specimens from both premenopausal and postmenopausal women except in the situation of marked atrophy in which metaplastic and endocervical cells often cannot be distinguished from parabasal-like cells.

A very important fact to remember is that a smear should never be called unsatisfactory for evaluation if an abnormality is identified. For example, if cells consistent with LSIL are present

TABLE 3–2.

The 1991 Bethesda System for Reporting Cervical/Vaginal Cytologic Diagnoses

I. Adequacy of the Specimen for Evaluation

Satisfactory for evaluation

Satisfactory but limited by . . . (specify reason)

Unsatisfactory for evaluation . . . (specify reason)

II. General Categorization

Within normal limits

Benign cellular findings: See descriptive diagnosis

Epithelial cell abnormality: See descriptive diagnosis

III. Descriptive Diagnoses

Benign Cellular Changes

Infection

- Trichomonas vaginalis
- Fungal organisms morphologically consistent with *Candida* spp.
- Predominance of coccobacilli consistent with shift in vaginal flora
- Bacteria morphologically consistent with *Actinomyces* spp.
- Cellular changes associated with Herpes simplex virus
- Other

Reactive Changes

Reactive cellular changes associated with:

- Inflammation (includes typical repair)
- Atrophy with inflammation (atrophic vaginitis)
- Radiation
- Intrauterine contraceptive device (IUD)
- Other

Epithelial Cell Abnormalities

Squamous Cell

- Atypical squamous cells of undetermined significance: Qualify*
- LSIL, encompassing: HPV† and mild dysplasia (CIN 1)
- High-grade SIL encompassing moderate and severe dysplasia (CIN 2 and CIN 3/CIS)
- Squamous cell carcinoma

Glandular Cell

- Endometrial cells, cytologically benign, in a postmenopausal woman
- Atypical glandular cells of undetermined significance: Qualify*
- Endocervical adenocarcinoma
- Endometrial adenocarcinoma
- Extrauterine adenocarcinoma
- Adenocarcinoma (unable to identify primary site of origin)

Other Malignant Neoplasms: Specify

Hormonal Evaluation (applies to vaginal smears only)

- Hormonal pattern compatible with age and history
- Hormonal pattern incompatible with age and history: Specify
- Hormonal evaluation not possible due to: Specify

* Atypical squamous or glandular cells of undetermined significance should be further qualified as to whether a reactive or a premalignant or malignant process is favored.

† Cellular changes secondary to HPV infection (previously termed koilocytosis, koilocytotic atypia, or condylomatous atypia) are included in the category of LSIL.

but there are only a few squamous cells the smear should not be considered unsatisfactory. It should be called "satisfactory for evaluation but limited by scant squamous component; changes consistent with LSIL are identified." Unsatisfactory implies that no diagnosis is possible, and no diagnosis should be made.

The next decision that is usually made is the general categorization. This is an optional category. It divides the findings into three types: within normal limits, benign cellular changes, and epithelial cell abnormalities. This category is often used as a triage route to separate those smears that are completely normal from those showing benign changes and those with epithelial cell abnormalities. The category of benign cellular changes may necessitate additional follow-up or sometimes a diagnostic procedure or treatment for infection. Most cytologic changes secondary to infection (but not HPV) are in the benign cellular change category. HPV is considered an epithelial cell abnormality and at least LSIL. The infectious and reactive processes causing benign cellular changes have been described in Chapter 2.

Epithelial cell abnormalities are divided into squamous cell abnormalities, glandular cell abnormalities, and other malignant neoplasms. The squamous cell category is divided into ASCUS, LSIL, HSIL, and squamous cell carcinoma. The ASCUS category should be separated further according to whether a reactive (Fig. 3–10) or a premalignant or malignant (Fig. 3–11) process is favored. Glandular cell abnormalities are separated into cytologically benign endometrial cells in a postmenopausal woman, atypical glandular cells of undetermined significance ([AGUS], which should be further qualified as to whether a reactive or premalignant-malignant process is favored), endocervical, endometrial, or extrauterine adenocarcinoma, and adenocarcinoma not otherwise specified. Figure 3–12 shows in schematic form the cells of ASCUS, LSIL, HPV/LSIL, and HSIL including moderate dysplasia, severe dysplasia, and CIS.

The criteria for LSIL include the presence of nuclear enlargement of at least three times the area of a normal intermediate cell nucleus in cells that have cytoplasm similar to that of a normal mature superficial cell (Fig. 3–13). This results in an increased nuclear to cytoplasmic ratio. There is moderate variation in nuclear size and shape. Hyperchromasia is present, and the chromatin is uniformly distributed.

Cells that are diagnostic for HPV infection demonstrate a well-defined, optically clear perinuclear cavity and peripheral dense rim of cytoplasm.

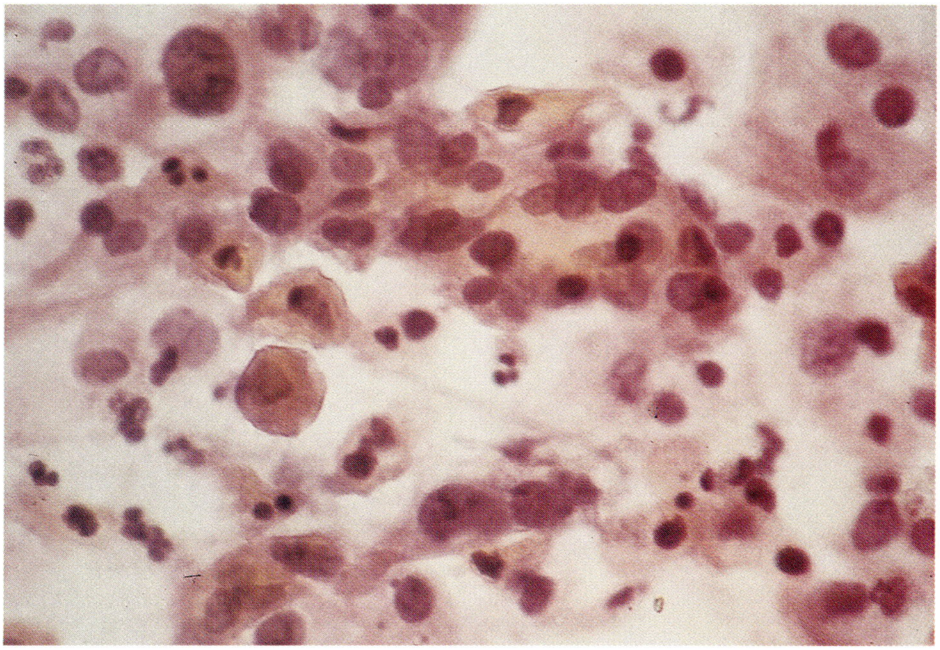

FIGURE 3-10
This cervical smear has numerous squamous cells, many of which have enlarged and hyperchromatic nuclei. However, the chromatin is smudged, and cell and nuclear borders are not crisp. This is consistent with degeneration and inflammatory changes. Leukocytes are present. This smear is diagnosed as ASCUS, favor a reactive process.

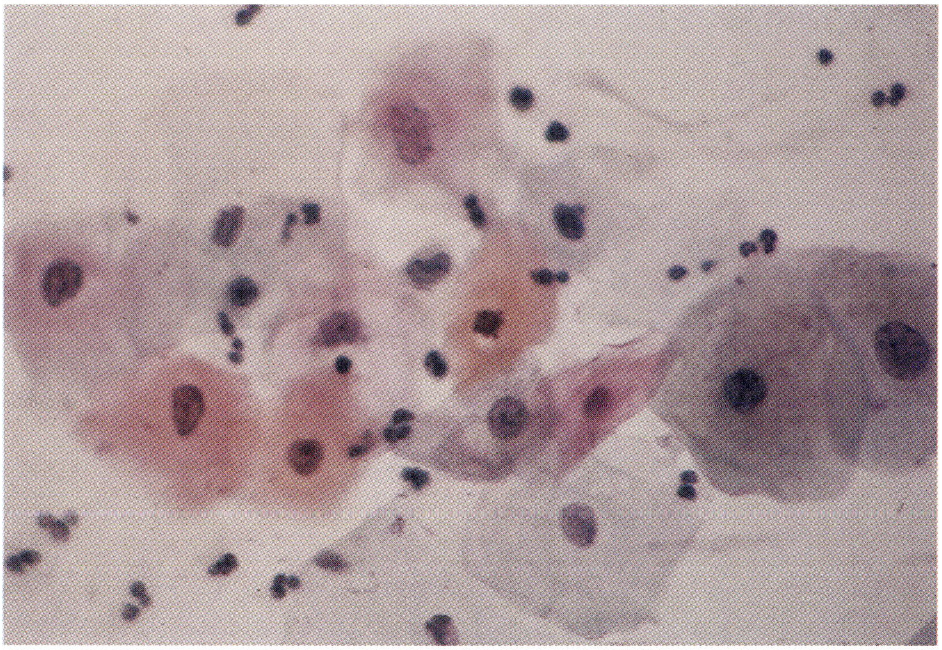

FIGURE 3-11
A normal intermediate cell is seen near the bottom center of this cervical smear. Three cells that have pink to orange cytoplasm and hyperchromatic nuclei are seen on the left. At the center there are three cells with degenerate nuclei. The one at the top center exhibits karyorrhexis. The three cells on the left would be best classified as ASCUS, favor LSIL, since the nuclear area is not three times that of a normal intermediate cell nucleus.

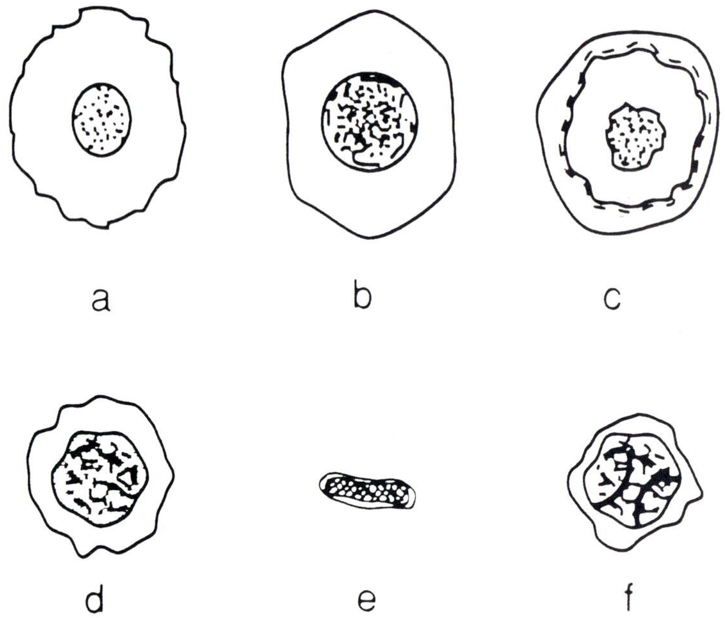

FIGURE 3-12
The cytologic appearance of all grades of squamous intraepithelial lesions is shown. The cells show increasing levels of abnormality from *a* to *f*. *a*, ASCUS. The cell is normal in size, but the nucleus is two to three times the size of a normal intermediate cell nucleus and the cytoplasmic borders are sometimes wrinkled. *b*, LSIL (CIN 1). The cell is normal in size, but the nucleus is more than three times the size of a normal intermediate cell nucleus and uniform hyperchromatism is seen. *c*, LSIL/HPV changes (CIN 1). Similar to *b*, but a wrinkled nucleus sits within a large cavity and there is cytoplasmic condensation around the edges of this cavity. *d*, HSIL (CIN 2). The size of the cell is about the size of a metaplastic cell, but the nucleus is larger and more hyperchromatic and has irregular shape. *e*, HSIL (CIN 3). The cell is small with scant cytoplasm, the nucleus is elongate, and the dense hyperchromatism has a sieve-like pattern. *f*, HSIL (CIN 3). The cell is smaller and has less cytoplasm than the one shown in *d*, and there is nuclear folding appearing as lines in the nucleus. Nucleoli are not seen in any of these cells.

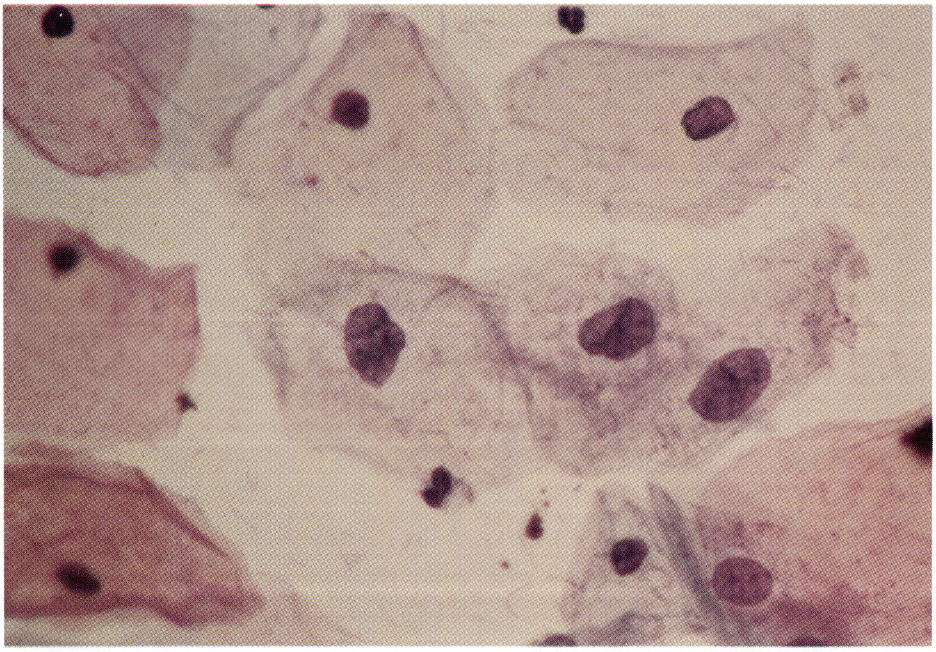

FIGURE 3-13
Three normal superficial cells are seen on the left. Three abnormal cells are seen in the center. The amount of cytoplasm in these cells is the same as that in an intermediate cell, but the size (area) of the nucleus is at least three times that of a normal intermediate cell nucleus. The nuclear borders are irregular, and lines secondary to folding are visible. There is hyperchromatism. These cells are diagnostic of LSIL (CIN 1).

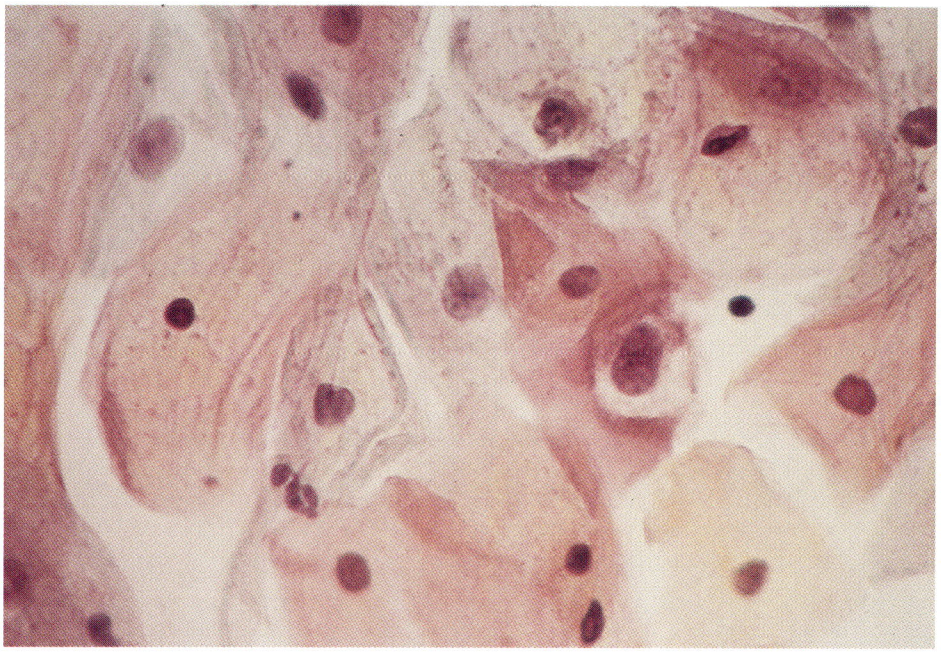

FIGURE 3–14
The fuchsia cell near the center is a koilocyte, diagnostic of LSIL/HPV. There is a large cavity within which two nuclei are seen. The cytoplasm surrounding the cavity is dense. To the left of the field there is a superficial cell that has a small pyknotic nucleus and abundant yellowish material, which is glycogen. The intermediate cell to its right is a glycogenated cell mimicking a koilocyte.

These cells are diagnostic of HPV infection and are called koilocytes only if they also have nuclear abnormalities (Fig. 3–14). These koilocytic cells may have slightly less nuclear enlargement than three times the area of a normal intermediate cell nucleus. However, the diagnosis of LSIL is still made.

The criteria for the diagnosis of HSIL are that the abnormal cells occur both singly and in either sheets or syncytial-like aggregates (Figs. 3–15, 3–16, and 3–17). The nuclear abnormalities occur predominantly in squamous cells that have cytoplasm characteristic of an immature or metaplastic cell. The chromatin may be lacy and delicate. Nuclear enlargement is in the size range of that seen in LSIL, but because the cytoplasmic area is decreased the nuclear enlargement results in a marked increase in the nuclear to cytoplasmic ratio. In HSIL the cell size is smaller than that seen in LSIL, and hyperchromasia is more evident. There may be finely or coarsely granular but evenly distributed chromatin. Nuclear outlines are irregular.

ASCUS is a lower category than LSIL. The defi-

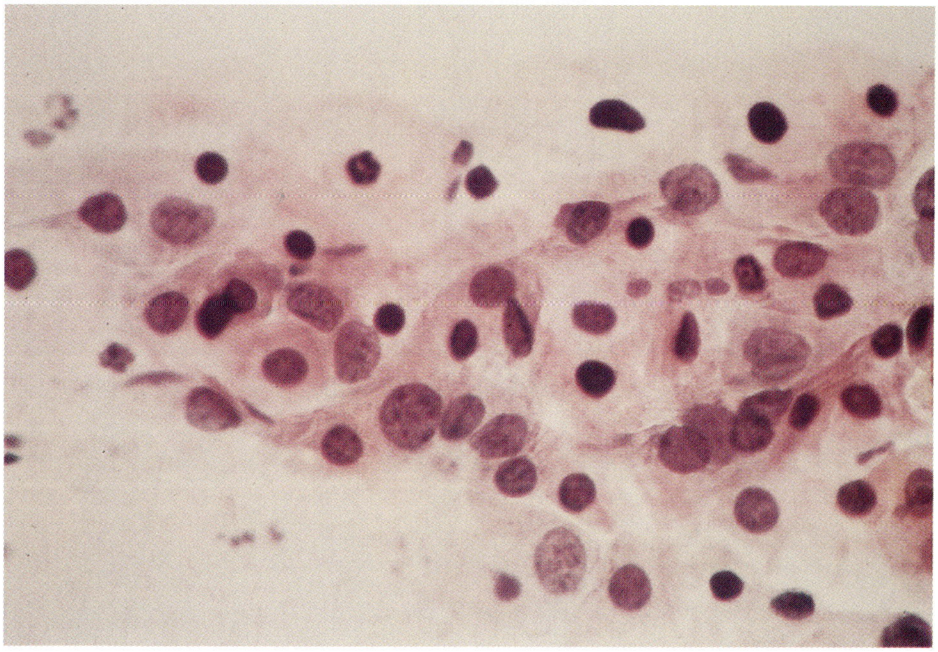

FIGURE 3–15
This smear shows many squamous cells with enlarged hyperchromatic nuclei. The cells at the top have a normal amount of cytoplasm and are consistent with LSIL, whereas many of the other cells have larger nuclei and scanter cytoplasm. These are diagnostic of HSIL (CIN 2).

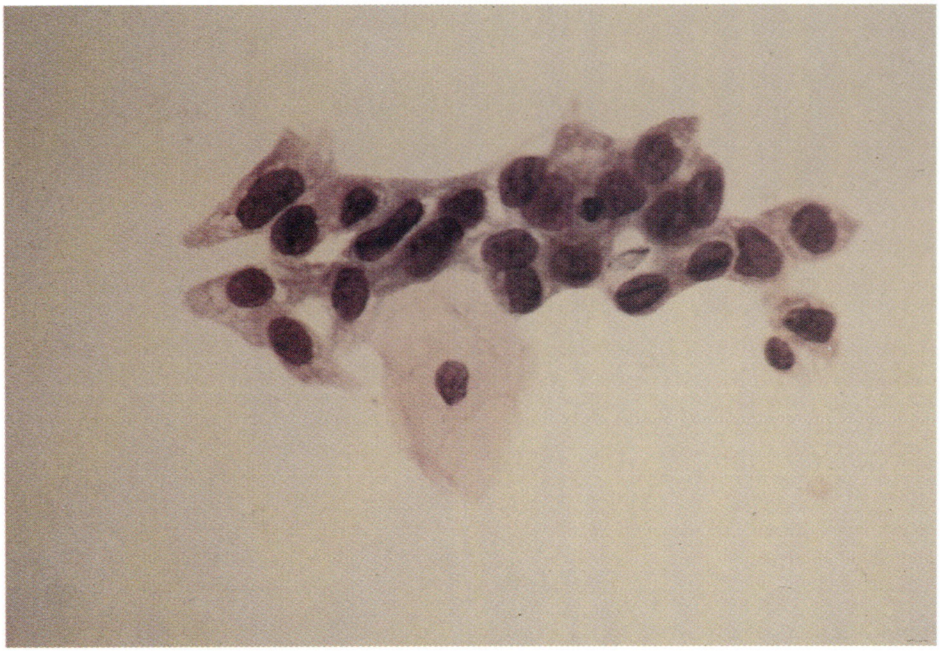

FIGURE 3-16
A sheet of abnormal squamous cells (syncytial group) is seen above a normal intermediate cell. The nuclei are enlarged and hyperchromatic. There is very scant cytoplasm in most of the cells. This is diagnostic of HSIL (CIN 3).

nition for ASCUS is that the cytologic changes are more marked than those classified as reactive, but quantitatively or qualitatively they are short of a definitive diagnosis of SIL. This category may have cells that reflect an exuberant benign change or a potentially serious lesion and should be used with care. Nuclear enlargement is generally two and a half to three times that of a normal intermediate squamous cell nucleus, but the cytoplasm is similar to that of a normal superficial cell. This leads to a slight increase in the nuclear to cytoplasmic ratio. Variations in nuclear size and shape and binucleation may be observed. Mild hyperchromasia may be present, but the chromatin remains evenly distributed without granularity. Nuclear outlines are generally smooth and regular.

The ASCUS category should not be overused. In any one laboratory no more than 10 percent of cervical-vaginal smears or 2 to 3 times the rate of LSIL plus HSIL diagnoses should be read as ASCUS. In our laboratory, which serves a high-risk inner city population, 1 percent of Papanicolaou smears are called ASCUS, 6 percent are

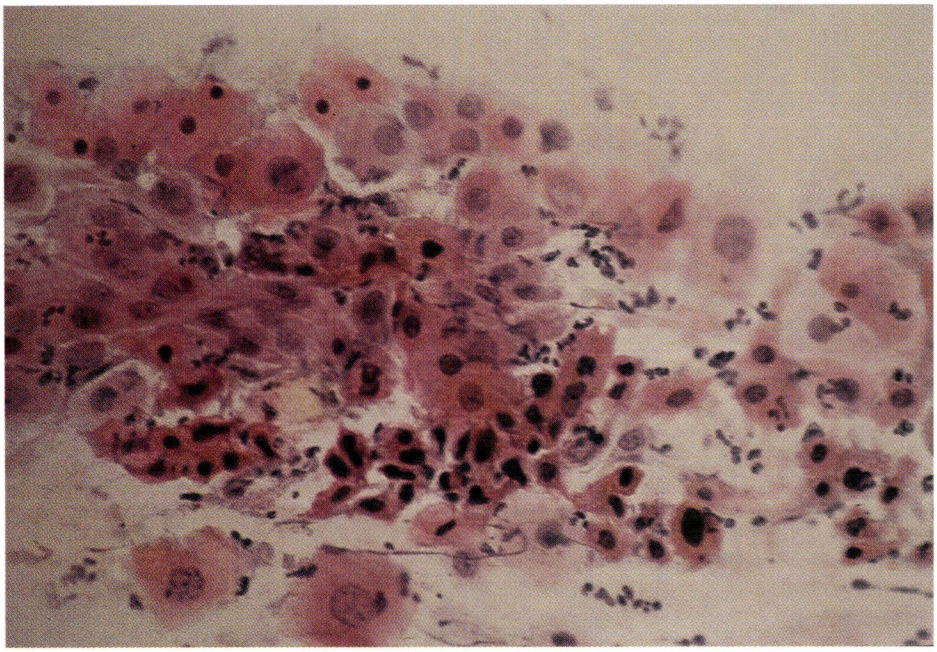

FIGURE 3-17
This smear shows a range of abnormal squamous cells from CIN 1 to keratinizing CIN 3. The cells with very hyperchromatic, often elongate, nuclei and scant hyperkeratinized (reddish) cytoplasm represent CIN 3.

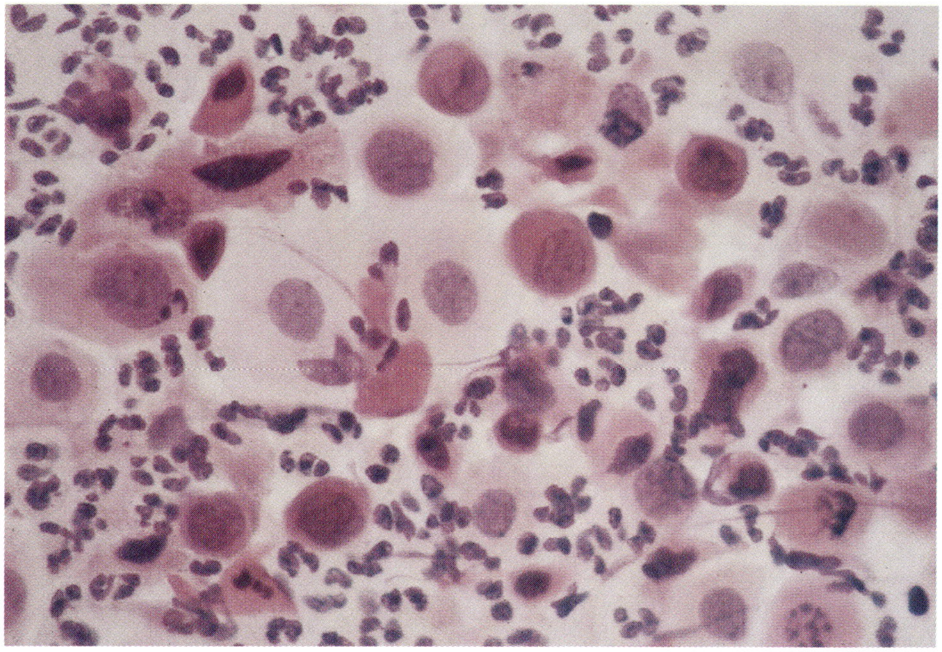

FIGURE 3-18
This cervical smear shows pleomorphic single squamous cells in a background of neutrophils. The nuclei vary in size, shape, and degree of hyperchromatism. The cytoplasm varies from very scant to abundant. Some of the cells have keratinized cytoplasm as seen by the dense texture and orangeophilic color. This smear was obtained from a patient who had cervical squamous cell carcinoma.

called ASCUS-favor reactive process, 4 percent ASCUS-favor LSIL, 4 percent LSIL, 1 percent HSIL, and 0.1 percent cancer. In the past it was shown that 20 to 30 percent of patients who had a cytologic diagnosis of ASCUS harbored CIN in their cervix.[71, 72] With the refinement of TBS we have found that this is now true in less than 15 percent of cases and that if a repeat Papanicolaou smear obtained 4 months after the initial ASCUS diagnosis is read as normal, we have found no patient with a significant abnormality identified by colposcopy and targeted biopsies.[73] Therefore, we no longer recommend colposcopic evaluation of patients who have a single Papanicolaou smear reading of ASCUS. These patients can be followed with Papanicolaou smears every 4 to 6 months until two or three normal smears are retrieved. Colposcopy is reserved for patients who have persistent ASCUS or a worse cytologic diagnosis.

A cytologic diagnosis of squamous cell carcinoma is rendered when abundant malignant cells are present. The background of the slide may be clean or, more often, degenerated blood and necrotic debris are present. This is considered a tumor diathesis. The malignant cells may be keratinized, nonkeratinized large cells, or small cells. Tumor cells are recognized by a marked pleomorphism of the single cells (Fig. 3-18) and of the cells within a single group. The nuclei show malignant features. These include hyperchromatism, irregular shape, and irregular chromatin clearing. Nucleoli may be present in carcinoma; they are not present in the cells of intraepithelial neoplasia. Malignant squamous cells usually have abundant cytoplasm. When the cells are keratinized they have pleomorphic shapes such as tadpole-like or fusiform.

The final aspect of the Bethesda system is the hormonal evaluation. As mentioned earlier, this evaluation should be done on a sample taken from the lateral vaginal wall. The hormonal patterns seen on a cervical or vaginal smear have been discussed in Chapter 2. Glandular intraepithelial lesions are discussed later in this chapter, and adenocarcinoma is discussed in Chapter 4.

COLPOSCOPY

The effectiveness of cervical cytology as a screening tool rests on its ability to detect abnormal cells in the surface epithelium of the cervical transformation zone in the asymptomatic woman. The revised Bethesda system reflects the current view of the biologic behavior of HPV infection and preinvasive cervical disease and can be used to standardize guidelines for clinical diagnosis and management.[74] An abnormal Papanicolaou smear identifies the woman who needs colposcopy. Colposcopy is the obligatory triage step after an abnormal result is found on screening cervical cytologic examination.

The colposcope is a binocular instrument capable of visualizing and magnifying the transformation zone of the cervix (Fig. 3-19). The skilled colposcopist can examine the cervix and vagina and then identify the most abnormal areas of the transformation zone for biopsy. This increases the specificity and sensitivity of the biopsy. As previ-

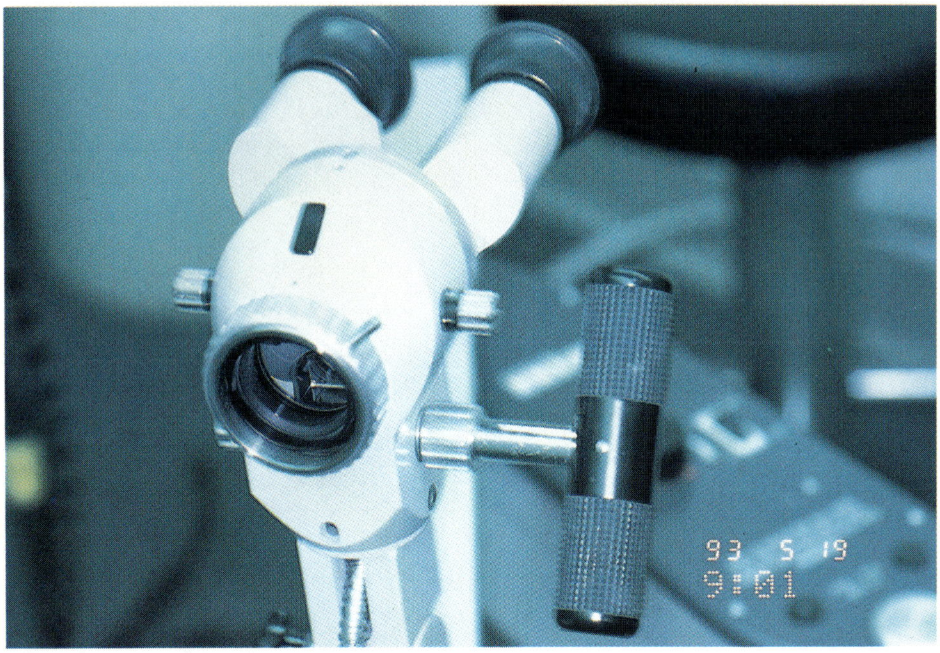

FIGURE 3-19
This colposcope has several levels of magnification that are controlled by the knobs on the sides. The black handle on the left is used to position the head of the colposcope.

ously described, squamous metaplasia is a dynamic and physiologic process that is subject to extrinsic and intrinsic factors that can alter the normal maturation of the transformation zone. Neoplastic changes in the cells in the transformation zone result in varying degrees of progression of CIN to carcinoma.[75] Thc primary goal of colposcopy is to exclude the presence of invasive cancer and to identify the extent of the lesion or lesions that were predicted by the screening cytologic examination. Indications for colposcopy are summarized in Table 3–3.

The Normal Transformation Zone

The anatomy and boundaries of the normal transformation zone were described earlier. The cephalad border of the transformation zone has mucin-secreting columnar epithelium. On colposcopic examination this area appears reddish owing to the single layer of cells covering the fine capillary loops that lie within the connective tissue. Squamous metaplasia lies between the glandular and the native squamous epithelium (Fig. 3–20). This immature squamous epithelium lines the surface of the transformation zone and fills the endocervical glands, changing the villous structure to a flattened and blunted surface. This squamous metaplasia appears smooth, pale, and it will turn white after application of dilute acetic acid solution (see below). It may resemble the abnormal epithelium of LSIL. The nuclei of LSIL and squamous metaplasia are relatively large and reflect the same amount of light, causing a similar acetowhite change. The most caudal border of the transformation zone is lined by fully mature squamous epithelium, which has multiple layers of cells with nuclei that are small relative to the cytoplasm. Normal squamous epithelium appears pink by absorbing light and reflecting the underlying subepithelial capillary network. This mature epithelium may be interspersed by cleft openings from the original columnar epithelium.

The Abnormal Transformation Zone

When there has been a malignant transformation of the cells of the cervix abnormalities in the transformation zone are visible on colposcopic examination. SIL or CIN results in an increase in the normal nuclear to cytoplasmic ratio owing to a progressive increase in the size of the nucleus and a loss of cytoplasm. Acetic acid (3% or 5%), which

TABLE 3–3.
Indications for Colposcopy

Clinical suspicion of invasive cancer
Epithelial cell abnormality on cytologic examination
Atypical squamous cells of undetermined significance
Low-grade squamous intraepithelial lesion
High-grade squamous intraepithelial lesion
Atypical glandular cells of undetermined significance
Squamous cell carcinoma, adenocarcinoma, and other malignant neoplasms
Clinical evidence of vaginal or vulvar condyloma, intraepithelial neoplasia, or cancer
In utero exposure to DES

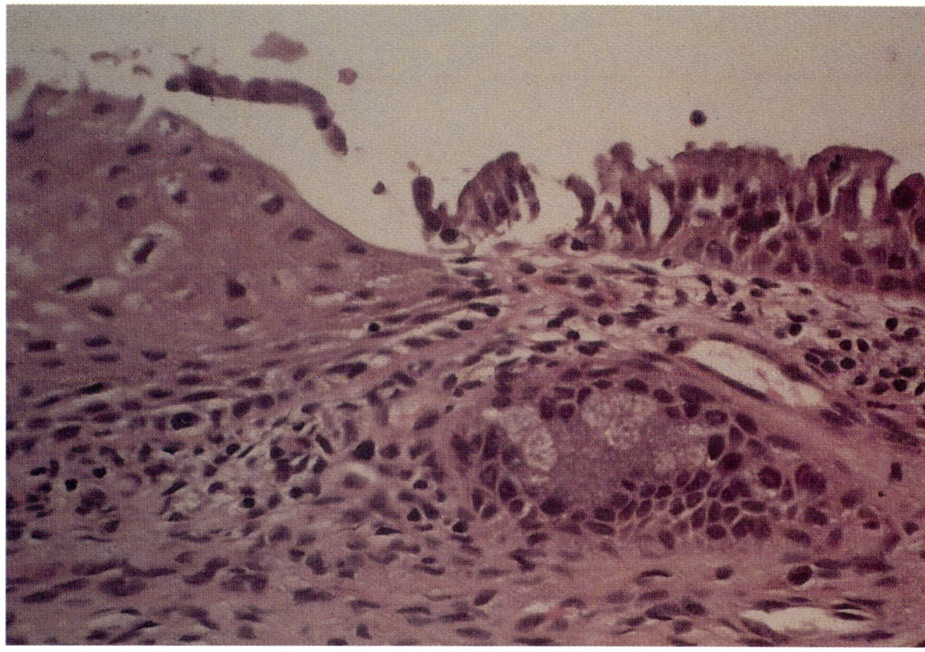

FIGURE 3-20
This is the transformation zone with immature squamous metaplasia on the left and glandular epithelium on the right. The glandular epithelium covers early stratification of the basal layer. This will eventually transform to squamous epithelium.

is applied to the cervix during the colposcopic examination, has a temporary dehydrating effect on the cells. This accentuates the abnormal nuclear to cytoplasmic ratio. The nucleus prevents transmission of light, making the abnormal epithelium appear white. This is known as acetowhite epithelium. It has also been postulated that the acetowhitening of CIN 1 lesions is attributable to a transient reaction between the acetic acid and abnormal envelope proteins in HPV-infected cells.[76]

Cervical Intraepithelial Neoplasia

Virtually all CIN lesions originate from and conform to the distribution of the transformation zone. Colpomicroscopic studies have shown that CIN occurs on the anterior lip of the cervix twice as commonly as on the posterior lip.[77] Although CIN lesions frequently extend into the endocervical canal, their caudal extension is well demarcated and rarely extends beyond the margin of the new SC junction. In contrast, subclinical HPV infection is not so limited and may transgress the SC junction onto the native squamous epithelium of the cervix. It sometimes extends into the vagina. Examination of the vulva may reveal HPV-associated changes in patients who have HPV changes on Papanicolaou smear and in whom no cervical lesions are identified.

By histopathology the grade of CIN is recognized by the proportion of epithelium between the basement membrane and the surface that is replaced by neoplastic cells. On colposcopy the degree of CIN is reflected by characteristic surface changes. The colposcopic features of CIN are varied, and most expert colposcopists emphasize evaluation of the following basic features when examining an abnormal transformation zone: the color tone relative to the normal epithelium (degree of whiteness), the lesion topography and surface contour (flat, raised, irregular, or papillary), and the vascular pattern (normal or abnormal) (Table 3–4).

Acetowhite Epithelium

An acetowhite lesion is the most frequent colposcopic finding in a patient who has CIN. However, it is important to recognize that the presence of acetowhite epithelium may also indicate only normal physiologic changes of squamous metaplasia (Table 3–5). Other features of acetowhite lesions range from well-demarcated, flat, and translucent lesions to raised, irregular, dull oyster-white le-

TABLE 3–4.
Colposcopic Terminology Used to Describe the Transformation Zone

Acetowhite epithelium
Vascular pattern
Punctation
Mosaicism
Atypical vessels
Surface contour
Margin of lesion
Leukoplakia

TABLE 3–5.
Conditions Causing Acetowhite Epithelium

Inflammation
Reactive or regenerative changes
CIN
HPV
Immature squamous metaplasia
Cervical adenocarcinoma in situ
Squamous cell carcinoma

sions, and any of these may or may not have abnormal capillary patterns (Fig. 3–21). There is a general correlation between an increasing degree of whiteness and an increasing grade of CIN.[78] In general, the more opaque and less translucent lesions coincide with a higher grade of CIN because the nuclear to cytoplasmic ratio is higher. Another variable feature of acetowhite epithelium is the characteristic of its margin with the surrounding normal epithelium—the sharper the border, the more abnormal the tissue.

Abnormal Vascular Pattern

When proliferation of neoplastic epithelium occurs there is an increased demand for nutritional and oxygen support, which leads to proliferation of the microvasculature. This is mediated in part by tumor angiogenesis factor (TAF), which is released by the neoplastic cells. TAF is responsible for the proliferation of microvessels, which in turn leads to an abnormal angioarchitecture of the superficial and subepithelial capillary network. As CIN progresses, the capillary loops of the SC junction undergo proliferation, dilatation, or ramifications.

Punctation and mosaic are descriptive terms referring to the abnormal vascular patterns that are usually found in acetowhite epithelium. *Punctation* refers to the appearance of a fine, delicate stippling pattern of the terminal vessels, which are arranged perpendicular to the surface in a translucent acetowhite lesion (Fig. 3–22). Coarse punctation refers to large caliber vessels. There is increased space between the capillaries. The vessels are frequently coiled, randomly directed, and sometimes raised. *Mosaic* patterns result from branching of vessels that are parallel to the surface epithelium. This leads to a characteristic partitioning of the acetowhite epithelium (Fig. 3–23). The vessels forming the mosaic pattern may form fine lines surrounding regularly shaped areas, or they may be coarse, dilated vessels that outline irregular areas of epithelium. The vessels responsible for the punctation and mosaic patterns may show wide variations in size, shape, arrangement, and intercapillary distance depending on the degree of CIN. Normal immature squamous metaplasia may appear as an acetowhite lesion and sometimes exhibits punctation or a mosaic pattern; however, such findings generally indicate that a significant lesion is present. In general, CIN is usually characterized by sharply demarcated acetowhite epithelium with coarse punctation or an irregular mosaic pattern. Typically, punctation and mosaic patterns coexist and are frequently adjacent to each other.

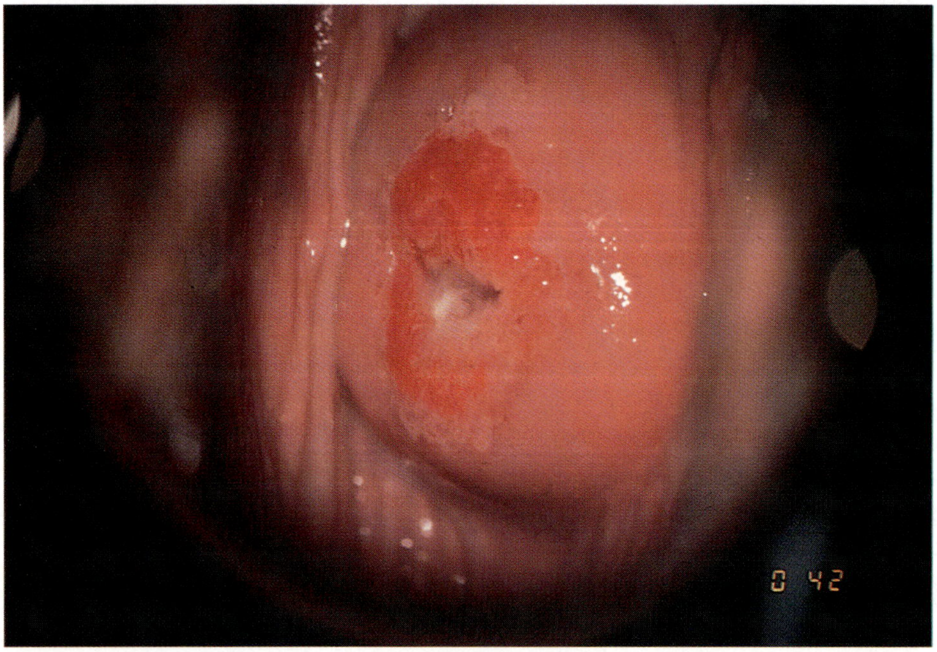

FIGURE 3–21
Faint acetowhite epithelium is seen at the 12 o'clock position within the transformation zone. The borders of the lesion are well demarcated. Multiple gland openings are present in this transformation zone. The junction of the endocervical epithelium (reddish) and the squamous epithelium (pink) is accentuated by a thin line of acetowhite epithelium. This represents squamous metaplasia.

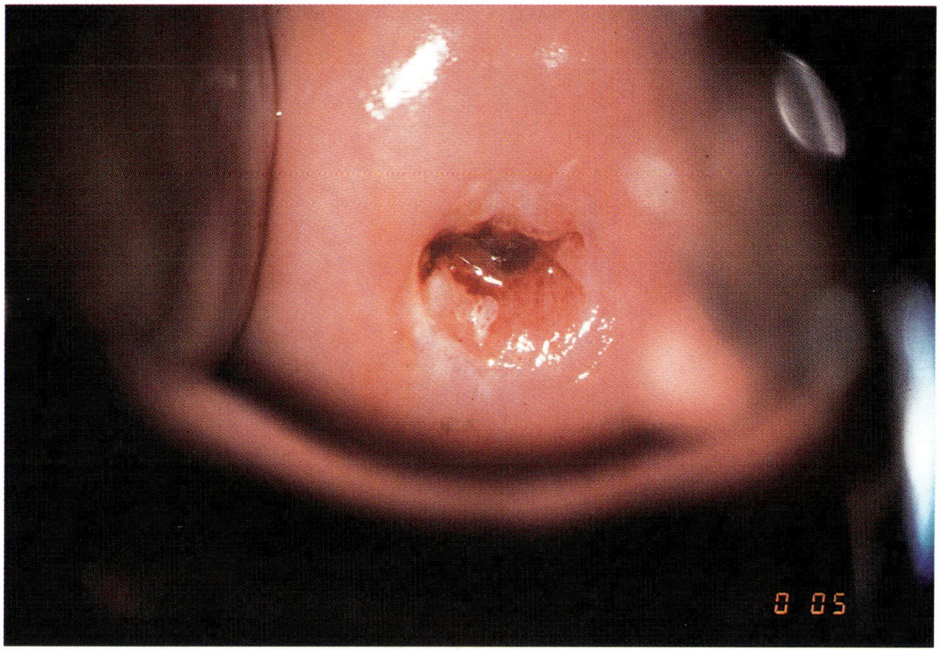

FIGURE 3-22
An acetowhite lesion with coarse punctations (red dots) is seen within the endocervical canal at the 7 o'clock position. There is faint acetowhite epithelium at the 12 and 1 o'clock positions.

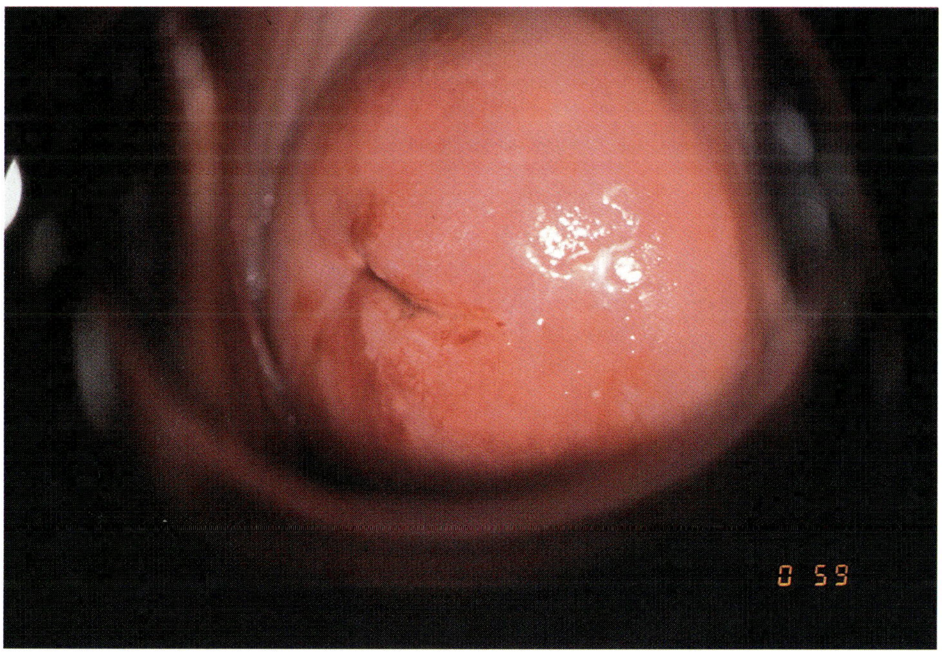

FIGURE 3-23
Several areas with mosaic patterns are seen in this colpophotograph. The most obvious is the one at the 5 o'clock position.

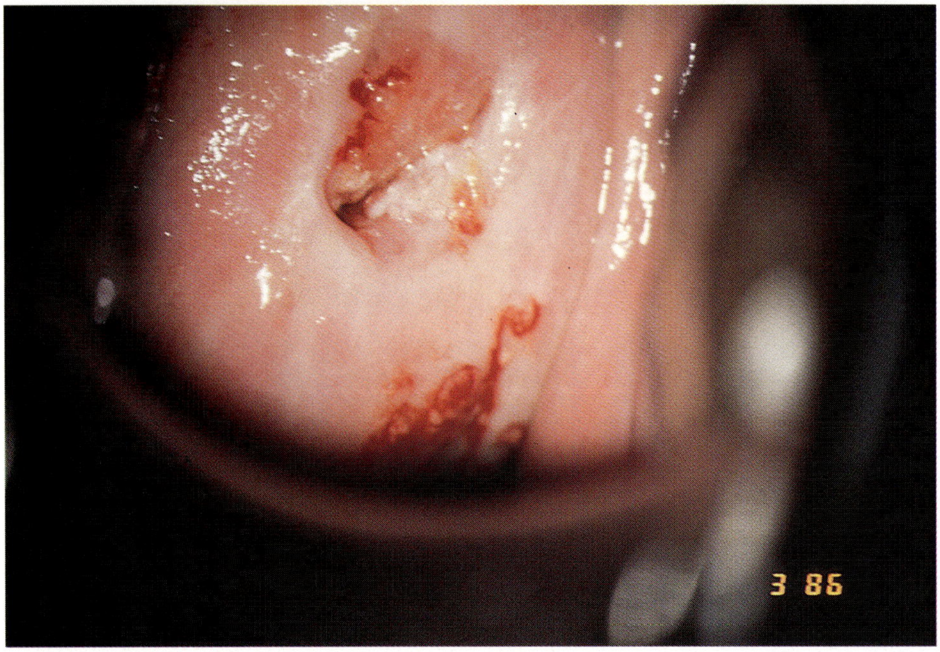

FIGURE 3–24
Markedly atypical, dilated vessels are seen on the posterior ectocervix. This proved to be a metastatic lesion from an endometrial carcinoma. An acetowhite lesion is seen at the 4 o'clock position within the transformation zone.

Atypical Vessels

Atypical vessels represent a progression of the severity of CIN. These vessels may be associated with CIN 3 lesions, but more commonly they are seen in microinvasive or frankly invasive carcinoma. The terminal vessels may appear coiled like a corkscrew or rounded like a comma. They may have an abnormal branching pattern characterized by a haphazard and distorted course, prominent caliber, and wide intercapillary distance (Fig. 3–24).

Surface Contours and Margins

In contrast to the normally smooth surface of the ectocervix, CIN lesions may be variable and may be flat, uneven, or exophytic. On colposcopic examination, HPV-associated lesions sometimes appear to have surface micropapillary projections. Higher grade CIN lesions may have a more convoluted or brainlike contour containing punctation and mosaicism. Acetowhite lesions with microexcresences and abnormal vessels of large caliber are more suspicious of early invasive cancer.[79] Exophytic lesions of HPV and benign lesions typically have an indistinct margin. In contrast, the majority of significant CIN lesions have a straight peripheral margin. In many cases of HSIL the line of demarcation between normal and dysplastic epithelium is quite striking (Fig. 3–25).

Leukoplakia

The normal mature squamous epithelium of the cervix is nonkeratinized, as described previously in Chapter 2. Leukoplakia is the descriptive term for the benign process of hyperkeratosis that affects the surface epithelium. This gives the epithelium a patchy, white, raised, and irregular appearance. These areas can be seen with the naked eye and appear white prior to the application of acetic acid (Fig. 3–26). Leukoplakia may be seen in patients with an HPV infection or as a response to chronic trauma resulting from prolapse or pessary use. Rarely, this thickened keratin layer may cover a dysplastic lesion or a carcinoma. Leukoplakia is more likely to be clinically significant when it coexists with areas of adjacent acetowhite epithelium that contains punctations and mosaicism.

Grading of Abnormal Colposcopic Findings

Various experts in the field of colposcopy promote the use of a grading system in the evaluation of an abnormal transformation zone. The purpose of this system is to eliminate subjective judgment and provide a meaningful standard of assessment that clinically predicts a histopathologic diagnosis. The increased prevalence of genital HPV infection caused Reid et al[79] to propose a scoring system to simplify the colposcopic differentiation of HPV and

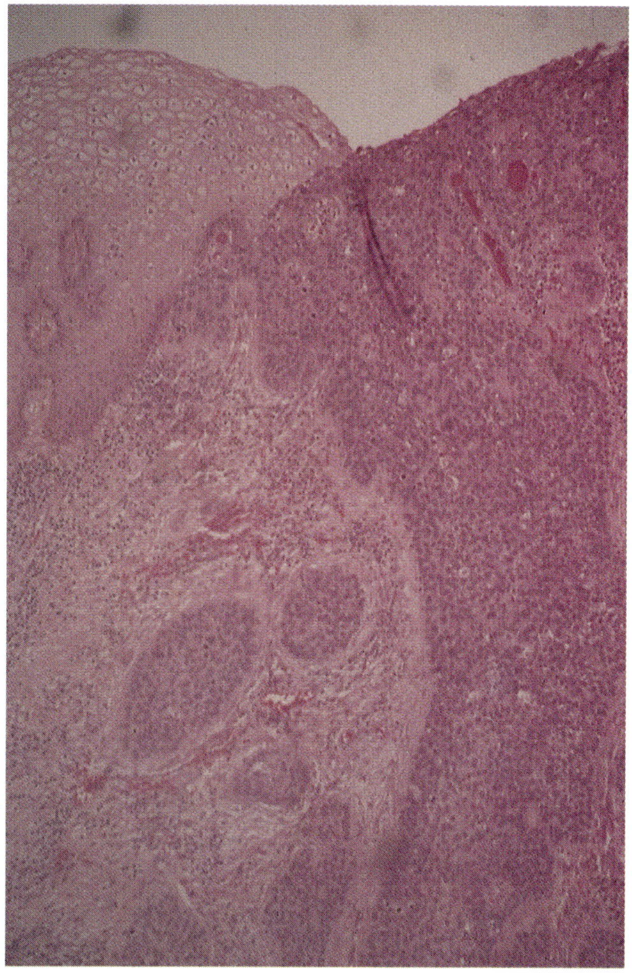

FIGURE 3-25
This cervical biopsy demonstrates a sharp demarcation between the normal squamous epithelium on the left and CIN 3 on the right. Several glands are filled with neoplastic squamous epithelium.

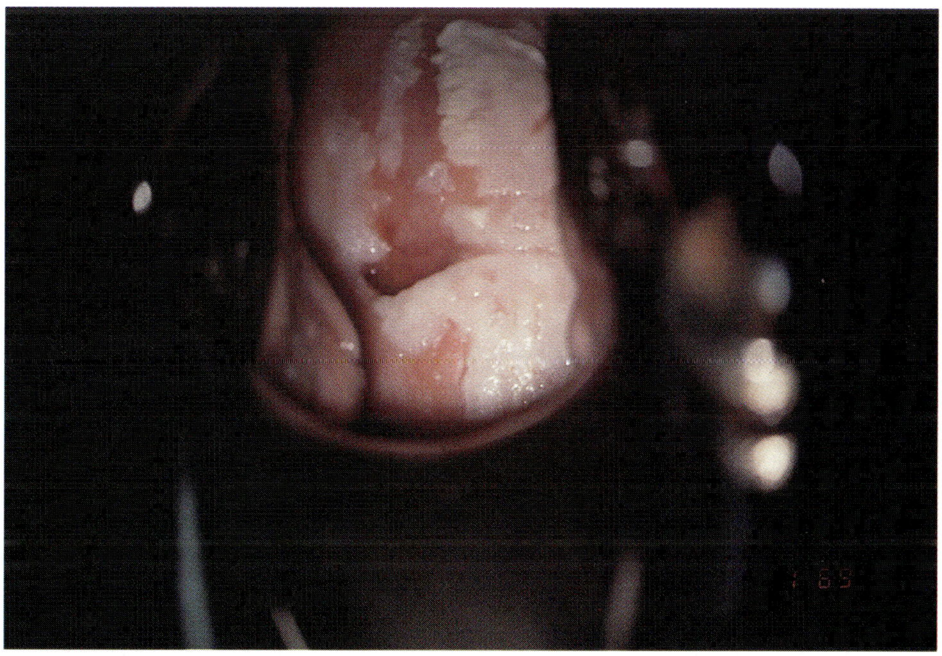

FIGURE 3-26
This cervix has extensive leukoplakia. These are areas of hyperkeratosis.

TABLE 3–6.
Colposcopic Index

Colposcopic Finding	0 Points	1 Point	2 Points
Margin	Condylomatous micropapillary contour, indistinct acetowhitening, flocculated or feathered margins, angular, jagged lesions. Satellite lesions and acetowhitening that extend beyond the transformation zone	Regular lesions with smooth, straight outlines	Rolled, peeling edges. Internal demarcations between areas of differing appearance
Color	Shiny, snow-white color. Indistinct acetowhitening	Intermediate shade (shiny gray)	Dull, oyster white
Vessels	Fine-caliber vessels, poorly formed patterns	No blood vessels seen	Definite punctations or mosaicism
Iodine reaction	Entire cervix stains dark brown	Some areas stain light brown	Nonstaining areas are present

Score: 0–2 points = HPV/CIN 1; 3–5 points = CIN 1–2; 6–8 points = CIN 2–3.
Modified from Reid R: Colposcopy of cervical preinvasive neoplasia. *In* Singer A (ed): Premalignant Lesions of the Lower Genital Tract. New York, Elsevier, 1990, p 106, with permission.

LSIL from HSIL. This system has been modified so that four colposcopic features—margin, color, vessels, and iodine response—are graded according to a weighted scoring system in an attempt to maximize the colposcopic and histopathologic correlation (Table 3–6).[80] The combined colposcopic index that results from this scoring system is reportedly better than 95 percent accurate in differentiating LSIL from HSIL. Although this colposcopic index is not formally employed by all colposcopy clinics, the relative clinical significance of its descriptive features provides a common and uniform terminology such that a well-trained colposcopist can predict which lesions are more likely to be associated with HSIL. The histopathologic diagnosis serves as the internal control for colposcopic assessment.

MANAGEMENT OF CERVICAL INTRAEPITHELIAL NEOPLASIA

The most important factor in the management of a patient with CIN is the pretreatment evaluation. As described previously, this evaluation includes the cytologic, colposcopic, and histopathologic diagnoses and how they are correlated. The indications for therapy have been established. Patients are categorized into four distinct groups: those who have invasive cancer; those who have HSIL (CIN 2 or CIN 3), both of which require treatment; those who have LSIL (HPV/CIN 1), who may be followed conservatively; and those in whom invasion has not been ruled out and who therefore require additional diagnostic procedures. Deviation from this protocol is the most common cause of treatment failure.

Treatment of HSIL involves destruction or excision of the transformation zone. This principle is based on colposcopic and histopathologic studies showing that the vast majority of CIN lesions develop in the transformation zone and the recurrence rate is high if the lesion alone is destroyed.[81–85] Although CIN often extends into the endocervical canal, it rarely extends out onto the native squamous epithelium of the portio unless invasive disease has developed. The most commonly employed methods of treatment of CIN are listed in Table 3–7. Hot cautery and cold coagulator are equally effective but have not gained popularity in the United States.

During the last two decades the management of CIN has evolved toward a more conservative approach with the use of local destructive (ablative) techniques and a decrease in the number of cervical conizations. More recently, observation without treatment of patients with LSIL has become acceptable. This is the result of prospective studies that have analyzed the natural history of CIN and the biologic behavior of HPV-associated cervical

TABLE 3–7.
Treatment Options for Patients with CIN

- Observation
- Destructive methods
  - Laser vaporization
  - Cryosurgery
- Excisional or diagnostic methods
  - "Cold" or "hot" knife cone biopsy
  - Laser cone biopsy
  - Loop electroexcision procedure
  - Hysterectomy

lesions. It is unequivocal that CIN 2 and CIN 3 lesions should be treated because there is a significant risk of progression to invasive disease with these lesions.[86, 87] More controversial is the treatment of CIN 1 or HPV-related lesions. Traditionally, patients who had a diagnosis of LSIL by cytologic examination and CIN 1 by histopathologic analysis were evaluated and treated exactly like patients who had HSIL. There is now a body of opinion that strongly favors conservative management, which could consist of clinical observation alone (i.e., by follow-up cytologic or colposcopic examination or both), for patients who have LSIL. Clinicians and researchers who favor this approach do so based on the knowledge that the regression rate for CIN 1 lesions is approximately 60 percent.[88] The progression rate from CIN 1 to CIN 3 (i.e., carcinoma in situ) is approximately 15 percent. Furthermore, local treatment of the transformation zone does not guarantee clearance of HPV infection because HPV infection consists of a ubiquitous distribution of the virus in the lower genital tract.[89, 90] Finally, all methods of treatment have inherent complications. In contrast, those who advocate treatment of low-grade lesions quote studies showing less favorable regression rates[91–93] and a progression rate from CIN 1 to CIN 3 of 26 percent.[91] They contend that destruction of the transformation zone for any CIN lesion is more than 90 percent effective in preventing progression and in addition eliminates the oncogenic potential of low-grade lesions infected with high-risk HPV genotypes (e.g., HPV 16, 18, and 33).[89, 94] Other considerations include the psychological implications for women who fear HPV or preneoplasia and the possible avoidance of the more expensive and time-consuming follow-up by colposcopy.

The management of patients with CIN should be further individualized according to associated factors including the patient's desire for fertility, compliance, pregnancy, and other coexisting gynecologic conditions. It is rare for general medical conditions to affect management decisions of patients who have CIN.

Prerequisites to Treatment

As mentioned previously, it is necessary to rule out an invasive process prior to treatment of a patient who has CIN. The criteria to be met prior to ablation of CIN are listed in Table 3–8. If these conditions are met, the patient may be treated by methods that destroy or ablate the transformation zone but do not produce a specimen for histopathologic evaluation. The ablative treatment techniques that will be described next include cryosurgery and carbon dioxide laser vaporization.

Cryosurgery

Cryosurgery is the most common technique used in the United States for the treatment of CIN. The popularity of cryosurgery is due to its high success rate, cost-effectiveness, safety, and low complication rate. It is technically simple and requires no anesthesia or analgesia. The technique employs the use of a refrigerant such as nitrous oxide or carbon dioxide delivered to a cryoprobe, which is then used to cover the transformation zone (Fig. 3–27). Different probes are available, and the one which conforms best to the anatomy of the particular cervix and the extent of the lesion is used. Freezing the cervical tissue to −70°C results in biochemical injury, cell destruction, and subsequent sloughing of necrotic tissue. A standard treatment protocol employs two 3-minute freeze intervals separated by an interim partial thaw of approximately 5 minutes. The depth of tissue destruction that occurs following cryotherapy is between 2 and 5 mm. The three factors that are critical for treatment success are that the iceball extend for at least 5 mm beyond the cryoprobe, that the transformation zone be entirely covered by the cryoprobe, and that the lesion does not extend into the endocervical canal.

Complications from cryotherapy are rare. Patients should be advised to expect a malodorous, watery vaginal discharge that may last up to 1 month following the procedure. Cryosurgery of the cervix has no adverse effects on the patient's reproductive capacity, and labor and delivery are unaffected.[95, 96] Infection occurs in less than 5 percent of cases. Healing is complete in 6 to 8 weeks. However, cytologic and colposcopic assessment of treatment efficacy should be delayed for 3 to 4 months because changes secondary to repair may be confused with CIN.

TABLE 3–8.

Criteria To Be Met Before Ablation of Cervical Transformation Zone

The transformation zone is visualized in its entirety
Endocervical curettings are negative for CIN or cancer
There is adequate correlation (within 1 degree) between cytopathology, histopathology, and colposcopy*
There is no cytopathologic or colposcopic suspicion of invasive cancer
There is no microinvasion or adenocarcinoma in situ on histopathology

* For example, patients with LSIL on cytopathologic examination have CIN 1 or 2 on colposcopically directed biopsies but not CIN 3.

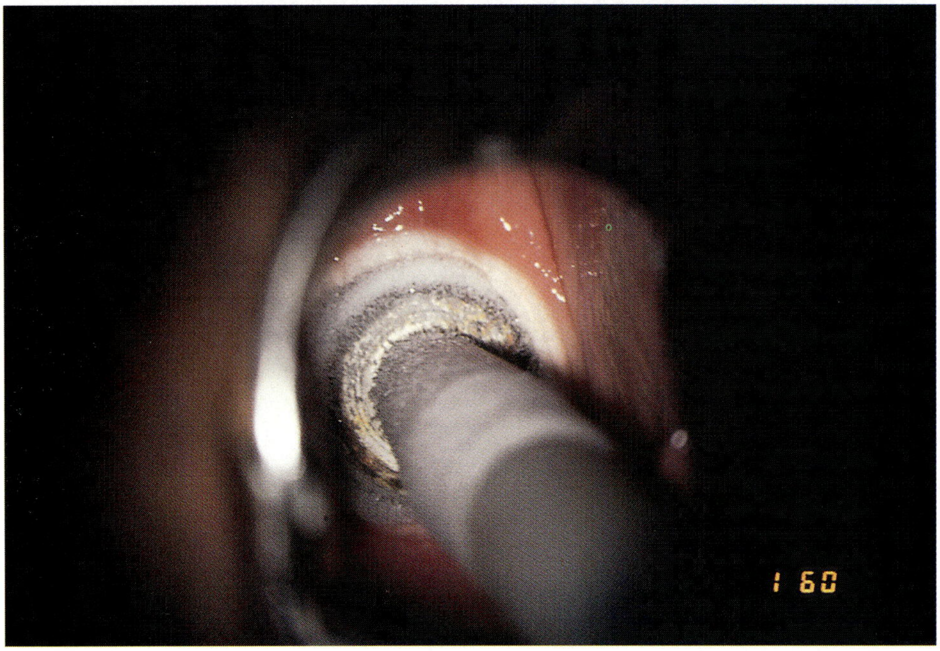

FIGURE 3-27
A cryotherapy probe *(silver disk)* is being applied to the cervix. An iceball *(peripheral white zone)* covers the transformation zone.

Carbon Dioxide Laser Vaporization

The CO_2 laser is the most efficient and commonly used laser in gynecologic surgery. When used for the treatment of CIN, the laser is attached to a colposcope so that the beam can be easily directed onto the target tissue by using a hand-held micromanipulator (Fig. 3–28). The surgeon visually controls the extent and depth of tissue destruction. The most effective technique for treating CIN with the laser involves vaporization of the entire transformation zone to a depth of 7 mm.[97] The laser beam results in the vaporization of intracellular and extracellular water to steam by converting light energy to heat.

Complications of laser vaporization of the cervix are minimal. It can be performed as an outpatient procedure, in which case it may produce mild to moderate pain in a few patients that may require local anesthesia with a paracervical block.[98] Bleeding may occur in 5 to 10 percent of cases but is less common if a vasoconstrictor is combined with the local anesthetic.[99] Infection following laser treatment is extremely rare.

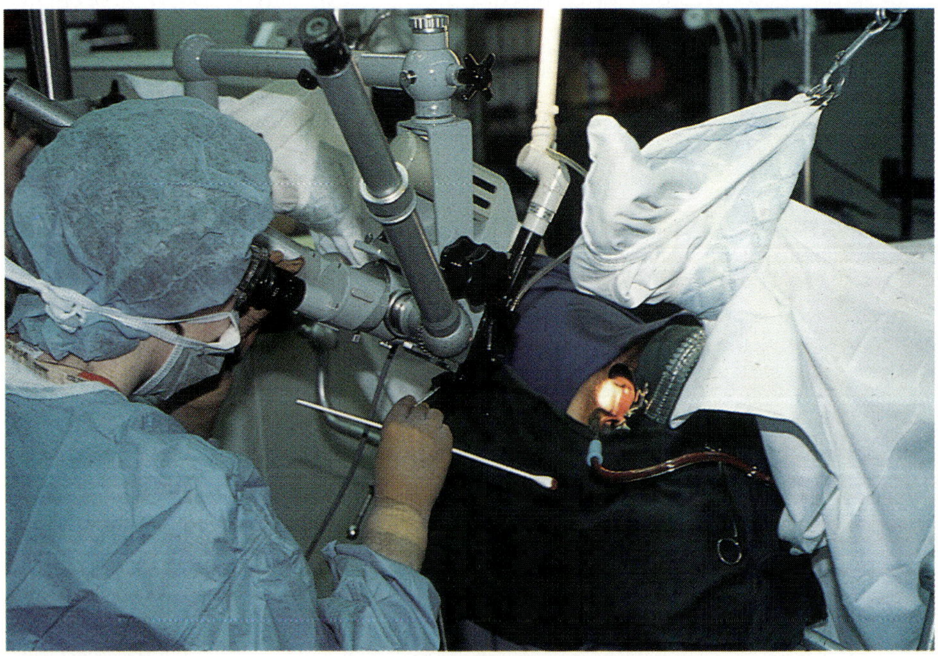

FIGURE 3-28
Laser vaporization of the cervix is performed using a colposcope. The laser beam is attached to the colposcope by the white tube at the top center. The surgeon is holding the micromanipulator and a cotton swab.

Compared with cryosurgery, laser vaporization of the cervix results in more rapid healing, no scarring, and less vaginal discharge.[100] Healing is complete within 3 to 4 weeks after laser vaporization. The new SC junction is usually visualized at the level of the external os, which allows satisfactory follow-up with colposcopic examinations. Laser vaporization of the cervix has no significant effects on subsequent reproductive function.[101]

The drawbacks of laser vaporization are few and are unrelated to treatment efficacy. The practice of laser surgery demands an apprenticeship on the part of the gynecologic surgeon. This includes an understanding of laser biophysics, development of good hand–eye coordination, and knowledge of the safe handling of the laser equipment. Learning this technique is significantly more time-consuming than the training required for performing successful cryosurgery. Another drawback is the high price of laser equipment.

Efficacy of Cryosurgery and CO_2 Laser Vaporization

As described previously, the treatment of patients with CIN by cryosurgery or laser vaporization is associated with minimal complications. Numerous studies have analyzed the recurrence of CIN after the use of these two treatment modalities. In two separate studies comparing laser and cryosurgery, the authors found the laser more effective in the treatment of patients with cervical lesions larger than 3 cm in diameter, high-grade lesions, or lesions extending into the endocervix.[102, 103] Specifically, Ferenczy[102] reported that for lesions greater than 3 cm, laser vaporization resulted in cure rates of 92 percent versus 62 percent with cryosurgery. Several studies have demonstrated that cryosurgery is very effective in the treatment of CIN 2 and CIN 3 lesions.[104,105] The general consensus is that failure to eradicate CIN with cryosurgery is a function of lesion size and endocervical extension rather than higher original histopathologic grade. Proponents of laser therapy argue that the laser is adaptable for all lesions and allows incomparable microsurgical precision in destroying the entire transformation zone to a desired depth. Overall, the body of evidence supports the conclusion that, when used correctly, cryosurgery and laser vaporization offer similarly good cure rates of better than 85 percent.[106–111]

In comparing these two treatment modalities, another area of concern is the post-treatment colposcopic appearance of the cervix. In one prospective randomized trial, patients treated with cryosurgery had a significantly higher incidence of retraction of the SC junction into the endocervical canal than did patients treated with laser. At follow-up colposcopy, satisfactory colposcopic visualization of the transformation zone occurred in 86 percent of the laser-treated group compared to 52 percent of patients treated with cryosurgery.[112] This means that a higher proportion of unsatisfactory follow-up colposcopic evaluations can be expected in cryosurgery-treated patients, and this may be a significant disadvantage if abnormal follow-up cytologic findings occur.

The benefit of colposcopic visualization of the post-treatment SC junction is debatable. Persistence of the transformation zone at the portio after treatment of CIN may in theory predispose to recurrence of CIN. The process of active squamous metaplasia may allow incorporation of viral and other carcinogens into the cells at the transformation zone. Following physical destruction of the transformation zone, healing could result in eversion of the endocervical columnar epithelium. Active squamous metaplasia follows in a manner similar to that seen at menarche, which may predispose to the development of recurrent CIN. Reinfection of the regenerating transformation zone by persistent HPV in the surrounding normal ectocervix has been documented.[113]

Long-term follow-up of patients undergoing destructive therapy for CIN is essential and is particularly important in the first 2 years following therapy because the majority of recurrences occur within this interval. We obtain follow-up cervical cytologic examinations every 4 months for the first year following treatment. If all these smears are normal, subsequent cervical cytologic follow-up is obtained annually. If any smear is abnormal, colposcopy is performed. It has been suggested that at least one colposcopic examination be performed during the first year of follow-up even if cervical cytologic results are normal.[114]

Critical analysis of patients in whom invasive cancer has developed following cryosurgery or laser vaporization consistently identifies a lack of expertise on the part of the clinician performing the colposcopy. Often there was a lack of recognition that the examination was unsatisfactory (because the transformation zone was not fully visualized) or that invasive disease was present. Inadequate follow-up after treatment has also been identified as a problem in these patients. Another reason for treatment failure is poor technique, which results in incomplete destruction of the transformation zone. Poor technique could be due to inadequate freezing with cryosurgery or insufficient breadth and depth of tissue destruction with the laser. In some cases recurrence is inevitable and is related to the association between HPV infection and CIN. Local destruction of the transformation zone does not eliminate the HPV reservoir of the lower genital tract. Higher rates of recurrence have been reported for lesions containing HPV types 16 and 18.[115]

Diagnostic and Excisional Procedures

A diagnostic excision is indicated when the colposcopic evaluation is unsatisfactory and cancer cannot be excluded on the basis of colposcopy and targeted biopsies (see Table 3–7). A specimen (Fig. 3–29) suitable for histopathologic evaluation can be obtained by scalpel excision or by performing an excisional biopsy using a laser or a loop electroexcisional procedure (LEEP).[116] In the majority of cases these procedures are also therapeutic. In general, only about 10 percent of patients evaluated for abnormal cervical cytologic results need to undergo a conization procedure.[117]

Processing of the Conization Specimen

Removal of the transformation zone with a scalpel, laser, or electrosurgical loop results in what is called a cone specimen (see Fig. 3–29). This specimen may have a conical shape but frequently it has the appearance of a cube. In the operating room the specimen is marked with a suture, which is placed generally at the 12 o'clock position in the ectocervix or at any other location that can be clearly identified in the pathology consultation request. The specimen should not be placed in formalin in the operating room and then sent to the pathology laboratory, since formalin will interfere with the proper inking and also cause the specimen to curl, making orientation difficult. In the pathology laboratory the specimen is opened longitudinally and is pinned flat open on a wax block. The endocervical and ectocervical margins are identified and marked with different colors of India ink. The specimen is then fixed in 10 percent formalin overnight. After fixation the cone is divided into 12 equal pieces as if dividing a clock face. Each piece is consecutively labeled (e.g., 1 o'clock, 2 o'clock). It is important for each piece to have a portion of the SC junction (Fig. 3–30). One histologic section is then prepared from each of the 12 tissue blocks.

Loop Electroexcision Procedure (LEEP)

Since the late 1980s LEEP has gained wide acceptance for the treatment of CIN. Like cryosurgery, LEEP can be safely and easily employed in an outpatient setting. The procedure is rapid (less than 1 minute) and is effectively carried out under either local anesthesia or no anesthesia. It offers the advantage of being a simple outpatient procedure that produces a surgical specimen for histopathologic diagnosis.

LEEP is done with a fine wire loop (Fig. 3–31) connected to an electrosurgical unit that delivers a high-frequency, low-voltage alternating current. The electrical generator can transmit a blend of

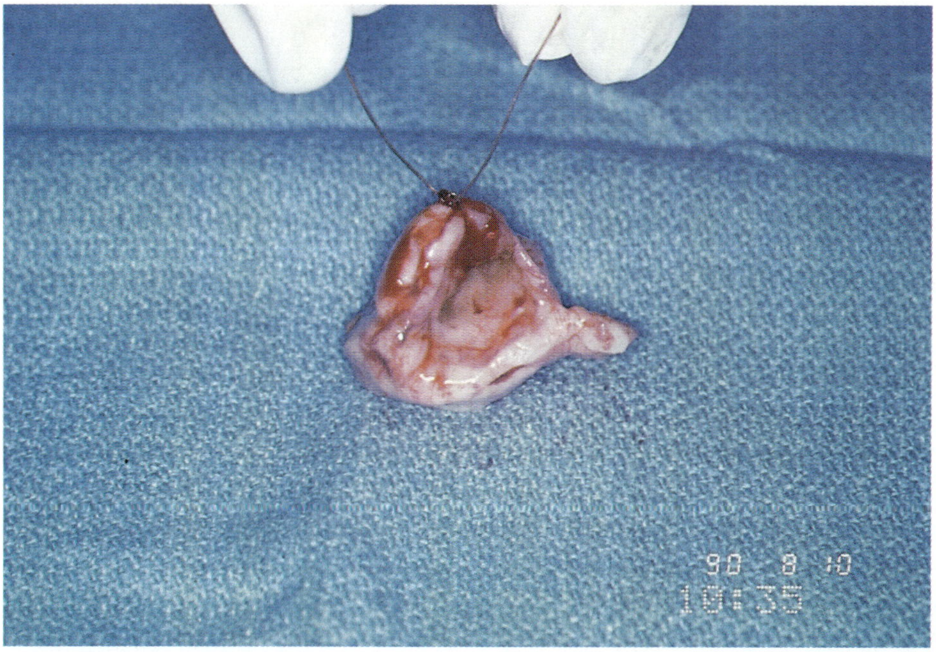

FIGURE 3–29
This cervical conization specimen is shown en face. The cervical os is in the middle and appears as a tan circle. The suture marks the 12 o'clock position. Only squamous epithelium is seen, since the lack of visualization of the squamocolumnar junction after an abnormal Papanicolaou smear was the indication for the procedure.

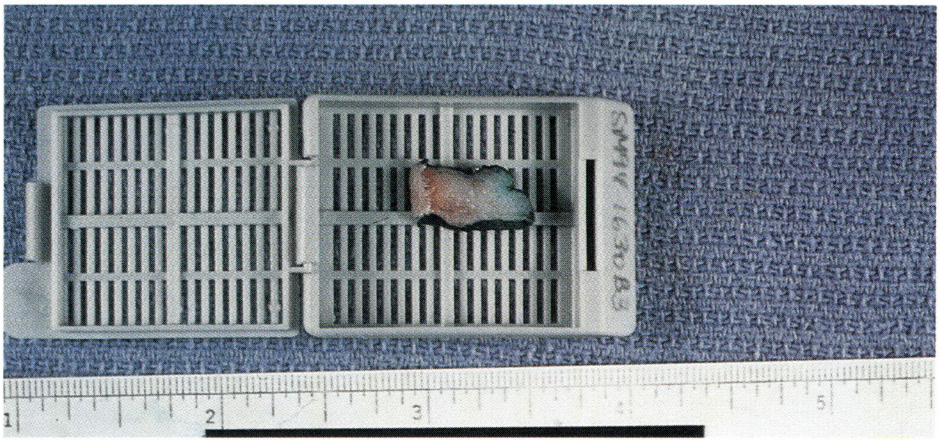

FIGURE 3-30
This tissue slice from a conization specimen has been laid flat in the cassette with the squamous epithelium on the left. The squamous epithelium appears smooth and pink. There is India ink on all the other edges. The squamocolumnar junction is at the top, and the endocervical margin is at the far top right.

both cutting and coagulation currents. Excision of the entire transformation zone can be accomplished, and only minimal bleeding and minimal thermal artifact occur. Specimens obtained by LEEP are satisfactory for histopathologic evaluation in over 90 percent of cases.[118] The loops are provided in various sizes to allow for different widths of the transformation zone and different depths of excision. An adequate excision incorporates a lateral margin of at least 3 mm beyond the abnormal transformation zone and a depth of 5 to 7 mm. In a patient with a very large transformation zone the procedure may need to be completed by using several passes of the wire loop (i.e., an anterior lip, a posterior lip, and an endocervical biopsy). The ectocervical and endocervical margins of the specimen (or specimens) should be clearly marked with a suture or surgical clip before sending them to the pathology laboratory. As described previously, the pathologist applies different colored India inks to these margins for easier identification during microscopic examination. There is some concern that in inexperienced hands LEEP results in fragmented specimens or specimens that may show significant thermal damage, which can preclude adequate evaluation of the surgical margin (Fig. 3-32).[119]

It is not necessary to meet all the criteria shown in Table 3-8 when LEEP is used. LEEP departs from this approach in several ways. With LEEP the limits of the lesion and the transformation zone do not have to be seen in their entirety prior to therapy because the tissue at risk for neoplasia will be excised for histopathologic evaluation. LEEP allows for diagnosis and treatment in the same visit.[120] However, the simplicity and expeditious nature of LEEP also accounts for its liability. Overtreatment with LEEP is a concern. Patients who have only minimally abnormal cervical cytologic findings (ASCUS or LSIL) may be man-

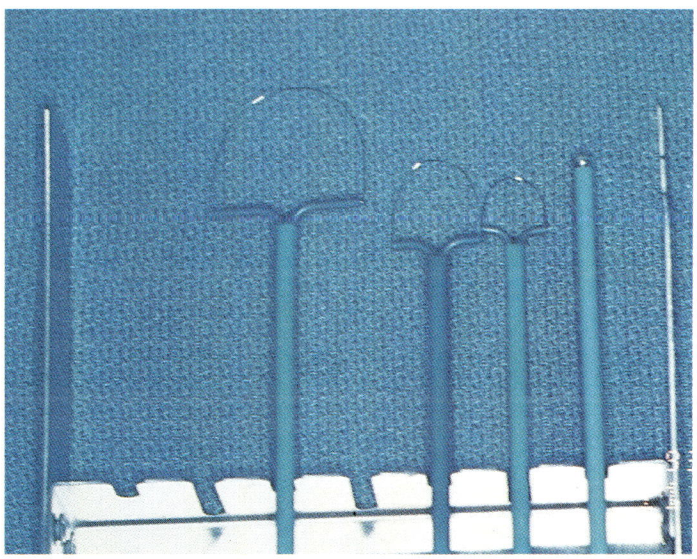

FIGURE 3-31
Several sizes of wire loops used to perform LEEP are shown on a stand. On the far right, a 5 mm ball used to cauterize the surgical bed is seen.

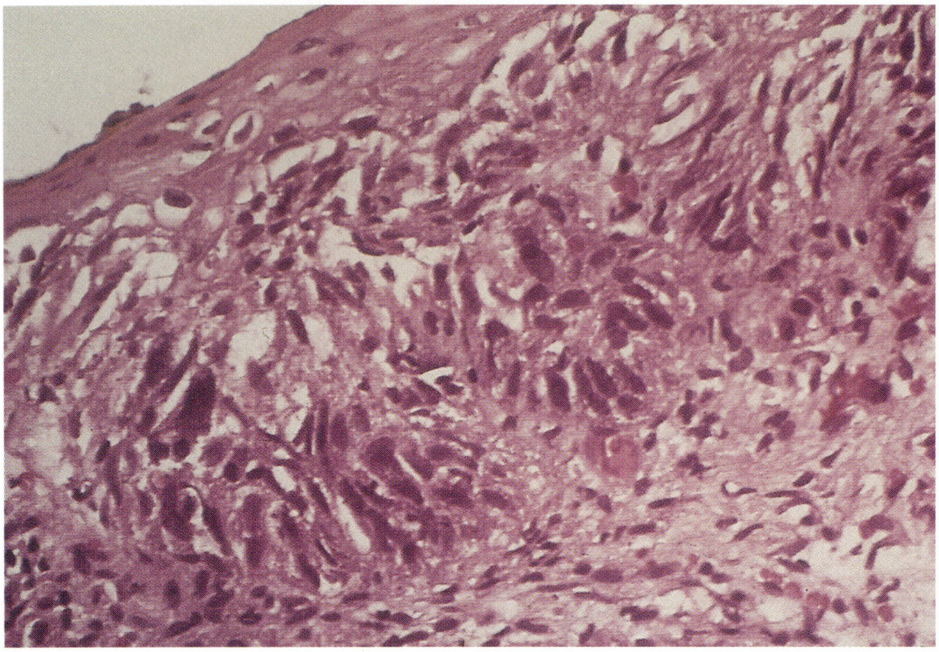

FIGURE 3-32
This is the excision margin of a LEEP specimen. The thermal damage is characterized by artifactual vacuolated spaces, loss of cellular borders, and nuclear detail. The basement membrane is obscured. The presence or absence of CIN cannot be determined on this specimen.

aged by colposcopic evaluation and followed by observation if the lesion is no worse than CIN 1 on targeted biopsies.

Complications due to LEEP are infrequent. Effects on reproductive function are thought to be insignificant, but reports on long-term follow-up are unavailable. Complications of delayed bleeding and cervical stenosis have been reported in about 1 percent of cases.[121,122] In a randomized study comparing LEEP with laser vaporization, cure rates were comparable and exceeded 90 percent in both groups.[123] The LEEP group experienced less postoperative hemorrhage, less discomfort, and shorter operative time. Two separate reports have documented a few cases of unsuspected microinvasive carcinoma in the LEEP specimens of patients whose colposcopically directed biopsies showed only CIN 2 or CIN 3.[124,125] Large series of patients undergoing LEEP for the treatment of CIN showed a cure rate of approximately 95 percent.[121,122] This figure is comparable to the results obtained with cold knife cone biopsy. Sometimes the surgical margins of a LEEP specimen are difficult to evaluate owing to fragmentation or thermal artifact. However, the cure rate is high even when the surgical margins are found to be involved with CIN. Murdoch et al[126] found that only 31 (12 percent) of 256 patients who had incomplete excisions with LEEP had residual CIN on follow-up. They recommended that a patient with CIN at the surgical margin of a LEEP specimen be followed closely with cervical cytologic and colposcopic evaluations.

Cold Knife Conization

Cases in which an invasive cancer has developed following destructive therapy for CIN have prompted an increased use of excisional methods for the treatment of CIN.[127] In the past the cold knife cone biopsy was the standard of care when a diagnostic procedure was indicated. Now that use of LEEP has increased, the decision to perform a cold knife conization has become more selective. Conization of the cervix still remains necessary in specific clinical settings: a postmenopausal patient whose cervix is flush with the vaginal fornices or the patient who has already undergone several surgical procedures on the cervix. In these cases the precision and control of the scalpel are necessary to avoid vaginal lacerations or inadvertent entry into the bowel or bladder. Conization procedures usually require general or regional anesthesia and thus are not suitable for the office.

Several large reviews have reported on the morbidity associated with cone biopsy. The most common complication is bleeding, which can be either intraoperative or delayed. One study reported that significant hemorrhage occurred in 9.9 percent of patients.[118] Other complications including sepsis, cervical stenosis, infertility, and cervical incompetence occur in 2 to 12 percent of patients depending on the depth of excision and the geometry of the excised specimen.[128–130]

Conization of the cervix is extremely effective in the diagnosis and treatment of CIN. The overall cure rate is over 95 percent. Recurrence of CIN following a cone biopsy has been found to be associated with the status of the endocervical margins of resection. Two Scandinavian studies reported a 98 percent cure rate in patients who had margins free of CIN.[131, 132] Another large study that had long-term follow-up found no recurrence or progression to invasive disease when the margins were not involved.[133] However, when the margins of resection are involved, the risk of persistent or recurrent CIN has been reported to range from 30 percent to 50 percent.[134–136] The management of a patient who has endocervical margins involved by CIN must be individualized. It is important to consider the patient's desire for future fertility, the patient's reliability with regard to long-term follow-up, and the need to ensure unequivocal exclusion of an invasive process. Repeat conization, which may have an adverse impact on fertility, should be recommended only when histopathologic assessment of the excision margins shows a neoplastic process and invasion cannot be excluded. Long-term follow-up by serial cervical cytology is a reasonable option in women who wish to maintain fertility. Abnormal exfoliative cytologic results have been shown to be a reliable predictor of persistent or recurrent CIN and eliminate the need to perform a repeat conization or hysterectomy.[136] We recommend that patients with CIN on the surgical margin of a cone biopsy who wish to retain their fertility be followed by cervical cytology evaluation every 4 months for 1 year. Colposcopy should be performed at least once during this period or if any of the cervical smears is found to be abnormal.

Hysterectomy

Hysterectomy is an option in the treatment of CIN. Cumulative data show that the incidence of recurrent neoplasia or cancer following hysterectomy is less than 1 percent. In contrast, in patients who have been treated by cold knife conization for CIN the incidence of recurrent neoplasia and of subsequent development of invasive cancer is 3 percent and 0.6 percent, respectively.[137,138] However, cone biopsy is 97 percent effective when the margins of resection are uninvolved. Conservative management consisting of frequent follow-up cytologic examination has been shown to be effective in the detection of recurrent CIN even when the margins are involved. Thus, hysterectomy with its associated morbidity probably represents an overtreatment in the majority of cases. The indication for hysterectomy in the treatment of CIN is limited and is usually related to some other gynecologic condition.

Several recent reports have reviewed the long-term follow-up of women after hysterectomy for CIN. Wiener et al[139] reported that 3 (1.6 percent) of 195 women showed abnormal cytologic findings within 10 years and 7 (3.5 percent) within 20 years following hysterectomy for CIN. The majority of these abnormal findings were detected within the first 2 years following hysterectomy. This suggests either incomplete excision of the cervix or the presence of preexisting vaginal intraepithelial neoplasia (VAIN). Continued close follow-up, particularly during the first 2 years following hysterectomy, is indicated to identify women who may have persistent or new disease. In another study, Schneider et al[140] evaluated the significance of vaginal HPV infection in women who had negative vaginal cytologic findings after undergoing hysterectomy for benign disease, CIN, or cancer. Patients with a history of cervical neoplasia had a significantly higher HPV infection rate than patients who had had a hysterectomy for benign disease alone (33 vs. 14 percent). VAIN was diagnosed by colposcopic-directed biopsies in 5 percent of the HPV-positive group. These results support the need to continue to obtain vaginal cytologic results in women who have undergone hysterectomy, particularly those who have a history of cervical neoplasia. In the experience of Schneider et al, HPV testing in conjunction with colposcopy was a better predictor of VAIN than vaginal cytologic examination alone. These and many other studies support continued and lifelong cytologic surveillance in women who have undergone a hysterectomy for CIN.

ADENOCARCINOMA IN SITU

An exhaustive body of literature has led to our current understanding of the epidemiology of CIN. Similar data on adenocarcinoma in situ (AIS) of the endocervix are scarce and reflect the lower incidence of this disease. AIS accounts for less than 5 percent of cervical intraepithelial lesions.[141] Recently, it has been suggested that the incidence of AIS is increasing, but it remains unclear whether this trend is real or represents a refinement of cytopathologic and histopathologic criteria for the diagnosis of AIS.[142,143]

AIS of the cervix is recognized as a possible precursor lesion of adenocarcinoma. The putative risk factors associated with AIS are assumed from the few epidemiologic studies on invasive adenocarcinoma of the cervix. Between 40 and 100 percent of AIS lesions are found concurrently with

CIN, which raises the possibility that there are common factors in their etiology. In a recent epidemiologic study by Brinton et al,[144] the strongest risk factors for development of cervical adenocarcinoma were the interval since the last Papanicolaou smear and the presence of DNA of HPV genotype 16 or 18 in cervical cells. In this same study oral contraceptive use was also found to be a risk factor. There has been a suggestion that long-term use of contraceptive steroids may affect the pathogenesis of AIS and cervical adenocarcinoma.[145, 146]

The natural history of AIS also remains unclear. There is not yet a uniformly accepted histopathologic continuum of endocervical intraepithelial neoplasia. A spectrum of glandular atypia of a lesser degree than AIS has been described and a grading system has been applied.[147, 148] The detection of glandular atypia is frequently associated with both high-grade CIN and AIS. One study looked at cone biopsy and hysterectomy specimens and found glandular atypia in 15 percent of the cases associated with squamous CIN 3 compared to only 1 percent in those with AIS.[147]

Endocervical glandular dysplasia, endodysplasia, cervical intraepithelial glandular neoplasia (CIGN), and atypical hyperplasia are all terms which have been used to describe glandular lesions of the endocervix that demonstrate less severe atypia than those seen in AIS. The histopathologic criteria for glandular dysplasia have not been well defined in the past, although Brown and Wells[147] devised a scheme in 1986 by which such lesions may be classified as low-grade or high-grade cervical glandular dysplasia based on the degree of nuclear stratification, nuclear pleomorphism, mitotic activity, and glandular irregularity exhibited. In an attempt to group glandular dysplasia and AIS together under one heading, Gloor and Hurlimann[149] proposed the designation CIGN in analogy with squamous CIN. According to this classification, atypical glandular lesions are divided into three grades (CIGN 1 to CIGN 3). In CIGN 1, the nuclei display slight hyperchromasia and are arranged in a single row along the base of the cells. Few if any mitoses are present. In comparison with normal columnar epithelium, the atypical epithelium appears reduced. Intracellular mucin may be either abundant or diminished. In CIGN 2, the nuclei are oval, hyperchromatic, and crowded, resulting in a slight degree of pseudostratification (two rows of nuclei). The epithelium is often thicker than that lining the normal glands. Mitotic figures are more common, and intracellular mucin is depleted. CIGN 3 corresponds to AIS, to be discussed later. Although some investigators contend that the changes seen in glandular dysplasia serve as precursors of the development of cervical adenocarcinoma, others argue that further studies of its biologic behavior are necessary to validate this terminology and grading system.[150]

Diagnosis

The accuracy of cervical cytologic examination for the screening of AIS is considered variable with detection rates reported to be between 40 and 90 percent.[151] The use of the endocervical brush is expected to improve detection by cytopathology.

Under TBS the diagnosis of atypical glandular cells of undetermined significance (AGUS) is used whenever cells of a glandular type display nuclear atypia that exceeds obvious reactive or reparative changes but lack the unequivocal features of invasive carcinoma. This is a very broad classification that embraces all glandular changes up to those highly suspicious for invasive adenocarcinoma. The kinds of lesions that should be considered when a cytologic diagnosis of AGUS is made include glandular intraepithelial lesions, microglandular hyperplasia, endocervical or endometrial polyps, tubal metaplasia (Fig. 3–33), atypical repair reactions, and adenocarcinoma. With a differential as broad as this, it is important to try to determine first whether the glandular cells are of endocervical, endometrial, or of other origin. This can sometimes be done based on the size of the individual cell.

Endometrial cells are normally smaller than endocervical cells, have scantier cytoplasm, and have a cuboidal to round shape rather than the columnar shape of the endocervical cells. As endocervical cells become malignant and less differentiated they become larger and more pleomorphic. Endometrial hyperplasia and grade 1 endometrial carcinoma both shed cells that are generally smaller than endocervical cells, whereas grade 2 and 3 lesions of endometrial adenocarcinoma shed cells that are in the same size range as endocervical cells. Tumor diathesis is more apt to be present with an invasive endocervical tumor, but cells of malignant endometrial tumors also may be shed with blood and necrotic debris. Often cells of malignant endometrial and ovarian tumors are shed on a clean background, and the balls of neoplastic cells look very out of place on a background of normal squamous and endocervical cells.

Although TBS does not currently subclassify AGUS it is hoped that in the future further categorization into more specific diagnoses will occur. We use the diagnosis "atypical endocervical cells, favor a reactive process" when there is evidence of

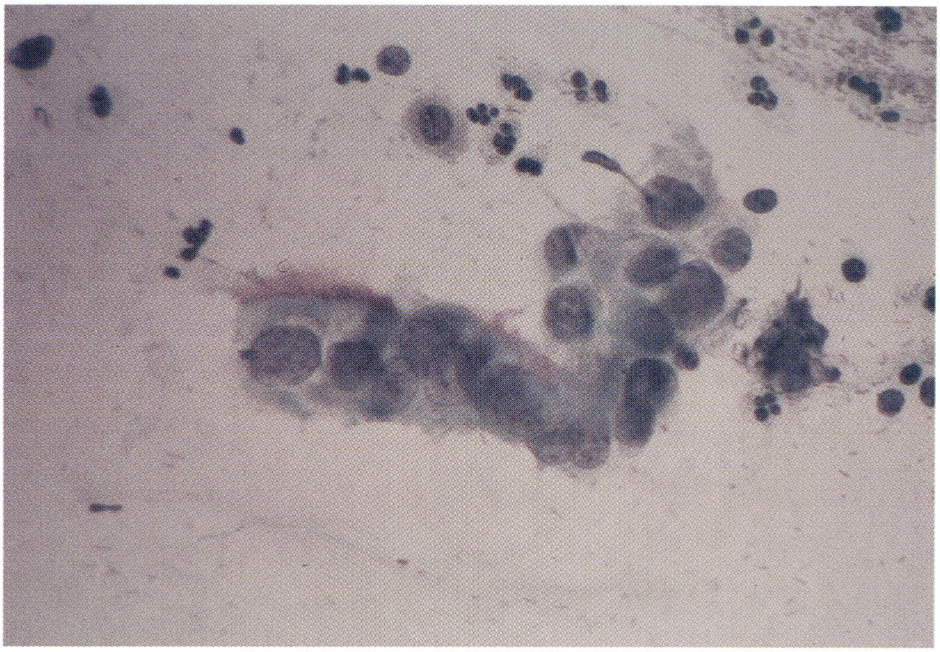

FIGURE 3-33
A strip of columnar ciliated cells is seen in this cervical smear. These are endocervical tubal metaplastic cells. The nuclei are enlarged and crowded, but in view of the tubal metaplasia this smear should not be labeled AGUS.

possible inflammatory effect but also a definite nuclear enlargement sometimes associated with variability or irregularity of the nuclear shape. The cells are usually in groups that maintain a strip-like or honeycomb organization (Fig. 3–34). There may be some variation to the cells within the group. The term AGUS favoring a dysplastic process is used when the cells have more abnormal nuclei and usually have hyperchromasia. Overlapping of nuclei usually occurs (Fig. 3–35). Additional features that may help distinguish endocervical glandular dysplasia from a reactive process are crowded sheets, elongated nuclei, a high nuclear to cytoplasmic ratio, and ill-defined cell borders. There is usually hyperchromatism. Cells diagnostic of AIS occur in sheets, strips, or rosettes (Fig. 3–36). Nuclear crowding and overlap is prominent. The decrease in cytoplasm is especially prominent. There are often ill-defined cell borders. A palisading nuclear arrangement is seen, and the nuclei protrude from the acinar cell clusters. This is termed feathering, and it is a characteristic feature of AIS. Nuclear enlargement with elongation is also seen and may lead to a colonic

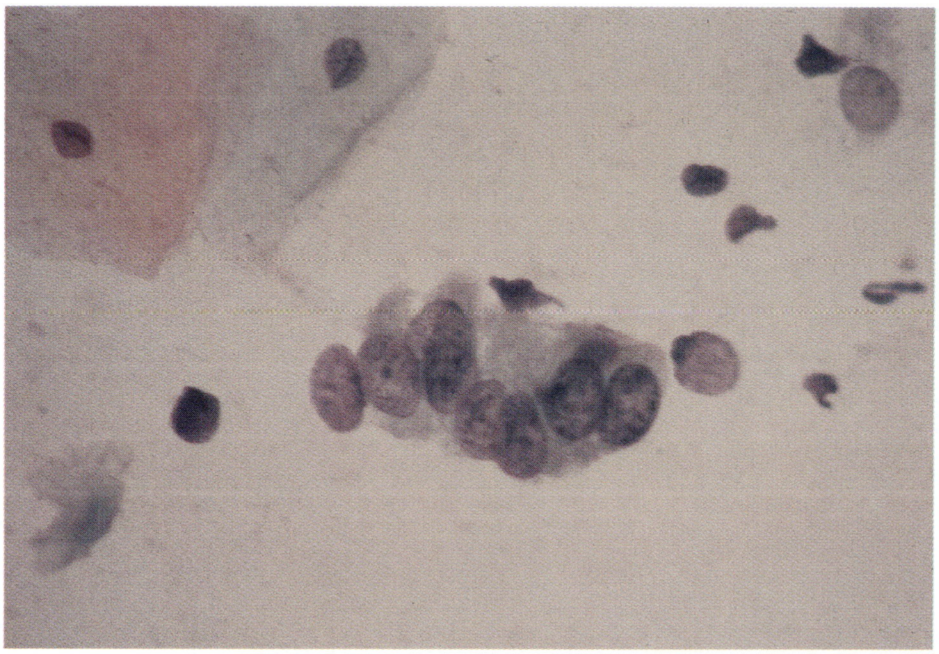

FIGURE 3-34
A strip of columnar cells with enlarged, hyperchromatic nuclei that show crowding is seen in this cervical smear. The cells are relatively uniform, and the top of the strip is straight. This suggests a minor degree of atypia, which is probably reactive, and possibly tubal metaplasia without the cilia. A cytologic diagnosis of atypical glandular cells, favor a reactive process, could be made.

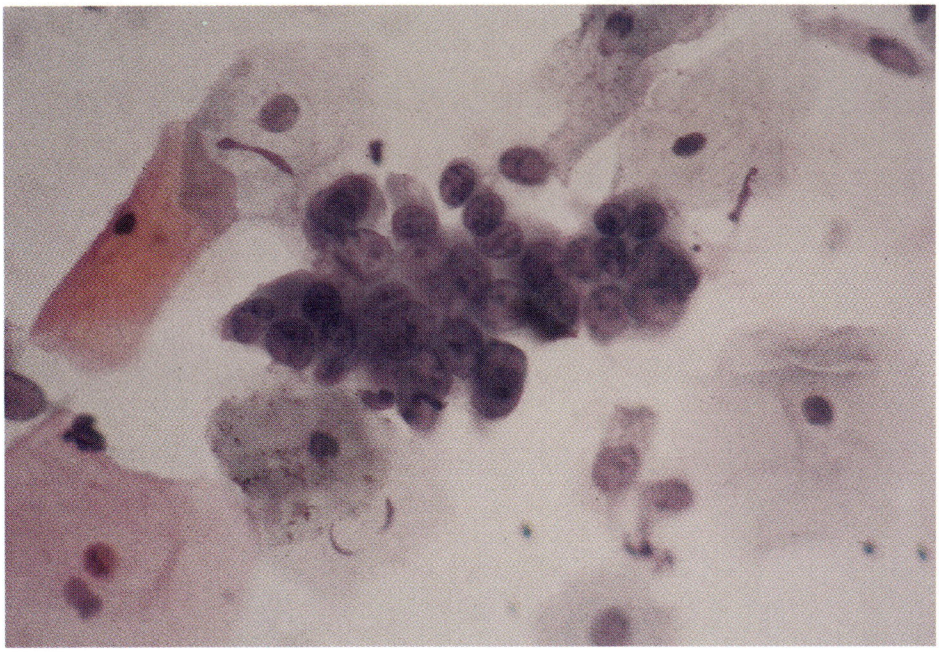

FIGURE 3-35
This cervical smear shows a normal endocervical cell close to the center on the right. A group of cells with hyperchromatism and slightly pleomorphic, enlarged nuclei that overlap is seen above the normal endocervical cell. Nucleoli are prominent in the largest nuclei. A diagnosis of atypical glandular cells, favor intraepithelial neoplasia, can be made.

cell-like appearance (Fig. 3–37). Stratification is also evident. More irregularly dispersed individual cells are present in invasive endocervical adenocarcinoma than in AIS, just as is true of invasive squamous carcinoma. In invasive endocervical adenocarcinoma the cells are larger and have more abundant cytoplasm than in AIS (Fig. 3–38). This leads to a smaller nuclear to cytoplasmic ratio than is typically seen in AIS. The cells of invasive adenocarcinoma are more pleomorphic than those of AIS. A dirty background may be seen.

The diagnosis and ultimately the treatment of the patient with AIS is complicated by the difficulty of making the correct diagnosis. Morphometric, histopathologic, and cytopathologic studies have shown the close similarity between AIS and invasive cervical adenocarcinoma.[152–154] Establishment of consistent histopathologic criteria may facilitate making the diagnosis. Cervical AIS is characterized by nuclear atypism, cellular stratification, and brisk mitotic activity of the endocervical epithelium. The epithelium is thicker than normal and the cells are densely packed around

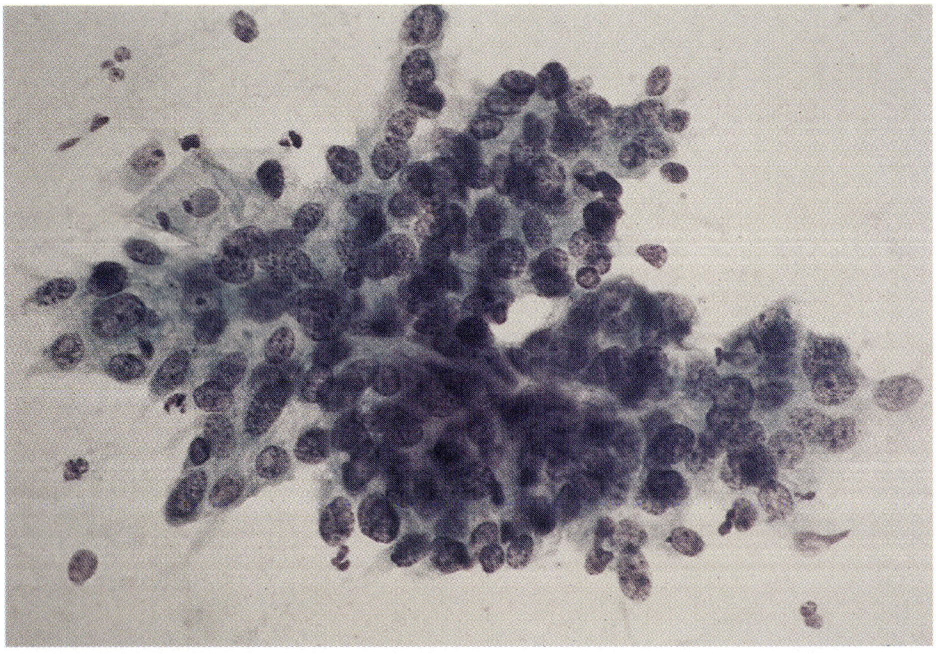

FIGURE 3-36
A large group of glandular cells is seen in this cervical smear. The center shows acinar formation with piling, crowding, and overlapping of the nuclei. There is pleomorphism. The cells are loosely cohesive at the periphery of the group. This is suggestive of AIS.

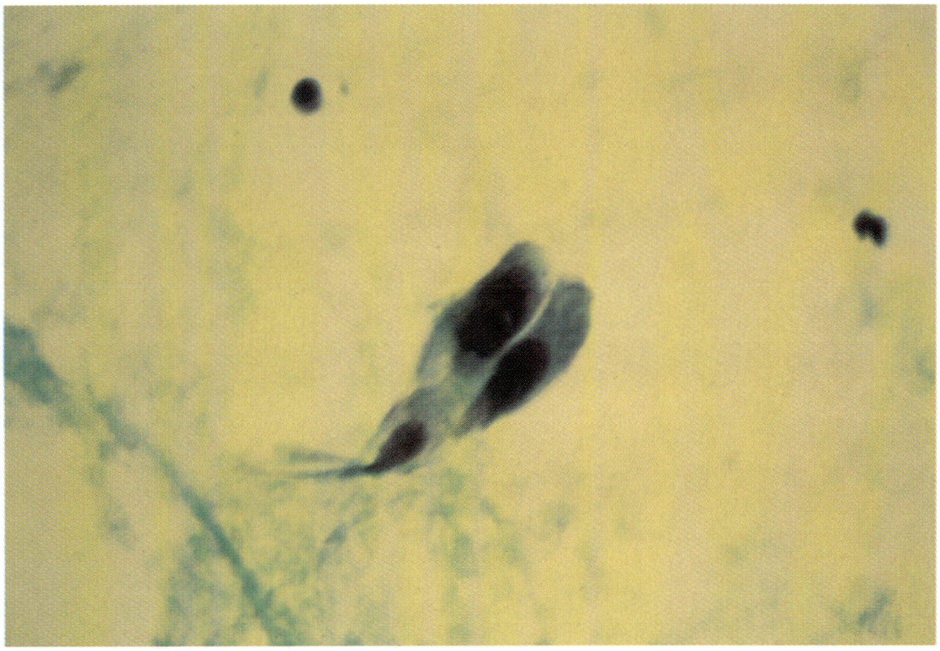

FIGURE 3-37
These cells retain their glandular shape. The nuclei are large, elongated, and very hyperchromatic. These cells come from the AIS shown in Figure 3–39.

the glandular lumens. Nuclei are enlarged and elongated and exhibit marked hyperchromasia. Nuclear pseudostratification is prominent because three or more tiers of nuclei may be seen; often they are positioned at the juxtaluminal region. Intracytoplasmic mucin is scant or completely absent. As the neoplastic cells proliferate, the affected glands develop buds or evaginations that may appear as clusters of small neoplastic glands when cut transversely. Papillary excrescences may be found protruding into the intraluminal spaces, and fusion of these projections gives rise to the formation of cribriform structures. The glands affected by AIS retain their smooth regular contours, however, and do not extend beyond the level of the normal endocervical glands. Cervical AIS, in contrast to invasive adenocarcinoma, is usually focal and is confined to superficial endocervical glands. A transition from normal endocervical epithelium to AIS is frequently identified (Fig. 3–39). There is no desmoplastic reaction of the cervical stroma surrounding the atypical glands, although an inflammatory infiltrate may be present. When these changes involve many glands or if the in-

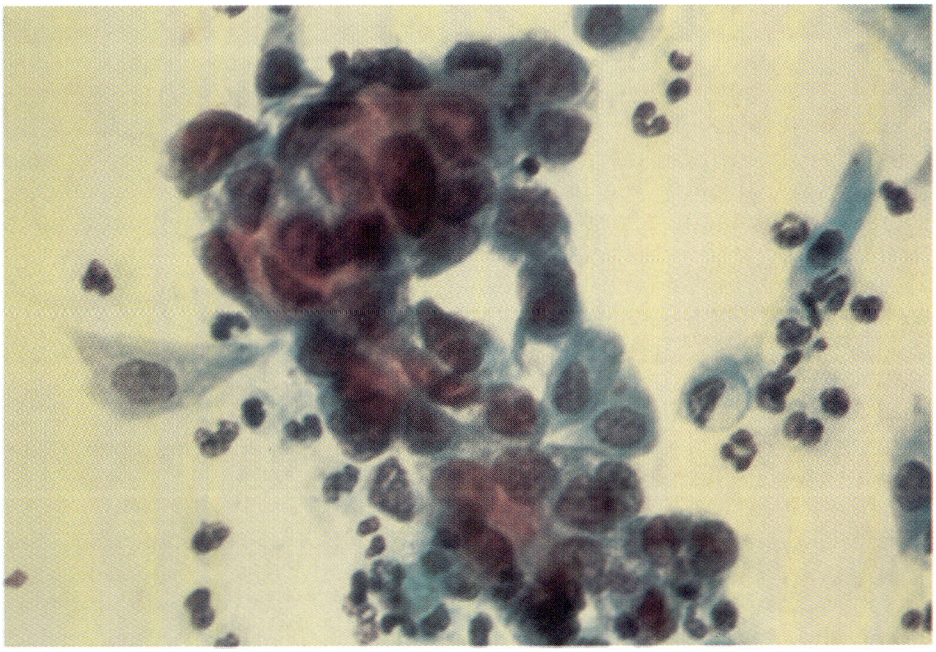

FIGURE 3-38
A group of highly pleomorphic malignant glandular cells is seen in this cervical smear. A solitary normal parabasal squamous cell is seen on the left. Some of the nuclei of the malignant glandular cells are three to four times larger than the nucleus of the basal squamous cell. Some of the malignant glandular cells have abundant cytoplasm. The cells at the top of the group form a ball-like structure, while those at the bottom form an acinus. The pink color in the cytoplasm is due to degeneration. These cells were shed from an endocervical adenocarcinoma.

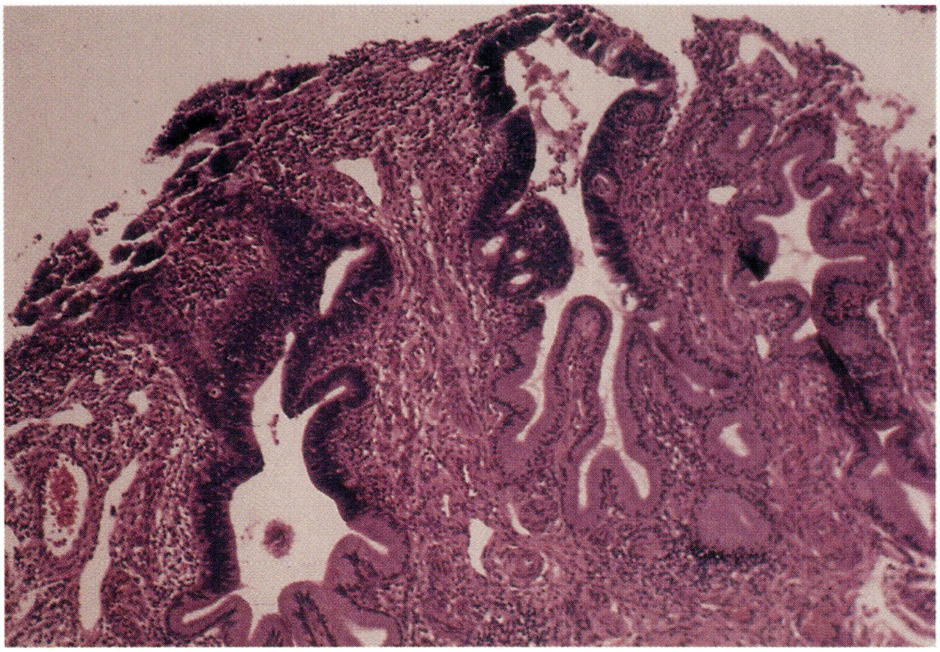

FIGURE 3-39
This adenocarcinoma in situ was present in superficial endocervical glands. The transition from normal to neoplastic epithelium is clearly seen. The normal endocervical epithelium has a single layer of nuclei that is located at the base of the cells. The neoplastic epithelium shows stratification and hyperchromatic nuclei. Mitotic activity is present but not appreciated at this magnification.

volved glands are deep in the cervical stroma, a diagnosis of adenocarcinoma should be considered because metastases have been reported from such lesions.[155]

Several histopathologic variants of AIS have been described. The endocervical or mucinous subtype is by far the most common pattern encountered and may be seen either in its pure form or in combination with other types. As its name implies, this type of endocervical AIS resembles the native glandular epithelium. AIS of the endometrioid subtype infrequently occurs in its pure form but is usually admixed with other variants. It shares many histopathologic features with the endocervical or mucinous type of AIS; however, nuclear pseudostratification is more exaggerated, and the neoplastic cells contain diminished amounts of cytoplasm devoid of any discernible intracellular mucin. A scant amount of mucicarminophilic material along the luminal border of the glands is occasionally demonstrable. Intestinal differentiation in AIS is reflected by the presence of absorptive enterocytes and prominent goblet cells within the involved glands; argentaffin and, uncommonly, Paneth cells may also be seen but are not a prerequisite for the designation of intestinal AIS. Rare cases of adenosquamous AIS have also been reported.[156]

Opinions vary about the ability of colposcopic examination to assess AIS effectively. Some think it is useful, but others think it is not helpful. Many authors think that the ability to diagnose AIS by colposcopy is hampered by the lack of specific colposcopic features.[157,158] AIS is sometimes multifocal, and some lesions are high in the canal and therefore beyond visualization with the colposcope.[159] Ueki et al contend that colposcopy is unreliable in the assessment of AIS and that colposcopically distinct lesions are only recognized once the lesion has become invasive.[160] Furthermore, because AIS and invasive adenocarcinoma share similar features, particularly at the surface epithelium, a small, colposcopically directed biopsy cannot exclude an invasive lesion. Coppleson and colleagues, on the other hand, contend that the majority of AIS lesions are located in the transformation zone or its vicinity and that they are colposcopically distinct.[161] Because of the limitations of colposcopy and targeted biopsies discussed earlier, cervical conization should be done in the patient whose cervical cytologic results show atypical glandular cells suggestive of cervical adenocarcinoma. Only on a cone biopsy or a hysterectomy specimen can invasion be excluded and the diagnosis of AIS made. The role of hysterectomy in this condition is discussed later.

Treatment

The management of the patient with cervical AIS is controversial and revolves around the debate on whether conservative therapy (i.e., cervical conization) is adequate to treat AIS effectively or whether a more radical approach (i.e., hysterectomy) is justified. A number of factors are important in making a management decision such as the patient's desire for future fertility, the status of conization margins, the adequacy of the conization specimen, and the findings obtained from endocervical curettage.

Arguments against conization as definitive therapy for cervical AIS include the possibility that multifocal disease, deep glandular involvement, or upper endocervical extension exists.[162, 163] Recent histopathologic reviews of cone and hysterectomy specimens have shown that the majority of AIS lesions are unifocal, however.[158, 164] These lesions usually occur within the transformation zone or in its vicinity.[165, 166] Bertrand et al[154] measured the distance from the transformation zone to the most cephalad focus of AIS and found that it never exceeded 25 mm. Ostor and associates[158] recorded similar results (30 mm maximum) and measured the depth of glandular involvement at between 0.5 and 4 mm. These data suggest that a very deep cone biopsy would encompass the majority of cervical AIS lesions.

Hysterectomy has been strongly recommended for the treatment of AIS when the conization margins are involved. This approach is suggested because of the studies documenting the high risk of persistent AIS after conization. Muntz et al[167] combined their data with those of other published series and found that 21 (62 percent) of 34 women who had AIS at the conization margin or abnormal endocervical curettings were found to have residual AIS in the hysterectomy specimen. In comparison, residual AIS was found in only 4 (8 percent) of 50 women who had uninvolved margins. In addition, occult invasive cancer was found in the hysterectomy specimens of some women who had AIS in the margins. Women who have cervical AIS and positive conization margins need at minimum a repeat conization and may need a hysterectomy.

The more recent literature supports the use of cervical conization as a definitive therapy for the patient who has cervical AIS and who desires preservation of fertility provided the conization margins and the endocervical curettings are uninvolved. Muntz et al[167] followed 18 women who had cervical AIS with uninvolved conization margins and reported that all are relapse free after a median follow-up of 3 years. Cullimore and colleagues[168] and Andersen and Arffmann,[169] respectively, reported no recurrences in their follow-up of patients who had AIS and uninvolved margins. Luesley et al[157] reported one case of persistent cervical AIS detected by cytology 13 months following a shallow conization (12 mm deep). Although long-term follow-up data are not available, close observation following an adequate cone biopsy seems to be a reasonable and safe management course in women with cervical AIS with uninvolved margins who desire future pregnancies.

VAGINAL INTRAEPITHELIAL NEOPLASIA (VAIN)

Epidemiology

The incidence of VAIN is increasing and parallels the epidemic increase of HPV-related lesions of the lower genital tract in women. Like its counterpart in the cervix, a dramatic increase in VAIN has also been detected in younger patients. However, VAIN still remains a much less common disease than other intraepithelial lesions of the lower genital tract. Its annual incidence in the United States is approximately 0.2 per 100,000 women.[170]

VAIN is strongly associated with CIN and multifocal lower genital tract neoplasia. About 60 percent of women with VAIN 3 lesions have a history of preexisting or synchronous cervical neoplasia.[171, 172] In fact, the majority of cases of VAIN are diagnosed in women who have undergone a hysterectomy for CIN. Patients who have VAIN share many of the epidemiologic characteristics associated with CIN. These include cigarette smoking, immunosuppression, a history of genital warts, and previous abnormal Papanicolaou smears. Approximately 2 percent of patients with CIN are found to have VAIN, but in more than half of these cases the vaginal lesions are in continuity with the cervical lesions.[173]

Although HPV infection occurs as frequently in the vagina as in the cervix, the prevalence of VAIN is significantly lower than CIN.[174, 175] This is probably due to the particular sensitivity of the transformation zone epithelium to carcinogens. Women exposed in utero to DES who have vaginal adenosis that undergoes the same process of metaplasia as occurs in the cervix have been reported to have an increased incidence of VAIN.[176] Even in DES-exposed women the increased risk of VAIN and CIN is highly associated with early onset of sexual activity and the number of sexual partners, which suggests a sexually transmitted etiology for VAIN similar to that found for CIN.

Diagnosis

Screening for VAIN and its detection and diagnosis is identical to that described for CIN. Patients with VAIN are usually asymptomatic, and the lesion is detected during evaluation of the patient who has an abnormal Papanicolaou smear. If a vaginal lesion is seen, a direct scrape of the lesion should be made and a separate slide submitted for cytologic evaluation. The cytologic and histopathologic criteria for diagnoses of vaginal smears or biopsies are essentially the same as those used for

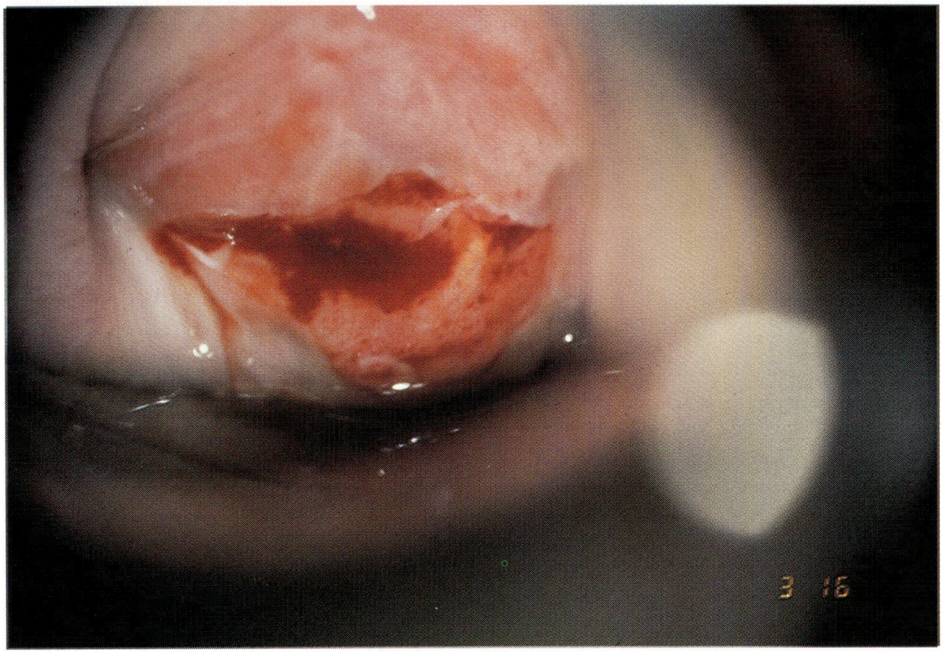

FIGURE 3-40
This postmenopausal patient developed VAIN several years after a hysterectomy for CIN 3. The atrophic mucosa at the apex of the vagina has been abraded by the speculum. Coarse punctations are seen in the lower aspect of the abrasion. Biopsy of this area revealed VAIN 2.

cervical lesions. The most common location of VAIN is the upper third of the vagina, and in most cases the lesions are unifocal.[177] On colposcopic examination VAIN lesions appear similar to CIN lesions (i.e., acetowhite epithelium, mosaicism, punctations, and abnormal vessels) (Fig. 3-40).

The use of topical estrogen cream is recommended prior to the colposcopic evaluation of a postmenopausal woman who has had an abnormal vaginal cytologic examination. The atrophic vaginal epithelium can be a source of misleading cytopathologic and colposcopic diagnoses secondary to degenerative and inflammatory changes in the parabasal cells.

Hybridization studies have now documented the fact that HPV type 16 can be detected in approximately 70 percent of VAIN lesions.[178] Progression of VAIN to invasive cancer has been reported,[179] but the natural history of VAIN lesions and the characteristics of those lesions at risk for progression are not known. This lack of information reflects the relative rarity of this condition.

Treatment

The treatment of VAIN must be individualized and must take into consideration several factors: the location of the lesion, the patient's age, whether the lesion is unifocal or multifocal, whether coexisting multicentric disease exists, and whether the uterus is still present. As described in the previous section on CIN, treatment must follow confirmation of the diagnosis by colposcopically directed biopsy. VAIN is more difficult to manage than CIN because it can be multifocal or diffuse and is commonly associated with other lower genital tract neoplasia including cervical and vulvar lesions. Higher failure rates are seen in patients treated for VAIN than in those treated for CIN. Treatment options for VAIN are listed in Table 3-9.

A key consideration in the choice of therapy is the extent of lower genital tract disease. Laser vaporization or the use of topical 5-fluorouracil is most successful in the treatment of patients in whom well-defined unifocal lesion is found at colposcopy and who have an intact uterus. In such cases the overall treatment efficacy exceeds 80 percent. One study reported an 11 percent failure rate in patients with unifocal VAIN compared with 28 percent in patients with multifocal disease.[180] The use of the ultrasonic surgical aspirator results in a failure rate of less than 20 percent.[181] In the treatment of patients with multifocal VAIN or multicentric squamous neoplasia it must be recognized that HPV infection in the lower genital tract is diffuse and carries the potential for reinfection and recurrent disease. We prefer to treat patients with multifocal VAIN with topical 5-fluorouracil.[182] Good results have also been reported by initial laser vaporization followed by weekly application of 5-fluorouracil for 6 months.[183] Radical laser vaporization of the entire vagina, cervix, and vulva with the intent to treat VAIN and reduce subclinical HPV infection does not improve outcome and results in significant morbidity.[184]

TABLE 3-9.
Treatment Options for Patients with VAIN

Laser vaporization
Intravaginal 5-fluorouracil
Ultrasonic surgical aspiration
Partial vaginectomy

Another important factor associated with the outcome of treatment of patients with VAIN is whether or not they have had a hysterectomy. Many women who have VAIN have had a hysterectomy for CIN.[185] This suggests that either there was a lack of recognition of CIN extension into the vaginal fornices or that there was synchronous upper VAIN at the time of hysterectomy.

Evaluation of abnormal vaginal cytologic findings in a patient who has had a hysterectomy can be compromised by inadequate colposcopic assessment of the vaginal scar because lesions can be "buried" in the folds of the vaginal cuff. Several series have reported the presence of occult invasive cancer in the excised vaginal vault of patients who had abnormal vaginal cytologic findings.[186, 187] Laser vaporization and intravaginal 5-fluorouracil can be used for treatment in these patients, but treatment failure rates are high. Surgical excision of the vault scar is the treatment of choice. Following treatment for VAIN a patient should be followed with frequent vaginal cytologic samples and colposcopic evaluation for any abnormal cytologic findings.

REFERENCES

1. Krantz KE: The anatomy of the human cervix, gross and microscopic. *In* Blandau RJ, Moghissi K (eds): The Biology of the Cervix. Chicago, University of Chicago Press, 1973, pp 57–69.
2. Robboy SJ, Taguchi O, Cunha D: Normal development of the human female reproductive tract and alterations resulting from experimental exposure to diethylstilbestrol. Hum Pathol 1982;13:190–198.
3. Crum CP, Nuovo G: The cervix. *In* Sternberg SS, Mills SE (eds): Surgical Pathology of the Female Reproductive System and Peritoneum. New York, Raven Press, 1991, pp 71–103.
4. Morrow CP, Townsend DE: Premalignant and related disorders of the lower genital tract. *In* Morrow CP, Townsend DE (eds.): Synopsis of Gynecologic Oncology. New York, Churchill Livingstone, 1987, pp 1–43.

4a. Carson HJ, DeMay RM: The mode ages of women with cervical dysplasia. Obstet Gynecol 1993;82:430–434.

5. Koss LG, Phillips A: Summary and recommendations of the workshop on uterine cancer. Cancer 1974;33:1753–1754.
6. Task Force of the Department of Health and Welfare of Canada: Cervical cancer screening programs: The Walton report. Can Med Assoc J 1982;127:581–589.
7. Sebastian JA, Leeb BO, See R: Cancer of the cervix—a sexually transmitted disease: Cytologic screening in a prostitute population. Am J Obstet Gynecol 1978;131: 620–623.
8. Vonka V, Kanka J, Hirsh I, et al: Prospective study on the relationship between cervical neoplasia and herpes simplex type 2 virus: II. Herpes simplex type 2 antibody presence in sera taken at enrollment. Int J Cancer 1984;33:61–66.
9. Vonka V, Kanka J, Jelinek I, et al: Prospective study on the relationship between cervical neoplasia and herpes simplex type 2 virus: I. Epidemiological characteristics. Int J Cancer 1984;33:49–60.
10. Rotkin ID, Cameron JR: Clusters of variables influencing the risk of cervical cancer. Cancer 1986;21:663–671.
11. Rotkin ID: Relation of the adolescent coitus to cervical cancer risk. JAMA 1962;179:486–491.
12. Thomas D: An epidemiologic study of carcinoma in situ and squamous dysplasia of the uterine cervix. Am J Epidemiol 1973;98:10–28.
13. La Vecchia C, Franceschi S, DeCarli A, et al: Sexual factors, venereal diseases, and the risk of intraepithelial and invasive cervical neoplasia. Cancer 1986;58:935–941.
14. La Vecchia C: The epidemiology of cervical neoplasia. Biomed Pharmacother 1985;39:426–433.
15. Cartwright RA, Simon JD: Carcinoma of the penis and cervix (letter). Lancet 1980;1:97.
16. MacGregor JE, Innes G: Carcinoma of the penis and cervix (letter). Lancet 1980;1:1246–1247.
17. Li J, Li FP, Blot WJ, Miller RW, Fraumeni JF: Correlation between cancers of the uterine cervix and penis in China. J Natl Cancer Inst 1982;69:1063–1065.
18. Graham S, Priore R, Graham M, Browne R, Burnett W, West D: Genital cancer in wives of penile cancer patients. Cancer 1979;44:1870–1874.
19. Martinez I: Relationship of squamous cell carcinoma of the cervix uteri to squamous cell carcinoma of the penis. Cancer 1969;24:777–780.
20. Smith PG, Kinlen LJ, White GC, Adelstein AM, Fox AJ: Mortality of wives of men dying with cancer of the penis. Br J Cancer 1980;41:422–428.
21. Kesler II: Human cervical cancer as venereal disease. Cancer Res 1976;36:783–791.
22. Pridan H, Lilienfeld AM: Carcinoma of the cervix in Jewish women in Israel, 1960–67: An epidemiological study. Isr J Med Sci 1971;7:1465–1470.
23. Buckley JD, Harris RWC, Doll R, Vessey MP, Williams PT: Case-control study of the husbands of women with dysplasia or carcinoma of the cervix uteri. Lancet 1981;2:1010–1015.
24. Zunzunegui MV, King MC, Coria CF, Charlet J: Male influence on cervical cancer risk. Am J Epidemiol 1986;123:302–307.
25. Agarwal SS, Sehgal A, Sardana S, Kumar A, Luthra UK: Role of male behavior in cervical carcinogenesis among women with one lifetime sexual partner. Cancer 1993; 72:1666–1669.
26. Winkelstein W: Smoking and cancer of the uterine cervix: Hypothesis. Am J Epidemiol 1977;106:257–259.
27. Harris RWC, Brinton LA, Cowdell RH, Skegg DCG, Smith PG, Vessey MP, Doll R: Characteristics of women with dysplasia or carcinoma in situ of the cervix uteri. Br J Cancer 1980;42:359–369.
28. Clarke EA, Morgan RW, Newman AM: Smoking as a risk factor in cancer of the cervix: Additional evidence from a case-control study. Am J Epidemiol 1982;115:59–66.
29. Lyon JL, Gardner JW, West DW, Stanish WM, Herbertson RM: Smoking and carcinoma in situ of the uterine cervix. Am J Public Health 1983;73:558–562.
30. Trevathan E, Layde P, Webster LA, Adams JB, Benigno BB, Ory H: Cigarette smoking and dysplasia and carcinoma in situ of the uterine cervix. JAMA 1983;250:499–502.
31. Brinton LA, Schairer C, Haenszel W, Stolley P, Lehman HF, Levine R, Savitz DA: Smoking and invasive cervical cancer. JAMA 1986;255:3265–3269.

32. Hellberg D, Nilson S, Haley NJ, Hoffman D, Wynder E: Smoking and cervical intraepithelial neoplasia: Nicotine and continine in serum and cervical mucus in smokers and non-smokers. Am J Obstet Gynecol 1988;158:910–913.
33. Holly EA, Petrakis NL, Friend NF, Sarles DL, Lee RE, Flander LB: Mutagenic mucus in the cervix of smokers. J Natl Cancer Inst 1986;76:983–986.
34. Barton SE, Maddox PH, Jenkins D, Edwards R, Cuzick J, Singer A: Effect of cigarette smoking on cervical epithelial immunity: A mechanism for neoplastic change? Lancet 1988;2:652–654.
35. Tay SK, Jenkins D, Maddox P, Singer A: Subpopulations of Langerhans cells in cervical intraepithelial neoplasia and human papillomavirus infection. Br J Obstet Gynaecol 1987;94:16–21.
36. Schiffman MH, Haley NJ, Felton JS, Andrews AW, Kaslow RA, Lancaster WD, Kurman RJ, Brinton LA, Lannom LB, Hoffman D: Biochemical epidemiology of cervical neoplasia: Measuring cigarette smoke constituents in the cervix. Cancer Res 1987;47:3886–3888.
37. Noffsinger A, White D, Fenoglio-Preiser CM: The relationship of human papillomaviruses to anorectal neoplasia. Cancer 1992;70:1276–1287.
38. Schneider A, Hotz M, Gissman L: Increased prevalence of human papilloma virus in the lower genital tract of pregnant women. Cancer 1987;40:198–201.
39. Feingold AR, Vermud SH, Burk RD, Kelley KF, Shrager LK, Shreiber K, Munk G, Friedland GH, Klein RS: Cervical cytologic abnormalities and papillomavirus in women infected with human immunodeficiency virus. J Acquir Immune Defic Syndr 1190;3:896–903.
40. Maiman M, Tarricone N, Vieira J, Suarez J, Serur E, Boyce JG: Colposcopic evaluation of human immunodeficiency virus seropositive women. Obstet Gynecol 1991; 78:84–88.
41. Vermud SH, Kelly KF, Klein RS, Feingold AR, Schreiber K, Munk G, Burk RD: High risk of human papillomavirus infection and cervical squamous intraepithelial lesions among women with symptomatic human immunodeficiency virus infection. Am J Obstet Gynecol 1991;165: 392–400.
42. Maiman M, Fruchter RG, Serur E, Levine PA, Arrastia CD, Sedlis A: Recurrent intraepithelial neoplasia in human immunodeficiency virus-seropositive women. Obstet Gynecol 1993;82:170–174.
43. Maiman M, Fruchter RG, Guy L, Cuthill S, Levine P, Serur E: Human immunodeficiency virus infection and invasive cervical carcinoma. Cancer 1993;71:402–406.
44. Spinillo A, Tenti P, Zappatore R, De Seta F, Silini E, Guaschino S: Langerhans' cell counts and cervical intraepithelial neoplasia in women with human immunodeficiency virus infection. Gynecol Oncol 1993;48:210–213.
45. Barrasso R, DeBrux J, Croissant O, Orth G: High prevalence of papillomavirus-associated penile intraepithelial neoplasia in sexual partners of women with cervical intraepithelial neoplasia. N Engl J Med 1987;317:916–923.
46. Oriel JD: Natural history of venereal warts. Br J Vener Dis 1971;47:1–13.
47. Koutsky L, Holmes K, Critchlow C, Stevens C, Paavonen J, Beckmann AM, DeRouen TA, Galloway DA, Vernon D, Kiviat NB: A cohort study of the risk of cervical intraepithelial neoplasia grade 2 or 3 in relation to papillomavirus infection. N Engl J Med 1992;327:1272–1278.
48. Reeves WC, Brinton LA, Garcia M, Brenes MM, Herrero R, Gaitan E, Tenorio F, de Britton RC, Rawls WE: Human papillomavirus infection and cervical cancer in Latin America. N Engl J Med 1989;320:1437–1441.
49. Meisels A, Fortin R: Condylomatous lesions of the cervix and vagina: I. Cytologic patterns. Acta Cytol 1976;20:505–509.
50. Koss LG, Durfee GR: Unusual patterns of squamous epithelium of the uterine cervix: Cytologic and pathologic study of koilocytotic atypia. Ann NY Acad Sci 1956; 63:1245–1261.
51. Lorincz AT, Temple GF, Kurman RJ, Jenson AB, Lancaster WD: Oncogenic association of specific human papillomavirus types with cervical neoplasia. J Natl Cancer Inst 1987;79:671–677.
52. Kreider JW, Howert MK, Wolfe SA, Bartlett GL, Zaino RJ, Sedlacek T, Mortel R: Morphologic transformation in vivo of human uterine cervix with papillomavirus from condylomatous acuminata. Nature 1985;317:639–641.
53. Pirisi L, Yasumoto S, Feller M, Doniger J, DiPaolo JA: Transformation of human fibroblasts and keratinocytes with human papillomavirus type 16 DNA. J Virol 1987; 61:1061–1066.
54. Lungu O, Sun WX, Felix J, Richart RM, Silverstein S, Wright TC Jr: Relationship of human papillomavirus type to grade of cervical intraepithelial neoplasia. JAMA 1992;276:2493–2496.
55. Schiffmann MH: Recent progress in defining the epidemiology of human papillomavirus infection and cervical neoplasia. J Natl Cancer Inst 1992;84:394–398.
56. Kjaer SK, deVilliers EM, Haugaard BJ, Christensen RB, Teisen C, Moller KA, Poll P, Jensen H, Vestergaard BF, Lynge E, Jensen OM: Human papillomavirus, herpes simplex virus and cervical cancer incidence in Greenland and Denmark: A population based cross-sectional study. Int J Cancer 1988;41:518–524.
56a. Kurman RJ, Henson DE, Herbst AL, Noller KL, Schiffman MH: Interim guidelines for management of abnormal cervical cytology. JAMA 1994;271:1866–1869.
57. Melchers W, van den Brule A, Walboomers J, de Bruin M, Burger M, Herbrink P, Meijer C, Lindeman J, Quint W: Increased detection rate of human papillomavirus in cervical scrapes by the polymerase chain reaction as compared to modified FISH and Southern blot analysis. J Med Virol 1989;27:329–335.
58. Young LS, Bevan IS, Johnson MA, Blomfield PI, Bromidge T, Maitland NJ, Woodman CB: The polymerase chain reaction: A new epidemiological tool for investigating cervical human papillomavirus infection. Br Med J 1989;298: 14–18.
59. Giuntoli R, Atkinson BF, Ernst CS, Rubin MM, Egan VS (eds): Atkinson's Correlative Atlas of Colposcopy, Cytology, and Histopathology. Philadelphia, JB Lippincott, 1987.
60. Kuman RJ, Solomon D: The Bethesda System for Reporting Cervical/Vaginal Cytologic Diagnoses. New York, Springer-Verlag, 1994, p 44.
61. McClatchey KD, Dawson JB, Bernackie EG, Kurtycz D, Lukerman JM, Noller KL, Perna VP, Plott AE, Plowden K, Richart R: Papanicolaou Technique: Proposed Guideline. Document GP 15-P. Villanova, PA, National Committee for Clinical Laboratory Standards (NCCLS), 1989.
62. Thompson D: Adequate Pap Smears: A Guide for Sampling Techniques in Screening for Abnormalities of the Uterine Cervix. Toronto, Laboratory Proficiency Testing Program, 1989.
63. Soost HJ: Comparative studies on the degree of proliferation of the vaginal and ectocervical epithelium in the hormonal evaluation of a patient by means of exfoliative cytology. Acta Cytol 1960;4:199–209.
64. Wied GL, Bahr GF: Vaginal, cervical and endocervical smears on a single slide. Obstet Gynecol 1959;14:362–367.
65. Bibbo M: Comprehensive Cytopathology. Philadelphia, WB Saunders, 1991, p 86.
66. Boon ME, deGraaf Guilloud JC, Rietveld WJ: Analysis of five sampling methods for the preparation of cervical smears. Acta Cytol 1989;33:843–848.
67. Harrison DD, Hernandez E, Dunton CJ: Endocervical brush versus cotton swab for obtaining cervical smears at a clinic: A cost comparison. J Reprod Med 1993;38:285–288.
68. Tyau L, Hernandez E, Anderson L, Heller P, Edmonds P: The Cell-Sweep: A new cervical cytology sampling device. J Reprod Med 1994;39:899–902.

69. College of American Pathologists/American Society of Clinical Pathologists: CLIA '88 Final Rules: A Summary of the Major Provisions of the Final Rules Implementing the Clinical Laboratory Improvement Amendment of 1988. Chicago, CAP Press, 1992.
70. Broder S: Rapid communication: The Bethesda System for reporting cervical/vaginal cytologic diagnoses: Report of the 1991 Bethesda workshop. JAMA 1992;267:1892.
71. Davis GL, Hernandez E, Davis JL, Miyazawa K: Atypical squamous cells in Papanicolaou smears. Obstet Gynecol 1987;69:43–46.
72. Hernandez E: Cervical cytology of atypical squamous cells: What does it mean and what to do about it? Clin Pract Sexuality 1992;7:21–24.
73. Gonzalez D, Hernandez E, Anderson L, Heller P, Atkinson BF: Clinical significance of a cervical cytology diagnosis of atypical squamous cells of undetermined significance favor reactive process or favor low grade squamous intraepithelial lesion. J Reprod Med (In press).
74. Ambros RA, Kurman RJ: Current concepts in the relationship of human papillomavirus infection to the pathogenesis and classification of precancerous squamous lesions of the uterine cervix. Semin Diagn Pathol 1990;7:158–172.
75. Coppleson M, Pixley EC: Colposcopy of cervix. *In* Coppleson M (ed): Gynecologic Oncology: Fundamental Principles and Clinical Practice, 2nd ed. London, Churchill Livingstone, 1992, pp 297–323.
76. Reid R, Herscham BR, Crum CP, Fu YS, Braun L, Shah KV, Agronov SJ, Stanhope CR: Genital warts and cervical cancer: V. The tissue basis of colposcopic change. Am J Obstet Gynecol 1984;149:293–303.
77. Richart RM: Colpomicroscopic studies of the distribution of dysplasia and carcinoma in situ on the exposed portion of the human uterine cervix. Cancer 1965;18: 950–954.
78. Sakuman T, Hasegawa T, Tsutsui F, Kurihara S: Quantitative analysis of the whiteness of the atypical cervical transformation zone. J Reprod Med 1985;30:773–776.
79. Reid R, Stanhope CR, Herschman BR, Crum CP, Agronow SJ: Genital warts and cervical cancer: IV. A colposcopic index for differentiating subclinical papillomaviral infection from cervical intraepithelial neoplasia. Am J Obstet Gynecol 1984;149:815–823.
80. Coppleson M, Pixley EC, Reid BL: Colposcopy: A Scientific and Practical Approach to the Cervix, Vagina and Vulva in Health and Disease, 3rd ed. Springfield, IL, Charles C Thomas, 1986.
81. Johnson LD, Easterday CL, Gore H, Hertig AT: The histogenesis of carcinoma in situ of the uterine cervix: A preliminary report of the origin of carcinoma in situ in subcylindrical cell anaplasia. Cancer 1964;17:213–229.
82. Wielenga G, Old JW,von Haam E: Squamous carcinoma in situ of the uterine cervix: II. Topography and clinical correlations. Cancer 1965;18:1612–1621.
83. Saito K, Saito A, Fu YS, Smotkin D, Gupta J, Shah K: Topographic study of cervical condyloma and intraepithelial neoplasia. Cancer 1987;59:2064–2070.
84. Abdul-Karim FW, Fu YS, Reagan JW, Wentz WB: Morphometric study of intraepithelial neoplasia of the uterine cervix. Obstet Gynecol 1982;60:210–214.
85. Richart RM: Colposcopic studies of cervical intraepithelial neoplasia. Cancer 1966;19:395–405.
86. Peterson O: Spontaneous course of cervical precancerous conditions. Am J Obstet Gynecol 1956;72:1063–1071.
87. Masterson JG: Analysis of untreated intraepithelial carcinoma of the cervix. Proceedings of the Third National Cancer Conference. Philadelphia, JB Lippincott, 1957.
88. Nasiell K, Roger V, Nasiell M: Behavior of mild cervical dysplasia during long-term follow-up. Obstet Gynecol 1986;67:665–669.
89. Reid R, Greenberg M, Jenson AB, Husain M, Willett J, Daoud Y, Temple G, Stanhope CR, Sherman AI, Phibbs GD, Lorincz AT: Sexually transmitted papillomaviral infections: I. The anatomic distribution and pathologic grade of lesions associated with different viral types. Am J Obstet Gynecol 1987;156:212–222.
90. Planner RS, Hobbs JB: Human papillomavirus infection and associated neoplasia of the cervix, vagina and vulva. Aust NZ J Obstet Gynecol 1987;27:132–135.
91. Campion MJ, McCance DJ, Cuzick J, Singer A: Progressive potential of mild cervical atypia: Prospective cytologic, colposcopic and virological study. Lancet 1986;2: 237–240.
92. Rome R, Chanen W, Pagano R: The natural history of human papillomavirus (HPV) atypia of the cervix. Aust NZ J Obstet Gynecol 1987;27:287–290.
93. Syrjanen K, Mlantyjlarvi R, Vlayrynen M, Syrjanen S, Parkkinen S, Yliskoski M, Castren O: Human papillomavirus (HPV) infections involved in the neoplastic process of the uterine cervix as established by prospective follow-up of 513 women for two years. Eur J Gynecol Oncol 1987;8:5–16.
94. Reid R: Human papillomavirus infection: The key to rational triage of cervical neoplasia. Obstet Gynecol Clin North Am 1987;14:407–429.
95. Popkin DR, Scali V, Ahmed MN: Cryosurgery for the treatment of cervical intraepithelial neoplasia. Am J Obstet Gynecol 1978;130:551–554.
96. Hemmingson E, Stendahl U, Stenson S: Cryosurgical treatment of cervical intraepithelial neoplasia with follow-up of five to eight years. Am J Obstet Gynecol 1981; 139:144–147.
97. Anderson MC, Hartley RB: Cervical crypt involvement by intraepithelial neoplasia. Obstet Gynecol 1980;55:546–550.
98. Stever MR, Hernandez E, Miyazawa K: Laser vaporization of cervical intraepithelial neoplasia. JAOA 1988;88: 1269–1272.
99. Lee ET, Ozumba EN, Bevan JR: A randomized trial of citanest with octopressin for relief of pain associated with the laser vaporization of the cervix. Br J Obstet Gynecol 1986;93:967–969.
100. Stafl A, Wilkinson EJ, Mattingly RF: Laser treatment of cervical and vaginal neoplasia. Am J Obstet Gynecol 1977;128:128–136.
101. Saunders N, Fenton DW, Soutter WP, Brown VA, Sharp F, Abernethy F: A case controlled study of the outcome of pregnancy following laser vaporization cone of the cervix. *In* Sharp F, Jordan JA (eds): Gynecological Laser Surgery. New York, Perinatology Press, 1986, pp 121–125.
102. Ferenczy A: Comparison of cryosurgery and carbon dioxide laser therapy for cervical intraepithelial neoplasia. Obstet Gynecol 1985;66:793–798.
103. Kurwan PH, Smith IR, Naftalin NJ: A study of cryosurgery and the CO_2 laser in the treatment of carcinoma in situ (CIN III) of the uterine cervix. Gynecol Oncol 1985;22:195–200.
104. Draeby-Kristiansen J, et al: Ten years after cryosurgical treatment of cervical intraepithelial neoplasia. Am J Obstet Gynecol 1991;165:43–45.
105. Richart RM, Townsend DE, Crisp W, De Petrillo A, Ferenczy A, Johnson G, Licrish G, Roy M, Villasanta U: An analysis of "long-term" follow-up results in patients with CIN treated by cryotherapy. Am J Obstet Gynecol 1980;137:823–826.
106. Walton LA, Edelman DA, Fowler WC Jr, Photopulos GJ: Cryosurgery for the treatment of cervical intraepithelial neoplasia during the reproductive years. Obstet Gynecol 1980;55:353–357.
107. Benedet JL, Miller DM, Nickerson KG: The results of cryosurgical treatment of cervical intraepithelial neoplasia at one, five, and ten years. Am J Obstet Gynecol 1987; 57:268–273.
108. Anderson ES, Thorup K, Larsen G: The results of cryosurgery for cervical intraepithelial neoplasia. Gynecol Oncol 1988;30:21–25.

109. Indman PD, Arndt BC: Laser treatment of cervical intraepithelial neoplasia in an office setting. Am J Obstet Gynecol 1985;152:674–676.
110. Wright VC: Carbon dioxide laser surgery for the cervix and vagina: Indications, complications, and results. Compr Ther 1988;14:54–64.
111. Baggish MS, Dorsey JH, Adelson M: A ten-year experience: Treatment of cervical intraepithelial neoplasia with the CO_2 laser. Am J Obstet Gynecol 1989;161:60–68.
112. Jobson VW, Homesley HD: Comparison of cryotherapy and CO_2 laser for cervical intraepithelial neoplasia. Colpo Gynecol Laser Surg 1984;1:176–180.
113. Ferenczy A, Mitao M, Nagai N, Silverstein SJ, Crum CP: Latent papillomavirus and recurring genital warts. N Engl J Med 1985;313:784–788.
114. Paraskevadis E, Jandial L, Mann EMF, Fisher PM, Kitchener HC: Pattern of treatment failure following laser for cervical intraepithelial neoplasia: Implications for follow-up protocol. Obstet Gynecol 1991;78:80–83.
115. Gloppinger A, Ikenberg H, Birmelin G, Hilgarth M, Pfleiderer A, Hillemanns HG: CO_2 laser therapy and typing of human papillomavirus in follow-up studies of cervix intraepithelial neoplasms (German). Geburtshilfe Frauenheilkd 1988;48:343–345.
116. American College of Obstetricians and Gynecologists: Cervical cytology: Evaluation and management of abnormalities. ACOG Tech Bull. 1993;83.
117. Jones HW III, Butler RE: The treatment of cervical intraepithelial neoplasia by cone biopsy. Am J Obstet Gynecol 1980;137:882–886.
118. Wright TC Jr, Richart RM, Ferenczy A, Koulos F: Comparison of specimens removed by CO_2 laser conization and the loop electrosurgical excision procedure. Obstet Gynecol 1992;79:147–153.
119. Krebs H-B, Pastore L, Helmkamp BF: Loop electrosurgical excision procedures for cervical dysplasia: Experience in a community hospital. Am J Obstet Gynecol 1993;169:289–295.
120. Keijser KGG, Kenemans P, van der Zander PHThH, Schijf CPT, Vooijs GP, Rolland R: Diathermy loop excision in the management of cervical intraepithelial neoplasia: Diagnosis and treatment in one procedure. Am J Obstet Gynecol 1992;166:1281–1287.
121. Luesley DM, Cullimore J, Redman CWE, Lawton FG, Emens JM, Rollason TP, Williams DR, Buxton EJ: Loop diathermy excision of the cervical transformation zone in patients with abnormal cervical smears. Br Med J 1990;300:1690–1693.
122. Wright TC Jr, Gagnon S, Richart RM, Ferenczy A: Treatment of cervical intraepithelial neoplasia using the loop electrosurgical excision procedure. Obstet Gynecol 1992; 79:173–178.
123. Gunasekers PC, Phipps JH, Lewis BV: Large loop excision of the transformation zone (LLETZ) compared to carbon dioxide laser in the treatment of CIN: A superior mode of treatment. Br J Obstet Gynaecol 1990;97:995–998.
124. Chappatte QA: Histologic difference between colposcopic-directed biopsy and loop excision of the transformation zone (LETZ): A cause for concern. Gynecol Oncol 1991; 43:46–50.
125. Turner MJ, Rasmussen MJ, Flannelly GM, Kelehan P, Lenehan P, Murphy JF: Outpatient loop diathermy conization as an alternative to inpatient knife conization of the cervix. J Reprod Med 1992;37:314–316.
126. Murdoch JB, Morgan PR, Lopes A, Monaghan JM: Histological incomplete excision of CIN after large loop excision of the transformation zone (LLETZ) merits careful follow-up, not retreatment. Br J Obstet Gynaecol 1992;99:990–993.
127. Townsend DE, Richart RM, Marks E, Nielsen J: Invasive cancer following outpatient evaluation and therapy for cervical disease. Obstet Gynecol 1981;57:145–149.
128. Luesley DM, McCrum A, Terry PB, Wade-Evans T: Complications of cone biopsy related to the dimensions of the cone and the influence of prior colposcopic assesment. Br J Obstet Gynaecol 1985;92:158–164.
129. Larson G, Gullberg B, Grundsell H: A comparison of laser and cold knife conization. Obstet Gynecol 1983;62:213–217.
130. Jordan JA: Symposium on cervical neoplasia: I. Excisional methods. Colpo Gynecol Laser Surg 1984;1:271.
131. Ahlgren M, Ingemarsson I, Lindberg LG, Nordqvist SRB: Conization as treatment of carcinoma in situ of the uterine cervix. Obstet Gynecol 1975;46:135–139.
132. Kullander S, Sjoberg NO: Treatment of carcinoma in situ of the cervix uteri by conization: a five year follow-up. Acta Obstet Gynecol Scand 1971;50:153–157.
133. Berghardt E, Hozler E: Treatment of carcinoma-in-situ: Evaluation of 1609 cases. Obstet Gynecol 1980;55:539–545.
134. Lubicz S, Ezekweche C, Allen A, Schiffer M: Significance of cone biopsy margins in the management of patients with cervical neoplasia. J Reprod Med 1984;29:179–184.
135. White C, Cooper W, Williams R: Cervical intraepithelial neoplasia extending to the margins of resection in conization of the cervix. J Reprod Med 1991;36:635–638.
136. Lapaquette TK, Dihn TV, Hannigan EV, Doherty MG, Yandell RB, Buchanan VS: Management of patient with positive margins after cervical conization. Obstet Gynecol 1993;82:440–443.
137. Boyes DA, Worth AJ, Fidler HK: The results of treatment of 4389 cases of preclinical cervical squamous carcinoma. J Obstet Gynaecol Br Commonw 1970;77:769–780.
138. Kolstad P, Klem V: Long-term follow-up of 1121 cases of carcinoma in situ. Am J Obstet Gynecol 1976;48:125–129.
139. Wiener JJ, Sweetnam PM, Jones JM: Long-term follow-up of women after hysterectomy with a history of pre-invasive cancer of the cervix. Br J Obstet Gynaecol 1992; 99:907–910.
140. Schneider A, de Villiers E-M, Schneider V: Multifocal squamous neoplasia of the female genital tract: Significance of human papillomavirus infection of the vagina after hysterectomy. Obstet Gynecol 1987;70:294–298.
141. Cristopherson WM, Nealon N, Gray LA: Non-invasive precursor lesions of adenocarcinoma and mixed adenosquamous carcinoma of the cervix uteri. Cancer 1979;44:975–983.
142. Bousfield L, Pacey F, Young Q: Expanded cytologic criteria for the diagnosis of adenocarcinoma in-situ of the cervix and related lesions. Acta Cytol 1980;24:283–295.
143. Maier RC, Norris HJ: Coexistence of cervical intraepithelial neoplasia with primary adenocarcinoma of the endocervix. Obstet Gynecol 1980;56:361–364.
144. Brinton LA, Herrero R, Reeves WC, de Britton RC, Gaitan E, Tenorio F: Risk factors for cervical cancer by histology. Gynecol Oncol 1993;51:301–306.
145. Persson E, Einhorn N, Pettersson F: A case control study of oral contraceptive use in women with adenocarcinoma of the uterine cervix. Eur J Obstet Gynecol Reprod Biol 1987;26:85–90.
146. Peters RK, Chao A, Mack TM, Thomas D, Bernstein L, Henderson BE: Increased frequency of adenocarcinoma of the uterine cervix in young women in Los Angeles County. J Natl Cancer Inst 1986;76:423–428.
147. Brown LJR, Wells M: Cervical glandular atypia associated with squamous intraepithelial neoplasia; a premalignant lesion? J Clin Pathol 1986;39:22–28.
148. Jaworski RC, Pacey N, Greenberg ML, Osborn RA: The histologic diagnosis of adenocarcinoma in situ and related lesions of the cervix uteri. Cancer 1988;61:1171–1181.
149. Gloor E, Hurlimann J: Cervical intraepithelial glandular neoplasia: Adenocarcinoma in situ and glandular dysplasia. A correlative study of 23 cases with histological grading, histochemical analysis of mucins, and immunohistochemical determination of the affinity for four lectins. Cancer 1986;58:1272–1280.

150. Kudo R: Cervical adenocarcinoma. Curr Top Pathol 1992;85:81–107.
151. Boon ME, Baak JPA, Kurver PJH, Overdiep SH, Verdonk GW: Adenocarcinoma in situ of the cervix: An under-diagnosed lesion. Cancer 1981;48:768–773.
152. Gloor E, Ruzicka J: Morphology of adenocarcinoma-in-situ of the uterine cervix: A study of 14 cases. Cancer 1982; 49:294–302.
153. Van Roon E, Boon ME, Kurver PJH, Baak JPA: The association between precancerous columnar and squamous lesions of the cervix: A morphometric study. Histopathology 1983;7:887–896.
154. Bertrand M, Lickrish GM, Colgan TJ: The anatomical distribution of cervical adenocarcinoma in situ: implications for treatment. Am J Obstet Gynecol 1987;157:21–25.
155. Buscema J, Woodruff JD: Significance of neoplastic atypicalities in endocervical epithelium. Gynecol Oncol 1984; 17:356–362.
156. Christopherson WM, Nealon N, Gray LA Sr: Noninvasive precursor lesions of adenocarcinoma and mixed adenosquamous carcinoma of the cervix uteri. Cancer 1979; 44:975–983.
157. Luesley DM, Jordan JA, Woodman CB, Watson N, Williams DR, Waddell C: A retrospective review of adenocarcinoma in situ and glandular atypia of the uterine cervix. Br J Obstet Gynaecol 1987;94:699–703.
158. Ostor Ag, Pagano R, Davoren RAM, Fortune DW, Chanen W, Rome R: Adenocarcinoma in situ of the cervix. Int J Gynecol Pathol 1984;3:179–190.
159. Nguynen GK, Jeannot ART: Exfoliative cytology of in-situ and microinvasive adenocarcinoma of the uterine cervix. Acta Cytol 1984;28:461–467.
160. Ueki M, Ueda M, Kitsuki K, et al: Colposcopy of cervical adenocarcinoma-in-situ and changes in findings associated with early invasion. J Exp Clin Cancer Res 1990;9 (Suppl):173.
161. Coppleson M, Atkinson KH, Dalrymple JC: Cervical squamous and glandular intraepithelial neoplasia: Clinical features and review of management. *In* Coppleson M (ed): Gynecologic Oncology: Fundamental Principles and Clinical Practice, 2nd ed. London, Churchill Livingstone, 1992, pp 571–607.
162. Wells M, Brown LJR: Glandular lesions of the uterine cervix: The present state of our knowledge. Histopathology 1986;10:777–792.
163. Cristopherson WM, Nealon N, Gray LA Sr: Noninvasive precursor lesions of adenocarcinoma and mixed adenosquamous carcinoma of the cervix uteri. Cancer 1979; 44:975–983.
164. Qizibash AH: In situ and microinvasive adenocarcinoma of the uterine cervix: A clinical, cytologic and histologic study of 14 cases. Am J Clin Pathol 1975;64:155–170.
165. Laverty CR, Farnsworth A, Thurloe J, Bowditch R: The reliability of a cytological prediction of cervical adenocarcinoma in situ. Aust NZ J Obstet Gynecol 1988;28:307–312.
166. Teshima S, Shimosato Y, Kishi K, Kasamatsu T, Ohmi K, Vei Y: Early stage adenocarcinoma of the uterine cervix: Histopathologic analysis with consideration of histogenesis. Cancer 1985;56:167–172.
167. Muntz HG, Bell DA, Lage JM, Goff BA, Feldman S, Rice LW: Adenocarcinoma in situ of the uterine cervix. Obstet Gynecol 1992;80:935–939.
168. Cullimore JE, Luesley DM, Rollason TP, Byrne P, Buckley CH, Anderson M, Williams DR, Waddell C, Hudson E, Shafi MI: A prospective study of conization of the cervix in the management of cervical intraepithelial glandular neoplasia (CIGN): A preliminary report. Br J Obstet Gynaecol 1992;99:314–318.
169. Andersen ES, Arffmann E: Adenocarcinoma in situ of the uterine cervix: A clinicopathologic study of 36 cases. Gynecol Oncol 1989;35:1–7.
170. Cramer DN, Cutler SJ: Incidence and histopathology of malignancies of the female genital organs in the U.S. Am J Obstet Gynecol 1974;118:443–460.
171. Hummer WK, Mussey F, Decker DG, Docherty MB: Carcinoma in situ of the vagina. Am J Obstet Gynecol 1970; 108:1109–1116.
172. Campion MJ, Clarkson P, McDance DJ: Squamous neoplasia of the cervix in relation to other genital tract neoplasia. *In* Singer A (ed): Clinical Obstetrics and Gynecology. London, WB Saunders, 1985, pp 265–280.
173. Nwabinell NJ, Monaghan JM: Vaginal epithelial abnormalities in patients with CIN: Clinical and pathological features and management. Br J Obstet Gynaecol 1991; 98:25–29.
174. Copenhaver EH, Salzman FA, Wright KA: Carcinoma in situ of the vagina. Am J Obstet Gynecol 1964;89: 962–969.
175. Gallup DG, Morley GW: Carcinoma in situ of the vagina: A study and review. Obstet Gynecol 1975;46:334–340.
176. Robboy SJ, Noller KL, O'Brien P, Kaufman RH, Townsend D, Barnes AB, Gundersen J, Lawrence WD, Bergstrahl E, McGorray Sl: Incidence of cervical and vaginal dysplasia in 3,980 diethylstilbestrol-exposed young women. JAMA 1984;252:2979–2983.
177. Benedet JL, Sanders BH: Carcinoma in situ of the vagina Am J Obstet Gynecol 1984;148:695–700.
178. McCance DJ, Clarkson PK, Dyson JL, Walker PG, Singer A: Human papillomavirus types 6 and 16 in multifocal intraepithelial neoplasia of the lower genital tract. Br J Obstet Gynaecol 1985;92:1093–1000.
179. Rutledge F: Cancer of the vagina. Am J Obstet Gynecol 1967;97:635–655.
180. Dorsey JH, Baggish MS: Multifocal vaginal intraepithelial neoplasia with uterus in situ. *In* Sharp F, Jordan JA (eds): Gynecological Laser Surgery: Proceedings of the 15th Study Group of the Royal College of Obstetricians and Gynecologists. Ithaca, NY, Perinatology Press, 1985, p 173.
181. Abbas F, Sert B, Fields A, Rosenshein N: The management of vaginal intraepithelial neoplasia by ultrasonic surgical aspiration (abstract). Gynecol Oncol 1993;49:142.
182. Caglar H, Hertzog RW, Hreshchyshyn MM: Topical 5-fluorouracil treatment of vaginal intraepithelial neoplasia. Obstet Gynecol 1981;58:580–583.
183. Krebs HB: Prophylactic topical 5-fluorouracil following treatment of human papillomavirus-associated lesions of the vulva and vagina. Obstet Gynecol 1986;68:837–841.
184. Riva JM, Sedlacek TV, Cunnane MF, Mangan CE: Extended carbon dioxide laser vaporization in the treatment of subclinical papillomavirus infection of the lower genital tract. Obstet Gynecol 1989;73:25–30.
185. Woodman CBJ, Jordan JA, Wade-Evans T: The management of VAIN after hysterectomy. Br J Obstet Gynaecol 1984;91:707–711.
186. Ireland D, Monaghan JM: The management of the patient with abnormal vaginal cytology following hysterectomy. Br J Obstet Gynaecol 1988;95:973–975.
187. Barclay DL: Carcinoma of the vagina after hysterectomy for severe dysplasia or carcinoma in situ of the cervix. Gynecol Oncol 1979;8:1–11.

4

Malignant Neoplasms of the Cervix and Vagina

Paul B. Heller / Enrique Hernandez / Barbara F. Atkinson

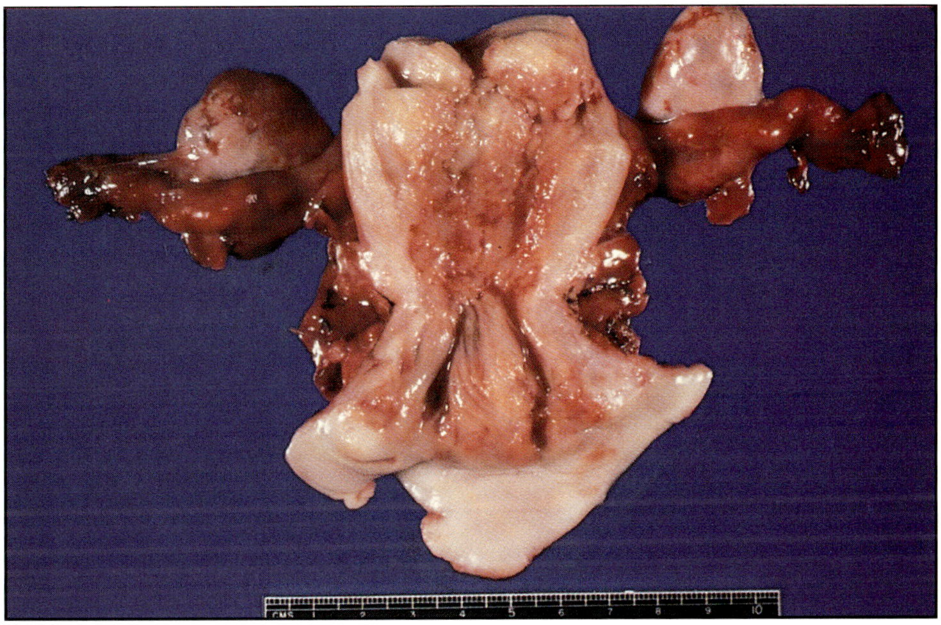

CERVICAL CANCER

The prevalence of invasive squamous cervical cancer in the United States has decreased over time. This is thought to be due to an increase in the detection and treatment of its precursor lesion, cervical intraepithelial neoplasia (CIN). Most cervical cancers are squamous cell carcinomas. Of 140 patients with cervical carcinoma recently treated with radiation therapy at the Medical College of Pennsylvania, 92 percent had squamous cell carcinomas.[1] Most of the remainder were adenocarcinomas. The proportion of cervical cancers that are adenocarcinomas has increased at many medical centers, and this histopathologic type now constitutes 10 to 20 percent of all cervical cancers in some series.[2] This increase is thought to be secondary to a decrease in the number of squamous cell carcinomas and not to an increase in the absolute number of adenocarcinomas.[3, 4] The clinical and pathologic characteristics of these two histopathologic cell types are different and therefore will be discussed separately.

Squamous Cell Carcinoma

Epidemiology and Clinical Presentation

Squamous cell carcinoma and CIN are a continuum and share the epidemiologic and etiologic features discussed in Chapter 3. This disease is rare in women younger than 20 years old and in those who have never been sexually active. The mean age at diagnosis is in the early sixth decade of life.[5] Of those treated with radiation therapy at the Medical College of Pennsylvania, the mean and median age was 57 years.[1] However, 86 percent of them had disease that extended outside of the cervix. The age of the patient correlates with the extent of the disease. Patients with more advanced cervical cancer tend to be older. Of 195 patients treated for cervical cancer at The Johns Hopkins Hospital between 1981 and 1983, the mean age was 47.5 years for those with stage I disease, 53.7 years for those with stage II, 57.8 years for those with stage III, and 60.7 years for those with stage IV (Neil B. Rosenshein, MD, personal communication). The age range of these 195 patients was 19 to 91 years.

The symptoms of cervical cancer are also variable and relate to the extent of the disease and the growth characteristics of the tumor (i.e., endophytic vs. exophytic). The patient may be asymptomatic and the carcinoma found during evaluation of an abnormal Papanicolaou smear. The symptomatic patient may complain only of a watery, mucoid, or purulent vaginal discharge that may be blood-tinged. Abnormal vaginal bleeding is also a frequent complaint. This can occur after intercourse but is frequently described as a heavy and prolonged menstrual flow or intermenstrual bleeding. The postmenopausal patient may present with postmenopausal vaginal bleeding. As the tumor grows and involves the adjacent structures or spreads to the regional lymphatics, the patient may complain of flank or leg pain, dysuria, hematuria, hematochezia, obstipation, and leg edema. When tumor growth and extension blocks both ureters, the patient may present in an obtunded state or even comatose secondary to uremia.

The gross appearance of squamous cell carci-

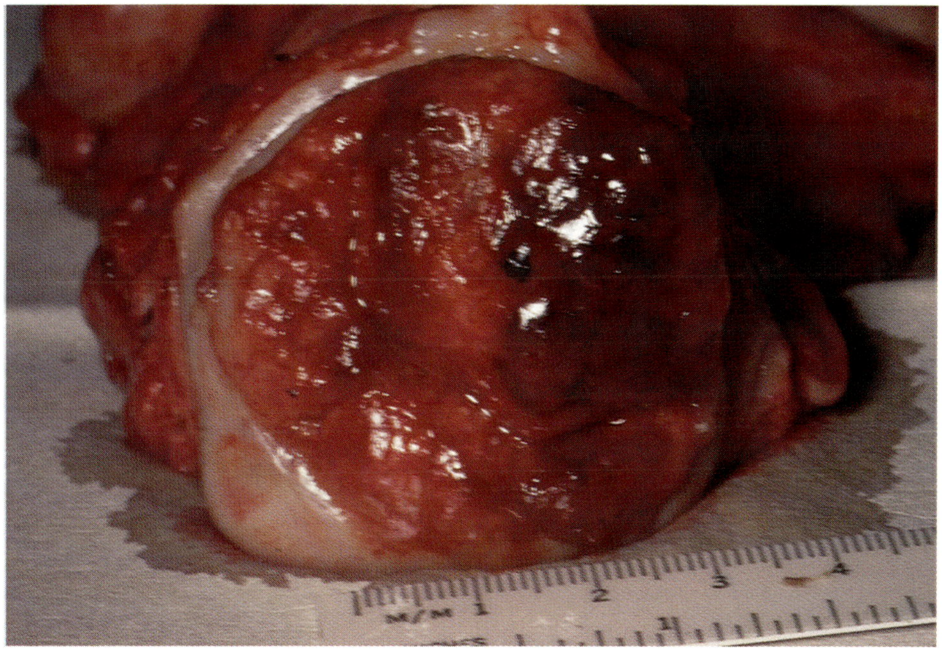

FIGURE 4-1
This is a radical hysterectomy specimen from a woman who had early stage IIA squamous cell carcinoma of the cervix. The cervix is replaced by a large, irregular, exophytic, friable tumor that touches the vaginal fornices. This view shows the cervix en face with a rim of vagina surrounding it.

noma is also variable. It may be an early lesion that is only recognizable by colposcopy (see Chapter 3), or it may be identified on a cervical biopsy. It can be a large, friable, exophytic lesion (Fig. 4-1) or an ulcerative lesion that destroys the cervix. The tumor may extend down the vagina and may involve one or both parametria. Invasion into the bladder and rectum can occur and is identifiable by endoscopy. The term microinvasive carcinoma is used to describe the earliest invasive lesion (discussed subsequently).

Microinvasive Squamous Cell Carcinoma

The International Federation of Obstetrics and Gynecology (FIGO) staging system divides early carcinoma of the cervix into stage IA1 and stage IA2 (Table 4-1).[6] Stage IA1 is defined as minimal microscopic evidence of invasion (i.e., a few neoplastic cells are seen to break through the basement membrane and infiltrate the underlying stroma). Stage IA2 comprises lesions that are more than minimal microscopic evidence, but the invasion does not exceed 5 mm in depth from the basement membrane from which it originates, be it from an endocervical gland or from the surface epithelium. The horizontal spread of stage IA2 lesions cannot exceed 7 mm. Lesions that exceed these measurements are classified as stage IB regardless of whether they are grossly evident or identifiable only by microscopy.

Microinvasive squamous cell carcinoma (i.e., stage IA) comprises 5 to 10 percent of all cervical cancers. In the Johns Hopkins series described previously, 5.6 percent of the patients had stage IA disease. A report from the Norwegian Radium Hospital shows that the proportion of stage IA cervical cancer has varied over a period of time.[7] In the interval between 1976 and 1978 patients with stage IA cervical cancer comprised 19.3 percent of all patients with cervical cancer treated at that institution. In the interval between 1982 and 1984 patients with stage IA disease comprised 8.6 percent. This decrease probably reflects earlier detection by cervical cytology screening. The Norwegian series is one of the largest reported, with 643 cases of stage IA cervical squamous cell carcinoma. The age of the patients ranged from 19 to 79 years. Eighty percent of the patients were between 30 and 59 years old. Although most patients with microinvasive squamous cell carcinoma of the cervix had no symptoms, 44 percent complained of abnormal vaginal bleeding or discharge.[7] Most patients with cervical microinvasive squamous cell carcinoma come to medical attention because of an abnormal Papanicolaou smear, the findings on which range from atypical squamous cells to cytopathologic changes consistent with carcinoma. The cytopathologic criteria for microinvasion that have been suggested include the presence of macronucleoli, irregular chromatin clumping and clearing, increased cell size with more abundant cytoplasm, and cellular and nuclear pleomorphism (Fig. 4-2). In contrast, cells from CIN lesions lack pleomorphism, have an even chromatin distribution, and do not have nucleoli. In actual practice we find that these criteria are good but are not specific for microinvasive lesions. The cells at the surface of

TABLE 4–1.

Staging of Carcinoma of the Cervix According to the International Federation of Gynecology and Obstetrics (FIGO) 1985 Classification

Stage I. The carcinoma is strictly confined to the cervix (extension to the corpus should be disregarded)

- **Stage IA.** Preclinical carcinomas of the cervix (those diagnosed only by microscopy)
  - **Stage IA1.** Minimally microscopically evident stromal invasion
  - **Stage IA2.** Lesions detected microscopically that can be measured. The upper limit of the measurement should not show a depth of invasion of more than 5 mm taken from the base of the epithelium, either surface or glandular, from which it originates. A second dimension, the horizontal spread, must not exceed 7 mm. Larger lesions should be staged as IB
- **Stage IB.** Lesions of greater dimensions than stage IA2, whether seen clinically or not. Preformed space involvement should not alter the staging but should be specifically recorded so as to determine whether it should affect treatment decisions in the future

Stage II. The carcinoma extends beyond the cervix but has not extended onto the pelvic wall. The carcinoma involves the vagina but not the lower third

- **Stage IIA.** No obvious parametrial involvement
- **Stage IIB.** Obvious parametrial involvement

Stage III. The carcinoma has extended to the pelvic wall. On rectal examination there is no cancer-free space between the tumor and the pelvic wall. The tumor involves the lower third of the vagina. All cases with hydronephrosis or nonfunctioning kidney

- **Stage IIIA.** No extension onto the pelvic wall
- **Stage IIIB.** Extension onto the pelvic wall and/or hydronephrosis or nonfunctioning kidney

Stage IV. The carcinoma has extended beyond the true pelvis or has clinically involved the mucosa of the bladder or rectum. Bullous edema as such does not permit a case to be allotted to stage IV

- **Stage IVA.** Spread of the growth to adjacent organs
- **Stage IVB.** Spread to distant organs

most microinvasive squamous cell carcinomas are those of the CIN 3 lesion from which the microinvasion arose. Because cytologic sampling retrieves cells only from the top two or three cell layers, the deeper invasive cells are often not obtained.

The colposcopic appearance of cervical microinvasive squamous cell carcinoma is consistent with microinvasive or invasive carcinoma in 48 percent of cases.[7] In the majority of the remaining cases the colposcopic appearance is consistent with CIN. As discussed in the previous chapter, if a colposcopically directed cervical biopsy shows microinvasion, a cone biopsy is mandatory to exclude more advanced disease.

Almost all cases of squamous cell carcinoma of the cervix originate from CIN 3 lesions. Therefore, a full-thickness neoplastic change of the cervical epithelium must occur before invasion occurs. A few rare cases of squamous cell cervical carcinoma not associated with CIN 3 have been reported.[8] The progression from CIN to carcinoma is usually slow,[9] but a more rapid progression may occur in some patients. In one study, 44 percent of women with cervical cancer that contained human papillomavirus (HPV) type 18 had a history of three normal Papanicolaou smears in the 3 years preceding the diagnosis of cervical cancer.[10] The progression from CIN 3 to invasive carcinoma is not universal. Of 131 patients with biopsy-proven carcinoma in situ of the cervix who continued to have abnormal cytologic findings, 29 (22 percent) developed invasive squamous cell carcinoma.[11] These patients had been followed for from 5 to 19 years.

The typical appearance of earliest invasive squamous cell carcinoma is that of a cervical epithelium showing a full-thickness neoplastic change consistent with CIN 3. The cells of the surface or glandular epithelium have a high nuclear to cytoplasmic ratio, the nuclei are atypical, and the cells' orientation is random. At the base of the epithelium the earliest invasive cells are seen breaking through the basement membrane. These cells have abundant eosinophilic cytoplasm (Fig. 4–3). Electron microscopic studies have identified actin and myosin microfibrils in these early invasive cells.[12] These microfibrils enable these cells to move, resulting in invasion of the underlying cervical stroma. The nuclei of these cells may be enlarged or pyknotic. Mitoses are infrequent. An inflammatory infiltrate is frequently found in the stroma at the site of invasion.

The diagnosis of an early invasive cervical cancer may be difficult owing to the small foci of invasion compared to the large area of the cervical epithelium that usually is involved in CIN. Confusion between the earliest invasive cancer and dysplastic epithelium that appears to have infiltrated the stroma may occur.[13, 14] Tangential sectioning and improper evaluation of a gland or glands involved with CIN 3 may lead to an erroneous diagnosis. Often the demarcation between the epithelium involved with CIN and the cervical stroma, which frequently has an inflammatory infiltrate, becomes distorted.[15] Sedlis et al[13] evaluated 265 cases diagnosed by the referring pathologist as microinvasive squamous cell carcinoma of the cervix. In 99 (37 percent) of these there was no evidence of invasion.

The diagnosis of early invasive squamous cell carcinoma of the cervix is difficult to make if identification of disruption of the basement membrane by the neoplastic cells is required. This basal lamina (basement membrane) is often difficult to identify.[14] Frequently the well-differentiated squamous cells of early invasion appear to create their own basement membrane. The basement mem-

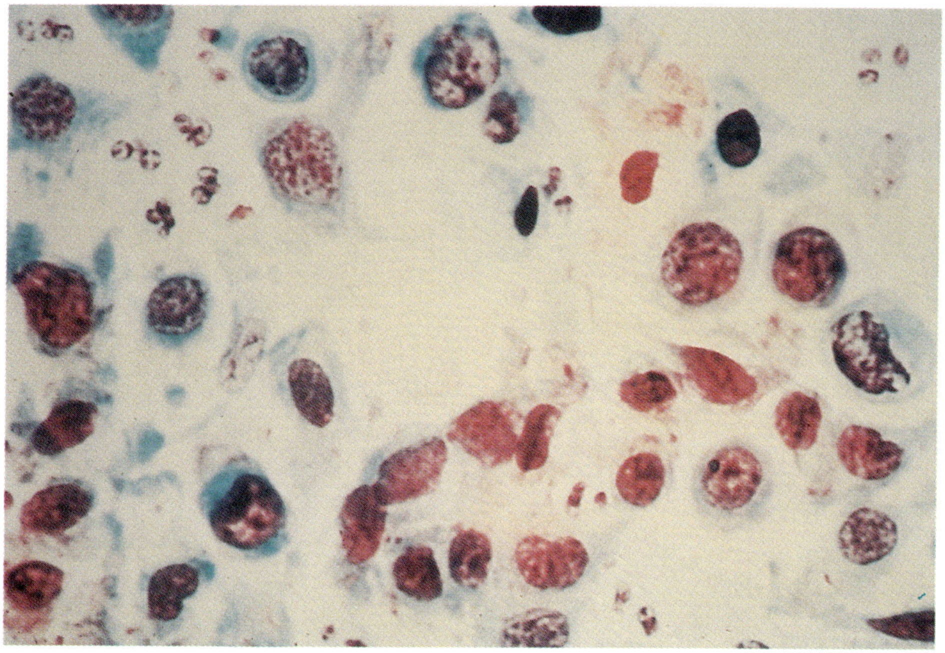

FIGURE 4-2
This is a Papanicolaou smear from a patient who had microinvasive squamous cell carcinoma of the cervix. The cells are pleomorphic. The cell in the lower left corner with dense blue cytoplasm has a macronucleolus. Irregular chromatin clumping is seen.

brane may not be visualized in areas of CIN and yet may be noted near the border of an area of invasion. The inflammatory infiltrate frequently seen with CIN can disrupt the appearance of the basement membrane. The inflammatory cells seen are plasma cells and lymphocytes and probably represent an immunologic response to neoplastic change.[16] Because of these factors, the solitary finding of a small area of disruption of the basement membrane is not considered by some authors to be a sign of invasion.[15] The typical early invasive cell described previously should also be identified. These early invasive cells are typically surrounded by a heavy infiltrate of lymphocytes.[17]

Microinvasive squamous cell carcinoma can be unifocal or multifocal. As these lesions grow from a few neoplastic cells infiltrating the cervical stroma to a measurable lesion, a decision must be made about the point when the lesion is no longer microinvasive. This decision is based on clinical-pathologic studies that correlate the incidence of nodal metastasis and recurrence with tumor volume and other pathologic factors to be discussed subsequently.

DEFINITION. The terminology previously used to describe early invasive carcinoma was confusing. To understand and accurately evaluate the literature on this subject a historical review is in order. Until the 1985 FIGO definition was formulated, descriptions of microinvasive squamous cell carcinoma of the cervix varied from author to author. The FIGO definition prior to 1985 was so vague that it forced individual investigators to set their own criteria. In some studies measurements were taken from the basement membrane to the deepest tumor cell, whereas other investigators used the epithelial surface as the point from which the maximum depth of invasion was measured. The depth of invasion that was considered microinvasive disease varied and could be as much as 1 cm. In 1977, Benson and Norris[18] reviewed 41 studies of early cervical cancer in an attempt to describe the depth of invasion at which metastatic disease became significant. The literature on the subject was so confusing and incomplete that they could find only three studies in which there was adequate detail to relate the depth of invasion to the risk of nodal metastasis.

Before 1985 FIGO defined stage IA cervical cancer as early stromal invasion. No objective criteria were given. In 1985 FIGO divided stage IA lesions into stage IA1 and IA2 as described earlier. Specific maximum tumor measurements were given for stage IA, above these the lesion is no longer considered microinvasive but stage IB. The specific measurements consist of a depth of invasion that does not exceed 5 mm. Depth of invasion is measured from the base of the epithelium from which the invasion originates, be it the surface epithelium or a gland. The width or horizontal spread should not exceed 7 mm.[1] A similar recommendation was made by the Ninth Study Group of the Royal College of Obstetricians and Gynaecologists, but the limit of the horizontal width in their recommendation is 10 mm.[19]

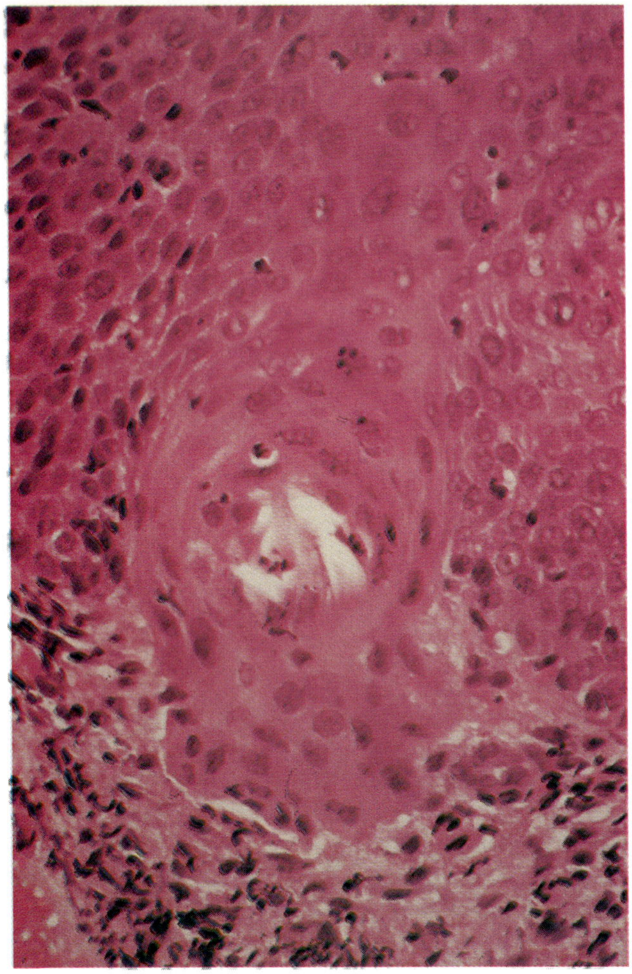

FIGURE 4-3
The earliest invasive squamous cells are shown here invading from the base of the intraepithelial neoplastic squamous epithelium of the cervix. These cells have abundant eosinophilic cytoplasm.

PROGNOSTIC FACTORS. Several factors have been identified as significant in predicting the outcome of microinvasive cervical squamous cell carcinoma. These include depth of invasion, tumor volume, lymphovascular space invasion, and tumor confluency. A depth of invasion of 5 mm or less was originally suggested as defining microinvasive disease.[20] However, the death of some patients who had apparently small lesions has led to further evaluation of this concept. The importance of measuring lateral spread also has been recognized.[13, 21] As lateral spread increases there is an increased incidence of nodal involvement. There is a direct relationship between the depth of invasion and lateral spread. As the depth of tumor penetration increases, lateral spread increases. Several investigators have approached this issue by measuring tumor volume and correlating it with nodal metastasis and risk of recurrence. The initial extensive tumor volume measurement studies concluded that below a tumor volume of 500 mm^3 metastasis did not occur.[22] More recently, a maximum tumor volume of 350 mm^3 (depth × length × width [of 5 × 7] × 10 mm^3) is considered a safer definition of microinvasive cervical carcinoma.[7] These tumor volume measurements were used to establish the current FIGO definition of microinvasive cervical carcinoma.

Lymphovascular space invasion in microinvasive cervical squamous cell carcinoma has been studied by many investigators.[13–16, 23] Lymphovascular space invasion is not considered important by some authors, but others suggest that it relates to metastatic potential.[13–15, 23] VanNagel et al,[23] in a study of 177 patients with microinvasive cervical cancer, found that 17 patients who had vascular space involvement associated with invasion of less than 3 mm did not have nodal metastasis. The FIGO classification does not exclude tumors with lymphovascular invasion from stage IA as long as the maximum measurements of depth of invasion and lateral spread are not exceeded. However, the presence of lymphovascular space involvement should be noted (Fig. 4–4). In contrast, the Society of Gynecologic Oncologists in the United States defines microinvasive squamous cell carcinoma as a lesion that does not invade deeper than 3 mm from the basement membrane and excludes all cases in which there is lymphovascular space involvement. A review of the available literature concludes that of all patients who have squamous cell carcinoma of the cervix that invades to a depth of less than 3 mm but is associated with lymphovascular space invasion, 2.6 and 4 percent of patients, respectively, have pelvic node metastases or develop recurrences.[24] If the depth of tumor invasion is more than 3 mm but less than 5 mm and lymphovascular space invasion is present, the proportion of patients who develop recurrences is 9 percent.

Several patterns of invasion in cases of cervical microinvasive squamous cell carcinoma have been described. These include drop invasion, finger-like invasion, bulky invasion, and confluent invasion.[25] Some consider a confluent pattern of invasion a risk factor for nodal metastasis and tumor recurrence.[25] The confluent pattern results as several foci of microinvasive carcinoma merge to form a meshwork (Fig. 4–5). The proportion of cases exhibiting a confluent pattern increases as the depth of invasion increases. Sedlis et al[13] found that 38 percent of tumors that invaded to a depth of greater than 3 mm showed confluence. With a depth of penetration of less than 1 mm, confluence occurred in 4 percent of cases. Although the confluent pattern is frequently present in microinva-

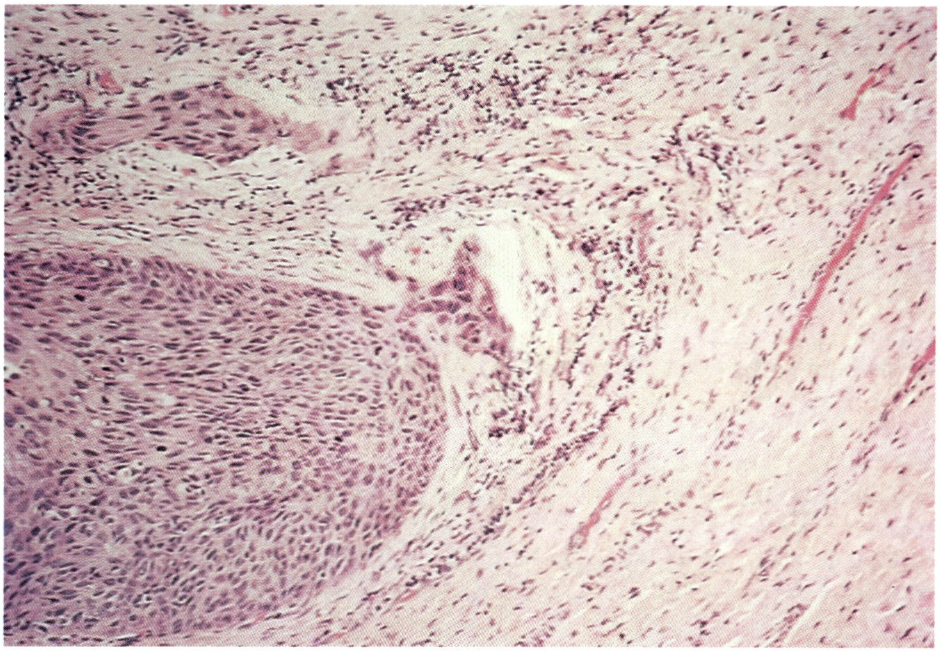

FIGURE 4-4
Early invasive squamous cell carcinoma is seen arising from an endocervical gland that has been replaced by abnormal squamous epithelium. The malignant cells invade what appears to be a preformed space.

sive carcinomas removed from patients who later develop recurrence, it is also frequently found in patients in whom the disease does not recur. Therefore, a confluent pattern in cervical microinvasive squamous cell carcinoma is considered a sensitive but not specific marker for recurrence.[26]

HISTOPATHOLOGIC EVALUATION. In the presence of CIN involving more than two quadrants of the cervix a microinvasive lesion may be missed unless a cone or equivalent biopsy is performed. The manner of examination of the conization specimen varies according to the pathologist. In many institutions in the United States the cone is divided into quadrants. Several tissue sections from each quadrant are examined. Questionable lesions are step-sectioned to find the worst possible disease in that location. Burghardt and Holzer[22] have reported a method of serial step-sectioning that produces 70 to 100 sections per cone specimen. This was the technique used to derive the data described previously on the association between tumor volume in early invasive cervical cancer and nodal metastases. However, in many institutions, including our own, the examination of 12 tissue sections per conization specimen is considered adequate. Our approach to the processing of a conization specimen was discussed in Chapter 3.

A variety of ways to measure and define microinvasive squamous cell carcinoma of the cervix have been suggested.[27–31] The members of the Society of Gynecologic Oncologists of the United States have recommended their own definition.[32] They define microinvasive cervical cancer as those lesions that invade to 3 mm or less as measured from the basement membrane and are not associated with lymphovascular space invasion. As discussed earlier, the present FIGO definition requires a two-dimensional evaluation. The first measurement is the maximum depth of invasion measured from the base of the epithelium from which the lesion originates. The second is the horizontal spread. These measurements may be multiplied to give a notation in millimeters squared. The most exhaustive method used to define microinvasion is the measurement of tumor volume.[22, 22, 33] The suggested technique involves extensive step-sectioning of the conization specimen at intervals of 100 to 300 microns. The serial sections are then placed in sequential order and the

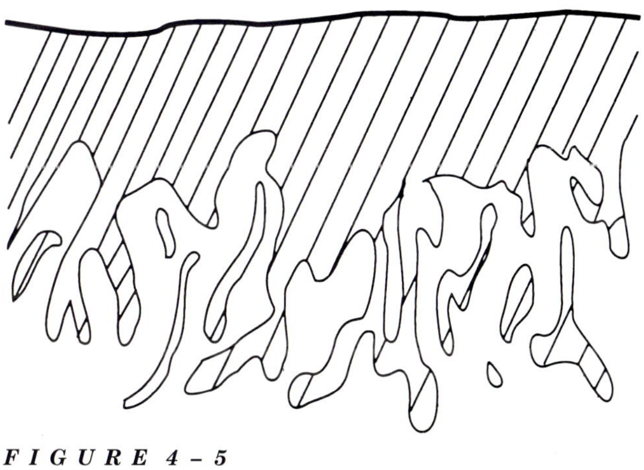

FIGURE 4-5
The confluent pattern of microinvasive squamous cell carcinoma is shown here.

lesion measured in three dimensions. This approach is not considered practical. Most pathologists evaluate approximately 12 tissue sections from the conization specimen and measure the two dimensions as suggested by FIGO.

TREATMENT. The treatment of patients who have stage IA squamous cell carcinoma is based on the prognostic factors previously discussed. Almost no patient with stage IA1 cervical squamous cell carcinoma is later found to have lymph node metastases or develops recurrence.[34] Total abdominal (extrafascial) hysterectomy is considered standard treatment in these cases.[35] Cervical conization with clear margins of resection in the compliant young patient who desires to preserve her fertility is adequate therapy. This approach may be satisfactory for all patients with stage IA1 cervical squamous cell carcinoma. Burghardt et al[26] reported on 93 patients who had stage IA1 cervical squamous cell carcinoma and were treated with cervical conization with clear resection margins. These patients were carefully followed for 5 years or more. No patient had recurrent disease. One patient who was not compliant with the follow-up instructions died of cervical cancer 12 years after the cone biopsy. This tumor was considered a secondary primary and not a recurrence.

Stage IA2 disease is approached in a stratified manner depending on the depth of invasion and the presence or absence of lymphovascular space involvement. The proportion of patients with tumors that invade to less than 3 mm and have no lymphovascular space involvement who later are found to have lymph node metastases or recurrent disease is less than 1 percent.[24, 34] These patients can be treated by total abdominal (extrafascial) hysterectomy. A few patients who meet these criteria and in whom the margins of resection are free of neoplasia have been successfully treated with cervical conization.[36] When lymphovascular space involvement is present the proportion of patients found to have lymph node metastases or recurrent tumors increases to approximately 4 percent.[24, 34] In these patients radical hysterectomy with bilateral pelvic node dissection is the most reasonable treatment alternative. This approach can also be used in cases in which multiple foci of microinvasion or confluency exist. However, the data in these situations are not conclusive. For cervical stage IA2 squamous carcinomas that have a depth of invasion greater than 3 mm radical hysterectomy and pelvic lymphadenectomy is the treatment of choice. In these cases the proportion of patients who have lymph node metastases or recurrent disease is between 5 and 9 percent.[24, 34] Radiation therapy has also been used in the treatment of selected patients with stage IA cervical carcinoma.[37]

Invasive (Stage IB–IVB) Squamous Cell Carcinoma

Any tumor volume that exceeds the FIGO definition of stage IA cervical cancer but is still confined to the cervix is considered stage IB. Stage IB tumors range from microscopic lesions to tumors measuring several centimeters in size. If the tumor extends to the vagina and involves its upper two-thirds without parametrial extension it is considered stage IIA. A tumor with unilateral or bilateral parametrial involvement that does not reach either pelvic sidewall is considered stage IIB. Stage IIIA exists when the cervical cancer reaches the lower third of the vagina and parametrial tumor, if present, does not reach the pelvic sidewall. A stage IIIB tumor extends to one or both pelvic sidewalls. Hydronephrosis or a nonfunctioning kidney secondary to ureteral obstruction by the cancer also places the lesion in stage IIIB. A stage IVA cervical carcinoma extends to the bladder or rectum and is proved by biopsy. Stage IVB connotes spread to distant organs. The lung and the liver are the distant organs most frequently involved with metastasis from cervical squamous cell carcinoma.[38, 39] This staging classification considers only clinically obtainable information. In contrast, the current FIGO staging classification of endometrial, ovarian, and vulvar cancer is surgical and pathologic. The surgical staging of cervical cancer is the source of disagreement. In approximately one-third of cases the clinical stage does not correspond to the surgical-pathologic findings. However, most patients with cervical cancer when treated with radiation do not undergo surgery. The morbidity of surgical staging is considered significant. Some of the proponents of surgical staging in cervical cancer have reversed themselves recently and have suggested that surgical staging should be used only when it is a component of a study protocol.[40,41]

HISTOPATHOLOGY AND PROGNOSTIC FACTORS. Squamous cell carcinoma is the most common cancer of the cervix. Broders[42] suggested a system of grading carcinoma according to the proportion of the lesion that is analogous to the normal benign counterpart. Broders' grading system uses the squamous epithelium of the skin as a model rather than that of the cervix. This grading system is based on the presence and amount of keratinization in tumor cells. The original four-grade system of Broders was reduced to three grades (well, moderately, and poorly differentiated) by Warren.[43] Grading systems based on Broders' classification have been used in cervical carcinoma. A well-differentiated squamous carcinoma has generous amounts of keratin in the form of epithelial pearls (Fig. 4–6). Necrotic keratinizing debris may be present. When this necrotic keratinizing debris is found in the center of the masses of infiltrating squamous carcinoma it may produce a pseudoglandular appearance (Fig. 4–7). There are prominent intercellular bridges. The nuclei are often hyperchromatic and pyknotic, and less than two mitoses per high power microscopic field are seen. Intracellular glycogen might be noted. This tumor has an infiltrating pattern, but an exophytic component may also be present. In a moderately differentiated tumor there is a lesser amount of keratin. Cells have individual cytoplasmic keratin, but epithelial pearls are absent. This tumor is composed of large cells, and there are less well defined intercellular bridges. There is cellular pleomorphism, and two to four mitoses per high power microscopic field are seen. The nuclei are enlarged and irregular in size and have coarse granular cytoplasm. The moderately differentiated squamous cell carcinoma pattern of infiltration generally consists of cellular masses with pushing, rounded borders. In poorly differentiated squamous cell carcinoma individual cell keratinization is absent. Cell size varies (Fig. 4–8), and the cytoplasm is scant. Intercellular bridges are scant or absent. The nuclei are pleomorphic, may be hyperchromatic, or may have a vesicular chromatin pattern. Nucleoli are present. The mitotic rate is more than four per high power field. In poorly differentiated squamous cell carcinoma the cervical stroma is infiltrated extensively by single cells, tumor cords, and small nests.

A different histopathologic classification of cervical squamous cell carcinoma was proposed by Martzloff[44] and further developed by others.[45] Squamous carcinoma of the cervix is classified as large cell keratinizing, large cell nonkeratinizing, and small cell. These categories essentially correspond to the descriptions of well, moderately, and poorly differentiated squamous cell carcinoma just given. Some studies suggest that there is an association between survival rate and cell type in patients with cervical squamous cell carcinoma. Small cell squamous carcinoma is associated with the worst prognosis, whereas patients with large cell nonkeratinizing squamous cell carcinoma fare best.[46] However, the literature is not consistent about the value of tumor grade and histopathologic type as prognostic indicators.[47] This lack of consistency may be due to tumor heterogeneity. We have treated patients who had a tumor that appeared to be of one cell type on a small cervical biopsy, but on extensive sampling of the hysterectomy specimen a different cell type was found to predominate. Many patients with cervical carcinoma are treated with radiation therapy, and the only specimen available for histopathologic examination in such patients is a small cervical biopsy. There is a poor correlation between tumor grade and survival rate when radiation has been used as therapy.[44,48]

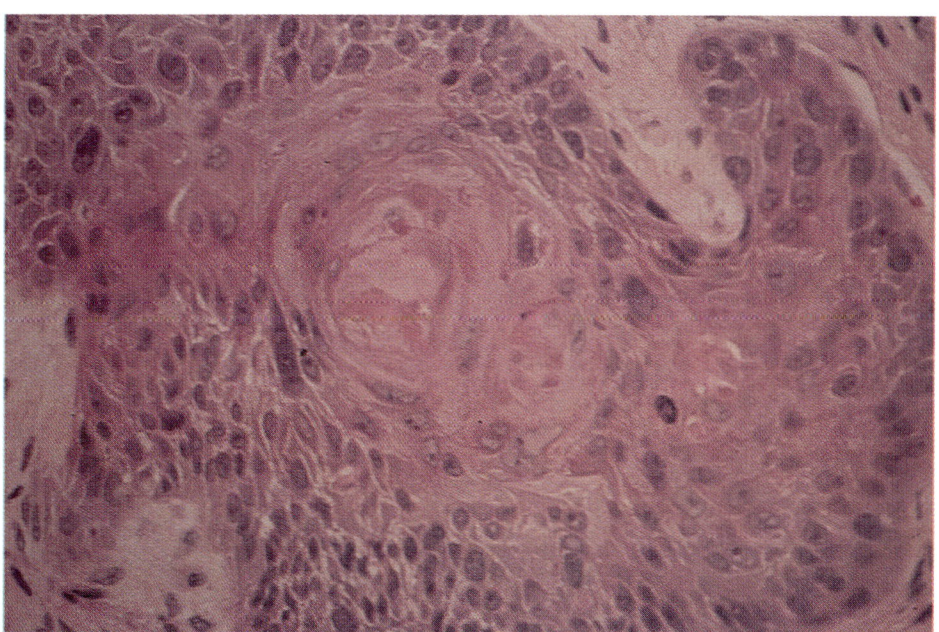

FIGURE 4–6
A well-differentiated squamous cell carcinoma that shows keratin pearl formation is seen. Intracytoplasmic keratin is seen as densely eosinophilic material. The cells surrounding the keratin pearl demonstrate prominent intercellular bridges and less cytoplasmic keratinization.

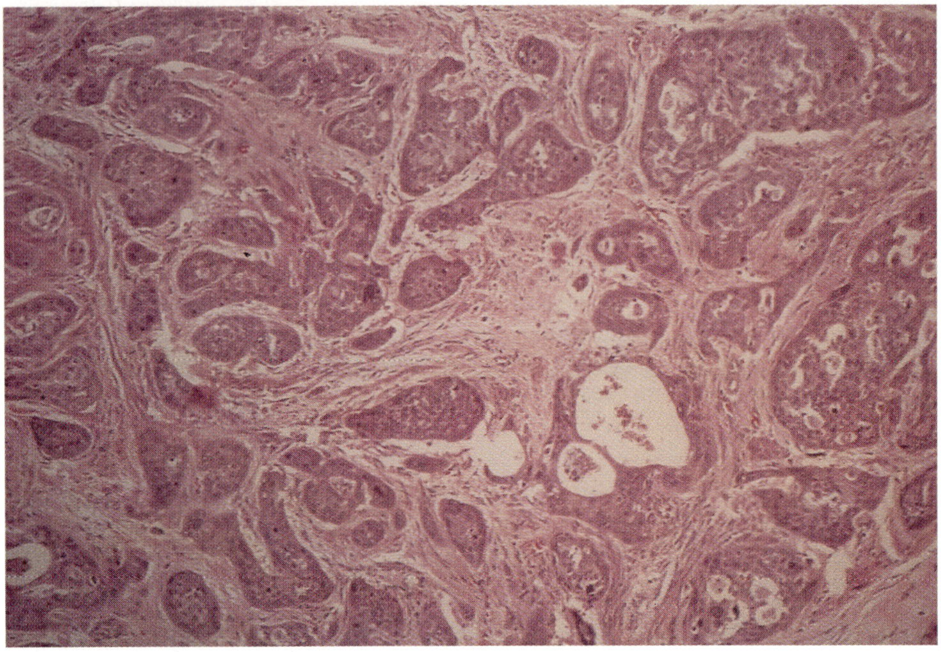

FIGURE 4-7
This squamous cell carcinoma forms cystic spaces filled with debris. This pseudoglandular appearance may be confused with adenosquamous carcinoma.

In addition to histopathologic type and tumor grade, investigators have tried to correlate different histopathologic factors with the prognosis of cervical cancer. These include tumor volume, depth of invasion, pattern of invasion, and lymphovascular permeation.[49] A Gynecologic Oncology Group study reviewed 195 specimens from patients who underwent radical hysterectomy and pelvic and aortic node dissection for stage IB squamous cell carcinoma of the cervix.[47] Nine histopathologic parameters were examined in an attempt to identify reproducible and prognostic indicators. The tumors were initially examined by a referring pathologist and subsequently were reviewed independently by two of the investigators. The parameters examined included the presence and amount of keratin, nuclear pleomorphism, mitotic activity, and "gestalt" grading. The tumor-stromal junction was examined for pattern of invasion. A tumor that produced large areas of infiltration without intervening stroma was designated as pushing. Tumor that demonstrated mul-

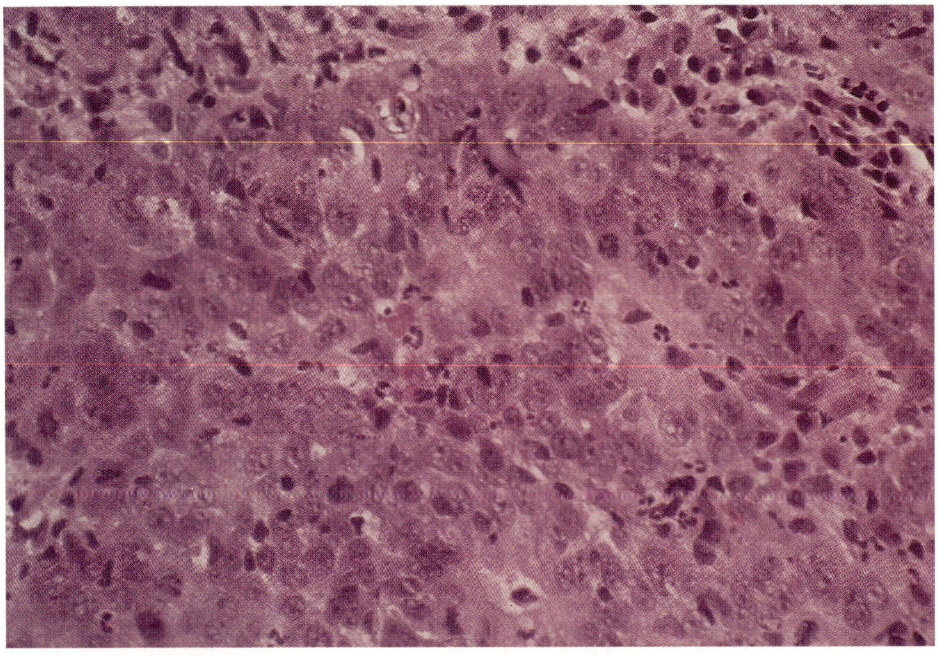

FIGURE 4-8
This poorly differentiated squamous cell carcinoma shows marked pleomorphism. Many of the cells have scant cytoplasm, and intercellular bridges are absent. The nuclei have a vesicular chromatin pattern and prominent nucleoli.

tiple small or intermediate nests within the intervening stroma was designated as infiltrating. The depth of invasion below the basement membrane and the density of the associated inflammatory infiltrate were recorded. The presence or absence of lymphovascular space involvement was noted. Lymphovascular invasion was diagnosed only when tumor cell nests were seen in spaces clearly lined by endothelial cells. It was concluded that the degree of reproducibility of all of the histopathologic grading methods was poor. This is inconsequential because lymph node metastases and disease-free survival were not associated with any of the tumor grading methods studied in this cohort of surgically treated patients. Depth of invasion was found to be highly predictive of lymph node metastases and disease-free survival. The 5-year disease-free survival rate for patients whose tumors were confined to the inner third of the cervical stroma was 98 percent. It was 81 percent when the tumor involved the middle third, and 63 percent when it invaded the outer third ($p <$ 0.0001). The presence of lymphovascular space involvement resulted in a 5-year disease-free survival rate of 70 percent compared with 83 percent when no lymphovascular space invasion was identified ($p < 0.05$).

More recently, the association of DNA index and c-*erb* B-2 oncoprotein expression with the outcome of cervical carcinoma has been studied. A clinical-pathologic study of 124 cases of staged IA and IB cervical carcinoma was undertaken by means of flow cytometry for DNA studies.[50] The median survival of patients whose tumors had a DNA index of 1.7 or greater was 36 months compared with 73.5 months when the DNA index was less than 1.7. It was confirmed by multivariate analysis that a DNA index of 1.7 in patients with early invasive cervical carcinoma is an independent prognostic indicator. In another study of biopsy specimens obtained from 192 patients with stage III cervical squamous cell carcinoma, cancer cells in tumors from 37 patients[51] stained positive with antibody to c-*erb* B-2 oncoprotein. In the remaining cases there was no staining (n = 143) or ambiguous staining (n = 12). The 5-year survival rate for the first group was 41 percent compared to 61 percent for patients whose tumors did not stain for c-*erb* B-2 oncoprotein. Confirmation of these two studies by other investigators is awaited.

The finding of HPV type 18 in cervical carcinoma has been associated with an aggressive clinical behavior.[52] A group of investigators from France has shown that patients with HPV DNA-negative cervical carcinoma have a poorer prognosis than those with HPV DNA-positive tumors.[53] They also found that overexpression of the c-*myc* oncogene was associated with a high risk of recurrence.

Positive peritoneal cytologic findings are obtained in 6 percent of patients who have squamous cell carcinoma of the cervix and are undergoing primary radical operation, surgical staging, or surgery for persistent or recurrent disease.[54] The peritoneal cytologic findings do not seem to be associated with prognosis in patients with cervical carcinoma.

Young age has also been advanced as a poor prognostic factor in squamous cell carcinoma of the cervix.[55] However, large population studies have failed to corroborate this contention.[56]

TREATMENT. Patients with stage IB and early IIA cervical carcinoma can be offered surgical therapy.[57, 58] The surgery involves radical hysterectomy and bilateral pelvic lymphadenectomy. The ovaries can be preserved if they appear grossly normal because metastasis to the ovaries from a cervical cancer is extremely rare. Of 990 patients with stage IB cervical carcinoma, only 4 (0.5 percent) of 770 patients with squamous cell carcinoma and 2 (1.7 percent) of 121 patients with adenocarcinoma were found to have ovarian metastases.[59] No patient with adenosquamous carcinoma (n = 82) or other histopathologic types (n = 17) was found to have tumor spread to the ovaries. Radical hysterectomy involves removing the uterus and the paracervical tissues (i.e., parametria). A cuff of vagina is also removed to guarantee complete removal of the lesion and to minimize the risk of local recurrence (Fig. 4–9). Some gynecologic oncologists also perform a paraaortic node dissection. However, paraaortic node metastasis occurs in only 5 percent of patients with stage IB cervical squamous cell carcinoma that at the time of surgical exploration is grossly confined to the cervix.[60] The 5-year survival rate of surgically treated patients with stage IB cervical squamous cell carcinoma is 90 percent.[57] Radiation therapy can also be used in the treatment of patients with stage IB and early stage IIA cervical carcinoma, especially in women who are considered to have a high surgical risk and in those who do not wish to preserve ovarian function and who do not desire surgery. The 5-year survival rate for patients with stage IB cervical cancer treated with radiation is similar to that for patients treated with surgery.[1] The complications of radical hysterectomy and bilateral pelvic lymphadenectomy include hemorrhage, infection, thromboembolism, bladder and rectal dysfunction, urinary-vaginal

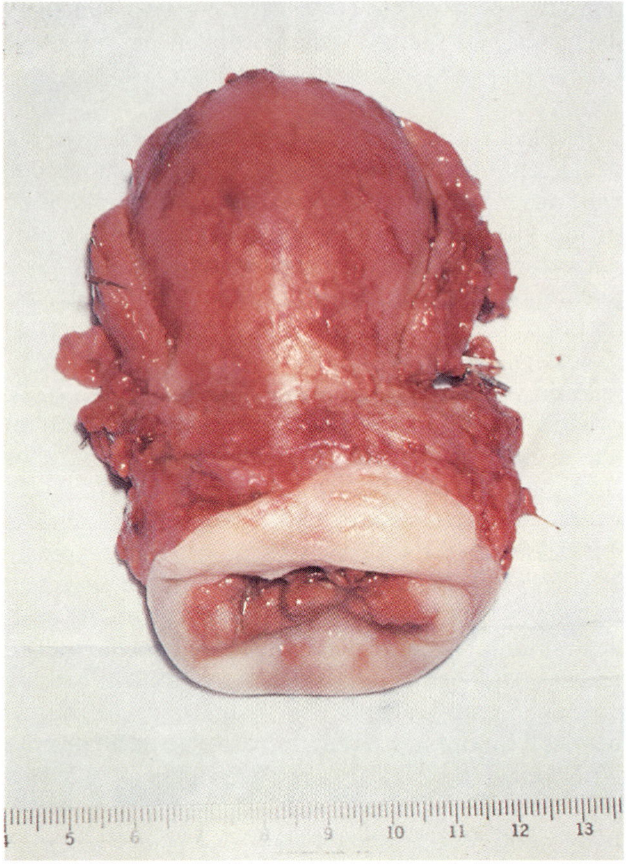

FIGURE 4–9
A radical hysterectomy specimen from a patient who had early stage IIA squamous cell carcinoma of the cervix demonstrates a rim of grossly uninvolved vagina that surrounds the tumor. The parametrial tissue is seen at either side of the cervix. Surgical clips are seen on this tissue. The adnexa were not removed. (From Hernandez E, Rosenshein NB: Manual of Gynecologic Oncology. New York, Churchill Livingstone, 1989.)

fistulae, lymphocyst, and possible nerve damage. The complications of radiation therapy include treatment-induced diarrhea and dysuria, hematotoxicity, radiation-induced menopause, reduction in vaginal caliber and vaginal wall pliability, enteritis, colitis, urinary-vaginal or enterovaginal fistulae, and hemorrhagic cystitis. The medical condition of the patient and the evaluation, with the assistance of the oncologist, of the possible risks and benefits determine the mode of therapy selected for the treatment of patients with squamous cell carcinoma at this early stage. When stage IIA lesions encroach on areas that could cause concern about a "close" margin or microscopic invasion of a surgical margin, the patient is offered radiation therapy rather than surgery.

A special situation is the subset of patients with so-called stage IB barrel or "bulky" lesions. The size of the tumors that fall into this category ranges from 4 cm to more than 6 cm. A high rate of central recurrence has been reported in this group of patients.[61] These patients are treated with radiation followed by a total abdominal (extrafascial) hysterectomy.[62–64] The addition of chemotherapy to the therapy of patients with stage IB bulky squamous cell carcinoma is being evaluated. The postradiation surgical specimen shows atrophy of the squamous epithelium. The cells of the endocervical epithelium show nuclear enlargement and decreased mucin content. The cervical stroma is fibrous and contains an inflammatory infiltrate and macrophages. Scattered atypical fibroblasts with fibrillar cytoplasm, a pyknotic nucleus, and several nucleoli are seen. Areas of necrosis may be present, and the vascular spaces may be obliterated by hyalinized tissue. Intimal thickening may be present. The endothelial cells may be enlarged and may contain hyperchromatic nuclei. These radiation-induced changes are typical of the uterus removed 6 weeks after radiation treatments. Extensive hyalinization of the cervical stroma and of many of the vascular channels occurs over time if the uterus is not removed after radiation therapy.

If parametrial or pelvic lymph node involvement is found in the surgical specimen of a patient who has undergone a radical hysterectomy and pelvic lymphadenectomy for early-stage cervical carcinoma, the prognosis is poorer. A study of 272 patients who had stage IB or IIA cervical carcinoma and were treated by radical hysterectomy and pelvic lymphadenectomy showed that the corrected 5-year survival rate was 90.3 percent in the absence of parametrial or lymph node involvement by tumor, 75 percent in the presence of tumor spread to the parametrium alone, 62.1 percent in the presence of lymph node metastases alone, and 50 percent when both the parametrium and the lymph nodes were involved by tumor.[65] Patients who have tumor spread to the parametrium or pelvic lymph nodes receive adjuvant whole pelvis irradiation in an effort to decrease the risk of local recurrence and improve survival.[66, 67] The vaginal margin at the time of radical hysterectomy is examined by frozen section. If tumor is found to extend to the margin, additional vagina is removed. If the vaginal margin proves to be involved by tumor on paraffin-embedded sections, intravaginal irradiation is delivered (i.e., brachytherapy).

Patients with stage IIB, IIIA, IIIB, and IVA cervical cancer are treated with radiation therapy. Chemotherapy can be added before, during, or after the radiation.[35] Patients with stage IVB cervical cancer usually receive palliative treatment with radiation or chemotherapy. Unfortunately, cervical squamous cell carcinoma cannot be cured with currently available cytotoxic drugs. Cisplatin is now the most active cytotoxic agent against cervical squamous cell carcinoma, with response rates on the order of 30 percent. These responses are short-lived. At the Medical College of Pennsylvania the actuarial 5-year survival rate of patients with cervical carcinoma treated with radiation therapy compares favorably with that reported by other centers.[1] It is 82 percent for patients with stage I disease, 62 percent for stage II disease, 53 percent for stage III, and 6 percent for stage IV.

As stated earlier, paraaortic lymph node metastases occur in 5 percent of patients with stage IB cervical squamous cell carcinoma that is grossly confined to the cervix as determined at the time of surgical exploration. Paraaortic node metastases occur in 21 percent of patients with stage IIB disease, 31 percent of those with stage III disease, and 13 percent of those with stage IV lesions.[68] If metastasis to the paraaortic lymph nodes is detected during evaluation and therapy of the patient with cervical carcinoma and there is no supraclavicular adenopathy, a left scalene fat pad biopsy is recommended prior to curative local therapy being considered. Tumor has been found in the scalene lymph nodes in approximately 10 percent of these cases.[69, 70] If the supraclavicular nodes are suspected of being involved, fine needle aspiration biopsy is performed. If the scalene lymph nodes are negative for tumor then a computed tomogram of the chest is obtained. In the absence of proven disease above the paraaortic lymph nodes, the field of radiation is extended to encompass the paraaortic region.[71,72]

Patients who have pelvic recurrence after radiation therapy are evaluated to ascertain the extent of disease. If the recurrence is thought to be confined to the pelvis and the tumor is not fixed to the pelvic bones, ultraradical surgery (exenteration) is considered (Fig. 4–10). This surgery is completed only if intraoperative evaluation confirms the findings on preoperative clinical examination. Recurrences that occur after radical hysterectomy can be controlled by radiation therapy. In one report of 28 such patients followed for at least 12 months, 35.7 percent remained free of disease.[73]

If invasive cervical carcinoma is found inadvertently in a simple hysterectomy specimen, the situation must be evaluated retrospectively to give appropriate adjunctive therapy if necessary. Proper staging is not possible at this time; however, a search for residual local disease and regional or distant spread should be undertaken. Adjunctive therapy is probably not necessary for lesions that have invaded to less than 3 mm.[74] For more advanced lesions that are considered equivalent to stage IB, radical parametrectomy or whole pelvis irradiation should be considered. For lesions considered equivalent to stage IIB radiation therapy is the treatment of choice.[75, 76] However, some of the older literature suggests ultraradical surgery in these cases.[77, 78] The survival rate of patients with lesions equivalent to stage IIB is better with adjunctive radiation therapy than with ultraradical surgery.[79]

Yet another special situation is that of cervical

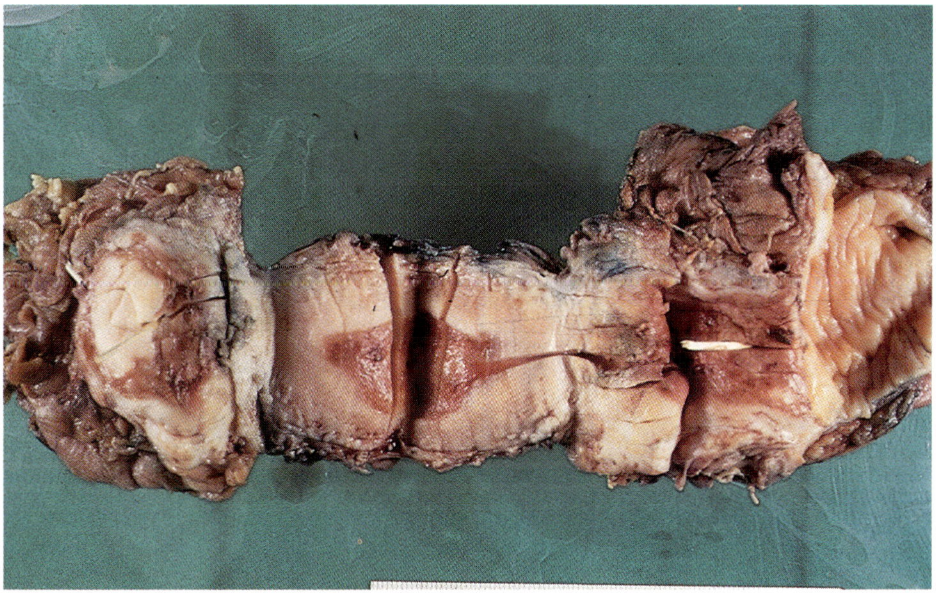

FIGURE 4–10
This is a total pelvic exenteration specimen from a woman who had recurrent squamous cell carcinoma of the cervix. The specimen has been bifurcated in the sagittal plane. The uterus *(center)* is flanked by the bladder *(left)* and the rectum *(right)*.

carcinoma found during pregnancy. The most appropriate therapy in this situation is determined not only by the stage of the disease but also by the gestational age of the fetus at the time of diagnosis. Patients who are diagnosed with early-stage cervical carcinoma during the first 20 weeks of gestation are offered pregnancy termination and immediate treatment of the carcinoma. If the diagnosis is made when the pregnancy is close to term, delivery of the fetus is accomplished as soon as fetal lung maturity is confirmed, after which therapy is instituted. There are differences of opinion about whether the abdominal or vaginal route should be used for delivery of the fetus whose mother has a cervical carcinoma. When a gross lesion is present, vaginal delivery may result in cervical trauma and uncontrollable bleeding. In these cases, delivery of the fetus by cesarean section is preferred. If the lesion is a microscopic finding there is concern that the tumor may gain access to the lymphovascular spaces during the process of cervical dilatation and vaginal delivery. However, this is only a theoretical consideration and has not been proved.[79a] Nonetheless, cesarean section and radical hysterectomy are frequently performed in patients with stage IB cervical carcinoma diagnosed during pregnancy. If frozen section evaluation of lymph nodes removed from these pregnant patients is performed, the decidualization of the tissues that occurs during pregnancy may be a source of confusion (Fig. 4–11). The most difficult therapeutic decision occurs when the gestational age of the fetus is greater than 20 weeks but still far less than the time at which fetal lung maturity is expected to occur (i.e., 36 to 38 weeks). A delay of several weeks before the institution of therapy is acceptable, but there is great concern when this interval is prolonged.[80,81,81a]

Follow-up of the patient treated for cervical carcinoma consists of pelvic examination every 3 months for the first 3 years and then every 6 months until the fifth anniversary of therapy. During this period a vaginal Papanicolaou smear is obtained every 6 months. The smear of the patient treated with radiation therapy may show a radiation effect for the lifetime of the patient. These changes are characterized by large, bizarrely shaped cells that retain a normal nuclear to cytoplasmic ratio. There may be smudging of the chromatin, vacuoles in the nucleus and cytoplasm, or cytoplasmic polychromasia (Fig. 4–12). Squamous intraepithelial lesion (SIL) is difficult to diagnose after radiation therapy. Dysplasia in a background of radiation effect (i.e., radiation dysplasia) may occur but is diagnosed only when cells meeting the criteria for high-grade squamous intraepithelial lesion (HSIL) are present. Owing to the appearance of radiation effect, low-grade squamous intraepithelial lesion (LSIL) should not be diagnosed in women who have been irradiated. In some patients postradiation necrosis of the vaginal mucosa may occur and must be differentiated from recurrence (Fig. 4–13). Colposcopic examination and biopsies are necessary in these cases. Hydrogen peroxide douches and estrogen cream are used to treat this condition. Clindamycin or metronidazole cream could also be used because the necro-

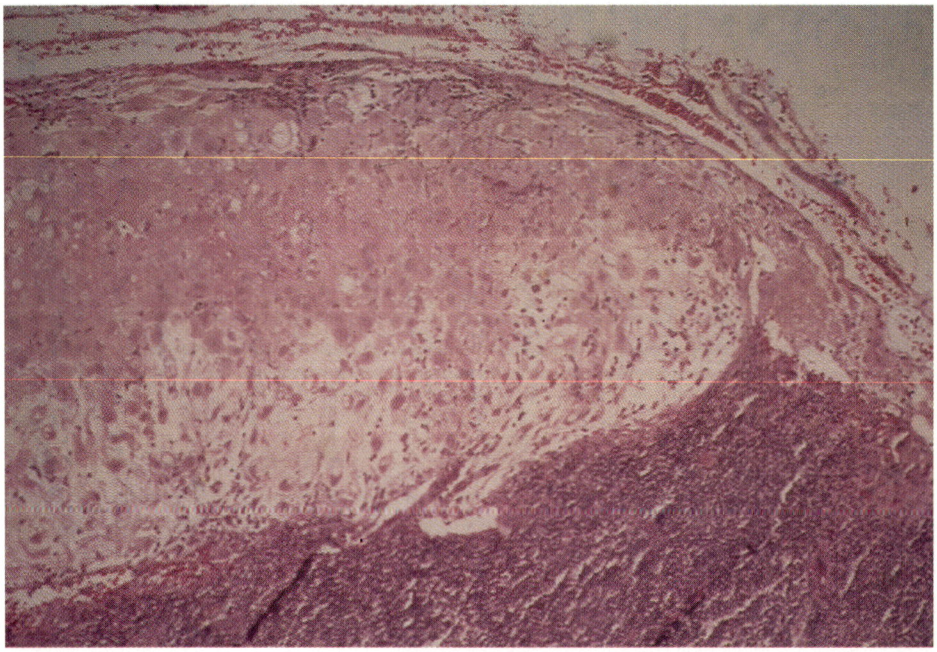

FIGURE 4–11
This pelvic lymph node was removed at the time of cesarean section/radical hysterectomy for cervical squamous cell carcinoma. The normal lymphoid tissue is seen at the bottom. The cells under the lymph node capsule *(top)* have abundant, lightly eosinophilic cytoplasm. These are decidualized cells of probable mesodermal origin. This could be confused with metastatic squamous cell carcinoma.

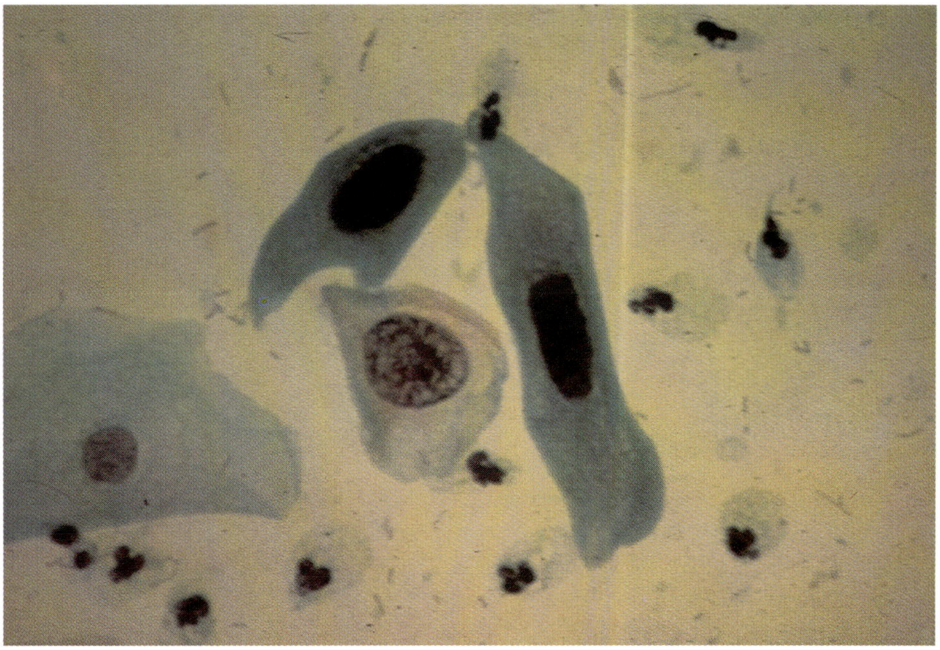

FIGURE 4-12
This Papanicolaou smear is from a patient who had prior radiation therapy to the pelvis. Very large cells are present. Some of the nuclei are enlarged and have abnormal, smudged, or degenerated chromatin patterns. The nuclear to cytoplasmic ratio is normal. The cell in the center shows polychromasia, which is a combination of pink and blue in the cytoplasm. This smear could be misinterpreted as diagnostic for LSIL if the history of radiation therapy is not given.

sis is usually associated with an anaerobic bacterial infection.

Adenocarcinoma

Adenocarcinoma of the uterine cervix has been reported to comprise approximately 5 percent of all cervical carcinomas. Although this figure has been the accepted standard, an even higher proportion (i.e., 10 to 20 percent) has been reported by several medical centers.[2,82]

Epidemiology

The mean age at diagnosis of patients with cervical adenocarcinoma is 49 years, and the range is between 23 and 79 years.[83, 84] In one study, 12 percent of patients with cervical adenocarcinoma were younger than 30 years. It is not known whether the same etiologic factors associated with cervical squamous carcinoma are relevant to adenocarcinoma. The relationship to onset of sexual activity, multiplicity of partners, and smoking is not as clear in this histopathologic type.[85] HPV

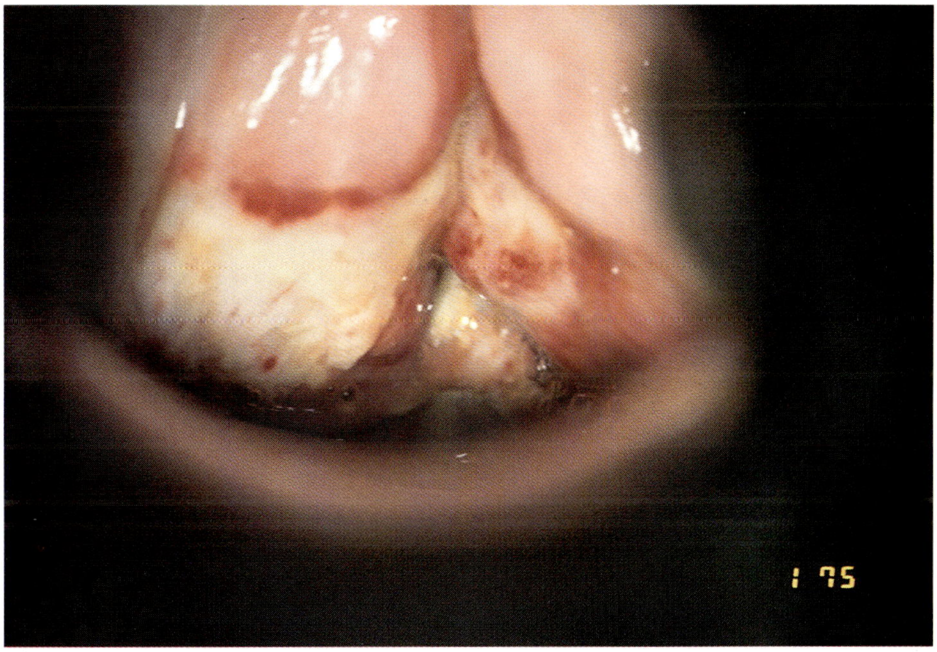

FIGURE 4-13
This colpophotograph was taken from a patient recently treated with radiation therapy for stage IIB squamous cell carcinoma of the cervix. The cervix is flush with the vagina and unrecognizable. The dark dimple in the center is the cervical os. A pseudomembrane of yellow-white tissue covers the upper vagina. Abnormal vessels are more prominent on the right. Multiple biopsies showed necrosis and radiation-induced changes.

types 16, 18, and 31 have recently been implicated in the development of squamous cell cervical carcinoma (see Chapter 3) as well as adenocarcinoma. HPV type 16 DNA was detected in one of two cervical adenocarcinomas, and HPV type 18 DNA was noted in four of five adenosquamous carcinomas.[86] In a study by Maier and Norris of 230 cases of cervical adenocarcinoma,[87] 99 instances of squamous intraepithelial lesions and 6 of squamous carcinoma were identified. These data suggest the possibility of a common causative factor or factors.

Clinical Presentation

Approximately half of the patients with cervical adenocarcinoma complain of abnormal vaginal bleeding at presentation.[88] Pain, vaginal discharge, or an abnormal Papanicolaou smear leads to the diagnosis in the remaining cases (Fig. 4–14). Colposcopic evaluation is of minimal value in early adenocarcinoma of the cervix. In one study only 6 of 24 cases presented with significant colposcopic changes (see Chapter 3).[89] Cytologic smears may be unrevealing as well. A large series reported that 51 percent of patients with adenocarcinoma had normal cytologic findings on evaluation of the cervix.[90] In the same report, only 20 percent of patients with a clinically observable lesion had a positive smear. Within 1 year of the diagnosis of cervical adenocarcinoma 27 percent of patients have had normal results on cervical cytologic examination; 40 percent have had a normal Papanicolaou smear in the 3 years prior to the diagnosis.[91]

Early Cervical Adenocarcinoma

As in squamous cell carcinoma, precursor lesions of adenocarcinoma have been recognized and have been termed glandular dysplasia or glandular intraepithelial lesions and adenocarcinoma in situ (see Chapter 3). The progression from a dysplastic lesion to an in situ carcinoma is not as easily identified as in the squamous lesion. Unlike the squamous lesion, a relatively low rate of preinvasive glandular disease of the cervix is reported. In situ lesions account for 2 to 7 percent of glandular lesions of the cervix, whereas they comprise 60 to 70 percent of squamous cell cervical neoplasia.[84]

A change in the glandular architecture and cytologically atypical cells rather than a breach in the basement membrane suggest invasion. There is still controversy about the definition of microinvasive adenocarcinoma of the cervix as a category of disease that exists between in situ and frankly invasive lesions. Some investigators believe that the term microinvasive adenocarcinoma should not be used because of the lack of agreement on a definition. The potential of nodal metastasis with respect to amount of cervical adenocarcinoma is not well established.[9] It is difficult to measure the depth of penetration of these lesions because the endocervical glands normally extend into the stroma. Tumors that extend only 3 mm into the stroma have been known to recur. To date the num-

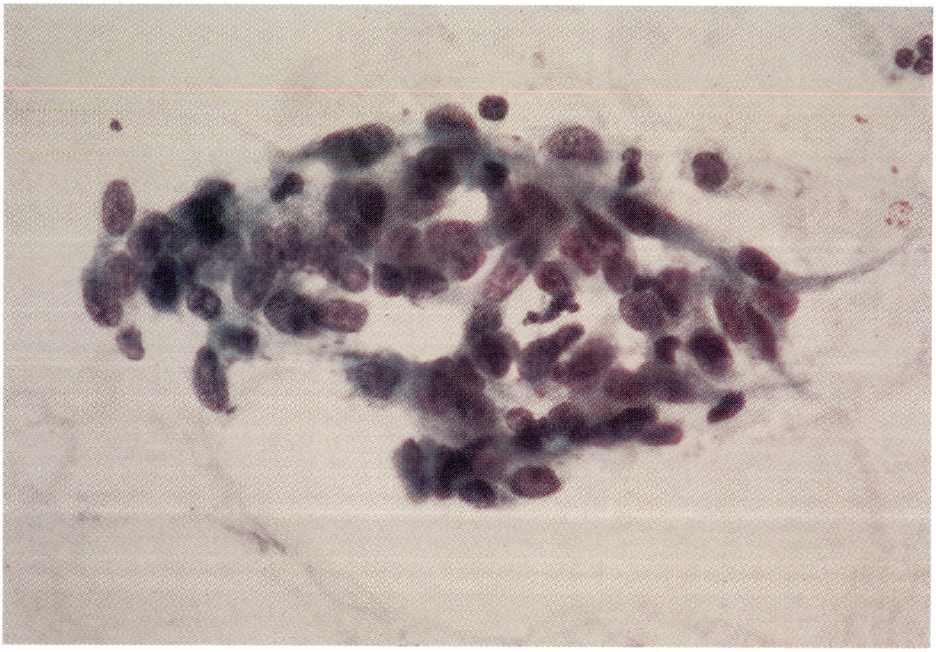

FIGURE 4–14
This Papanicolaou smear was taken from a patient who has cervical adenocarcinoma. A loose cluster of cells is seen. Some of the cells are elongated and have nucleoli suggesting an origin from columnar epithelium. A group of cells *(upper left)* form an acinus. Clear spaces suggesting lumens are seen. The nuclei are pleomorphic and there is no organization to the orientation of the cells. The arrangement of loose cells at the periphery of the cluster is known as feathering, which is a cytopathologic criterion for adenocarcinoma in situ.

ber of reported cases of microinvasive cervical adenocarcinoma is small.

The criteria for diagnosis of early cervical adenocarcinoma or microinvasive adenocarcinoma have been defined by several authors. These criteria include (1) proliferation of atypical cells and glands that have normal endocervical architecture and infiltration into the stroma as tiny buds or nests that each measure less than 1 mm, (2) large size of the atypical cells, which are larger than normal endocervical columnar cells, and (3) the presence of hyperchromatic nuclei with an increased nuclear to cytoplasmic ratio and mitoses. Squamous carcinoma in situ can accompany this process, but if invasive squamous cell carcinoma is present, that is the major diagnosis.[89, 92] Since the histopathologic criteria for distinguishing invasive from microinvasive adenocarcinoma of the cervix are still under development, some prefer to follow the definition established for squamous microinvasive tumors, which was discussed previously. Other authors suggest a depth of no more than 2 mm and a horizontal spread of 7 mm or less as the limit of what should be considered microinvasive adenocarcinoma.[92]

Tumor volume measurements have been evaluated in early endocervical adenocarcinoma. The technique of Burghardt and Holzer[22] has been adapted to the evaluation of adenocarcinoma of the cervix. Five hundred cubic millimeters has been established as the size below which the observed rate of recurrence is minimal. In a study by Kaspar et al, the clinical outcomes of 36 patients with early adenocarcinoma of the cervix were studied in relation to tumor volume.[93] Thirty-two of these patients underwent radical hysterectomy and pelvic lymph node dissection. Fourteen of this group ultimately received additional radiation therapy. Two patients had an extrafascial hysterectomy and pelvic lymphadenectomy followed by radiation therapy. Two patients were treated by radiation after cervical conization and pelvic lymph node biopsy. Neither lymph node spread nor recurrence was found in patients who had tumor volumes equal to or less than 500 mm^3. Tumor volumes were estimated from the section with the largest tumor surface area by multiplying the measurement of tumor depth by horizontal spread by a third dimension. The third dimension was calculated by multiplying the largest measured tumor depth or spread by 1.5 (Fig. 4–15). In contrast to clinical outcomes associated with a tumor volume of less than 500 mm^3, when the deepest malignant gland measured from the surface of the closest normal epithelium was less than 5 mm deep, 8 percent of patients with adenocarcinoma of the cervix were found to have lymph node metastases and 8 percent developed recurrence. Therefore, tumor volume was thought to be a better predictor of clinical outcome than depth of glandular involvement by tumor in patients with early adenocarcinoma of the cervix.

The location of the adenocarcinoma may vary. It may originate at the squamocolumnar junction or within the columnar epithelium above this area (i.e., higher in the endocervical canal). The transformation from adenocarcinoma in situ to microinvasive adenocarcinoma of the cervix may be difficult to identify. Infolding and formation of intraglandular papillae demonstrate proliferative activity associated with invasion. Loosened stroma with edema and round cell infiltration may be another indicator of invasion. In the absence of these associated changes, invasion is not likely to be present.

The cells in microinvasive adenocarcinoma of the cervix may resemble normal columnar endocervical or endometrial epithelium. In many cases there is a comingling of these two cell types, but the most predominant type determines the histopathologic classification. An early invasive adenocarcinoma of the cervix that exhibited hobnail cells as seen in clear cell carcinoma was reported by Teshima et al.[89]

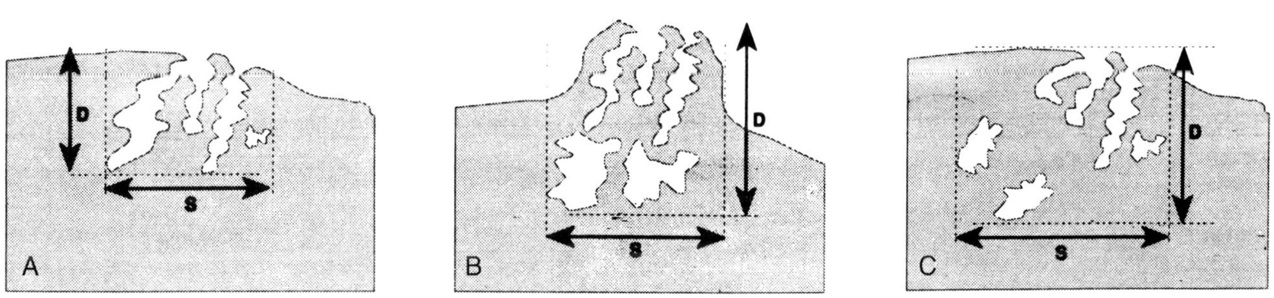

FIGURE 4–15
This is a chart that outlines the measurement of tumor depth (D) and spread (S) in cases of early cervical adenocarcinoma. (From Kaspar HG, Dinh TV, Doherty MG, Hannigan EV, Kumar D: Clinical implications of tumor volume measurements in stage I adenocarcinoma of the cervix. Obstet Gynecol 1993;81:296–300.)

The average age of patients with early adenocarcinoma of the cervix is in the late forties.[89, 93] This lesion may be recognized by an abnormal Papanicolaou smear. There may be no symptoms or vaginal discharge, or vaginal bleeding may be present.

Deciding on the best treatment for patients with early adenocarcinoma of the cervix is as difficult as differentiating between in situ, microinvasive, and invasive adenocarcinoma. Most series report only a few cases, and therefore a sound judgment about management cannot be made. Opinions range from simple to radical hysterectomy. Radiation therapy can also be used; however, it is thought that surgery is as good as or better than radiation. Burghardt suggests that surgical therapy should be similar to that recommended for similar squamous lesions.[93a] His series includes patients treated by either simple or radical hysterectomy according to size of the lesion. There were no recurrences. One of the 30 patients reported by Teshima et al[89] developed tumor recurrence after radical hysterectomy performed for the treatment of a 3-mm deep adenocarcinoma of the cervix. At the Medical College of Pennsylvania we make no distinction between microinvasive and invasive cervical adenocarcinoma. If there are no contraindications to surgery, we recommend radical hysterectomy and pelvic lymphadenectomy. If desired by the patient, the ovaries are conserved because the proportion of patients with cervical adenocarcinoma with microscopic spread to the ovaries is less than 2 percent.[59]

Gross Pathology

The gross appearance of adenocarcinoma of the cervix is variable. These lesions often present as exophytic or fungating masses (Fig. 4–16). They may also manifest as ulcerative or endophytic lesions. Nearly 15 percent of patients with adenocarcinoma of the cervix do not have visible lesions. These lesions may infiltrate deeply and yet remain entirely within the endocervical canal and thus are not visible during vaginal inspection.

Cytopathology

The diagnosis of glandular malignancy is suggested when balls, sheets, or single pleomorphic glandular cells are seen on a cytologic specimen from the cervix or vagina. It is important to determine whether the cells are of endocervical, endometrial, or other origin. Endometrial cells are normally smaller than endocervical cells, have scant cytoplasm, and are cuboidal to round rather than columnar like endocervical cells. As endocervical cells become less differentiated they become larger and more pleomorphic. Some well-differentiated endometrial carcinomas are composed of relatively small cells. On cervical or vaginal cytologic specimens they are usually present in large balls or small glandular clusters. A helpful feature in cells from endometrial carcinoma is the presence of variably sized vacuoles in the cytoplasm. These often distort the nuclei. Sometimes polymorphonuclear leukocytes are present in these vacuoles. This feature is also associated with some reactive

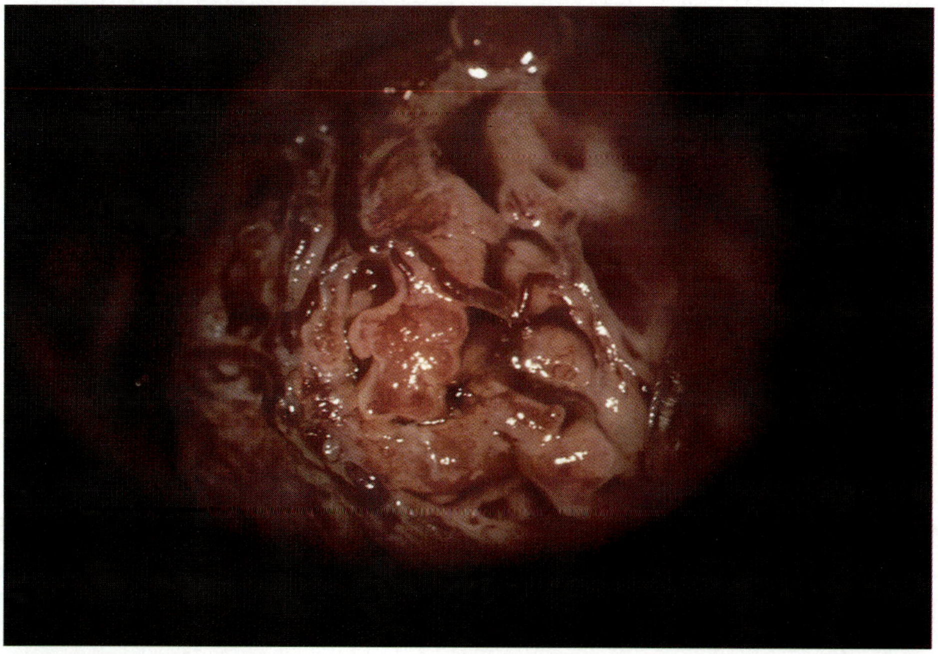

FIGURE 4–16
This is a colpophotograph of a fungating cervical adenocarcinoma. Markedly dilated abnormal vessels are seen on the surface of the tumor, which has a cerebriform appearance.

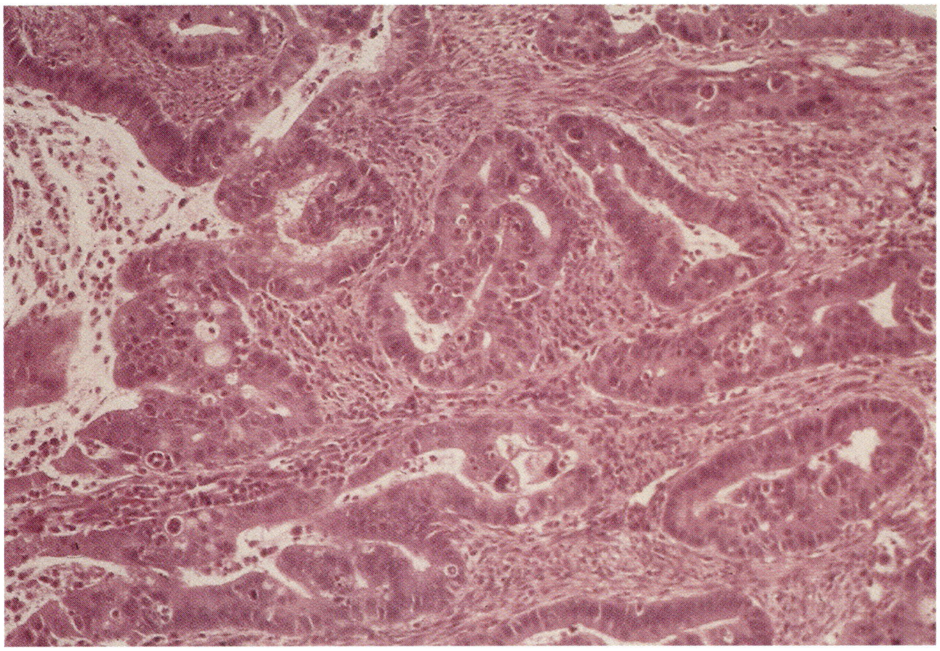

FIGURE 4-17
A moderately differentiated endocervical adenocarcinoma is seen. Infiltrating glandular structures are present, and a cribriform pattern is prominent in the large gland *(left)*. In some of the glands the cells have nuclei at the base and eosinophilic cytoplasm oriented toward the lumen.

conditions such as the use of an intrauterine device (IUD) and marked endocervicitis, but it should always raise the question of the possibility of endometrial carcinoma. The more poorly differentiated endometrial carcinomas often have a ball-like configuration and may have vacuoles. Invasive endocervical adenocarcinoma is usually composed of pleomorphic cells seen singly and in sheets. There may be some vacuolization of the cytoplasm but usually the glandular differentiation is recognized because the cells retain some columnar shape or there is acinar or rosette-like formations. Nucleoli are usually prominent. These are not a feature of squamous intraepithelial lesions but may be a feature of cells of invasive squamous carcinoma, usually of the nonkeratinizing type. Prominent nucleoli are usually found in most tumor cells in adenocarcinoma.

Histopathology

The most frequent histopathologic form of adenocarcinoma of the cervix is the endocervical variety. It accounts for approximately 70 percent of all cervical adenocarcinomas. Other histopathologic types of adenocarcinoma of the cervix are classified by their predominant cell type, including serous, endometrioid, clear cell, and villoglandular adenocarcinoma. A mixed-type adenocarcinoma of the cervix is diagnosed when more than 20 percent of a secondary histopathologic type is present.

Endocervical adenocarcinoma can appear as well-differentiated mucin-containing glands or poorly differentiated solid sheets of cells. Most endocervical-type adenocarcinomas are well to moderately differentiated and form glandular structures lined by cells that resemble those of the normal endocervical epithelium. The cells contain atypical nuclei that show mitotic activity. The complex glands may have a cribriform pattern and extensively infiltrate the cervical stroma (Fig. 4–17). As the carcinoma becomes less differentiated mucin production is lost. Poorly differentiated endocervical adenocarcinomas are composed of back-to-back glands forming almost solid sheets of malignant cells. The lumens may be unrecognizable or may be represented only by slits. It may be impossible to distinguish a poorly differentiated adenocarcinoma from a squamous carcinoma. The components of differentiation of an adenocarcinoma are the presence of intracellular mucin and the tendency to form glands and acini. In the absence of these characteristics the tumor is usually classified as a poorly differentiated carcinoma that is most often assumed to be squamous.

Clinical Correlation

Patients with adenocarcinoma of the cervix have been reported to have a worse survival rate than those with cervical squamous cell carcinoma. Because of its endophytic growth, adenocarcinoma of the cervix may reach a higher stage on presentation than the exophytic squamous lesion. However, in many reported series the stage by stage survival rate is poorer for patients with adenocarcinoma of the cervix compared with those with squamous cell carcinoma.[4] In one large series the actuarial 5-year survival of patients with cervical adenocarcinoma by stage was: stage I, 60 percent; stage II, 47 percent; stage III, 8 percent; and stage IV, 0 percent.[94] The reasons for this poorer survival are not clear. Tumor biology is one possibility, larger size at the time of discovery owing to endophytic growth that escapes earlier detection is another. Endocervical growth may allow earlier spread to the parametria and discovery of the disease at a later stage. There is also controversy about whether there is a relative lack of radiation sensitivity of adenocarcinoma of the cervix.

Some investigators have found no difference in survival rate between patients with adenocarcinoma of the cervix and those with cervical squamous cell carcinoma.[95] Other authors have reported that there appears to be an identical survival for both squamous carcinoma and adenocarcinoma of the cervix when patients with stage IB disease are considered, but when treatment results for stages II to IV were reviewed, the 5-year survival rate was found to be 51 percent for patients with squamous cell carcinoma and 24 percent for those with adenocarcinoma of the cervix.[96]

Factors other than stage and depth of invasion that are associated with prognosis include tumor size and grade, lymph node status, and patient's age.[94, 97] It has been suggested that patients with bulky lesions are more likely to have recurrence after primary therapy. The proportion of paraaortic lymph node metastasis in patients with adenocarcinoma of the cervix that exceeds 4 cm in diameter has been reported to be 82 percent.[97] In patients with adenocarcinoma of the cervix who underwent primary surgical therapy, lymph node metastases were present in 5 percent of those with a grade 1 tumor, 11 percent of those with grade 2 tumors, and 50 percent of those with grade 3 lesions.[97] In the series reported from the University of Michigan Medical Center, lymph node metastases were found in 65 percent of patients less than 40 years of age who had cervical adenocarcinoma, in 46 percent of those between 40 and 60 years old, and in 30 percent of those older than 60 years.[94]

When radical hysterectomy and pelvic lymphadenectomy are used for the treatment of patients with stage I adenocarcinoma of the cervix the 5- and 10-year survival is 85 percent.[98] Some practitioners have reported similar results using radiation therapy as the only form of therapy for stage I disease.[99] However, others have reported a poorer survival of patients with stage I disease treated with radiation therapy only when these results are compared to the results of radical surgery or radiation therapy followed by simple hysterectomy.[100] This discrepancy is probably explained by differences in distribution of tumor size among the different series. Survival of patients with stage I adenocarcinoma of the cervix is excellent when tumor size is less than 2 cm regardless of treatment modality employed.[98] Therefore, patients with small stage I adenocarcinoma of the cervix can be treated by radical hysterectomy and pelvic lymphadenectomy or by radiation therapy. Patients with large lesions are best treated by radical hysterectomy or radiation therapy followed by simple hysterectomy.

Villoglandular Papillary Adenocarcinoma

This form of well-differentiated adenocarcinoma of the cervix has been reported only recently. The disease occurs in younger women, most of whom are less than 40 years of age. One study observed that the mean age was 33 years.[101] In none of the few cases reported has spread occurred beyond the contiguous uterus. The clinical presentation is similar to that described earlier for the endocervical type of adenocarcinoma. The majority of patients complain of abnormal vaginal bleeding. The gross lesion in most cases appears to be exophytic, and descriptions range from polyps to a warty or fungating mass.

The histopathologic appearance is usually of tall, thin papillae (Fig. 4–18), but the papillae can also be broad and short. The papillae contain a fibrous central core in which numerous inflammatory cells are found. The pattern may be elaborate and may resemble an embellishment of the normal endocervical epithelium. Small papillae budding off the larger villous papillae are rarely seen, but this is a common feature of papillary serous adenocarcinoma, which is rarely found in the cervix. The invasive portion of the villoglandular papillary adenocarcinoma is composed of enlongated branching glands that are separated by fibrous stroma and may extend from the surface of the mucosa to deep within the cervical tissue. The tumor is sharply limited at the edges, and only scattered foci of invasion into the cervical stroma beyond the main mass are seen. The tumor cells are stratified or pseudostratified columnar cells without mucin. A small number of glands may be lined by columnar cells that do contain mucin. Mild to moderate nuclear atypicality and few mitotic figures are noted in these tumor cells.

Villoglandular papillary adenocarcinoma appears to have a better prognosis than other adenocarcinomas of the cervix. The absence of recurrence among 13 patients in one series implies

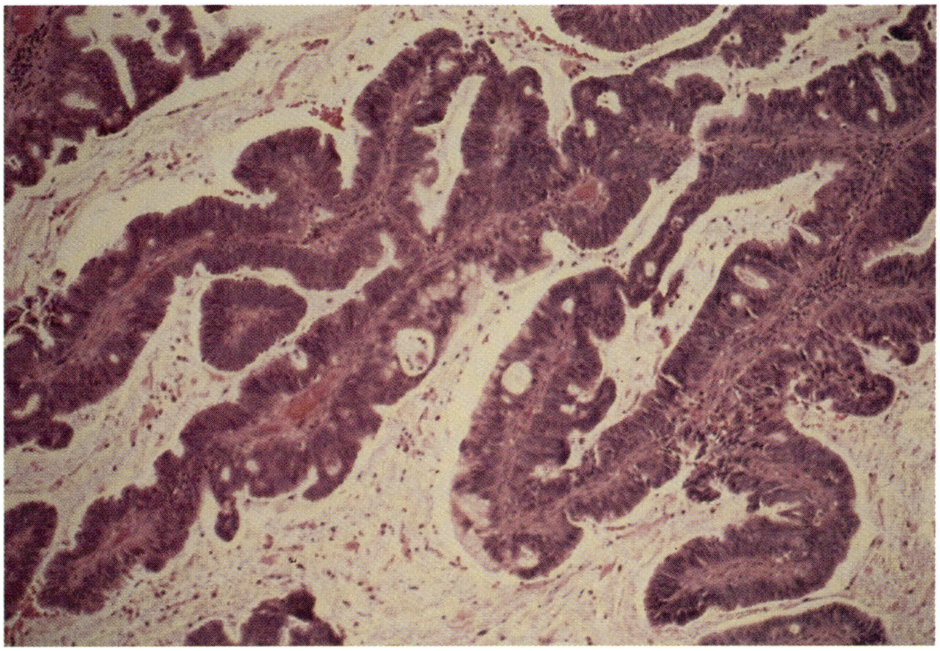

FIGURE 4-18
A villoglandular papillary adenocarcinoma of the cervix has long, thin papillae lined by malignant cells. These cells have long spindle-shaped nuclei and scant cytoplasm. Occasional cells *(bottom center)* have mucin.

that only conservative treatment methods are needed.[101] Rather than radical hysterectomy or radiation therapy, simple surgical procedures have been suggested. Cone biopsy with clear resection margins has been recommended as definitive therapy in selected cases. In the series by Young and Scully, 4 of 12 hysterectomy specimens had no residual disease and one cervical conization specimen had no residual tumor after punch biopsy of a small lesion.[101] There were no tumor recurrences. Because only a few studies on a small number of patients have been reported, more aggressive therapy may be considered until more information is available.

Papillary Serous Carcinoma

Papillary serous carcinoma, like the tumor that occurs in the ovaries and endometrium, is a rare entity in the cervix. As at other sites, extracervical spread or multifocal disease is frequent. This tumor should not be confused with villoglandular papillary adenocarcinoma.[101] Whereas the prognosis of patients with villoglandular papillary adenocarcinoma of the cervix is excellent, that of patients with papillary serous carcinoma is poor, especially if extracervical disease is present.

Adenosquamous Carcinoma

As implied by its name, adenosquamous carcinoma of the cervix is a tumor composed of both glandular and squamous malignant elements. One of the first series of cases found in the literature is that of 195 patients reported by Glücksman and Cherry in 1956.[102] These authors suggested that the tumor arose in the endocervix, had a relatively poor prognosis, and was associated with pregnancy in 17 percent of cases. They also suggested classifying this group of tumors as mixed carcinomas of the uterine cervix.

These lesions present at all ages of adult life; however, the mean age at presentation is in the late fifth and early sixth decades.[103, 104] In a more recent report of 20 patients who had adenosquamous cell carcinoma the mean age was 41 years, and 50 percent of patients were 40 years old or younger.[105] In approximately one-sixth of the patients in the series of Glücksman and Cherry the disease was diagnosed at the time of pregnancy or within 18 months post partum.[102] The findings of Julian et al were different in that only 1 of their 32 patients presented at the time of or immediately after pregnancy.[103] The patients often present with an endophytic lesion that eventually produces a barrel-shaped cervix (Fig. 4–19). On inspection, no lesion is seen, but palpation reveals expansion of the upper cervix, induration, and thickening.[105] Other patients present with exophytic lesions, often associated with abnormal vaginal bleeding. In one report of 49 cases of adenosquamous carcinoma of the cervix 41 patients had a cervical mass.[106] Some of the larger tumors also showed ulceration.

Microscopically, this tumor consists of both malignant glandular and malignant squamous elements that infiltrate and intermingle. A theory has been proposed that both the squamous and

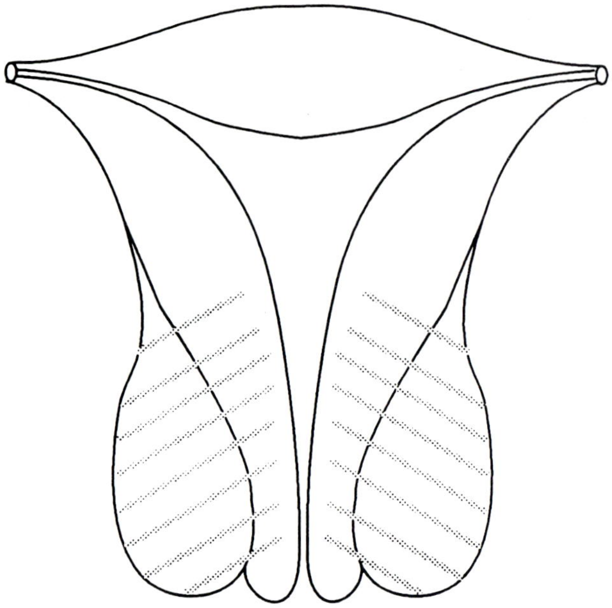

FIGURE 4-19
This diagram depicts how an endophytic adenocarcinoma of the cervix could expand the cervix to the size of the uterine fundus, resulting in a barrel shape.

glandular cells arise from a single precursor, the subcylindrical or reserve cell.[107] The cells in the glands can appear mucinous or endometrioid, and some may have a signet ring appearance. There may be acinar structures or sheets and nests of poorly differentiated cells with occasional slits where the gland lumens have been overgrown by the tumor (Fig. 4–20). The signet ring variety of adenocarcinoma has cells with clear cytoplasm with a crescent-shaped nucleus pushed against the cell wall by a large mucinous vacuole. When admixed with squamous cells the signet ring cells may be difficult to visualize using low power. Special stains can be used to demonstrate intracytoplasmic mucin (Fig. 4–21). A diagnosis of mucoepidermoid carcinoma has been made when special stains of a squamous cell carcinoma demonstrate intracytoplasmic mucin. This tumor is considered an adenosquamous carcinoma in the World Health Organization (WHO) classification. The squamous portion of adenosquamous carcinomas is often reported to be nonkeratinizing and can vary from well to poorly differentiated. The glassy cell carcinoma of the cervix is a type of adenosquamous cell carcinoma whose unique features merit discussion under a separate heading.

The prognosis of patients with adenosquamous carcinoma of the cervix is reported in almost all series as worse than that of patients with squamous cell carcinoma. Julian et al noted a 38.5 percent survival rate for patients with all stages of disease excluding those with in situ lesions.[103] Wheeless et al[108] reported an overall 5-year survival rate of 41 percent and suggested that better results occurred when patients with early disease were treated by surgery rather than radiation. They reported no survivors among patients with stage III or IV disease and a 61 percent survival rate among those with stage I or II disease treated by surgery as opposed to 45 percent among those treated with radiation. In a more recent series of 127 patients with cervical carcinoma the survival rate for patients with squamous cell and adenocarcinoma of the cervix was 78 percent and 70

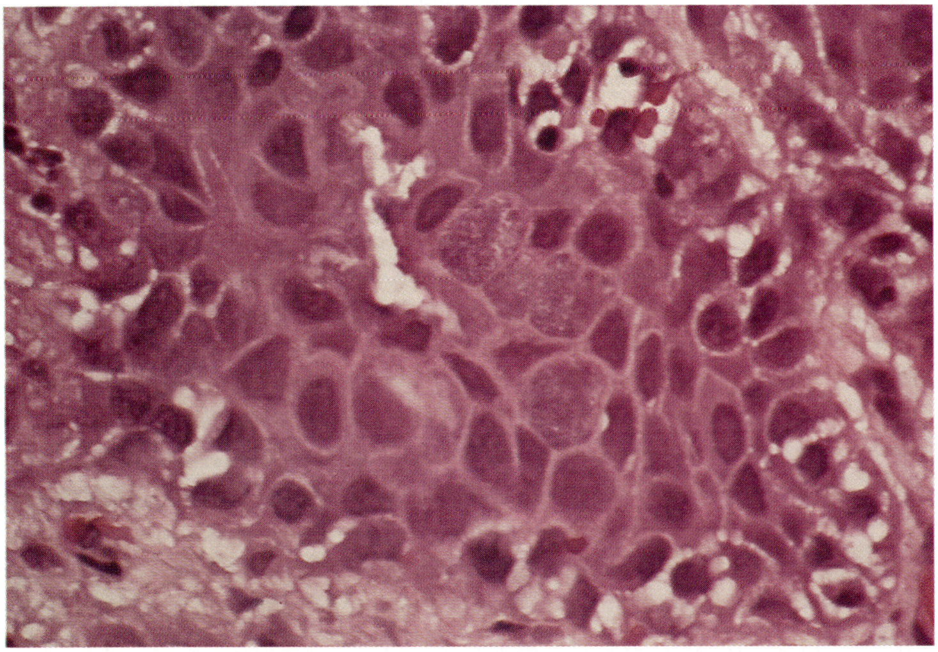

FIGURE 4-20
This high-power view of an adenosquamous carcinoma of the cervix has squamous cells surrounding a slitlike lumen. Intercellular bridges are seen best in the lower right and upper left. Four large cells near the center contain purplish mucin. This was confirmed by mucicarmine stain.

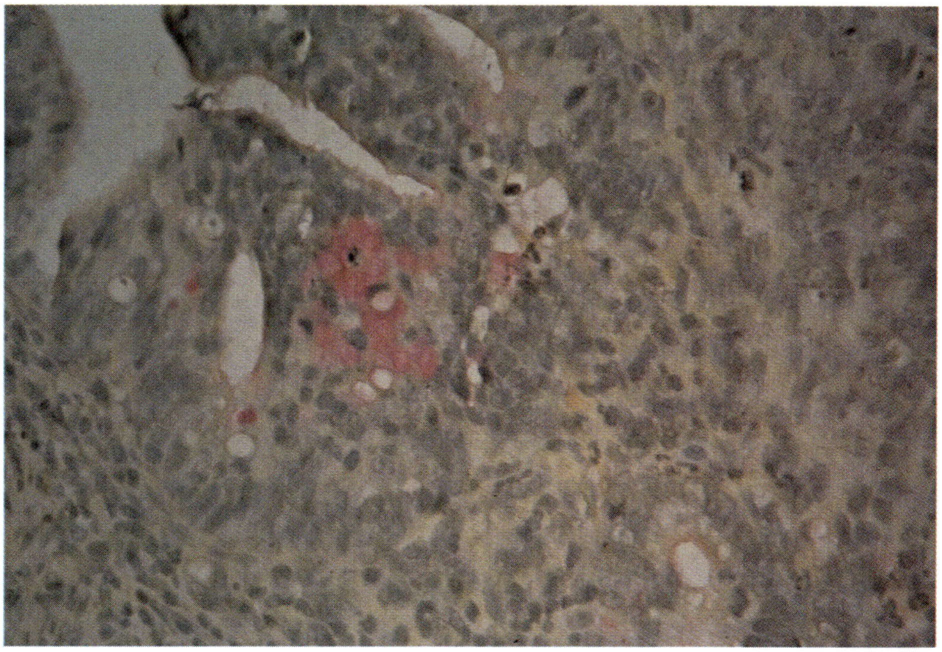

FIGURE 4-21
This mucicarmine stain of an adenosquamous carcinoma of the cervix shows intracytoplasmic mucin that stains red. A pink luminal stain *(bottom right)* is not considered positive.

percent, respectively. In contrast, the survival rate for the 20 patients with adenosquamous cell carcinoma was only 20 percent even though 75 percent had stage IB disease. The majority (87.5 percent) of patients with adenosquamous cell carcinoma who died from cancer developed distant metastasis (e.g., lung, bone).

Glassy Cell Carcinoma

This tumor is considered a poorly differentiated form of adenosquamous carcinoma. It was originally described by Glücksman and Cherry[102] and reexamined by Littman.[109] Glassy cell carcinoma represents only about 1 to 2 percent of all cervical cancers but approximately 10 percent of the category of cervical adenocarcinoma. Patients who have this tumor are usually in the age range from the middle of the third to the end of the seventh decade. In three reports the mean age of the patients was 43 years.[109-111] Most patients present with vaginal discharge or vaginal bleeding. In the majority of instances a bulky exophytic lesion is observed.

Glassy cell carcinoma is characterized by compact sheets and nests of tumor cells that invade the cervical stroma extensively. The stroma has an inflammatory infiltrate of lymphocytes and plasma cells. The tumor cells are large and polygonal with eosinophilic or amphophilic cytoplasm. The cytoplasm has a "ground-glass" or granular appearance. The cells contain a large nucleus, which has one or more conspicuous nucleoli. Cell borders are well defined (Fig. 4-22). There may be an occasional whorl that is reminiscent of squamous pearl formation. In some specimens obtained at hysterectomy, squamous carcinoma in situ is also found.[111, 112] Other histopathologic types of adenocarcinoma are often mixed with glassy cell carcinoma. To consider the glassy cell component significant it must comprise at least one-third of the tumor.

Electron microscopy of the glassy cells has demonstrated that these are cohesive epithelial cells. The cells have interdigitating cytoplasmic projections or microvilli. Cohesiveness is maintained by desmosomes, which may be rare[112] or numerous.[113] There is abundant cytoplasmic material that has an increased nuclear to cytoplasmic ratio. Nucleoli are prominent and often multiple. Intracellular organelles such as Golgi apparatus, mitochondria, and dilated cisternae of endoplasmic reticulum are present in variable amounts. The combination of dilated rough endoplasmic reticulum and cytoplasmic filaments may lead to the granular appearance of the cells.[112]

Response to treatment, whether surgery or radiation, has been reported as poor. The small number of cases reported in the available articles makes a determination of prognosis difficult. There is one report of a 42 percent overall 4-year survival.[110] However, a review of glassy cell carcinoma summarized the overall survival of 60 patients as 11 percent.[114] In one series patients with lesions that were more advanced than stage II did not survive.[110] Another report suggested that patients with all stages of this tumor have a uniformly poor outcome.[109]

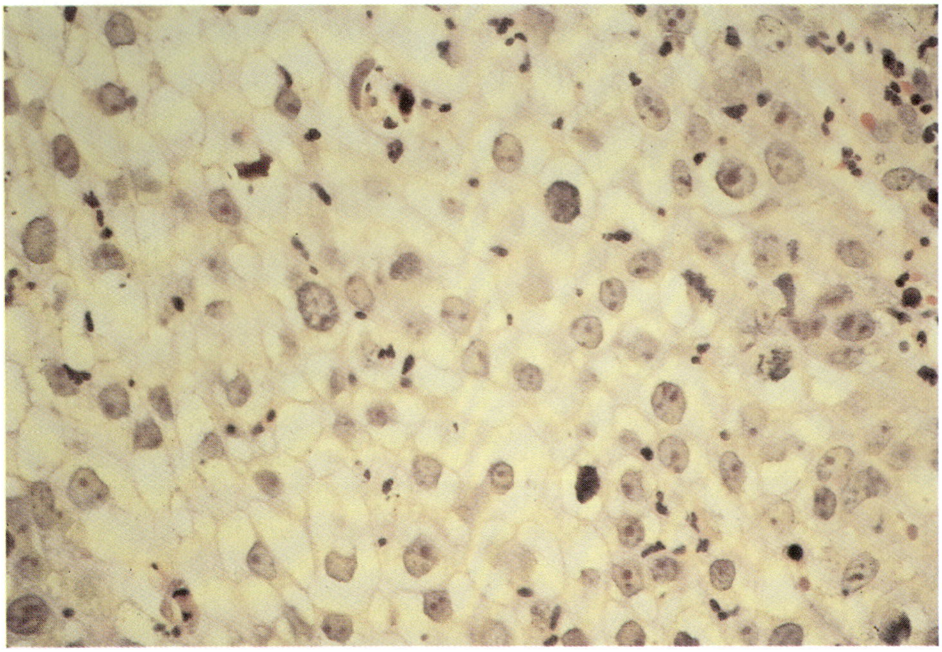

FIGURE 4-22
This tumor was present in the cervix of a 22-year-old woman. Solid sheets of malignant cells with well-defined borders are seen. Granular, amphophilic cytoplasm is present in some of the cells *(right)*, while most of the cells appear to have clear cytoplasm. The nuclei are large and contain one or more nucleoli. This is a glassy cell carcinoma.

Adenoid Cystic Carcinoma

Adenoid cystic carcinoma comprises approximately 1 percent of all cervical adenocarcinomas. This variety of cervical cancer was originally described in 1949.[115] It usually occurs in older women whose average age is in the middle sixties. Few patients are under the age of 40 years. The distribution by stage is similar to that of adenocarcinoma of the cervix, approximately 60 percent of tumors occurring as stage I lesions.

The presentation of this lesion is most often abnormal vaginal bleeding. Because of the usual age of the patients, the bleeding is frequently postmenopausal. On clinical examination a mass involving the cervix is found. This may be small and polypoid or large, friable, and exophytic or endophytic. An associated uterine prolapse has been seen in some patients.[116,117]

This tumor consists of clusters or nests of round or ovoid uniform cells. The nuclei are dark staining. The amount of cytoplasm varies. The cells are arranged in sheets, solid masses, or anastomosing cords around centrally located cystic cavities that contain an acellular eosinophilic substance (Fig. 4–23).[118] The histopathologic appearance is similar to that of adenoid cystic carcinomas located in salivary glands, skin, breast, bronchus, and Bartholin gland. These tumors are often admixed with squamous cell carcinoma or adenocarcinoma or associated with squamous carcinoma in situ. All of these tumors may arise from one totipotential-type cell.[119] The adenoid cystic pattern may be found within the more common squamous or glandular cancer of the cervix.[120]

Adenoid cystic carcinoma of the cervix is an aggressive tumor associated with frequent lymph node metastases and late pulmonary metastases. Treatment modalities for this tumor are difficult to assess because of the small number of reported cases. Treatment may consist of surgery, radiation, or a combination of surgery and radiation. According to one report, radiation rather than surgery is the therapy of choice for stage I disease; there was a reported survival rate of 71 percent when patients received radiation versus 50 percent when they underwent surgery. The survival rate for all patients with stage I adenoid cystic carcinoma of the cervix in that report was 56 percent for stage I, 27 percent for stage II, and 0 percent when the disease was diagnosed at stage III or IV.[121]

Adenoid Basal Carcinoma

Baggish and Woodruff first made the distinction between adenoid basal carcinoma and adenoid cystic carcinoma of the cervix.[122] The term cylindroma has been used to designate the low-grade form of adenoid cystic carcinoma characterized by local infiltration and lack of metastasis. The tumor consists of nests of uniform round to oval cells with dark-staining nuclei (Fig. 4–24). There is palisading of cells at the periphery of the nests. Pseudoglandular formation is rarely seen. Neither cellular anaplasia nor mitosis is noted. There is a paucity of desmoplastic reaction or lymphocytic infiltration. Surface epithelium has shown changes associated with CIN 3. The cluster of adenoid

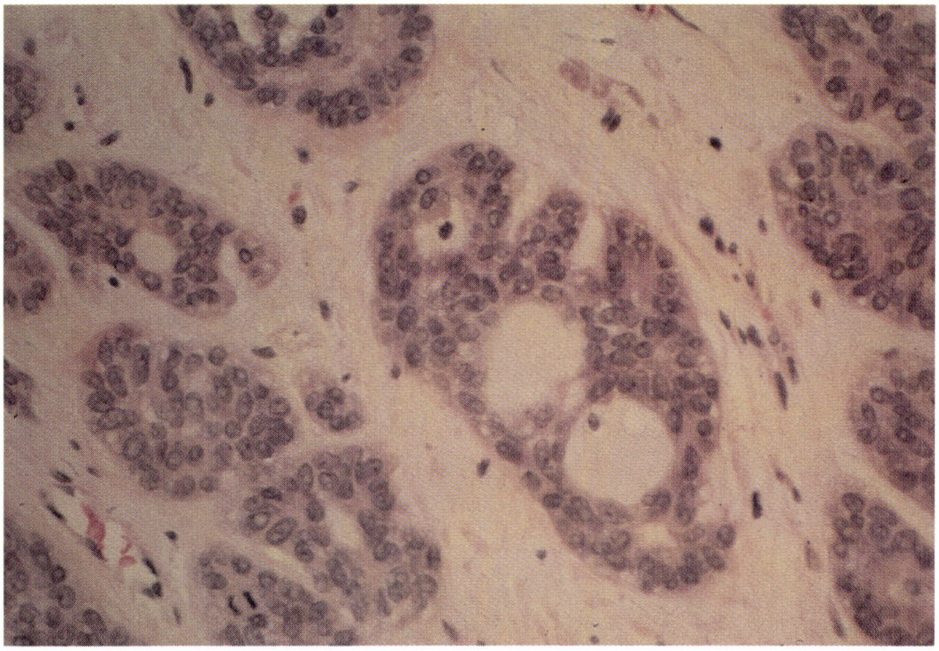

FIGURE 4–23
This adenoid cystic carcinoma shows nests of cells that have small nuclei and scant cytoplasm. The cells surround globules of eosinophilic, acellular material. This results in a cribriform appearance.

basal cells in some cases has been noted to arise directly from the base of the overlying dysplastic surface epithelium. Squamous differentiation is noted in some of the nests of adenoid basal carcinoma cells nearer to the surface.[117]

The separation of adenoid basal carcinoma of the cervix from the more aggressive adenoid cystic carcinoma allows consideration of more conservative therapy for patients with adenoid basal carcinoma. One death from sepsis secondary to uterine perforation at curettage occurred among five patients with adenoid basal carcinoma of the cervix.[118] The other four had stage IB disease and underwent a simple hysterectomy. They were alive 2, 3, 9, and 12 years after hysterectomy. Total abdominal hysterectomy with or without ovarian conservation is considered the treatment of choice for this disease. The frequent association of adenoid basal carcinoma of the cervix with other cervical carcinomas makes it mandatory to perform a cone biopsy when a punch biopsy reveals that type of tumor. If a more aggressive tumor coexists with the adenoid basal carcinoma, a conservative surgical approach is no longer appropriate.

Clear Cell Carcinoma

Cases of clear cell carcinoma account for 3 percent of all cases of adenocarcinoma of the cervix.[123] The greatest portion of these patients have had intrauterine exposure to diethylstilbestrol (DES). Before 1970 the finding of a clear cell carcinoma of the cervix was unusual. Exposure of the fetus in utero to DES or a related nonsteroidal estrogen has led to an increased incidence of this type of adenocarcinoma. However, 25 percent of patients with clear cell carcinoma have no history of exposure to DES. The age of those who have had no exposure is usually 45 years or older. Clear cell carcinoma related to DES exposure appears to be most commonly discovered in the late teens to early twenties.[124] This tumor may arise in either the cervix or vagina (see later discussion). Many patients seek medical care because of a knowledge of their antenatal history. Others have symptoms of abnormal vaginal bleeding or discharge.[125] The clinical presentation is similar whether the patient had antenatal DES exposure or not. The tumor may be polypoid and fungating or ulcerative.[123, 125] On some occasions there is no visible lesion. On palpation the cervix may be indurated and firm.

A tumor caused by antenatal DES exposure is microscopically identical to one that is not related to that etiologic event. The cells are large and polygonal and have abundant clear to eosinophilic cytoplasm. Cells often have a "hobnail" shape, in which there is minimal cytoplasm so that the nucleus appears to protrude toward the surface (Fig. 4–25). Nuclei are often large and distinct with irregular borders. Multiple nucleoli are present. Chromatin is often condensed near the edge of the nuclear membrane. Four growth patterns have been observed. These are papillary, microcystic, tubular, and solid. All of the patterns may exist simultaneously, but often one type prevails. The tubular pattern resembles various-sized tubules lined by cuboidal flattened cells

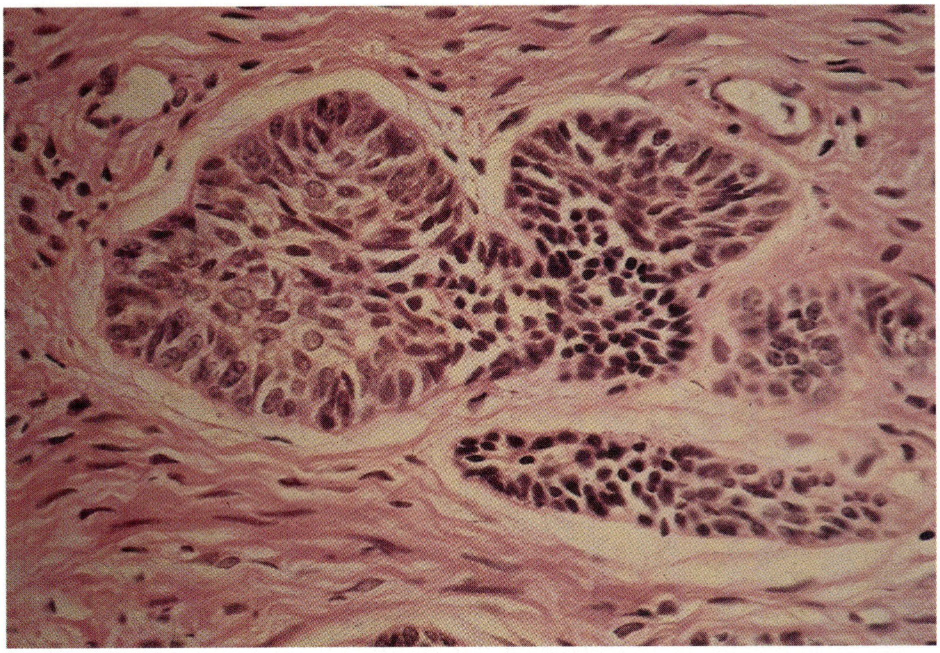

FIGURE 4-24
An adenoid basal carcinoma is seen here. There are nests of uniform cells with oval to elongate nuclei, most of which are dark-staining. There is palisading of nuclei at the periphery of the large nest. (Courtesy of Dr. Tung Van Dinh, Galveston, Texas.)

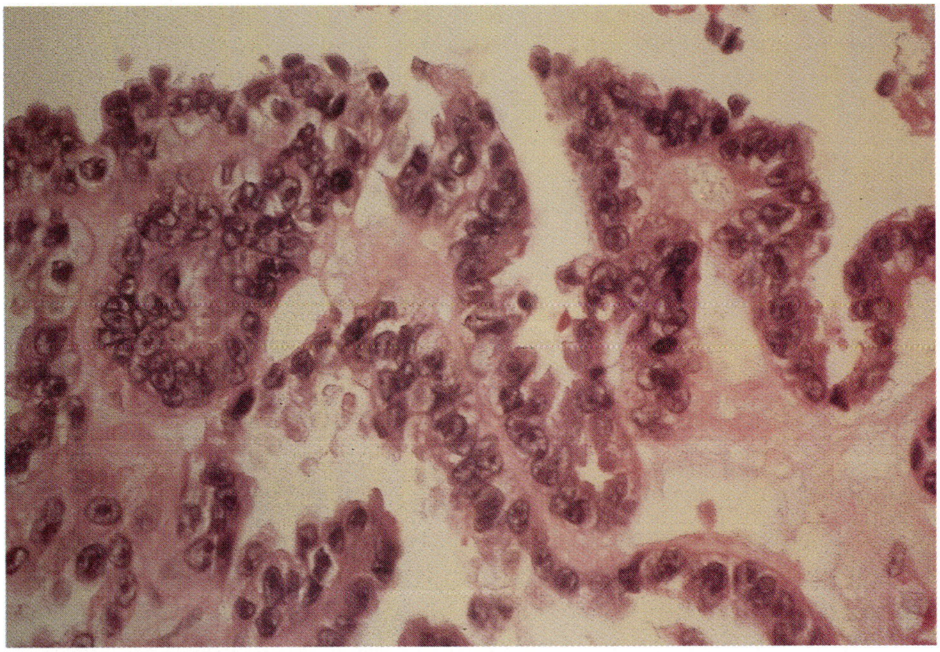

FIGURE 4-25
In this clear cell adenocarcinoma the papillary projections are lined by hobnail cells. The hobnail cells have scant cytoplasm and an irregular nucleus that protrudes toward the surface. Prominent nucleoli are present.

or hobnail cells. The microcystic pattern is composed of larger tubules that are also lined by cuboidal to flattened cells or hobnail cells. In the papillary pattern thin fibrovascular cores are covered by hobnail or clear cells. The nests of cells in the preceding patterns are often separated by fibrous connective tissue. Psammoma bodies may be present in any of these patterns. The solid pattern of the tumor consists of sheets of clear cells (Fig. 4–26).[123,125]

In a report of 23 patients with non–DES-related clear cell carcinoma of the cervix, 20 patients with stage I and II disease were treated with surgery, a combination of radiation and surgery, and occasionally with radiation only.[125] Three patients with stage III or IV disease received palliative radiation. All three died within 1 year. The reported survival rate was reasonable for patients with early-stage disease. Of the 20 patients who had early-stage disease, two were lost to follow-up. Twelve (67 percent) of the remaining 18 are alive 4 to 23 years after diagnosis. Among patients exposed to DES in utero, those who develop the cancer at the age of 15 years or younger do not fare as well as those who are 19 years or older.[124] The tubulocystic pattern also appears to be associated with a better prognosis than the papillary, solid, or combination patterns. However, the older patients with better survival also are more likely to have a tumor with a tubulocystic pattern, which in itself is associated with a better outcome.

Endometrioid Adenocarcinoma

Endometrioid adenocarcinoma is so named because the cells and glands resemble those typical of endometrial adenocarcinoma. By convention, if such a tumor is present in the cervix it is considered an extension from an endometrial primary until proved otherwise. Once this clinical consideration is eliminated, the diagnosis of endometrioid adenocarcinoma of the cervix can be made. Endometrioid adenocarcinoma is the second most frequent adenocarcinoma of the cervix after the endocervical type.

Characteristics of patients with endometrioid adenocarcinoma of the cervix do not differ from those of patients with cervical adenocarcinoma of other histopathologic types. The clinical presentation is similar to that described previously for cervical adenocarcinoma of the endocervical type. Most patients who have this type of adenocarcinoma of the cervix are in their middle forties to middle fifties. The tumor may be polypoid or fungating in 50 percent of cases and may not be visible in up to 15 percent of cases.

Endometrioid adenocarcinoma of the cervix is usually a well-differentiated lesion. The glands form complex patterns with a gland-within-gland configuration and intraluminal budding. The gland lumens often contain neutrophils.[126] The cellular cytoplasm is amphophilic and dense. It is rare to see vacuolated or clear cytoplasm. Glycogen particles are seen in the cytoplasm of some of the tumor cells as demonstrated by periodic acid–Schiff stain. Mucicarmine-positive material is present in the glands but not in the cytoplasm in contrast to endocervical-type adenocarcinoma, in which mucicarmine-positive material is found in the cytoplasm in 90 percent of cases.[104]

The survival of patients with endometrioid ade-

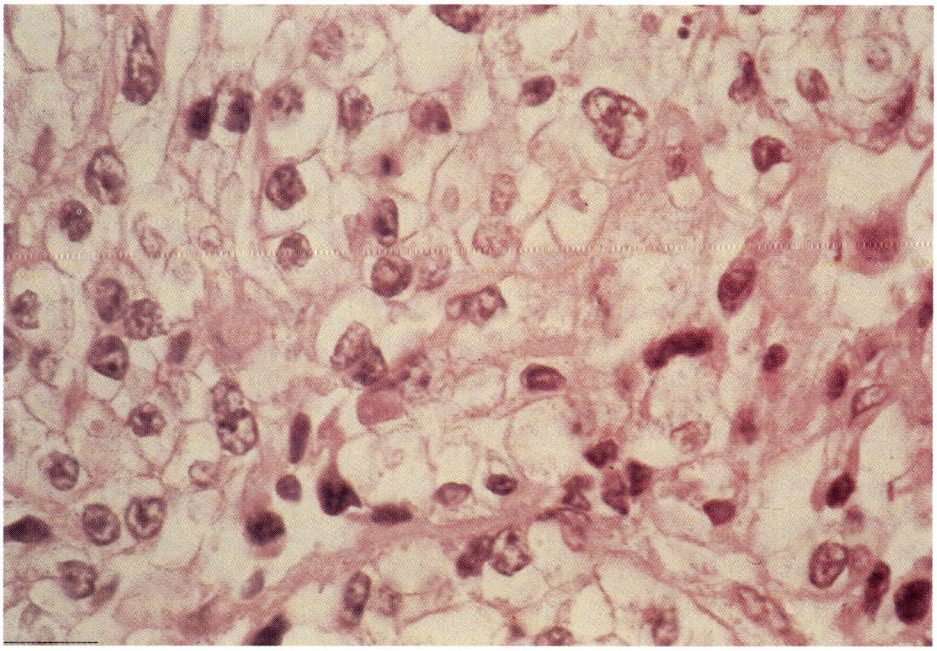

FIGURE 4–26
This demonstrates the clear cell pattern of a clear cell carcinoma of the cervix.

nocarcinoma of the cervix has been reported to be better than that of patients with other histopathologic types. One study reported a 5-year survival rate of 85 percent for patients with endometrioid adenocarcinoma of the cervix compared to 51 percent for patients with the mucinous type, 64 percent for those with clear cell adenocarcinoma, and 39 percent for those with the adenosquamous type.[84] Hurt et al also reported a relatively good prognosis for patients with endometrioid adenocarcinoma of the cervix.[127] The 5-year survival rate for these patients was 67 percent compared to 40 percent for patients with clear cell or endocervical-type adenocarcinoma.

Minimal Deviation Carcinoma (Adenoma Malignum)

This type of adenocarcinoma of the cervix is extremely rare. Silverberg and Hurt proposed the term minimal deviation adenocarcinoma (MDC) for this tumor.[128] Although the microscopic appearance is bland, the outcome is poor. The disease appears to metastasize rapidly and is not easily treated.

Cases of MDC constitute 1 to 3 percent of all cases of adenocarcinoma of the cervix. Although an association between adenocarcinoma of the cervix and ovarian neoplasms has been reported, patients with this specific histopathologic type have a higher prevalence of associated ovarian neoplasms.[129, 130] The ovarian tumor may be found at the same time or after the diagnosis of MDC has been made. The ovarian tumor is usually mucinous or, rarely, of specialized gonadal stromal origin. MDC has been associated with Peutz-Jeghers syndrome.[131]

In the report by Kaminski and Norris the patients' ages were between 31 and 76 years, and the mean age was 46 years.[131] The presenting symptoms were similar to those described earlier for patients with other histopathologic types of adenocarcinoma of the cervix. Patients with MDC may present with abnormal vaginal bleeding, vaginal discharge, and occasionally an abnormal Papanicolaou smear. The tumor may be ulcerative or exophytic. The physical examination findings may be subtle such as a laceration on the cervical portio. The cervix may appear completely normal, or cervical stenosis may be present.

On microscopic examination there are well-formed glands that show minimal if any cellular stratification. The most frequent cell type is mucinous. Other histopathologic cell types that may be seen include clear cell and endometrioid adenocarcinoma. The endocervical-type cells line the glands in a single layer. Nuclei are basally oriented, and nucleoli are not prominent. There is a paucity of nuclear atypia. The nuclear to cytoplasmic ratio is normal. Reports about the amount of mitotic activity indicate that it varies from minimal to an increased level. The glands are increased in number and invade more deeply into the stroma than do normal endocervical glands (Figs. 4–27 and 4–28). They have a variety of sizes and shapes. Some are round, whereas others have deformed shapes and angular projections. There is some desmoplasia in the adjacent stroma.

The differential diagnosis of MDC includes mi-

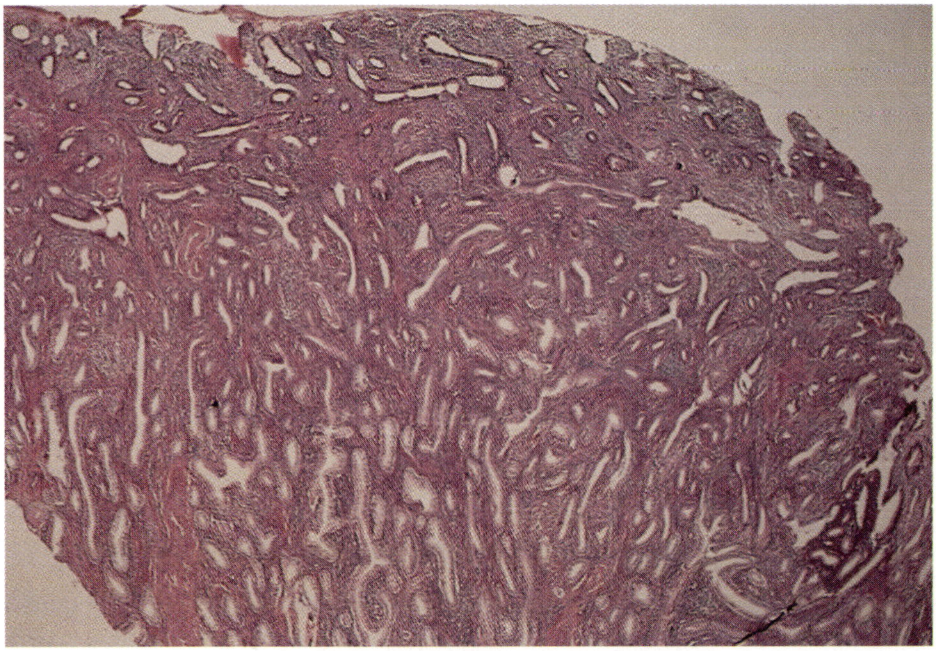

FIGURE 4-27
Irregular, elongated endocervical glands are present throughout the entire cervical stroma in this case of adenoma malignum. Even at this low-power magnification a single row of basally oriented nuclei are seen to line the glands. (Courtesy of Dr. Paul Kaminski, Hershey Medical Center, Hershey, PA.)

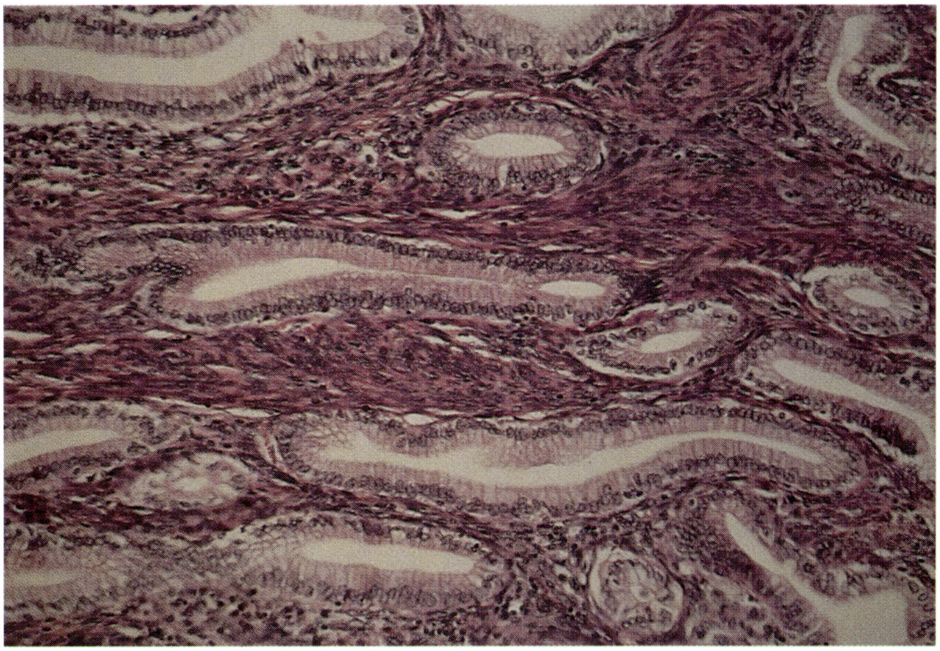

FIGURE 4-28
This is a high-power microphotograph of adenoma malignum. The cytologic appearance is that of normal endocervical epithelium. (Courtesy of Dr. Paul Kaminski, Hershey Medical Center, Hershey, PA.)

croglandular hyperplasia (see Chapter 2). MDC differs from microglandular hyperplasia by the great variety of glandular size and shape characteristic of MDC and the depth to which MDC invades the stroma. Microglandular hyperplasia is superficial and does not extend below the level of the endocervical glands. The glands of microglandular hyperplasia are more dense, and squamous metaplasia is frequently present. A heavy inflammatory infiltrate is more frequently seen in microglandular hyperplasia than in MDC. Nodular clustering (tunnel clusters) may be confused with MDC; however, the irregularity of glandular size and shape characteristic of MDC but not of nodular clustering (Fig. 4–29) should lead to the correct diagnosis. MDC has a greater depth of gland penetration than does nodular clustering.

Primary radiation therapy is rarely used for this disease process. The lesion is usually not discovered until after hysterectomy has been performed. Because MDC invades deeply but is not overt, there may be extensive spread before therapy is begun. The patient is often understaged, and the therapy may not encompass the tumor volume. This leads to an unfavorable outcome. Kaminski and Norris reported improved survival with radical hysterectomy and pelvic lymphadenectomy.[131]

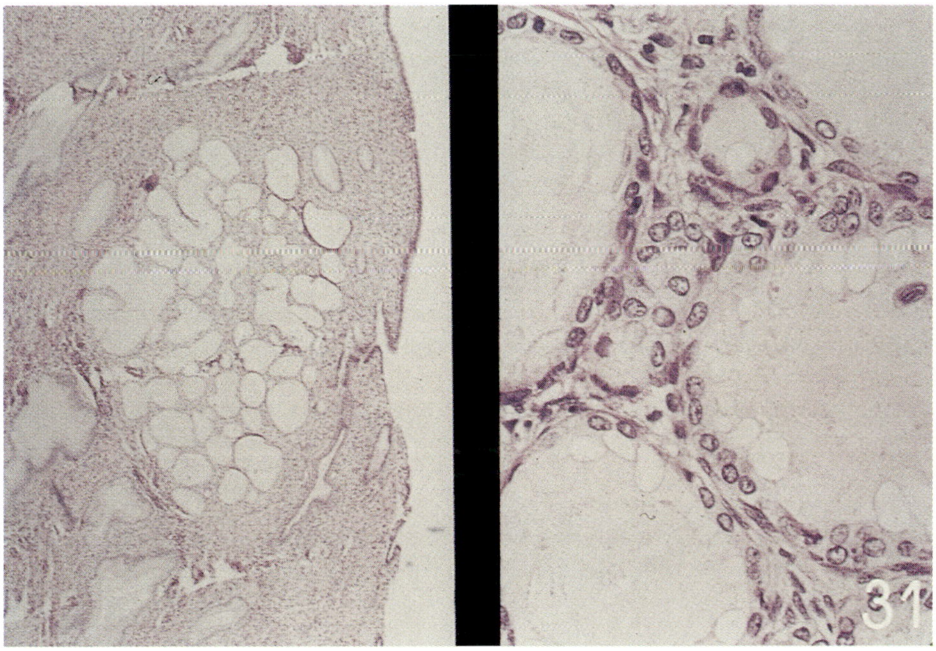

FIGURE 4-29
A cluster of dilated endocervical glands close to the surface characterizes nodular clustering. The high-power view shows that the glands are lined by flattened epithelium. (Courtesy of Dr. David C. Wilbur, University of Rochester, Rochester, NY.)

OTHER RARE CERVICAL MALIGNANT NEOPLASMS

Verrucous Carcinoma

This is an extremely rare variant of cervical cancer. This nomenclature was first used by Ackerman in 1948 to refer to lesions in the oral cavity.[132] Verrucous carcinoma is an unusual type of squamous carcinoma that has a gross appearance of a large exophytic lesion that may resemble condyloma acuminatum. An entity called giant condyloma may be confused with verrucous carcinoma, but usually there is no cytologic atypia in this whereas disordered architecture and cytologic atypia are typical of verrucous carcinoma. Verrucous carcinoma may also be confused with well-differentiated squamous carcinoma. The invasion of well-differentiated squamous carcinoma usually takes the form of finger-like projections or nests of invading cells in contrast to the invading front of verrucous carcinoma, which is blunt and broad.

On microscopic examination verrucous carcinoma is arranged in rounded fronds that do not have a central fibrovascular core. These fronds compress the surrounding tissue and underlying stroma. The basement membrane appears to be intact. The tumor fronds are composed of benign-appearing squamous cells. Often there are associated keratin whorls admixed with the epithelium. There is minimal nuclear or cytologic atypia. Mitotic activity is also limited. Koilocytosis is not seen. However, owing to its papillary appearance and similarity to condyloma acuminatum as well as to its minimally aggressive nature, a common etiologic factor has been suggested. DNA hybridization studies have identified HPV type 6 in verrucous carcinoma of the vagina[133] and vulva.[134]

An adequate biopsy is necessary to make this diagnosis because the lesion is exophytic and stromal invasion may not be identified if the biopsy is superficial. Local recurrences are frequent after surgical removal. Extension into the surrounding pelvic structures is frequent. This may compromise bladder, rectal, or ureteral function, which ultimately causes the patient's demise. Metastatic disease is rare. Enlarged regional lymph nodes are often present.[135] However, they usually represent an inflammatory reaction to the tumor. Although the bland microscopic appearance and lack of distant metastasis suggest that this tumor is not aggressive, the reported survival rate for patients with verrucous carcinoma of the cervix is only 40 percent at 2 years. In contrast, when this tumor occurs on the vulva the 2-year survival rate is 75 percent.[136]

Some practitioners think that radiation therapy is contraindicated for this condition. However, some patients with verrucous carcinoma of the cervix have benefited from radiation therapy. Wide surgical excision, which in some cases may require a total pelvic exenteration, yields the best results.[136]

Neuroendocrine (Oat Cell) Carcinoma

Tumors of the cervix, described as "small cell cancers," have included several other tumor types such as poorly differentiated small cell squamous cell carcinoma. Small cell squamous carcinoma can usually be recognized by focal keratinization. The cells of the adenoid cystic and adenoid basal carcinomas are also small, but these tumors have unique characteristics that were described previously. Another small cell cancer, the neuroendocrine small cell carcinoma of the cervix, has unique electron microscopic and immunohistochemical characteristics and is associated with an extremely poor prognosis. At one medical center, 2 percent of all cervical cancer cases were neuroendocrine small cell carcinomas.[137] The mean age of patients with neuroendocrine small cell carcinoma of the cervix is in the middle forties.

This neuroendocrine tumor is composed of cells that are uniform in size and shape, causing it to have a rather monotonous appearance (Fig. 4–30). The cells are small and round. They invade the cervical stroma in solid sheets. The cellular cytoplasm is scant, and the cellular borders are indistinct. The nuclear to cytoplasmic ratio is high. The nucleus contains coarse granular chromatin. The nucleolus is inconspicuous. Electron microscopy reveals dense-core, membrane-bound cytoplasmic neurosecretory granules that are 80 to 140 nm in diameter (Fig. 4–31). Immunocytochemistry can be used to demonstrate the presence of neuron-specific enolase and chromogranin in this tumor but not cytokeratin or epithelial membrane antigen, which are characteristically found in small cell squamous carcinomas.[138]

The prognosis for patients with neuroendocrine small cell carcinoma of the cervix is extremely poor. Of 14 patients with stage IB or IIA disease reported by Sheets et al,[137] all developed tumor recurrence, and 12 died of cancer 8 to 31 months after diagnosis. Common sites of extrapelvic metastases include the bone, brain, liver, lung, supraclavicular lymph nodes, adrenal gland, and breast. Currently, the treatment of this disease follows guidelines used for the treatment of small cell (oat cell) carcinoma of the lung, which it closely resembles both cytologically and clinically.

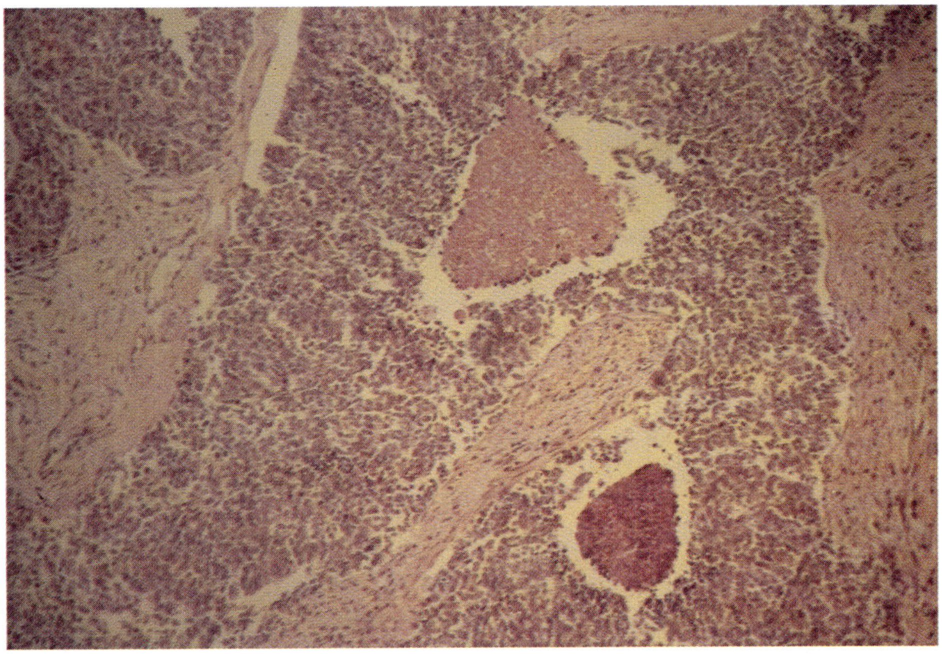

FIGURE 4-30
This neuroendocrine carcinoma is composed of a uniform population of small cells, which results in a monotonous appearance. They are arranged in solid sheets, some of which have necrotic debris in the center.

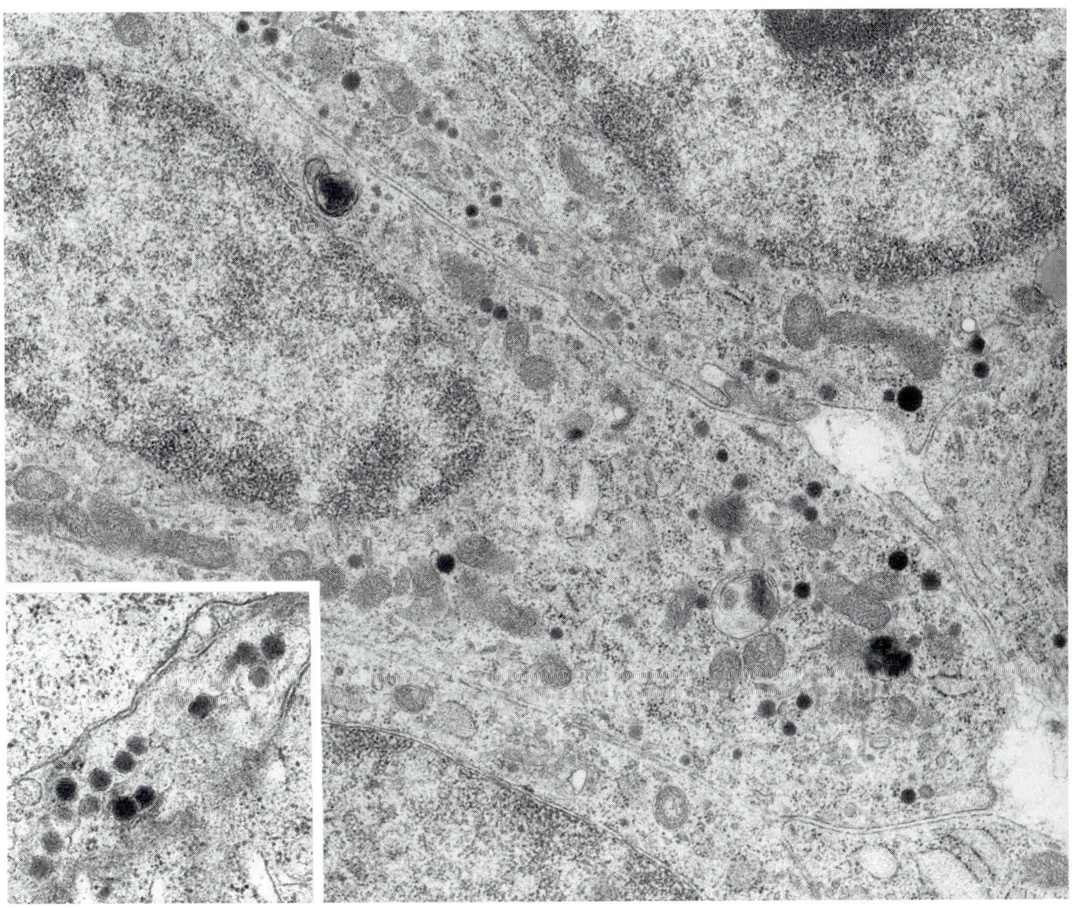

FIGURE 4-31
This electron micrograph shows a portion of three cells from a neuroendocrine carcinoma. The neurosecretory granules are dense black round bodies in the cytoplasm. The inset *(bottom left)* shows that the granules are surrounded by a membrane. The nucleus at the right corner has a prominent nucleolus. (Courtesy of Dr. Roberto Nicosia and Mr. James Diven, Medical College of Pennsylvania and Hahnemann University School of Medicine, Philadelphia, PA.)

In early-stage disease radical hysterectomy and bilateral pelvic lymphadenectomy are performed, followed by chemotherapy and radiation therapy. In one regimen whole pelvis irradiation is delivered between four courses of cisplatin and etoposide.

Sarcoma

Uterine sarcoma in general is an extremely rare malignancy, constituting between 1 and 2 percent of all gynecologic tumors. There have been only a few reports of a sarcoma primary of the cervix. The types reported include stromal sarcoma, malignant mixed mesodermal tumor (carcinosarcoma), leiomyosarcoma, and rhabdomyosarcoma. The most frequent sarcoma of the cervix is the stromal sarcoma. The average age of patients with cervical sarcoma is 54 years.

The criteria for the diagnosis of sarcoma of the cervix were established by Abell and Ramirez.[139] There should be no involvement of the body of the uterus. The body of the uterus should not be enlarged, and the endometrial curettings should not show sarcoma (hysteroscopy may allow better identification of the primary site). If the sarcoma arises in a cervical stump, the previously resected uterus must have been free of a similar neoplasm.

Rotmensch et al reviewed the subject of cervical sarcomas and suggested a modification of Ober's classification of uterine sarcomas that could be applied to sarcomas arising in the cervix.[140] They divided cervical sarcomas into leiomyosarcomas and stromal sarcomas. The stromal sarcomas include homologous tumors, heterologous sarcomas, sarcoma botryoides, adenosarcoma, and malignant mixed müllerian tumor or carcinosarcoma.

Endocervical stromal sarcoma usually has a gross appearance similar to that of a cervical polyp. Microscopic examination reveals cells that are round to fusiform in shape and contain large, dark nuclei. Normal endocervical glands are seen scattered among the tumor cells. Mitotic activity is brisk.[141]

Mixed mesodermal tumor of the cervix has been reported. This tumor is also known as carcinosarcoma. Like its counterpart in the uterus, it is composed of epithelial and stromal elements (see Chapter 7). The epithelial elements may be adenocarcinoma or squamous cell carcinoma. The sarcomatous component may be represented by homologous or heterologous tissue or both. The sarcomatous cells are often large and pleomorphic and are arranged in sheets or cords. The cytoplasm is eosinophilic and foamy. The nuclei are hyperchromatic. Brisk mitotic activity is present. The carcinomatous component may show increased cellularity, nuclear pleomorphism, and increased mitotic activity (Fig. 4–32).[142]

Sarcoma botryoides is a subtype of embryonal rhabdomyosarcoma that arises beneath the cervical mucosa and produces an edematous polypoid mass. This rare tumor can also arise in the nasopharynx, nasal cavity, bile duct, anus, and eyelid. Rhabdomyosarcoma is the most common malignancy of the lower genital tract in young girls.

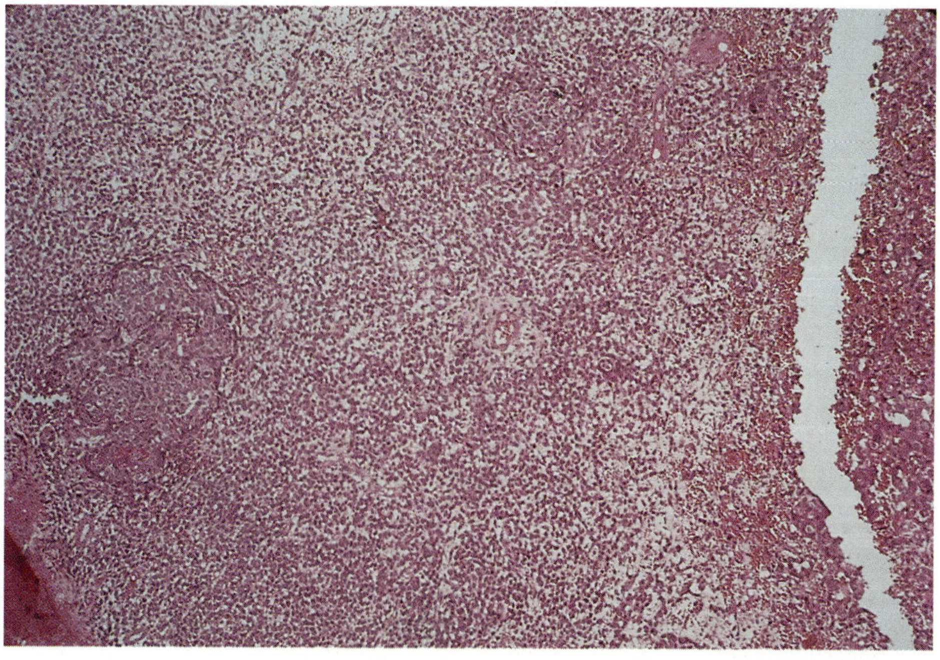

FIGURE 4–32
This is a cervical biopsy from a patient who had carcinosarcoma of the cervix. An island of poorly differentiated carcinoma is seen *(left)* in a background of undifferentiated sarcomatous cells.

This tumor arises in the vagina five times more often than in the cervix. Patients with sarcoma botryoides arising in the cervix tend to be older than those whose tumor arises in the vagina (see later discussion). The age of patients with sarcoma botryoides of the cervix ranges from 5 months to 48 years, but most patients are in their second decade of life.[143, 144] Symptoms include either vaginal bleeding or "something coming out of the vagina" or both. Physical examination reveals a smooth, glistening, focally hemorrhagic polypoid mass that arises from the cervix. The polypoid mass may have a stalk or pedicle and may have the gross appearance of an endocervical polyp.

Sarcoma botryoides is characterized by a normal mucosal covering that may show focal ulceration. Beneath the mucosa the cambium layer of Nicholson is visible (Fig. 4–33). This is a cellular zone of primitive rhabdomyoblasts, which are plump, spindle-shaped cells with hyperchromatic nuclei and scant cytoplasm. Below the cambium layer, fusiform cells with eosinophilic cytoplasm, with or without cross striations, are found within an edematous and vascular stroma. Cellular atypicality varies from mild to marked. Mitotic activity is moderate. Focal areas of mature cartilage may be present. Immunohistochemical staining for myoglobin is focally positive. Electron microscopy reveals myofilaments within the cytoplasm of the primitive rhabdomyoblast.

The therapeutic modalities employed in patients with sarcoma botryoides of the cervix range from polypectomy to anterior exenteration. Adjunctive radiation therapy has been used, but it is now thought that chemotherapy that contains vincristine and dactinomycin is more effective. In most patients the tumor is confined to the cervix. It has been suggested that initial therapy should consist of vincristine- and dactinomycin-based chemotherapy.[144] Therapy should be guided by the response to chemotherapy and should attempt to preserve ovarian, vaginal, bladder, and rectal function. In a series of 13 patients who were followed for from 1 to 8 (average 3.5) years, all but one are alive and without evidence of recurrence.[143] Three of these patients had had polypectomy only. One had been followed for 1 year and the other two followed for 5 years. None had tumor recurrence. The survival rate of patients who underwent complete resection of disease that was confined to the cervix is 88 percent.[144]

Leiomyosarcoma of the cervix is similar to that found in the uterine corpus and is described in Chapter 7. There are atypical smooth muscle cells that often have large hyperchromatic nuclei. The cells are arranged in interlacing bundles. The mitotic rate is high.

With the exception of sarcoma botryoides, the best therapeutic approach to cervical sarcomas has not been established. For stage IB lesions, radical hysterectomy and surgical staging seems appropriate. Adjuvant therapy with radiation or chemotherapy may be used, but the results are generally poor when extracervical disease is present.

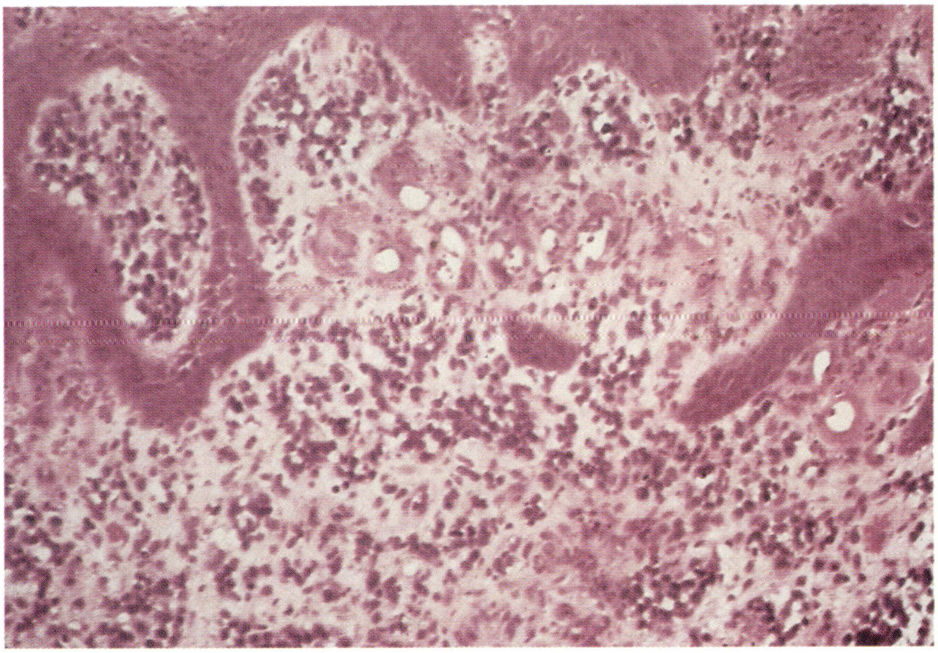

FIGURE 4–33
This is sarcoma botryoides. Normal squamous epithelium is present *(top)*. Small cells with dark nuclei infiltrate the submucosal stroma. These are immature rhabdomyoblasts. (Courtesy of Dr. J. Donald Woodruff, The Johns Hopkins Hospital, Baltimore, MD.)

Lymphoma

Involvement of the female reproductive tract by disseminated lymphoma is a frequent occurrence. In a review of 1269 autopsies of patients who had widespread lymphoma or leukemia, genital tract involvement was found in 40 percent.[145] However, primary cervical lymphoma is extremely rare. Only a handful of cases are found in the literature.[146, 147] The age range of these patients is between 20 and 80 years with the mean and median age in the early forties. Over two-thirds of the reported cases of cervical lymphoma occurred in premenopausal patients. The majority of patients complain of abnormal vaginal bleeding (e.g., postcoital or postmenopausal bleeding, menometrorrhagia). Other common complaints include perineal discomfort and vaginal discharge. Some patients have no symptoms, and cervical lymphoma is discovered on routine physical examination or is an incidental finding in a hysterectomy specimen. The typical lesion exceeds 4 cm at the time of diagnosis (Fig. 4–34). However, tumor growth is usually endophytic, which may result in cervical expansion and parametrial extension without mucosal changes. Cervical cytologic findings are usually normal. The distribution of tumors at presentation by FIGO stage is 48 percent stage I, 28 percent stage II, 15 percent stage III, and 9 percent stage IV.[146] However, most patients are classified as having stage IE extranodal lymphoma using the Ann Arbor Staging System (i.e., involvement of a single extralymphatic organ or site without lymph node involvement).[147]

Cervical lymphoma arises in the cervical stroma, and preservation of the overlying cervical mucosa is seen in early lesions. The most common lymphomas are those with a follicular pattern (Fig. 4–35). However, diffuse large cell (Working Formulation) or diffuse histiocytic (Rappaport classification) comprise most cases of cervical lymphoma.[147] They most commonly present as local disease, but if untreated, rapid dissemination and aggressive locally destructive growth occur. In contrast, follicular lymphomas are often disseminated at presentation but follow an indolent course. Therefore, the treatment of patients with cervical lymphoma is dependent on the stage and the histopathologic type. Surgical staging followed by individualized treatment is suggested. Most patients with cervical lymphoma have been treated with radiation, which is an effective modality of therapy for this disease. The reported overall 5-year survival rate is 73 percent.[146] Aggressive chemotherapy in young patients with high-grade lymphomas has been used in an effort to preserve fertility. Experience with this approach for the treatment of cervical lymphoma is limited, but the results of radiation therapy used alone or in combination with hysterectomy are excellent in patients with Ann Arbor stage IE disease.[147]

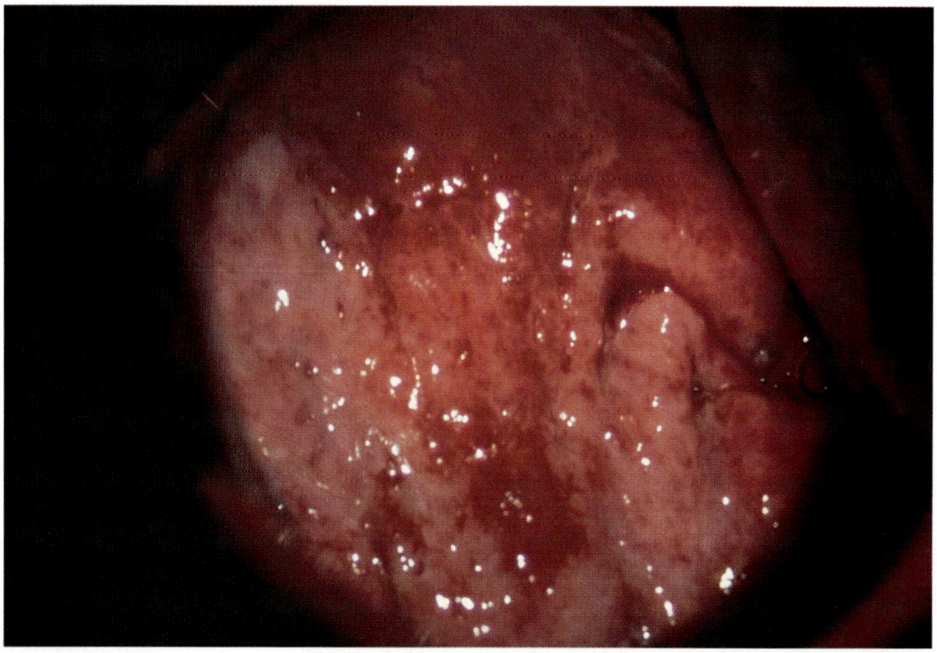

FIGURE 4–34
This colpophotograph of the cervix was taken from a 15-year-old girl who had a 2-month history of vaginal bleeding. The cervix was replaced by a 5 to 6 cm fleshy tumor with prominent vasculature. Biopsy showed a malignant lymphoma, small noncleaved cell type.

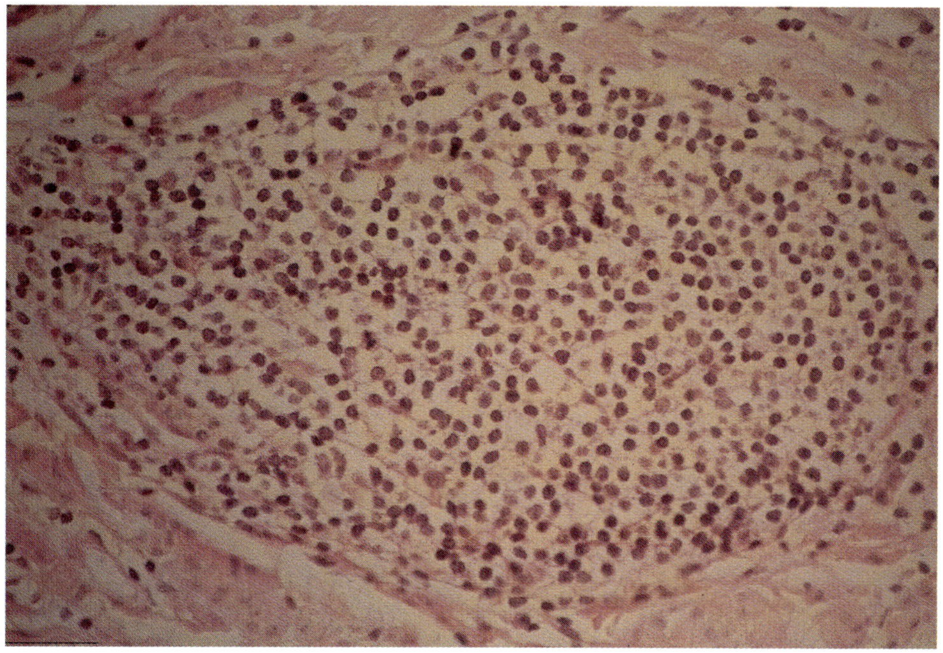

FIGURE 4-35
This cervix had multiple nodules in the stroma like the one shown here. This nodule consists of a uniform population of small lymphocytes. The nodule is the size of a normal germinal center, but it does not have the normal mixture of activated lymphocytes. This patient had follicular lymphoma of the cervix.

Metastatic Cancer to the Cervix

Metastatic tumors to the cervix are rare. The most frequent source of metastasis is other organs in the pelvis. These include the bladder, endometrium, and rectum. The majority of other metastases arise from the breast or gastrointestinal tract, especially the stomach and colon. Way reported eight cases of metastatic disease of the cervix.[148] This report included four patients who had metastatic disease from proximal organs: two from the ovary, one from the fallopian tube, and one from the sigmoid colon. Three others had spread from distant sites including two patients with gastric carcinoma and one with breast carcinoma. One tumor appeared to be metastatic from a primary peritoneal carcinoma. In another study of 208 patients with adenocarcinoma of the cervix, 45 tumors were considered to be metastases to the cervix.[149] Thirty-one of these were of endometrial origin. However, the distinction between an endometrial and an endocervical primary is often difficult because tumors with similar histopathologic and immunohistochemical features can arise at either site. Melanoma, lymphoma, pancreatic carcinoma, and choriocarcinoma have been reported as metastatic lesions to the cervix. It has been suggested that when the lesion in the cervix is metastatic from another genital organ, the primary and the metastasis are usually discovered at the same time. In contrast, lesions that are metastatic from nongenital organs were detected 4 to 38 (average 14) months after the diagnosis of the primary cancer in one study.[146]

PROCESSING OF A RADICAL HYSTERECTOMY SPECIMEN AND LYMPH NODES

A radical hysterectomy specimen consists of the uterus and cervix, which have been removed en bloc with the paracervical tissue (parametrium) and a cuff of vagina (Fig. 4–36). The fallopian tubes and ovaries may or may not accompany the specimen. The gross description of the specimen should include its weight and dimensions, paying special attention to the size of the cervix and the tumor. The vaginal cuff and parametrium are evaluated for the presence of tumor. The uterus is opened anteriorly, as described in Chapter 7, and the endometrium is assessed for the presence of tumor extension to it. It has been suggested that endometrial extension of cervical carcinoma is associated with a poorer prognosis.[150] We amputate the cervix and parametria from the uterus and the vaginal cuff from the cervix. The lateral borders of the parametria are marked with India ink to identify the resection margin when the microscopic examination is performed. Each parametrium is then sliced into pieces perpendicular to the uterus and placed in cassettes. This allows the pathologist to evaluate the entire width of the parametrium from the medial to the lateral side; if tumor is found its location can be identified as the medial or lateral

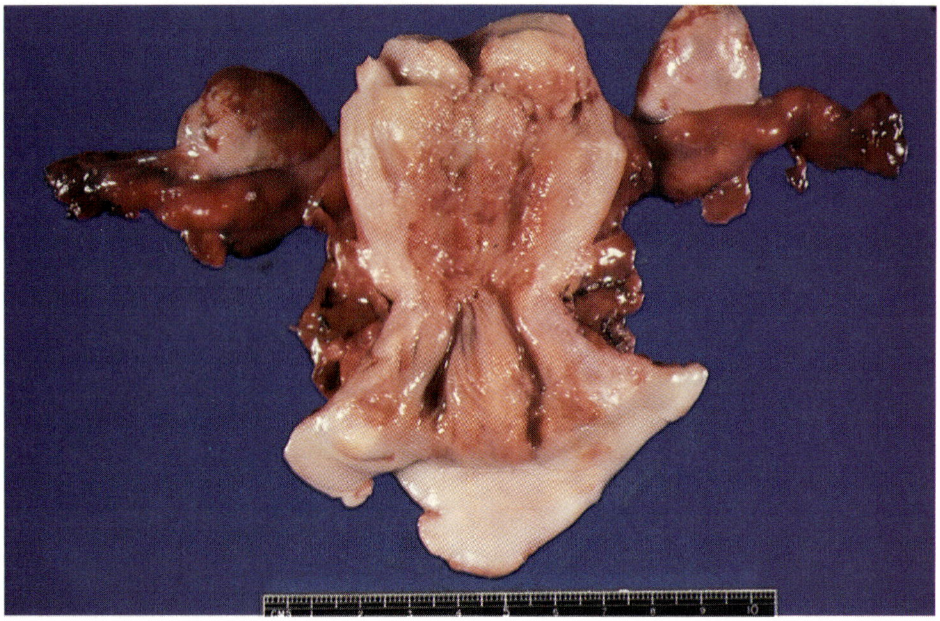

FIGURE 4-36
The uterus in this radical hysterectomy specimen has been opened anteriorly. This patient had a small endocervical adenocarcinoma but was found to have metastasis to the endometrium. Normal tubes and ovaries are attached to the uterus. A wide vaginal margin was removed. The parametrial tissue is seen on either side of the cervix and lower uterine segment.

parametrium, and it will be clear whether or not it involves the resection margin. The cervix is processed in a fashion similar to that described in Chapter 3 for the cervical conization specimen. The caudal vaginal mucosa is also stained with India ink. Like the cervix, it is also sliced into 12 pieces and embedded so that both the cephalic and caudal vaginal mucosa are present on the tissue sections. Frequently, frozen section evaluation of the vaginal resection margin is requested. Sections from each quadrant and from any suspicious areas are submitted for this evaluation. Again, the caudal mucosal margin should be inked, and the tissue section should show both the cephalic and caudal vaginal mucosa. Representative sections from the lower uterine segment, fundal endometrium, and myometrium are also submitted.

The nodes in the lymphadenectomy specimen should be labeled as left or right pelvic lymph nodes or by the specific nodal chains involved (e.g., right external iliac, left obturator). The fat should be carefully examined to remove all nodal tissue. The lymph nodes are brown-gray in color and can be smaller than a pea, which makes gross identification difficult. At least six nodes should be found in the specimen from each side of the pelvis. The extra fat should also be submitted because very small nodes are frequently found by microscopic examination. The grossly identified nodes are each divided into four pieces and placed in tissue cassettes, alternating the cut surface that is placed down (Fig. 4–37). This allows a larger area of the node to be evaluated by microscopy.

The pathology report of the radical hysterectomy and pelvic lymphadenectomy specimens should include a gross description of the tumor, including its dimensions and whether or not it extends to adjacent organs. The summary of the microscopic findings should include the histopathologic type and grade of the tumor, the depth of stromal invasion, the presence or absence of lymphovascular invasion, whether there is extension of the tumor to the vagina, parametrium, or endometrium, and the status of the resection margins. The number of lymph nodes recovered from each nodal chain and the number and size of the nodes that are involved by metastatic disease are also reported (Fig. 4–38).[151–153]

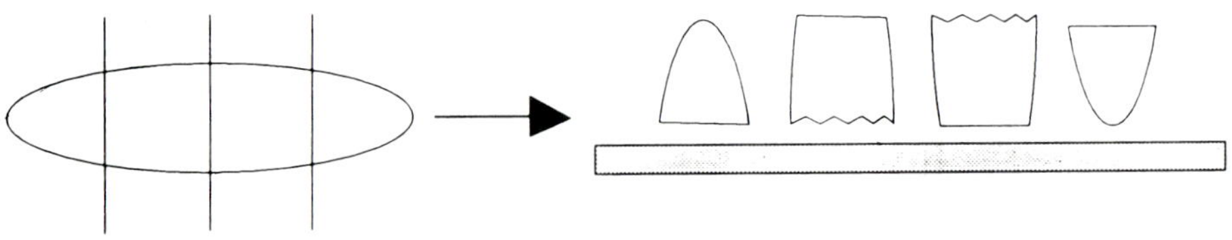

FIGURE 4-37
This is a diagram of the optimal way of processing large lymph nodes.

Radiation therapy is considered the cornerstone of therapy for patients with vaginal adenocarcinoma. Radical surgical excision has also been used in selected patients (those with a small vaginal apex or distal vaginal lesions). In one report it was suggested that the 5-year survival of patients with adenocarcinoma was better than that of patients with vaginal squamous cell carcinoma (60 versus 48 percent).[154]

Clear Cell Adenocarcinoma

Most cases of clear cell adenocarcinoma of the vagina and cervix are associated with in utero exposure to DES and other nonsteroidal estrogens prior to the 18th week of intrauterine life. The total dose of DES taken by mothers of patients who developed clear cell adenocarcinoma of the vagina or cervix was between 131 and 21,400 mg; no clear association between maternal DES dose and subsequent malignancy in the offspring has been found.[165] The incidence of clear cell carcinoma of the vagina seemed to increase incrementally after 1970 as the daughters of women who took DES during pregnancy grew older.[124] However, now that most of these women are over 40 years of age, these tumors are again rare. Most patients with DES-related clear cell adenocarcinoma of the vagina or cervix were between 18 and 24 years old at the time of diagnosis. However, this diagnosis has been made in girls as young as 7 years and in women in their early thirties.[166, 167] Abnormal vaginal bleeding or discharge is the most frequent complaint. In a few patients the diagnosis is made during evaluation of abnormal cervical or vaginal cytologic findings. In one study, 21 percent of patients with clear cell adenocarcinoma of the vagina or cervix had negative Papanicolaou smears, however.[165]

The most frequent location of clear cell adenocarcinoma is the upper third of the vagina.[166] The early lesion frequently presents as a submucosal nodule in the anterior upper vaginal wall.[167] As the tumor grows, it may ulcerate the vaginal mucosa, or it may grow as a polypoid, fungating lesion similar to the lesion described in the cervix. The histopathologic features are identical to those previously described in the cervix.

The stage of disease is the most important prognostic parameter in this disease. The 5-year survival rate for patients with clear cell adenocarcinoma of the vagina is 87 percent for stage I, 76 percent for stage II, 30 percent for stage III, and 0 percent for stage IV.[168] Patients with stage I disease have traditionally been treated by vaginectomy combined with radical hysterectomy and pelvic lymphadenectomy. Wide local excision and staging laparotomy with retroperitoneal node dissection followed by local irradiation has been suggested as an alternative treatment for patients who have stage I disease and who desire to preserve their reproductive function.[166] Patients who have stage II or III disease are treated with external and interstitial radiation. Exenteration is reserved for patients whose tumors are not controlled by radiation therapy. The results of chemotherapy in the treatment of patients with advanced or recurrent clear cell adenocarcinoma of the vagina are disappointing.

Endodermal Sinus Tumor

Endodermal sinus tumor is a germ cell tumor that rarely occurs in the vagina of infants. Cases of endodermal sinus tumor of the vagina have been called mesonephroma, mesonephric carcinoma, clear cell carcinoma, and yolk sac carcinoma.[169] The terminology is a source of confusion when reviewing the literature. Because of the rarity of this tumor, most of the literature on endodermal sinus tumor of the vagina consists of case reports and reviews.

This tumor occurs in infants under the age of 3 years. The clinical presentation is usually a bloody or blood-tinged vaginal discharge. Examination reveals a friable polypoid mass that is frequently confused with embryonal rhabdomyosarcoma (sarcoma botryoides).[170] The histopathologic appearance is identical to that of the endodermal sinus tumor of the ovary (see Chapter 10). Each tumor may have one or more of the histopathologic types, which include festoon, reticular, and solid growth patterns. The festoon pattern is one of anastomosing channels and tubules lined by cuboidal cells that have vacuolated cytoplasm and hyperchromatic nuclei. Schiller-Duval bodies identical to those found in the ovarian endodermal sinus tumor are seen. Hyaline globules are often present. These spherical bodies stain positive for PAS and contain α-fetoprotein, which is a marker for this tumor. The reticular pattern is a network of cystic spaces lined by flattened epithelial cells. Solid sheets of undifferentiated cells are also seen in some areas of the tumor. The polyvesicular pattern, which is rare in the ovary, is also rare when the endodermal sinus tumor arises in the vagina.

In the past, when infants who had endodermal sinus tumor of the vagina were treated by radiation or radical surgery, the results were poor.[171] In one report, only 3 of 13 patients treated by these modalities were alive 2 years after diagnosis.[171] More recent reports have emphasized the importance of modern multiagent chemotherapy in the management of this disease. The sensitivity of this tumor to vincristine, actinomycin-D, and cyclophosphamide has been demonstrated. A report of six patients with endodermal sinus tumor of the cervix or vagina who received chemotherapy after surgery noted that four of the six were known to be alive between 2 and 23 years after diagnosis.[170] It has been suggested that after diagnostic biopsy the use of multiagent chemotherapy may result in a complete response and the need for either no surgery or conservative surgery in cases of partial response.[169,172]

Melanoma

Melanoma of the vagina is a rare entity. According to one study it accounts for only 0.5 percent of all vaginal malignancies.[173] In another series primary melanoma of the vagina comprised 2.6 percent of all primary vaginal cancers.[174] Only 3 percent of all melanomas in women occur in the vagina.[175] In the past, primary melanoma of the vagina was not considered possible owing to the lack of pigmentation of this organ. When melanoma was found in the vagina it was considered metastatic from another site. However, Das Gupta and D'Ursa in 1964 reported the presence of melanocytes in the vagina.[176] Chung et al[174] reported that the age of patients with primary vaginal melanoma was between 37 and 72 years with a mean of 60 years. Vaginal bleeding and discharge are the common symptoms of patients who have vaginal melanoma.

The melanoma may appear as a nodule elevated above the surrounding mucosa, or it may be a nearly flat plaque. Frequently there is ulceration with an associated inflammatory response that results in a foul-smelling vaginal discharge. The lesion is often blue-black or black-brown; however, some lesions are nonpigmented, and other colors are possible.[177] The majority of primary vaginal melanomas are located in the lower third of the vagina.

Although the microscopic appearance of primary vaginal melanoma may be similar to that of melanoma at other sites, in one report of 15 cases of primary vaginal melanoma, all were of the nodular type.[178] The lesions are characteristically very cellular and exhibit marked cellular and nuclear pleomorphism (Fig. 4–40). Melanin granules are present in the cytoplasm of some of the cells. The cells may be nevoid, epithelioid, or spindle-shaped in appearance. The malignant melanocytes may migrate up into the more superficial layers of the overlying epithelium or may spread radially to the adjacent epithelium. The lateral spread can be extensive and in some cases may reach the vulva.

Most patients with primary vaginal melanoma are treated by radical excision. However, the type of surgery (conservative versus radical) or the addition of radiation therapy does not seem to affect survival. The 5-year survival rate of patients with primary vaginal melanoma is only 17.4 percent.[178] The survival rate is better for patients who have lesions smaller than 3 cm but is not influenced by the patient's age or the tumor thickness, location, or stage. Distant recurrences are as frequent as local recurrences. Once recurrence occurs,

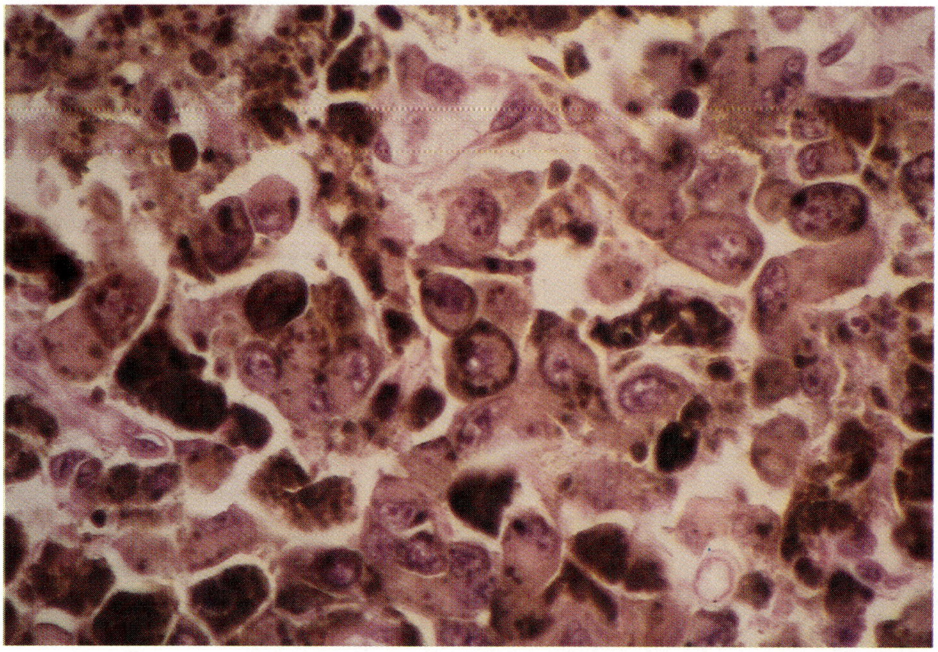

FIGURE 4–40
The cells of this melanoma are pleomorphic and contain fine to coarse melanin granules. The cells are round and epithelioid in appearance.

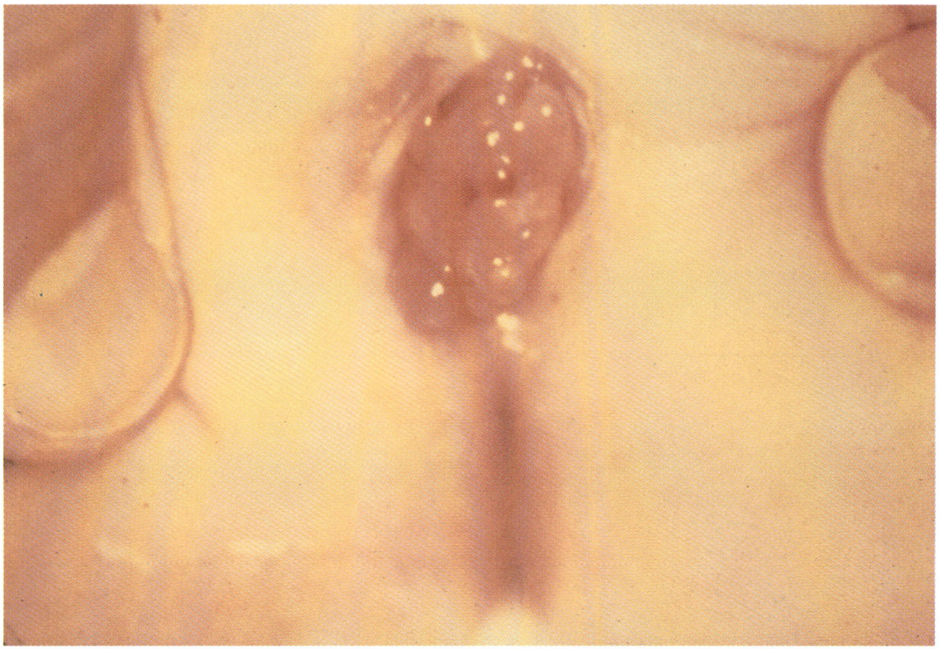

FIGURE 4-41
Multiple, coalescent, shiny, pink polypoid structures are seen protruding from this infant's vagina. This is embryonal rhabdomyosarcoma (sarcoma botryoides). (Courtesy of Dr. J. Donald Woodruff, The Johns Hopkins Hospital, Baltimore, MD.)

the prognosis is extremely poor. At present there is no effective chemotherapy for melanoma. The mean interval from recurrence to death is 8.5 months.

Embryonal Rhabdomyosarcoma (Sarcoma Botryoides)

Sarcoma botryoides is the most frequent neoplasm arising in the vagina of girls less than 5 years old. The most frequent presenting symptom is vaginal bleeding. This lesion appears as one or more polypoid tumors arising from the mucosa of the vagina. The polypoid structures are translucent and have a pink-white unblemished surface (Fig. 4–41). This tumor is composed of rhabdomyoblasts, which are round to spindle-shaped cells that have scant cytoplasm and hyperchromatic nuclei. The rhabdomyoblasts may grow in one or more patterns.[179] These have been classified as alveolar, botryoid, embryonal, and pleomorphic.[180] The polypoid appearance of the tumor gave this tumor the botryoid name. Seventy-five percent of patients who have the botryoid type of embryonal rhabdomyosarcoma have genitourinary lesions.[181] In sarcoma botryoides the primitive rhabdomyoblasts are located in a subepithelial zone known as the cambium layer of Nicholson. Fusiform cells that may or may not have cross striations typical of skeletal muscle are found within an edematous and vascular stroma below the cambium layer (Fig. 4–42). Mitotic activity is moderate. The vaginal mucosa that covers the neoplasm is normal but may show focal ulceration.

The gross appearance of sarcoma botryoides can be confused with that of endodermal sinus tumor, benign vaginal polyps, and benign rhabdomyoma. Vaginal polyps occur in women between the ages of 17 and 50 years; the median age is 35 years. Atypical cells have been noted in the stroma of benign vaginal polyps, but mitotic figures are rarely seen. A cambium layer is not present.[182]

Treatment of sarcoma botryoides in the past consisted of ultraradical and radical surgery.[183] Recent results using multiagent chemotherapy combined with less extensive surgery or radiation therapy have been promising, and this is now the preferred treatment approach.[144, 179]

Leiomyosarcoma

Leiomyosarcoma is rare but is the most common malignant mesenchymal tumor in the vagina. It accounts for 3 percent of all vaginal malignancies registered at the Swedish Cancer Registry.[184] A report from that country included five patients whose ages ranged from 31 to 69 years. The mean age of eight patients reported by Malkasian et al[185] was 42 years. The most frequent presenting symptoms were an enlarging mass, vaginal and rectal pain, and vaginal bleeding or purulent discharge. The tumor is between 0.5 and 15 cm in size and is usually firm but may be soft. The tumor margin is circumscribed in the majority of cases, but some are infiltrating.[186, 187] The lesion is composed of malignant smooth muscle cells. Tavassoli and Norris[187] reviewed a series of 60 smooth muscle tumors of the vagina and sug-

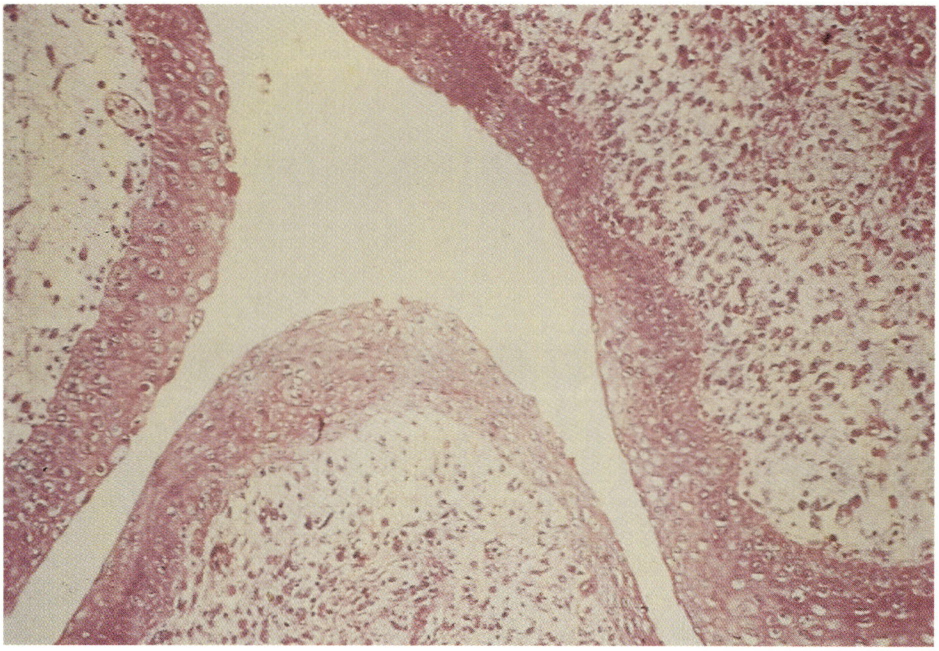

FIGURE 4-42
The microscopic view of the tumor shown in Figure 4-41 exhibits a normal squamous epithelium covering edematous polypoid stroma. Small malignant cells are seen scattered throughout the submucosal stroma. A few cells *(left)* have abundant eosinophilic cytoplasm. Some of the cells are fusiform. (Courtesy of Dr. J. Donald Woodruff, The Johns Hopkins Hospital, Baltimore, MD.)

gested that lesions that have five or more mitotic figures per 10 high power microscope fields and a moderate to marked cellular atypia should be classified as leiomyosarcoma. The cells are elongated, spindle-shaped, and arranged in interweaving bundles. The nuclei are hyperchromatic and have blunted ends and prominent nucleoli. There is moderate nuclear pleomorphism.[188] Bizarre mitotic figures may be seen. As in leiomyosarcoma of the uterus (see Chapter 6), myxoid changes may be present. If an epithelioid appearance is present it may be necessary to use immunocytochemical stains to help distinguish the smooth muscle origin from a poorly differentiated carcinoma. A leiomyosarcoma stains positive for vimentin and desmin but not for keratin or epithelial membrane antigen.

Treatment of patients with vaginal leiomyosarcoma has varied from local excision to some form of ultraradical surgery. Radiation has been occasionally used as adjunctive therapy. The recurrence rate and frequency of metastases appears to be associated with the degree of cellular atypia, the mitotic rate, and the presence or absence of an infiltrative tumor margin. It has been suggested that pelvic exenteration produces the best treatment results.[189]

Other Sarcomas

There are several less common types of primary vaginal sarcomas.[189] Carcinosarcoma can occur in the vagina. As when it arises in other structures of müllerian origin, it can be homologous or heterologous. The prognosis of primary vaginal carcinosarcoma is extremely poor. Other sarcomas that have been reported to arise in the vagina are fibrosarcoma, angiosarcoma, neurofibrosarcoma, alveolar soft-part sarcoma, hemangiopericytoma, malignant fibrous histiocytoma, and rhabdomyosarcoma of the adult variety.[189-194]

Neuroendocrine (Small Cell) Carcinoma

The small cell carcinoma of the vagina and cervix is related to the neuroendocrine small cell undifferentiated (oat cell) carcinoma that arises in the lung. As noted in the discussion of this tumor in the cervix, the tumor is extremely aggressive. Chafe reported on two patients who had small cell carcinoma of the vagina, both of whom were in their eighth decade of life.[195] They both succumbed to the disease within 1 year from diagnosis.

This tumor is composed of sheets of closely packed small cells. Most of the cells are undifferentiated. Some may have a squamoid or glandular appearance.[196] The nucleus is relatively large and the cytoplasm is scant, which leads to a high nuclear to cytoplasmic ratio. The hyperchromatic nucleus is round to elongated. Mitotic figures are abundant. Capillary-like space involvement is seen. Neurosecretory granules can be seen in the cytoplasm on electron microscopic examination.

Because there is rapid and widespread progression of this disease, it is necessary to use chemotherapy after radiation or surgery even if the

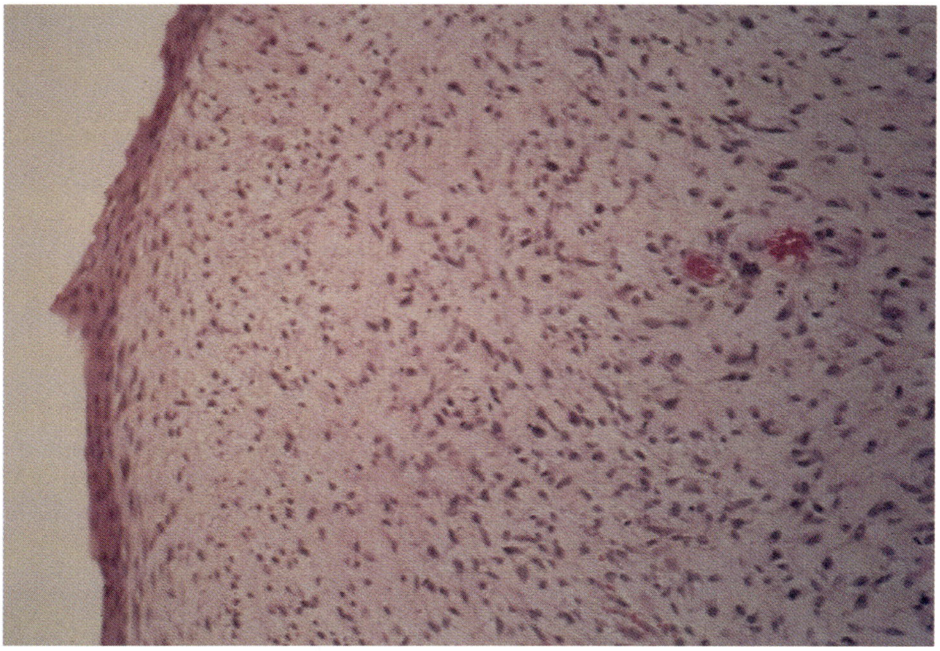

FIGURE 4–43
Normal atrophic vaginal epithelium is seen *(left)*. The submucosal stroma has been replaced by metastatic endometrial stromal sarcoma. The nuclei are dark, pleomorphic, and spindle-shaped.

tumor appears to be localized.[30] The cytotoxic agents currently known to be most active against this neoplasm are etoposide and cisplatin.

Metastatic Tumors to the Vagina

The most common tumors metastatic to the vagina arise in the cervix and endometrium (Fig. 4–43). Tumors of the rectum and ovary are next in frequency. Cases of renal cancer metastatic to the vagina have been reported. These can have a clear cell component and may be confused with clear cell carcinoma of the vagina. Breast carcinoma also metastasizes to the vagina.

Metastatic choriocarcinoma in the vagina appears as a bluish nodule that may have satellite lesions. The characteristic biphasic picture of syncytiotrophoblast and cytotrophoblast is characteristic (see Chapter 12). If the patient is known to have a choriocarcinoma, biopsy of a vaginal lesion is not necessary and should not be performed because it can result in profuse hemorrhage.

REFERENCES

1. Magos S, Ottinger M, Parker J, Dunton CJ, Hernandez E: Treatment of cervical carcinoma with ionizing irradiation using moving fields. J Natl Med Assoc 1991;83:986–990.
2. Brand E, Berek J, Hacker N: Controversies in the management of cervical adenocarcinoma. Obstet Gynecol 1988;71:261–269.
3. Hernandez E, Miyazawa K, Berenberg J: Cervical adenocarcinoma among cytologically screened and unscreened women. Am J Gynecol Health 1988;2:134–137.
4. Hopkins MP, Morley GW: A comparison of adenocarcinoma and squamous cell carcinoma of the cervix. Obstet Gynecol 1991;77:912–917.
5. Carson HJ, DeMay RM: The mode ages of women with cervical dysplasia. Obstet Gynecol 1993;82:430–434.
6. International Federation of Obstetrics and Gynecology: FIGO News. Int J Gynecol Obstet 1987;25:87–88.
7. Kolstadt P: Follow-up study of 232 patients with stage IA1 and 411 patients with stage IA2 squamous cell carcinoma of the cervix (microinvasive carcinoma). Gynecol Oncol 1989;33:265–272.
8. Morrow CP, Townsend DE: Synopsis of Gynecologic Oncology, 3rd ed. New York, John Wiley & Sons, 1987, p 112.
9. Briggs RM: Dysplasia and early neoplasia of the uterine cervix; a review. Obstet Gynecol Surv 1979;34:70–99.
10. Walker J, Bloss JD, Liao S-Y, Berman M, Bergen S, Wilczynski SP: Human papillomavirus genotype as a prognostic indicator in carcinoma of the uterine cervix. Obstet Gynecol 1989;74:781–785.
11. McIndoe WA, McLean M, Jones RW, Mullins PR: The invasive potential of carcinoma in situ of the cervix. Obstet Gynecol 1984;64:451–458.
12. Genadry R, Olson J, Parmley T, Woodruff JD: The morphology of the earliest invasive cell in low genital tract epidermoid neoplasia. Obstet Gynecol 1978:51:718–722.
13. Sedlis A, Sall S, Tsukada Y, Park RC, Mangan C, Shingleton H, Blessing JA: Microinvasive carcinoma of the uterine cervix: A clinical-pathologic study. Am J Obstet Gynecol 1979;133:64–74.
14. Leman MH, Benson WL, Kurman RJ, Park RC: Microinvasive carcinoma of the cervix. Obstet Gynecol 1976; 48:571–578.
15. Simon NL, Gore H, Shingleton HM, Seng-Jaw S, Orr JW, Hatch KD: Study of superficially invasive carcinoma of the cervix. Obstet Gynecol 1986;68:19–24.
16. Burghardt E: Diagnostic and prognostic criteria in cervical microcarcinoma. Clin Oncol 1982;1:323–333.
17. Fox H: Stages in the evolution of squamous cell carcinoma of the uterine cervix: A critique of the concepts of "dysplasia" and "cancer." Pathol Res Pract 1985;180:665–669.
18. Benson WL, Norris HJ: A critical review of the frequency of lymph node metastasis and death from microinvasive carcinoma of the cervix. Obstet Gynecol 1977;49:632–638.

19. Jordan JA, Sharp F, Singer A (eds): Preclinical Neoplasia of the Cervix: Proceedings of the Ninth Study Group of the Royal College of Obstetricians and Gynaecologists. London, Royal College of Obstetricians and Gynaecologists, 1982.
20. Mestwerdt G: Die Frühdiagnose des Kollumkarzinoms. Zentralbl Gynäkol 1947;69:198–202.
21. Maiman MA, Fruchter RG, DiMaio TM, Boyce JG: Superficially invasive squamous carcinoma of the cervix. Obstet Gynecol 1988;72:399–403.
22. Burghardt E, Holzer E: Diagnosis and treatment of microinvasive carcinoma of the cervix uteri. Obstet Gynecol 1977;49:641–653.
23. Van Nagell JR, Greenwell N, Powell DF, Donaldson ES, Hanson MB, Gay EC: Microinvasive carcinoma of the cervix. Obstet Gynecol 1983;145:981–991.
24. Copeland LJ, Silva EG, Gershenson DM, Morris M, Young DC, Wharton JT: Superficially invasive squamous cell carcinoma of the cervix. Gynecol Oncol 1992;45:307–312.
25. Tsukamoto N, Kaku T, Matsukuma K, Matsuyama T, Kamura T, Saito T, Suenaga T: The problem of stage IA (FIGO, 1985) carcinoma of the uterine cervix. Gynecol Oncol 1989;34:1–6.
26. Burghardt E, Girardi F, Lahousen M, Pickel H, Tamussino K: Microinvasive carcinoma of the uterine cervix (International Federation of Gynecology and Obstetrics stage IA). Cancer 1991;67:1037–1045.
27. Nelson JH, Averette H, Richart RM: Detection, diagnostic evaluation and treatment of dysplasia and early carcinoma of the cervix. Cancer 1975;25:134–151.
28. Ullery JC, Boutselis JG, Botschner AC: Microinvasive carcinoma of the cervix. Obstet Gynecol 1965;26:866–875.
29. Creasman WT, Parker RT: Microinvasive carcinoma of the cervix. Clin Obstet Gynecol 1973;16:261–275.
30. Park RC, Patow WE, Rogers RE, Zimmerman EA: Treatment of stage I carcinoma of the cervix. Obstet Gynecol 1973;41:117–122.
31. Roche WD, Norris HJ: Microinvasive carcinoma of the cervix: The significance of lymphatic invasion and confluent patterns of stromal growth. Cancer 1975;36:180–186.
32. Seski JC, Murray RA, Morley G: Microinvasive carcinoma of the cervix: Definition, histologic analysis, late results of treatment. Obstet Gynecol 1977;50:410–414.
33. Lohe KJ: Early squamous cell carcinoma of the uterine cervix: I. Definition and histology. Gynecol Oncol 1978; 6:10–30.
34. Sevin B-U, Nadji M, Averette HE, Hilsenbeck S, Smith D, Lampe B: Microinvasive carcinoma of the cervix. Cancer 1992;70:2121–2128.
35. Dunton CJ, Rebane BA, Hernandez E: Treatment of early invasive (IA) and advanced-stage (IIB-IVA) cervical carcinoma. Am J Gynecol Health 1990;4:192–194.
36. Morris M, Mitchell MF, Silva EG, Copeland LJ, Gershenson DM: Cervical conization as definitive therapy of early invasive squamous carcinoma of the cervix. Gynecol Oncol 1993;51:193–196.
37. Jones EB, Mercer GO, Lewis JL Jr, Rubin SC, Hoskins WJ: Early invasive carcinoma of the cervix. Gynecol Oncol 1993;51:26–32.
38. Imachi M, Tsukamoto N, Matsuyama T, Nakano H: Pulmonary metastasis from carcinoma of the uterine cervix. Gynecol Oncol 1989;33:189–192.
39. Kaseki H, Yasui K, Niwa K, Mizuno K, Inoue T, Ota M: Hepatic resection for squamous cell carcinoma from the uterine cervix. Gynecol Oncol 1992;44:284–287.
40. Averette HE, Dudan RC, Ford JH: Exploratory ceilotomy for surgical staging of cervical cancer. Am J Obstet Gynecol 1972;113:1090–1096.
41. Averette HE, Donato DM, Lovecchio JL, Sevin B-U: Surgical staging of gynecologic malignancies. Cancer 1987; 60:2010–2020.
42. Broders AC: Carcinoma: Grading and practical application. Arch Pathol Lab Med 1926;2:376–381.
43. Warren S: The grading of carcinoma of the cervix uteri as checked at autopsy. Arch Pathol 1931;12:783–786.
44. Martzloff KH: Carcinoma of the cervix uteri: A pathological and clinical study with particular reference to the relative malignancy of the neoplastic process as indicated by the predominant type of cancer cells. Bull Johns Hopkins Hosp 1923;34:141–149.
45. Wentz WB, Regan JW: Survival in cervical cancer with respect to cell type. Cancer 1959;12:384–388.
46. Ng APB, Atkin NB: Histological cell types and DNA value in the prognosis of squamous cell cancer of the uterine cervix. Br J Cancer 1973;28:322–331.
47. Zaino RJ, Ward S, Delgado G, Bundy B, Gore H, Fetter G, Ganjei P, Frauenhoffer E: Histopathologic predictors of the behavior of surgically treated Stage IB squamous cell carcinoma of the cervix. Cancer 1992;69:1750–1758.
48. Reagan JW: Microscopic grading and radiosensitivity. Clinical Conference Monograph: Carcinoma of the Uterine Cervix, Endometrium and Ovary. Houston, M.D. Anderson Hospital and Tumor Institute, 1960, pp 31–40.
49. Crissman JD, Makuch R, Budhraja M: Histopathologic grading of squamous cell carcinoma of the uterine cervix. Cancer 1985;55:1590–1596.
50. Nguyen HA, Sevin B-U, Averette HE, Ganjei P, Perras J, Ramos R, Angioli R, Donato D, Penalver M: The role of DNA index as a prognostic factor in early cervical carcinoma. Gynecol Oncol 1993;50:54–59.
51. Oka K, Nakano T, Arai T: c-*erb*B-2 oncoprotein expression is associated with poor prognosis in squamous cell carcinoma of the cervix. Cancer 1994;73:668–671.
52. Walker J, Bloss JD, Liao S-Y, Berman M, Bergen S, Wilczynski SP: Human papillomavirus genotype as a prognostic indicator in carcinoma of the uterine cervix. Obstet Gynecol 1989;74:781–785.
53. Riou G, Jeannel D, Bourhis J, Favre M, Lê M, Orth G: High risk of distant metastasis for early-stage invasive cervical cancers with HPV-negative status and c-*myc* gene overexpression. Proc Am Soc Clin Oncol 1991;10:184.
54. Abu-Ghazaleh S, Johnston W, Creasman WT: The significance of peritoneal cytology in patients with carcinoma of the cervix. Gynecol Oncol 1984;17:139–148.
55. Prempree T, Patanaphan V, Sewchand W, Scott RM: The influence of patients' age and tumor grade on the prognosis of carcinoma of the cervix. Cancer 1983;51:1764–1771.
56. Meanwell CA, Kelly KA, Wilson S, Roginski C, Woodman C, Griffiths R, Blackledge G: Young age as a prognostic factor in cervical cancer: Analysis of population based data from 10022 cases. Br Med J 1988;296:386–391.
57. Artman LE, Hoskins WJ, Bibro MC, Heller PB, Weiser EB, Barnhill DR, Park RC: Radical hysterectomy and pelvic lymphadenectomy for stage IB carcinoma of the cervix: 21 years experience. Gynecol Oncol 1987;28:8–13.
58. Hoskins WJ, Ford JH, Lutz MH, Averette HE: Radical hysterectomy and pelvic lymphadenectomy for the management of early invasive cancer of the cervix. Gynecol Oncol 1976;4:272–290.
59. Sutton GP, Bundy BN, Delgado G, Sevin B-U, Creasman WT, Major FJ, Zaino R: Ovarian metastases in stage IB carcinoma of the cervix: A Gynecologic Oncology Group study. Am J Obstet Gynecol 1992;166:50–53.
60. Delgado G, Bundy BN, Fowler WC Jr, Stehman FB, Sevin B, Creasman WT, Major F, DiSaia P, Zaino R: A prospective surgical pathological study of stage I squamous carcinoma of the cervix: A Gynecologic Oncology Group study. Gynecol Oncol 1989;35:314–320.
61. Gallion HH, van Nagell JR, Donaldson ES, Hanson MB, Powell DE, Maruyama Y, Yoneda J: Combined radiation therapy and extrafascial hysterectomy in the treatment of stage IB barrel-shaped cervical cancer. Cancer 1985; 56:262–265.
62. Durrance FY, Fletcher GH, Rutledge FN: Analysis of central recurrent disease in stages I and II squamous cell carcinomas of the cervix on intact uterus. AJR 1969;106:831–838.

63. Jampolis S, Andras J, Fletcher GH: Analysis of sites and causes of failure of irradiation in invasive squamous cell carcinoma of the intact uterine cervix. Radiology 1975;115:681–685.
64. Andras AJ, Fletcher GH, Wharton JT: Indications for adjunctive conservative extrafascial hysterectomy in selected cases of carcinoma of the uterine cervix. AJR 1975; 123:91–99.
65. Bleker OP, Ketting BW, van Wayjen-Eecen B, Kloosterman GJ: The significance of microscopic involvement of the parametrium and/or pelvic lymph nodes in cervical cancer stages IB and IIA. Gynecol Oncol 1983;16:56–62.
66. Larson DM, Stringer CA, Copeland LJ, Gershenson DM, Malone JM Jr, Rutledge FN: Stage IB cervical carcinoma treated with radical hysterectomy and pelvic lymphadenectomy: Role of adjuvant radiotherapy. Obstet Gynecol 1987;69:378–381.
67. Soisson AP, Soper JT, Clarke-Pearson D, Berchuck A, Montana G, Creasman WT: Adjuvant radiotherapy following radical hysterectomy for patients with stage IB and IIA cervical cancer. Gynecol Oncol 1990;37:390–395.
68. Heller PB, Malfetano JH, Bundy BN, Barnhill DR, Okagaki T: Clinical-pathologic study of stage IIB, III, and IVA carcinoma of the cervix: Extended diagnostic evaluation for paraaortic node metastasis: A Gynecologic Oncology Group study. Gynecol Oncol 1990;38:425–430.
69. Burke TW, Heller PB, Hoskins WJ, Weiser EB, Nash JD, Park RC: Evaluation of the scalene lymph nodes in primary and recurrent cervical carcinoma. Gynecol Oncol 1987;28:312–317.
70. Stehman FB, Bundy BN, Hanjani P, Fowler WC, Abdulhay G, Whitney CW: Biopsy of the scalene fat pad in carcinoma of the cervix uteri metastatic to the periaortic lymph nodes. Surg Gynecol Obstet 1987;165:503–506.
71. Lovecchio JL, Averette HE, Donato D, Bell J: 5-year survival of patients with periaortic nodal metastases in clinical stage IB and IIA cervical carcinoma. Gynecol Oncol 1989;34:43–45.
72. Terada KY, Morley GW, Roberts JA: Stage IB carcinoma of the cervix with lymph node metastases. Gynecol Oncol 1988;31:389–395.
73. Potter ME, Alvarez RD, Gay FL, Shingleton HM, Soong S-J, Hatch KD: Optimal therapy for pelvic recurrence after radical hysterectomy for early-stage cervical cancer. Gynecol Oncol 1990;37:74–77.
74. Heller PB, Barnhill DR, Mayer AR, Fontaine TP, Hoskins WJ, Park RC: Cervical carcinoma found incidentally in a uterus removed for benign indications. Obstet Gynecol 1986;67:167–190.
75. Orr JW, Ball C, Soong SJ, Hatch KD, Partidge EE, Austin JM: Surgical treatment of women found to have invasive cervix cancer at the time of total hysterectomy. Obstet Gynecol 1986;68:353–356.
76. Hopkins MP, Peter WA, Anderson W, Morley GW: Invasive cervical cancer treated initially by standard hysterectomy. Gynecol Oncol 1990;36:7–12.
77. Barber HRK, Pece GV, Brunschwig A: Operative management of patients previously operated upon for a benign lesion with cervical cancer as a surprise finding. Am J Obstet Gynecol 1968;101:959–965.
78. Green TH, Morse WJ: Management of invasive cervical cancer following inadvertent simple hysterectomy. Obstet Gynecol 1969;33:763–769.
79. Andras EJ, Fletcher GH, Rutledge F: Radiotherapy of carcinoma of the cervix following simple hysterectomy. Am J Obstet Gynecol 1973;115:647–655.
79a. Hopkins MP, Morley GW: The prognosis and management of cervical cancer associated with pregnancy. Obstet Gynecol 1992;80:9–13.
80. Hacker NF, Berek JS, Lagasse LD: Carcinoma of the cervix associated with pregnancy. Obstet Gynecol 1982;59: 735–747.
81. Lee RB, Neglia W, Park RC: Cervical carcinoma in pregnancy. Obstet Gynecol 1981;58:584–589.
81a. Greer BE, Easterling TR, McLennan DA, Benedetti TJ, Cain JM, Figge DC, Tamimi HK, Jackson JC: Fetal and maternal considerations in the management of stage I-B cervical cancer during pregnancy. Gynecol Oncol 1989; 34:61–65.
82. Davis JR, Moon LB: Increased incidence of adenocarcinoma of the uterine cervix. Obstet Gynecol 1975;45:79–83.
83. Weiss RJ, Lucas WE: Adenocarcinoma of the uterine cervix. Cancer 1986;57:1996–2001.
84. Saigo PE, Cain JM, Kim WS, Gaynor JJ, Johnson K, Lewis JL Jr: Prognostic factors in adenocarcinoma of the cervix. Cancer 1986;57:1584–1593.
85. Brinton LA, Herrero R, Reeves W, de Britton RC, Gaitan E, Tenorio F: Risk factors for cervical cancer by histology. Gynecol Oncol 1993;51:301–306.
86. Smotkin D, Berek JS, Fu YS: Human papillomavirus deoxyribonucleic acid in adenocarcinoma and adenosquamous carcinoma of the uterine cervix. Obstet Gynecol 1986;68:241–244.
87. Maier RC, Norris HJ: Coexistence of cervical intraepithelial neoplasia with primary adenocarcinoma of the cervix. Obstet Gynecol 1980;56:361–364.
88. Miller BE, Flax SD, Arheart K, Photopulos G: The presentation of adenocarcinoma of the uterine cervix. Cancer 1993;72:1281–1285.
89. Teshima S, Shimosato Y, Kasamatsu T, Ohmi K, Uei Y: Early stage adenocarcinoma of the uterine cervix. Cancer 1985;56:167–172.
90. Hurt GW, Silverberg SG, Frable WJ, Belgrad R, Crooks LD: Adenocarcinoma of the cervix: histopathologic and clinical features. Am J Obstet Gynecol 1977;129:304–315.
91. Benoit AG, Krepart GV, Lotocki RJ: Results of prior cytologic screening in patients with a diagnosis of Stage I carcinoma of the cervix. Am J Obstet Gynecol 1984; 148:690–694.
92. Matsuma K, Tsukamoto N, Kaku T, Matsumura M, Toki N, Toh N, Nakano H: Early adenocarcinoma of the uterine cervix: Its histologic and immunohistologic study. Gynecol Oncol 1989;35:38–43.
93. Kaspar H, Dinh TV, Doherty MG, Hannigan EV, Kumar D: Clinical implications of tumor volume measurement in stage I adenocarcinoma of the cervix. Obstet Gynecol 1993;81:296–300.
93a. Coppleson M: Early invasive squamous and adenocarcinoma of cervix: (FIGO stage IA) clinical features and management. *In* Coppleson M (ed): Gynecologic Oncology: Fundamental Principles and Clinical Practice. London, Churchill Livingstone, 1992, p 644.
94. Hopkins MP, Schmidt RW, Roberts JA, Morley GW: Gland cell carcinoma (adenocarcinoma) of the cervix. Obstet Gynecol 1988;72:789–795.
95. Davidson SE, Symonds RP, Lamont D, Watson ER: Does adenocarcinoma of uterine cervix have a worse prognosis than squamous carcinoma when treated by radiotherapy? Gynecol Oncol 1989;33:23–26.
96. Kjorstad KE, Bond B: Stage IB adenocarcinoma of the cervix: Metastatic potential and patterns of dissemination. Am J Obstet Gynecol 1984;150:297–299.
97. Berek JS, Hacker NF, Fu YS, Sokale JR, Leuchter RC, Lagasse LD: Adenocarcinoma of the uterine cervix: Histologic variables associated with lymph node metastasis and survival. Obstet Gynecol 1985;65:46–52.
98. McLellan R, Dillon MB, Woodruff JD, Heatley GJ, Fields A, Rosenshein NB: Long-term follow-up of stage I cervical adenocarcinoma treated by radical surgery. Gynecol Oncol 1994;52:253–259.
99. Prempree T, Amornmarn R, Wizenberg MJ: A therapeutic approach to primary adenocarcinoma of the cervix. Cancer 1985;56:1264–1268.
100. Berek JS, Castaldo TW, Hacker NF, Petrilli ES, Lagasse LD, Moore JG: Adenocarcinoma of the uterine cervix. Cancer 1981;48:2734–2741.

101. Young RH, Scully RE: Villoglandular papillary adenocarcinoma of the uterine cervix. Cancer 1989;63:1773–1779.
102. Glücksman A, Cherry CP: Incidence, histology, and response to radiation of mixed carcinomas (adenocanthomas) of the uterine cervix. Cancer 1956;9:971–979.
103. Julian CG, Daikoku NH, Gillespie A: Adenoepidermoid and adenosquamous carcinoma of the uterus. Am J Obstet Gynecol 1977;128:106–116.
104. Fu YS, Reagan JW, Hsiu JG, Storaasli JP, Wentz B: Adenocarcinoma and mixed carcinoma of the cervix. Cancer 1966;49:2560–2570.
105. Gallup DG, Harper RH, Stock RJ: Poor prognosis in patients with adenosquamous cell carcinoma of the cervix. Obstet Gynecol 1985;65:416–422.
106. Dougherty CM, Cotten N: Mixed squamous-cell and adenocarcinoma of the cervix. Cancer 1964;17:1132–1143.
107. Alva J, Lauchlan SC: The histogenesis of mixed cervical carcinomas. Am J Clin Pathol 1975;64:20–25.
108. Wheeless CR, Graham R, Graham JB: Prognosis and treatment of adenoepidermoid carcinoma of the cervix. Obstet Gynecol 1970;35:928–932.
109. Littman P, Clement PB, Henriksen B, Wang CC, Robboy SJ, Taft PD, Ulfelder H, Scully RE: Glassy cell carcinoma of the cervix. Cancer 1976;37:2238–2246.
110. Maier RC, Norris HJ: Glassy cell carcinoma of the cervix. Obstet Gynecol 1982;60:219–224.
111. Ulbright TM, Gersell DJ: Glassy cell carcinoma of the uterine cervix. Cancer 1983;51:2255–2263.
112. Richard L, Guralnick M, Ferenczy A: Ultrastructure of glassy cell carcinoma of the cervix. Diagn Gynecol Obstet 1981;3:31–38.
113. Paulsen SM, Hansen KC, Nielsen VT: Glassy-cell carcinoma of the cervix: Case report with a light and electron microscopy study. Ultrastruct Pathol 1980;1:377–384.
114. Zaino RJ, Nahas WA, Mortel R: Glassy cell carcinoma of the uterine cervix. Arch Pathol Lab Med 1982;106:250–254.
115. Paalman RJ, Counsellor VS: Cylindroma of the cervix with procidentia. Am J Obstet Gynecol 1949;58:184–187.
116. Hoskins WJ, Averette HE, Ng ABP, Yon JL: Adenoid cystic carcinoma of the cervix uteri: Report of six cases and review of the literature. Gynecol Oncol 1979;7:371–384.
117. Ferry JA, Scully RE: "Adenoid cystic" carcinoma and adenoid basal carcinoma of the uterine cervix. Am J Surg Pathol 1988;12:134–144.
118. Dinh TV, Woodruff JD: Adenoid cystic and adenoid basal carcinomas of the cervix. Obstet Gynecol 1985;65:705–709.
119. Miles PA, Norris HJ: Adenoid cystic carcinoma of the cervix. Obstet Gynecol 1970;38:103–110.
120. Shingleton H, Lawrence WD, Gore H: Cervical carcinoma with adenoid cystic pattern. Cancer 1977;40:1112–1121.
121. Prempree T, Villasanta U, Tang C-K: Management of adenoid cystic carcinoma of the uterine cervix (cylindroma). Cancer 1980;46:1631–1635.
122. Baggish MS, Woodruff JD: Adenoid-basal carcinoma of the cervix. Obstet Gynecol 1966;28:213–218.
123. Hart WR, Norris HJ: Mesonephric adenocarcinomas of the cervix. Cancer 1972;29:106–113.
124. Herbst AL, Cole P, Norusis MJ, Welch WR, Scully RE: Epidemiologic aspects and factors related to survival in 384 registry cases of clear cell adenocarcinoma of the vagina and cervix. Am J Obstet Gynecol 1979;135:876–886.
125. Kaminski PF, Maier RC: Clear cell adenocarcinoma of the cervix unrelated to diethylstilbestrol exposure. Obstet Gynecol 1983;62:720–727.
126. Rombaut RP, Charles D, Murphy A: Adenocarcinoma of the cervix. Cancer 1966;19:891–900.
127. Hurt WG, Silverberg SG, Frable WJ, Belgrad R, Crooks LD: Adenocarcinoma of the cervix: Histopathologic and clinical features. Am J Obstet Gynecol 1977;129:304–315.
128. Silverberg SG, Hurt WG: Minimal deviation adenocarcinoma ("adenoma malignum") of the cervix: A reappraisal. Am J Obstet Gynecol 1975;121:971–975.
129. Kaminski PF, Norris HJ: Coexistence of ovarian neoplasms and endocervical adenocarcinoma. Obstet Gynecol 1984;64:553–556.
130. LiVolsi VA, Merino MJ, Schwartz PE: Coexistent endocervical adenocarcinoma and mucinous adenocarcinoma of ovary: A clinicopathologic study of four cases. Int J Gynecol Pathol 1983;1:391–402.
131. Kaminski PF, Norris HJ: Minimal deviation carcinoma (adenoma malignum) of the cervix. Int J Gynecol Pathol 1983;2:141–152.
132. Ackerman LL: Verrucous carcinoma of the oral cavity. Surgery 1948;23:670–678.
133. Okagaki T, Clark BA, Zachow KR, Twiggs LB, Ostrow RB, Pass RB, Faras AJ: Presence of human papillomavirus in verrucous carcinoma (Ackerman) of the vagina. Arch Pathol Lab Med 1984;108:567–570.
134. Rando RF, Sedlacek TV, Hunt J, Jenson AB, Kurman RJ, Lancaster WD: Verrucous carcinoma of the vulva associated with an unusual type 6 human papillomavirus. Obstet Gynecol 1986;67:70S–75S.
135. Raheja A, Katz DA, Dermer MS: Verrucous carcinoma of the endocervix. Obstet Gynecol 1983;62:535–538.
136. Degefu S, O'Quinn AG, Lacey CG, Merkel M, Barnard DE: Verrucous carcinoma of the cervix: A report of two cases and literature review. Gynecol Oncol 1986;25:37–47.
137. Sheets EE, Berman ML, Hrountas CK, Liao SY, DiSaia PJ: Surgically treated, early-stage neuroendocrine small-cell cervical carcinoma. Obstet Gynecol 1988;71:10–14.
138. van Nagell JR, Powell DE, Gallion HH, Elliot DG, Donaldson ES, Carpenter AE, Higgins RV, Kryscio R, Pavlik EJ: Small cell carcinoma of the uterine cervix. Cancer 1988;62:1586–1593.
139. Abell MR, Ramirez JA: Sarcomas and carcinosarcomas of the uterine cervix. Cancer 1973;31:1176–1192.
140. Rotmensch J, Rosenshein NB, Woodruff JD: Cervical sarcoma: A review. Obstet Gynecol Surv 1983;38:456–460.
141. Jaffe R, Altaras M, Bernheim J, Ben Aderet N: Endocervical stromal sarcoma: A case report. Gynecol Oncol 1985;22:105–108.
142. Miyazawa K, Hernandez E: Cervical carcinosarcoma: A case report. Gynecol Oncol 1986;23:376–380.
143. Daya DA, Scully RE: Sarcoma botryoides of the uterine cervix in young women: A clinicopathological study of 13 cases. Gynecol Oncol 1988;29:290–304.
144. Brand E, Berek JS, Nieberg RK, Hacker NF: Rhabdomyosarcoma of the uterine cervix. Cancer 1987;60:1552–1560.
145. Rosenberg SA, Diamond HD, Jaslowitz B, Craver LF: Lymphosarcoma: A review of 1269 cases. Medicine 1961;40:31–84.
146. Andrews SJ, Hernandez E, Woods J, Cook B: Burkitt's-like lymphoma presenting as a gynecologic tumor. Gynecol Oncol 1988;30:131–136.
147. Muntz HG, Ferry JA, Flynn D, Fuller AF, Tarraza HM: Stage IE primary malignant lymphomas of the uterine cervix. Cancer 1991:68:2023–2032.
148. Way S: Carcinoma metastatic in the cervix. Gynecol Oncol 1980;9:298–302.
149. Korhonen M, Stenbäck F: Adenocarcinoma metastatic to the uterine cervix. Gynecol Obstet Invest 1984;17:57–65.
150. Grimard L, Genest P, Girard A, Gerig L, Prefontaine M, Drouin P, Nair RC, Stats M: Prognostic significance of endometrial extension in carcinoma of the cervix. Gynecol Oncol 1988;31:301–309.
151. Burghardt E, Pickel H, Haas J, Lahousen M: Prognostic factors and operative treatment of stages IB and IIb cervical cancer. Am J Obstet Gynecol 1987;156:988–996.
152. Inoue T, Chihara T, Morita K: The prognostic significance of the size of the largest nodes in metastatic carcinoma from the uterine cervix. Gynecol Oncol 1984;19:187–193.
153. Inoue T, Morita K: The prognostic significance of number of positive nodes in cervical carcinoma stages IB, IIA, and IIB. Cancer 1990;65:1923–1927.
154. Ball HG, Berman ML: Management of primary vaginal carcinoma. Gynecol Oncol 1982;14:154–163.

155. Frick HC, Jacox HW, Taylor HC: Primary carcinoma of the vagina. Am J Obstet Gynecol 1968;101:695–703.
156. Benedet JL, Murphy KL, Fairly RN, Boyes DA: Primary invasive carcinoma of the vagina. Obstet Gynecol 1983;62:715–719.
157. Johnston GA, Klotz J, Boutselis JG: Primary invasive carcinoma of the vagina. Surg Gynecol Obstet 1983;156:34–40.
158. Pride GL, Buchler DA: Carcinoma of the vagina 10 or more years following pelvic irradiation therapy. Am J Obstet Gynecol 1977;127:513–517.
159. Spirtos NM, Doshi BP, Kapp DS, Teng N: Radiation therapy for primary squamous cell carcinoma of the vagina: Stanford University experience. Gynecol Oncol 1989;35:20–26.
160. Gallup DG, Talledo E, Shah KJ, Hayes C: Invasive squamous cell carcinoma of the vagina: A 14-year study. Obstet Gynecol 1987;69:782–785.
161. Rubin SC, Young J, Mikuta JJ: Squamous carcinoma of the vagina: Treatment, complications, and long-term follow-up. Gynecol Oncol 1985;20:346–353.
162. Kucera H, Vavra N: Radiation management of primary carcinoma of the vagina: Clinical and histopathological variables associated with survival. Gynecol Oncol 1991;40:12–16.
163. Peters WA, Kumar NB, Morley GW: Carcinoma of the vagina. Cancer 1985;55:892–897.
164. Rhatigan RM, Mojadidi Q: Adenosquamous carcinomas of the vulva and vagina. Am J Clin Pathol 1973;59:208–217.
165. Herbst AL, Robboy SJ, Scully RE, Poskanzer DC: Clear-cell adenocarcinoma of the vagina and cervix in girls: Analysis of 170 registry cases. Am J Obstet Gynecol 1974;119:713–724.
166. Senekjian EK, Frey KW, Anderson D, Herbst AL: Local therapy in stage I clear cell adenocarcinoma of the vagina. Cancer 1987;60:1319–1324.
167. Hanselaar AGJM, Van Leusen NDM, De Wilde PCM, Vooijs GP: Clear cell adenocarcinoma of the vagina and cervix. Cancer 1991;67:1971–1978.
168. Herbst AL, Norusis MJ, Rosenow PJ, Welch WR, Scully RE: An analysis of 346 cases of clear cell adenocarcinoma of the vagina and cervix with an emphasis on recurrence and survival. Gynecol Oncol 1979;7:111–122.
169. Andersen WA, Sabio H, Durso N, Mills SE, Levein M, Underwood PB: Endodermal sinus tumor of the vagina. Cancer 1985;56:1025–1027.
170. Copeland LJ, Sneige N, Ordonez NG, Hancock KC, Gershenson DM, Saul PB, Kavanagh JJ: Endodermal sinus tumor of the vagina and cervix. Cancer 1985;55:2558–2565.
171. Allyn DL, Silverberg SG, Salzberg AM: Endodermal sinus tumor of the vagina. Cancer 1971;27:1231–1238.
172. Collins HS, Burke TW, Heller PB, Olson TA, Woodward JE, Park RC: Endodermal sinus tumor of the infant vagina treated exclusively by chemotherapy. Obstet Gynecol 1989;73:507–509.
173. Sulak P, Barnhill D, Heller P, Weiser E, Hoskins W, Park R, Woodward J: Nonsquamous cancer of the vagina. Gynecol Oncol 1988;29:309–320.
174. Chung AF, Casey MJ, Flannery JT, Woodruff JM, Lewis JL: Malignant melanoma of the vagina: Report of 19 cases. Obstet Gynecol 1980;55:720–727.
175. Ariel IM: Malignant melanoma of the female genital system: A report of 48 patients and review of the literature. J Surg Oncol 1981;16:371–383.
176. Das Gupta T, D'Ursa J: Melanoma of the female genitalia. Surg Gynecol Obstet 1964;119:1074–1078.
177. Laufe LE, Bernstein ED: Primary malignant melanoma of the vagina. Obstet Gynecol 1971;37:148–154.
178. Reid GC, Schmidt RW, Roberts JA, Hopkins MP, Barrett RJ, Morley GW: Primary melanoma of the vagina: A clinicopathologic analysis. Obstet Gynecol 1989;74:190–199.
179. Copeland LJ, Gershenson DM, Saul PB, Sniege N, Stringer A, Edwards CL: Sarcoma botryoides of the female genital tract. Obstet Gynecol 1985;66:262–266.
180. Horn RC, Enterline HT: Rhabdomyosarcoma: A clinicopathological study and classification of 39 cases. Cancer 1958;11:181–199.
181. Maurer HM, Moon T, Donaldson M, Fernandez C, Gehan EA, Hammond D, Hays DM, Lawrence W, Newton W, Ragab A, Raney B, Soule EH, Sutow WW, Tefft M: The intergroup rhabdomyosarcoma study. Cancer 1977;40:2015–2026.
182. Norris HJ, Taylor HB: Polyps of the vagina. Cancer 1966;19:227–232.
183. Hilgers RD, Malkasian GD, Soule EH: Embryonal rhabdomyosarcoma (botryoid type) of the vagina. Am J Obstet Gynecol 1970;107:484–502.
184. Rastogi BL, Bergman B, Angervall L: Primary leiomyosarcoma of the vagina: A study of five cases. Gynecol Oncol 1984;18:77–86.
185. Malkasian GD, Welch JS, Soule EH: Primary leiomyosarcoma of the vagina. Am J Obstet Gynecol 1963;86:730–736.
186. Davos I, Abell MR: Sarcomas of the vagina. Obstet Gynecol 1976;47:342–350.
187. Tavassoli FA, Norris HJ: Smooth muscle tumors of the vagina. Obstet Gynecol 1979;53:689–693.
188. Tobon H, Murphy AI, Salazar H: Primary leiomyosarcoma of the vagina. Cancer 1973;32:450–457.
189. Peters WA III, Kumar NB, Andersen WA, Morley GW: Primary sarcoma of the adult vagina: A clinicopathologic study. Obstet Gynecol 1985;65:699–704.
190. Chang H-C, Hsueh S, Ho Y-S, Chang M-Y, Soong Y-K: Alveolar soft part sarcoma of the vagina: A case report. J Reprod Med 1994;39:121–125.
191. Tohya T, Katabuchi H, Fukuma K, Fujisaki S, Okamura H: Angiosarcoma of the vagina: A light and electronmicroscopy study. Acta Obstet Gynecol Scand 1991;70:169–172.
192. Chan WWY, SenGupta SK: Postirradiation angiosarcoma of the vaginal vault. Arch Pathol Lab Med 1991;115:527–528.
193. Buscema J, Rosenshein NB, Taqi F, Woodruff JD: Vaginal hemangiopericytoma: A histopathologic and ultrastructural evaluation. Obstet Gynecol 1985;66:82S–85S.
194. Webb MJ, Symmonds RE, Weiland LH: Malignant fibrous histiocytoma of the vagina. Am J Obstet Gynecol 1974;119:190–192.
195. Chafe W: Neuroepithelial small cell carcinoma of the vagina. Cancer 1989;64:1948–1951.
196. Ulich TR, Liao S-, Layfield L, Romansky S, Cheng L, Lewin KJ: Endocrine and tumor differentiation markers in poorly differentiated small-cell carcinoids of the cervix and vagina. Arch Pathol Lab Med 1986;110:1054–1057.

5

Benign Conditions of the Uterus

Paul F. Kaminski / Edward S. Podczaski

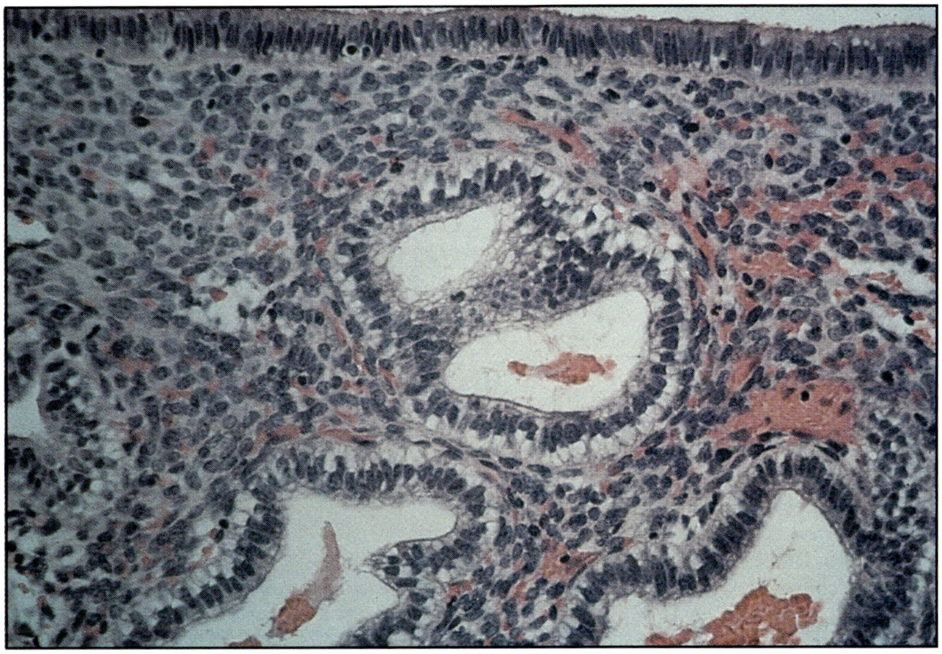

THE NORMAL UTERUS

Gross Anatomy

The uterus in women of reproductive age is a pear-shaped organ divided into cervix and corpus. The uterus is normally a pelvic structure, lying dorsal to the urinary bladder. Behind the normal uterus is the peritoneum-lined cul de sac, or pouch of Douglas. The peritoneum then reflects onto the rectosigmoid colon. The supports of the uterus include the uterosacral ligaments, which attach posterolaterally to the cervix and insert into the sacrum. The cardinal ligaments, also known as Mackenrodt ligaments, are lateral supports of the cervix and lower uterine segment. They attach to the pelvic sidewall laterally and to the pelvic diaphragm inferiorly. The uterine vessels are found in the cardinal ligaments, and the ureter lies below the uterine vessels within the cardinal ligaments. The cardinal ligaments are the major support of the uterus and cervix. They maintain the uterus in its anatomic position. Laterally the infundibulopelvic ligament (mostly a neurovascular bundle) attaches the uterine fundus to the pelvic sidewall. Lastly, the round ligament is a muscular structure that attaches to the cornual region of the uterine corpus anterior to the fallopian tube and courses through the inguinal canal to insert in the labium majus. Its counterpart in the male is the gubernaculum testis.

The normal uterus is brownish pink. The serosal surface is smooth and glistening. On cut section the myometrium appears as whorls and interdigitating bundles of muscle. The endometrium is yellow-tan and creamy in consistency (Fig. 5–1). The endometrial cavity is triangular and has a volume of approximately 7 to 10 ml in the woman of reproductive age. The size and dimensions of the normal uterus can vary depending on the age, hormonal status, and pregnancy history of the individual, with the nulliparous uterus being smaller and the parous uterus somewhat larger.[1] The length of the fundus is twice that of the cervix during the reproductive years. The average linear dimensions of the nulligravid uterus are 7.7 cm in length from cervix to fundus, 4.7 cm in width between the uterine cornua, and 2.9 cm in depth. The weight of the nulligravid uterus ranges from 46 to 71 gm. The primiparous uterus averages 8.6 cm in length, 5.0 cm in width, and 3.5 cm in depth. The weight ranges from 86 to 101 gm. The multiparous uterus averages 9.4 cm in length, 5.8 cm in width, and 4.2 cm in depth. The weight ranges from 100 to 152 gm.[1]

Premenarchal and postmenopausal uteri are smaller than uteri during the reproductive years. During the prepubertal years and the postmenopausal years the cervix is approximately two to four times longer than the fundus. The average weight of the adolescent uterus is 63 gm. The average adolescent uterus measures 8.0 cm in length, 5.0 cm in width, and 2.8 cm in depth. The average postmenopausal uterus weighs 60 gm. The average postmenopausal uterus measures 8.0 cm in length, 4.5 cm in width, and 2.8 cm in depth.[1]

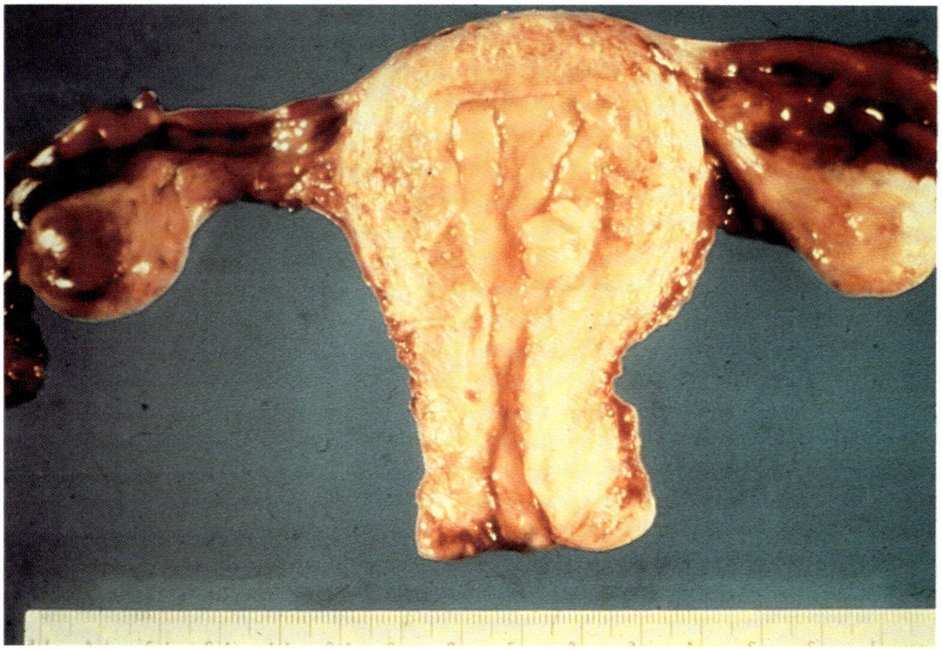

FIGURE 5-1
This is a normal uterus with attached adnexa. The triangular endometrial cavity has lush, cream-colored endometrium. This hysterectomy was performed in late luteal phase of cycle.

The endometrium varies in thickness depending on the day of the menstrual cycle and grossly can measure as much as 12 mm in thickness in a normal uterus as menses approaches. Likewise, the myometrium can vary in thickness up to 3 cm in greatest diameter. Myometrial thickness is dependent on age, hormonal status, and pregnancy history.

The blood supply of the uterus derives from the uterine artery, a branch of the anterior division of the hypogastric artery. This uterine artery on each side divides near the uterus into an ascending branch that joins with the ovarian vessels, while a descending branch joins with the vaginal arteries. The arteries freely anastomose in the infundibulopelvic and cardinal ligaments and send branches at regular intervals into the myometrium. These branches penetrate the myometrium at right angles, divide and supply the myometrium, and penetrate to the endometrium. In the endomyometrial region the vessels divide into horizontal and vertical branches. The horizontal branches supply the basal endometrium (basalis), while the vertical branches supply the more superficial endometrium or the functionalis. The vertical vessels during the luteal phase of the cycle become the spiral arterioles. The coiling of the spiral arterioles during the menstrual cycle occurs under the influence of ovarian steroid hormones and prostaglandin. Venous and lymphatic vessels closely follow the course of the arteries. Lymphatic drainage is to the pelvic and paraaortic lymph nodes.

Embryology

The adult uterus is mesodermal in origin. The uterus is part of the müllerian system, derived embryologically from the müllerian duct. The müllerian duct develops as an invagination on the dorsal wall of the parietal peritoneum, lateral to the simultaneously developing genital ridge. Thus the müllerian duct derivatives, genital ridge structures, and closely related mesonephric (wolffian) duct structures derive from mesothelium with its adjacent primitive mesenchymal tissue. Metanephric structures are also developing in close relation and proximity. Thus, the term "müllerian epithelium" is an embryologic misnomer, as this "epithelium" is truly mesenchyme. The common embryologic origin of the genital ridge, müllerian duct, wolffian duct, and parietal peritoneum helps explain the wide capacity of metaplastic differentiation of müllerian "epithelial" cells. Müllerian epithelium and the müllerian mesenchyme both have a common origin from the coelom.[2] The müllerian epithelium is typically glandular and can appear as an endometrioid cell, ciliated cell, mucinous cell, or clear cell and by a process of metaplasia can undergo squamous change.

Decidual change, endometriosis, and endosalpingosis are easier to understand when one realizes the embryologic origin of the müllerian mesenchyme. An understanding of the embryologic origin of these tissues also helps explain those pathologic conditions and neoplasms that are a combination of endometrial stroma and smooth muscle.

The distal portion of the müllerian ducts fuse at approximately 10 weeks of gestation. The fused müllerian duct forms the uterus and upper vagina. Initially the endometrium consists of a single layer of columnar epithelium supported by a dense fibroblastic stroma. After 20 weeks of gestation the surface epithelium invaginates into the underlying fibroblastic stroma, forming glandular structures. The endometrial stroma and the myometrium also develop from this primitive fibroblastic stromal tissue.

In the newborn the uterus measures about 4 cm in length. Approximately 80 percent of this represents cervix. The endometrium may have some proliferative activity secondary to intrauterine stimulation by maternal levels of estrogen and progesterone. At birth the maternal hormones are no longer present. At times a slight amount of withdrawal bleeding may occur. The endometrium then quickly regresses to an inactive state. The absence of proliferative or secretory activity characterizes the endometrium from the newborn period to puberty.

Hormonal Interactions

The response of the endometrium to stimulation by endogenous or exogenous steroid hormones is predictable. Endometrial response is a reflection of the hypothalamic-pituitary-ovarian axis.[3] To understand this, a brief summary of the complex interaction of the relationship between these structures is appropriate. Gonadotropin releasing hormone (GnRH) is a product of the hypothalamus. It is a peptide hormone. Released into the hypothalamic pituitary portal circulation, GnRH stimulates the pituitary gland to secrete follicle stimulating hormone (FSH) and luteinizing hormone (LH). FSH stimulates the theca cells in the developing follicles to secrete unaromatized androgenic precursors. The granulosa cells aromatize these steroids to the active hormone estradiol.[4] This process occurs through the presence of FSH and LH receptors in the appropriate cells of the developing follicle. Following ovulation, the luteinized cells of the corpus luteum produce progesterone. Estrogen and progesterone produce both a positive and a negative feedback to the hypothalamus and the pituitary.[4] Estrogen and progesterone both have a positive effect on the endometrium. Estrogen causes proliferation, and progesterone promotes differentiation. The purpose of this complex cycle is to prepare the endometrium for implantation and nourishment of a pregnancy.

Estrogen and Progesterone Receptors

Circulating steroid hormones rapidly cross cell membranes through a process of simple diffusion. At the cellular level, estrogen receptor (ER) and progesterone receptor (PR) in the endometrial epithelial and stromal cells are important in steroid hormone control of the endometrium. These steroid receptors are specific proteins concentrated in the nuclei of endometrial glandular and stromal cells.[5–7] Cytosol assays for these receptors measure binding proteins released from the nucleus during tissue processing. Immunocytochemical studies indicate that antibodies to ER interact only with the nuclei of human endometrium.[5, 6] ER and PR have a high affinity for estradiol and progesterone.[8] Chemically similar steroids from either an endogenous or an exogenous source can also compete for the same binding sites. This includes both steroidal and nonsteroidal estrogens. Diethylstilbestrol is an example of a nonsteroidal estrogen. The principal effect of estrogen on endometrial tissue is cellular proliferation and an increase in the concentration of receptors for estrogen and progesterone. Increased ER renders the endometrium increasingly responsive to estrogen. The principal effect of progesterone on endometrium is differentiation. The PR complex appears to influence the replenishment of cytoplasmic ER.[9] Progesterone administration reduces the level of ER in the uterus. This may occur by interference with ER resynthesis or recycling, which thereby decreases the ability of uterine tissue to respond to estrogen.[10] Thus, estradiol promotes the synthesis of estrogen and progesterone receptors, while progesterone inhibits synthesis of estrogen receptors.[8]

Quantification of estrogen and progesterone receptors is possible and reflects their binding capacity to tritiated estradiol and synthetic reference progestins. Units used to express the results are femtomoles (fmol/mg cytoplasmic protein). The concentration of estrogen and progesterone receptors varies widely throughout the normal menstrual cycle. Highest values occur in the midproliferative phase of the cycle. This value for estrogen receptor is in the order of 400 fmol/mg tissue. Progesterone receptor values approach 1000 fmol/mg tissue.[11]

Histology

The serosal surface of the uterus consists of a single layer of flattened mesothelial cells. These have elongated nuclei and scant cytoplasm. The myometrium consists of interlacing bundles of smooth muscle in a fibrovascular stroma. A typical smooth

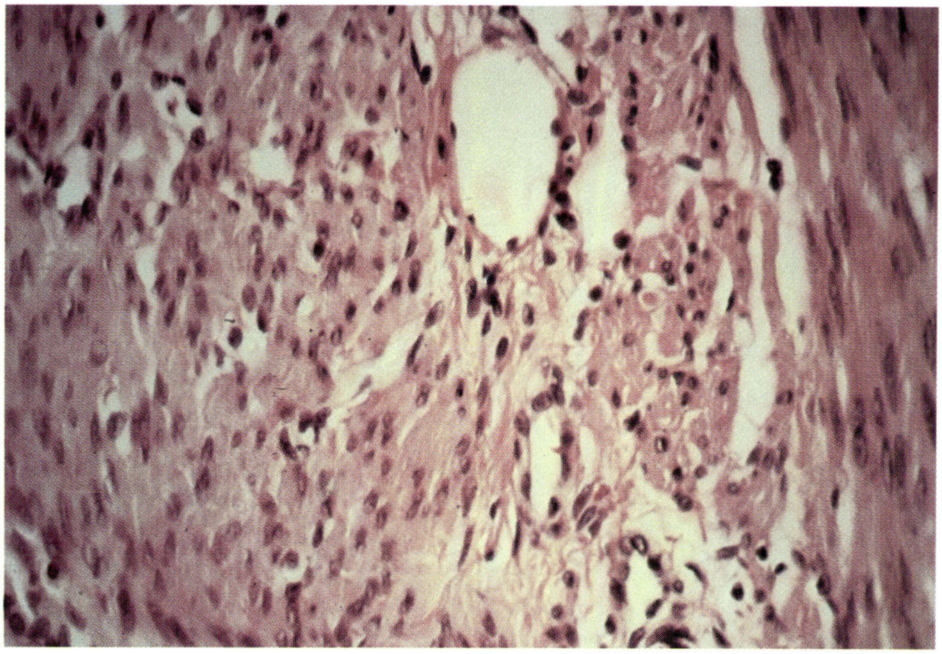

FIGURE 5-2
This normal myometrium has uterine smooth muscle with elongated cells containing eosinophilic cytoplasm. Cell borders are indistinct. Nuclei are ovoid and fusiform. Muscle bundles intertwine and interweave. Most of the muscle fibers have been cut on cross section. Longitudinal fibers are seen on the right side. Vascular channels are prominent across the center.

muscle cell is fusiform with indistinct cell borders. The cytoplasm is eosinophilic and fibrillar. The nucleus is fusiform, and the chromatin is finely granular and uniform. A small nucleolus may be present (Fig. 5-2).

The endometrium consists of glands and stroma (Fig. 5-3). The endometrium has two functional subdivisions, a deeper basalis and a superficial functionalis. The basalis responds minimally to hormones, while the functionalis responds to estrogen and progesterone and is the layer of endometrium that sheds at the time of menstruation. In the basalis layer the endometrial glands are simple tubules. Individual cells have a basophilic cytoplasm and oval nuclei with dispersed chromatin. The only positive features of the endometrial stroma in the proliferative phase or in the basalis layer of the endometrium are a monotonous cytologic uniformity of relatively small cells with cytoplasm difficult to discern and an arborizing vasculature.[12] In the basalis layer the endometrial stroma tends to be more compact. The individual stromal cell has densely basophilic cytoplasm, and the nuclei are oval with dense chromatin.

The histology of the functionalis varies with the hormonal milieu. The normal cyclic hormonal influence divides the endometrial cycle into a preovulatory, proliferative or estrogenic phase under the influence of estrogen alone, and a postovulatory, secretory or luteal phase under the influence of estrogen and progesterone. The length of the proliferative phase of the cycle is variable. Under the influence of estrogen the endometrium grows. If pregnancy does not occur, the postovulatory or secretory phase is relatively constant at approximately 14 days. The histology of the secretory phase reflects the influence of progesterone, which causes differentiation. Throughout the typical cycle, endometrial glands increase in size 144 percent from the early proliferative to the late secretory phase. The increase in glandular mass occurs at the expense of the lumen, while the epithelial thickness grows by a factor of two.[13] An understanding of the histologic changes in the functionalis throughout the cycle is necessary.

Proliferative Phase Endometrium

Under the influence of estrogen the endometrium grows. Initially the gland to stroma ratio favors the endometrial stroma. The glands are straight and tubular. The epithelium is pseudostratified (Fig. 5-4). Cilia may or may not be present. Mitotic activity is present in both the endometrial glands and the endometrial stroma. The glands gradually elongate and become tortuous as the estrogenic stimulation increases. During the midproliferative phase of the cycle a minor degree of stromal edema appears (Fig. 5-5).

Fifteen to 20 percent of normal endometria contain lymphoid aggregates, which, if they are large enough, resemble normal lymphoid follicles and may even have germinal centers. They include both T cells and macrophages.[14] Plasma cells are not normally present. Although the B lymphocytes stain for IgA, IgM, or IgG, we currently do not

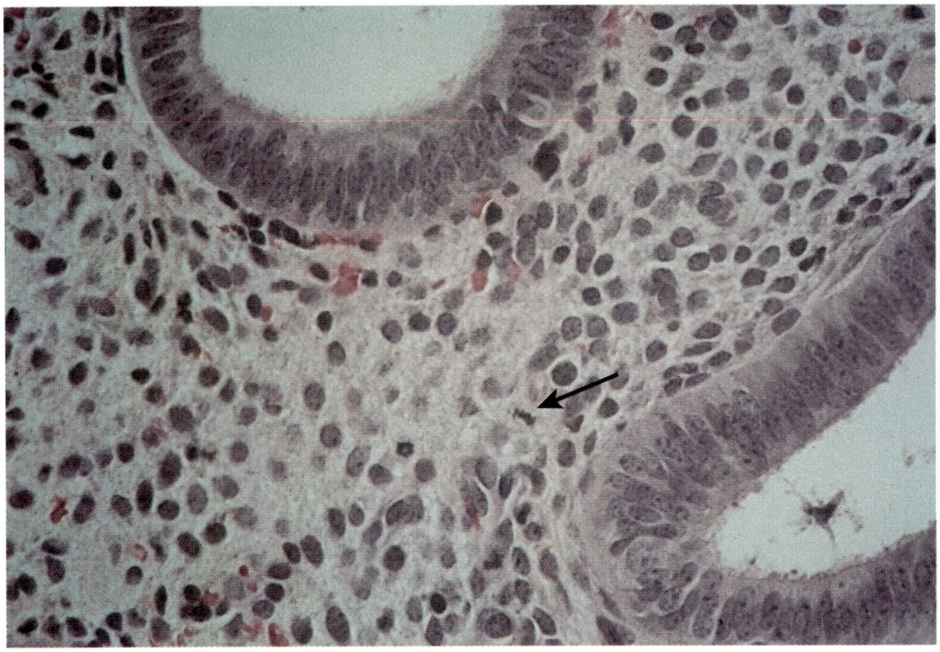

FIGURE 5-3
This proliferative endometrium exhibits a compact stroma with mitotic figures *(arrow)* and tubular glands with pseudostratification.

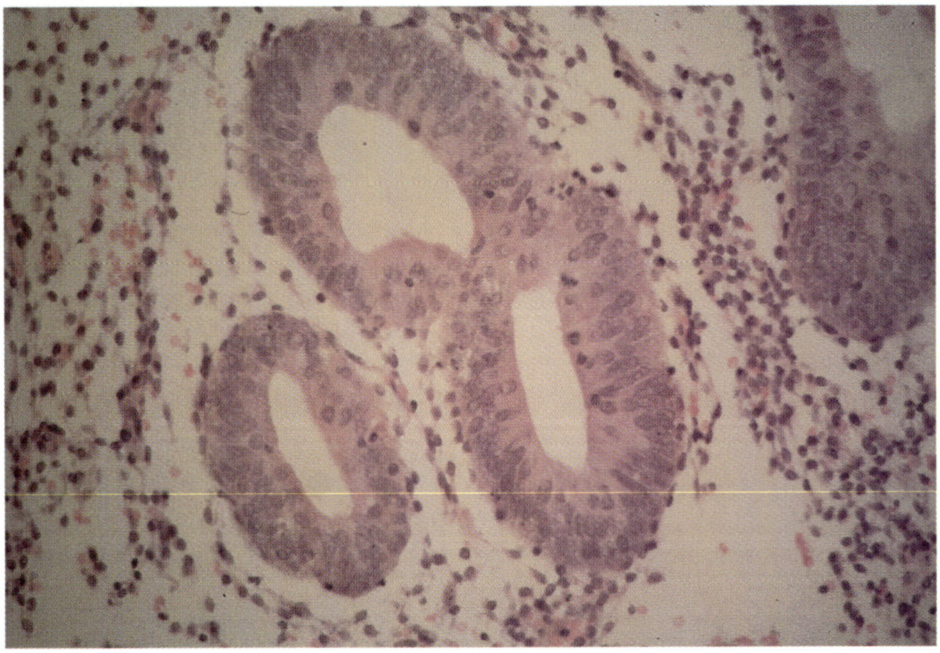

FIGURE 5-4
In this proliferative endometrium it is possible to see pseudostratified glandular epithelium. Multiple mitotic figures are present in the glandular epithelium. This is a curettage specimen.

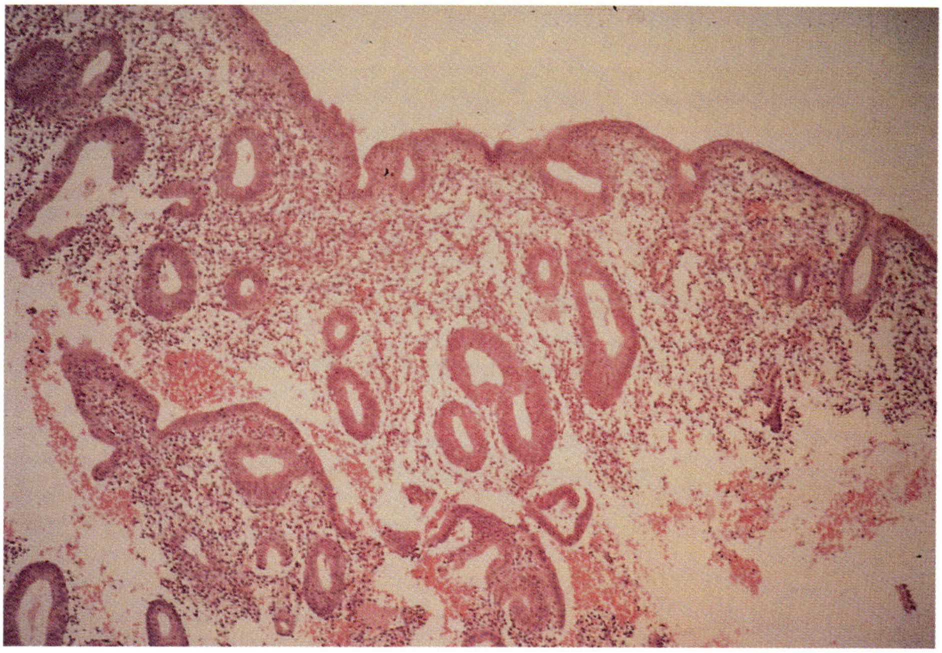

FIGURE 5-5
This curettage specimen shows midproliferative endometrium with tubular glands present. The stroma is loose; the blood is secondary to the curettage; the surface endometrium is seen.

understand their role, if any, in the immunology of the endometrium.[14]

Secretory Phase Endometrium

This phase begins at ovulation, typically on day 14 of an ideal 28-day cycle. The endometrial histology begins to reflect the influence of progesterone along with estrogen. A period of quantifiable differentiation begins. The histology changes daily as the endometrium prepares itself for implantation and early nourishment of a pregnancy (Fig. 5–6). While estrogen stimulates mitotic activity, progesterone produces mitotic arrest. At the beginning of the luteal phase, a pseudostratified columnar epithelium lines the endometrial glands. The gland to stroma ratio, while initially favoring the endometrial stroma, shifts and favors the endometrial glands. Vacuoles containing glycogen appear in the endometrial glandular epithelium. Active secretion occurs into the gland lumens, and the glands become secretorily exhausted. Progesterone stimulates the endometrial stroma to undergo pseudodecidual change. Hertig and Rock have delineated these histologic changes by day of the cycle.[3, 15] These changes are reproducible and may be used to date endometrial biopsies. The findings correlate well with the onset of the next menses. Pathologists' concordance is 50 percent for identical day, and is within 2 days in 80 percent of instances.[15] To be able to accurately date the secretory endometrium, the sample being examined should contain surface endometrium, since the basalis responds minimally to hormones.

One can best understand the postovulatory changes when this phase of the menstrual cycle is conceptually divided into thirds.

The *first third* of the secretory, ovulatory, or progestogenic phase of the cycle begins on day 16 (postovulatory day 2) and ends on day 20 (postovulatory day 6). Ovulation typically occurs on the 14th day of a 28-day cycle. Progesterone is absent until ovulation, and the plasma concentration gradually increases until late in the luteal phase. There are no distinct histologic changes in the endometrium during the first 24 hours following ovulation. The earliest histologic changes become apparent on the second day after ovulation. Changes in the endometrial glands characterize this phase of the cycle. The earliest histologic change, first recognized on day 16 (postovulatory day 2), is the presence of subnuclear vacuoles in the glandular epithelial cells. These are present in most of the endometrial glands. By day 17 (postovulatory day 3) subnuclear vacuoles are present in practically all endometrial glands (Fig. 5–7). These subnuclear vacuoles contain glycogen. Mitotic activity, characteristic of estrogenic stimulation, becomes less apparent in both the endometrial glands and the stroma and is no longer seen by day 18 (postovulatory day 4). By day 18, the vacuoles become larger and are now present both basally and luminally (sub- and supranuclearly) (Fig. 5–8). Bubbles of secretion begin to appear in the gland lumens at this time, and by day 20 (postovulatory day 6) the glands exhibit secretory exhaustion. Secretory material is now present entirely within the gland lumens. The endometrial

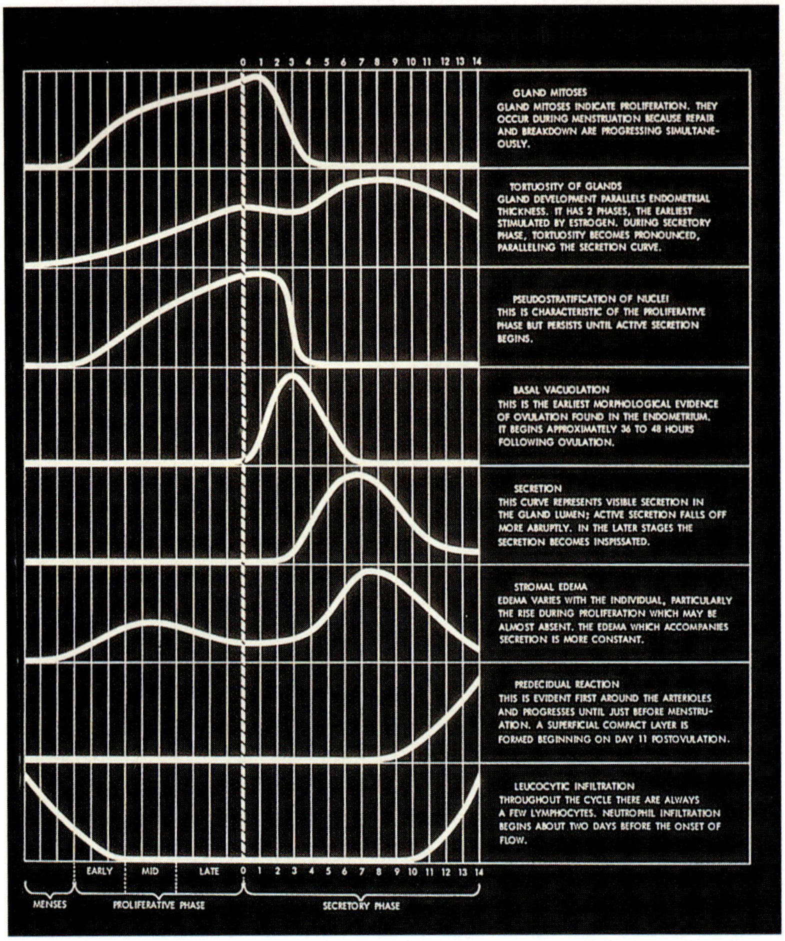

FIGURE 5-6
This figure shows criteria for histologically dating the endometrium. (From Noyes RW, Hertig AT, Rock J: Dating the endometrial biopsy. Fertil Steril 1950; 1:3–25.)

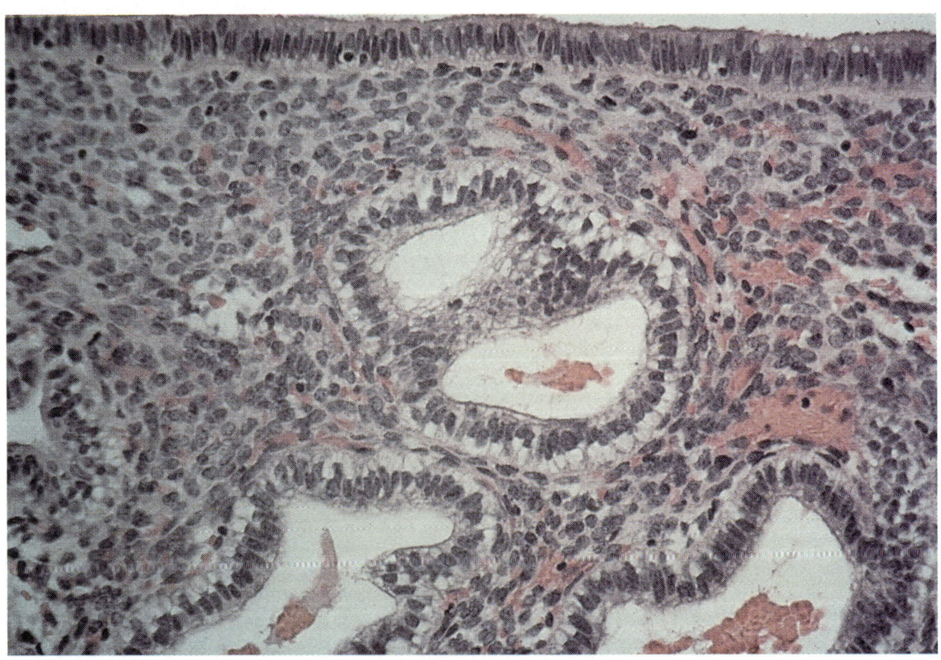

FIGURE 5-7
This is an early secretory endometrium, approximately 2 to 3 days post ovulation (day 16 to 17 of cycle). Glands have subnuclear vacuoles. There is no secretion in gland lumen yet. The stroma is compact. Few vacuoles are present in surface endometrium.

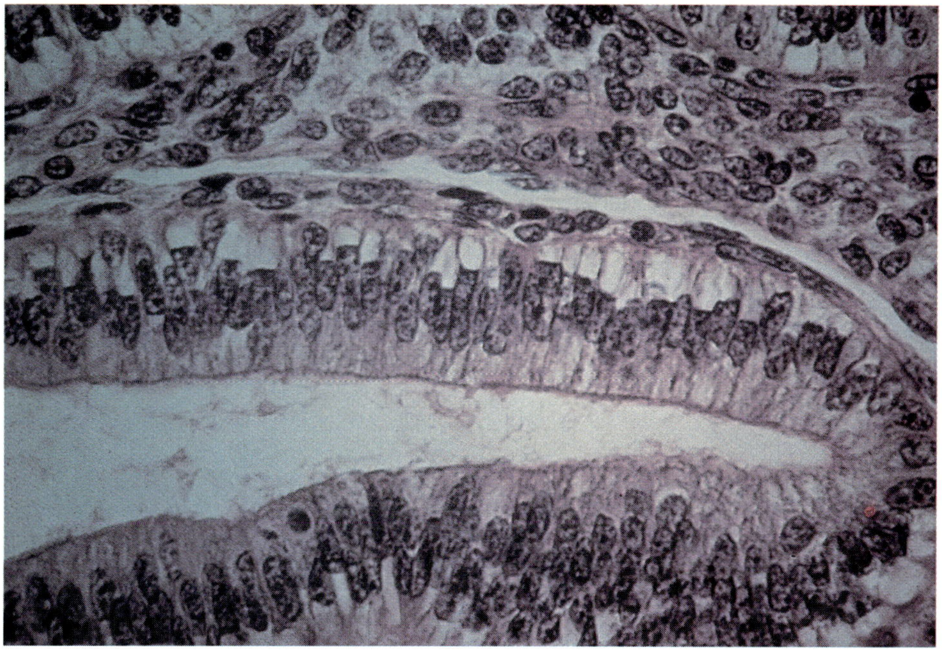

FIGURE 5-8
This is an early secretory endometrium, approximately 4 days post ovulation (day 18 of cycle). High-power view of endometrial gland lined by pseudostratified columnar epithelium. Secretion is present in both subnuclear and supranuclear locations. Secretions are beginning to appear as bubbles at gland lumen.

glands continue to elongate and become more tortuous during this phase of the cycle. Thus the proportion of the glands to endometrial stroma becomes greater.

The *middle third* of the ovulatory, progestogenic, or secretory phase of the cycle encompasses cycle days 21 to 23 (postovulatory days 7 to 9). If fertilization has taken place, implantation of the blastocyst occurs at this time. Histologic changes now begin in the endometrial stroma, and the distinctive histologic changes for accurate dating focus on the stroma throughout the remainder of the cycle. On day 21 (postovulatory day 7) there is the abrupt onset of stromal edema. Stromal edema reaches its peak on day 22 (postovulatory day 8) (Fig. 5–9). Naked stromal nuclei are characteristic on this day. The cytoplasm of the endometrial stromal cells appears indistinct. On day 23 (postovulatory day 9), there is an increase in mitotic activity in the endometrial stromal cells. Predecid-

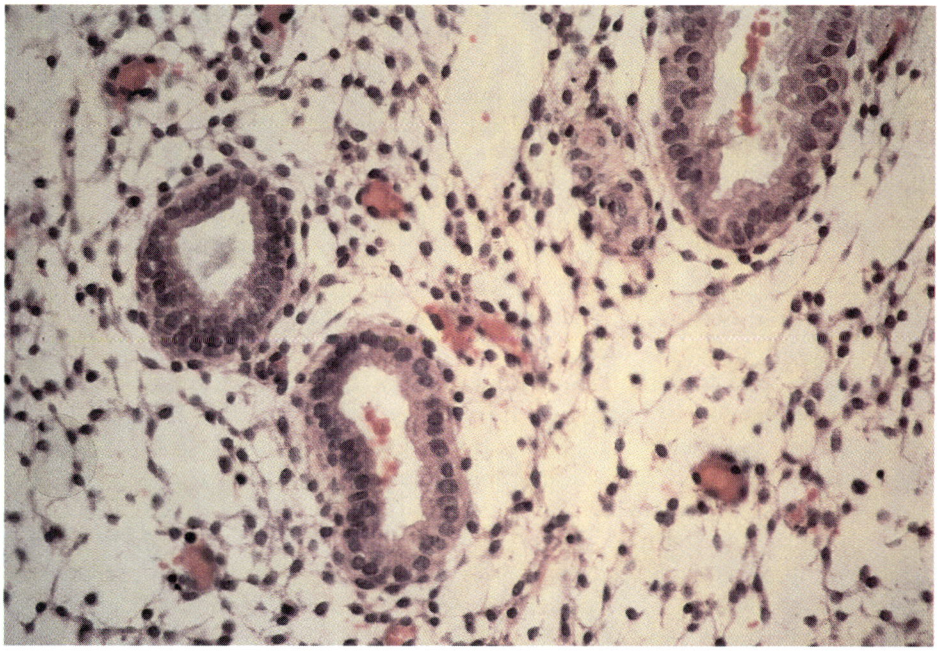

FIGURE 5-9
This is a midsecretory endometrium, approximately 7 to 8 days postovulatory (day 21 to 22 of cycle). Peak stromal edema is present with naked stromal nuclei. Glands are secretorily exhausted. A little secretion is present in gland lumen. There is no predecidual change around spiral arterioles yet.

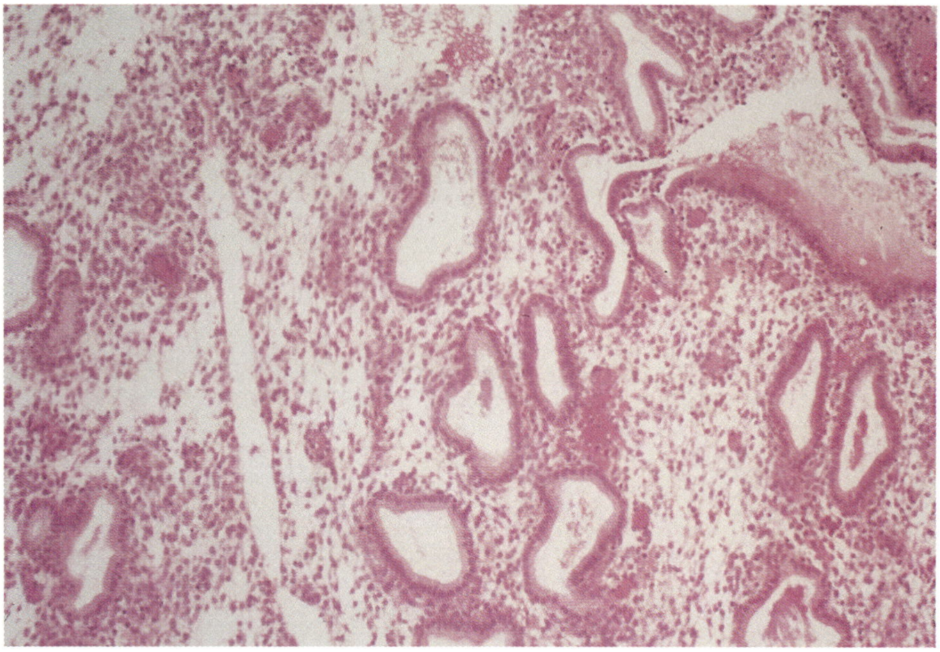

FIGURE 5-10
This is a midsecretory endometrium, approximately 9 days post ovulation (day 23 of cycle). Periarteriolar cuffing (i.e., decidualized stromal cells surrounding arterioles) is seen.

ual changes, known as periarteriolar cuffing (Fig. 5–10), also begin to occur around the spiral arterioles. The predecidual cells are precursors to true decidual cells that occur in pregnancy, and they contain glycogen.

The *last third* of the ovulatory, progestogenic, or secretory phase encompasses days 24 to 28 (postovulatory days 10 to 14). Two distinct histologic changes occur simultaneously during this last phase of the cycle. The first is an increase in predecidual cells. On day 24 (postovulatory day 10), predecidual change, also known as subcapsular decidualization, appears beneath the surface endometrium. As the cycle continues, the predecidual change gradually progresses. By day 28 (postovulatory day 14), the predecidual change is present throughout the functionalis. The second histologic marker is the presence of inflammatory cells. On day 25 (postovulatory day 11), an inflammatory infiltrate begins to occur within the endometrial stroma, becoming more pronounced with each passing day. By day 28 the entire functionalis is decidualized and peppered by a granulocytic inflammatory infiltrate (Fig. 5–11). Glandular changes are nonspecific. Secretion within the glands becomes inspissated. The glands assume a saw-toothed appearance. Late in the cycle the ratio of the endometrial glands to endometrial stroma reverses to favor the endometrial glands. Morphometrically, the nuclear area of the endometrial glandular cells increases in the late luteal phase of the cycle.[16] This may be a requirement for later endometrial regeneration.

It has been postulated that in the luteal phase of the cycle the endometrial stromal cell differentiates along two pathways, the first pathway being the predecidual cell and the second the endometrial stromal granulocyte. Thus the premenstrual endometrial stromal inflammatory infiltrate may originate in large part directly from the endometrial stromal cell. As menses approaches, the endometrium begins to undergo breakdown. At this time some polymorphonuclear leukocytes obtain entrance to the endometrial stroma by diapedesis.[17]

The foregoing cyclic histologic changes occur in the corpus of the uterus. In the isthmic region or lower uterine segment, the endometrial lining is thinner. The glands frequently contain ciliated cells. There is a gradual transition to endocervical glands. The endometrial stroma becomes more fibrous. Glands and stroma in this area respond weakly to hormonal stimulation. When it is necessary to histologically assign a postovulatory date to the endometrium, a lower segment endometrial biopsy is not useful.

On day 28 of a typical cycle, menses begins unless the woman is pregnant. Histologic characteristics of menstrual endometrium include collapse of the stroma about the endometrial glands, fragmentation of the endometrial glands, and the presence of fibrin thrombi within the endometrial stroma (Fig. 5–12). These are hallmarks of a bleeding endometrium. The glands are exhausted of secretions, and because of the collapse of the stroma the glands may appear increased in proportion to the stroma. At times the glands may assume a papillary appearance. It is easy to con-

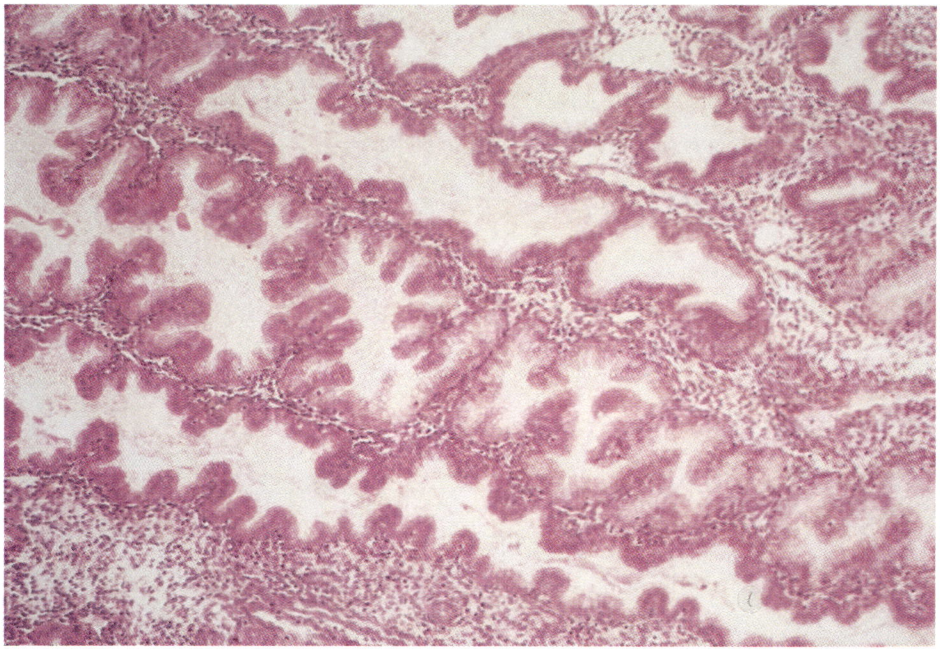

FIGURE 5-11
This is a late secretory endometrium approximately 13 days postovulatory (day 27 of cycle). The glands are tortuous with inspissated secretions within the lumen. The stroma shows a heavy granulocytic infiltrate.

fuse a menstrual endometrium with hyperplasia or at times even carcinoma. The lack of mitotic activity and the lack of cytologic atypia in menstrual endometrium may help in arriving at the correct diagnosis.

Mechanical artifacts and the quality of tissue processing or slide preparation may sometimes complicate the recognition of normal endometrial changes throughout the menstrual cycle. The lack of endometrial surface epithelium may render histologic dating impossible.

Endometrial Changes in Pregnancy

When pregnancy occurs, the endometrium assumes characteristic changes consistent with increased levels of the hormones: estrogen, progesterone, and human chorionic gonadotropin (hCG). Collectively the term gestational endometrium describes these histologic changes. Microscopically this includes a combination of decidual change with hypersecretory change. Decidual change occurs in other anatomic locations besides the en-

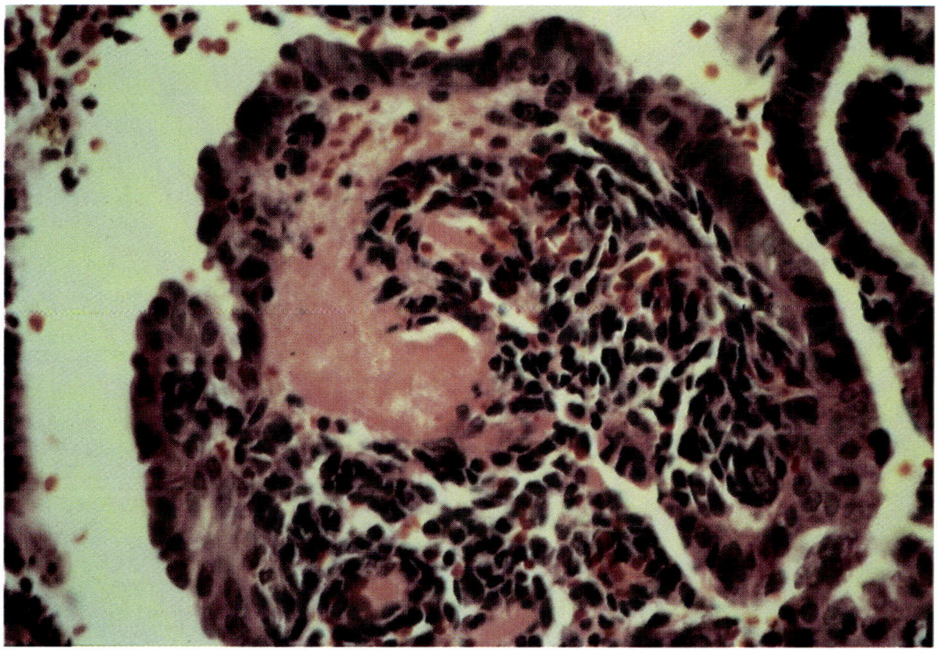

FIGURE 5-12
This is a menstrual endometrium in a high-power magnification to demonstrate compact collapsed stroma, disrupted glandular epithelium with a tendency to papillary changes, and fibrin thrombi. This is a curettage specimen.

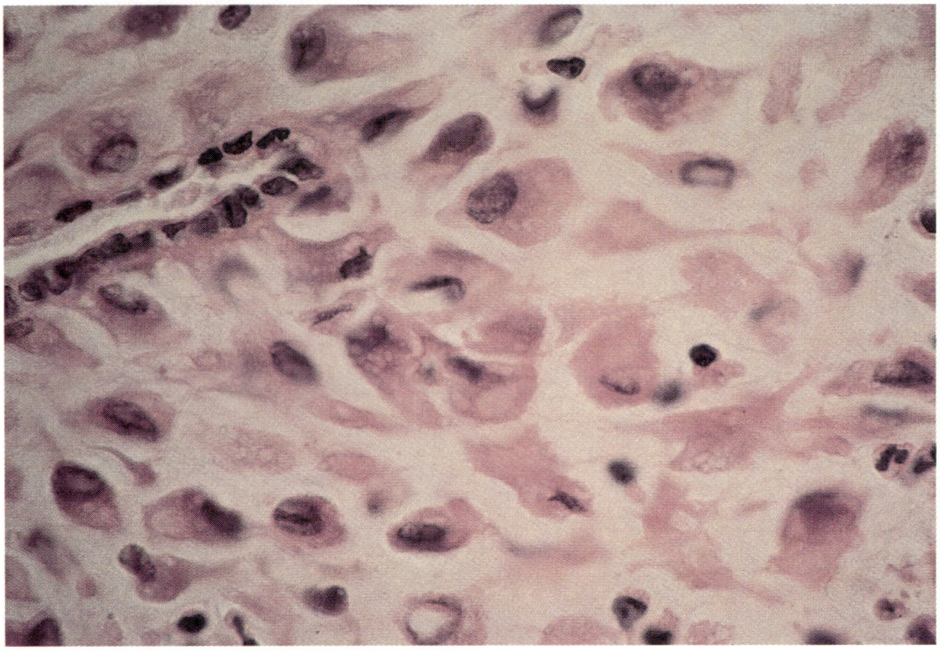

FIGURE 5-13
This is an endometrium with decidual changes. Cells appear almost pavement-like, with eosinophilic cytoplasm. Nuclei are regular. The gland in upper left corner is lined by cuboidal epithelium. An occasional inflammatory cell is present.

dometrium. The nuclei of decidualized cells are oval and have a granular chromatin pattern. The eosinophilia and the abundant cytoplasm are useful distinguishing features. Decidual cells are rich in glycogen. Sheets of decidual cells have a pavement-like appearance caused by the accentuation of the cytoplasmic borders and the space between the cells. In decidualized endometrium the endometrial glandular epithelium appears atrophic. The glands themselves may appear merely as narrow slits in the sheets of decidualized stroma. These glands are lined by columnar, cuboidal, or flattened epithelium (Fig. 5–13). Secretory activity is absent. Decidual change may be widespread throughout the endometrium or may be more focal. The other characteristic histologic finding is hypersecretory endometrium (Fig. 5–14). The glands appear more crowded than in a normal endometrium but fall short of back-to-back crowding. Stroma is present between all endometrial glands. The glands themselves exhibit secretory exhaustion and a peculiar appearance of individual cells

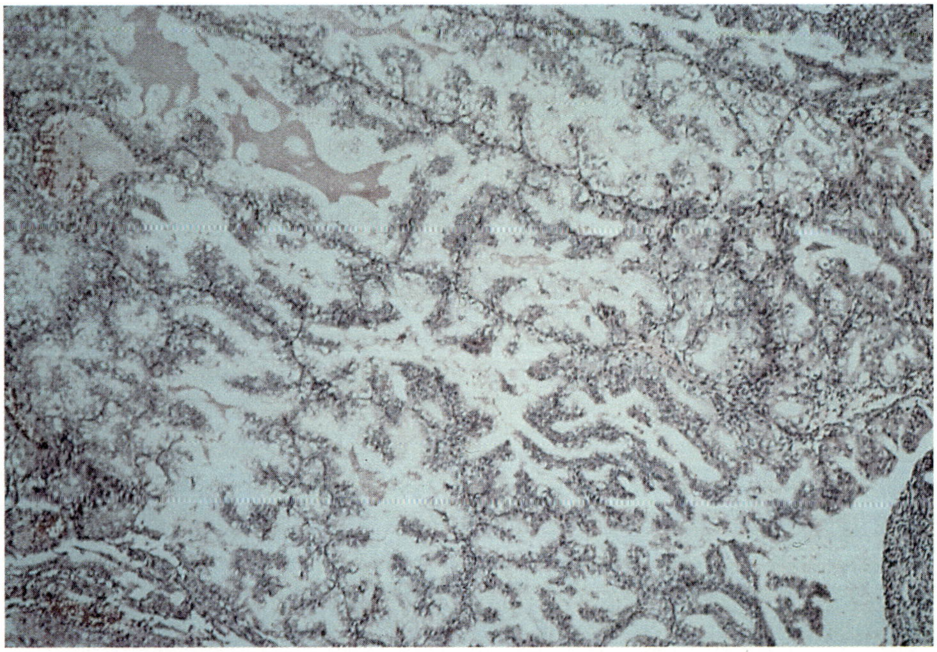

FIGURE 5-14
This is a gestational endometrium with hypersecretory glands with epithelial tufting. Glands are crowded with little intervening stroma. The presence of secretory activity and the lack of mitotic activity differentiate this state from hyperplasia.

containing bulbous nuclei that protrude into the gland lumens. This phenomenon is known as the Arias-Stella reaction. These cells have a striking similarity to the hobnail cell that is characteristic of clear cell carcinoma. However, they lack cytologic atypia and the mitotic activity characteristic of carcinoma.

In abnormal gestation, either ectopic pregnancy or a nonviable intrauterine pregnancy, the endometrial histology is extremely variable. Decidual change with or without gestational endometrium is present in most instances, but normal proliferative, secretory, or menstrual endometrium may be present. Additionally, chronic inflammatory changes, characterized by the presence of plasma cells, are not uncommon. The finding of placental tissue or fetal parts in an endometrial specimen readily identifies an intrauterine pregnancy. The presence of decidua and hypersecretory endometrium without chorionic villi or fetal parts, along with a positive pregnancy test, is excellent evidence of pregnancy but does not identify the location as intrauterine or extrauterine. In the absence of chorionic villi or fetal tissue an extrauterine pregnancy must be considered and excluded clinically.[18]

The Prepubertal Endometrium

In late pregnancy the high maternal concentration of estrogen and progesterone has an effect on the endometrium of the fetus. The endometrium in the newborn is histologically active and reflects maternal hormone levels. Following delivery, the estrogen and progesterone level of the newborn quickly falls to negligible amounts. Occasionally a small amount of withdrawal bleeding will occur. Rapidly, in the absence of hormonal stimulus, the endometrium regresses. Then until puberty it consists of inactive glands and stroma. At puberty, under the influence of ovarian hormones, cyclic endometrial stimulation and proliferation become apparent.

The Postmenopausal Endometrium

The histology of the endometrium in a postmenopausal woman lacks the cyclic changes induced by estrogen and progesterone. The glands are simple tubules lined with cuboidal to low columnar epithelium. The stroma becomes more fibrous. Mitotic activity is not present in either glands or stroma. The gland to stroma ratio favors the stroma. Sometimes, individual glands or groups of glands may appear cystically dilated, with the epithelium assuming a flattened to low cuboidal appearance. This is cystic atrophy (Fig. 5–15). Cystic atrophy differs from simple hyperplasia because in hyperplasia the glands and stroma are actively proliferating. Mitotic figures, while not necessarily abundant, are present.[19]

Endometrial Changes Induced by Oral Contraceptive Steroids

The histology of the endometrium under the influence of oral contraceptives is variable and depends upon the following: the dose of estrogen and pro-

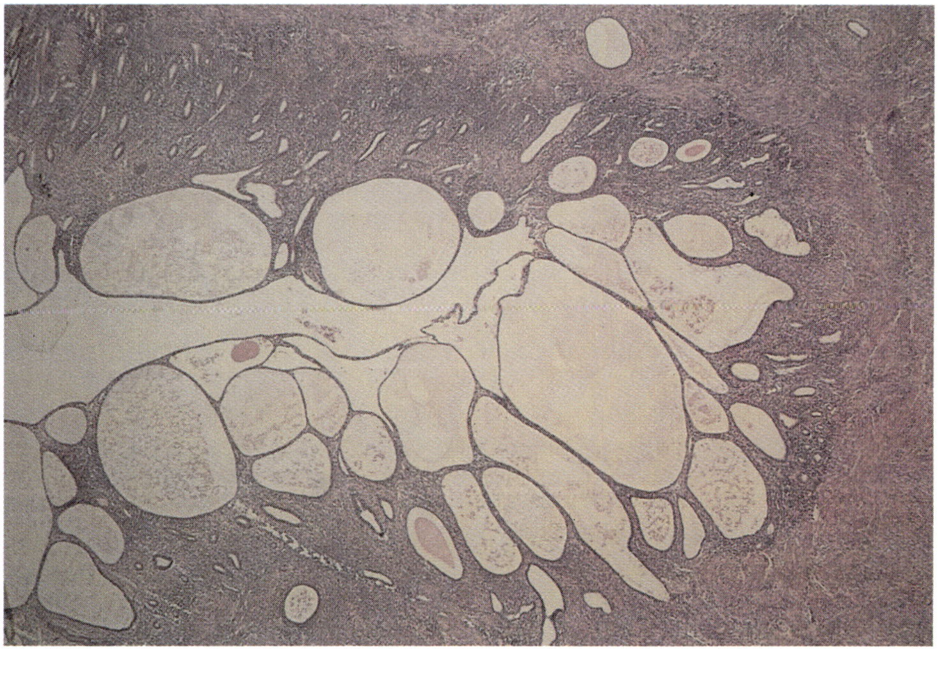

FIGURE 5–15
This is cystic atrophy in a postmenopausal endometrium which demonstrates retrogressive changes. The endometrium is inactive, with the individual glands being cystically dilated and lined with low columnar to flattened epithelium. This is a hysterectomy specimen; myometrium surrounds the endometrium.

gestogen in the oral contraceptive preparation, the day of the cycle on which the specimen is obtained, the interval that the patient has been on oral contraceptives, and the histology of the endometrium before starting oral contraceptives. Until the mid-1970s, the use of sequential oral contraceptive pills was common. These pills administered 20 days of estrogen alone, followed by 5 days of estrogen and a weak progestogen. An association with endometrial hyperplasia and neoplasia became apparent in some young women.[20]

Today the typical oral contraceptive preparation is a "combined" pill, with each pill containing a combination of estrogen and progestogen. The dosage of hormones has become lower over the years, and the progestogens of today differ from those used in the past. The estrogen in all combined oral contraceptive pills today is ethinyl estradiol. In the past mestranol was the estrogen in some preparations. The liver converts mestranol to ethinyl estradiol. Progestogens in today's oral contraceptives include the following: norethindrone, norgestrel, levonorgestrel, and, more recently, norgestimate and desogestrel. Typically a woman takes both the estrogen and the progestogen continuously for 21 days of the month. Three dosage regimens are available. The simplest consists of both estrogen and progestogen in the same dose administered for 21 days with 7 days of placebo or iron pills. The other combinations include a biphasic and triphasic dosage schedule. These regimens vary the dose of progestogen throughout, either in two or three steps. In some triphasic oral contraceptives the dose of the estrogen also varies along with the dose of the progestogen.

Because progestogen is present beginning with the first pill, the combined-regimen contraceptive steroids cause premature endometrial secretion to appear within the endometrial glandular cells. The effects of the first pills begin to appear within 48 hours of taking the first active pill. As the cycle progresses, endometrial involution occurs, leading to a suppressed endometrium with small tubular glands. Spiral arterioles fail to develop. Decidua-like changes in the stroma are dose related.[21] The gland to stroma ratio favors greatly the stroma later in the cycle. Dilatation of venules in the superficial endometrium is also a progestogen-related change. Thrombosis of these venules, perhaps estrogen mediated, leads to local tissue infarction and may be the proximate cause of breakthrough bleeding.[21] Typically, specimens from cycle days 9 through 12 demonstrate prominent subnuclear vacuoles and supranuclear vacuoles, resembling a normal cycling day 16 to day 18 endometrium. Biopsy obtained later in the cycle shows regression of the secretory reaction.[21] By cycle day 20, the endometrial glandular epithelium appears exhausted and inactive. By the end of a 3-week contraceptive cycle, the histologic appearance of the endometrium is one of inactivity and suppression. Decidua-like stromal reaction may occur as early as day 17 and appears to be related to the dose and biologic activity of the progestogen. At a dose of 10 mg of progestogen, stromal decidual change will be present and variable in amount from patient to patient. At a dose of 5 mg of progestogen, decidua-like stromal reaction becomes weak and infrequent. At a dose equal to or less than 2.5 mg of progestogen, small endometrial glands with a low cuboidal to columnar epithelium without mitotic activity are present.[21] Secretory activity is absent. The endometrial stroma is loosely reticular, and many of the nuclei appear naked. A decidua-like stromal reaction at this low dose of progestogen is extremely uncommon. There is no development of spiral arterioles. Dilatation of superficial venules is absent.[21]

The medical treatment of endometriosis sometimes utilizes continuous oral contraceptives. The dose of progestogen is high and can approach 40 mg daily. At this dosage level a diffuse intense decidual reaction that resembles the decidua vera of pregnancy occurs. The decidual cells align in a typical pavement pattern, and the gland lumens appear slit-like, easily mistaken for small blood vessels.[21] Similar histologic changes occur with intramuscular injection of medroxyprogesterone acetate (e.g., Depo-Provera).[21] After two or three injections the endometrium will be thin and atrophic. Small hyperinvoluted glands in a compact stroma without vascular development are present.

The subcutaneous implantation of six capsules containing a total of 36 mg levonorgestrel, 6 mg in each capsule, is a method of reversible contraception that is gaining in popularity. For the first 9 months the release of levonorgestrel is approximately 85 mg per day. This decreases to approximately 35 mg per day by the third year. A bothersome side effect is breakthrough bleeding. Amenorrhea occurs in some individuals. Although description of histologic changes in the endometrium is lacking, changes produced by exogenous progestogen should occur.

Besides histologic changes in the endometrium, oral contraceptive agents have an association with thromboembolic disease. Thrombi and lesions of the vascular wall are commonplace in women using these preparations, and proliferative intimal lesions may occur in healthy women using them. Moderate to severe cellular proliferation of the intimal layer is present in 82 percent of women exposed to exogenous contraceptive steroids.[22] The severity of involvement correlates with duration of exposure and decreases in patients who stop steroid use, as documented from examination of surgical specimens.[22] On microscopic examination this intimal proliferation appears as a proliferation of endothelial cells that have tightly packed nuclei. In some vessels the intercellular stroma is more prominent, varying from loose and myxomatous or mucinous to dense and fibrous. Such proliferations can partially or totally occlude vessels.[23]

Endometrial Changes Induced by Estrogen Replacement Therapy

Postmenopausal women benefit from estrogen replacement therapy. These benefits include both long- and short-term effects. Long-term effects are a delay or prevention of osteoporosis[24] and a reduction in heart disease.[25] The short-term effects include relief of vasomotor symptoms, improvement in vaginal dryness and dyspareunia due to atrophic changes in the vaginal mucosa, and decrease of other genitourinary symptoms such as urinary stress incontinence. Other problems related to insomnia, depression, and libido are ameliorated in some women.[26] Some physicians, in response to fear of litigation and concern about detecting preexisting endometrial cancer, routinely perform endometrial sampling on every woman before beginning estrogen replacement therapy. Endometrial sampling in asymptomatic women, however, has a low detection rate for abnormalities. Occult endometrial carcinoma is found in fewer than 7 out of 1000 asymptomatic postmenopausal women who undergo endometrial sampling.[27] On the other hand, the increased risk of endometrial cancer and its precursors in patients exposed to high levels of endogenous or unopposed exogenous estrogen[28] may warrant endometrial sampling. Any abnormal vaginal bleeding warrants a histopathologic diagnosis before hormone replacement therapy is begun.[29]

In the 1970s an association between prolonged use of estrogens by postmenopausal women and an increased risk of endometrial cancer was suggested.[10] Two types of data appeared: data reporting a possible increase in the overall incidence of endometrial carcinoma; and epidemiologic studies showing a possible association between estrogen use and endometrial cancer. An in-depth review of the available literature suggested the following conclusions.[30] The annual incidence of endometrial cancer is 0.06 to 0.08 percent. Prolonged use of estrogen may raise this incidence to 0.3 percent; thus the increase related to estrogen therapy is 0.23 percent. Most of these cancers represent localized disease, with a survival rate exceeding 90 percent. The estimated risk of dying from an estrogen-induced endometrial carcinoma has been calculated to be 1 in 4347 for women who have a history of estrogen replacement therapy.[30]

Currently, two dissimilar regimens account for most estrogen replacement therapy— a cyclic and a continous approach. The first consists of estrogen administered for 25 to 30 days of the month, with a progestogen administered for 10 to 14 days of each cycle. With this regimen, withdrawal bleeding usually occurs after cessation of the progestogen. Data derived from the use of sequential oral contraceptives in younger women were applied to estrogen replacement in postmenopausal women. Sequential oral contraceptives were estrogen dominant and became associated with the development of endometrial hyperplasia and endometrial carcinoma.[20] This, in turn, became a concern for women on estrogen replacement therapy. To deter osteoporosis, a dose of 0.625 mg of conjugated equine estrogen or its equivalent has been shown to be sufficient.[24] This dose is biologically less than the dose of estrogen in sequential oral contraceptive pills. Lengthening the time of administration of the progestogen to 13 days each month drastically reduces the prevalence of endometrial hyperplasia and endometrial carcinoma.[10]

The dose of estrogen, the dose of progestogen, the length of time the patient has been taking the medication, the date of the biopsy, and the previous underlying histology of the endometrium will each influence the microscopic appearance of any endometrial sample. The goal of the cyclic method of therapy is to diminish both estrogenic stimulation and the progestogenic changes in the endometrium. Estrogen will cause endometrial proliferation to some degree. Microscopically these changes should be similar to the changes in a normal proliferative endometrium. With the addition of a progestogen, the histology will demonstrate secretory change, and possibly decidual change, depending on the dose of the progestogen. At a high dose of progestogen (such as 10 mg of medroxyprogesterone acetate) decidual change commonly occurs, whereas it is infrequent at a dose of 2.5 mg. Histopathologic changes in women receiving estrogen replacement therapy may include endometrial polyps, simple hyperplasia, rarely atypical hyperplasia,[28] and even more uncommonly endometrial carcinoma.

A combined method of daily administration of estrogen and progestogen is becoming more common.[31] The dose of estrogen is 0.625 to 1.25 mg of conjugated equine estrogen or its equivalent; the dose of progestogen varies from 2.5 to 10 mg of medroxyprogesterone acetate. The most commonly prescribed regimen is 0.625 mg conjugated equine estrogen and 2.5 mg of medroxyprogesterone acetate daily. This results in a lower monthly total dosage of progestogen. Women using this regimen enjoy the benefit of estrogen replacement without the inconvenience of regular progestogen-induced withdrawal bleeding. After troublesome spotting early in the regimen, women develop amenorrhea. However, 12 to 14 percent of women drop out of treatment because of symptoms of breakthrough spotting and bleeding during the first 3 months of therapy.[32, 33] If bleeding occurs after the development of amenorrhea, it requires further investigation.

Endometrial histology in women using a combined estrogen-progestogen regimen currently lacks substantial documentation. In a small series of 41 women using this regimen, 6 experienced breakthrough bleeding after achieving amenorrhea. At this time the endometrial biopsy demonstrated that two patients each had endometrial polyps, endometrial adenocarcinoma, and atrophic endometrium.[32] The cancer diagnoses were made 2 years and more than 4 years after the beginning of the combined hormone replacement therapy. One of the women who developed endometrial carcinoma had previously been on long-term unopposed estrogen and had an earlier diagnosis of complex atypical endometrial hyperplasia.[32]

In another small study of 36 women who received 0.625 mg of conjugated equine estrogen continuously with either 2.5 mg or 5 mg of medroxyprogesterone acetate or placebo, endometrial sampling after 3 months in the combined treatment groups revealed inactive or atrophic endometrium.[31] In the unopposed estrogen group, the diagnosis in nine of the endometria was atrophy; one had a mixture of secretory endometrium plus adenomatous change and one endometrium demonstrated complex hyperplasia.[31]

Using conjugated equine estrogens in either a 0.625 or 1.25 mg dose along with norethisterone as the progestogen in a dose of 0.35 to 2.1 mg daily, the lower dose of estrogen and progestogen produces amenorrhea in 65 percent of patients.[33] Fifty-six percent of women had an endometrial biopsy after 6 months of combined treatment. The biopsy revealed atrophic endometrium regardless of the dose of estrogen.[33]

In a study that compared cyclic hormonal replacement with continuous therapy using estrogen and 10 mg of medroxyprogesterone acetate, the women in the combined treatment group had inactive endometrium, whereas in the cyclic group there was one patient with complex hyperplasia and a few examples of proliferative endometrium.[34] Another recently described variation of the combined regimen proposes 0.625 mg conjugated equine estrogen and 2.5 mg medroxyprogesterone acetate daily Monday through Friday with no treatment on the weekend. Endometrial histology at the end of 6 months revealed minimal growth of the endometrial glands and stroma.[35] The amount of progestational activity was barely identifiable. None of the biopsy specimens was totally atrophic, but none showed proliferative endometrium, hyperplasia, or carcinoma.[35]

Thus far, all studies of endometrial histology in patients on combined estrogen and progestogens have only a small number of subjects. However, there appear to be no adverse effects of the regimen on the endometrium.

Endometrial Changes Following GnRH Agonists

Gonadotropin releasing hormone (GnRH) agonists are useful for the treatment of endometriosis. They are also useful for preoperative preparation of the endometrium for endometrial ablation and other operative hysteroscopic procedures. Following a depot injection of GnRH agonist, the endometrium on gross examination appears smooth, pale, flat, and hypovascular.[36] Microscopically, the endometrium is thin and inactive, with little or no edema. The gland to stroma ratio favors the stroma. Smaller endometrial glands in reduced numbers are present. The size and number of blood vessels decrease. Endometrial stromal cells appear decreased in number, and the endometrial stroma is compact.[36] These endometrial changes are reversible. Resumption of cyclic menses occurs following discontinuation of GnRH therapy.

Endometrial Changes Associated with Intrauterine Contraceptive Devices

There are two intrauterine contraceptive devices (IUDs) currently available in the United States. One contains copper, and the other contains 38 mg of progesterone. In Europe, some IUDs contain L-norgestrel. Intrauterine devices can cause pressure changes with focal crowding of the glands and stroma directly beneath the endometrium, where there is physical contact with the device. An inflammatory response, both acute and chronic, may be responsible for bleeding, pain, and vaginal discharge. When an IUD is in place for more than 3 years, chronic inflammation with plasma cells is present in 40 percent of patients.[21] Squamous metaplasia of the underlying endometrium may also occur, and, rarely, foreign body giant cells may be present.[21]

Copper-containing IUDs initiate an inflammatory response in the endometrium. Histologically this varies from mild to severe. A common pattern is the presence of polymorphonuclear leukocytes in the glandular lumens.[21] A thin layer of exudate may be present on the surface but without leukocytic infiltration in the stroma. These findings correlate with the length of time the device has been in contact with the endometrium.[21]

The L-norgestrel–releasing IUDs produce glandular atrophy and a focal decidualized stroma. A focal inflammatory response with necrosis may also be present.[37] The prominence of the stromal decidual change is generally inversely proportional to the length of time the device has been in place. The stromal leukocytic infiltrates sometimes contain plasma cells.[37] After 3 years of continued use, focal calcifications may be present. Thick-walled fibrotic vessels similar to those found in endometrial polyps also occur on rare occasions.[37]

The endometritis associated with an IUD is self-limited. Menorrhagia and intermenstrual bleeding are common symptoms associated with these devices. The chronic inflammatory changes disappear and symptoms also usually resolve following removal of the device.

Intrauterine contraceptive devices have long been known to cause shedding of glandular cells, which may be detected on a Pap smear. Sometimes these cells and cellular groupings can be quite atypical and have led to an overdiagnosis of adenocarcinoma.[37a] The irritation of the device in the endometrial cavity allows for shedding of endometrial cells, often in papillary type groups. These cells have a degenerate and inflammatory appearance that can be suggestive of endometrial carcinoma.[37b] Likewise, the IUD string may cause irritation and inflammation of the endocervical canal and may lead to shedding of atypical endocervical cells. The only way for these cells to be correctly characterized is for the cytopathologist to know of the presence of an IUD. If the cells are very suspicious, it may be necessary to remove the device. This should cause the abnormal cells to disappear. If they do not, additional studies (e.g., curettage) are necessary.

The Endometrial Biopsy in the Infertility Patient

Approximately 14 percent of women attempting to conceive are infertile. The definition of infertility is the inability of a couple to conceive after 1 year of unprotected intercourse. Determination of whether ovulation has occurred is one important component of any infertility evaluation. Pregnancy and direct observation of ovulation at laparoscopy or with ultrasound are the only definitive indications of ovulation. All other methods are presumptive and indirect. The indirect methods include basal body temperature charts, serum progesterone levels, and endometrial sampling. The presence of a secretory endometrium implies that ovulation occurred at an earlier time in the cycle. Histologic dating of the endometrium using the criteria described earlier is an important part of every infertility evaluation. Comparison of the assigned histologic date and the date of onset of the next menstrual period is important in determining whether a luteal phase defect is present.

As discussed earlier, histologic dating of the endometrium is at best approximate. For an endometrial biopsy to be "in phase," the assigned date should agree within 48 hours with the calculated date as determined by the onset of the next menses. This is done since the proliferative phase of the cycle may be of variable length, while the secretory phase is consistently 14 days. If there is a greater than 48 hour lag, the biopsy is "out of phase" and may indicate a luteal phase defect. For example, an assigned histologic day 23 with onset of menses 2 days later, i.e., bleeding from a histologic day 25 endometrium, is inappropriate. Clinically this may correspond to a decreased progesterone level for the cycle in question. Documentation of a low serum progesterone along with the endometrial biopsy may be helpful. Luteal phase deficiency is present in approximately 3 percent of women with infertility.[38] To make the diagnosis, an "out of phase" endometrial biopsy must persist for at least two consecutive cycles, since this finding may occur sporadically in normal cycling women. The pathogenesis of luteal phase defect is uncertain, and some clinicians do not believe that this entity exists. Twenty-nine percent of biopsies are "out of phase" in any given cycle, but only 10.9 percent are out of phase in two cycles.[39]

Other common abnormal histopathologic findings in the endometrial biopsy from infertility patients include chronic endometritis (2.1 percent), hyperplasia (1.1 percent), and endometrial polyps (0.2 percent).[39]

Three different approaches to the treatment of luteal phase deficiency are currently employed. Clomiphene citrate is used if it is believed that poor follicle maturation results in a deficient corpus luteum. The administration of clomiphene citrate begins between cycle days 3 and 5 and continues through cycle day 7 or 9. This causes an elevation of FSH and stimulation of the dominant follicle. Histologic changes in infertility patients treated with clomiphene citrate differ subtly from the normal cycling endometrium.[38] The glands tend to be straight, narrow, and less tortuous than usual. As with normal endometrium, the gland to stroma ratio favors the stroma. Secretions are not as abundant throughout the secretory phase. Luminal secretions appear inspissated earlier in the cycle. Although predecidualization occurs, the decidualized cells are often smaller. These features suggest a hypoestrogenic effect.[38] A second method of treatment involves midcycle administration of hCG, which is similar to luteinizing hormone. This stimulates progesterone production and conversion of the proliferative endometrium to a normal secretory endometrium. This is usually not given alone but as an adjunct to clomiphene treatment. A third method of treatment is the administration of progesterone vaginal suppositories or the use of micronized oral progesterone. Administration begins following the midcycle temperature rise. If pregnancy occurs, progesterone administration continues until the placenta takes over progesterone production. The goal of treating luteal phase deficiency is pregnancy. Endometrial sampling obtained during a cycle of therapy should be histologically in phase and otherwise normal.

Approximately 1.5 percent of endometrial biopsies done for infertility evaluation occur in the cycle of conception. Most implantations occur in the uterine fundus or its posterior wall. To avoid disruption of the implantation site, some recommend that the endometrial biopsy be obtained only from the anterior portion of the endometrium. Spontaneous abortion occurs in 22.2 percent of women whose endometrial sampling is done in the cycle of conception.[39] This is not significantly different from the spontaneous abortion rate of the general population. Sampling of the actual implantation site is rare (Fig. 5–16). The implantation site was present on the histopathology slides prepared from endometrial biopsies of 0.6 percent of infertility patients.[40] Some of these pregnancies have gone to term with the delivery of a normal infant.[39] In those pregnancies that do not progress, the sampling of the implantation site probably represented an excisional biopsy of the site.[40]

Immunocytochemistry of the Endometrium

Immunocytochemistry has become an integral part of pathology. Immunocytochemical staining identifies specific proteins in both normal and abnormal tissues. In normal endometrium, the number of proteins that can be demonstrated in fresh and paraffin-embedded tissue increases daily.

Immunocytochemical staining for estrogen receptors has demonstrated localized staining in the nuclei of the epithelial and stromal cells. Secretory endometrium stains less intensely than proliferative endometrium, but both estrogen and progesterone receptors are present in normal endome-

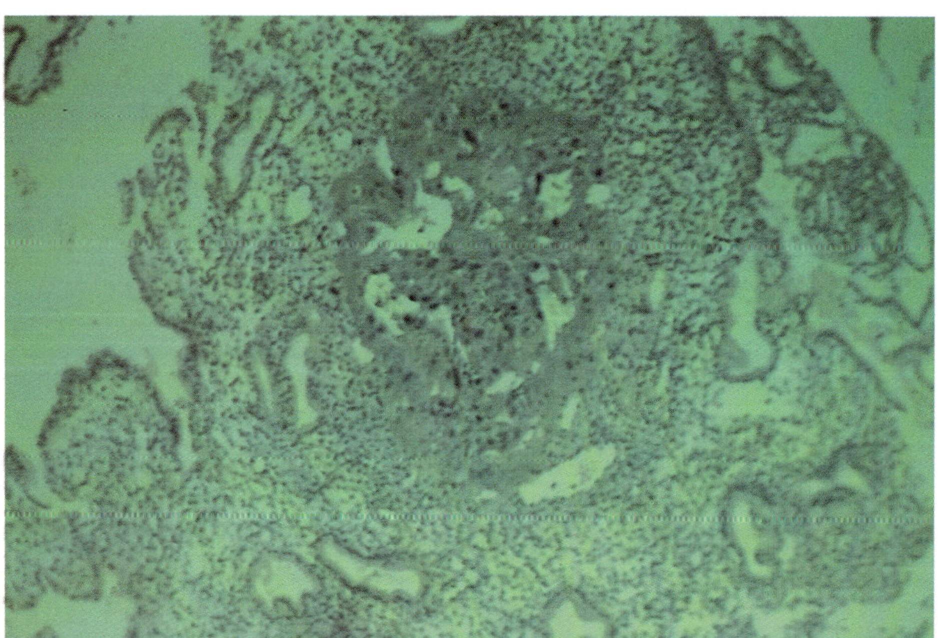

FIGURE 5–16
This endometrial biopsy demonstrates a day 24 to 25 endometrium with an early implantation site. Trophoblasts *(center)* are proliferating, attempting to invade individual endometrial vessels.

trium throughout the menstrual cycle.[41] Squamous cells in normal and abnormal endometrium do not stain for estrogen receptor.[42]

Although initially used to monitor disease activity in patients with ovarian carcinoma, elevated serum levels of CA 125 occur in some patients with endometrial carcinoma. This tumor-associated antigen is also present in the glandular epithelium of normal cycling endometrium.[43] CA 125 is most prominent during the secretory phase. Positive staining, particularly at the base and apex of proliferative endometrial glands, occurred in all nine patients whose biopsies were tested. Staining was focal and involved less than half the glandular epithelium.[43] Positive staining was also present in biopsies from all 11 patients who had secretory endometrium (Fig. 5–17). In late secretory endometrium more than 50 percent of the glandular epithelium stained positive for CA 125.[43]

CA 19-9 was present in 4 of 20 patients with normal endometrium; 2 of 9 patients with proliferative endometrium, and 2 of 11 with secretory endometrium. Staining was focal and limited to the apical cell surface.[43] Although the monoclonal antibody to this antigen was originally produced by immunization with a colon carcinoma cell line, the antibody recognizes the sialylated Lewis a antigen, a member of the Lewis blood group.[43] The expression of such carbohydrates in most normal endometria and in sera relates to the genetic status of the individual, i.e., ABO and Lewis type, as well as saliva secretor status.[44]

Tumor-associated glycoprotein 72 (TAG 72) is a glycoprotein originally associated with metastatic breast cancer. It is present in almost 100 percent of fundal secretory endometrium. Expression is weaker in endometrium from the lower uterine segment.[45] It is absent in proliferative and inactive endometrium.

Other proteins that can be demonstrated by immunocytochemistry in the endometrial glandular epithelium include serotonin, somatostatin, pancreatic polypeptide, an apocrine epithelial membrane antigen directed against human milk fat globules (EMA), immunoreactive secretory polypeptide, and IgA.[46–48] Alpha-1-antitrypsin and α-1-antichymotrypsin granules are present in the stromal cells of normal endometrium. They are also present in macrophages and in some uterine sarcomas.[49] Insulin-like growth factor-1 and its receptor are demonstrable in normal cycling endometrium in both the glandular epithelium and the endometrial stroma.[50]

CONGENITAL ANOMALIES

Congenital anomalies of the uterus represent anomalies in the müllerian system. They are of three basic types: congenital absence of all or part of the müllerian system, fusion anomalies, and changes associated with in utero exposure to diethylstilbestrol and other nonsteroidal estrogens. Arteriovascular anomalies may occur, but these anomalies are extremely rare.

The development of the female genital system

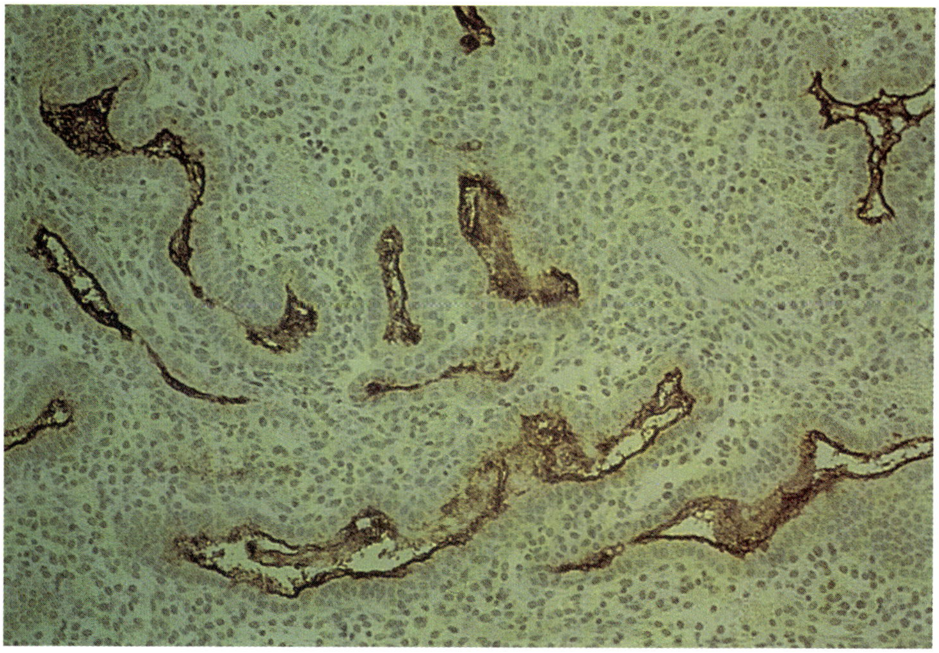

FIGURE 5–17
This is a late secretory endometrium demonstrating intense staining for CA 125 at the luminal surface of the cells and staining of secretions within the lumen. (From Podczaski E, Kaminski PF, Zaino R: CA 125 and CA 19-9 immunolocalization in normal, hyperplastic and carcinomatous endometrium. Cancer 1993; 71:2551–2556.)

begins early in pregnancy with fusion of the paired müllerian ducts, which occurs at approximately 8 weeks of gestation. Development continues throughout the first half of pregnancy.

Congenital Absence

Congenital absence of the uterus is a rare occurrence. Mayer-Rokitansky-Küster-Hauser syndrome or some combination of this eponym refers to this anatomic phenomenon. When present, the ovaries and fallopian tubes are normal, but the latter end in a rudimentary central bud, which may contain endometrium. If endometrium is present, a pelvic abdominal mass can develop from the resulting cryptomenorrhea.[51] The vagina fails to develop and appears as a dimple. If there is no cervix, salvage of the uterine bud for reproduction is not successful. Creation of a neovagina is necessary for satisfactory sexual function.[52] This can be achieved by either the Frank procedure, i.e., dilatation with graduated dilators,[52] or the McIndoe vaginoplasty.[53] In patients with müllerian agenesis, a search for associated abnormalities of the lumbar spine and the urinary system is appropriate.[54] Intravenous pyelogram, ultrasound, computed tomography (CT), and magnetic resonance imaging (MRI) are the methods currently employed to evaluate for these anomalies.

Fusion Anomalies

Fusion anomalies produce a variety of uterine anatomic configurations. These include, at one extreme, complete duplication of the müllerian system (Fig. 5–18), and, at the other extreme, a small uterine septum in the fundus or a bicornuate uterus (Fig. 5–19). The frequency of fusion anomalies is unknown. The majority of these anomalies are asymptomatic and cause no reproductive difficulties.[55] Detection of fusion anomalies is usually incidental. The most common methods of diagnosis are hysterosalpingography, hysteroscopy, and laparoscopy during an infertility investigation.[56, 57] Sometimes a uterine fusion anomaly first becomes manifest during routine obstetric care or delivery. Pregnancy in one horn of a bicornuate uterus can result in premature labor and delivery. Early pregnancy loss may result from a unicornuate uterus or from a septate uterus. In theory, this may happen when implantation occurs on the relatively avascular septum rather than the normal uterine wall. Rarely, one of the horns of a bicornuate uterus will fail to communicate with the remainder of the endometrial cavity, resulting in cryptomenorrhea. This causes cyclic abdominal pain and may produce an abdominopelvic mass, i.e., hematometria (Fig. 5–20). Approximately 2 percent of women undergoing transcervical sterilization were found to have abnormal uteri, later confirmed by hysterosalpingogram.[56] By far the most common anomalous finding was a bicornuate uterus or a septate uterus. Unicornuate uteri accounted for 6 percent of the anomalies.[56] When there is complete duplication of the müllerian system, a longitudinal vaginal septum is present. The presence of a longitudinal vaginal septum on ex-

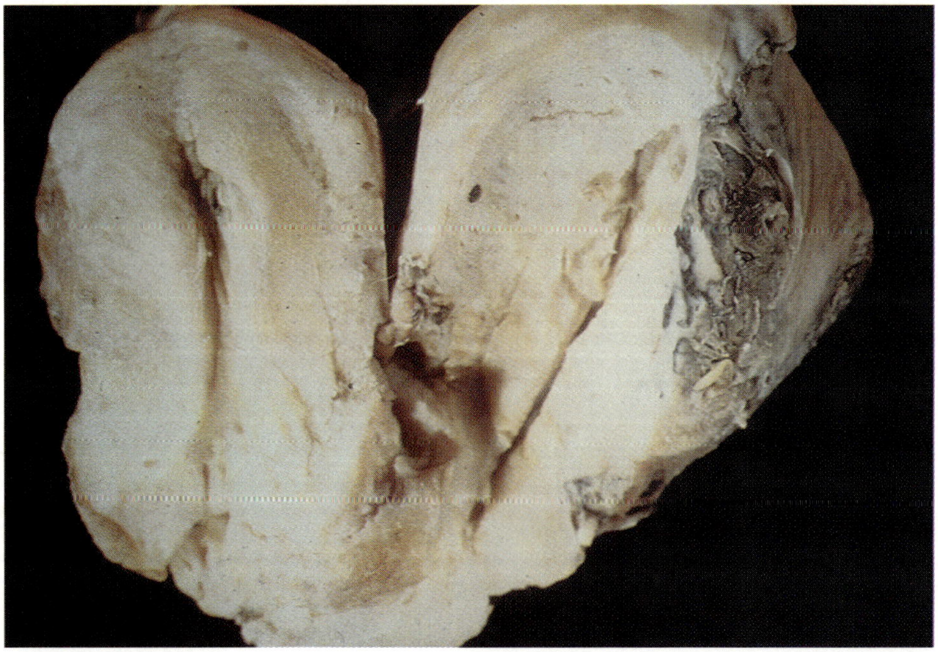

FIGURE 5–18
This is a uterus didelphys. Two separate cervices are present. They share some stromal tissues; the cavities are independent.

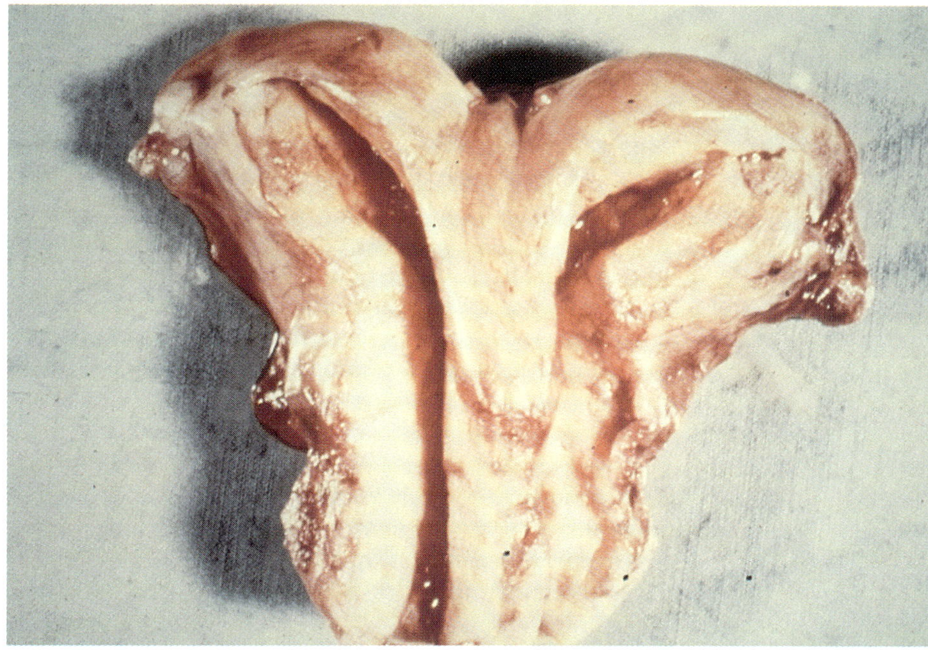

FIGURE 5-19
This bicornuate uterus has one cervix. There are two distinct uterine fundi, which differentiates this anomaly from a septate uterus. The latter would not have the fundal indentation. On pelvic examination the uterus may be perceived as heart-shaped. A fibromuscular septum extends almost to the cervix in this specimen.

amination should prompt further evaluation for complete duplication of the müllerian system.

Treatment of uterine anomalies may not be necessary unless there is a history of pregnancy loss. However, in women with pregnancy loss that may be attributable to a uterine anomaly, correction of the anatomic defect should be accomplished. This may include hysteroscopic excision of a uterine septum or unification of a bicornuate uterus by an abdominal metroplasty. In those rare patients who have a noncommunicating horn, treatment consists of resection of the horn and conservative treatment of the frequently associated endometriosis.

Impaired reproductive performance occurs in some women exposed in utero to diethylstilbestrol and other nonsteroidal estrogens. The pregnancy wastage rate in these women approaches 58 percent, while the live birth rate is 42 percent.[58] Some of these births are premature. In those women with reproductive failure, 30.6 percent abort in the first trimester, 4.8 percent have tubal

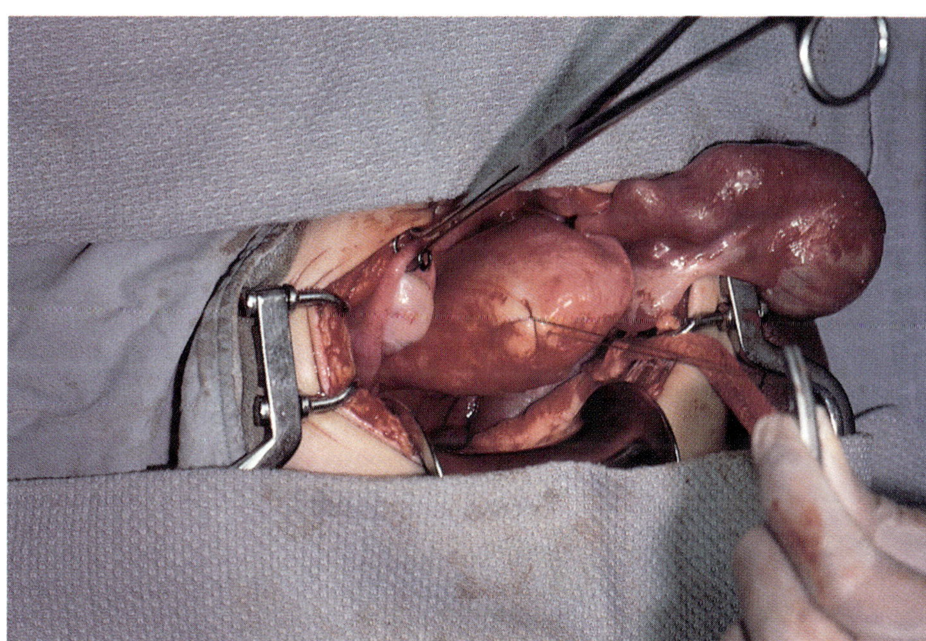

FIGURE 5-20
A 13-year-old with cyclic abdominal pain and an irregular right sided pelvic mass has a hematosalpinx on the right, and an enlarged uterine horn of a bicornuate uterus in the center. The normal-sized left uterine horn is not seen, but a normal left fallopian tube is identified.

pregnancies, and 17.7 percent have spontaneous midtrimester losses. An additional 12.9 percent of women will deliver prematurely, i.e., before 35 weeks.[58] A hysterosalpingogram in these women reveals changes that vary from a T-shaped endometrial cavity to a markedly hypoplastic uterus and cervix.[59] Investigation of women with reproductive loss should include a history of possible in utero exposure to diethylstilbestrol or other nonsteroidal estrogens. Hysterosalpingography is an indicated procedure in women with this history, particularly if they also have a history of reproductive wastage. A cervical cerclage to prevent premature delivery may be necessary in some cases.[58]

Clinically significant arteriovenous malformations are rare. These patients present with menorrhagia. This is the one clinical situation in which curettage is not helpful and may exaggerate the bleeding. Arteriovenous malformation is a rare cause of fetal wastage. The gross appearance of the uterus depends on the caliber of the vessels and the extent of involvement of the uterus. The vessels range from medium-sized irregular vessels to large thick-walled vessels. The malformations consist of a mixture of muscular and thin-walled capillary-like vessels in varying proportions. Most vessels appear to be intermediate between arteries and veins, and distinction between arteries and veins is difficult in some instances. Prominent intimal thickening is present in many vessels. In other instances the vessels resemble a cavernous hemangioma. Uterine angiography has successfully diagnosed malformations.[60] Refractory bleeding, unresponsive to or aggravated by endometrial curettage strongly suggests an arteriovenous malformation.[61] Treatment in most instances is hysterectomy, sometimes as an emergency because of heavy bleeding. Embolization of arteriovenous anomalies using invasive radiologic techniques could control the bleeding.[60] There are reports of successful pregnancy following embolization.[62]

BENIGN CONDITIONS

The classification of endometrial pathology relies largely on a subjective and qualitative system of diagnosis that includes alterations due to metaplasia, inflammation or infection, hormonal changes, hyperplasia, and neoplasia.[63]

Endometrial Metaplasia

Hendrickson and Kempson introduced this concept in 1980.[64] They defined non-neoplastic epithelial metaplasia as the replacement of normal epithelium in a given site with a mature benign epithelium that is inappropriate for that site.[64] The endometrial epithelium manifests metaplastic changes by a replacement of the typical endometrial glandular epithelium with an epithelium that is normally present in another müllerian organ, such as the fallopian tube or endocervix. These metaplastic changes may occur in normal, hyperplastic, and neoplastic endometrium. Metaplastic changes are important to recognize, because confusion occurs between benign metaplastic changes and neoplasia.*

Metaplastic changes identified in normal endometrium and the frequency of these changes are as follows: ciliated or tubal metaplasia (58 percent), mucinous metaplasia (24 percent), clear cell and hobnail cell metaplasia (10 percent), squamous metaplasia morules (34 percent), papillary metaplasia (12 percent), and eosinophilic, oxyphil, or pink cell metaplasia (48 percent).[64] More than one type of metaplasia may be present in any given endometrium.

Ciliated Metaplasia

Ciliated metaplasia (tubal metaplasia) is most common around the fallopian tube ostia but may occur in other areas of the endometrium (Fig. 5–21). Ciliated metaplasia appears as large numbers of cytologically bland ciliated cells occurring either singly or in small pear-shaped aggregates. These cells have an eosinophilic cytoplasm. The glandular epithelium often appears stratified. Halo cells are common. Occasional mitoses are present. The differential diagnosis includes hyperplasia with severe atypia, ciliated cell adenocarcinoma, and papillary serous carcinoma.

Mucinous Metaplasia

Mucinous metaplasia typically occurs toward the lower uterine segment, near the junction with the endocervix. Unlike the squamocolumnar junction in the cervix, the junction of the lower uterine segment and endocervix is not distinct, either grossly or microscopically. Cells that have undergone mucinous metaplasia contain intracytoplasmic mucin. They have cytologically bland nuclei

* The definitions and descriptions of endometrial metaplasias presented above were modified from: Hendrickson MR, Kempson RL: Endometrial epithelial metaplasias: report of 89 cases and proposed classification. Am J Surg Pathol 1980; 4:525–542, with permission of the authors and publisher, Raven Press.

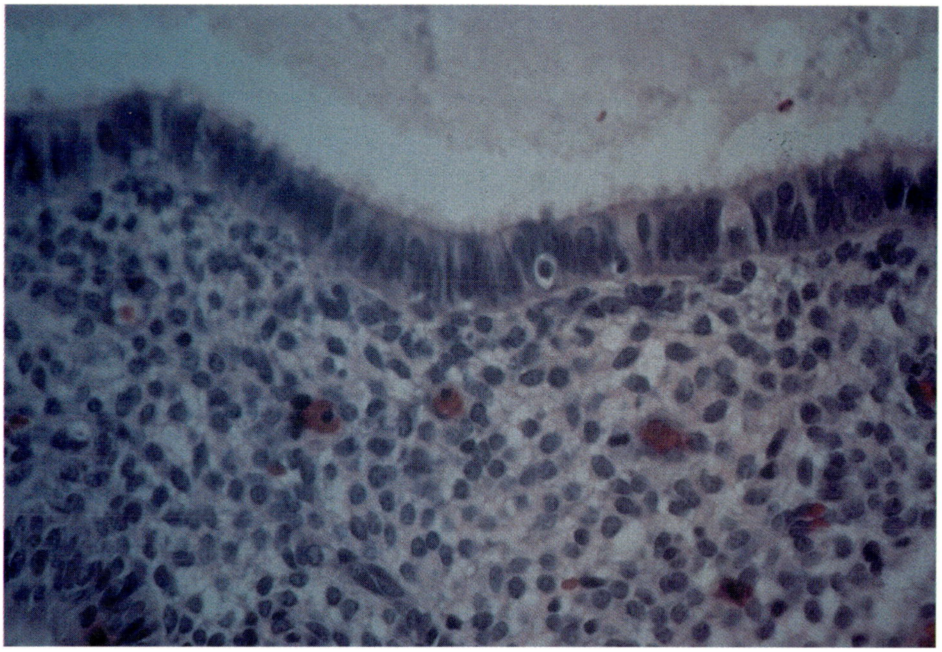

FIGURE 5-21
This is an endometrial gland with tubal type metaplasia. The gland contains ciliated and secretory type epithelia similar to those found in the normal fallopian tube.

that may be pyknotic or vesicular. Mitotic figures are rare. Stratification is lacking (Fig. 5–22). The differential diagnosis includes normal endocervix, cervical microglandular hyperplasia, mucinous endometrial adenocarcinoma, endocervical adenocarcinoma with extension to the corpus, and metastatic colon carcinoma.

Clear Cell Metaplasia

Clear cell metaplasia is the least common type. The clear cell and the hobnail cell are variants of the endometrioid cell. Clear cells are cytologically bland, and there is no mitotic activity. Nuclear pleomorphism is minimal to absent. Hobnail metaplasia contains cytologically bland cells with rare mitotic figures and minimal nuclear pleomorphism. The cells are pear-shaped with rounded atypical luminal projections. The bulbous nucleus protrudes into the lumen and resembles the hobnails of a boot. The cytoplasm is either clear or slightly eosinophilic. The differential diagnosis includes clear cell carcinoma, Arias-Stella phenomenon, and metastatic renal carcinoma.

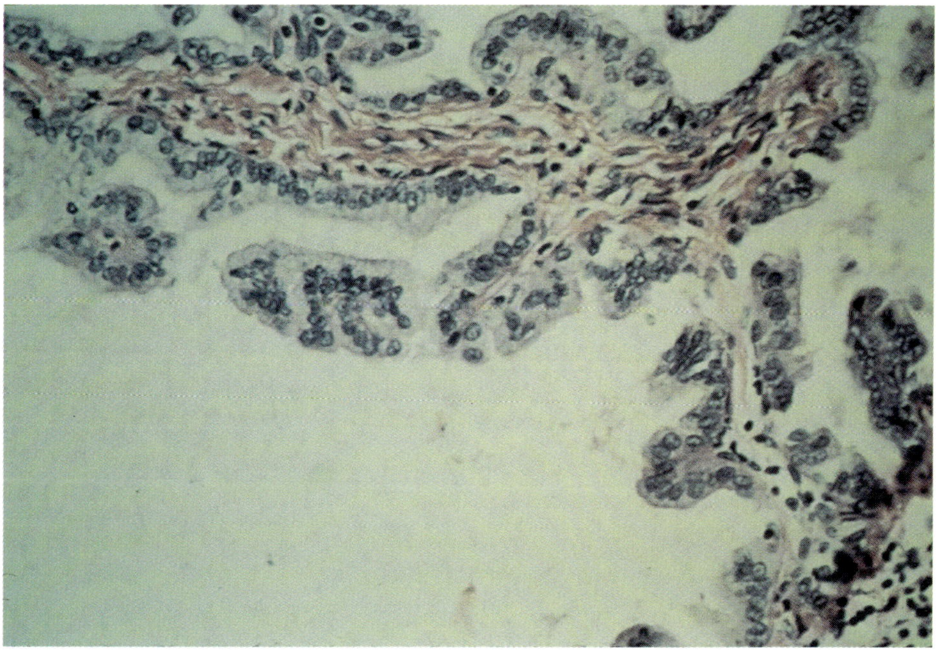

FIGURE 5-22
This is papillary mucinous epithelium occurring in a hyperplastic endometrial gland.

Squamous Metaplasia

Squamous metaplasia occurs commonly in hyperplasia and endometrial adenocarcinoma but may also arise in benign endometrium. Squamous change in benign endometrium occurs as morules, seen in a background that is otherwise proliferative or occasionally secretory (Fig. 5–23). Morules are round aggregates of epithelial cells that are often in continuity with the endometrial gland lining. The cells are cytologically bland and demonstrate abundant keratinized cytoplasm; intercellular bridges are frequently present. Mitotic activity is sparse, and nuclear pleomorphism is minimal. The differential diagnosis of squamous change in the endometrium includes granulomas, disintegrating endometrial stroma, poorly differentiated endometrial adenocarcinoma, metastatic adenocarcinoma, and uterine sarcoma.

Papillary Changes

Papillary changes are common. They are usually present on the endometrial surface but may involve portions of the deeper glands. The cells form a syncytium-like mass that has cells with indistinct cytoplasmic borders. The nuclei are shrunken, pyknotic, and degenerated. However, they are uniform and cytologically bland. An infiltration with polymorphonuclear leukocytes is frequent. Papillary metaplasia is common in menstrual endometrium. The collapse of the endometrial stroma and the presence of fibrin thrombi help identify the process as benign. The differential diagnosis includes papillary adenocarcinoma and fragmented endometrioid adenocarcinoma.

Eosinophilic Metaplasia

Eosinophilic metaplasia (oxyphil metaplasia, or pink cell metaplasia) has distinguishing staining characteristics. The cytoplasm of these cells is copious and eosinophilic, much paler than the surrounding endometrium (Fig. 5–24). The cells themselves are cytologically bland with uniform vesicular nuclei. Nuclear pleomorphism is not present. Mitotic figures are rare. Usually these cells are nonstratified, but minor degrees of stratification may be present. In the past pathologists associated these changes with hyperplasia (Fig. 5–25) or carcinoma, but eosinophilic changes also occur in benign endometrium, similar to the changes that occur in the fallopian tube. The differential diagnosis includes complex atypical hyperplasia, typical endometrial adenocarcinoma, and secretory endometrium.

Ninety percent of women with metaplastic changes in the endometrium are perimenopausal or postmenopausal. Seventy-five percent had taken estrogen replacement therapy within 1 month of the curettage or biopsy.[64]

Endometritis

Acute Endometritis

Acute endometritis is common post partum and post abortion. Prolonged rupture of the fetal mem-

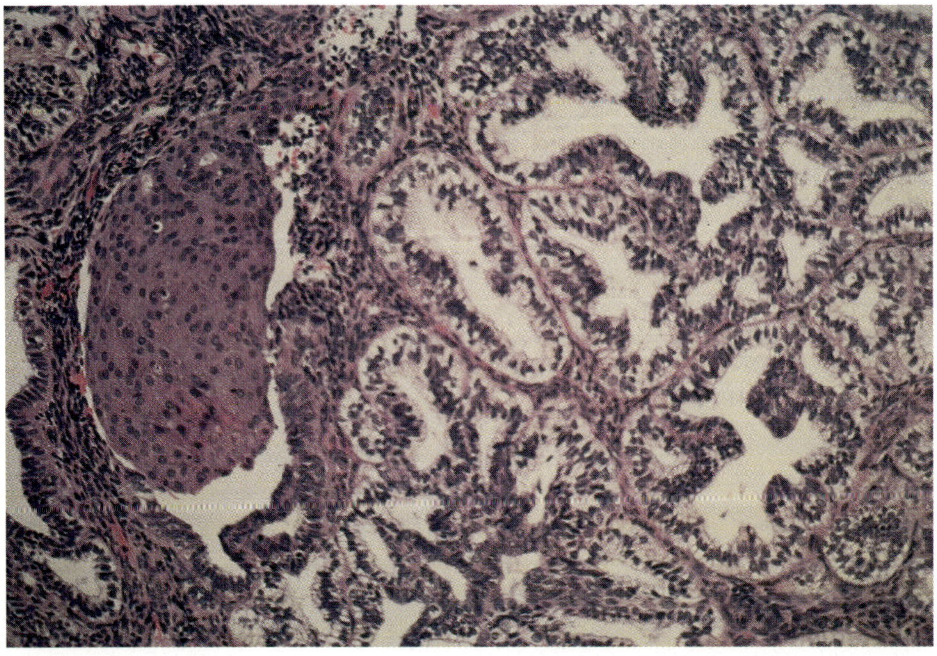

FIGURE 5–23
This squamous morule partially fills the gland lumen in normal early secretory endometrium.

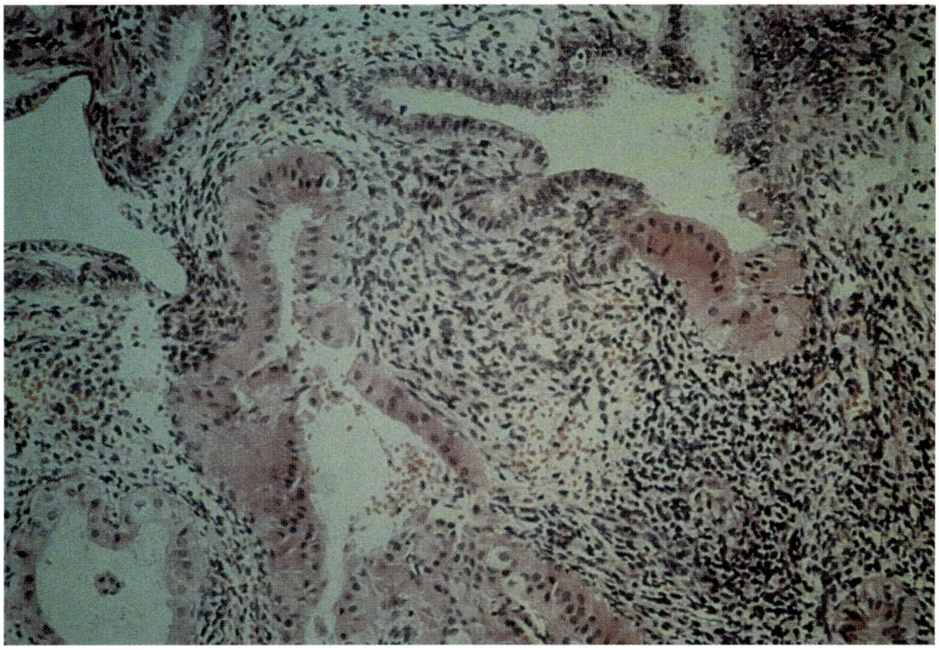

F I G U R E 5 - 2 4
Eosinophilic metaplasia is seen here. The endometrium demonstrates simple hyperplasia with eosinophilic changes in the cytoplasm of some cells.

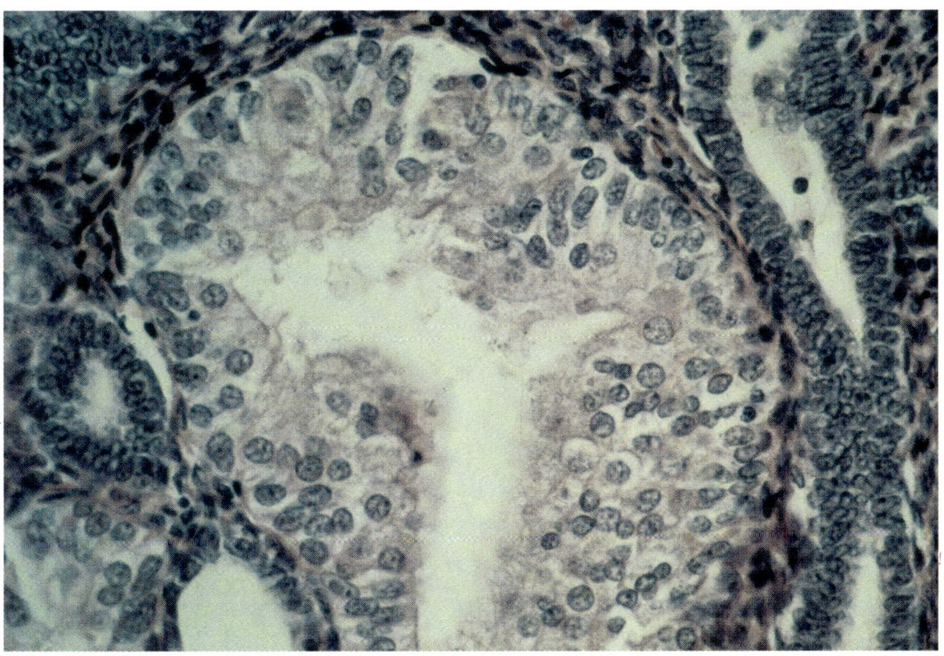

F I G U R E 5 - 2 5
This hyperplastic gland demonstrates eosinophilic metaplasia. The pink color of the cytoplasm is characteristic. This glandular epithelium is stratified to at least three cell layers and is cytologically atypical.

branes is a predisposing factor in many cases; retained placental tissue is the cause in other instances. When the inflammatory process involves the parametrium, it causes abdominopelvic pain, fever, and a foul yellow discharge from the cervix. Cervical motion tenderness is the cardinal physical finding. Usually the clinician will institute antibiotic therapy; only on occasion, when the diagnosis is uncertain or profuse hemorrhage occurs from retained placental tissue, will he or she obtain an endometrial sample or perform a curettage. Polymorphonuclear leukocytes generally are present in proportion to the degree of inflammation. These fill gland lumens as well as infiltrate the endometrial stroma. In severe infections, polymorphonuclear leukocytes even infiltrate the myometrium. Treatment is removal of any retained products of conception or other foreign material along with antibiotic coverage for aerobic and anaerobic organisms, as the infection is usually polymicrobial.

An *eosinophilic endomyometritis* occurs rarely following curettage. To produce this phenomenon, a circumferential mucosal injury, together with at least a focal myometrial lesion with an occluding blood clot, is necessary. There is individual variability in the number of eosinophils. The process occurs 18 hours to 24 days after curettage.[65] Acute suppurative changes significantly diminish the eosinophilic response. A lymphocytic infiltrate will eventually accompany the eosinophilia. Dense areas of eosinophils are seen in the central portion of the uterus but may also be interspersed throughout the myometrium.[65] This process appears to be self-limiting.

Chronic Endometritis

Chronic endometritis refers specifically to the presence of plasma cells within the endometrial stroma (Fig. 5–26). Chronic endometritis is present in approximately 7 percent of endometrial samples from patients who have abnormal uterine bleeding.[29] Chronic endometritis does not refer to the presence of lymphoid aggregates, which may be present in up to 20 percent of normal cycling endometria. Symptoms of chronic endometritis are usually heavy menses and intermenstrual bleeding. Chronic endometritis is common in the following circumstances: postpartum or postabortal; in association with an IUD; next to or admixed in the stroma of endometrial polyps, endometrial hyperplasia, or endometrial neoplasia. In these conditions plasma cells will be present, and, in addition, the surrounding endometrium histologically will not appear to be cycling properly. The stroma is denser, and evidence of bleeding and fibrin thrombi may be seen. Treatment consists of removal of the offending cause and/or specific treatment of the underlying condition. In many instances curettage is necessary.

Rarely, an inflammatory reaction may be so florid that the possibility of malignant lymphoma arises. The microscopic distinction of malignant lymphoma from benign lymphoid infiltrates in the uterus can be difficult at times.[66] The major dis-

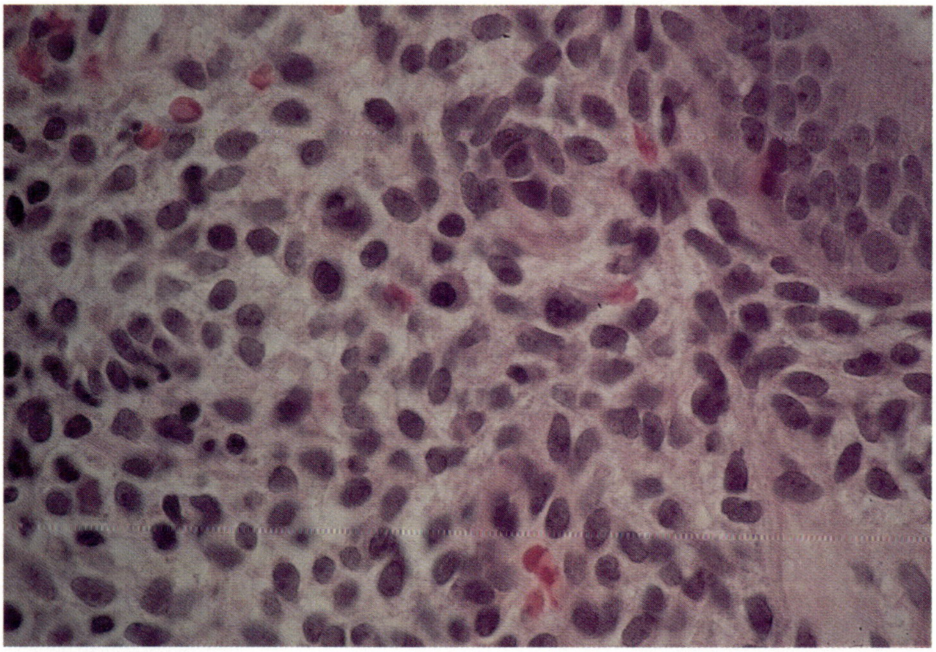

FIGURE 5–26
This is chronic endometritis. The presence of a plasma cell (in center of field) with eccentric nuclei and basophilic cytoplasm is diagnostic.

tinguishing point is that in a reactive process there is a mixed population of lymphocytes. There are variable-sized cells ranging from small mature lymphocytes to germinal center reactive lymphocytes with large immunoblasts and tingible-body macrophages. On the other hand, in malignant lymphoma there is usually a relatively uniform population of atypical-appearing lymphocytes. Benign lymphoid aggregates can measure up to 2.5 mm in diameter.[66] When an inflammatory reaction becomes florid, involvement of the surface endometrium is almost universal. Ulceration is commonly present. Florid inflammatory reactions contain only rare plasma cells and polymorphonuclear leukocytes. Plasma cells are often prominent at the periphery of lymphoid aggregates. Nuclear debris and histiocytes containing phagocytized debris are prominent features.[66] Most of the aggregates resemble reactive germinal centers, but they lack a peripheral mantle of mature lymphocytes.[66] No significant sequelae have been observed in patients with such florid chronic inflammation of the uterus.

A specific type of chronic endometritis occurs in the presence of tuberculosis. Typical granulomas form, but caseation necrosis is usually not present, since the functionalis of the endometrium sheds monthly (Fig. 5–27). Epithelioid type granulomas, disseminated throughout the endometrial layers, are prominent. However, their density is highest in the superficial layers. Involvement of the basal portion of the endometrium occurs in only 40 percent of cases.[67] A dense cuff of lymphocytes surrounds these granulomas. Occasionally, the granulomatous inflammation erodes the glandular epithelium and is discharged into the glandular lumens. A neutrophilic infiltrate accompanies this process, and microabscesses are seen.[67] Adjacent endometrial glands have altered features and do not appear to cycle properly. Superficial myometrial involvement by granulomas is present in 20 percent of patients.[67]

Tuberculous involvement of the endometrium is usually secondary to spread from the fallopian tubes. Definitive diagnosis consists of identification of the acid-fast microorganisms. A chest radiograph will identify the primary source in most individuals. Tuberculosis is resurgent today, secondary to the increase in the number of immunosuppressed individuals. Infertility occurs in almost all women with pelvic tuberculosis.[67] While rare in the United States, the clinician occasionally encounters pelvic tuberculosis as a cause of infertility.

Rarely, chronic inflammation in the endometrium is the result of pinworm or *Ascaris* infestation of the endometrium. In some areas of the world, schistosome ova may be present in the endometrium and cause chronic inflammation.

Malacoplakia involving the endometrium is extremely rare. This is an unusual chronic granulomatous inflammation. A histiocytic infiltrate (von Hansemann cells) with intra- and extracellular calcified bodies (Michaelis-Gutmann bodies) characterizes this condition.[68] Sheets of large, pale, round or polygonal von Hansemann cells with a

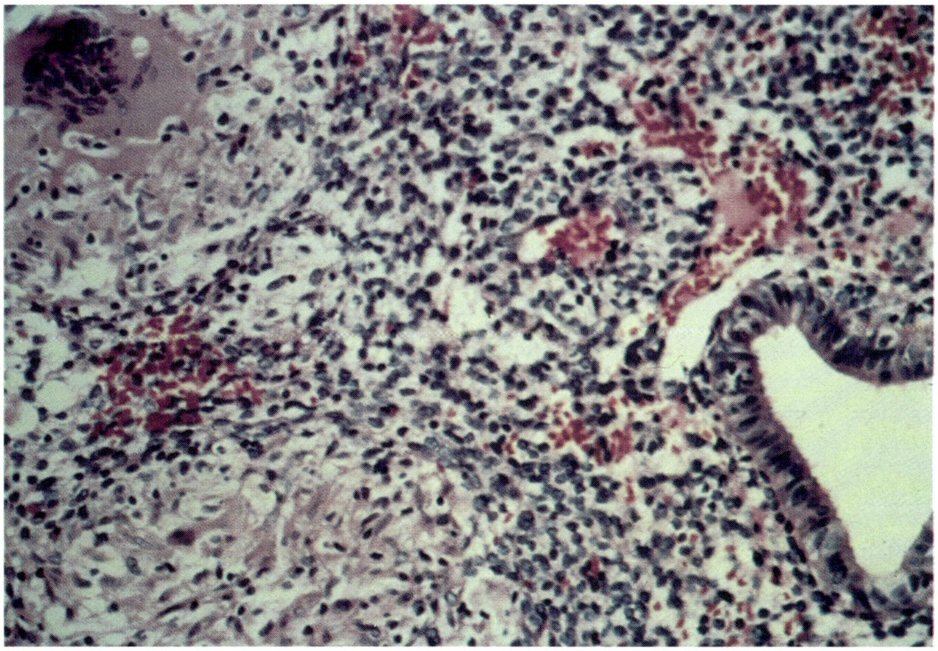

FIGURE 5–27
In this granulomatous endometritis, two granulomas are present, and the one in the upper left has a Langhans type giant cell. The endometrium rarely shows caseation.

coarsely granular cytoplasm are seen on microscopic examination.

Although involvement of the cervix with human papillomavirus (HPV) is common, involvement of the endometrium with *papillomatous lesions* is rare. However, diffuse uterine papillomatosis involving the endometrium with extension into endometrial glands does occur. Immunoperoxidase staining for HPV may be positive.[69] However, ultrastructural studies have been unable to identify intranuclear viral particles.[69] With the use of the polymerase chain reaction, HPV DNA sequences have been identified in both benign and neoplastic endometrium. The HPV type 16 genome may be present in up to 70 percent of benign endometria.[70] Although inoculation of viral particles into the upper genital tract may not be that uncommon, infection of the endometrium with HPV is rare. The method of spread may be transluminal, translymphatic, or hematogenous.[70]

Dysfunctional Uterine Bleeding

Dysfunctional uterine bleeding refers to abnormal uterine bleeding in the presence of a normal pelvic examination, after exclusion of all organic causes. Dysfunctional uterine bleeding is therefore a diagnosis of exclusion. It is not appropriate to include bleeding secondary to the withdrawal of exogenous estrogen or progestogen. Such bleeding is not dysfunctional bleeding. The most common cause of dysfunctional bleeding is anovulation. The proximate cause of bleeding is usually endogenous estrogen withdrawal. The term disordered proliferation describes specific histologic changes in the endometrium; it is commonly seen in association with anovulatory bleeding. When ovulation does not occur, the endometrium continues to proliferate. As the endometrial glands proliferate, the gland lumens dilate and show irregularity, and the gland to stroma ratio begins to favor the glands. The glandular epithelium becomes pseudostratified. Cilia may be present. Mitotic figures are seen in both the endometrial glandular epithelium and the stroma.

The histologic changes present in an anovulatory endometrium differ subtly from those of a normal proliferative endometrium. At the onset of bleeding, the endometrium becomes fragmented and the stroma collapses. Fibrin thrombi, indicative of bleeding, are present. Secretory exhaustion of the glands is absent. Treatment of anovulatory bleeding is progestogen therapy, orally or intramuscularly. This will convert the proliferative endometrium to a secretory endometrium. At the withdrawal of the progestogen support, bleeding will recur. However, it will be lighter in amount and of short duration. Anovulatory bleeding can be extremely heavy, requiring curettage for control. Patients with long-term anovulation resulting in unopposed estrogen stimulation of the endometrium are at risk for developing hyperplasia or cancer. Patients 40 years of age or younger who do not respond to progestogens, and those older than 40 years, should have histologic evaluation of the endometrium to exclude hyperplasia or cancer.

In some women with unexplained menorrhagia, endometrial biopsy will reveal secretory endometrium. After exclusion of all other causes, changes in fibrinolytic activity and prostaglandin production seem to explain some cases.[71] Endothelial defects, as seen at the ultrastructural level, are more common and last longer. Hemostatic plugs may or may not be present. These women have unexplained menorrhagia in the presence of secretory endometrium. Regeneration of the surface epithelium tends to be irregular and prolonged.[71]

Irregular Shedding

Irregular shedding refers to uterine bleeding that results from a persistent corpus luteum (Halban's syndrome). Menses begin at the appropriate time, but the flow lasts longer and is heavier than usual. If the diagnosis is clinically suspected, an endometrial biopsy on day five to eight of the cycle will confirm it. The endometrium consists of an admixture of proliferative and secretory glands. Many of the secretory glands have a peculiar star-shaped appearance. The endometrial stroma is more compact than that of the typical endometrium. Fibrin thrombi, indicative of bleeding, are present. The treatment of irregular shedding is administration of estrogen, which will stabilize the endometrium and promote growth of the endometrial lining.

Uterine Changes Following Endometrial Ablation

Endometrial ablation is becoming a common procedure for the treatment of premenopausal women with abnormal uterine bleeding. Some patients may then avoid hysterectomy. Technically, the ability to perform endometrial ablation requires either a neodymium:yttrium-aluminum-garnet (Nd:YAG) laser or a urologic resectoscope. The "rollerball" of the urologic resectoscope creates a furrow, destroying the basalis layer of endometrium. Most gynecologists who perform endometrial ablation prepare the endometrium preoperatively. Most prefer a GnRH agonist as a single dose of a long-acting preparation,[36] but some perform suction curettage immediately before ablation to reduce the amount of endometrium.[72, 73] Both methods seem to be effective, but GnRH agonists result in the highest percentage of women with complete amenorrhea (approximately 67 percent).[37]

We are just beginning to understand uterine healing after endometrial ablation. Within 3 months of endometrial ablation by Nd:YAG laser the amount of tissue obtained at endometrial biopsy is scanty and contains large amounts of blood, mucus, and fibrin. Variable amounts of viable endometrial tissue may be present.[74] After 3 months, biopsy specimens remain scanty. Fibroconnective tissue predominates, but there may be variable amounts of endometrial tissue exhibiting cyclic activity.[74] In uteri removed following endometrial ablation, the endometrium for the most part is less than 1 mm in thickness.[74] Attenuated cuboidal epithelium closely approximates itself to the underlying myometrium in most areas. The endometrial stroma is cellular in some areas and edematous in others, with prominent telangiectatic vascular spaces. At the endometrial-myometrial interface, there may be centrally necrotic palisaded granulomas centered on nondegradable residue.[74] When menorrhagia persists or recurs after endometrial ablation, cycling glands up to 3 mm in thickness may be seen. Usually this cycling endometrium is present in the uterine cornua.[74] When endometrial ablation fails, this could be due either to technical failure of the procedure itself or to regeneration of the endometrial epithelium from the region of the tubal ostia or perhaps the isthmus. Endometrial ablation produces complete amenorrhea in the majority of patients. Laser coagulation of the endometrium is successful in up to 94 percent of women when the operator is experienced.[72] "Rollerball" coagulation achieves complete amenorrhea in 29 to 67 percent of women for at least 12 months; 30 to 60 percent continue with spotting or light flow.[74–76] Some patients, however, will be treatment failures. The "rollerball" technique fails in up to 19 percent of patients.[77] A documented reason for failure is deep adenomyosis.[78] Two women undergoing intrauterine surgery with the Nd:YAG laser delivered by the artificial sapphire tip have had catastrophic air embolism leading to cardiovascular collapse and death during the procedure.[79] Long-term studies of women following endometrial ablation are lacking at this time. The potential for subsequent pregnancy or the development of endometrial adenocarcinoma may exist, as some portion of endometrium may remain.

Heterotopic Tissue

Heterotopic tissue refers to the presence of what appears to be normal tissue in a location where it is not normally seen. Heterotopic tissue is rarely present in the endometrium. Persistent chronic irritation of the endometrium can result in metaplasia of the normal endometrial stroma into bone and cartilage (Fig. 5–28). When bone and cartilage are present, differentiation from retained products of conception must be made. The majority of women with bone and cartilage in the uterus are multiparous and have a history of therapeutic or midtrimester abortion. A history of pregnancy may antedate, in many instances by years, spontaneous passage of fetal bones and cartilage.[80] Most authors favor the theory that glial tissue, when present in the uterus, represents fetal tissue implanted during interruption of a pregnancy.[80] The persistence, growth, and occasional recurrence of such glial tissue after excision are difficult to explain on this basis alone. Rarely, a benign teratoma of the uterus occurs.[81] These may contain bone and cartilage along with the ectodermal and endodermal tissues typical of a teratoma. There is a case report of a glioma of the uterus in a 15-year-old girl.[82]

Endometrial Polyps

A polyp is a benign tumor attached by a stem or pedicle. Polyps in the endometrium are rare in the prepubertal female and common in the postmenopausal female. The peak incidence occurs at about the age of 50 years. Endometrial polyps arise in a milieu of estrogen excess and represent local overgrowth of the endometrium. Usually, polyps are incidental findings at the time of hysterectomy, hysteroscopy, or endometrial sampling. When they are symptomatic, the most common presenting complaint is abnormal uterine bleeding.[83] Premenopausal woman will typically have menorrhagia or intermenstrual bleeding, whereas postmenopausal women typically will have spotting or light bleeding. In symptomatic postmenopausal patients the incidence of endometrial polyps may exceed 20 percent.[83]

By gross examination, polyps are tan to yellow, pedunculated, smooth, spherical, or cylindrical structures. A fibrous stalk attaches the polyp to the underlying endometrium and myometrium. Some polyps, particularly in the postmenopausal

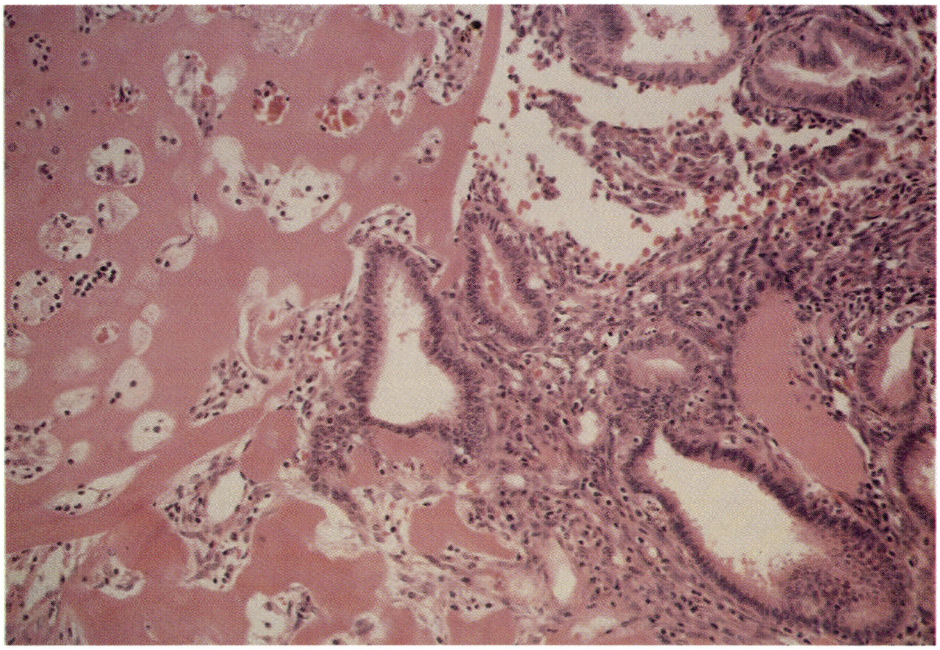

FIGURE 5-28
This benign endometrium has heterotopic osteoid tissue. Heterotopic tissue occurs uncommonly in a normal endometrium.

woman, have a broad base (Fig. 5–29). Polyps may be singular or multiple (Fig. 5–30). Uncommonly, endometrial polyps will protrude through the cervical os and be visible on speculum examination (Fig. 5–31). The overlying epithelium of the exposed surface of the polyp may ulcerate and bleed.

By microscopic examination, the presence of epithelium on three sides, a dense fibrous stroma, and a central fibrovascular core differentiates an endometrial polyp from surrounding normal endometrium. The glandular epithelium in endometrial polyps may or may not respond to estrogen and only occasionally responds to progesterone. In the presence of endometrial polyps, the background endometrium varies considerably, ranging from normal cycling endometrium to simple hyperplasia or at times to a more complex endometrial histology, and, rarely, to endometrial adenocarcinoma. The relative frequency of various histopathologic patterns in endometrial polyps is proliferative endometrium, 44 percent; normal secretory endometrium, 3.6 percent; lower uterine segment endometrium, 4.2 percent; basal endometrium, 19.9

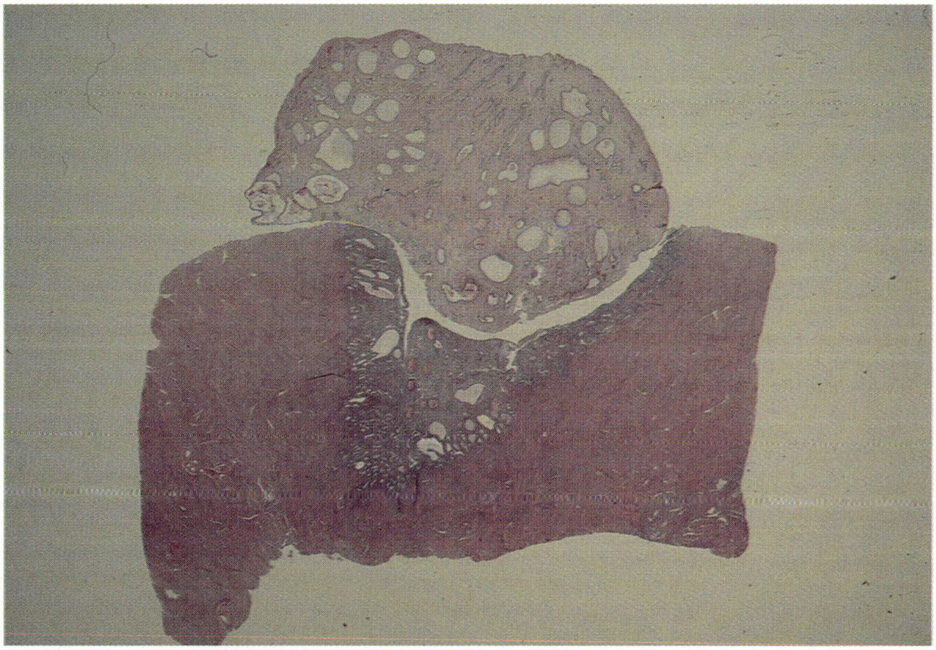

FIGURE 5-29
This is a normal uterus and endometrium with a broad-based endometrial polyp. There is artifactual separation of the polyp from its base.

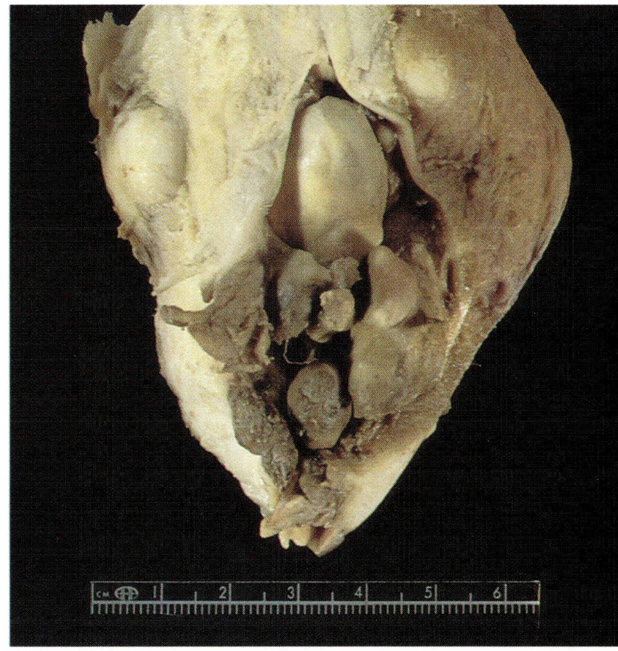

FIGURE 5-30
The endometrial cavity demonstrates multiple endometrial polyps. Intramural leiomyomas are also present. This is a formalin-fixed specimen.

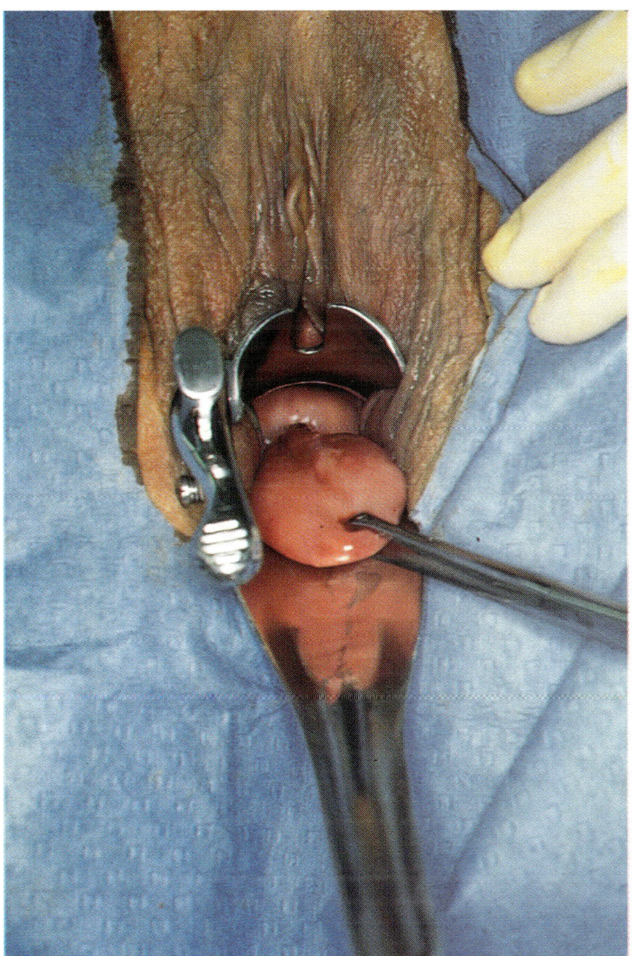

FIGURE 5-31
This large endometrial polyp protrudes through the cervical os in a postmenopausal woman.

percent; cystic atrophy in postmenopausal women, 1.3 percent; hyperplasia, 6.8 percent; secretory change out of phase with the adjacent normal endometrium, 13 percent; progestogen effect, 4.8 percent; and adenocarcinoma, 0.6 percent.[83] The presence of active dilated glands, occasionally with focal crowding, suggests endogenous or exogenous estrogen stimulation of the polyp. The stroma in a polyp is more fibrous than the typical endometrial stroma. In many polyps, dilated blood vessels are present beneath the epithelial surface. Rupture of these dilated capillaries may account for intermenstrual and postmenopausal spotting.[76] Foci of necrosis and thrombosis may be present. In areas of ulceration and necrosis, there is an infiltrate of acute and chronic inflammatory cells.

The differential diagnosis includes normal cycling endometrium and endocervical polyp. The thick-walled blood vessels and the dense fibrotic stroma serve to distinguish endometrial polyps from normal cycling endometrium. Endocervical polyps contain a mucinous epithelial lining.

On rare occasions, postmenopausal women develop a polypoid and necrotic endometrium. Because of the abundant quantity of endometrial tissue, confusion with a neoplastic process is possible, but this tissue shows complete or nearly complete decidualization.[84] Mitotic activity is lacking in these specimens. Many of these women have been receiving exogenous progestogen therapy. However, these changes apparently can occur without exogenous progestogen stimulation.[84]

Currently available endometrial sampling techniques, including curettage, commonly miss endometrial polyps. This is particularly true in postmenopausal women.[85, 86] Hysteroscopic identification is the most reliable method of diagnosis, and resection or curettage under direct vision ensures both removal of all polyps and resection of the stalk at the base. In the woman with persistent uterine bleeding after curettage showing a benign condition, hysteroscopy may prove useful.

Endometrial Changes Induced by Long-Term Tamoxifen Therapy

Approximately 3 million breast cancer patients have received or are currently receiving tamoxifen therapy. There are ongoing clinical trials testing tamoxifen for the prevention of breast cancer in high-risk women.[87, 87a, 87b, 87c] Its beneficial effect on the breast is attributable to its antiestrogen effect. However, recent reports suggest an increase in the occurrence of endometrial polyps, hyperplasia, and cancer in women receiving long-term tamoxifen therapy.[85, 88]

Many postmenopausal women receiving tamoxifen have a thickened endometrial stripe by transvaginal ultrasound.[89, 90] In some, the endometrial stripe has measured over 10 mm.[85] Hysteroscopy performed in 51 breast cancer patients receiving tamoxifen and in 52 breast cancer patients not receiving hormones revealed atrophic endometrium in only 28 percent of women on tamoxifen, compared with 87 percent of women in the control group.[85] Endometrial polyps were present in 40 percent of women receiving tamoxifen who had an endometrial thickness over 5 mm, compared with 10 percent of controls. These polyps measured up to 3 cm in diameter. Histologically these polyps have an epithelium that varies from flattened or cuboidal to columnar pseudostratified, with two or three cell layers. This corresponds to glands ranging from inactive, atrophic to hyperplastic. Typical endocervical polyps also occurred with twice the frequency in the tamoxifen-treated patients compared with the controls. Simple and complex hyperplasia were also present, as was adenocarcinoma. However, these findings appeared with equal frequency in the tamoxifen and the no-tamoxifen groups.[85]

Some of the endometrial polyps in postmenopausal women receiving tamoxifen therapy for breast cancer have unusual histopathology. These patients have been symptomatic and present with postmenopausal bleeding.[91] These polyps are large, the largest measuring more than 9 cm, and broad-based. Microscopically the stroma is edematous and may exhibit a prominent decidual reaction. Lymphocytes are present focally, and there may be small areas of stromal necrosis. The glands themselves appear cystically dilated, and at times markedly plump columnar epithelium lines the gland lumens. In some cases cytologic atypia of mild to moderate degree is present. Mitotic figures are rare. Abundant luminal secretion may be present.[92] Focal crowding may cause confusion with adenocarcinoma.

Several large studies have shown an increased risk of developing endometrial carcinoma among women with breast cancer who took tamoxifen versus those who did not.[85, 87a, 87b, 87c] The relative risk is higher in women who took 40 mg per day of tamoxifen as compared with those who took 20 mg per day.[87c] At present, the best estimate of risk for women with an intact uterus who take 20 mg of tamoxifen per day is based on the fact that the annual hazard rate doubles. In the National Surgical Adjuvant Breast and Bowel Project, the annual hazard rate among women who took tamoxifen was 1.2/1000.[87b] Although most endometrial carcinomas occurring after tamoxifen therapy are stage I, grade 1 or 2, advanced-stage and grade 3 tumors have also occurred.[87b, 87c, 87d]

The primary known action of tamoxifen is competitive binding to estrogen receptors.[93] It also demonstrates agonist properties, possibly activating one of the estrogen receptor's domains.[94] Tamoxifen, although antiestrogenic in its effect on the breast, acts as a partial estrogen receptor agonist in the endometrium.[91] The cause of the endometrial decidualization in patients taking tamoxifen is unknown. Tamoxifen is not a progestational agent. However, experimental studies have shown that estrogens can influence prostaglandin and leukotriene metabolism. This may cause endometrial decidual changes in some patients.[95, 96]

Atypical Polypoid Adenomyoma

Mazur originally described this distinctive lesion in 1981.[97] Although uncommon, over 35 examples of this neoplasm have been reported in the literature. This is a biphasic neoplasm with histologically benign, but atypical, endometrial glands and a smooth muscle stroma. It usually occurs in women of reproductive age. The average age is 39 years. Three cases occurring in association with Turner syndrome have been reported.[98] Two of these three women were on long-term estrogen therapy. This would seemingly implicate estrogen stimulation in the epidemiology of this lesion. The presenting complaint is usually abnormal uterine bleeding. On physical examination an exophytic mass may protrude through the cervical os and clinically suggests a malignant neoplasm.

The gross appearance is that of a polypoid growth projecting into the endometrial cavity. The average size is 2 cm. Many of these lesions arise from the lower uterine segment. The part of the polypoid lesion which on occasion protrudes through the cervical os is frequently necrotic. A broad stalk attaches the neoplasm to the uterus. There is a sharp demarcation between this lesion and the underlying myometrium or cervical wall. Its color is yellow, tan, or red and on cut section the neoplasm is firm, solid, and fleshy. Fragments of neoplasm removed at curettage are firm, irregular, and tan in color.

Microscopic examination shows endometrial glands with varying degrees of stratification, dilatation and architectural atypia. Architecturally the glands, though histologically benign, exhibit marked variation in size and shape. Focal crowding with little intervening stroma may be present. The individual glands resemble proliferative endometrium. Squamous metaplasia seen as morules is often present. Mucinous metaplasia is less common. Mitotic activity is variable but can be brisk in the glandular epithelium. Cytologic atypia, if present, is usually mild. The nucleus of the epithelial cells contains a small nucleolus and finely granular and evenly dispersed chromatin. The stroma of these neoplasms is cellular, and composed of smooth muscle rather than endometrial stroma. The smooth muscle cells have a typical histopathologic appearance. They appear as intersecting fascicles, but are more cellular and more disorganized than normal uterine muscle. Mild to moderate nuclear pleomorphism may be present in the smooth muscle cells. Mitotic activity in the smooth muscle is present, but generally is less than two mitotic figures per 10 high power fields (HPF) in the most active areas. There is only one reported case with increased stromal mitotic activity. This neoplasm contained nine mitotic figures per 10 HPF and recurred outside the uterus six years after hysterectomy.[100]

In at least one case, keratin granulomas 0.3 to 0.7 cm in diameter occurred in the peritoneum in association with this type of polyp. They were present on the surface of the ovary and the fallopian tube as well. They consisted of laminated deposits of keratin surrounded by foam cells and foreign body giant cells.[99]

Although adenocarcinoma may exist adjacent to or within an atypical polypoid adenomyoma, malignant sequelae have not occurred, with the exception of the stromal neoplasm mentioned above.[100]

Many of these neoplasms are incidental findings at hysterectomy for other indications. The diagnosis of polypoid lesions protruding through the cervical os requires histopathologic examination. The differential diagnosis of an atypical polypoid adenomyoma includes endometrial and endocervical polyp, prolapsed leiomyoma, polypoid adenocarcinoma, or sarcoma. The smooth muscle stroma differentiates this neoplasm from a typical endometrial polyp. The mild degree of glandular cytologic and architectural atypia differentiate this lesion from both adenocarcinoma and sarcoma.

Treatment consists of excision. Excision under hysteroscopic guidance allows for inspection of the entire endometrial cavity and ensures removal of the entire lesion, including the base of the stalk.

Placental Polyps

True polyps arising from the placenta are extremely rare. Most commonly these lesions represent large polypoid fragments of retained placental tissue. Placental polyps may arise from a focal area of placenta accreta that went unrecognized.[101]

As with retained placental tissue, patients present with heavy vaginal bleeding. Bleeding may be so heavy that hysterectomy is necessary in some patients. At the time of hysterectomy these polypoid lesions are found to contain hemorrhage and necrosis and grossly resemble gestational choriocarcinoma.

Pyometra

Pyometra refers to an endometrial cavity that contains frankly purulent material. For pyometra to occur, cervical stenosis or occlusion must be present. A common cause of cervical stenosis is scarring from laser therapy, cryotherapy, or conization of the cervix. In postmenopausal women, sterile pyometra secondary to cervical stenosis is the most common cause of an intrauterine fluid collection. With the increasing use of pelvic ultrasound and computed tomography pyometra presenting as an intrauterine fluid collection has become a more common incidental finding. The most frequent presenting complaint is vaginal spotting. In every postmenopausal woman there is the concern that pyometra is secondary to obstruction of the cervical canal by a malignant process. Thus, any postmenopausal patient with an intrauterine fluid collection requires endometrial evaluation. Outpatient endometrial sampling or hysteroscopy is necessary to exclude a neoplastic etiology. Dilatation of the cervix and drainage is adequate treatment for those pyometra that are the result of cervical stenosis and scarring. The endometrial cavity can harbor several hundred milliliters of pus. In the rare instance of a symptomatic infection the patient will be febrile with an enlarged and tender uterus. This represents an abscess that requires surgical drainage, usually transcervically by cervical dilatation.

Myometritis

Myometrial inflammation may occur in conjunction with any endometrial inflammatory conditions. Rarely, hematogenous spread of bacteria can produce inflammation and microabscess formation within the myometrium. An endometritis with extension to the myometrium is the usual presentation. Pain, fever, and serosanguineous yellow vaginal discharge are the presenting complaint. The most common clinical scenario is postpartum or postabortal endomyometritis. The uterus appears boggy and edematous. Both the endometrium and the myometrium have an infiltration of leukocytes. The degree of inflammation parallels the severity of the infection.

In any endometrial condition in which chronic inflammation occurs, secondary involvement of the underlying myometrium may be present. These women usually present with heavy vaginal bleeding. The uterus is boggy and enlarged. Microscopically the myometrium contains an infiltrate of plasma cells between muscle bundles. As with chronic endometritis, treatment should address the underlying cause.

Myometrial Hypertrophy

The absence of pathology in an enlarged but otherwise normal uterus indicates hypertrophy of the myometrium. The size and weight of the normal uterus varies with the age and parity of the patient.[1] In women of reproductive age, the range of normal uterine weight varies from 46 to 137 gm. There is documentation of normal uteri in parous women as large as 243 gm.[1] Thus, in the presence of histologically normal endometrium and myometrium, a uterus weighing more than 250 gm is abnormal. Women whose uteri weigh 250 gm or more may bleed profusely, and may present with anemia. If medical therapy with oral contraceptive agents or progestogens does not control the menorrhagia, hysterectomy may be necessary. Endometrial ablation may play a role in the treatment of these patients.

Uterine Subinvolution

Uterine subinvolution is a common cause of postpartum hemorrhage. To make this diagnosis, retained products of conception must not be present. In normal pregnancy, the spiral arterioles of the endometrium distend to become vessels of low resistance and high conductance. In early pregnancy, intermediate trophoblasts migrate along and into the spiral arterioles, where they replace the endothelium. The musculoelastic layer of these vessels is absent or not well developed, and deposits of fibrinoid material occur.[102] Post partum the uteroplacental arteries undergo thrombosis and organization. The placental site rapidly decreases in size, and epithelial regeneration occurs.[103] As the uterine musculature and vascular bed regress, this process may be incomplete in the placental site. This can cause delayed hemorrhage, even after an early pregnancy loss that requires surgical intervention.[104] In a term pregnancy these vessels may remain widely dilated and tortuous. The lumen of the vessels contain organized thrombi and red blood cells. Completely involuted vessels and incompletely involuted vessels may exist side by side.[105] Immunocytochemical observation suggests that the subinvoluted vessels lack an endothelial lining and show persistence of perivascular and intravascular trophoblasts.[106] Recent observations further suggest an association between complement activation and deposition through the classical pathway and the normal involution of uteroplacental arteries.[106] A deficiency of this immunologic reaction in the subinvoluted vessels, together with a deficiency in the vascular endothelium, suggests that the failure of re-endothelialization of uteroplacental arteries may be the basis for the pathology of subinvolution of the placental bed spiral arterioles and its subsequent delayed hemorrhage.[106]

Placenta Accreta

Placenta accreta clinically refers to the abnormal adherence of the placenta to the uterine wall so that normal separation of the placenta does not occur after delivery. This reflects partial or complete absence of Nitabuch layer in the endometrial decidua,[107] which results in placental villi adhering directly or growing into and between the uterine muscle fibers. The generic term for this condition is placenta accreta. Two subdivisions exist: Placenta increta refers to placental invasion of the myometrium (Fig. 5–32), and placenta percreta refers to penetration of placental tissue through the full thickness of the myometrium. In the latter instance the placenta can secondarily invade extrauterine structures such as fallopian tube, ovary, bowel, or parietal peritoneum. Placenta accreta is uncommon. However, it occurs in up to 64 percent of women with placenta previa,[108] often in areas of previous cesarean section scars.[109–111] The entire placenta may be adherent, or it may be adherent only focally and limited to the cesarean section scar.[112] Other predisposing factors for placenta accreta include previous curettage and intrauterine synechiae. Placenta accreta causes no specific symptoms during pregnancy. Patients with placenta accreta and placenta previa present with third trimester bleeding. Placenta accreta does not become manifest until the placenta fails to separate following delivery of the infant.

Microscopically, the decidua basalis is absent.[113] Placental villi are in direct contact with and may invade the myometrium without intervening decidua. Heavy and even life-threatening bleeding may occur. Treatment usually consists of hysterectomy because of the profuse hemorrhage, but occasionally conservative measures are effective. Conservative measures include uterine artery ligation and hypogastric artery ligation. If the area of placenta accreta is small, injection of prostaglandin F2-α and uterine massage may control bleeding.

Trophoblastic Myometritis

Trophoblastic myometritis is a term for a normal phenomenon that occurs in pregnancy. When hysterectomy is necessary in a term gestation, microscopic examination of the uterine smooth muscle reveals cytotrophoblasts and syncytiotrophoblasts singly and in groups distant from the placental bed and seemingly "invading" the myometrium.

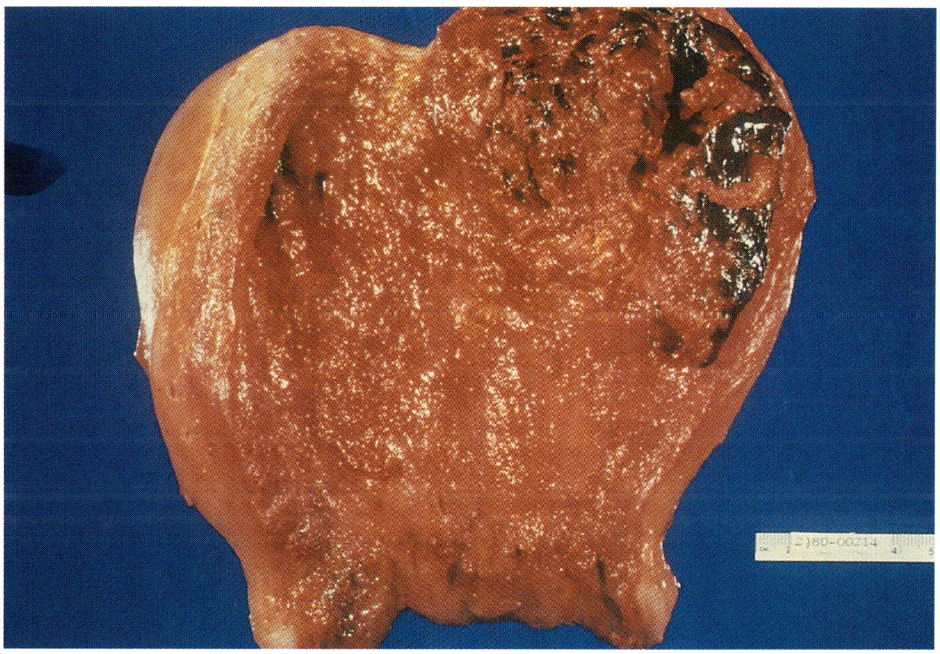

FIGURE 5–32
This hysterectomy was performed after inability to completely remove the placenta from the left cornu. The patient had persistent profuse bleeding. The placenta is implanted deep in the myometrium, almost reaching the serosa.

Such a microscopic observation has no clinical significance. (See also Chapter 12.)

Leiomyoma (Fibroid Tumor)

Leiomyomas, the most common tumors of the uterus, are benign tumors of smooth muscle cells. They occur in 20 to 40 percent of women of reproductive age.[114] Smooth muscle tumors probably arise as clones from a single smooth muscle cell. Genetic rearrangements occur frequently in uterine smooth muscle tumors. These genetic rearrangements tend to be uniform within a given neoplasm. Translocations between chromosomes 12 and 14 are particularly common.[115, 116]

Up to 50 percent of leiomyomas produce symptoms, including pelvic pain and pressure, excessive uterine bleeding, recurrent pregnancy loss, and, uncommonly, infertility.[114, 117] The likelihood of leiomyomas being symptomatic depends upon their number, size, and location. Small leiomyomas may be quite symptomatic, and large ones may be asymptomatic. Leiomyomas arise anywhere within the myometrium (Fig. 5–33). Submucosal leiomyomas compress the overlying endometrium. As they enlarge, they bulge into the endometrial cavity and occasionally protrude through the cervical os (Figs. 5–33 and 5–34). Intramural leiomyomas grow within the myometrium, the most common location (Fig. 5–35). Subserosal leiomyomas can become pedunculated, may undergo torsion with necrosis of the pedicle, and may rarely lose their connection entirely with the uterus, becoming attached and receiving their blood supply from an adjacent structure (parasitic leiomyomas).

If a patient presents with uterine bleeding, the leiomyoma is usually an incidental finding rather than the cause.[118] Excess bleeding from a submucosal leiomyoma occurs because of the attenuation of the overlying endometrium and the ulceration with focal areas of necrosis. This necrosis occurs as leiomyomas in this anatomic location enlarge. Another explanation for the excess bleeding that can occur in patients with leiomyomas may be the increased surface area of the endometrium as the tumors enlarge and distort the endometrial cavity. The surface area of a normal endometrial cavity is approximately 15 cm^2.[1] In a patient who has large intramural leiomyomas, the endometrial surface area may be more than 200 cm^2. Hemorrhage and necrosis can occur in larger leiomyomas (see Fig. 5–35). Patients with torsion of a leiomyoma or a hemorrhagic leiomyoma will present with acute abdominal pain. Degenerative changes within a leiomyoma are common. Besides hemorrhage, there may be hyalinization, calcification, and cystic change.

The incidence of obstetric complications when leiomyomas are present in the gravid uterus may be as high as 37 percent (Fig. 5–36).[119] These complications consist mainly of premature onset of labor and preterm delivery. Rarely, a leiomyoma can cause an obstructed labor, if the leiomyoma is located within the true pelvis. In these instances, cesarean section is necessary for delivery of the infant.

On abdominal or pelvic examination the uterus is firm and irregularly enlarged. A subserosal or pedunculated leiomyoma may occupy the position of the adnexa. This may make evaluation of the

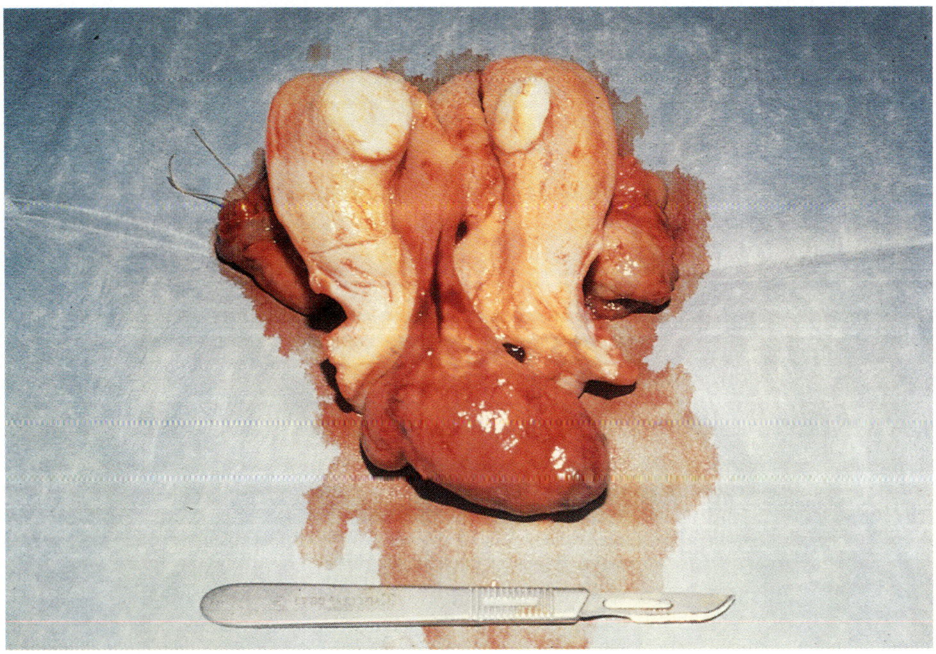

FIGURE 5–33
This is a uterus with a pedunculated prolapsed submucous leiomyoma. An intramural leiomyoma is also present. (Courtesy of Dr. John Wheelock.)

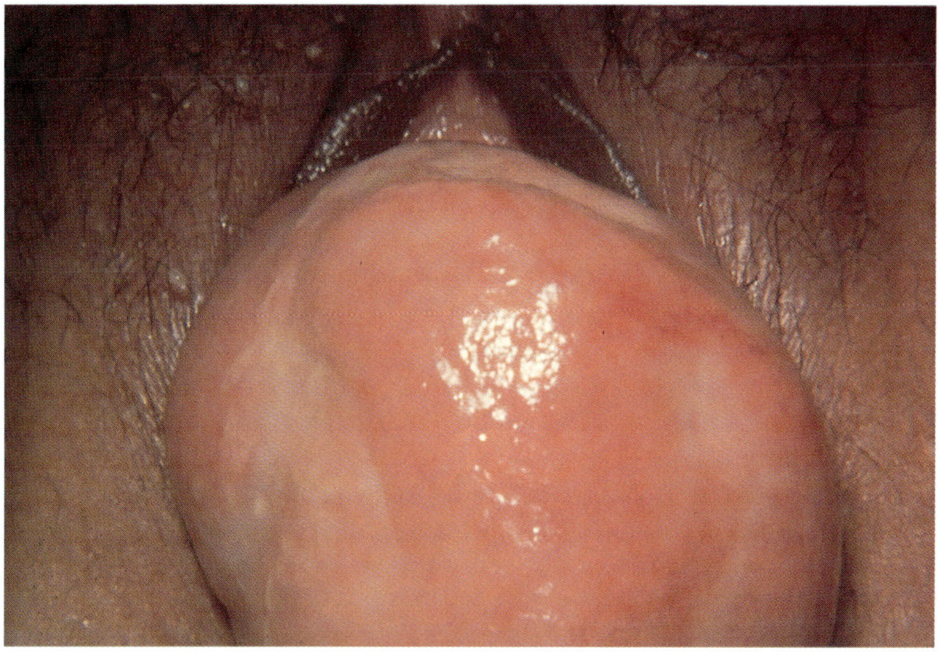

FIGURE 5–34
A prolapsed submucous fibroid outside the introitus is seen here. Compromise of venous return caused rapid expansion of this tumor. A combined abdominal and vaginal approach was necessary for its removal.

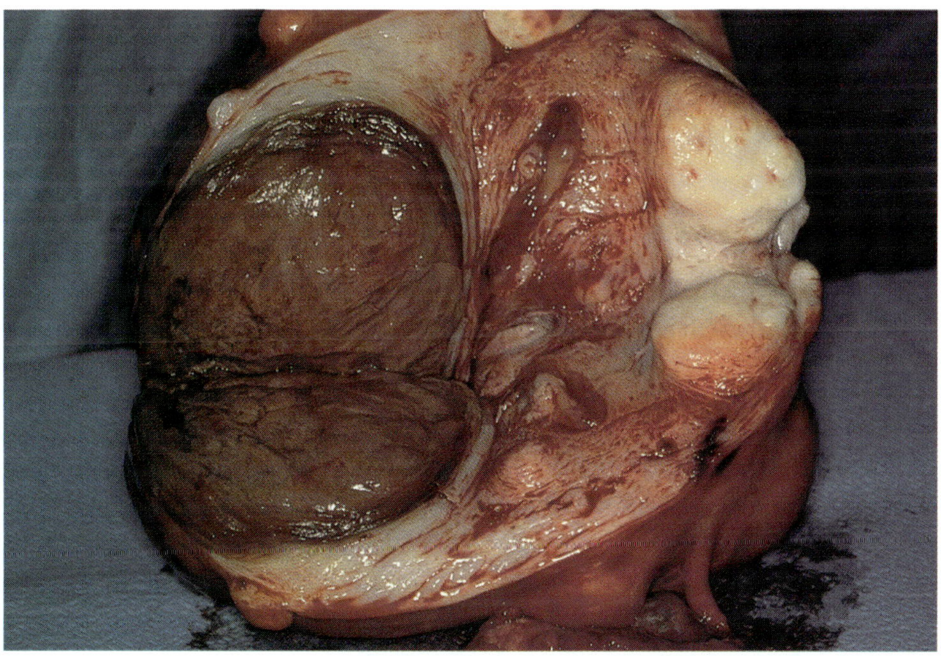

FIGURE 5–35
This uterus has multiple leiomyomas. The large leiomyoma on the left shows hemorrhagic (i.e., carneous) degeneration.

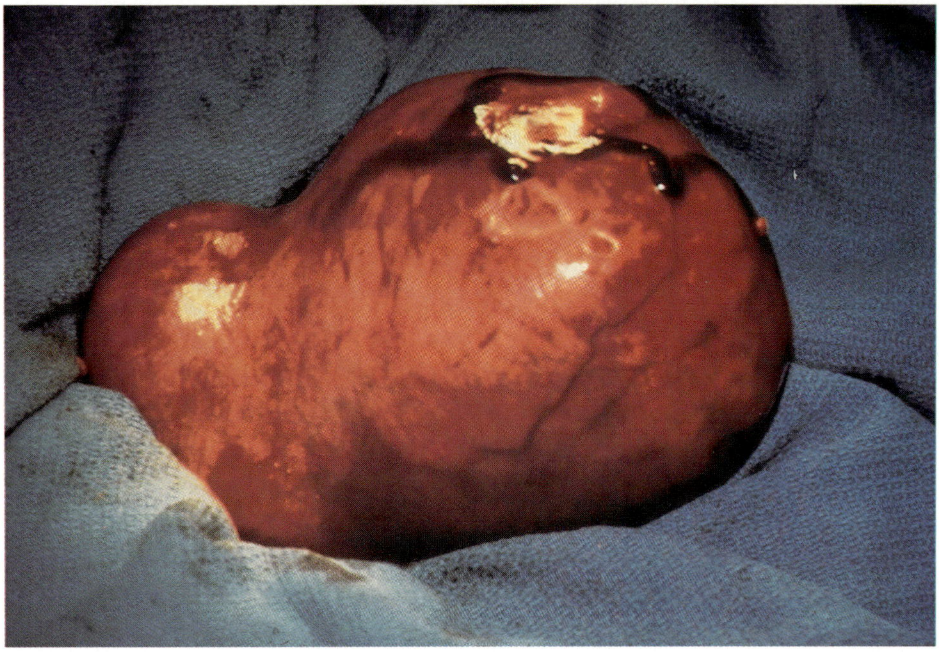

FIGURE 5–36
This woman with an intrauterine pregnancy at 16 weeks had a large right-sided fibroid that on pelvic examination was thought to be an adnexal mass. (Courtesy of Dr. John Wheelock.)

adnexa by physical examination difficult and at times impossible. Clinicians compare the size of a leiomyomatous uterus to weeks of gestation. A physician's estimate of uterine size generally correlates well with the weight of the hysterectomy specimen. Uteri of approximately 12-week gestational size weigh approximately 280 gm.[118]

Ultrasound commonly detects small asymptomatic leiomyomas and is useful in delineating the number, size, and location of leiomyomas in symptomatic patients. Ultrasound criteria for the diagnosis of leiomyoma include a spherical mass, distortion of the myometrial contour by the mass, and differentiation of the mass from the surrounding myometrium by different acoustic texture. To make the diagnosis of leiomyoma during pregnancy a spherical mass measuring at least 3 cm in diameter should be identified.[120] Cystic degeneration may also be apparent on ultrasound or CT. Dystrophic calcification within a leiomyoma produces "popcorn" radiodensities on pelvic radiographs (Fig. 5–37).

By gross examination leiomyomas have a characteristic appearance. They are well-circumscribed

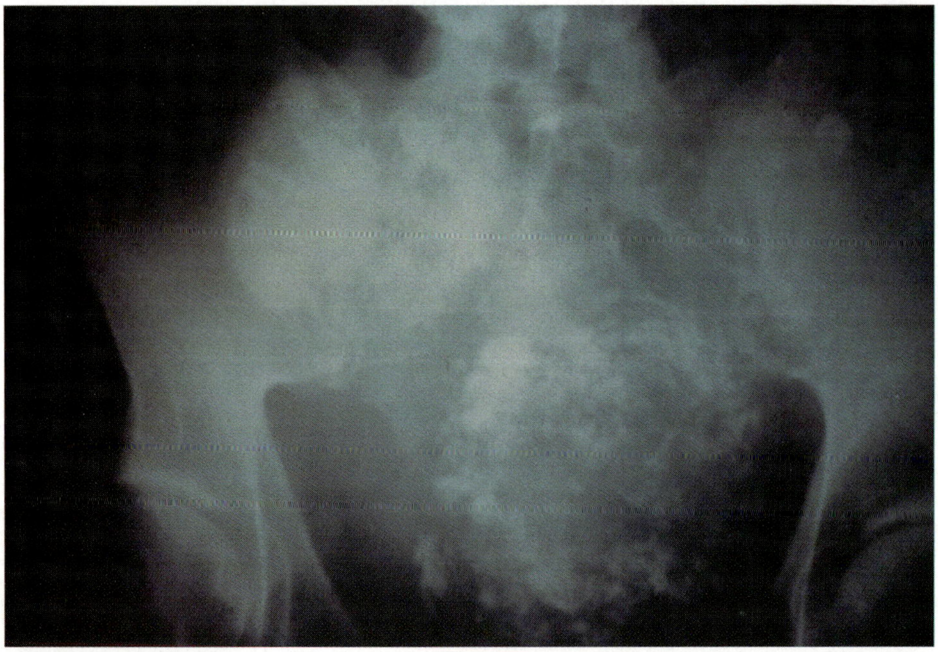

FIGURE 5–37
This is a flat plate radiograph of the pelvis in a patient with calcified leiomyomas. (Courtesy of Dr. John Wheelock.)

nodules of white to gray, whorled, firm tissue (see Fig. 5–34). Occasionally the texture will be soft. They bulge above the surrounding myometrium on cut section. A pseudocapsule of compressed adjacent normal myometrium circumscribes the typical leiomyoma. One to two percent of leiomyomas contain areas of visible hemorrhage. This increases to 8 percent in women on oral contraceptives.[121] Hemorrhage is grossly visible in 30 percent of leiomyomas associated with pregnancy.[121] Areas of degeneration are commonly seen and appear as soft, red or yellow, necrotic areas. Other degenerative changes include hyalinization and calcification. Leiomyomas generally feel firm. Hyalinized leiomyomas are more homogeneous on cut section. They lose some of the whorled fascicular pattern. Calcified leiomyomas have a gritty feeling when sectioned.

Microscopically a typical whorled pattern of smooth muscle cells is present. The cellularity of the central region is greater than that of the outer regions. Typical smooth muscle cells are spindle-shaped (Fig. 5–38). If fibrosis is present it usually occupies the central area of the nodule. Multinucleate cells with cytologic atypia are not uncommon.[117, 121] They are present in up to 23 percent of benign leiomyomas.[117] Some leiomyomas demonstrate decreased cellularity, whereas others may have an increased cellularity. Microscopic comparison of a leiomyoma with the adjacent normal myometrium gives a good estimate of its cellularity. The number of nuclei in a unit area is sometimes a useful indicator to grade the cellularity in a leiomyoma.[121] In a small leiomyoma the centrally located cells are ultrastructurally less mature than those occupying the outer layers.[122] Mast cells are present in some smooth muscle tumors, particularly the smaller and more cellular neoplasms.[117, 123] When mast cells are present, they are within the fibrous connective tissue septa, between the muscle bundles.[123] Leiomyomas in patients who had undergone treatment with GnRH analogs have a higher mast cell count. The increased number of mast cells reflects either the degree of cellularity of the tumor or the degree of atrophy of the surrounding tissue.[123] Histiocytes may also be present and may be either focal or diffuse.[124] Histiocytes contain Factor XIII, which is known to induce fibroblast proliferation and stimulate the growth of vascular smooth muscle and is important for wound healing. An occasional leiomyoma contains a prominent lymphoid infiltrate.[125] This infiltrate may be focal or diffuse and can be moderately to markedly dense. There may be a scattering of plasma cells and a rare eosinophil. Occasionally, prominent germinal centers are present.[125] Areas of sclerosis are common.

Pyomyoma, or leiomyoma with acute inflammation and abscess formation, may occur secondary to bacterial infection. A dense acute inflammatory cell infiltrate, consisting mainly of neutrophils, is present. The involved smooth muscle is necrotic. This condition may also complicate cystic degeneration of a leiomyoma. The inflammation can result in suppuration with the formation of abscess cavities. In a subserosal location, dense adhesions between the leiomyoma and the surrounding in-

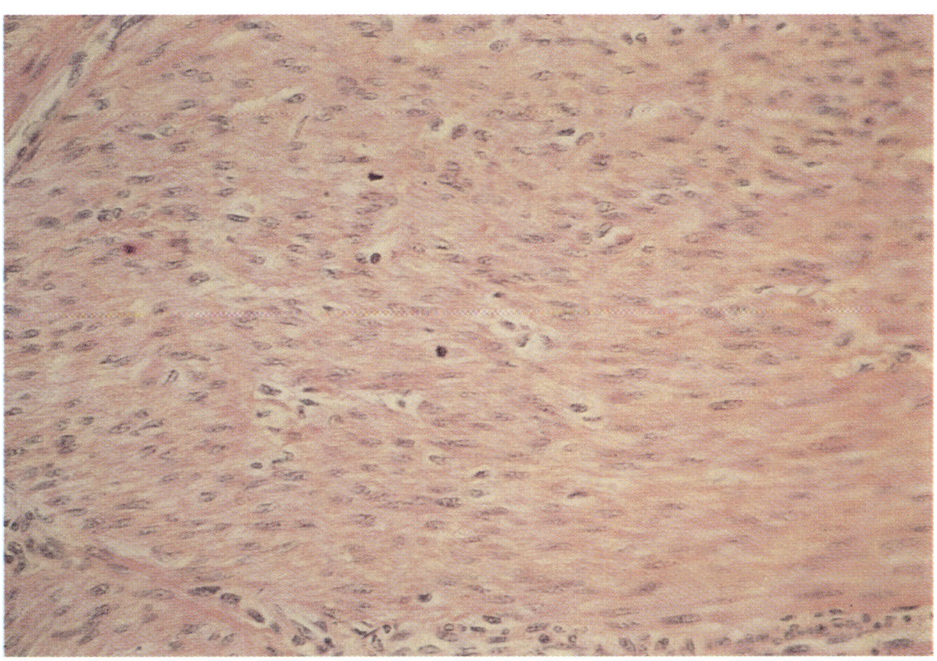

FIGURE 5–38
This is typical smooth muscle in a benign leiomyoma. The muscle fibers are seen in longitudinal bundles. The cells are spindle-shaped with uniform ovoid to spindle-shaped nuclei.

traabdominal contents may occur. Dystrophic calcification is a common sequel.

Mitotic count is the traditional histopathologic method used to distinguish benign from malignant smooth muscle tumors. It has been criticized, however. Some suggest that mitotic figures may disappear after surgery, reflecting "completion" of the mitoses after the uterus is removed.[126] Another argument is that mitotic counting is subjective and subject to gerrymandering of microscopic fields that may result in either an overestimate or an underestimate of the number of mitotic figures per unit area. Other variables to consider in the differential diagnosis include the degree of cellularity of the neoplasm, the hormonal milieu including the phase of the menstrual cycle, and tissue preservation.[127] Despite these potential shortcomings, mitotic counts are generally reproducible and correlate well with clinical outcome. The traditional approach is to express mitotic activity as the number of mitotic figures per 10 HPF as counted in the most active areas of the neoplasm. Table 5–1 presents a useful guide to help distinguish between benign and malignant smooth muscle tumors.[128]

Drugs, particularly steroids, have an effect on the histopathologic appearance of leiomyomas that can be deceptive to the unwary. A common finding in women receiving exogenous steroids, or in leiomyomas removed during pregnancy, is red or carneous degeneration.[129] Ordinary leiomyomas in pregnancy contain microscopic hemorrhage in 70 percent of examples. These degenerating neoplasms exhibit increased cellularity with bizarre, hyperchromatic nuclei or multinucleate cells.[130] They may also exhibit increased mitotic activity. Confusion with malignancy is not uncommon. The increased mitotic activity should not be surprising, since uterine smooth muscle contains estrogen and progesterone receptors. The increased mitotic activity of smooth muscle tumors in the presence of progestogen may be a function of the progestogen itself or a function of adjacent necrosis.[128] In nonpregnant women, mitotic activity appears to be highest in those using preparations that contain only progestogen, particularly the long-acting depo-medroxyprogesterone acetate. Focal areas that contain up to 8 mitotic figures per 10 HPF are seen.[128] However, the mitotic count in pregnancy or with the presence of exogenous progestogens rarely exceeds 10 mitotic figures per 10 HPF.[129] Neoplasms with an increased mitotic count in this hormonal milieu generally do not contain cells with significant nuclear pleomorphism. Women using estrogen-progestogen oral contraceptives have the same mitotic rate in their leiomyomas as do controls.[129]

Distinguishing between a benign smooth muscle tumor and leiomyosarcoma is sometimes difficult. Leiomyosarcoma is rare before the age of 40 years. Unlike leiomyomas, which tend to be multiple, leiomyosarcomas are usually single. The incidence of incidental leiomyosarcoma discovered in uteri removed for presumed leiomyoma is approximately 1 in 2000.[131, 132] The prognosis for leiomyosarcoma diagnosed in premenopausal women appears to be generally favorable when it is an incidental finding.[133]

Attention to detail in sampling and examining these tumors is necessary in order to distinguish benign from malignant. Thorough sampling of suspicious smooth muscle tumors should include one block per cm of greatest tumor diameter. Careful mitotic counting should include at least five sets of 10 HPF per slide. Leiomyosarcoma is discussed in further detail in Chapter 6.

The definitive treatment of symptomatic leiomyomas in a woman who has completed childbearing is hysterectomy. Myomectomy is an alternative for the symptomatic woman who desires preservation of childbearing ability. Myomectomy may be either a transabdominal or a transcervical procedure depending on the size and location of the lesion. Operative laparoscopy is an approach to some leiomyomas that in the past required laparotomy. It is possible to remove pedunculated leiomyomas and some subserous leiomyomas laparoscopically without resorting to laparotomy. Injection of vasopressin into the operative site reduces bleeding. Careful surgical technique and tissue handling are necessary to prevent adhesion formation, particularly if the leiomyoma is near the tubal ostia.

Transcervical surgery represents an alternative

TABLE 5–1.

Metastatic Potential of Smooth Muscle Tumors of the Uterus

Mitoses/ 10 HPF	Atypia	Diagnosis	Metastatic Potential
1–4	Any degree	Leiomyoma	Very low
5–9	None	Leiomyoma with high mitotic activity	Very low
5–9	Grade 1	Smooth muscle tumor of uncertain malignant potential	Low
5–9	Grade 2 or 3	Leiomyosarcoma	Moderate
10 or more	Grade 1	Leiomyosarcoma	High
10 or more	Grade 2 or 3	Leiomyosarcoma	Very high

Modified from O'Connor DM, Norris HJ: Mitotically active leiomyomas of the uterus. Hum Pathol 1990; 21:223–227.

to hysterectomy when surgical intervention is necessary because of menorrhagia. Resection of a submucous leiomyoma using a urologic resectoscope offers the possibility of histopathologic examination of the leiomyoma and the adjacent and overlying endometrium.[134] Using this technique, leiomyomas can be resected to the plane of the uterine wall. A curette and forceps can remove tissue chips.[135] Uterine perforation occurs in 3 percent of patients, and hyponatremia with nausea, vomiting, and mental confusion can occur secondary to fluid overload caused by absorption of the operative medium during a lengthy procedure.[135]

The hormonal manipulation of leiomyomas as an adjunct to surgery may prove useful. GnRH agonists can reduce the size of leiomyomas. This can allow some patients who traditionally would have undergone an abdominal procedure to undergo a vaginal or a laparoscopically assisted vaginal procedure. Additionally, transabdominal myomectomy may be easier to perform. Blood loss and other surgical morbidity may be less severe. However, this approach is in the process of being evaluated with regard to benefits and potential risks.

The use of oral contraceptives or the use of estrogen replacement therapy in women with asymptomatic leiomyomas is controversial. Leiomyomas contain estrogen and progesterone receptors. They also rapidly increase in size during pregnancy. Hence, there is the theoretical and, at times, real possibility that leiomyomas will increase in size in women using these medications.[121, 126] So when oral contraceptive agents and estrogen replacement therapy are used in patients with symptomatic leiomyomas, this requires follow-up in order to monitor the size of the neoplasms.

The treatment of asymptomatic large leiomyomas continues to be controversial. Removal of the leiomyomas has traditionally been the standard of care. The rationale for removal of large asymptomatic leiomyomas is (1) inability to adequately evaluate the adnexa, (2) the increased complication rate with surgical removal of a larger uterus, and (3) the concern for sarcomatous degeneration in the leiomyoma.[118] However, there appears to be no significant increase in perioperative complications with uteri clinically larger than 12-week size compared with those smaller than 12-week size. In asymptomatic women with large uteri, hysterectomy need not be routine prophylaxis against increased operative morbidity associated with further growth.[118] Ultrasonography may prove helpful in evaluating the adnexa in women with large myomatous uteri. Rapid increase in uterine size, however, leaves concern that sarcomatous change may have occurred.

There are several histopathologic variants of leiomyoma that deserve special consideration. These include bizarre leiomyoma, hemorrhagic cellular leiomyoma, mitotically active leiomyoma, lipoleiomyoma, intravenous leiomyoma, and benign metastasizing leiomyoma.

Bizarre or Symplastic Leiomyoma, Pleomorphic Leiomyoma

These names refer to neoplasms that contain areas of giant cells and bizarre-appearing cells (Fig. 5–39). The average age of patients who have this variation of leiomyoma is 45.6 years.[136] From a purely cytologic viewpoint, these lesions are so pleomorphic and so cellular as to make one seriously consider leiomyosarcoma. They contain multinucleate cells and cells that have large red nucleoli and even larger inclusions. However, they lack significant mitotic activity. If there are 5 or more mitotic figures per 10 HPF in the most active area of the neoplasm, the neoplasm is a leiomyosarcoma.[128] All women with bizarre leiomyomas meeting the criteria outlined above and followed for an average of 11.2 years survived.[136] These microscopic changes may rarely occur following hormonal therapy, but bizarre leiomyomas also exist without exogenous hormonal therapy or pregnancy.

Hemorrhagic Cellular Leiomyomas (Apoplectic Leiomyoma)

This is a term used to denote changes seen specifically in a subset of leiomyomas that develop in association with pregnancy or oral contraceptive use. Over 75 percent arise in women taking oral contraceptive agents. The remainder occur during pregnancy or in the immediate postpartum period.[121] The progestogen is probably responsible for the hemorrhagic cellular changes, because this tumor is not seen in postmenopausal women taking estrogen. Of those occurring in pregnancy, only one has arisen in the last trimester, when estrogen levels are highest.[121] All patients who have this neoplasm are in the reproductive age group; the median age is 37 years.[121] Some patients present with hemoperitoneum due to erosion or rupture of the vascular leiomyoma into the abdominal cavity.[121] In nonpregnant women the most common complaint is abnormal uterine bleeding. Pain localized to the abdomen or pelvic area occurs in many nonpregnant women. One half of the women have rapidly enlarging neoplasms.[121]

These neoplasms have unusual gross and histopathologic findings. At surgery the uterus appears irregularly enlarged, and both gross and micro-

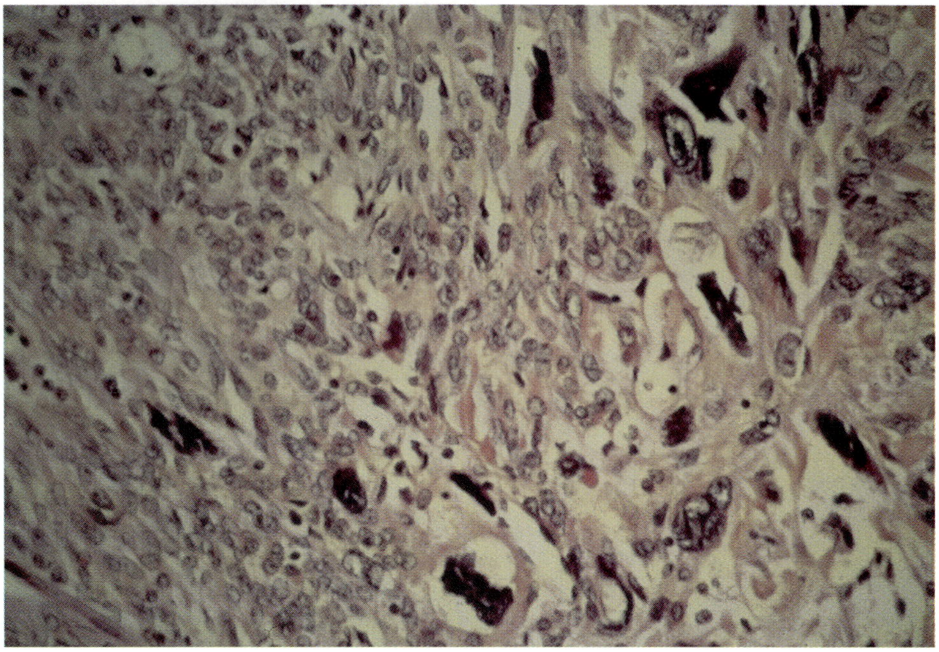

FIGURE 5-39
A bizarre (symplastic) leiomyoma is shown. Cells with markedly atypical nuclei in a smooth muscle tumor are shown. Several pink to red intracytoplasmic inclusions are seen on the right-hand side. Mitotic count is crucial in these neoplasms, since if more than 5 mitotic figures per 10 HPF are seen a diagnosis of leiomyosarcoma should be made.

scopic hemorrhage and edema are present. This may be particularly apparent in those leiomyomas that occupy a subserosal location. Although the size and location are variable, the majority of these neoplasms are subserosal. Some may be hemorrhagic or necrotic to the point that cystic degeneration occurs.

Microscopically these lesions appear as circumscribed, densely cellular proliferations of oval and spindle-shaped smooth muscle cells that have areas of central hemorrhage and edema. Cellularity is most noticeable around areas of hemorrhage. The individual cells are small. The nuclei appear elongated and narrow but not enlarged. Mild cytologic atypia is common. This manifests as slight nuclear enlargement and hyperchromasia. A few neoplasms contain scattered multinucleate giant cells.[121] Mitotic activity is evident in most neoplasms and is most noticeable in the longitudinal muscle fascicles next to areas of shearing artifact.[121] Mitotic activity should not exceed 4 mitotic figures per 10 HPF in the most active areas of the neoplasm. Indication of recent hemorrhage is the hallmark of these lesions. This is present in the most densely cellular areas and often in the areas where there is shearing or tearing artifact.[121] These artifacts probably result from separation of the cellular areas by edema and hemorrhage; the tearing occurs during processing. Focal edema is present in all neoplasms. Fibrin deposits are present near areas of hemorrhage.[121] The adjacent myometrium generally demonstrates hypertrophy. Abnormal arteries that have fibrosis of the intima and medial hypertrophy, similar to those described in women on oral contraceptives, are present in half of these neoplasms.[22] These vascular abnormalities occur within or next to the hemorrhagic cellular leiomyomas.[121]

Hemorrhagic cellular leiomyomas must be distinguished from leiomyosarcomas. Leiomyosarcomas are generally single, whereas hemorrhagic cellular leiomyomas are usually small and multiple. The increased mitotic activity in hemorrhagic cellular leiomyomas is present only along a narrow area next to the areas of hemorrhage.[119] In addition, leiomyosarcomas are cytologically more abnormal and demonstrate a higher mitotic rate than do hemorrhagic cellular leiomyomas.

Mitotically Active Smooth Muscle Tumors of the Uterus

This term refers to neoplasms that contain 5 to 9 mitotic figures per 10 HPF in the most active areas but that lack cytologic atypia (Fig. 5–40). In the past the term smooth muscle tumor of uncertain malignant potential was used to describe these neoplasms. Mitotically active smooth muscle tumors occur in women of all ages, but the majority are 35 to 45 years old. The mean age is 39 years.[128] Eighty-three percent of women with these tumors are white. Sixteen percent are nulliparous. Twenty-eight percent have a history of taking combined oral contraceptives.[128]

The location of these neoplasms within the uterus varies, as does their size. As with typical leiomyomas, they may arise from the endocervix and, rarely, extend into the parametrium or broad

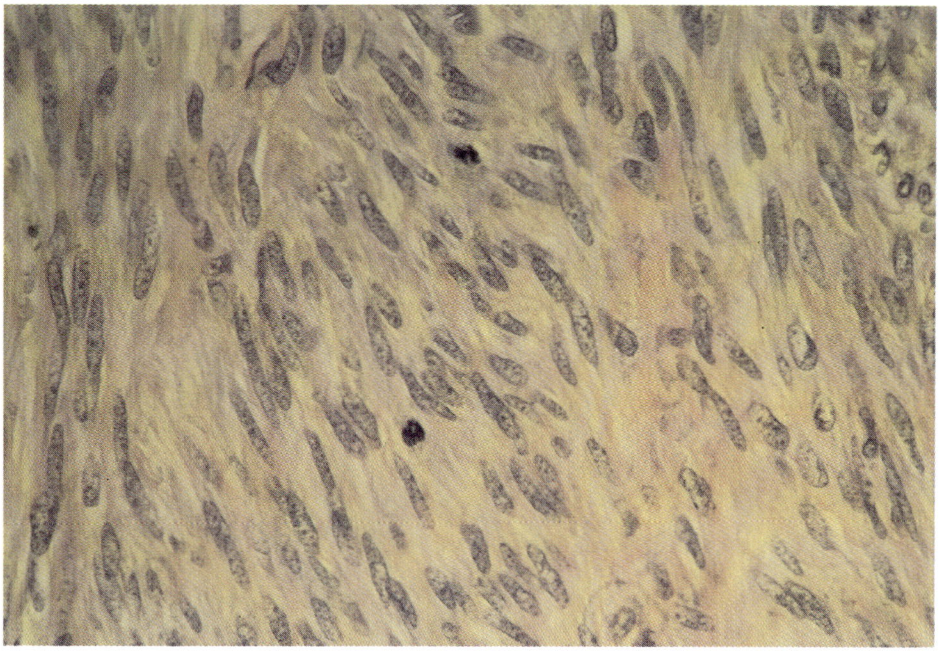

FIGURE 5-40
This leiomyoma demonstrates two mitotic figures. There is no cytologic atypia, but the cellularity is increased. This neoplasm proved to be a mitotically active leiomyoma.

ligament. They are usually single but may be multiple. Microscopically they have a pushing border and compress the adjacent myometrium, but they rarely infiltrate the adjacent myometrium. Hyalinization, focal hemorrhage, and necrosis are common. Fifteen percent of these neoplasms contain one or more areas of vascular intrusion by tumor. This is seen as finger-like or bulbous intrusions into vascular channels.[128] As size and number of mitotic figures increase, the likelihood of vascular intrusion increases. Focal areas that demonstrate enlarged and multiple nuclei may be present.[128]

Mitotically active leiomyomas are not leiomyosarcomas. Distinction from sarcoma is mandatory and is based largely on degree of nuclear atypia. Women who have mitotically active leiomyomas are younger than those who have leiomyosarcoma. The younger age and the common use of oral contraceptive agents coincide with observations that patients who are premenopausal or who have taken hormones preoperatively may have stimulation of otherwise benign leiomyomas.[121, 126] The simultaneous presence of multiple leiomyomas that have increased mitotic activity suggests a benign process, because it is unlikely for two or more independent sarcomas to arise in the uterus at the same time.[137] To exclude sarcoma in these neoplasms, careful sampling and microscopic evaluation, as mentioned above, is necessary. Cytologic atypia in a smooth muscle tumor with a mitotic count exceeding 4 per 10 HPF in the most active areas of the neoplasm meets the histologic criteria for leiomyosarcoma.[128]

There have been no recurrences in women who have mitotically active leiomyomas treated by hysterectomy. In 14 women treated with myomectomy, there was one recurrence 8 years after myomectomy.[128] Smooth muscle tumors that have mitotic activity, between 5 and 9 mitoses per 10 HPF, but lack cytologic atypia have negligible metastatic potential. They behave biologically as benign leiomyomas.

Lipoleiomyoma

Lipomatous change is occasionally present in leiomyomas. Lipoleiomyoma is the term used for neoplasms that result from metamorphosis of uterine smooth muscle that can form mature adipose tissue, either focally or diffusely, in a leiomyoma.[138] Lipoleiomyomas characteristically occur in perimenopausal or postmenopausal women. The presenting complaint is menorrhagia or abdominal pain. Occasionally lipoleiomyomas present as an asymptomatic pelvic mass discovered on routine pelvic examination.

Just as typical leiomyomas, these neoplasms vary in size and location within the uterus. Grossly these tumors are well circumscribed and have a distinct rim of normal tissue around the whole circumference. They are gray-white and firm, with some yellow soft areas. The color and consistency depend on the amount of adipose tissue present within the neoplasm. When a preponderance of adipose tissue is present, they may appear as coarsely lobulated fatty tissue.[138]

Microscopic examination reveals smooth muscle cells and fibrous connective tissue admixed with irregularly arranged aggregates of adipose tissue (Fig. 5–41). Either type of tissue may predominate. Lipomatous changes may be diffuse or circumscribed. Atypia and pleomorphism are absent. Both mature and small lipocytes may be present. Hyalinized stroma is common. The whole mass may contain thin-walled blood vessels, and in places a round cell infiltrate composed mainly of lymphocytes, a few plasma cells, eosinophils, histiocytes, and some mast cells is present. Focal hyaline degeneration and hyalinized fibrous tissue are common.[127, 138]

The estimated frequency of lipomatous change in leiomyomas is 0.2 percent.[138] All women described have been overweight.[136]

Intravenous Leiomyomatosis

Intravenous leiomyomatosis is an uncommon neoplasm. It is characterized by nodular masses of histopathologically benign projections of smooth muscle growing within uterine veins. The intravascular growth takes the form of wormlike projections that may extend a variable distance outside the confines of a myometrial leiomyoma and sometimes into extrauterine veins.[139, 140]

The age of women with intravenous leiomyomatosis ranges from 28 to 76 years, the median being 42 to 45 years.[139, 140] Over 75 percent of the patients are white.[139] All have been premenopausal. One patient was pregnant at the time of diagnosis. Approximately 40 percent present with abnormal vaginal bleeding, either menorrhagia or polymenorrhea[139, 140]; a similar number present with pelvic pain and the remainder with vague pelvic discomfort or a sensation of pelvic pressure. Rarely, the initial complaint is the result of obstruction of the right atrium. This neoplasm has been an incidental finding at autopsy.[141] Half the women have coexisting leiomyomas. A lower abdominal mass consistent with a uterus enlarged by leiomyomas is the usual finding on pelvic examination.[139, 142]

At surgery, spread beyond the uterus is commonly seen. The uterus appears irregularly enlarged and may weigh as much as 750 gm.[141] Characteristically, intravenous leiomyomatosis presents as coiled or nodular well-demarcated masses in the myometrium with convoluted, often mobile, wormlike extensions into the uterine veins. In one third of patients the surgeon does not recognize the intravenous growth intraoperatively.[140, 141]

Growth beyond the uterus occurs in many instances.[140] Uterine, vaginal, and ovarian veins may contain protrusions of tumor; there is extension to the iliac vessels in some cases and, infrequently, to the vena cava. Rarely, a huge pelvic mass replaces the uterus, extends to both parametria, and becomes adherent to adjacent pelvic structures. Within the uterus, the tumor is located either within or in continuity with dilated veins. The former type presents as tentacular and cordlike projections, whereas the latter forms nodules and compresses but does not invade the intact uterine smooth muscle.[140] The involved veins are distinct within layers of apparently normal uterine smooth muscle. Some of the venous masses appear mobile. Sharp demarcation separates these neoplasms from the surrounding myometrium.[140] The

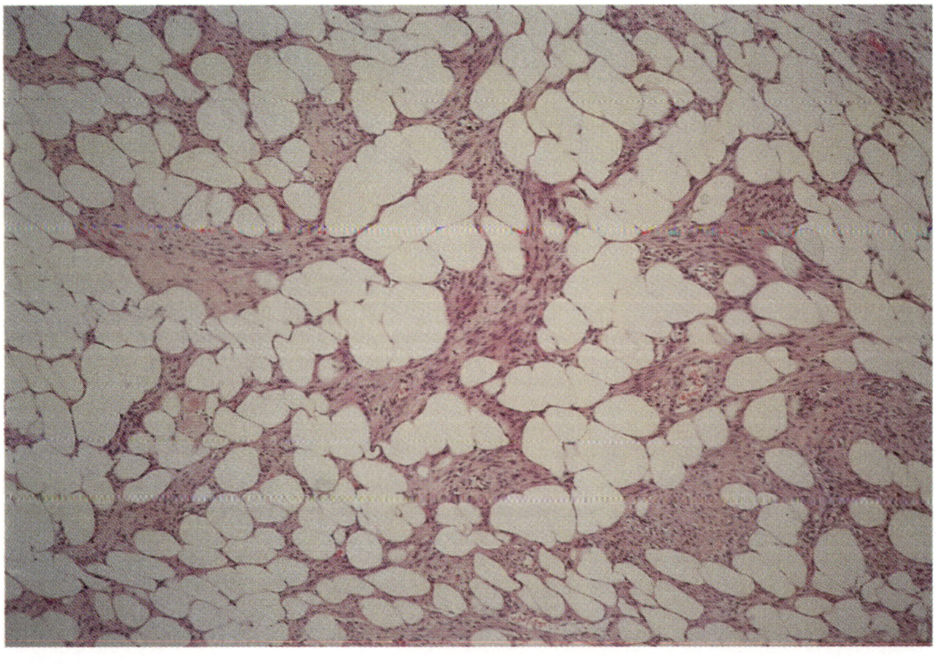

FIGURE 5–41
This lipoleiomyoma has smooth muscle fibers interspersed with large clear spaces that represent the adipose tissue.

consistency of the cut surface is variable. It may be soft and spongy or rubbery and firm. The color tends to be pinkish white, tan, gray, or reddish blue. Focal cystic degeneration may be present. When tumor is grossly visible within dilated veins, the neoplasm has the appearance of plugs within the involved vessels.

The microscopic appearance is of cytologically benign smooth muscle cells that are present within veins and endothelium-lined spaces. There have been no reported cases arising in arteries. Naked eye inspection of the histopathologic sections (i.e., glass slides) usually reveals visible tumor within vascular channels. The most common microscopic appearance is that of normal-appearing smooth muscle cells arranged in the whorled pattern typical of a leiomyoma but present in an abnormal location. The cells are fusiform and have eosinophilic cytoplasm, an ovoid nucleus, and a small nucleolus. Mitotic figures are uncommon. Most of these neoplasms average less than 1 mitotic figure per 10 HPF in the most active areas.[141] A variable amount of fibrosis may be present. Hyaline degeneration is present in some, forming collars around the vessels. Origin from a vessel wall is readily identifiable in most instances. In some examples the intravascular tumor is seemingly unattached and free-floating. In the typical case, an intimal attachment, which may be thin and delicate or broad-based, is present. Endometrial stroma is usually absent; only one reported case contained endometrial stroma.[141] The intravascular tumor itself contains numerous blood vessels. Moderate nuclear atypia may be present. An estimate of the amount of tumor filling each vein lumen varies from 5 to 100 percent.[140, 141]

All the histopathologic variants of leiomyoma may occur in intravenous leiomyomatosis.[140, 141] Epithelioid features in particular should prompt a closer look for intravascular growth (Fig. 5–42).[140] The diagnosis of intravenous leiomyomatosis requires the presence of histologically benign smooth muscle with multiple intravascular protrusions. Although the intravascular growth should be grossly evident, microscopic examination is necessary to confirm the diagnosis, especially when the process is intramural or the examiner does not recognize the gross features.[140]

There have been descriptions of over 20 cases that had direct extension of tumor to the right heart.[143, 144] In some of these cases the outcome has been fatal.[142] The cardiac mass appears whitish, elastic, soft, and irregularly shaped and is connected by a tail to the inferior vena cava. The tail may measure as much as 25 cm in length.[143] Deportation to the lung can occur with intravenous leiomyomatosis.[140, 141]

Two theories have been proposed for the origin of this neoplasm: (1) It originates from the smooth muscle component of uterine veins within the myometrium, or (2) it is the result of unusually extensive vascular invasion from a leiomyoma originating in the myometrium. Both views are necessary to explain all cases.

This neoplasm differs from leiomyoma because there is vascular invasion. Arbitrarily, the designation of leiomyoma with vascular invasion specif-

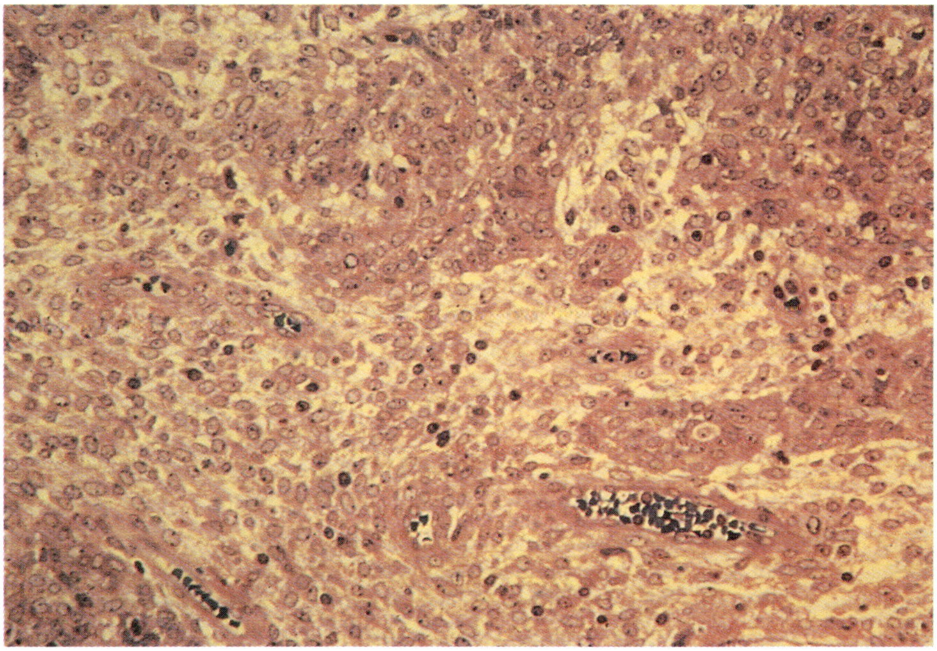

FIGURE 5–42
This epithelioid leiomyoma has two populations of smooth muscle cells. Those with abundant dark pink cytoplasm are the epitholioid cells in nests and cords. The nuclei in both populations are round to oval. There is no intravascular involvement on this section.

ically designates those neoplasms in which the vascular growth is a microscopic finding only, and the vascular growth is confined within the leiomyoma itself. The differential diagnosis also includes leiomyosarcoma, endometrial stromal sarcoma, and leiomyomatosis peritonealis disseminata. The increased mitotic activity of leiomyosarcoma is diagnostic. Endometrial stroma is not present in intravenous leiomyomatosis. The location of leiomyomatosis peritonealis disseminata on the serosal surface of the uterus and adjacent pelvic organs should serve to distinguish this condition.

Intravenous leiomyomatosis is underdiagnosed. Surgeons and pathologists frequently do not appreciate the gross features on initial examination. Its variable appearance on histopathologic examination may obscure recognition of its smooth muscle nature and intravenous location.[141]

The goal of treatment is complete surgical removal of the uterine tumor, usually by hysterectomy with removal of the adnexa if extrauterine extension occurs into these vessels.[140, 142] Pelvic recurrence and intravenous deportation may occur when there is extrauterine extension of the process and there has been incomplete surgical removal. There is persistence in as many as 30 percent of patients.[140–142] This happens most often after incomplete excision. Two instances of vaginal recurrence 24 and 26 months after initial excision have been reported.[140, 141] One patient experienced recurrence in the lung 9 years after excision.[141] Estrogen and progesterone receptors are present in most cases.[140, 142] Thus, some recommend oophorectomy and avoidance of estrogen replacement therapy, especially if the neoplasm is incompletely resected. Tamoxifen may be useful in controlling the growth of unresectable tumor.[144] Although this lesion is histopathologically benign, it is potentially fatal.

Benign Metastasizing Leiomyoma

Rarely, benign smooth muscle tumors are found in abnormal locations, usually the lung. In almost all instances the patient has a history of prior myomectomy or subtotal or total hysterectomy. In leiomyoma of the lung, virtually 100 percent of the patients are women. To qualify as benign metastasizing leiomyoma, origin from a vessel wall in the lung must not be present, either grossly or microscopically. Only then may one presume "metastases" or deportation from a leiomyoma in another location, which is usually the uterus. The existence of the rare "benign metastasizing leiomyoma" indicates that few leiomyomas can metastasize. Myomectomy, cesarean section, and possibly curettage may predispose to the spread of otherwise benign smooth muscle tumors of the uterus. The absence of significant mitotic activity and lack of cytologic atypia differentiates benign metastasizing leiomyoma from leiomyosarcoma.

Adenofibroma

This is an uncommon müllerian mixed tumor of the uterus, which is also known as papillary adenofibroma and papillary cystadenofibroma. More than 30 examples are documented in the medical literature.[145–148] The first description of this neoplasm arising in the uterine corpus was in 1973.[145] The patient presents with complaints of abdominal pain and abnormal or postmenopausal vaginal bleeding. These neoplasms may occur at any age, but most occur in the fifth and sixth decades. On physical examination a pelvic-abdominal mass may be present.

By gross examination this neoplasm is usually a polypoid mass that fills the endometrial cavity. Cut section reveals a yellow-gray neoplasm. Cystic spaces up to 1.5 cm are visible in the tumor. There is an intimate admixture of a glandular epithelial component with a fibromatous stromal component. Although the stromal component predominates, the glands are an integral part of this neoplasm. Both appear benign. The surface of the tumor usually appears as broad leaflike papillae. Glands vary in size from the simple tubular glands of an early proliferative endometrium to cystically dilated spaces corresponding to the gross appearance.[146–147] The glands are round and evenly spaced throughout the neoplasm. Slight degrees of architectural and nuclear atypia may be present. The epithelium is typically endometrioid in appearance, and glands are lined by a single layer of focally pseudostratified, uniform columnar cells, which may also appear flattened or show squamous, mucinous, or other metaplastic changes. Mild nuclear atypia may be present. Eosinophilic secretion may be present in the gland lumens. The stroma consists of benign fibroblasts or endometrial stromal cells or a mixture of these cell types. Stromal cellularity varies from minimal to marked. Stromal atypia is absent. Cuffs of dense cellular stroma around the glands are absent.[146] Varying amounts of collagen and hyalinization often separate the stromal cells. Small thin-walled blood vessels are apparent throughout the stroma. Mitotic activity is usually less than 1 mitotic figure per 10 HPF. In distinguishing this neoplasm from adenosarcoma, Clement and Scully allow 2 mitotic figures per 10 HPF,[146] while Zaloudek and Norris allow 4 mitotic figures per 10 HPF.[147]

There are two examples of adenofibroma that exhibited invasion of the myometrium and pelvic veins.[148] In one patient, uterine rupture occurred. As with the usual adenofibroma, a polypoid mass filled the uterus. However, deep myometrial invasion was obvious. Wormlike plugs of tumor appearing as gelatinous material were present within veins in the broad ligaments.[148] The microscopic appearance of these two neoplasms was benign. Mitotic activity was less than 1 mitotic figure per 10 HPF in both the glandular and the stromal components. To consider a benign diagnosis in the presence of myometrial invasion, the stroma must be virtually devoid of mitotic activity, lack marked stromal cellularity, and exhibit no more than mild stromal cell atypia.[148]

The differential diagnosis of adenofibroma includes benign endometrial polyp and adenosarcoma. Polyps generally lack the leaflike papillae of adenofibroma and show considerable heterogeneity from field to field, whereas adenofibroma is monotonous. Adenosarcoma can be differentiated by moderate stromal atypia and increased mitotic activity. Adenofibroma is much less common than its malignant counterpart, the müllerian adenosarcoma (see Chapter 6).[146]

The treatment of adenofibroma is hysterectomy. If a young woman wishes to preserve childbearing capacity, excision of the tumor under hysteroscopic guidance may prove useful.[146] However, these tumors may recur after local excision.

Adenomyosis

Adenomyosis is a common disorder. It refers to the presence of endometrial glands and stroma within the myometrium. This process may or may not represent "myometrial invasion," i.e., invaginations of endometrial glands and stroma to variable depths within the myometrium but still connected to the surface endometrium.

Sixty-five percent of women with adenomyosis experience symptoms, most commonly acquired dysmenorrhea and menorrhagia. The severity of the symptoms directly correlates with the extent of myometrial penetration. Pelvic examination is usually normal, but a globular enlarged uterus may be present. The weight of a uterus that contains diffuse adenomyosis can be as much as 340 gm.[118] The globular enlargement is a result of smooth muscle hypertrophy that surrounds areas of adenomyosis. Adenomyosis can be either focal and well circumscribed or diffuse throughout many microscopic fields. Focal adenomyosis may present as an intramyometrial or, less frequently, a subserosal mass. Rarely, adenomyosis can present as a polypoid mass projecting into the endometrial cavity.[149]

By gross examination the uterus with adenomyosis usually appears normal, although a globular enlargement of the fundus may be present (Fig. 5–43). By microscopic examination there are both benign endometrial glands and normal-appearing endometrial stroma at least one HPF below the endometrial-myometrial junction (Fig. 5–44). The glands in adenomyosis are usually proliferative or inactive. Smooth muscle hypertrophy may surround areas of adenomyosis.

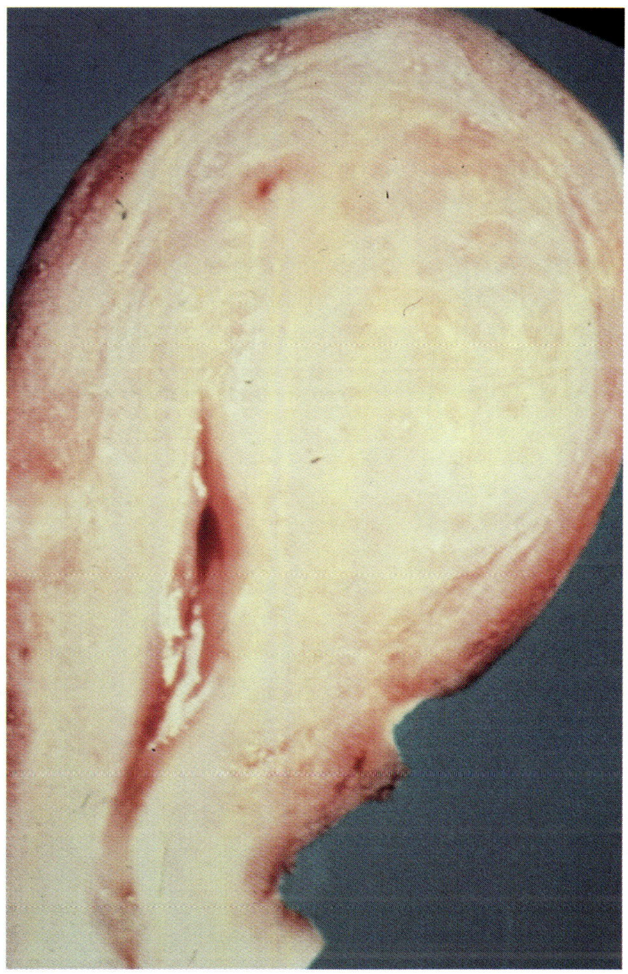

FIGURE 5–43
Diffuse enlargement of the uterine fundus is a frequent finding in uteri with adenomyosis. There are pink islands within the white muscle bundles and one small hemorrhagic area.

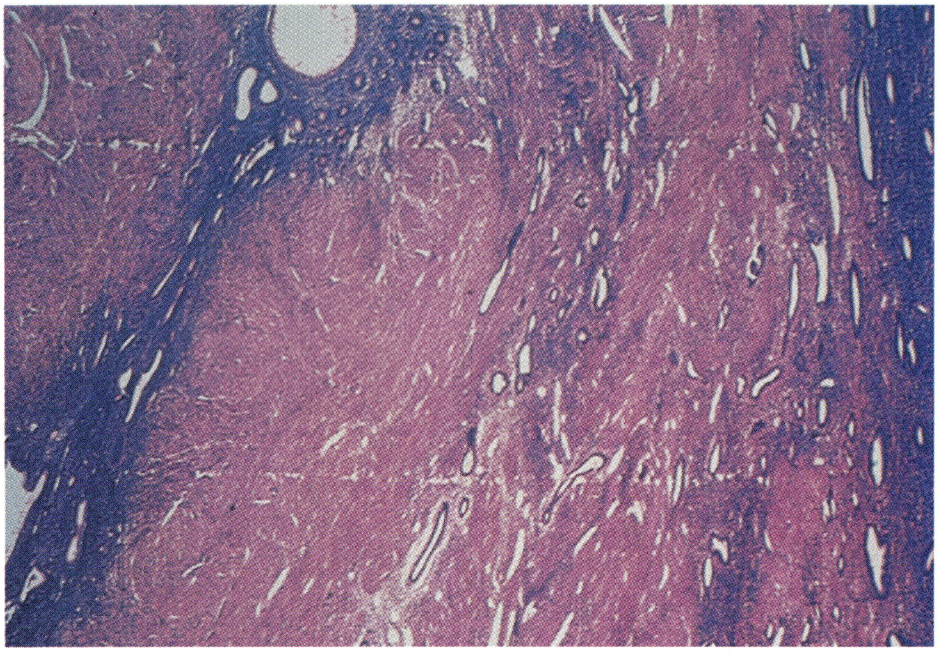

FIGURE 5-44
This shows normal endometrial glands and stroma within the myometrium.

In uteri with adenomyosis removed at the time of menstruation, fragments of endometrial tissue may be present within myometrial vessels. This tissue consists either of stromal cells or of stromal cells plus endometrial glands. The frequency of this occurrence is approximately 18 percent.[150] A possible origin of endometrial tissue from perivascular cells, or cutting and processing artifact, may account for this histopathologic phenomenon.

Steroid receptors are present in foci of adenomyosis. Estrogen receptors are more commonly present, while progesterone receptors are present in 60 percent of cases.[151] Thus there is a limited clinical response to progestational agents, owing to the inconsistent presence of receptors. The presence and severity of pain appear to be related to the total volume of adenomyotic foci and the depth of myometrial invasion. Adenomyosis and endometriosis are relatively common histopathologic findings, coexisting in 6 to 20 percent of patients. Endometriosis interna is the name that some apply to adenomyosis, while endometriosis externa refers to typical endometriosis, i.e., endometrial glands and stroma at an extrauterine site. Clinical and pathologic diagnosis is impossible without hysterectomy, except when a "myomectomy" specimen proves histologically to be an adenomyoma or adenomyosis rather than a leiomyoma.[152] The term *adenomyoma* refers to benign polypoid tumors of the uterus in which a benign endometrial glandular component exists in a stroma composed largely or exclusively of smooth muscle rather than endometrial stroma. The glands show no architectural complexity or cytologic atypia. Adenomyomas can vary in size. The gross appearance of an adenomyoma is similar to that of a leiomyoma (see Fig. 5-43).

Hysterosalpingography in patients with adenomyosis sometimes demonstrates a spiculated pattern, but this is not diagnostic. Ultrasonography exhibits a higher degree of diagnostic accuracy, but the specificity is poor. MRI is the noninvasive technique with the best diagnostic accuracy.[153]

Although adenomyosis is not a clinical diagnosis, history and physical findings may lead one to correctly suspect the correct diagnosis. No form of therapy short of hysterectomy has been consistently successful in controlling patients' symptoms.

Endometrial Stromal Nodule

Endometrial stromal nodule is an unusual benign neoplasm. It is the least common form of the endometrial stromal neoplasm, accounting for only 3.5 to 18 percent.[154, 155] These lesions are interesting mainly because of the diagnostic difficulties they pose when they are large or when they are present in a curettage specimen.[154] A well-circumscribed proliferation of endometrial stromal cells without endometrial glands characterizes an endometrial stromal nodule (Fig. 5-45). Invasion of surrounding tissue is not present, and involvement of endothelial spaces is absent. The margin of the tumor is the main feature that identifies whether an endometrial stromal tumor is benign or malig-

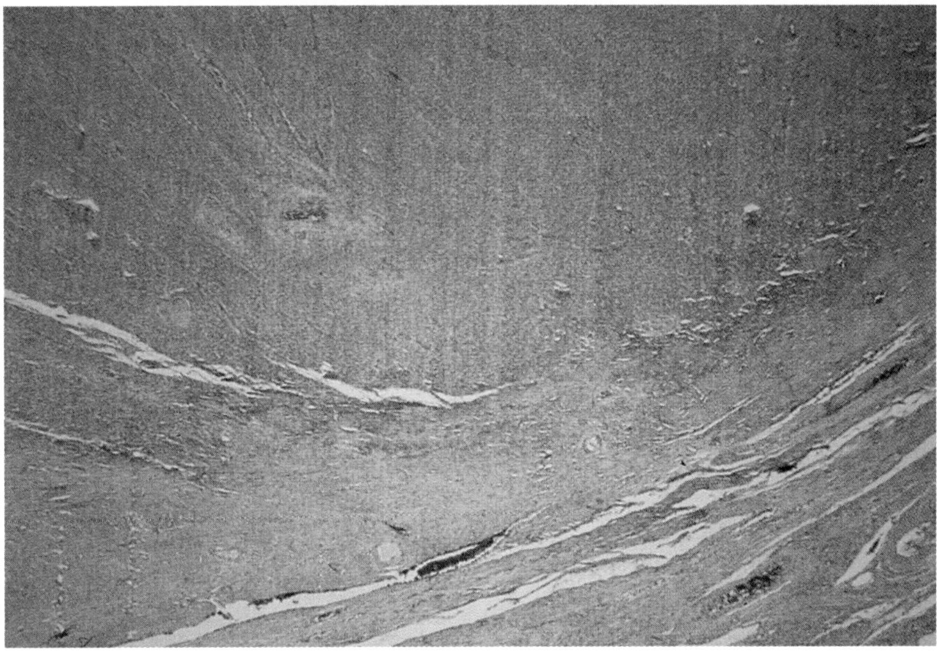

FIGURE 5-45
A low-power photomicrograph of an endometrial stromal nodule. The pushing margin with compression of the surrounding myometrium *(bottom)* is characteristic.

nant.[156] Mitotic activity is not a criterion in this neoplasm.[154]

The median age of patients with endometrial stromal nodules is 47 years; the range is 23 to 75 years.[154–156] Over 90 percent of cases occur in white women. Twenty-five percent of women are postmenopausal. Abnormal uterine bleeding and menorrhagia are the most common presenting complaints, occurring in two thirds of patients. Some women present with pelvic or abdominal pain. Approximately 25 percent of the cases are found incidentally in hysterectomy specimens.[154] Uterine enlargement or a uterine mass is the most common objective finding. Clinicians usually interpret this enlargement as either a leiomyoma or an adnexal mass.[156]

Endometrial stromal nodules are solitary, round or oval, fleshy, yellow or tan, and well circumscribed. The cut surface varies from whitish gray to bright orange. They have a discrete rounded contour and bulge above the surrounding myometrium when sectioned.[156] Some nodules are microscopic, while others may be as large as 15 cm.[152, 154] Cysts that range in size from 0.5 to 5 cm are seen in 18 percent of endometrial stromal nodules.[156] Another 18 percent present as polypoid lesions that project into the endometrial cavity. Occasionally endometrial stromal nodules may be multiple and at times lobulated rather than round. Necrosis and hemorrhage are uncommon findings. Rarely, a gelatinous degenerative change occurs.[156] In 6 percent of cases the lesion is located entirely within the endometrium; in 31 percent the endometrium and myometrium are involved; 63 percent are within the myometrium (intramural or subserosal) without any apparent connection to the endometrium.[154, 156]

On microscopic examination all nodules consist of normal-appearing stromal cells identical to or closely resembling those seen in proliferative endometrial stroma. The cells have scant cytoplasm with ill-defined borders and a uniform, round to oval nucleus that occasionally has a prominent nucleolus. The cells are uniform in size, shape, and staining qualities. The interface between the myometrium, the endometrium, and the neoplastic endometrial stromal cells is either smooth or shows, at most, minor microscopic interdigitation without an accompanying inflammatory response.[154] The margins are pushing, expansile, and noninfiltrative, compressing the adjacent myometrium and endometrium (Fig. 5–46). The mitotic rate is usually less than 10 mitotic figures per 10 HPF. The average is 4 mitotic figures per 10 HPF, but counts may be as high as 15 mitotic figures per 10 HPF.[156] In half the cases no mitoses are present.[156] Cytologic atypia is, at most, mild. Endometrial stromal nodules have a highly vascular supportive stroma. These tumors do not invade blood vessels.[156] Reticulin stain is useful to demonstrate the arborizing vasculature.

Occasionally, epithelial or sex cord–like structures may be present within an endometrial stromal nodule.[157] Collagen with areas of hyalinization is present in a minority of neoplasms. Calcium deposits are rare.[156] Cysts are present in approximately 15 percent and smooth muscle, as a minor component, in a similar number of examples.[156, 158]

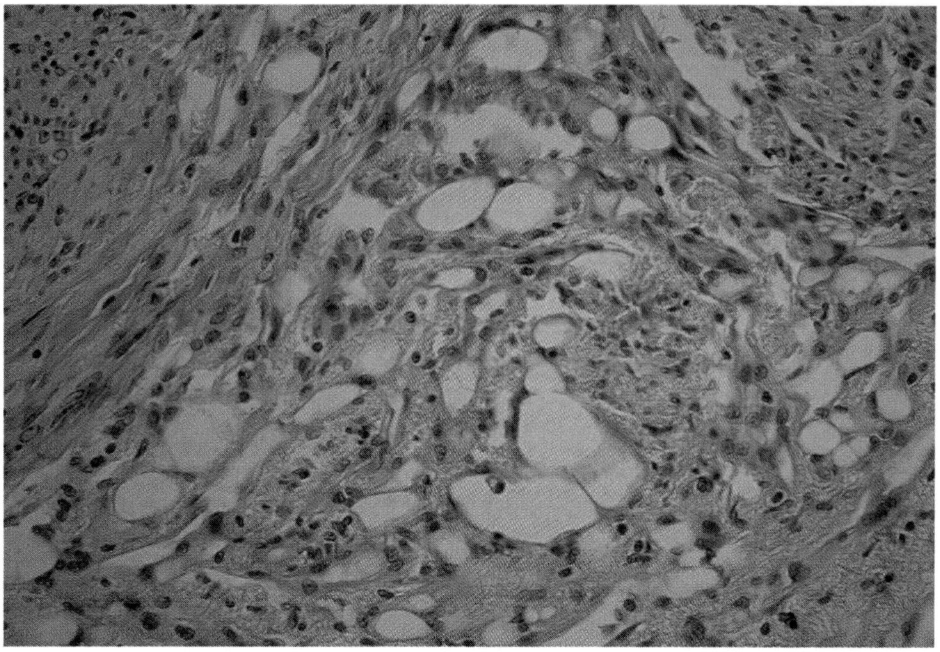

FIGURE 5-46
This adenomatoid tumor has flattened and cuboidal cells form cystic spaces. Cordlike growth is seen between muscle fibers *(upper left)*. These neoplasms connect in most cases with the peritoneal surface.

Areas of plexiform, trabecular, and tubular arrangements are prominent in some cases and are focal in many other tumors. Findings in endometrial stromal nodules indicate a capacity for neoplastic endometrial stromal cells to arrange themselves in epithelium-like formations and to form smooth muscle.[156, 159] The tumor lacks blood vessel invasion. The circumscribed margin and the prominent vascularity are the common characteristics of all endometrial stromal nodules.[156]

Diagnosis is difficult when endometrial stroma without glands is present either in a curettage or in a specimen thought to be a leiomyoma and removed by myomectomy.[154] Hysterectomy may be necessary to establish the diagnosis in such instances. The follow-up for a young woman who wishes to retain capacity for future childbearing when endometrial stromal nodule is strongly suspected, but not absolutely proved, could be done by ultrasound and CT. This may allow evaluation of the endometrium, myometrium, and other pelvic organs.[154] However, differentiation from a low-grade endometrial stromal sarcoma by these methods is impossible. Even histopathologically, this neoplasm is virtually identical to a low-grade endometrial stromal sarcoma. The sole differentiating feature is the well-delineated expansile growth pattern of its margin. Mitotic count is not a good predictor of clinical behavior. Although uncommon, endometrial stromal nodules may have mitotic counts that exceed 10 per 10 HPF. Low-grade endometrial stromal sarcoma, on the other hand, frequently has fewer than 3 mitotic figures per 10 HPF. All endometrial stromal nodules behave in a benign manner.

Hysterectomy has been the treatment in 90 percent of the reported cases.[154–156] Most endometrial stromal nodules have been incidental findings in uteri removed for other indications. None has recurred. The mitotic count, the presence of irregularities in the margin, or special histopathologic patterns do not affect outcome.

Uterine Tumor Resembling Ovarian Sex Cord Tumor

Uterine tumors resembling ovarian sex cord tumors are of uncertain histogenesis. Clement and Scully originally reported this distinctive neoplasm in 1976.[157] They divided these tumors into two groups. The first group was endometrial stromal tumors showing focal sex cord–like differentiation. These tumors often recurred. The second group showed diffuse or predominant sex cord–like differentiation. They behaved in a benign fashion. These authors postulated an origin from endometrial stroma. Grossly these neoplasms appear as yellow nodules with well-circumscribed borders, varying in diameter from 2 to 15 cm. Microscopically they contain epithelial nests, cords, trabeculae, and glandlike aggregates of cells, in close association with endometrial stroma. Strands of small tumor cells may form clefts, possibly representing rudimentary gland structures. Cytologic atypia and mitotic figures are not prominent features, and vascular invasion is not present. Reticulin fibers surround cords or nests of cells as well as single cells. In one example there was an intimate admixture of cells resembling endometrial foam cells, and numerous cells having variable amounts of clear or foamy cytoplasm intermediate in appearance between endometrial stroma and foam cells.[159]

Uterine tumors resembling sex cords and plexiform tumors appear to represent distinct variations of a related pathologic entity. The explanation may be the apparent capacity of endometrial stroma to undergo smooth muscle differentiation.[160]

The term stromomyoma refers specifically to a mixed endometrial stroma and smooth muscle neoplasm in which at least one third of the tumor bulk is smooth muscle.[156, 161]

Leiomyomatosis Peritonealis Disseminata (Peritoneal Leiomyomatosis)

This is an uncommon clinicopathologic entity. Over 60 cases have been documented.[139, 162–164] On gross examination these lesions appear malignant. However, the histopathology is benign, and the clinical course is favorable.[162] In most cases the women have been either pregnant or on oral contraceptives. In only a few reported cases was neither situation present.[162] Leiomyomatosis peritonealis disseminata is usually an incidental finding in women undergoing cesarean section or in women on oral contraceptives undergoing laparotomy, typically for myomectomy or tubal sterilization.[163] The peak incidence is in the third and fourth decades, (i.e., 22 to 41 years). All reported cases have been in women of reproductive age.[163] Sixty-five percent of them are white. One half were diagnosed during pregnancy or immediately post partum.[163] In a nonpregnant woman, the presenting complaint typically is pelvic discomfort or pain. All patients have coexistent leiomyomas.

On gross examination, multiple white-gray peritoneal nodules measuring 1 to 3 cm in diameter are present, which to the unwary may suggest a disseminated malignant neoplasm. Tens to hundreds of nodules may be present along peritoneal surfaces. This includes the peritoneal surface of the uterus, omentum, serosal surfaces of large and small intestine, urinary bladder, liver, mesentery, the peritoneal surface of the fallopian tubes, cul de sac, and surface of the ovaries.[163] The nodules are always subperitoneal. They seldom exceed 3 cm in diameter, but nodules up to 10 cm may occur.[162] In the few nonhormonally stimulated cases, the uterus is large and at surgery multiple small subserosal nodules, usually less than 1 cm in diameter, are present.[162] The lesions appear well circumscribed. They may be sessile or pedunculated with short stalks. Prominent vascularity is visible on the surface. On cut section they are white to gray, sometimes with areas of central hemorrhage.[164]

The nodules consist of uniform, spindle-shaped cells with eosinophilic cytoplasm and parallel longitudinal intracytoplasmic fibrils, typical of smooth muscle. Cellularity within each nodule is variable. Nodules contain a mixture of altered smooth muscle cells or myofibroblasts and fibroblasts.[163] Zones of hemorrhage may be present. The nuclei are fusiform and have the small distinct nucleoli characteristic of smooth muscle cells. Cytologic atypia and mitotic activity are uncommon. The stroma of the nodule is scanty and contains small blood vessels. In the pregnant woman, decidual cells may be conspicuous on light microscopic and ultrastructural studies. Decidual cells contain glycogen and exist in varying proportion with smooth muscle cells and fibroblasts.[164] Numerous microscopic nodules in early stages of development may be present. Adipose tissue or mesothelium surrounds these nodules.[139] Nodules regress or remain static on follow-up.[139] Estrogen and progesterone receptors are demonstrable in nearly all cells.[165]

Nodules do not have a uniform composition. The mixed composition results from varied stimuli, from the differences in the quality and degree of host response to the stimulus, and from sampling at different stages of development.[163] These nodules most likely result from proliferation of a mesenchymal stem cell. Opinions differ as to the pathways and type of differentiation. There are three theories: derivation from a primitive stem cell through a process of metaplasia[166]; derivation from stem cells that differentiate predominantly to myofibroblasts[167]; and decidual transformation of cells in the subcoelomic mesenchyme, replacement with fibroblasts or myofibroblasts, and differentiation into smooth muscle cells.[163, 168] However, endometrial stromal cells can also transform into smooth muscle cells.[160] The occurrence of leiomyomatosis peritonealis disseminata in women who are neither pregnant nor on contraceptive steroids suggests an unusual predisposition, or selective sensitivity, of the subperitoneal mesenchymal cells to undergo metaplasia and differentiation in some women. The high level of estrogen and progesterone binding in these nodules compared with normal myometrium supports this hypothesis.[165, 169]

The differential diagnosis includes leiomyosarcoma and benign metastasizing leiomyoma. Primary leiomyosarcomas arising from the peritoneal surface are usually larger than 5 cm, are accompanied by satellite lesions, and have a high mitotic rate and significant cytologic atypia. Distinguishing leiomyomatosis peritonealis disseminata from benign metastasizing leiomyoma is more difficult, but the latter generally presents as one or more pulmonary nodules. When it occurs in the pelvis, it is near the round ligaments or the iliac veins.[163]

No patient has had complete excision of disease, yet none has developed progressive disease.[163] At least four women who have had second-look laparotomy have demonstrated complete or partial regression; two women had a cesarean section, at which time persistence or recurrence of disease was documented.[163] A conservative approach is prudent, as this condition does not progress despite incomplete excision.

Adenomatoid Tumor (Adenomatoid Mesothelioma)

Adenomatoid tumor is a special variant of benign mesothelioma that occurs almost exclusively in the genital tract. This tumor is extremely rare.[170] In the past, the term lymphangioma often denoted this neoplasm.[171] Although it is the most common benign tumor of the fallopian tube, it arises with almost equal frequency in the uterus. These neoplasms are usually incidental findings at hysterectomy or at autopsy. Most are asymptomatic. They are small, averaging 0.5 cm to 3.5 cm in diameter. The largest reported adenomatoid tumor was 7.5 cm in diameter.[171] On gross examination these neoplasms are gray-white or yellow and have a pushing border. Generally they occupy a subserosal location. On microscopic examination, "glandular areas" are seen that are actually small cystic spaces lined with flattened or cuboidal endothelial type cells (see Fig. 5–46). Nuclei are small and uniform. Another component is solid areas composed of a proliferation of plump epithelioid cells that are arranged in nests or cords. These cells have abundant eosinophilic cytoplasm and round to oval eccentric nuclei. Cytoplasmic vacuoles are prominent. At first glance these cells resemble signet ring cells. If this tumor is serially sectioned, the connection with the serosal surface becomes apparent.

At least two examples have been reported that resembled cystic mesothelioma and that diffusely infiltrated the myometrium.[172, 173] These tumors contained clear yellow fluid. Microscopically a single layer of flattened cells with round to oval nuclei lined the cystic spaces. Fine connective tissue septa were present. The solid portions resembled the typical adenomatoid tumor. Cystic mesothelioma is a rare neoplasm thought to fall within the spectrum between adenomatoid tumor and malignant mesothelioma of the peritoneum. It occurs in the pelvis of adult women. Although cystic mesothelioma does not metastasize, some lesions may recur.[172]

Retroperitoneal Fibrosis

This is a condition unrelated to the uterus. Anatomic and histopathologic confusion with a leiomyomatous uterus is common. The process of retroperitoneal fibrosis is not understood. Grossly and microscopically, dense retroperitoneal accumulations of hyaline connective tissue occupy a retroperitoneal location in the pelvis. Retroperitoneal fibrosis may manifest as a pelvic mass. Rarely, a patient may present with ureteral obstruction. The most commonly accepted theories for the cause of retroperitoneal fibrosis are either a collagen vascular disease or a hypersensitivity reaction.[174] The condition may respond to progestogen therapy, e.g., megestrol acetate.

Hemangioma

Hemangiomas of the uterus are extremely rare. They appear to be benign by both gross and microscopic examination. They are predominantly of the capillary type. Immunocytochemistry and special stains may be important in establishing the diagnosis.

Hemangiopericytoma

Hemangiopericytoma is an unusual combined stromal and vascular neoplasm derived from the myoepithelial pericyte. The most common location for this neoplasm is in the extremities and the pelvic retroperitoneum. It is a locally aggressive neoplasm with a propensity for late and distant metastases.

The age range of patients is between 23 and 81 years with a mean of 45 years.[175] The most common presenting complaint is an abdominopelvic mass, followed by abnormal uterine bleeding. The uterine fundus is the most common location for this neoplasm among the müllerian-derived organs.[175] Most hemangiopericytomas arise within the myometrium or project as polypoid growths into the endometrial cavity. Gross lesions appear gray with a yellow or blue hue. In half these patients the neoplasm appears encapsulated. The consistency varies from semicystic, doughy or rubbery, to firm and fleshy. Hemorrhage may be present. The tumors may be as large as 24 cm.[174]

A proliferating stromal cellular component and a prominent vascular network characterize this neoplasm. The multiplying elements distribute in a concentric array, with the vascular compartments at the center. Tumor cell nesting is present. A whorling pattern is seen in most neoplasms. Vascular spaces range in size from microcapillaries to staghorn configurations.[175] The borders are expansile and usually encapsulated. Individual cells appear elongated with abundant pale cytoplasm. Nuclei are large and oval. Mitotic activity is uncommon.[175]

Approximately 25 percent of these neoplasms recur in the pelvis, abdomen, and lungs. In neoplasms that occur outside the müllerian system, the recurrence and metastasis rates are doubled.[176] The tendency to encapsulation in uterine lesions may play a role in the improved outcome. Histopathologic features do not correlate with recurrence.[175]

Epithelioid Leiomyoma (Plexiform Leiomyoma Including Plexiform Tumorlet)

The term epithelioid leiomyoma includes leiomyoblastoma, clear cell leiomyoma, plexiform leiomyoma, and plexiform tumorlet. The median age of patients is 48 years.[177] These neoplasms do not differ from other benign myometrial tumors, nor from their counterparts in other parts of the body. Microscopically, the cells are round or polygonal and arranged in clusters or cords.[177] The leiomyoblastoma has rounded "epithelioid type" cells with eosinophilic cytoplasm. As the name implies, the cells of clear cell leiomyoma have a clear cytoplasm. The clear cells contain glycogen. Plexiform leiomyomas contain rounded cells arranged in cords, trabeculae, and nests.[178] The behavior of these histopathologic variants, as with their behavior elsewhere in the body, is uncertain. Besides the usual criteria for malignant smooth muscle tumors, those epithelioid leiomyomas larger than 6 cm with mitotic activity exceeding 2 per 10 HPF recur with enough frequency to be of concern.[177]

Plexiform tumorlets are unique to the uterus. They behave in a benign fashion.[139, 178] As their name implies, these neoplasms are microscopic findings.[178] Borghard-Erdle and Hirsch were the first to describe this neoplasm.[179] Tumorlets have a distinct light microscopic appearance (Fig. 5–47). The median age of women with this finding is 45 years.[178] These lesions are usually incidental findings in uteri removed for other conditions. On retrospective analysis, the tumorlet was evident grossly in approximately 25 percent of examples.[178] The gross appearance is the same as that of a small leiomyoma. Tumorlets may be present anywhere in the uterus, but they generally occupy an intramyometrial location. Some tumorlets are within the endometrial stroma or within the myometrium in proximity to endometrial stroma or areas of adenomyosis. Tumorlets are multiple in 25 percent of instances.[178] Most tumorlets are less than 1 cm in greatest diameter. The margins of some tumorlets appear sharply circumscribed, but most have ill-defined margins. Multifocal tumorlets are particularly irregular in their shape and outline. Two distinct histopathologic patterns occur with equal frequency.[178] In the first, small

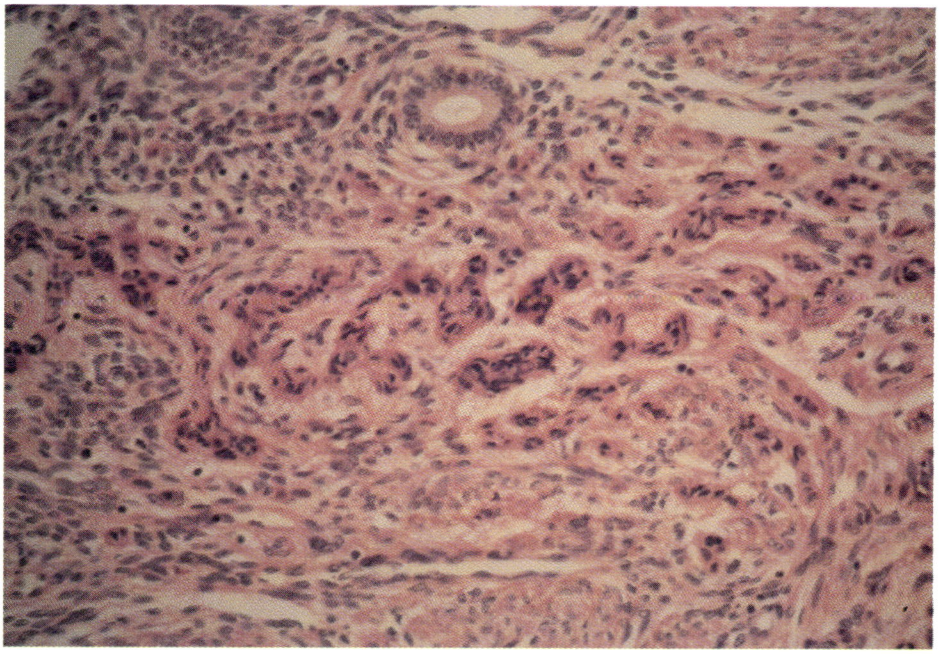

FIGURE 5–47
This is a plexiform tumorlet. Smooth muscle cells are in a plexiform or cordlike arrangement adjacent to benign endometrial gland and stroma. The cells are small, with hyperchromatic nuclei and purple cytoplasm.

nests of cells are interspersed in a hyalinized stroma containing occasional spindle cells (see Fig. 5–47). In the second, the cells have a trabecular pattern, forming branching cords one to three cells thick, separated by a similar hyalinized stroma. The pattern of narrow anastomosing cords of small cells is monotonous. These two histopathologic patterns frequently coexist. Blood vessels and capillaries occasionally are evident between cords and clusters of cells or at the periphery of well-circumscribed tumorlets. A relationship to adenomyosis may be evident.[178] Individual cells are oval or polygonal with indistinct cell margins. The cytoplasm is eosinophilic and granular or appears vacuolated. Nuclei are round to oval, often contain grooves with nuclear folds, and have finely distributed chromatin and occasionally a small nucleolus. Pleomorphism, atypia, necrosis, and mitotic activity are absent. Ultrastructural studies suggest a smooth muscle origin for these lesions.[178] Lesions larger than 1 cm (gross lesions) by definition are not tumorlets.

THE ROUND LIGAMENT

The round ligament arises anterolaterally from the cornual region of the uterus and traverses a course that leads beneath the inguinal ligament and through the inguinal canal to its terminus in the labium majus. Involvement of the round ligament in disease processes is infrequent. By 1962, Breen and Neubecker[180] had identified 224 cases in the world literature of such neoplasms. Neoplasms of the round ligament may be either primary or secondary (metastatic) and may be either solid or cystic. Additionally, the location of the neoplasm may be within the pelvis or extraperitoneal.

Striated muscle is present in 2.8 percent of round ligaments.[181] This does not appear to have any clinical or pathologic significance. Its origin is probably from aberrant persistence, differentiation, and maturation of gubernacular rhabdomyoblasts, which usually undergo involution in the female fetus.[181] The round ligament smooth muscle contains estrogen and progesterone receptors.[182]

Cystic lesions of the round ligament include mesothelial cysts and cysts of the canal of Nuck. Both the mesothelial cyst and the cyst of the canal of Nuck are lined by a single layer of flattened mesothelial cells that have bland nuclei and rare to absent mitoses. The only distinguishing feature is their location. A cyst of the canal of Nuck is a peritoneum-lined cystic structure that occurs in the extraperitoneal portion of the round ligament. Treatment is simple excision.

Solid neoplasms of the round ligament include typical leiomyomas, endometriosis including endometriomas, and adenomyomas. Leiomyomas account for approximately one half of the neoplasms involving the round ligament.[180] They have the histopathologic appearance of typical smooth muscle tumors described earlier. They may undergo the same degenerative changes. The leiomyoma can be located anywhere along the course of the round ligament. Intraabdominal round ligament leiomyomas usually cause no symptoms. The patient may present with an asymptomatic mass found on pelvic examination. Pain is the most common symptom in symptomatic patients. A mass in the inguinal or labial region is the typical presentation in patients who have a leiomyoma of the round ligament arising in an extraabdominal location. Leiomyomas of the round ligament are usually single. However, most patient have other leiomyomas in the uterus.[180]

Endometriosis and endometriomas of the round ligament are uncommon. The location may be either within the pelvis or along the extrapelvic portion of the ligament. Endometriosis of the round ligament is usually associated with pelvic endometriosis. Isolated round ligament endometriosis is rare. Over 30 cases of endometriosis involving the extraperitoneal portion of the round ligament have been reported.[184] In this location the clinical presentation is usually that of a painful mass that changes in size in association with the menstrual cycle.[184–186] It can be confused with an inguinal hernia,[185] and it can cause referred hip pain.[187] The histopathology of round ligament endometriosis is the same as that of endometriosis at other sites. If a significant amount of smooth muscle is present the term adenomyoma is used (see above). There is a single case report of carcinoma in the inguinal region arising in endometriosis.[188] The treatment of endometriosis originating in an extrapelvic location is the same as when it is found in the pelvis.

A number of other neoplasms have been reported to occur in the round ligament. These include benign mesenchymomas,[189] capillary hemangioma, fibroma, and teratoma.[180] Treatment is excision. Secondary involvement of the round ligament by neoplasia is common and is usually part of a generalized disease process.

OBTAINING ENDOMETRIAL BIOPSIES

Dilatation and curettage (D&C) has long been the standard for obtaining endometrial samples in women with both abnormal uterine bleeding and infertility. Despite extensive use of the D&C, critical evaluation of the tissue yield and diagnostic accuracy was not available until recently. In 1982, the estimated cost of this procedure in the United States approached 1 billion dollars.[190] A critical evaluation of D&C took place in 1985 under the direction of Smith and Schulman.[191] It involved a 10-year experience and included 1383 surgical specimens. These investigators found that the detection of uterine cancer did not increase until the patient was above the age of 50 years. No significant pathologic findings were present in 60 percent or more of women until age 70 years. Hyperplasia and atypical hyperplasia increased from 4 percent in the women 29 years of age or younger to 16 percent in the 45- to 49-year group. The authors concluded that the indications for this procedure were too broad and that outpatient procedures could replace formal D&C in most instances.[191]

Outpatient endometrial sampling has gradually replaced D&C. Endometrial sampling as an outpatient procedure causes minimal patient discomfort in most instances. Paracervical block may be helpful in some women. Newer sampling devices obtain a core of endometrium, usually 3 mm in diameter, for pathologic analysis (Fig. 5–48). Endometrial histopathology is necessary primarily in two broad areas of gynecology—evaluation of the infertile patient and evaluation of women with abnormal or postmenopausal uterine bleeding. Both indications have certain features in common. In every endometrial sampling, three items of information are important: the depth of the endometrial cavity, the contour of the endometrial cavity (smooth versus irregular), and the quantity of tissue removed.[86, 191, 192]

The technique of endometrial sampling is similar regardless of the instrument used. Most instruments currently in use rely on some means of suction to obtain the tissue sample. Before performing the procedure, a thorough pelvic examination is necessary. This allows the operator knowledge of the approximate size of the uterus and the position of the fundus in relation to the cervix: anteverted, anteflexed, midposition, retroflexed, or retroverted. As the position of the uterus changes, slight alteration in technique may be necessary. The operator inserts a speculum into the vagina and visualizes the cervix. Antiseptic solution removes mucus and cleanses the cervical os. For traction, a single tooth tenaculum or similar instrument grasps the anterior or posterior lip of the cervix. Insertion of a uterine sound will determine the depth of the endometrial cavity. Prior knowledge of the uterine position determines the direction of the sound. The depth of the uterine cavity in centimeters is noted. A normal uterus is approximately 6 to 8 cm in depth, measured from the external cervical os to the fundus.

Devices currently in use to obtain endometrial samples include the Novak curette, the Vabra aspirator, the endometrial Pipelle, and the endometrial Z-sampler. Each of these devices has advantages and disadvantages. The Novak curette is a hollow metal device. It has a curve culminating in a tip with a serrated opening just proximal to the distal tip. This device uses a syringe to obtain suction (see Fig. 5–48). The Vabra aspiration device consists of a plastic collection cylinder, which attaches at the patient end to a 3 or 4 mm hollow metal curette, similar to the Novak curette. The other end of the cylinder connects to an electrical suction pump, which helps collect the specimen into the hollow cylinder. A similar device is the

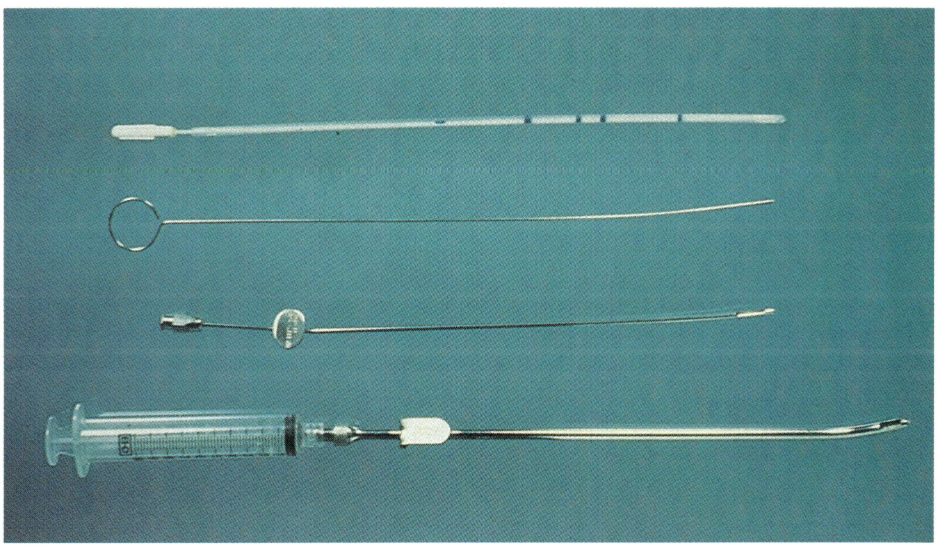

FIGURE 5–48
Several endometrial sampling devices are shown. *Top,* The plastic Pipelle. *Bottom,* A Novak curette attached to a syringe. *Center,* The Hofmeister curette and stylet.

Masterson curette (a hand-held pump instead of an electrical one) (Fig. 5–49). The endometrial Pipelle and the Z-sampler are similar. They are plastic, disposable, 3 mm, hollow tubes with a 25 cm long stylet. The endometrial Pipelle has markings at 3, 4, 7, 8, 11, and 14 cm. The operator inserts the sampling device into the endometrial cavity to the fundus. Once the device is within the endometrial cavity, the operator withdraws the stylet approximately 75 to 80 percent of the length of the instrument. This creates a suction. The operator rotates the sampling device in a circular fashion and samples the endometrium from fundus to lower uterine segment. The specimen collects in the hollow core of the instrument or in the appropriate container. The contents of the sampling device are then placed in a preservative-filled (e.g., formalin) container for subsequent processing. All the aforementioned devices obtain a satisfactory specimen. The endometrial sample appears as a long core of tissue in the specimen container. Microscopic architecture is of good quality. The Vabra aspirator obtains a sufficient quantity of tissue, but the tissue tends to fragment and is sometimes more difficult for the pathologist to interpret.

In women with abnormal uterine bleeding or postmenopausal bleeding, we recommend simultaneous endocervical curettage. This will diagnose endocervical pathology that might go unrecognized if only an endometrial sample were obtained. A Duncan curette or similar device is appropriate for obtaining endocervical specimens.

In the evaluation of the infertility patient, the desired information is the documentation of ovulation and histologic date of the endometrium to exclude luteal phase defect. One or two swipes from the anterior fundal portion of the uterus will easily obtain this information. As these samples are purposely obtained after suspected ovulation, the sampling technique should attempt to avoid disruption of a possible pregnancy. Most pregnancies implant in the fundus or posterior uterine wall. Interruption of a pregnancy is uncommon, occurring in approximately 0.6 percent of endometrial samples obtained for the evaluation of infertility.[40]

In the evaluation of women with abnormal or postmenopausal uterine bleeding, the main purpose of the sampling is to exclude neoplasia. Thus in these patients, thorough sampling of the endometrial cavity is desirable to obtain as representative a sample as possible for histopathologic analysis.

In premenopausal women with abnormal uterine bleeding, most diagnoses are benign. The prevalence of malignant diagnoses is about 0.5 percent. Approximately one half the neoplasms are primary in the endometrium. The remainder are primary in the endocervix or are metastatic, usually from the ovary. Hyperplasia, atypical hyperplasia, and endometrial polyps, which occur in a setting of estrogen excess, likewise are uncommon. These conditions are present in 2.6 percent of women sampled under 40 years of age and in 7.8 percent of premenopausal women over 40 years.[29]

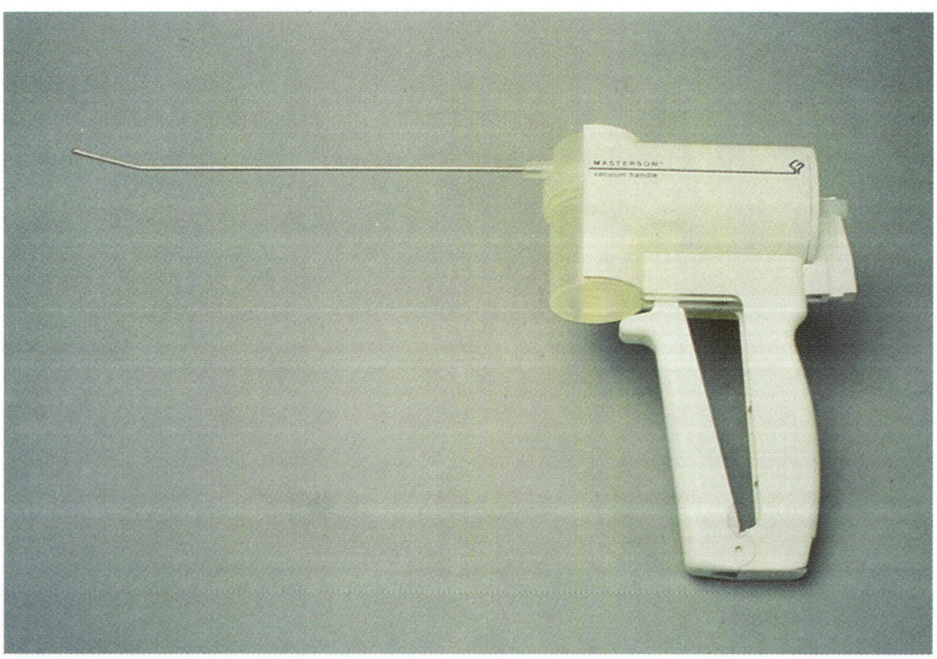

FIGURE 5–49
A Masterson curette attached to a hand-held vacuum pump is seen here. The metal curette (2 or 3 mm in external diameter) has a slightly bent tip and centimeter markings along its length. The tissue is collected in the plastic container that attaches to the pump.

Even in women who have postmenopausal bleeding the endometrium in most cases is benign. Obtaining sufficient tissue for histopathologic diagnosis, however, may be a problem. Eighty percent of endometria in postmenopausal women look atrophic on microscopic examination.[28, 86] All methods and devices used to obtain endometrial samples are unable to obtain suitable tissue for histopathologic evaluation in some patients.[28] This may be as high as 15 percent for D&C and 12 percent for specimens obtained with outpatient sampling devices.[28] In women of all ages, the Vabra aspirator obtains insufficient tissue in 3.1 percent of cases. The Novak curette averages 6.3 percent.[193] Atrophic endometrium yields little to no tissue on sampling. If the clinician is confident that the sampling instrument was in the uterine cavity beyond the internal cervical os and that there was strict adherence to proper technique, a presumptive diagnosis of atrophy is appropriate and there is no need to perform a D&C.[28, 193] The accuracy of tissue diagnosis is comparable for all currently used devices, but the instruments with smaller diameters cause less patient discomfort.[194–196] When comparing instruments by obtaining samples on the same day, the device used first is more likely to be associated with the correct diagnosis.[194, 196]

Many gynecologists routinely perform endometrial sampling before hysterectomy, supposedly to detect occult endometrial malignancy. In a study of prehysterectomy endometrial sampling there were 30 instances among 619 patients in which endometrial sampling failed to identify either endometrial hyperplasia or carcinoma. In the two cases of endometrial carcinoma, D&C was the sampling method used.[193] All techniques proved equal in their diagnostic capabilities. Only patients with postmenopausal bleeding or women older than 35 years with abnormal uterine bleeding appear to benefit from prehysterectomy endometrial sampling.[193] The most likely pathology to be missed by any of the sampling techniques is endometrial polyps.[86, 193, 194]

Uterine fluid collections in postmenopausal women are a cause for concern. When a pelvic examination, ultrasound, or MRI discovers an intrauterine fluid collection, endometrial sampling is mandatory. Findings on sampling include cancer of ovarian, tubal, endometrial, or cervical origin in 20 percent of women.[192]

Hysteroscopy is an invaluable adjunct in the evaluation of women with recurrent uterine bleeding unexplained by endometrial sampling. Even in this clinical setting, carcinoma is uncommon. Since the most common pathologic lesion that outpatient sampling fails to detect is an endometrial polyp, hysteroscopy with excision of the polyp under direct vision, followed by examination of the remainder of the endometrial cavity, is appropriate.[28, 86, 190, 197]

The newer hysteroscopes are proving to be useful for diagnostic purposes in the outpatient setting. Little or no anesthesia or analgesia is necessary with the smaller 3 to 4 mm instruments. If necessary, a paracervical block may be used. Beside the ability to obtain directed endometrial samples, hysteroscopy is invaluable in diagnosing anatomic lesions such as intrauterine synechiae, uterine septa, and submucous leiomyomas. Hysteroscopic findings are similar to the histopathologic findings at endometrial sampling. Hysteroscopic findings in 377 women with premenopausal abnormal uterine bleeding were as follows: normal cavity, 42.7 percent; endometrial polyp, 11.9 percent; cervical polyp, 5.6 percent; hyperplasia, 5.3 percent; submucous fibroid, 2.9 percent; and endometrial carcinoma, 1.3 percent.[197] The findings in 259 infertility patients were as follows: normal cavity, 49.8 percent; endometrial polyp, 9.7 percent; uterine malformation, 7.3 percent; intrauterine synechiae, 5.0 percent; cervical polyp, 2.3 percent; and hyperplasia, 2.3 percent.[197] Together with the histopathology, a permanent record on videotape of the hysteroscopic findings is useful for patient education, teaching, and follow-up of minor intrauterine lesions.

EXAMINATION AND PROCESSING OF UTERINE SPECIMENS

Gross and microscopic examination of the surgical specimen is an important adjunct to any gynecologic surgical procedure. Pathologists excel at examining, evaluating, measuring, and describing. A careful measurement and a thorough description of normal and abnormal findings are an important part of any pathology report. The pathology report should include all pathologic features that are important in prognosis and treatment. We will divide this section into three separate parts: curettings and endometrial contents, leiomyoma and other tumors separately removed, and the uterus.

Curettings

Curettings include both endocervical and endometrial specimens. Endocervical curettage can exclude or include the presence of primary endocervical disease, or the extension of disease from either the endometrium or the ectocervix. On gross examination both endometrial and endocervical curettage specimens consist of blood, tissue fragments, and mucus. After obtaining the specimen the gynecologist should avoid placing it on a surgical sponge or gauze pad, which has a tendency to absorb and hide small fragments of tissue. After examination the pathologist places the entire specimen, wrapped in nonabsorbent tissue paper, into a cassette. This is then dropped into a container with fixative (e.g., formalin) for further processing.

The gynecologist should submit the entire endometrial or endocervical specimen from all diagnostic procedures for pathology examination. The pathologist may process representative samples from large volumes of tissue (e.g., placental tissue) obtained from therapeutic procedures. The pathologist measures and weighs these tissues as an aggregate. In spontaneous or elective abortion, the pathologist should attempt to find fetal tissue or the gestational sac. Examination of the products of conception may show an intact empty sac, a ruptured empty sac with or without a cord stump, a normal fetus with intact or ruptured sac, or a focally abnormal or grossly abnormal fetus with an intact or empty sac. A description of the fetus along with its measurements (e.g., crown-rump length) is appropriate. If the initial samples of tissue do not reveal fetal or placental tissue on gross examination, the entire specimen should be submitted for histopathologic evaluation. In specimens from an elective termination of pregnancy, the pathologist should attempt to identify fetal parts or placental tissue and should immediately notify the clinician if none is found so that the patient can be evaluated for the possibility of an ectopic pregnancy.

Uterine Tumors

Leiomyomas, polyps, and other neoplasms require a separate description and examination of each specimen. Accurate measurement and a gross description of all lesions are important. The surgeon or pathologist should annotate the number and location of all neoplasms, if possible. The pathologist may describe the appearance of multiple typical leiomyomas as a group. The description should include color and consistency of the lesions plus documentation of areas of hemorrhage and necrosis. The surgeon or pathologist should open or bisect large specimens to allow proper and thorough fixation. The specimens are placed in a container with ample fixative and allowed to stand overnight. After proper fixation, one tissue section for each 2 cm of greatest diameter of the neoplasm is appropriate for lesions presumed grossly to be benign. For multiple leiomyomas that have a typical gross appearance, one tissue section per leiomyoma is adequate. For suspicious or malignant neoplasms, one tissue block for each centimeter of greatest diameter of neoplasm is prepared. If, after examination of the initial specimen, doubt remains as to the proper diagnosis, the pathologist should submit and examine additional representative tissue sections.

Uterus

Examination of the simple hysterectomy specimen differs depending on the indication for the surgery, i.e., whether benign or malignant (the processing of the radical hysterectomy specimen is discussed in Chapter 4). For benign functional disease, such as intractable dysfunctional bleeding, chronic pelvic pain, or uterine prolapse, the description should begin with whether the cervix and adnexa are present and attached to the specimen. To orient the surgical specimen anteriorly and posteriorly, the pathologist must identify the round ligaments, fallopian tubes, and peritoneal reflections. The round ligaments are anterior to the fallopian tubes. Posteriorly the peritoneal reflection extends below the lower uterine segment or isthmus, whereas anteriorly there is less peritoneum owing to the higher bladder flap that was surgically developed. The pathologist records the weight of the uterus and obtains the following uterine measurements: (1) length measured from cervix to fundus, (2) width measured from cornu to cornu, and (3) thickness measured from the anterior to posterior surface of the uterus. Other useful measurements include the length and width of the cervix, and the depth of the uterine cavity as measured from the external cervical os. The pathologist examines the outer surface of the uterus for evidence of adhesions, endometriosis, or other lesions. The patency of the cervical canal and endometrial cavity is determined with a probe. The cervix is examined for gross lesions such as lacerations, ulcerations, and cysts. The pathologist then opens the uterus and measures endometrial and myometrial thickness (Fig. 5–50). Any endometrial lesions are described and measured. A description of any intramyometrial lesions should follow. Sections from 12 o'clock

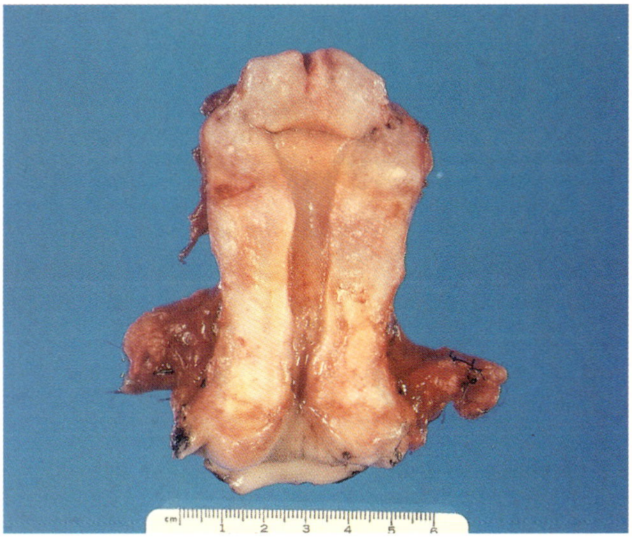

FIGURE 5-50
This is a radical hysterectomy specimen. The uterus has been opened anteriorly. The incision extends from the cervix to the fundus, where it is carried toward each corner in a Y shape. The parametrium is seen on either side of the cervix. Black ink has been applied to the vaginal cuff margin.

and 6 o'clock are adequate in grossly normal cervices. These sections should include the squamocolumnar junction, ectocervix, and endocervix. Sections through the body of the uterus should extend from the endometrial cavity to the serosal surface. From a grossly normal uterus, sections from the anterior and posterior endometrial surfaces are sufficient.

For benign disease such as a leiomyoma, endometrial hyperplasia, or endometrial polyp, the procedure outlined above is appropriate with some modifications. In the uterus removed for leiomyomas, the pathologist records the number, location (e.g., subserous, intramural, submucous), and size of all lesions. Distortion of the endometrial cavity is an important finding to document. Submission of sections as described above for the myomectomy specimen is done. In uteri removed for endometrial hyperplasia, the pathologist should submit multiple full-thickness sections of endometrium and myometrium. Multiple sections are necessary to exclude adenocarcinoma. Sections should be at least 2 cm long. It may be necessary to process the entire endometrium.

In uteri removed for malignant uterine disease, the pathologist should examine the surgical specimen for the presence of residual disease. The gross description of any lesion includes a description of the lesion itself, such as polypoid or plaquelike, focal or diffuse. The color, consistency, and location of the lesion are important, as is the presence of hemorrhage and necrosis. If invasion of the myometrium is grossly apparent, the depth of invasion is documented. It is important that the sections taken from these areas allow for accurate determination of the maximum depth of invasion. Extension to the cervix or the presence of cervical abnormalities requires documentation, as does involvement of the surgical margin. When taking a sample from a margin (e.g., vagina), it is important to take a piece that is perpendicular to the margin. In this way the paraffin block containing the tissue will be oriented correctly and allow for measuring the distance from the tumor to the margin. Ink placed on the surgical margin helps in its identification during microscopic evaluation.

The final report should include a histopathologic diagnosis that includes cell type and organ of origin of the neoplasm. Tumor grade, cervical involvement, depth of cervical involvement (e.g., involving superficial glands or deep into the stroma), depth of myometrial invasion (e.g., no invasion, less than 50 percent, more than 50 percent), and the presence of lymphovascular space involvement require documentation, as they affect staging and/or prognosis. Involvement or lack of involvement of margins should be noted. If a lymph node dissection or sampling accompanies the specimen, a description of the number, location, and gross appearance and microscopic involvement is necessary.

REFERENCES

1. Langlois PL: The size of the normal uterus. J Reprod Med 1970; 4:220–228.
2. Mazur MT, Kraus FT: Histogenesis of morphologic variations in tumors of the uterine wall. Am J Surg Pathol 1980; 4:59–74.
3. Noyes RW, Hertig AT, Rock J: Dating the endometrial biopsy. Fertil Steril 1950; 1:3–25.
4. Speroff L, Glass RH, Kase NG: Clinical Gynecologic Endocrinology and Infertility, 4th ed. Baltimore, Williams & Wilkins, 1989, pp 14–15.
5. Gorski J, Welshons WV, Sakai D, Hansen J, Walent J, Kassis J, Shull J, Stack G, Campen C: Evolution of a model of estrogen action. Recent Prog Horm Res 1986; 42:297–329.
6. King WJ, Greene GL: Monoclonal antibodies localize oestrogen receptor in the nuclei of target cells. Nature 1984; 307:745–747.
7. Welshons WV, Lieberman ME, Gorski J: Nuclear localization of unoccupied oestrogen receptors. Nature 1984; 307:747–749.
8. Katzenellenbogen BS: Dynamics of steroid hormone receptor action. Annu Rev Physiol 1980; 42:17–35.
9. Speroff L, Glass RH, Kase NG: Clinical Gynecologic Endocrinology and Infertility, 4th ed. Baltimore, Williams & Wilkins, 1989, pp 24–29.

10. Gambrell RD Jr, Bagnell CA, Greenblatt RB: Role of estrogens and progesterone in the etiology and prevention of endometrial cancer: review. Am J Obstet Gynecol 1983; 146:696–703.
11. Bayard F, Damilano S, Robel P, Beaulieu E-E: Cytoplasmic and nuclear estradiol and progesterone receptors in human endometrium. J Clin Endocrinol Metab 1978; 46:635–648.
12. Chang KL, Crabtree GS, Lim-Tan SK, Kempson RL, Hendrickson MR: Primary uterine endometrial stromal neoplasms: a clinicopathologic study of 117 cases. Am J Surg Pathol 1990; 14:415–438.
13. Artacho-Perula E, Roldan-Villalobos R, Roldan-Villalobos A-M, Vaamonde-Lemos R: Histomorphometry of normal and abnormal endometrial samples. Int J Gynecol Pathol 1993; 12:172–179.
14. Tabibzadeh SS, Mortillo S, Gerber MA: Immunoultrastructural localization of Ia antigens in human endometrium. Arch Pathol Lab Med 1987; 111:32–37.
15. Noyes RW, Haman JO: Accuracy of endometrial dating. Fertil Steril 1954; 4:504–517.
16. Roberts DK, Lavia LA, Horbelt DV, Walker NJ: Changes in nuclear and nucleolar areas of endometrial glandular cells throughout the menstrual cycle. Int J Gynecol Pathol 1989; 8:36–45.
17. Poropatich C, Rojas M, Silverberg SG: Polymorphonuclear leukocytes in the endometrium during the normal menstrual cycle. Int J Gynecol Pathol 1987; 6:230–234.
18. Stock RJ, Chao A, Slomka CV: The value of endometrial histology in suggesting the presence of ectopic gestation. J Reprod Med 1983; 28:330–334.
19. Kurman RJ, Kaminski PF, Norris HJ: The behavior of endometrial hyperplasia. A long term study of "untreated" hyperplasia in 170 patients. Cancer 1985; 56:403–412.
20. Silverberg SG, Makowski EL: Endometrial carcinoma in young women taking oral contraceptive agents. Obstet Gynecol 1975; 46:503–506.
21. Ober WB: Effects of oral and intrauterine administration of contraceptives on the uterus. Hum Pathol 1977; 8:513–527.
22. Osterholzer HO, Grillo D, Kruger PS, Dunnihoo DR: The effect of oral contraceptive steroids on branches of the uterine artery. Obstet Gynecol 1977; 49:227–232.
23. Irey NS, Norris HJ: Intimal vascular lesions associated with reproductive steroids. Arch Pathol 1973; 96:227–234.
24. Lindsay R: Estrogen, bone mass, and osteoporotic fracture. Am J Med 1991; 91:105–135.
25. Stampfer MJ, Colditz GA, Willett WC, Manson JE, Rosner B, Speizer FE, Hennekens CH: Postmenopausal estrogen therapy and cardiovascular disease: ten year follow-up from the Nurses' Health Study. N Engl J Med 1991; 325:756–762.
26. Sarrel PM: Sexuality and menopause. Obstet Gynecol 1990; 75:26S–30S.
27. Koss LG, Schreiber K, Oberlander SG, Moussouris HF, Lesser M: Detection of endometrial carcinoma and hyperplasia in asymptomatic women. Obstet Gynecol 1984; 64:1–11.
28. Garner WL, Wheelock JB, Kaminski PF: Postmenopausal bleeding: an outpatient approach. Am J Gynecol Health 1989; 3:165–168.
29. Kaminski PF, Stevens CW Jr: The value of endometrial sampling in abnormal uterine bleeding. Am J Gynecol Health 1988; 2:130–133.
30. Judd HL, Cleary RE, Creasman WT, Figge DC, Kase N, Rosenwaks Z, Tagatz GE: Estrogen replacement therapy. Obstet Gynecol 1981; 58:267–275.
31. Weinstein L: Efficacy of a continuous estrogen-progestin regimen in the menopausal patient. Obstet Gynecol 1987; 69:929–932.
32. Leather AT, Savvas M, Studd JWW: Endometrial histology and bleeding patterns after 8 years of continuous combined estrogen and progestogen therapy in postmenopausal women. Obstet Gynecol 1991; 78:1008–1010.
33. Magos AL, Brincat M, Studd JWW, Wardle P, Schlesinger P, O'Dowd T: Amenorrhea and endometrial atrophy with continuous oral estrogen and progestogen therapy in postmenopausal women. Obstet Gynecol 1985; 65:496–499.
34. Luciano AA, Turksoy RN, Carleo J, Hendrix JW: Clinical and metabolic response of menopausal women to sequential versus continuous estrogen and progestin replacement therapy. Obstet Gynecol 1987; 71:39–43.
35. Mishell DR, Shoupe D, Moyer DL, Roy S, Page MA: Postmenopausal hormone replacement with a combination estrogen-progestin regimen for five days per week. J Reprod Med 1991; 36:351–355.
36. Brooks PG, Serden SP: Preparation of endometrium for ablation with a single dose of leuprolide acetate depot. J Reprod Med 1991; 36:477–478.
37. Silverberg SG, Haukkamaa M, Arko H, Nilsson CG, Luukkainen T: Endometrial morphology during long-term use of levonorgestrel-releasing intrauterine devices. Int J Gynecol Pathol 1986; 5:235–241.
37a. Bibbo M: Comprehensive Cytopathology. Philadelphia, WB Saunders, 1991, p 126.
37b. Atkinson BF: Atlas of Diagnostic Cytopathology. Philadelphia, WB Saunders, 1992, p 126.
38. Benda JA: Clomiphene's effect on endometrium in infertility. Int J Gynecol Pathol 1992; 11:273–282.
39. Wild RA, Sanfilippo JS, Toledo AA: Endometrial biopsy in the infertility investigation. J Reprod Med 1986; 31:954–957.
40. Kaminski PF, Lyon DS: Implications of sampling the implantation site in the endometrial biopsy for infertility. J Reprod Med 1990; 38:208–210.
41. Janne O, Kauppila A, Kontula K, Syrjala P, Vihko R: Female sex steroid receptors in normal, hyperplastic and carcinomatous endometrium: the relationship to serum steroid hormones and gonadotropins and changes during medroxyprogesterone acetate administration. Int J Cancer 1979; 24:545–554.
42. Charpin C, Martin PM, Lavaut MN, Pourreau-Schneider N, Toga M: Estrogen receptor immunocytochemical assay (ER-ICA) in human endometrium. Int J Gynecol Pathol 1986; 5:119–131.
43. Podczaski E, Kaminski PF, Zaino R: CA 125 and CA 19-9 immunolocalization in normal, hyperplastic and carcinomatous endometrium. Cancer 1993; 71:2551–2556.
44. Ravn V, Teglbjaerg S, Mandel U, Dabelsteen E: The distribution of type 1 chain ABH and related histo-blood group antigens in normal cycling human endometrium. Int J Gynecol Pathol 1993; 12:70–79.
45. Osteen KG, Anderson TL, Schwartz K, Hargrove JT, Gorstein F: Distribution of tumor-associated glycoprotein-72 (TAG-72) expression throughout the normal female reproductive tract. Int J Gynecol Pathol 1992; 11:216–220.
46. Fetissof F, Dubois MP, Heitz PU, Lansac J, Arbeille-Brassart B, Jobard P: Endocrine cells in the female genital tract. Int J Gynecol Pathol 1986; 5:75–87.
47. Forsman LM, Autero M, Wahlstrom T, Gahmberg CG, Anderson LC: Hormonally regulated expression of an apocrine epithelial antigen in the cell membranes of endometrial glands. Int J Gynecol Pathol 1985; 4:355–361.
48. Arends JW, Groniowski MM, Gans HJdeK, Bosman FT: Immunohistochemical study of the distribution of secretory component and IgA in the normal and diseased uterine mucosa. J Gynecol Pathol 1983; 2:171–181.
49. Marshall RJ, Braye SG: A-1-antitrypsin, α-1-antichymotrypsin, actin and myosin in uterine sarcomas. Int J Gynecol Pathol 1985; 4:346–354.
50. Villeneuve MG, Plouffe L Jr, Pantazis CG, Smith MT, Thompson WO, McDonough PG: Immunocytochemical study of insulin-like growth factor I and insulin-like growth factor I receptor in human endometrium during the normal menstrual cycle. Int J Gynecol Pathol 1993; 12:180–185.
51. Vainright JR Jr, Fulp CJ Jr, Schiebler ML: MR imaging

of vaginal agenesis with hematocolpos. J Comput Assist Tomogr 1988: 12:891–893.
52. Frank RT: The formation of an artificial vagina without operation. Am J Obstet Gynecol 1932; 23:256–258.
53. McIndoe A: The treatment of congenital absence and obliterative conditions of the vagina. Br J Plast Surg 1950; 2:254–259.
54. Fedele L, Dorta M, Brioschi D, Giudici MN, Candiani GB: Magnetic resonance imaging in Mayer-Rokitansky-Kuster-Hauser syndrome. Obstet Gynecol 1990; 76:593–596.
55. Hunt JE, Wallach EE: Uterine factors in infertility: an overview. Clin Obstet Gynecol 1974; 17:44–64.
56. Ashton D, Amin HK, Richart RM, Neuwirth RS: The incidence of asymptomatic uterine anomalies in women undergoing transcervical tubal sterilization. Obstet Gynecol 1988; 77:28–30.
57. Siegler AM, Kemmann E, Gentile GP: Hysteroscopic procedures in 257 patients. Fertil Steril 1976; 27:1267–1273.
58. Berger MJ, Goldstein DP: Impaired reproductive performance in DES-exposed women. Obstet Gynecol 1980; 55:25–27.
59. Kaufman RH, Binder GL, Gray RM, Adam E: Upper genital tract changes associated with exposure in utero to diethylstilbestrol. Am J Obstet Gynecol 1977; 128:51–59.
60. Markoff G, Quagliarello J, Rosen RJ, Beckman EM: Uterine arteriovenous malformation successfully embolized with a liquid polymer, isobutyl 2-cyanoacrylate. Am J Obstet Gynecol 1986; 155:659–660.
61. Fleming H, Ostor AG, Pickel H, Fortune DW: Arteriovenous malformations of the uterus. Obstet Gynecol 1989; 73:209–214.
62. Poppe W, Van Assche FA, Wilms G, Favril A, Baert A: Pregnancy after transcatheter embolization of a uterine arteriovenous malformation. Am J Obstet Gynecol 1987; 156:1179–1180.
63. Winkler B, Alvarez S, Richart RM, Crum CP: Pitfalls in the diagnosis of endometrial neoplasia. Obstet Gynecol 1984; 64:185–194.
64. Hendrickson MR, Kempson RL: Endometrial epithelial metaplasias: proliferations frequently misdiagnosed as adenocarcinoma: report of 89 cases and proposed classification. Am J Surg Pathol 1980; 4:525–542.
65. Miko TL, Lampe LG, Thomazy VA, Molnar P, Endes P: Eosinophilic endomyometritis associated with diagnostic curettage. Int J Gynecol Pathol 1988; 7:162–172.
66. Young RH, Harris NL, Scully RE: Lymphoma-like lesions of the lower female genital tract: a report of 16 cases. Int J Gynecol Pathol 1985; 4:289–299.
67. Nogales-Ortiz F, Tarancon I, Nogales FF Jr: The pathology of female genital tract tuberculosis: a 31 year study of 1436 cases. Obstet Gynecol 1979; 53:422–428.
68. Willen R, Stendahl U, Willen H, Trope C: Malacoplakia of the cervix and corpus uteri: a light microscopic, electron microscopic, and x-ray microprobe analysis of a case. Int J Gynecol Pathol 1982; 2:201–208.
69. Venkataseshan VS, Woo TH: Diffuse viral papillomatosis (condyloma) of the uterine cavity. Int J Gynecol Pathol 1985; 4:370–377.
70. Lai C-H, Hsueh S, Lin C-Y, Huang M-Y, You G-B, Chang II-C, Pao CC: Human papillomavirus in benign and malignant ovarian and endometrial tissues. Int J Gynecol Pathol 1992; 11:210–215.
71. Hourihan HM, Sheppard BL, Bonnar J: The morphologic characteristics of menstrual hemostasis in patients with unexplained menorrhagia. Int J Gynecol Pathol 1989; 8:221–229.
72. Lefler HT Jr, Sullivan GH, Hulka JF: Modified endometrial ablation: electrocoagulation with vasopressin and suction curettage preparation. Obstet Gynecol 1991; 77:949–953.
73. Gimpelson RJ, Kaigh J: Mechanical preparation of the endometrium prior to endometrial ablation. J Reprod Med 1992; 37:691–694.
74. Reid PC, Thurrell W, Smith JHF, Kennedy A, Sharp F: Nd:YAG Laser endometrial ablation: histologic aspects of uterine healing. Int J Gynecol Pathol 1992; 11:174–179.
75. Townsend DE, Richart RM, Paskowitz RA, Woolfork RE: "Rollerball" coagulation of the endometrium. Obstet Gynecol 1990; 76:310-313.
76. McLucas B: Endometrial ablation with the roller ball electrode. J Reprod Med 1990; 35:1055–1058.
77. Daniell JF, Kurtz BR, Ke RW: Hysteroscopic endometrial ablation using the rollerball electrode. Obstet Gynecol 1992; 80:329–332.
78. Vancaillie TG: Electrocoagulation of the endometrium with the ball-end resectoscope. Obstet Gynecol 1989; 74:425–427.
79. Baggish MS, Daniell JF: Death caused by air-embolism associated with neodymium: yttrium-aluminum-garnet laser surgery and artificial sapphire tips. Am J Obstet Gynecol 1989; 161:877–878.
80. Gronroos M, Meurman L, Kahra K: Proliferating glia and other heterotopic tissues in the uterus: fetal homografts? Obstet Gynecol 1983; 61:261–266.
81. Martin E, Scholcs J, Richart RM, Fenoglio CM: Benign cystic teratoma of the uterus. Am J Obstet Gynecol 1979; 135:429–431.
82. Young RH, Kleinman GM, Scully RE: Glioma of the uterus: report of a case with comment on histogenesis. Am J Surg Pathol 1981; 5:695–699.
83. Van Bogaert L-J: Clinicopathologic findings in endometrial polyps. Obstet Gynecol 1988; 71:771–773.
84. Clement PB, Scully RE: Idiopathic postmenopausal decidual reaction of the endometrium. Int J Gynecol Pathol 1988; 7:152–161.
85. Lahti E, Blanco G, Kauppila A, Alaja-Sarkkinen M, Taskinen PJ, Laatikainen T: Endometrial changes in postmenopausal breast cancer patients receiving tamoxifen. Obstet Gynecol 1993; 81:660–664.
86. Choo YC, Mak KC, Hsu C, Wong TS, Ma HK: Postmenopausal uterine bleeding of nonorganic cause. Obstet Gynecol 1985; 66:225–228.
87. Powles TJ: The case for clinical trials of tamoxifen for prevention of breast cancer. Lancet 1992; 340:1145–1147.
87a. Fornander T, Cedermark B, Mattsson A, Skoog L, Theve T, Askergren J, Rutqvist LE, Glas U, Silfersward C, Someli A, Wilking N, Hjalmar M-L: Adjuvant tamoxifen in early breast cancer: occurrence of new primary cancers. Lancet 1989; 1(8630):117–120.
87b. Fisher B, Costatino JP, Redmond CK, Fisher ER, Wickerham L, Cronin WM, and other NSABP contributors: Endometrial cancer in tamoxifen-treated breast cancer patients: findings from the National Surgical Adjuvant Breast and Bowel Project (NSABP) B 14. J Natl Cancer Inst 1994; 86:527–537.
87c. Fornander T, Hellstrom A-C, Moberger B: Descriptive clinicopathologic study of 17 patients with endometrial cancer during or after adjuvant tamoxifen in early breast cancer. J Natl Cancer Inst 1993; 85:1850–1854.
87d. Magriples U, Naftolin F, Schwartz PE, Carcangiu ML: High-grade endometrial carcinoma in tamoxifen-treated breast cancer patients. J Clin Oncol 1993; 11:485–490.
88. Gal D, Kopel S, Bashevkin M, Lebowicz L, Lev R, Tancer M: Oncogenic potential of tamoxifen on endometria of postmenopausal women with breast cancer: preliminary report. Gynecol Oncol 1991; 42:120–123.
89. Nasri M, Coast G: Correlation of ultrasound findings and endometrial histopathology in postmenopausal women. Br J Obstet Gynaecol 1989; 96:1333–1338.
90. Nasri MN, Shepherd JH, Setchell ME, Lowe DG, Chard T: The role of vaginal scan in measurement of endometrial thickness in postmenopausal women. Br J Obstet Gynaecol 1991; 98:470–475.
91. Nuovo MA, Nuovo GJ, McCaffrey RM, Levine RU, Baron B, Winkler B: Endometrial polyps in postmenopausal patients receiving tamoxifen. Int J Gynecol Pathol 1989; 8:125–131.

92. Corley D, Rowe J, Curtis MT, Hogan M, Noumoff JS, Livolsi VA: Postmenopausal bleeding from unusual endometrial polyps in women on chronic tamoxifen therapy. Obstet Gynecol 1992; 79:111–116.
93. Branham WS, Zehr DR, Chen JJ, Sheehab DM: Alterations in developing rat uterine cell populations after neonatal exposure to estrogen and antiestrogens. Teratology 1988; 38:271–279.
94. Lees JA, Fawell SE, Parker MG: Identification of constitutive and steroid-dependent transactivation domains in the mouse oestrogen receptor. J Steroid Biochem 1989; 34:33–39.
95. Tawfik OW, Huet YM, Malathy PV, Johnson DC, Dey SK: Release of prostaglandins and leukotrienes from the rat uterus is an early estrogenic response. Prostaglandins 1987; 34:805–814.
96. Tawfik OW, Sagrillo C, Johnson DC, Dey SK: Decidualization in the rat. Role of leukotrienes and prostaglandins. Prostaglandins Leukot Med 1987; 29:221–227.
97. Mazur MT: Atypical polypoid adenomyoma of the endometrium. Am J Surg Pathol 1981; 5:473–482.
98. Clement PB, Young RH: Atypical polypoid adenomyoma of the uterus associated with Turner's syndrome: a report of three cases, including a review of "estrogen-associated" endometrial neoplasms and neoplasms associated with Turner's syndrome. Int J Gynecol Pathol 1987; 6:104–113.
99. Kim K-R, Scully RE: Peritoneal keratin granulomas with carcinomas of endometrium and ovary and atypical polypoid adenomyoma of endometrium: a clinicopathological analysis of 22 cases. Am J Surg Pathol 1990; 14:925–932.
100. Kaku T, Silverberg SG, Major FJ, Miller A, Fetter B, Brady MF: Adenosarcoma of the uterus: a Gynecologic Oncology Group clinicopathologic study of 31 cases. Int J Gynecol Pathol 1992; 11:75–88.
101. Dyer I, Bradburn DM: An inquiry into the etiology of placental polyps. Am J Obstet Gynecol 1971; 109:858–867.
102. Pignenborg R, Dixon G, Robertson WB, Brosens I: Trophoblast invasion of human decidua from 8–18 weeks of pregnancy. Placenta 1980; 1:3–19.
103. Ober WB, Grady HG: Subinvolution of the placental site. Bull NY Acad Med 1961; 37:713–730.
104. Lee ETC, Marley NJE, Bevan JR: A rare late complication of first trimester induced abortion requiring hysterectomy —subinvolution of the placental bed. Br J Obstet Gynaecol 1986; 93:777–781.
105. Andrew AC, Bulmer JN, Wells M, Morrison L, Buckley CH: Subinvolution of the uteroplacental arteries in the human placental bed. Histopathology 1989; 15:395–405.
106. Andrew A, Bulmer JN, Morrison L, Wells M, Buckley CH: Subinvolution of the uteroplacental arteries. An immunohistochemical study. Int J Gynecol Pathol 1993; 12:28–33.
107. Millar WG: A clinical and pathological study of placenta accreta. J Obstet Gynaecol Br Emp 1959; 66:353–364.
108. Breen JL, Neubecker R, Gregori CA, Franklin JE: Placenta accreta, increta, and percreta. Obstet Gynecol 1977; 49:43–47.
109. Naeye RL: Causes and consequences of chorioamnionitis. N Engl J Med 1975; 293:40–41.
110. Sumawoong V, Nondasuta A, Thanapath S, Budthimedhee V: Placenta accreta: a review of the literature and summary of 10 cases. Obstet Gynecol 1966; 27:511–516.
111. Read J, Cotton D, Miller F: Placenta accreta: changing clinical aspects and outcome. Obstet Gynecol 1980; 56:31–34.
112. Irving FC, Hertig AT: A study of placenta accreta. Surg Gynecol Obstet 1937; 64:178–200.
113. Meyer B: Placenta accreta: an analysis based on an unusual case. Acta Obstet Gynecol Scand 1955; 34:189–201.
114. Buttram VC, Reiter RC: Uterine leiomyomata: etiology, symptomatology and management. Fertil Steril 1981; 36:433–445.
115. AupSait SN, Dal-Cin P, Ovanessoff S, Sanberg AA: A uterine leiomyoma showing both t(12q-14) and del 7 abnormalities. Cancer Genet Cytogenet 1989; 37:157–161.
116. Nibert M, Heim S, Mandahl N, Floderus UM, Willen H, Mitelman F: Karyotypic rearrangement in 20 uterine leiomyomas. Cytogenet Cell Genet 1988; 49:300–304.
117. Hart WR, Billman JK Jr: A reassessment of uterine neoplasms originally diagnosed as leiomyosarcomas. Cancer 1978; 41:1902–1910.
118. Reiter RC, Wagner PL, Gambone JC: Routine hysterectomy for large asymptomatic uterine leiomyomata: a reappraisal. Obstet Gynecol 1992; 79:481–484.
119. Davis JL, Ray-Mazumder S, Hobel CJ, Baley K, Sassoon D: Uterine leiomyomas in pregnancy: a prospective study. Obstet Gynecol 1990; 75:41–44.
120. Muram D, Gillieson M, Walters JH: Myomas of the uterus in pregnancy: ultrasonographic follow-up. Am J Obstet Gynecol 1980; 138:16–19.
121. Norris HJ, Hilliard GD, Irey NS. Hemorrhagic cellular leiomyomas ("apoplectic leiomyoma") of the uterus associated with pregnancy and oral contraceptives. Int J Gynecol Pathol 1988; 7:212–224.
122. Konishi I, Fujii S, Ban C, Okuda Y, Okamura H, Tojo S: Ultrastructural study of minute leiomyomas. Int J Gynecol Pathol 1983; 2:113–120.
123. Crow J, Wilkens M, Howe S, More L, Helliwell P: Mast cells in the female genital tract. Int J Gynecol Pathol 1991; 10:230–237.
124. Adany R, Fodor F, Ablion RJ, Muszbek L: Increased density of histiocytes in uterine leiomyomas. Int J Gynecol Pathol 1990; 9:137–144.
125. Ferry JA, Harris NL, Scully RE: Uterine leiomyomas with lymphoid infiltration simulating lymphoma: a report of seven cases. Int J Gynecol Pathol 1989; 8:263–270.
126. Scully RG, Kempson RL, Norris HJ: Mitosis counting I–III. Hum Pathol 1976; 7:481–484.
127. Sieinski W: Lipomatous neometaplasia of the uterus: report of 11 cases with discussion of the histogenesis and pathogenesis. Int J Gynecol Pathol 1989; 8:357–363.
128. O'Connor DM, Norris HJ: Mitotically active leiomyomas of the uterus. Hum Pathol 1990; 21:223–227.
129. Tiltman AJ: The effect of progestins on the activity of uterine fibromyomas. Int J Gynecol Pathol 1985; 4:89–96.
130. Goldziehr JW, Maqueo M, Ricaus L, Aguilar JA, Canales E: Induction of degenerative changes in uterine myomas by high dose progestin therapy. Am J Obstet Gynecol 1966; 96:1078–1087.
131. Dicker RC, Greenspan JR: Complications of abdominal and vaginal hysterectomy among women of reproductive age in the United States. Am J Obstet Gynecol 1982; 144:841–848.
132. Gambone JC, Reiter RC, Lench JB, Moore JG: The impact of a quality assurance process on the frequency and confirmation rate of hysterectomy. Am J Obstet Gynecol 1990; 163:545–550.
133. Hannigan EV, Gomez KG: Uterine leiomyosarcoma: a review of prognostic clinical and pathological features. Am J Obstet Gynecol 1979; 134:557–567.
134. Istre O, Schiotz H, Vormdal J, Sadik L, Vangen O, Forman A: Transcervical resection of endometrium and fibroids: Initial complications. Acta Obstet Gynecol Scand 1992; 70:363–366.
135. Istre O, Skajaa K, Schjoensby AP, Forman A: Changes in serum electrolytes after transcervical: resection of endometrium and submucous fibroids with use of glycine 1.5% for uterine irrigation. Obstet Gynecol 1992; 80:218–222.
136. Christopherson WM, Williamson EO, Gray LA: Leiomyosarcoma of the uterus. Cancer 1971; 29:1512–1517.
137. Perrone T, Dehner LP: Prognostically favorable "mitotically active" smooth muscle tumors of the uterus. Am J Surg Pathol 1988; 12:1–8.
138. Willen R, Gad A, Willen H: Lipomatous lesions of the uterus. Virchows Arch[A] 1978; 377:351–361.
139. Evans HL, Chawla SP, Simpson C, Finn KP: Smooth muscle neoplasms of the uterus other than ordinary leio-

myoma: a study of 46 cases, with emphasis on diagnostic criteria and prognostic factors. Cancer 1988; 62:2239–2247.
140. Norris HJ, Parmley T: Mesenchymal tumors of the uterus: V. Intravenous leiomyomatosis. Cancer 1975; 36:2164–2178.
141. Clement PB, Young RH, Scully RE: Intravenous leiomyomatosis of the uterus: a clinicopathological analysis of 16 cases with unusual histologic features. Am J Surg Pathol 1988; 12:932–945.
142. Bahary CM, Gorodeski IG, Nilly M, Neri A, Avidor I, Garti I: Intravenous leiomyomatosis. Obstet Gynecol 1982; 59:73S–77S.
143. Sugiinami H, Kaura R, Ochi H, Matsuura S: Intravenous leiomyomatosis with cardiac extension: Successful surgical management and histopathologic study. Obstet Gynecol 1990; 76:527–529.
144. Tierney WM, Ehrlich CE, Bailey JC, King RD, Roth LM, Wann LS: Intravenous leiomyomatosis of the uterus with extension to the heart. Am J Med 1980; 69:471–475.
145. Vellios F, Ng ABP, Reagan JW: Papillary adenofibroma of the uterus: a benign mesodermal mixed tumor of Müllerian origin. Am J Clin Pathol 1973; 60:543–551.
146. Clement PB, Scully RE: Müllerian adenosarcoma of the uterus: a clinicopathologic analysis of 100 cases with a review of the literature. Hum Pathol 1990; 21:363–381.
147. Zaloudek CJ, Norris HJ: Adenofibroma and adenosarcoma of the uterus: a clinicopathologic study of 35 cases. Cancer 1981; 48:354–366.
148. Clement PB, Scully RE: Müllerian adenofibroma of the uterus with invasions of myometrium and pelvic veins. Int J Gynecol Pathol 1990; 9:363–371.
149. Dobashi Y, Fiedler PN, Carcangiu ML: Polypoid cystic adenomyosis of the uterus: report of a case. Int J Gynecol Pathol 1992; 11:240–243.
150. Sahin AA, Silva EG, Landon G, Ordonez NG, Gershenson DM: Endometrial tissue in myometrial vessels not associated with menstruation. Int J Gynecol Pathol 1989; 8:139–146.
151. Tamaya T, Motoyama T, Ohono Y, Ide N, Tsurusaki T, Okada H: Steroid receptor levels and histology of endometriosis and adenomyosis. Fertil Steril 1979; 31:396–400.
152. Nelson JR, Corson SL: Long term management of adenomyosis with a gonadotropin-releasing hormone agonist: a case report. Fertil Steril 1993; 59:441–443.
153. Togashi K, Nishimura K, Itah K, Fujizawa I, Noma S, Kanaoka M, Nakanoy Y, Itoh H, Ozasa H, Fujii S: Adenomyosis: diagnosis with MR imaging. Radiology 1988; 166:111–114.
154. Chang KL, Crabtree GS, Lim-Tan SK, Kempson RL, Hendrickson MR: Primary uterine endometrial stromal neoplasms: a clinicopathologic study of 117 cases. Am J Surg Pathol 1990; 14:415–438.
155. Thatcher SS, Woodruff JD: Uterine stromatosis: A report of 33 cases. Obstet Gynecol 1982; 59:428–434.
156. Tavassoli FA, Norris HJ: Mesenchymal tumors of the uterus: VII. A clinicopathologic study of 60 endometrial stromal nodules. Histopathology 1981; 5:1–10.
157. Clement PB, Scully RF: Uterine tumors resembling ovarian sex-cord tumors: clinicopathologic analysis of fourteen cases. Am J Clin Pathol 1976; 66:512–525.
158. Lloreta J, Prat J: Endometrial stromal nodule with smooth and skeletal muscle components simulating stromal sarcoma. Int J Gynecol Pathol 1992; 11:293–298.
159. Fekete PS, Vellios F, Patterson BD: Uterine tumor resembling an ovarian sex-cord tumor: report of a case of an endometrial stromal tumor with foam cells and ultrastructural evidence of epithelial differentiation. Int J Gynecol Pathol 1985; 4:378–387.
160. Bird CC, Willis RA: The production of smooth muscle by the endometrial stroma of the adult human uterus. J Pathol Bacteriol 1965; 90:75–81.
161. Tang CK, Toker C, Ances IG: Stromomyoma of the uterus. Cancer 1979; 43:308–316.
162. Goldberg MF, Hurt WG, Frable WJ: Leiomyomatosis peritonealis disseminata: report of a case and review of the literature. Obstet Gynecol 1977; 49:46S–52S.
163. Tavassoli FA, Norris HJ: Peritoneal leiomyomatosis (leiomyomatosis peritonealis disseminata): a clinicopathologic study of 20 cases with ultrastructural observations. Int J Gynecol Pathol 1982; 1:59–74.
164. Nogales FF, Matilla A, Carrascal E: Leiomyomatosis peritonealis disseminata: an ultrastructural study. Am J Clin Pathol 1978; 69:452–457.
165. Due W, Pickartz H: Immunohistologic detection of estrogen and progesterone receptors in disseminated peritoneal leiomyomatosis. Int J Gynecol Pathol 1989; 8:46–53.
166. Kuo TT, London SN, Dinh TV: Endometriosis occurring in leiomyomatosis peritonealis disseminata. Ultrastructural study and histogenetic consideration. Am J Surg Pathol 1980; 4:197–204.
167. Pieslor PC, Orenstein JM, Hogan DL, Breslow A: Ultrastructure of myofibroblasts and decidualized cells in leiomyomatosis peritonealis disseminata. Am J Clin Pathol 1979; 72:875–882.
168. Winn KJ, Woodruff JD, Parmley TH: Electron microscopic studies of leiomyomatosis peritonealis disseminata. Obstet Gynecol 1976; 48:225–227.
169. Sutherland JA, Wilson EA, Edger DE, Powell D: Ultrastructure and steroid binding studies in leiomyomatosis peritonealis disseminata. Am J Obstet Gynecol 1980; 138:992–998.
170. Tiltman AJ: Adenomatoid tumors of the uterus. Histopathology 1980; 4:437–443.
171. Young LA, Taylor HB: Adenomatoid tumors of the uterus and the fallopian tube. Am J Clin Pathol 1967; 48:537–545.
172. Livingston EG, Guis MS, Pearl ML, Stern JL, Brescia RJ: Diffuse adenomatoid tumor of the uterus with a serosal papillary cystic component. Int J Gynecol Pathol 1992; 11:288–292.
173. Palacios J, Manrique AS, Villaespesa AR, Lizaldez EB, Amat CG: Cystic adenomatoid tumor of the uterus. Int J Gynecol Pathol 1991; 10:296–310.
174. Ormond JK: Idiopathic retroperitoneal fibrosis. An established clinical entity. JAMA 1960; 174:1561–1568.
175. Buscema J, Klein V, Rotmensch J, Rosenshein N, Woodruff JD: Uterine hemangiopericytoma. Obstet Gynecol 1987; 69:104–108.
176. Fisher JH: Hemangiopericytoma: review of 20 cases. Can Med Assoc J 1960; 83:1136–1139.
177. Kurman RJ, Norris HJ: Mesenchymal tumors of the uterus: VI. Epithelioid smooth muscle tumors including leiomyoblastoma and clear-cell leiomyoma. A clinical and pathologic study of 26 cases. Cancer 1976; 37:1853–1865.
178. Kaminski PF, Tavassoli FA: Plexiform tumorlet: a clinical and pathologic study of 15 cases with ultrastructural observations. Int J Gynecol Pathol 1984; 3:124–134.
179. Borghard-Erdle AM, Hirsch EF: Glomus tumors of the uterus. Arch Pathol 1958; 65:244–246.
180. Breen JL, Neubecker RD: Tumors of the round ligament: a review of the literature and a report of 25 cases. Obstet Gynecol 1962; 19:771–780.
181. Honore LH, Manickavel V: Striated muscle heteroplasia in the uterine round ligament. Arch Pathol Lab Med 1991; 115:223–225.
182. Smith P, Heimer G, Norgrem A, Ulmsyen U: Steroid hormone receptors in pelvic muscles and ligaments in women. Gynecol Obstet Invest 1990; 30:27–30.
183. Jenkins S, Olive DL, Haney AF: Endometriosis: pathogenic implications of the anatomic distribution. Obstet Gynecol 1986; 67:335–338.
184. Clausen I, Nielson KI: Endometriosis in the groin. Int J Gynaecol Obstet 1987; 25:469–471.
185. Candiani GB, Vercellini P, Fedele L, Vendola N, Carinelli S, Scaglione V: Inguinal endometriosis: pathogenic and clinical implications. Obstet Gynecol 1991; 78:191–194.

186. Strasser EJ, Davis RM: Extraperitoneal inguinal endometriosis. J Am Surg 1977; 43:421–422.
187. Pelligrini VD Jr, Pasternak HS, Macauley WP: Endometrioma of the pubis: a differential diagnosis of hip pain: a report of two cases. J Bone Joint Surg [A]1981; 63:1333–1334.
188. Elemenoglou J, Skopelitou A, Nomikos I: Carcinoma of the inguinal region arising from endometriosis of the round ligament: report of a case. Eur J Gynaecol Oncol 1993; 14:28–32.
189. Nuovo MA, Nuovo GJ, Smith D, Lewis SH: Benign mesenchymoma of the round ligament: report of two cases with immunochemistry. Am J Clin Pathol 1990; 93:421–424.
190. Grimes DA: Diagnostic dilation and curettage: a reappraisal. Am J Obstet Gynecol 1982; 142:1–6.
191. Smith JJ, Schulman H: Current dilatation and curettage practice: a need for revision. Obstet Gynecol 1985; 65:516–518.
192. Carlson JA Jr, Arger P, Thompson S, Carlson EJ: Clinical and pathologic correlation of endometrial cavity fluid detected by ultrasound in the postmenopausal patient. Obstet Gynecol 1991; 77:119–123.
193. Stovall TG, Solomon SK, Ling FW: Endometrial sampling prior to hysterectomy. Obstet Gynecol 1989; 73:405–409.
194. Stovall TG, Photopulos GJ, Poston WM, Ling FW, Sandles G: Pipelle endometrial sampling in patients with known endometrial carcinoma. Obstet Gynecol 1991; 77:954–956.
195. Silver MM, Miles P, Rosa C: Comparison of Novak and Pipelle endometrial biopsy instruments. Obstet Gynecol 1991; 78:828–830.
196. Kaunitz AM, Maciello A, Ostrowski M, Rovira EZ: Comparison of endometrial biopsy with the endometrial Pipelle and Vabra aspirator. J Reprod Med 1988; 33:427–431.
197. Loin B-L, Iwata Y, Liu KH, Valle RF: The Fujinon diagnostic fiber optic hysteroscope: experience with 1,503 patients. J Reprod Med 1990; 35:685–689.

6

Premalignant and Malignant Conditions of the Uterus

Paul F. Kaminski / Edward S. Podczaski

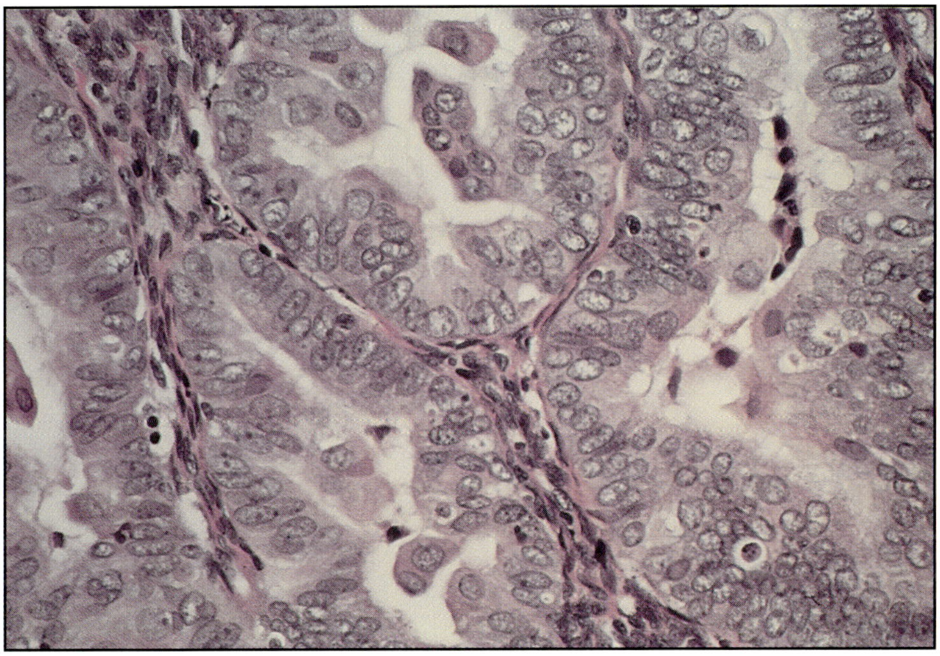

ENDOMETRIAL HYPERPLASIA

Endometrial hyperplasia is a histopathologic entity that has been a source of confusion. In reviewing the literature on this topic, it is important to realize that similar terms have different meanings for different authors. The multitude of nomenclature systems used to describe this entity is responsible for some of the confusion. The clinician faces a seemingly endless number of variations in terminology that almost precludes a rational approach to management. Although some authors use similar diagnostic terms, those terms may have significantly different meanings in different classification systems. Furthermore, not only do authors differ in their use of terminology, they also differ in their definition of hyperplasia, the criteria for which may range from a simple increase in the amount or volume of endometrial tissue to a complex histologic definition that attempts to correlate the glandular architecture to biologic potential.[1–6] In 1987 the International Society of Gynecologic Pathologists adopted a terminology for endometrial hyperplasia based on its architectural and cytologic characteristics. This classification was derived from a follow-up study of patients with untreated endometrial hyperplasia.[7] Table 6–1 presents a historical summary of the terms used to describe endometrial hyperplasia and includes the recommended terminology of the International Society of Gynecologic Pathologists. The latter is the classification preferred by us and is used in this textbook.

Studies that involve nuclear deoxyribonucleic acid (DNA) content,[8] cell biology, immunocytochemistry,[9] morphometric measurements,[10–12] and

TABLE 6–1.
The Terminology of Endometrial Hyperplasia

International Society of Gynecologic Pathologists	Simple	Complex	Atypical	
Vellios, Campbell, and Barter	Cystic Benign	Adenomatous Atypical type I	Atypical Atypical type II	CIS Atypical type III
Hertig and Sommers	Cystic	Adenomatous	Anaplasia	CIS
Gusberg	Cystic	Adenomatous G I	Adenomatous G II	Adenomatous G III
Beutler and Dockerty	Cystic	Glandular	Glandular atypia	

ultrastructure[13] imply that although hyperplasia may have a morphologic spectrum, it does not have a corresponding biologic spectrum. Prediction of the malignant potential and clinical behavior of hyperplasia is based on the presence or absence of cytologic atypia (Table 6–2).

Teleologically, the progression from proliferative endometrium through hyperplasia to adenocarcinoma is a continuum. Differentiation between the various subsets is arbitrary. Recently, the focus of attention has centered on the differentiation of hyperplasia from well-differentiated adenocarcinoma. In cases in which the hyperplasia is more complex, particularly if cytologic atypia is also present, progression to endometrial cancer is more likely.[7] Likewise, as hyperplasia becomes more complex and cytologically atypical, clinicians become more aggressive in their treatment. A histopathologic diagnosis of some degree of hyperplasia should open the channels of communication between pathologist and clinician.[14] The intent of the pathologist should be to communicate to the clinician his or her impression of the biologic potential of the particular endometrial proliferation. This will result in therapeutic interventions based on the pathologist's best judgment.

Epidemiology

Hyperplasia develops in a setting of unopposed estrogen. Estrogen stimulates the growth and proliferation of endometrial glands and stroma. Without endogenous (i.e., ovulation) or exogenous progesterone, continued estrogen stimulation results in hyperplasia. Hyperplasia is a histologic progression that starts with normal proliferative endometrium, continues to benign proliferations and atypical hyperplasia, and ultimately progresses to well-differentiated adenocarcinoma.[15] This progression can occur with endogenous estrogen production, e.g., polycystic ovaries or estrogen-producing tumors.[15, 16] It can also occur with exogenous unopposed estrogen ingestion.

TABLE 6–2.
Follow-up of Patients with Hyperplasia

Degree of Hyperplasia	*Number of Patients*	*Regressed*	*Persisted*	*Progressed to Carcinoma*
Simple	92	74 (80%)	17 (19%)	1 (1%)
Complex	29	23 (80%)	5 (17%)	1 (3%)
Simple atypical	13	9 (69%)	3 (23%)	1 (8%)
Complex atypical	35	20 (57%)	5 (14%)	10 (29%)

From Kurman RJ, Kaminski PF, Norris HJ: The behavior of endometrial hyperplasia. A long-term study of "untreated" hyperplasia in 170 patients. Cancer 1985; 56: 403–412.

Any condition associated with chronic anovulation and continuous unopposed estrogen will eventually produce endometrial hyperplasia. Potentially reversible hyperplasia is relatively common in the early perimenarchal and in perimenopausal menstrual cycles. Early menarche, because of the immaturity of the hypothalamic-pituitary-ovarian axis and the anovulation that results, is a risk factor for hyperplasia. With maturation of the hypothalamic-pituitary-ovarian axis, regular ovulation maintains a cycling endometrium, and hyperplasia does not develop. As a woman approaches menopause, anovulatory cycles again become more common, and hyperplasia may occur because of the endogenous unopposed estrogen. At menopause, plasma levels of estradiol fall, and plasma levels of estrone may remain elevated.[17] The main source of estrone is the peripheral conversion of adrenal and ovarian androstenedione to estrone. In a slender woman this amounts to 40 μg per day. Obesity magnifies this process. Thus, obesity, particularly morbid obesity of more than 50 percent over ideal body weight, is a risk factor for the development of endometrial hyperplasia. Estrone production in these women may exceed 200 μg per day.[17]

Signs and Symptoms

The presenting complaint of a woman of reproductive age with endometrial hyperplasia is menorrhagia, metrorrhagia, prolonged menses, or a combination of these. Postmenopausal vaginal bleeding is the cardinal symptom in postmenopausal women. The general physical examination may show signs of androgen excess such as increased facial hair, chest hair, and a male type of escutcheon. This is typical of the patient with polycystic ovaries. Acne may also be present. The pelvic examination is normal except for the presence of blood. In the postmenopausal woman the expected clinical signs of vaginal atrophy may be absent.

Diagnosis depends on the histologic examination of an endometrial biopsy or curettage specimen. This is mandatory to exclude endometrial adenocarcinoma. The clinical differential diagnosis includes, besides endometrial adenocarcinoma, endometrial polyps, submucous leiomyoma, chronic endometritis, and, uncommonly, complications of pregnancy. There are no distinguishing features of endometrial hyperplasia that can be identified on gross examination. There may be a subjective impression of an increased amount of tissue removed

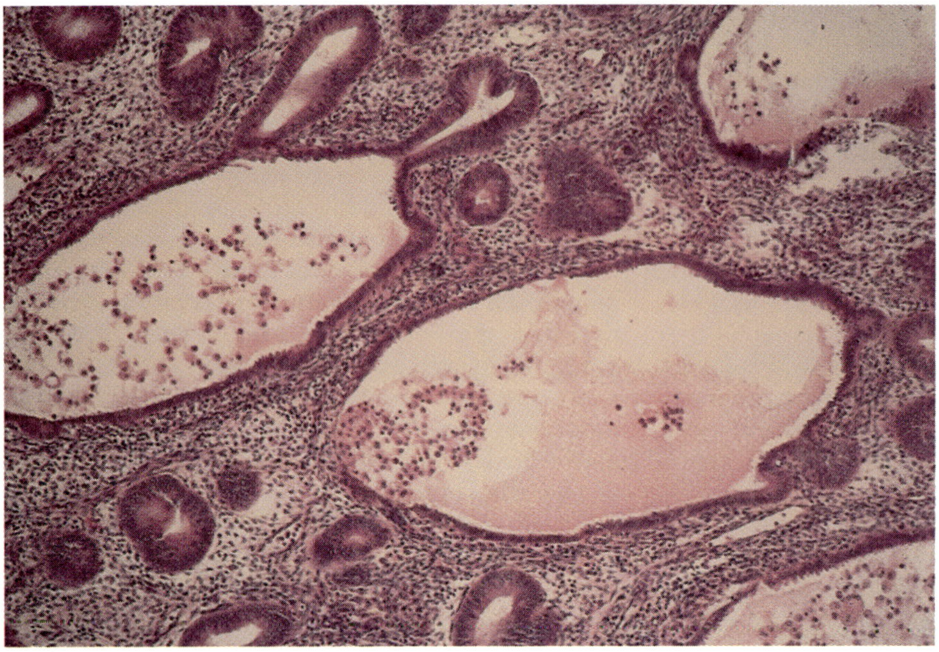

FIGURE 6-1
Cystically dilated glands lined by attenuated epithelium are seen in this case of simple hyperplasia. There is an increase in the number of glands with the gland to stroma ratio favoring the glands. This should not be confused with cystic atrophy (see Chapter 5), in which the glands are dilated but the gland to stroma ratio still favors the stroma.

at the time of endometrial biopsy or curettage. The thickness of the endometrial stripe on transvaginal ultrasound examination may suggest the presence of an endometrial proliferative condition,[18] but this is not a very specific finding.

In the evaluation of abnormal uterine bleeding, some degree of hyperplasia is present in 1 to 2 percent of endometrial tissue samples obtained from women under the age of 40 years. Hyperplasia is present in 8 percent of endometrial samples obtained from premenopausal women older than 40 years.[19] Likewise, endometrial sampling in postmenopausal women identifies hyperplasia in 8 to 9 percent.[20]

Definitions

In 1987 the International Society of Gynecologic Pathologists formulated a nomenclature for endometrial hyperplasia based on the presence of architectural and cytologic atypia.[7] According to this nomenclature, hyperplasia can be simple or complex and may or may not demonstrate cytologic atypia. The definitions presented here are adapted with permission from Kurman and associates.* *Simple hyperplasia* represents a benign proliferation of endometrial glands. The gland to stroma ratio favors the glands. The glands may appear dilated and show little crowding (Fig. 6–1), or they may have an irregular outline and exhibit crowding (to be described subsequently). Cytologic atypia is absent. *Complex hyperplasia* represents an endometrial proliferation in which glands with irregular outlines demonstrate marked structural complexity with unfolding of the glandular epithelium into its lumen and back-to-back crowding. However, normal endometrial stroma between the glands is identified. Cytologic atypia is also absent.

Atypical hyperplasia designates a proliferation of glands exhibiting cytologic atypia. The degree of atypia is variable. Loss of cellular polarity may be present. When atypia is not present, the cells are tall columnar cells and the nuclei are elongated. *Mild cytologic atypia* refers to the presence of enlarged and round nuclei. The chromatin is fine and evenly dispersed. *Moderate cytologic atypia* refers to an additional increase in nuclear size with greater pleomorphism and prominent nucleoli. The chromatin appears irregularly dispersed and clumped.

Simple atypical hyperplasia represents a proliferation of glands demonstrating cytologic atypia without architectural complexity. If architectural complexity is present, it falls short of back-to-back glandular crowding. *Complex atypical hyperplasia* represents an architecturally complex proliferation of endometrial glands demonstrating back-to-back crowding with cytologic atypia as defined earlier. However, endometrial stroma is still present between the glands.

Microscopic Findings

Microscopic findings in hyperplasia represent a continuum that begins histologically just beyond

* Kurman RJ, Kaminski PF, Norris HJ: The behavior of endometrial hyperplasia. A long-term study of "untreated" hyperplasia in 170 patients. Cancer 1985;56:403–412.

normal proliferative endometrium and ends just short of well-differentiated endometrial adenocarcinoma. As a continuum, the diagnostic term applied to any particular histopathologic specimen is arbitrary. It is mandatory for the clinician and the pathologist to have the same understanding of the terms used.[14] According to the terminology just listed, simple hyperplasia includes focal or diffuse architectural glandular irregularity (Fig. 6–2). The gland to stroma ratio favors the glands. The glandular epithelium appears pseudostratified or stratified. Mitotic activity is variable and frequently does not exceed that seen in normal proliferative endometrium.[7] As hyperplasia becomes more complex, glandular crowding and irregularity with epithelial protrusions, budding, and infolding become apparent (Fig. 6–3). The crowding at some point assumes a back-to-back appearance. The gland to stroma ratio increases further, but endometrial stroma remains between the endometrial glands. The glandular epithelium continues to be pseudostratified or stratified to two or three cell layers.[7] Mitotic activity remains variable but is readily identifiable in both the glands and the stroma. Further progression of hyperplasia involves cytologic atypia. This begins as rounding of the nuclei and nuclear enlargement. The chromatin is initially fine and evenly dispersed. Greater variability in nuclear size is seen as cytologic atypia increases (Fig. 6–4). Dispersed clumped chromatin becomes apparent, and the nucleoli become prominent.

Stratification of glandular epithelial cells may be present with any degree of hyperplasia. The degree of stratification is generally increased in the more complex proliferations. Mitotic activity is variable and may not be a prominent feature. Mitotic activity is not used to differentiate proliferative endometrium from hyperplastic endometrium or adenocarcinoma because it is present in all. Ciliated cells are commonly present in the milder degrees of hyperplasia but tend to decrease in number or disappear completely as the degree of hyperplasia becomes more complex. Squamous changes may be present with any degree of hyperplasia (Fig. 6–5). Squamous foci typically lack keratinization. Small glands that seem to extend as buds from the periphery typically surround the squamous foci.[21] Areas of central necrosis may be present in some of the squamous nests. Endometrial stromal foam cells are occasionally associated with hyperplasia.

At the benign end of the histologic spectrum of endometrial proliferations the term *disordered proliferation* designates those proliferations that exceed the histologic changes of normal proliferative endometrium but fall short of the definition of simple hyperplasia. At the complex end of the histologic spectrum, the lack of endometrial stromal invasion differentiates endometrial hyperplasia (Fig. 6–6) from well-differentiated endometrial adenocarcinoma.

Although the diagnosis of well-differentiated endometrial adenocarcinoma can be readily made in

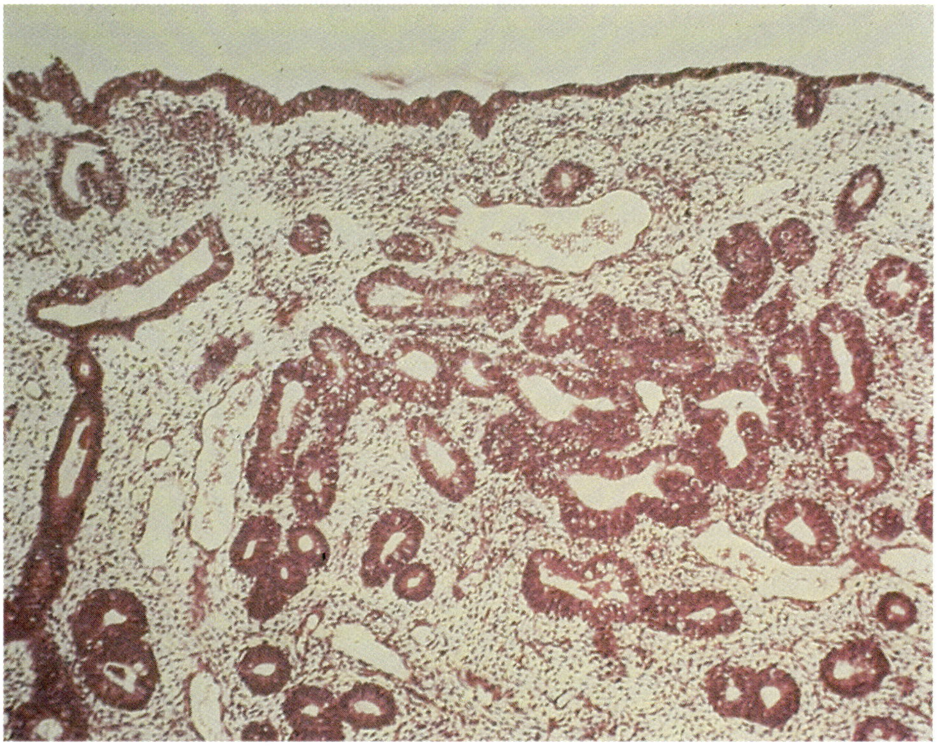

FIGURE 6–2
This area of focal glandular crowding represents simple hyperplasia (adenomatous hyperplasia) in an otherwise normal endometrium.

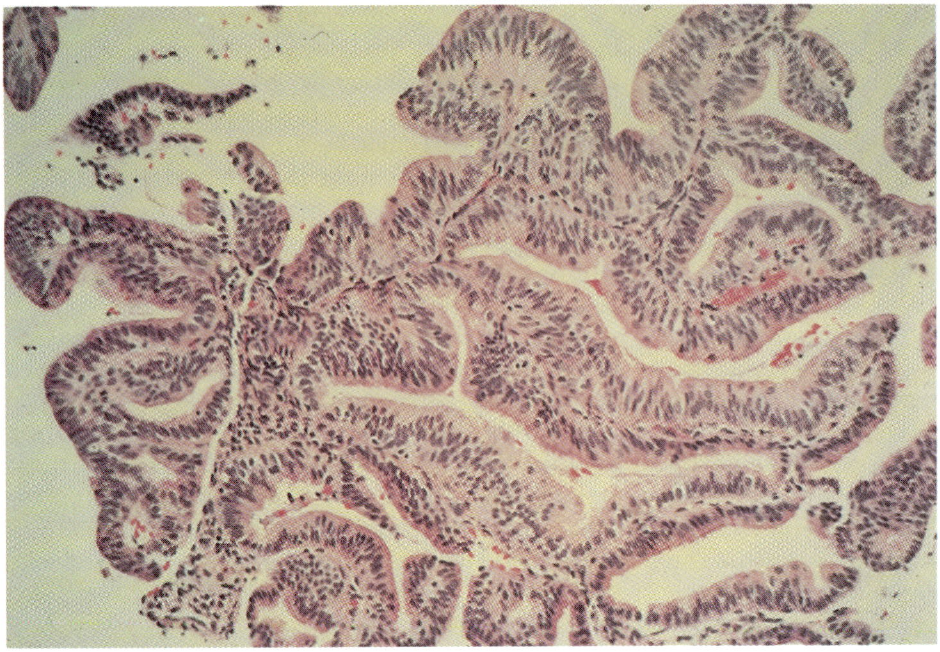

FIGURE 6–3
A complex papillary pattern (with some intervening stroma), which approaches back-to-back glandular crowding, is seen in this case of complex hyperplasia. Minimal cytologic atypia is present.

a hysterectomy specimen when myometrial invasion is present, such a diagnosis may prove elusive when one is evaluating endometrial curettings. The presence of endometrial stromal invasion is used to differentiate complex atypical hyperplasia from well-differentiated adenocarcinoma. Endometrial stromal invasion is the term used to describe the epithelial and stromal alterations seen in the endometrial curettings of patients who have adenocarcinoma. When any one of the following histologic criteria is present, a diagnosis of adenocarcinoma is rendered.[22]

DESMOPLASTIC RESPONSE. The interaction of the invasive endometrial glands and their stroma produces a fibrotic stromal response, also known as a desmoplastic reaction. The desmoplastic stroma appears denser than normal stroma because it has been infiltrated by fibroblasts and the collagen they deposit. Although the stromal cells of proliferative or hyperplastic endometrium have basophilic nuclei and ill-defined cell borders (Fig. 6–4), the cells of the desmoplastic stroma have elongated nuclei, and the surrounding collagen gives the cells an eosinophilic wavy appearance. The

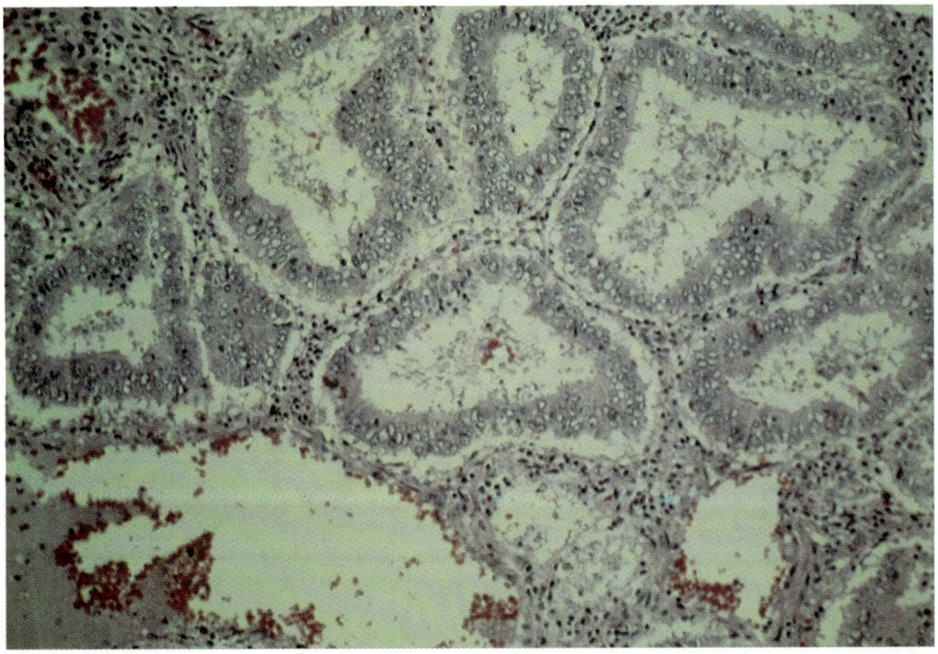

FIGURE 6–4
This complex atypical hyperplasia has back-to-back glandular crowding with little intervening stroma. Significant cytologic atypia with rounded vesicular nuclei is present. The presence of intervening stroma and the lack of desmoplastic response differentiate this from adenocarcinoma.

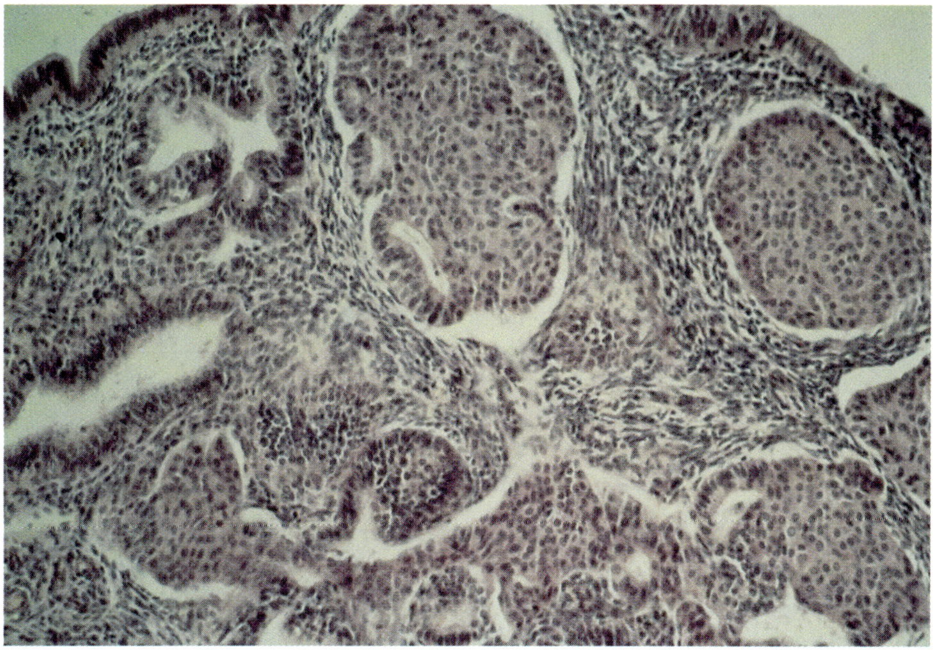

FIGURE 6-5
Simple atypical hyperplasia with squamous differentiation as morules is seen. Mild nuclear atypia is present. The glands fall short of back-to-back crowding.

presence of complex atypical endometrial glands in a desmoplastic stroma is, therefore, diagnostic of adenocarcinoma.

COMPLEX PATTERN. A complex glandular pattern without intervening stroma that occupies at least half (2.1 mm) of a low-power microscope field is considered diagnostic of adenocarcinoma. These glands seem to interconnect and in some cases grow in a cribriform arrangement (see Fig. 6–6).

PAPILLARY PATTERN. An extensive papillary pattern without endometrial stroma that occupies at least half of a low-power microscope field is also diagnostic of adenocarcinoma.

SQUAMOUS PATTERN. A complex squamous pattern that replaces the stroma, which is usually desmoplastic, is considered indicative of invasive carcinoma of the endometrium if it occupies more than half of a low-power microscope field (2.1 mm).

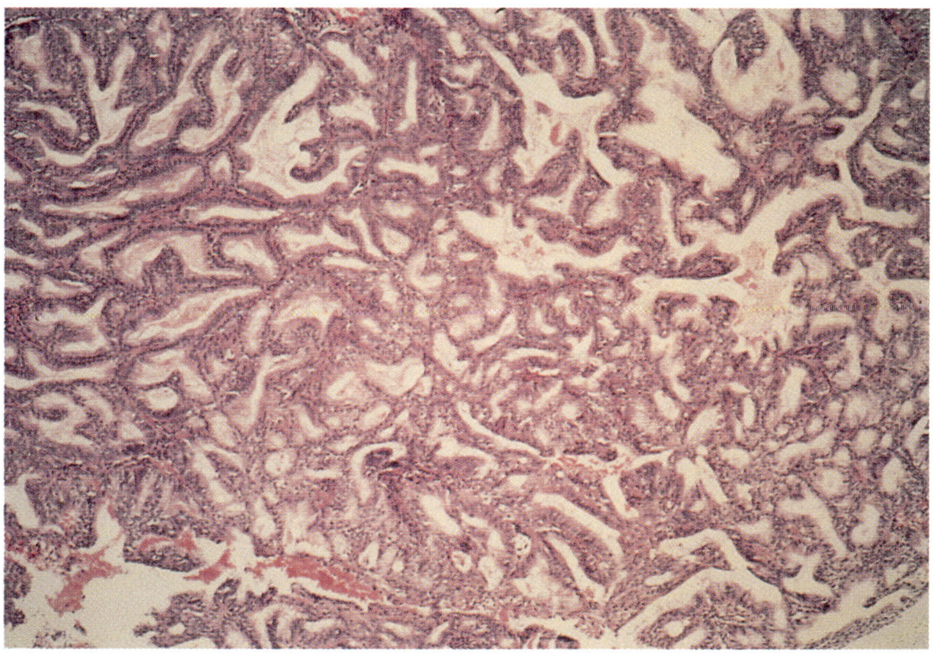

FIGURE 6-6
Well-differentiated endometrial adenocarcinoma demonstrates little to no intervening stroma in this complex glandular pattern. The glands seem to interconnect.

Biologic Behavior

Recognition of the biologic potential of any endometrial proliferation will influence treatment decisions. Cytologic atypia is the most useful single criterion for predicting the likelihood of progression to endometrial adenocarcinoma. The biologic behavior of complex hyperplasia without atypia is similar to that of simple hyperplasia (see Table 6–2). In addition, with increasing cytologic atypia there is an increased risk of progression to carcinoma. The presence of concomitant architectural complexity identifies a particularly high risk group.[7] In this high-risk group, progression to well-differentiated adenocarcinoma occurs in 25 percent of women despite medical therapy with progestogens.[23] Because the progression to well-differentiated adenocarcinoma is sometimes difficult to assess accurately by light microscopy, some investigators have used other methods to better identify those lesions with premalignant potential. Nuclear morphometry is one useful technique in delineating the biologic potential of questionable cases of atypical hyperplasia. However, the use of morphometry is not available to all pathologists. In specific instances in which preservation of reproductive function is important and the biologic potential of the endometrial proliferation is questionable by light microscopy, the additional time and expense required for nuclear morphometry may prove useful.[10] The nuclei in cases that progress to carcinoma are larger and more pleomorphic than those that do not.[10] The mean and standard deviation of the maximal nuclear diameter as measured by morphometry can accurately predict progression in over 80 percent of cases.[11]

The tumor markers CA 125 and CA 19-9 are both demonstrable focally in paraffin-fixed samples taken from endometrial hyperplastic tissue. CA 19-9, however, was absent in a limited series of patients with simple hyperplasia but was present in two-thirds of women with complex or atypical hyperplasia.[9] At present, immunocytochemistry has not proved useful in differentiating hyperplasia from normal endometrium or from well-differentiated adenocarcinoma.

Clinical Management

Any decision to intervene medically or surgically should include an evaluation of the risks versus benefits. Hyperplasia that is not treated results in continued abnormal uterine bleeding. In some women, progression to well-differentiated adenocarcinoma occurs (see Table 6–2). Factors influencing the decision regarding therapeutic intervention in women with endometrial hyperplasia include the patient's age, amount and duration of bleeding, associated anemia, desire for future childbearing, presence or absence of cytologic atypia, and the degree of cytologic atypia. The most important of these factors is cytologic atypia. Among women with cytologically atypical endometrial hyperplasia in a curettage specimen who underwent hysterectomy within 1 month, 17 percent were found to have an adenocarcinoma in the uterus that had not been detected in the curettage specimen.[22] These, however, were well-differentiated neoplasms and did not demonstrate more than 4 mm of myometrial invasion.[22] In patients with endometrial proliferations demonstrating cytologic atypia in whom follow-up consisted of observation or treatment with medroxyprogesterone acetate, progression to adenocarcinoma occurred in 25 to 40 percent.[7, 23]

The therapy for endometrial hyperplasia can be medical or surgical. Medical therapy may include the following: progestins, oral contraceptives, ovulation induction with clomiphene citrate, gonadotropin-releasing hormone analogs, and danazol. Surgical therapy includes curettage, hysteroscopy, endometrial ablation, and hysterectomy.

Hyperplasia can occur at any age from the teens[24] to the postmenopausal years.[20] Counseling of women with hyperplasia is important. Counseling should address the factors that apply to the individual patient. Dietary counseling and weight loss are appropriate in obese patients. Patients whose disease progresses to cancer tend to be obese, weighing more than 90 kilograms.[23] Some women who develop adenocarcinoma are also diabetic and hypertensive. Screening of selected women for diabetes mellitus is appropriate. This approach identifies previously undetected cases of diabetes.[17] In the younger woman who desires pregnancy, ovulation induction and pregnancy will treat the hyperplasia.[7] The simplest method of stimulating a surge of luteinizing hormone (LH) and ovulation is preferable. Clomiphene citrate is satisfactory in most cases. If pregnancy is not an immediate issue, treatment with oral contraceptives will suppress the endometrium and control the effects of androgen excess that are present in some patients. Progestin therapy, in the form of medroxyprogesterone acetate or megestrol acetate, may be appropriate for some women.[23] Oral therapy with medroxyprogesterone acetate suppresses 80 percent of the milder degrees of hyperplasia. In patients with more advanced degrees of hyperplasia associated with cytologic atypia, regression occurs in only 25 percent of women treated with medroxyprogesterone acetate.[23] If menorrhagia and anemia are present, suppression of menses with large doses of intramuscular progestin (i.e., depomedroxyprogesterone acetate) is appropriate. Women who develop hyperplasia while using unopposed estrogen should discontinue it.[7] Exclusion of the presence of an estrogen-secreting ovarian neoplasm may be necessary in some patients. In obese women or women with concomitant leiomyomas, ultrasound may be necessary to evaluate the adnexa adequately. Gonadotropin-releasing hormone analogs and danazol may be appropriate choices for selected patients. Both produce a menopausal-like state, which is reversible on discontinuation of the medication. However, the expense of these drugs, the side effects, and the paucity of data documenting their long-term effectiveness in treating hyperplasia argue against their routine use for this indication.

Many patients require surgical management in conjunction with medical management. Curettage may be necessary to control acute bleeding. In addition, in women with more complex and atypical lesions who wish to preserve childbearing potential, curettage as well as hysteroscopy may be necessary to exclude adenocarcinoma. In women who have completed childbearing, hysterectomy is the definitive treatment.[7, 23] Retention of the ovaries may be appropriate if endometrial adenocarcinoma and intrinsic ovarian pathology have been excluded. The role of endometrial ablation in treating hyperplasia is at present uncertain. This new technique is useful in controlling menorrhagia.[25] Appropriate follow-up of women treated with endometrial ablation for atypical endometrial hyperplasia is unknown. Failure to destroy all the endometrial tissue in most patients leaves room for doubt about this form of therapy.[25]

Other associated factors may influence treatment decisions. The presence of diabetes may complicate surgery and wound healing. The medical therapy of hyperplasia carries the risk of possible adverse drug reactions and side effects. Intramuscular progestin therapy can cause breast soreness, weight gain, fluid retention, bloating, nervousness, irritability, and other bothersome side effects. These side effects appear to be dose related. Oral therapy with progestogens causes a lower incidence of the same problems. Oral contraceptive agents can produce estrogen-related side effects in addition to the progestin side effects. Gonadotropin-releasing hormone analogs and danazol cause menopausal symptoms. Thus, hot flashes and vaginal dryness may be an immediate problem, and changes in serum lipid profile, effects on the coronary arteries, and bone loss are potential long-term effects. Danazol and, to a lesser extent, the gonadotropin-releasing analogs can cause an increase in androgenic side effects such as hirsutism, acne, and weight gain.

Follow-Up

Careful follow-up of patients with endometrial hyperplasia is important. Repeat endometrial sampling is necessary to follow the histologic changes.[7, 23] In the milder degrees of hyperplasia, endometrial sampling at 6-month intervals is appropriate, whereas in the more severe forms of hyperplasia (i.e., complex atypical hyperplasia) endometrial sampling at 3-month intervals has been recommended.[7] Follow-up is necessary until the hyperplasia regresses. After the hyperplasia regresses the patient may have to be maintained on cyclic progestogens (i.e., 14 days out of each month) or on oral contraceptives, depending on her age. Persistence of hyperplasia without cytologic atypia is worrisome but may continue to be followed in the young woman. Proliferations that progress to a more advanced degree of hyperplasia, particularly those with associated cytologic atypia, or that progress to adenocarcinoma are indications for definitive treatment.

ENDOMETRIAL CARCINOMA

Epidemiology

Endometrial adenocarcinoma is the most common female genital tract malignancy in the United States. Morphologically, it represents a heterogeneous group of neoplasms. Although the great majority are typical endometrioid endometrial adenocarcinomas, other epithelial neoplasms that arise more frequently at other sites of the so-called extended müllerian system are also seen.[26] Treatment of patients with this neoplasm in a community hospital is more likely than with any other gynecologic malignancy.[27] Thus, it is important for the practicing pathologist to be familiar with the features of this disease that are of therapeutic and prognostic significance. In 1993, approximately 31,000 new cases of endometrial cancer were diagnosed in the United States, and it accounted for 5700 deaths.[28] The estimated prevalence in asymptomatic postmenopausal women is 7 per 100,000.[29] Survival rates remain relatively constant at approximately 75 percent 5-year survival for patients with tumors clinically confined to the uterus at the time of diagnosis. The incidence of this disease is reportedly higher in Western nations. There appears to be an association between dietary fat intake and the development of endometrial carcinoma.[30] There is a significant reduction in endometrial cancer risk among cigarette smokers.[31] Endometrial atrophy, even in women taking estrogen replacement therapy, is frequently seen in smokers. However, the risk of developing endometrial cancer in women who are thin and smoke is increased by the use of exogenous estrogen.[32, 33] Other factors associated with endometrial carcinoma include obesity, nulliparity, early menarche, and late menopause. Of these, obesity of more than 50 pounds over ideal body weight may pose the greatest risk.[34, 35] Women who are 21 to 50 pounds overweight carry three times the normal risk of developing uterine corpus cancer; this risk increases to ten times in women more than 50 pounds overweight.[34, 35] In women under the age of 40 years who developed endometrial carcinoma, 81 percent were obese.[36] Sixty-three percent weighed more than 90 kilograms.[36] This increased risk of endometrial carcinoma may be due to increased circulating estrogen levels caused by aromatization of androstenedione to estrone that occurs in the fibroblasts in peripheral fat.[37] The association with diabetes mellitus and an abnormal glucose tolerance test is less clear. Overt diabetes occurs in 2 to 40 percent of women.[27] Abnormal glucose tolerance tests occur in 10 to 65 percent of women in whom endometrial carcinoma is diagnosed. However, a retrospective study in a large number of diabetic women showed fewer cases of endometrial carcinoma than expected.[38] Diabetes and hypertension appear to be more related to the exogenous obesity and are probably not directly associated with endometrial carcinoma.

Familial occurrence of endometrial cancer also exists. Lynch syndrome type II is a hereditary predisposition to colon, breast, ovarian, and endometrial cancer.[39] In addition, a history of prior pelvic radiation is present in 5 to 7 percent of women who subsequently develop endometrial carcinoma. The carcinoma develops 10 or more years after pelvic irradiation treatment. However, this risk does not differ statistically from that in the general population.[40]

The role of unopposed estrogen stimulation of the endometrium in the development of endometrial carcinoma deserves discussion in detail. In the United States there is epidemiologic evidence linking the prevalence of endometrial cancer with the number of prescriptions for estrogen replacement therapy.[41] Unopposed estrogen appears to be an important risk factor for the development of endometrial hyperplasia. Exposure to estrogen may be either exogenous or endogenous. There are four groups of women who appear to be at risk of developing endometrial carcinoma from endogenous estrogen sources. The first is a small group of women who have granulosa cell tumors, theca cell tumors, or other estrogen-secreting ovarian tumors. The estimated risk of these women developing endometrial carcinoma ranges from 3.5 to 27 percent.[42, 43] The second and largest group comprises women with chronic anovulation. Chronic anovulation has been identified in 19 to 25 percent of women under the age of 40 years who developed endometrial carcinoma.[44–47] These women have consistently elevated estrone levels, largely derived from peripheral conversion of androgens to estrogens. The third group is a group of obese postmenopausal women. Women who are extremely obese may convert as much as 12 percent of androstenedione to estrone.[41] The fourth group of women includes those with severe liver disease. The cause in these women is presumably the inability to metabolize androstenedione in the liver. Excessive circulating androstenedione leads to excessive peripheral conversion to estrone and thus chronic unopposed estrogen stimulation of the endometrium.[41]

Exogenous estrogen therapy is used for one of three reasons. Women who have gonadal dysgenesis receive unopposed estrogen therapy or, in a few instances, estrogen and progestogen therapy beginning at puberty. Case reports have documented the development of endometrial adenocarcinoma in these women.[48–57] The second situation is that of a group of women who in the 1970s used sequential oral contraceptives containing 100 μg of ethinyl estradiol. There were only 5 days per cycle when 25 mg of a weak progestogen was given. This proved to be insufficient progestogen to prevent progression to carcinoma in some of these women.[58–61] All carcinomas that occurred in women using sequential oral contraceptive pills occurred in those who were under the age of 40 years.[59] As a group, these patients tended not to be obese, and none were diabetic. Most of these cancers developed in women with a background of endometrial hyperplasia. The cell type was generally endometrioid. Deep myometrial invasion and spread beyond the uterus have been uncommon in this clinical setting.[58–61] The prognosis of these patients is excellent. The third situation is that of postmenopausal women who received estrogen replacement therapy unopposed by a progestogen. There is a historical association between the use of estrogen replacement therapy and the development of endometrial carcinoma. This method of therapy was common in the 1960s and 1970s until the association of endometrial carcinoma with unopposed estrogen therapy became apparent and the protective effect of progestogens was documented.[62] However, hospital-based studies reporting this association may suffer from selection bias.[63–72] This bias arises from the pattern of hospital referral. It is suggested that women who have endometrial carcinoma who take estrogens are more likely to bleed than nonestrogen users. Vaginal bleeding should prompt a referral for diagnostic testing. The final result is an increase in the number of hospital patients with endometrial carcinoma who have been exposed to estrogen and, therefore, a higher odds ratio.[72] Using a control group of women (i.e., those without endometrial carcinoma) who are also being evaluated for uterine bleeding may compensate for the possible bias introduced in the case group, since some of the control group may have bleeding secondary to exogenous estrogen.[72, 73] When such a control group is used, the odds ratio is no different than 1.[72] The conclusion is that there is no increased risk of developing endometrial adenocarcinoma among estrogen users.

In a case-control study involving postmenopausal women who have newly diagnosed endometrial carcinoma it was found that both the pattern of estrogen use and patient characteristics affected risk.[74] The use of progestogens in association with estrogen reduced the risk of developing endometrial carcinoma. The group with the highest risk were the current estrogen users, but the increased risk persisted even in women who had discontinued estrogen use for more than 5 years. Thirty-one percent of women with endometrial carcinoma reported using conjugated equine estrogens, whereas only 15 percent of controls used conjugated equine estrogens. The relative risk of developing endometrial adenocarcinoma associated with estrogen use in this study was 3.5. If use lasted at least 1 year, the relative risk estimate for early stage endometrial carcinoma, stage I or II, was 5.2, and for late stage endometrial carcinoma, stage III and IV, it was 3.1. Among women who had used estrogen for at least 1 year and then discontinued it, the risk of endometrial carcinoma remained significantly elevated even after an estrogen-free interval of more than 10 years. Prior use of oral contraceptive agents protects against endometrial cancer.[75] The use of combined estrogen and progestogen replacement therapy has a favorable effect on endometrial histology.

The studies just presented support the following statement: Estrogen stimulation unopposed by progesterone, if at a low level, must be present over a long period of time to produce endometrial carcinoma; estrogen stimulation at a high level may produce endometrial carcinoma even with a short exposure time.[41]

Unopposed estrogen stimulation of the endometrium explains only some cases of endometrial carcinoma. Epidemiologic and clinicopathologic evidence supports the hypothesis that there are two distinct forms of endometrial cancer. There is the type of endometrial cancer that occurs in a milieu of unopposed estrogen excess on a background of endometrial hyperplasia. This form occurs in younger women, and the neoplasms are usually of low histopathologic grade. The prognosis for patients with this type of endometrial carcinoma is excellent. The second type of endometrial carcinoma occurs predominantly in older women and appears to arise de novo.[76] The histopathologic grade tends to be high. Histopathologic types associated with aggressive behavior (e.g., clear cell, papillary serous) are common. Myometrial invasion is frequently deep. The prognosis for patients with this type of endometrial cancer is poorer. This type of endometrial cancer has little relationship to estrogen use and does not develop on a background of endometrial hyperplasia.

Signs and Symptoms

The almost universal presenting symptom of endometrial cancer is abnormal uterine bleeding. Any patient with abnormal uterine bleeding who is in the perimenopausal years or who has postmenopausal bleeding should be presumed to have endometrial cancer until proved otherwise. Evaluation should begin with a pelvic examination and a Papanicolaou smear that includes sampling of the endocervix. A biopsy should be performed of any obvious lesion in the cervix or vagina. Endometrial biopsy is mandatory. Usually these measures are all that is necessary to establish a diagnosis. Occasionally these methods fail or physical factors such as cervical stenosis preclude outpatient endometrial biopsy. Dilatation and curettage, preferably with hysteroscopy, then becomes necessary. In women with recurrent bleeding and a normal or inadequate office biopsy, hysteroscopy with directed biopsy will establish the diagnosis.

Superficially invasive, well-differentiated endometrial adenocarcinoma is found in 17 percent of women who have complex atypical hyperplasia.[22] In these women, if uterine preservation is desired, hysteroscopy and curettage is recommended.

Gross Findings

Gross findings in endometrial carcinoma are nonspecific. The endometrium may appear normal. It is not uncommon after outpatient endometrial sampling or curettage for the uterus to have no residual neoplasm.[22] In some cases the surface of

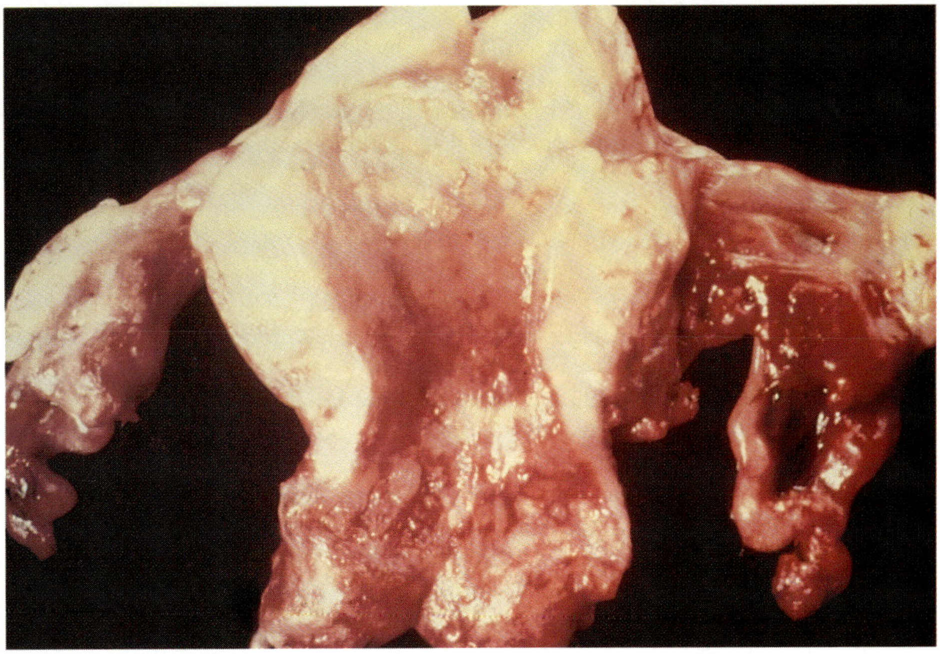

FIGURE 6–7
This uterus has been opened anteriorly. Normal-appearing adnexa are still attached. An irregular plaque is seen in the uterine fundus. This proved to be superficially invasive endometrial adenocarcinoma.

the endometrium is irregular (Fig. 6–7). Focal areas of hemorrhage and necrosis may be visible. Hemorrhage and necrosis are more common in high-grade neoplasms. If myometrial invasion by tumor is grossly visible it appears either as fingerlike or broad-based extensions beneath an exophytic neoplasm (Fig. 6–8). These extensions are firm, well demarcated, and lighter in color than the adjacent myometrium. At times, an invasive tumor contains yellowish areas indicating necrosis.

In 1988 the International Federation of Gynecology and Obstetrics (FIGO) revised the staging of endometrial cancer.[77] This staging system requires information obtained from surgical pathologic examination (Table 6–3). Some gynecologists may modify the surgical approach in the presence of deep myometrial invasion or cervical involvement. Therefore, intraoperative pathology consultation may be requested. Extrauterine spread may or may not be evident to the operating surgeon. If gross extrauterine disease is present, surgical debulking is appropriate.

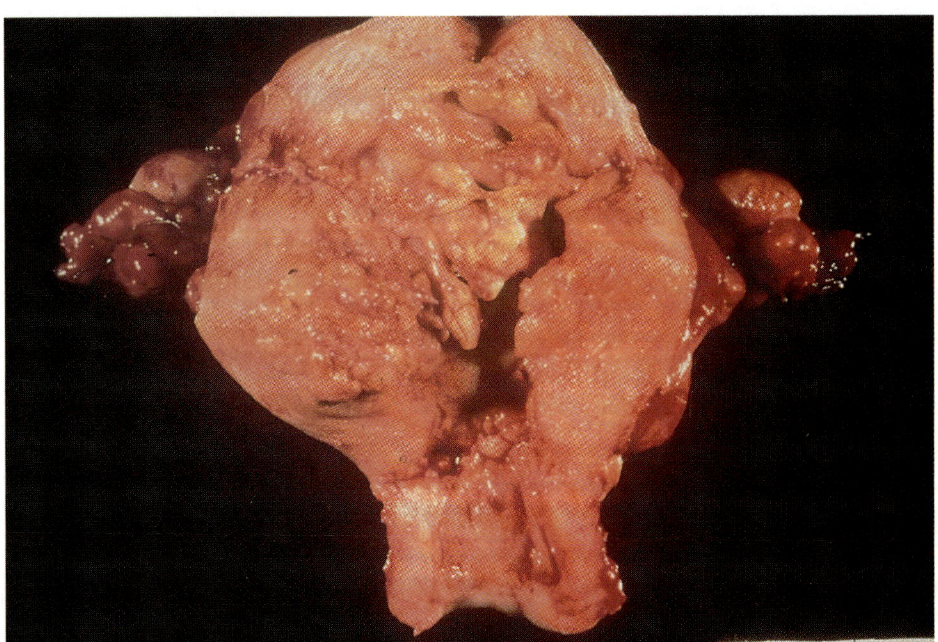

FIGURE 6–8
This uterus has been opened anteriorly. The tubes and ovaries are still attached and appear normal. A large exophytic tumor mass with yellow tones fills the endometrial cavity. Broad-based deep myometrial invasion is seen on the left. (From Hernandez E, Rosenshein NB: Manual of Gynecologic Oncology. New York, Churchill Livingstone, 1989).

TABLE 6–3.

Staging of Uterine Corpus Cancer According to the 1988 International Federation of Gynecology and Obstetrics (FIGO) Classification

Stages	
IA, G 123	Tumor limited to endometrium
IB, G 123	Invasion to less than half the myometrium
IC, G 123	Invasion to less than half the myometrium
IIA, G 123	Endocervical glandular involvement only
IIB, G 123	Cervical stromal invasion
IIIA, G 123	Tumor invades serosa and/or adnexa and/or positive peritoneal cytology
IIIB, G 123	Vaginal metastases
IIIC, G 123	Metastases to pelvic and/or paraaortic lymph nodes
IVA, G 123	Tumor invasion of bladder and/or bowel mucosa
IVB, G 123	Distant metastases including intraabdominal and/or inguinal lymph nodes.

Histopathology (Degree of Differentiation)

Grade 1: Less than 5% solid areas

Grade 2: 6–50% solid areas

Grade 3: More than 50% solid areas

Notes on Pathologic Grading

A. Notable nuclear atypia, inappropriate for the architectural grade, raises the grade of a grade 1 or grade 2 tumor by one grade.

B. In serous adenocarcinoma, clear cell adenocarcinoma, and squamous cell carcinoma nuclear grading takes precedence.

C. In adenocarcinoma with squamous differentiation, the nuclear grade of the glandular component determines the histologic grade.

Rules Related to Staging

A. Because surgery determines the stage of corpus cancer, procedures such as fractional dilation and curettage to differentiate between stage I and II are no longer applicable.

B. There may be a small number of patients with corpus cancer treated primarily with radiation therapy. In these patients the clinical staging adopted by FIGO in 1971 would still apply, but a notation designating use of that staging system is necessary.

C. Ideally, the pathologist should measure the width of the myometrium along with the width of tumor invasion.

Adapted from FIGO stages—1988 revision. Gynecol Oncol 1989; 35: 125.

Microscopic Findings

Endometrial carcinoma is a heterogeneous group of neoplasms. A variety of histopathologic subtypes exists. Any of the cell types normally found in the müllerian system can be seen. Table 6–4 presents a classification of the histopathologic subtypes of endometrial carcinoma. The majority of endometrial carcinomas are endometrioid type. Other commonly encountered cell types include (1) serous, which resembles the epithelium of the fallopian tube; (2) mucinous, which resembles the epithelium of the endocervix or, less commonly, that of the colon; and (3) clear cell, which is a variant of the endometrioid type of endometrial carcinoma.[78] Squamous change is also common in endometrial carcinoma. A detailed discussion of each of the histopathologic variants of endometrial carcinoma follows. Most patients who have endometrial carcinoma have a favorable prognosis. Those subtypes that behave aggressively include papillary serous carcinoma, clear cell carcinoma, poorly differentiated endometrioid adenocarcinoma, poorly differentiated adenocarcinoma with squamous differentiation, and some of the rare variants of endometrial carcinoma.

The diagnosis of endometrial carcinoma is usually self-evident when myometrial invasion is present. However, in the absence of invasion, differentiation of well-differentiated adenocarcinoma from complex atypical hyperplasia is sometimes difficult. The presence of endometrial stromal invasion distinguishes well-differentiated endometrial carcinoma (grade 1) from endometrial hyperplasia.[22] Distinguishing complex atypical hyperplasia from well-differentiated adenocarcinoma is of such importance that although it was previously described in the section on endometrial hyperplasia, revisiting it here is appropriate. There are four histopathologic features of stromal invasion, any one of which, when present, results in a diagnosis of carcinoma.[22] First is the presence of an altered endometrial stroma. This stroma has a desmoplastic or fibrous appearance (Fig. 6–9). The stromal cells are more spindle-shaped and their

TABLE 6–4.

Histopathologic Classification of Endometrial Carcinoma

A. Endometrioid adenocarcinoma
   1. Papillary
   2. Secretory
   3. Ciliated cell
   4. Adenocarcinoma with squamous differentiation
      a. With squamous metaplasia
      b. Adenosquamous adenocarcinoma

B. Mucinous carcinoma

C. Serous carcinoma

D. Clear cell carcinoma

E. Squamous carcinoma

F. Undifferentiated carcinoma

G. Mixed carcinoma

H. Metastatic carcinoma

From Sidawy MR, Silverberg SG: Endometrial carcinoma: Pathologic factors of therapeutic and prognostic significance. Pathol Annu 1992; 27: 153–185.

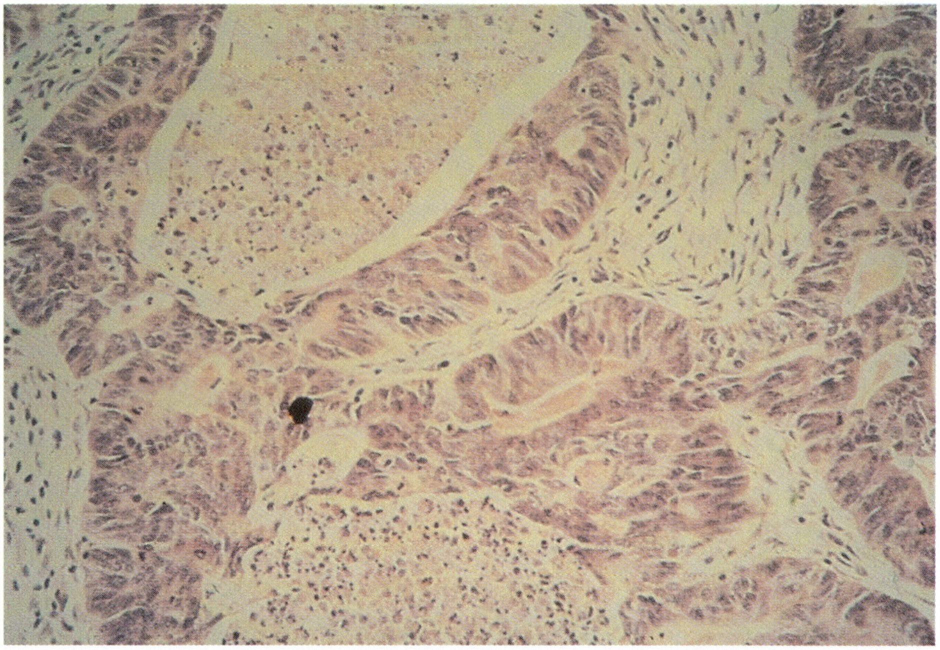

FIGURE 6-9
This is a well-differentiated endometrial adenocarcinoma with a desmoplastic stromal response. The stroma is infiltrated by fibroblasts. The endometrial stromal cells have elongated nuclei and an eosinophilic wavy appearance. This is indicative of stromal invasion. The glands are complex and have atypical stratified epithelium. Some of the nuclei are round, while others are elongated. There is focal loss of polarity.

nuclei more elongated. Stromal foam cells may be present. Second is the presence of a complex confluent gland-to-gland pattern with no intervening stroma and involving half of a low-power microscope field (2.1 mm) or more. Third is the presence of a complex papillary pattern with multiple epithelial-lined branching fibrous processes occupying at least half of a low-power microscope field (2.1 mm). Fourth is a proliferation of squamous cells forming solid sheets of cells replacing the stroma and occupying at least half of a low-power field (2.1 mm).[22]

A diagnosis of well-differentiated adenocarcinoma from a curettage specimen is associated with residual carcinoma in 50 percent of excised uteri.[22] Thirteen to 50 percent of these carcinomas are of a higher grade; in 25 percent deep myometrial invasion is present.[22, 79, 80] Increasing degrees of cytologic atypia, mitotic activity and stratification are poor discriminators for endometrial carcinoma. These histopathologic findings are frequently present but are of limited predictive value. Even with mild atypia, low mitotic activity, and little stratification, 20 percent of residual carcinomas are of high grade, and 10 percent demonstrate deep myometrial invasion.[22,79,80]

A number of possibilities must be considered in the differential diagnosis of well-differentiated endometrial adenocarcinoma in a curettage specimen. Complex hyperplasia may have a focally confluent pattern or may display squamous metaplasia, but these changes should not occupy more than half a low-power microscope field. Endometrial polyps and lower segment endometrium may be associated with a fibrous stroma. When endometrial polyps or lower segment endometrium are possible, criteria other than an altered stroma must be present to make a diagnosis of carcinoma. Metaplastic changes are common and can lead to confusion with neoplasia.[21] Endometrial metaplasia frequently coexists with abnormal proliferations but may also be present in normal endometrium. Thirty-two percent of stage I endometrial adenocarcinomas contain an admixture of adenocarcinomatous and metaplastic changes.[81] When metaplasia and carcinoma coexist, the carcinoma is more likely to be low grade. The most common metaplasia coexisting with endometrial carcinoma is eosinophilic metaplasia, followed closely by tubal metaplasia.[81] Normal menstrual endometrium, because of the collapse of the endometrial stroma and fragmentation of the endometrial glands, can at times appear as a complex back-to-back glandular pattern. The lack of mitotic activity and the presence of fibrin thrombi serve to separate normal menstrual endometrium from adenocarcinoma.

Before the recognition that endometrial stromal invasion was the best histopathologic predictor of carcinoma in a curettage specimen, the histologic characteristics used to separate complex atypical endometrial hyperplasia from well-differentiated endometrial adenocarcinoma were imprecise. In over 15 percent of reviewed cases of well-differentiated carcinoma the revised diagnosis was hyperplasia.[82] Overdiagnosis may occur in as many as 25 percent of cases. Thus, interpretation of the older literature should take into account the possible overdiagnosis of well-differentiated carcinoma.[82]

At the other extreme, the distinction of a poorly differentiated carcinoma from a uterine sarcoma may also be difficult. Uterine sarcoma will be discussed in detail in a subsequent section.

Typical (Endometrioid) Endometrial Carcinoma

Epidemiology

Endometrioid adenocarcinoma is by far the most common histologic type of endometrial carcinoma, accounting for more than 80 percent of all cases.[78, 82–85] When limited to "early" disease, studies report an even higher frequency of the endometrioid type of carcinoma.[86, 87] Because of its frequency, it is also known as typical endometrial adenocarcinoma or simply as endometrial adenocarcinoma. The age of patients with endometrioid adenocarcinoma of the endometrium ranges from the second to the ninth decades of life. Most patients are in their fifth or sixth decade. Only 10 percent of women are under age 40, and 12 percent are premenopausal. The average age of women with newly diagnosed endometrial adenocarcinoma is approximately 60 years.[82, 83] Thirty-five to 50 percent of women who develop typical endometrial adenocarcinoma are nulliparous.[82, 83] African-American women constitute approximately 13 percent of those with typical endometrial carcinoma.[88] They appear to have a lower incidence of the disease than expected in most series. Approximately half of the women who have endometrioid adenocarcinoma are obese. Fifteen percent have diabetes mellitus. Hypertension is present in as many as 45 percent.[82]

Histopathology

Although focal areas of a mixture of cells with other histopathologic types may be present, the endometrioid type of endometrial adenocarcinoma shows malignant-appearing endometrial glands with stromal invasion. On low-power microscopic examination, glandular crowding and irregularity with epithelial protrusions, budding, and infolding into the gland lumen are evident (Fig. 6–10). The glands may be confluent, cribriform, or separated by an altered focally necrotic stroma. Epithelial cells bridging across glands may be present.

If less than 5 percent of the tumor shows solid areas it is classified as grade 1. If more than 50 percent of the tumor is solid it is classified as grade 3. Grade 2 tumors have between 6 and 50 percent solid areas. The cells may be pseudostratified or stratified to two or more cell layers. They demonstrate a haphazard proliferation and loss of polarity. In a grade 1 tumor the individual cells are usually fairly uniform in size and shape. There is rounding of the nucleus and dispersed chromatin. Nucleoli are not prominent. A perpendicular orientation of the cells along the basement membrane is seen (Fig. 6–11). Mitotic activity is vari-

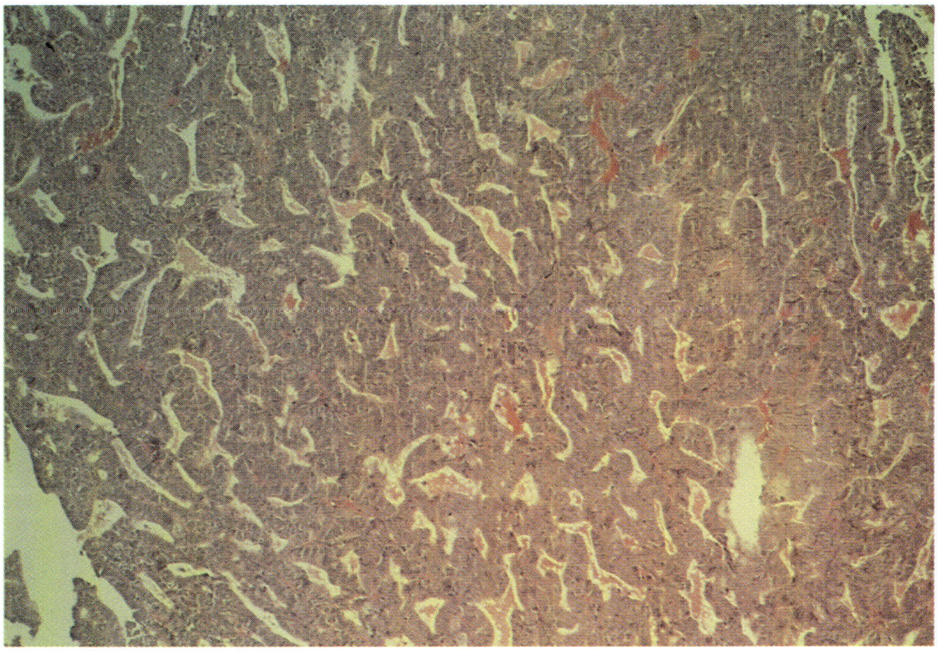

FIGURE 6–10
In this well-differentiated endometrial adenocarcinoma glands are back to back without intervening stroma. There are no solid areas.

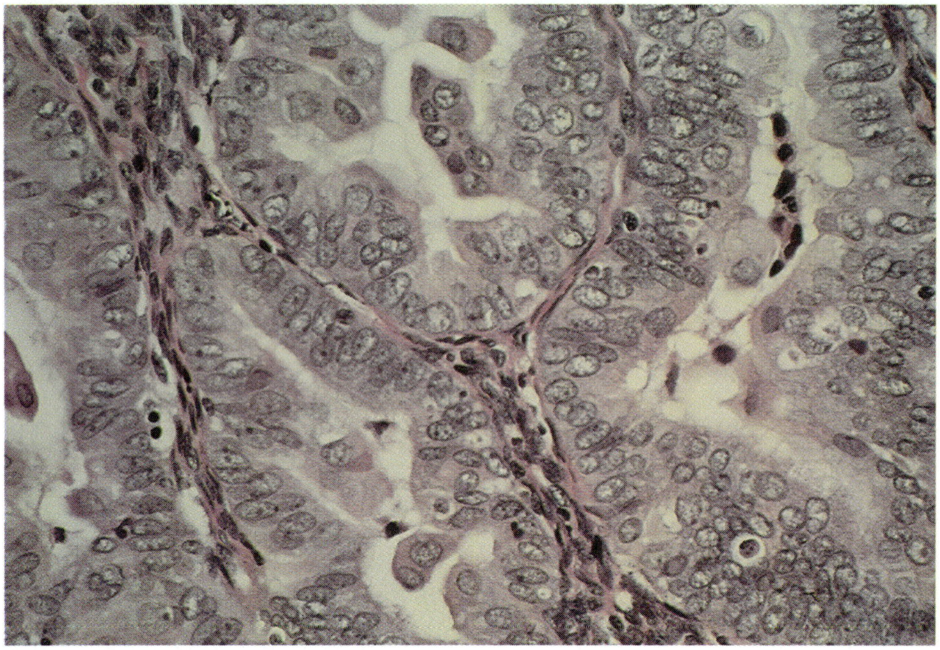

FIGURE 6-11
This is a high-power view of well-differentiated or grade 1 endometrial adenocarcinoma. There is stratification, loss of polarity, and cytologic atypia. Some nuclei are elongated, with their long axis oriented perpendicular to the basement membrane. Other nuclei are round with central clearing. Nucleoli are seen in some of the cells. The glands are back to back with little intervening stroma.

able and frequently does not exceed that of proliferative endometrium. Mitotic activity should not be used to distinguish well-differentiated endometrial adenocarcinoma from complex atypical hyperplasia. As the histopathologic grade becomes higher, an architecturally solid growth pattern becomes apparent (Fig. 6–12). Nuclear pleomorphism becomes more pronounced with prominent nucleoli and chromatin clumping.

According to FIGO, tumor grading in endometrial endometrioid adenocarcinoma makes use of architectural as well as nuclear grading (see Table 6–3). Significant nuclear atypia that is otherwise inappropriate for the architectural grade increases the tumor grade by one. Cells that have oval to rounded nuclei, an irregular nuclear membrane, minimal nuclear enlargement, and fine, evenly dispersed chromatin are considered to be nuclear grade 1. These cells do not have prominent nucleoli. Large rounded hyperchromatic nuclei that

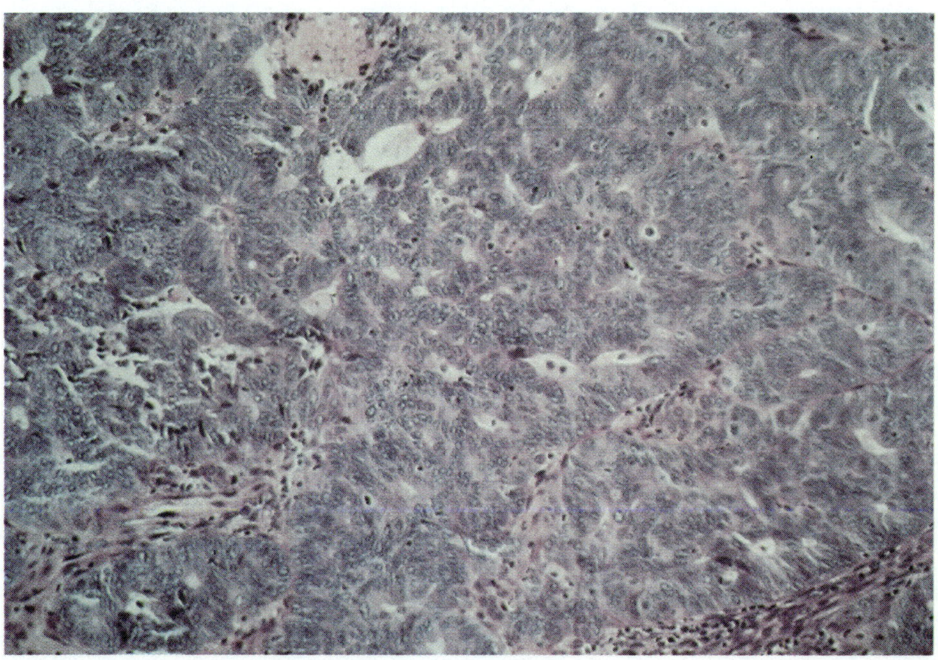

FIGURE 6-12
In this tumor the glands have overgrown the stroma and the gland lumen. An almost solid epithelial growth is present. However, suggestions of gland lumen are seen causing a cribriform pattern. This is a grade 2 endometrial adenocarcinoma.

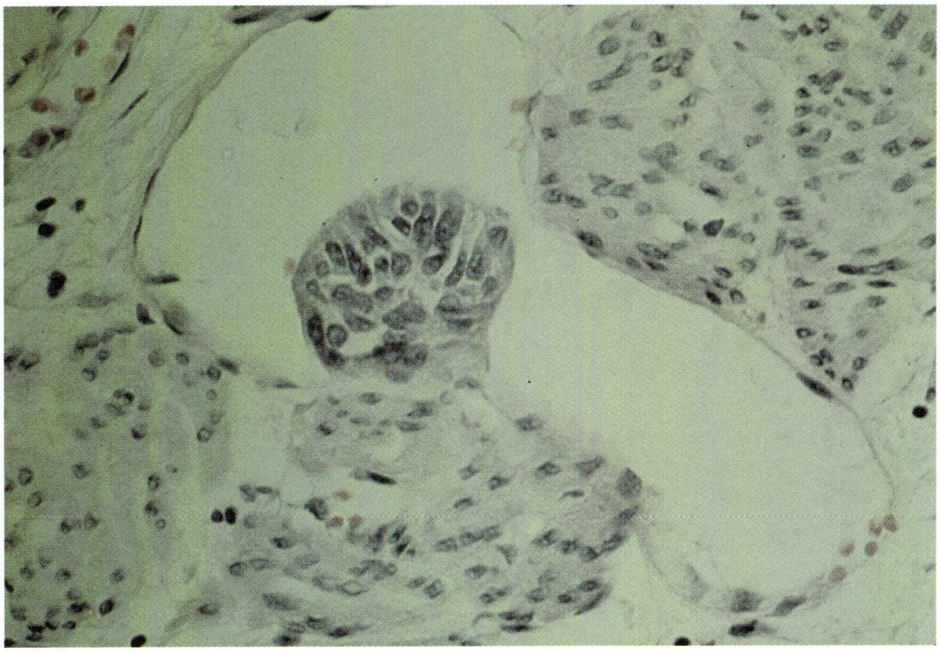

FIGURE 6–13
A cluster of endometrial adenocarcinoma cells in a vascular channel deep within the myometrium is seen here.

display significant pleomorphism, coarse chromatin clumping, a thick, irregular nuclear membrane, and prominent nucleoli are classified as nuclear grade 3. Mitoses are frequent in nuclear grade 3 neoplasms. Tumors that have cells that display intermediate nuclear characteristics are classified as nuclear grade 2.[88]

Lymphocytic infiltration may be seen when the tumor invades the myometrium.[83] The lymphocytes may be found at the junction of the myometrium and tumor nests or around myometrial vessels close to the tumor. The term vascular invasion-associated changes (VIAC) was recently coined to describe the presence of perivascular lymphocytes or intravascular nests of tumor cells (Fig. 6–13).[83] These changes are associated with an increased incidence of nodal metastases and a poorer prognosis.[83a]

A diffuse infiltrating pattern consisting of individual glands scattered throughout the myometrium is present in some tumors.[89] If this histologic pattern accounts for more than 50 percent of the neoplasm, the prognosis is worse. A 5-year mortality of 40 percent has been reported for patients with this histopathologic pattern.[89] This pattern should not be confused with that of an adenocarcinoma, which arises in adenomyosis and then diffusely involves the myometrium.[89a] This topic will be discussed in more detail later.

A typical endometrioid carcinoma spreads by direct extension to contiguous organs (Fig. 6–14) and by lymphatic or vascular dissemination (Figs. 6–15, 6–16). Spread to the cervix with involve-

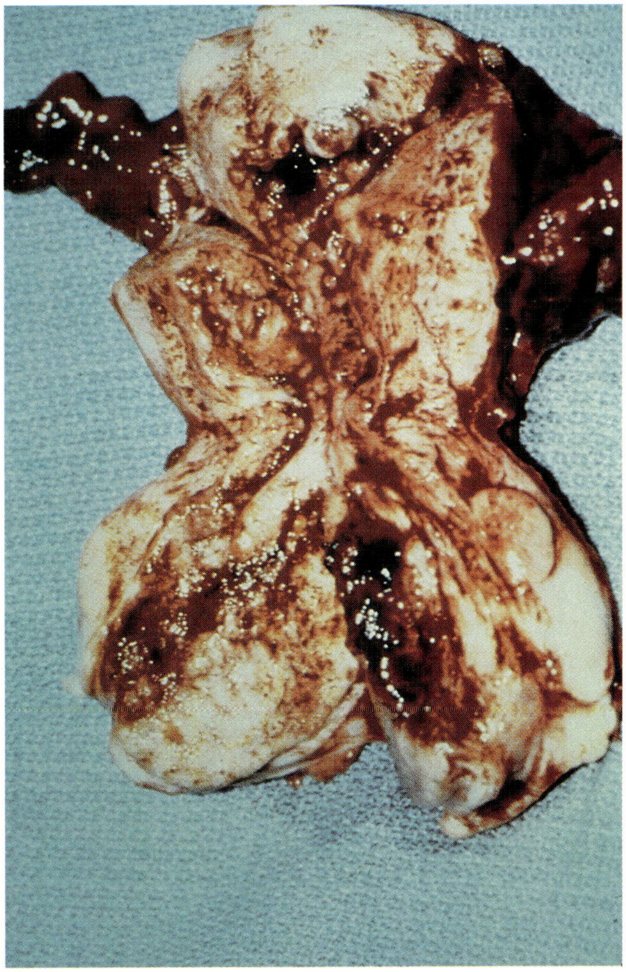

FIGURE 6–14
This is an endometrial carcinoma with gross extension to the cervix. (Courtesy of Dr. John Wheelock.)

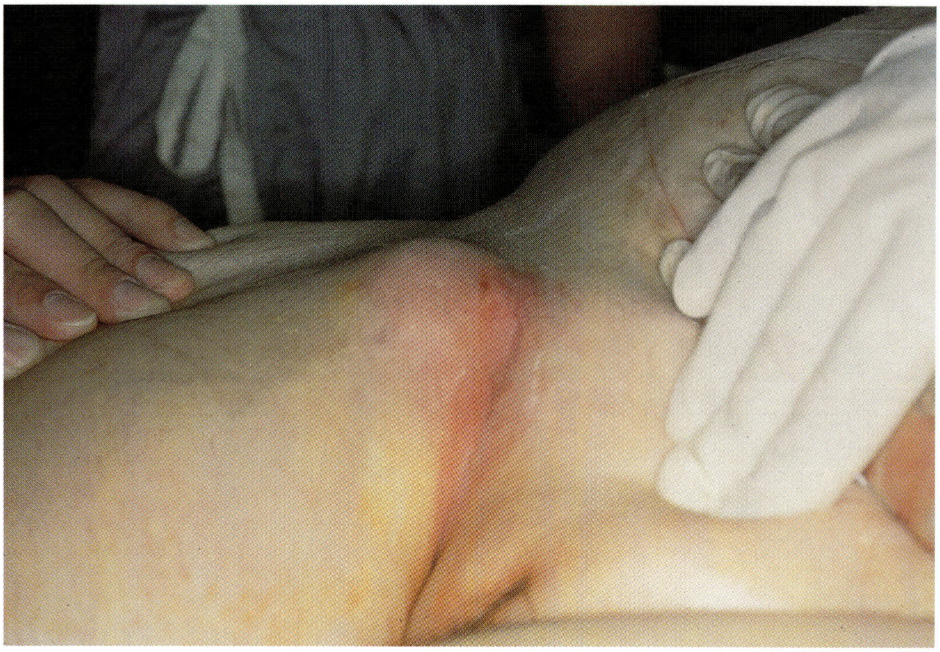

FIGURE 6-15
This is an example of stage IVB endometrial adenocarcinoma with groin metastasis. Spread of the tumor through the round ligament lymphatics can result in inguinal node metastasis.

ment only of the endocervical surface glandular epithelium usually occurs by direct continuity. However, in patients who have involvement of the endocervical stroma, tumor spread usually represents lymphatic metastases.[90–91] Endocervical gland involvement without stromal tumor occurs in approximately one-quarter of patients who have endometrial adenocarcinoma with cervical involvement. Both surface and underlying stroma contain tumor in two-thirds of cases; only the endocervical stroma contains tumor in 5 percent (Fig. 6–17).[92] Superficial cervical involvement tends to be associated with tumors of a lower histopathologic grade and less myometrial invasion.[92] Patients who have stage IIA endometrial adenocarcinoma (cervical glandular involvement only) have a prognosis similar to that of patients with stage I disease. When the spread of endometrial carcinoma involves the cervical stroma, deep myometrial invasion is usually present.[92]

In most patients, tumor spread to the pelvic lymph nodes occurs before spread to the periaortic nodes. In surgical stage I disease, when the surgeon performs pelvic and periaortic lymphadenectomy, 6.8 percent of patients are found to have pelvic node metastases and 2.5 percent have periaortic node metastases.[93] If the pelvic lymph nodes do not contain tumor, the incidence of periaortic node metastasis is extremely low. It has been suggested that for periaortic lymph node metastasis to occur, one or more of the following must be present: gross involvement of pelvic lymph nodes, uterine adnexa with tumor spread

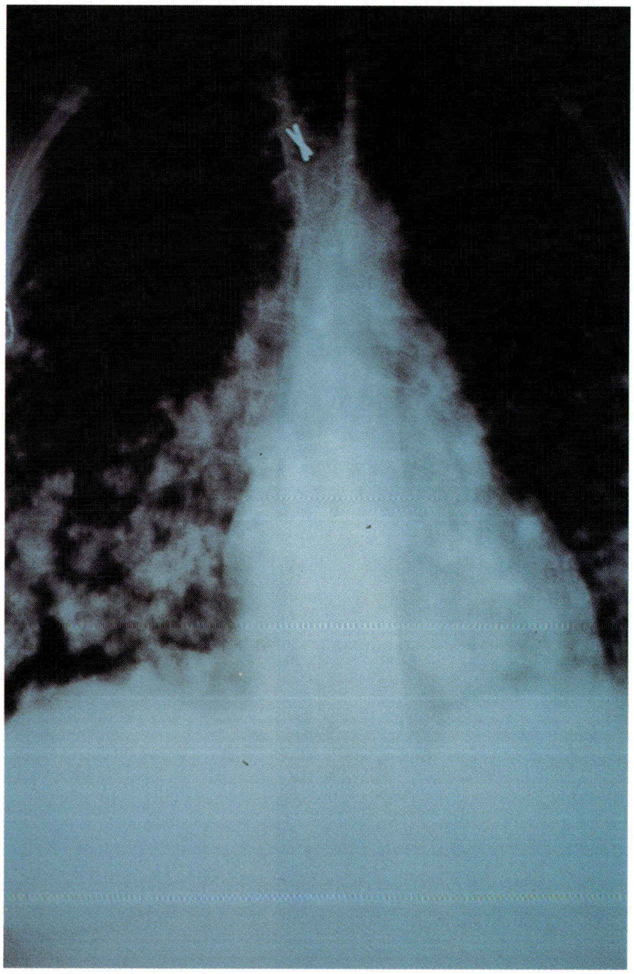

FIGURE 6-16
This chest radiograph demonstrates multiple "cotton-ball" densities on both lower lung fields. This is the result of hematogenous spread of endometrial adenocarcinoma.

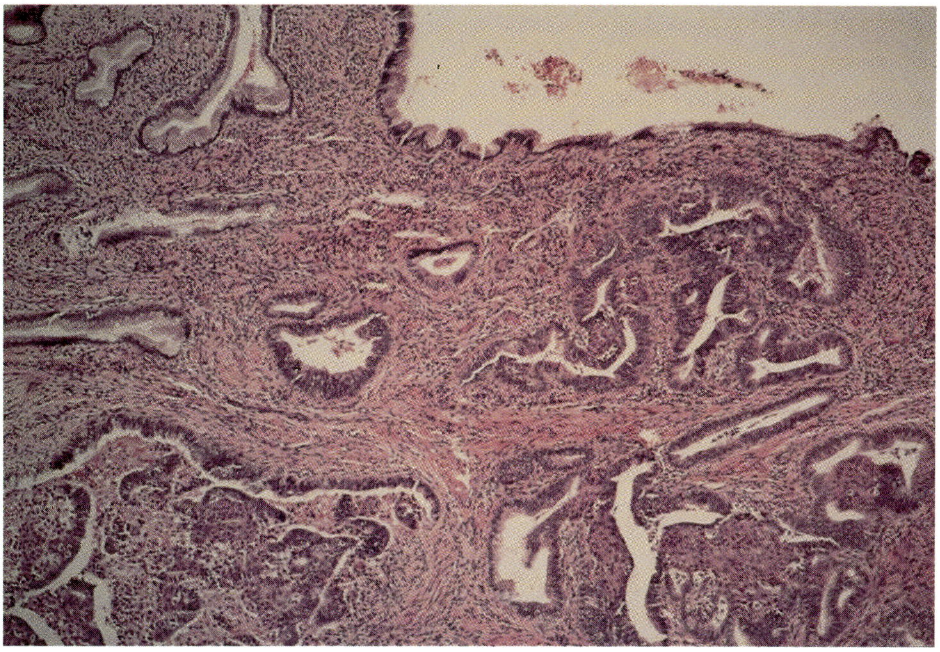

FIGURE 6-17
This section through the cervix shows normal endocervical epithelium on the surface. Glands with features consistent with endometrial adenocarcinoma are found in the cervical stroma. Normal endocervical glands are seen at the upper left.

(Fig. 6–18), or invasion to the outer third of the myometrium.[94]

Recurrence of typical endometrial carcinoma is either pelvic (25 percent), distant (61 percent), or both (9 percent). Tumor grade, depth of myometrial invasion, and surgical stage are each significant predictors of disease-free survival in this histopathologic subtype.[94–96]

Papillary Endometrioid Adenocarcinoma

This histopathologic subtype is uncommon. A review of the literature suggests that two variants may be included under this designation. There is one group of neoplasms that some designate simply as papillary adenocarcinoma or well-differentiated papillary carcinoma.[97] Another name for this histopathologic variant is villoglandular papillary adenocarcinoma.[27, 98] A second histopathologic pattern may represent a midpoint between endometrial endometrioid adenocarcinoma and the more aggressive papillary serous neoplasm.[99] This variant of papillary endometrioid adenocarcinoma is easy to confuse with papillary serous carcinoma or clear cell carcinoma. Both histopathologic variants of papillary endometrioid adenocarcinoma

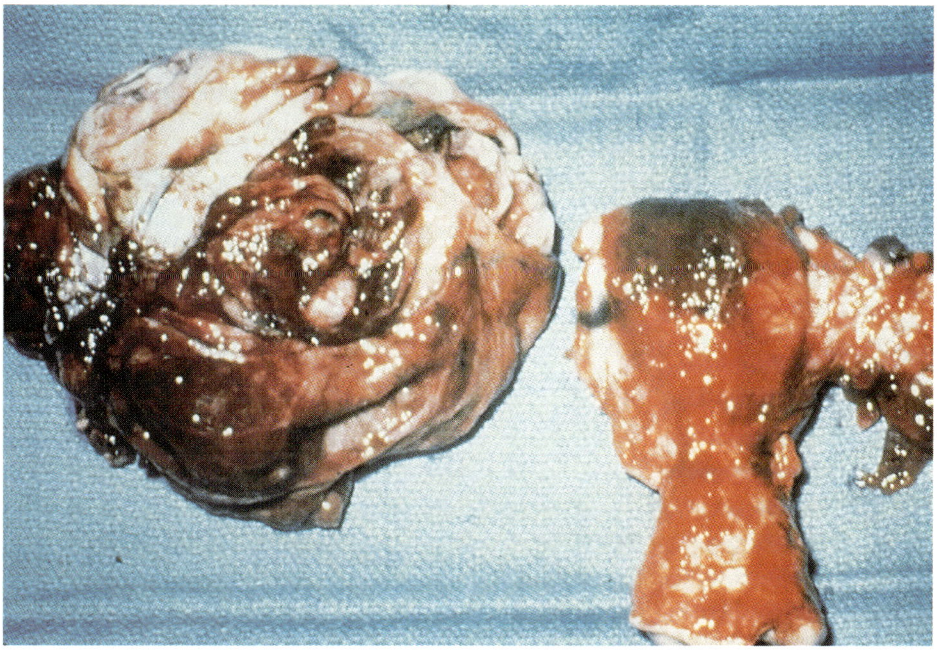

FIGURE 6-18
Endometrial carcinoma with gross adnexal involvement is seen here. Grossly one cannot differentiate ovarian metastases from a separate primary neoplasm in the ovary. (Courtesy of Dr. John Wheelock.)

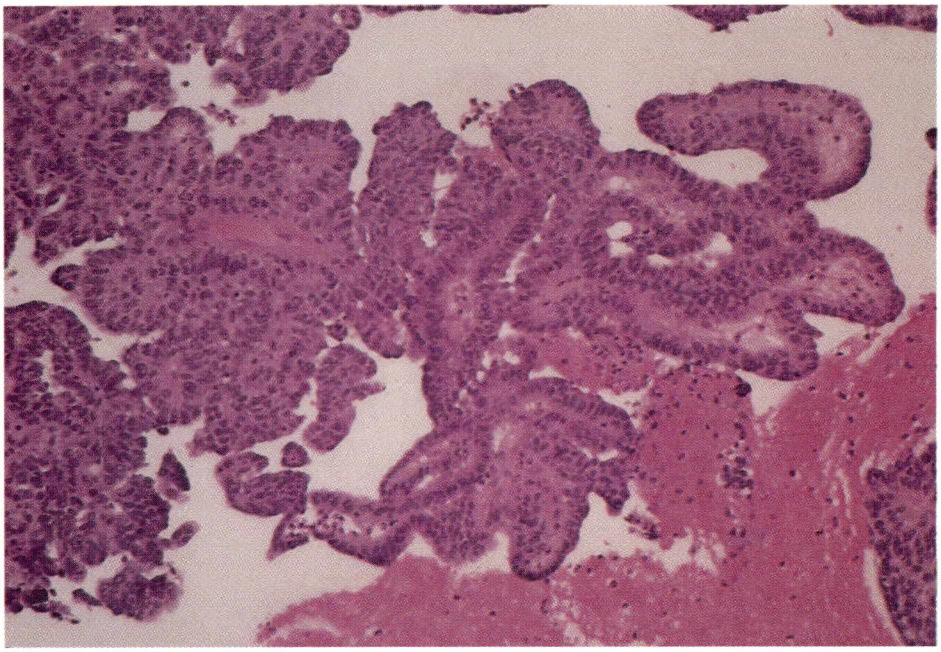

FIGURE 6-19
This is a well-differentiated endometrial adenocarcinoma with papillary architecture ("villoglandular"). The papillae are simple and have smooth profiles without cell tufts. The nuclear atypia is mild. Compare this with Figure 6-21, which represents a uterine papillary serous carcinoma.

account for less than 1 percent of all endometrial carcinomas.

The literature is sparse with data concerning their biologic behavior. The villoglandular or well-differentiated papillary pattern has epidemiologic characteristics similar to those associated with endometrial endometrioid adenocarcinoma (i.e., patients' age and ethnicity, associated hypertension or diabetes, nulliparity, obesity, and history of unopposed estrogen use.[98] The most common presenting complaint is abnormal or postmenopausal uterine bleeding. On microscopic examination, uniform neoplastic epithelium lines elongated slender papillae. Stratification is minimal, and the individual cells are cuboidal or columnar in shape. The nuclei are oval to round and are basally located. The nuclear grade of these neoplasms is low (i.e., grade 1 and occasionally grade 2).[27, 98] Hyperchromatism and nuclear pleomorphism are minimal. Nucleoli are small or of intermediate size. Mitotic figures vary but are less than those seen in papillary serous tumors, but this factor should not be used to distinguish between the two[98, 100] (Fig. 6-19). This histopathologic variant seems to have a better prognosis than typical endometrioid endometrial carcinoma. A patient with stage IV disease survived 5 years following this diagnosis.[98]

The second variant of papillary endometrioid adenocarcinoma has a more aggressive behavior than typical endometrial adenocarcinoma or the variant just described but is less aggressive than uterine papillary serous carcinoma. The neoplastic cells line delicate fibrovascular stalks. Stratification is minimal. The individual cells are elongated. Architecturally, most of these neoplasms are grade 1, whereas the nuclear grade is more likely to be grade 2 or 3.[99] To qualify as a papillary endometrioid adenocarcinoma, at least 20 percent of the tumor volume must have these histopathologic characteristics.[99] At the time of surgical staging extrauterine disease is present in 23 percent of women who have papillary endometrioid adenocarcinoma compared to 10 percent of women who have typical endometrioid adenocarcinoma.[99] Deep myometrial invasion is present in 36 percent.[99] This percentage is not significantly different from that seen in typical endometrial carcinoma. Recurrences tend to be local. Women who have recurrent or advanced papillary endometrioid adenocarcinoma have elevated serum levels of CA 125.[99]

The histopathologic differences between the two variants of papillary endometrioid adenocarcinoma as described in the literature seem to be based mostly on nuclear grade. As expected, the higher the nuclear grade, the more aggressive the tumor's clinical behavior. The important distinction is not between the variants of papillary endometrioid adenocarcinoma discussed earlier but between them and uterine papillary serous carcinoma, to be discussed subsequently (Table 6-5). To avoid confusion, we prefer to use the term endometrial endometrioid adenocarcinoma with papillary architecture to describe neoplasms demonstrating the features described in this section.[99a]

Secretory Adenocarcinoma

Secretory endometrial adenocarcinoma is a rare but distinct histopathologic variant. It represents

TABLE 6–5.

Histopathologic Features Distinguishing the Papillary Endometrioid and Papillary Serous Types of Endometrial Adenocarcinoma

	Papillary Endometrioid ("Villoglandular")	*Papillary Serous ("Serous")*
General architecture	Predominantly papillary; other areas tend to be cribriform, sometimes with squamous differentiation	Predominantly papillary (resembling ovarian type); other areas tend to be solid and anaplastic, sometimes with clear cell and squamous features. Frequent tumor necrosis
Papillae Arborization	More often simple	Often multiple branches and papillary fragments. Papillae may fuse to be "compressed or spongiform"
Profile of epithelial lining of papillae	Slender with straight sides. More orderly stratification and pseudostratification of nuclei	Broader with ragged sides; disordered stratification, and frequent cell tufts
Malignant epithelial cells Pleomorphism Nuclear atypia	More uniform cells Less nuclear atypia, usually nuclear grade 1 to 2. Nuclei are often oval and basally located within the cancer cells	Highly pleomorphic cells, sometimes large and bizarre. More nuclear atypia, usually nuclear grade 3, denoted by: 1. Marked abnormalities and variation in nuclear size, shape, chromatin, and location within the cells 2. Hyperchromasia 3. High nuclear to cytoplasmic ratio
Nucleoli	Small to medium size nucleoli	Macronucleoli are usually prominent
Mitotic activity	Variable mitotic rate, usually low	Prominent mitotic activity, abnormal mitotic spindles
Psammoma bodies	None (according to most recent studies)	Seen in 12–33% of cases
Myometrial and lymphatic invasion	Infrequent except in poorly differentiated and clinically advanced disease	Frequent even in cases of clinically early stage disease (preoperatively assessed) and normal-sized uterus. Invasion into myometrium forms "gaping glands with unfolding tufts"

From Dunton CJ, Balsara G, McFarland M, Hernandez E: Uterine papillary serous carcinoma: A review. Obstet Gynecol Surv 1991; 46: 97–102.

less than 1 percent of all endometrial carcinomas.[101] The epidemiologic features are similar to those of the typical endometrial carcinoma. The age range of patients who have this histopathologic variant is 36 to 79 years, with a mean age of 55 years.[101, 102] The patients usually present with postmenopausal or abnormal uterine bleeding. As with typical endometrial carcinoma, 15 to 25 percent of patients are nulliparous, and nearly half are obese. Diabetes and hypertension are present in approximately 10 percent of patients.[101] There are no distinguishing gross features. On microscopic examination the neoplastic glands appear well differentiated and have the appearance of an early secretory endometrium, similar to those of normal cycle days 17 to 22 (see Chapter 5).[101, 102] Varying numbers of subnuclear and supranuclear vacuoles may be present (Fig. 6–20). Squamous metaplasia is present in 22 percent of these tumors.[101] Over half of the cases reveal changes in the adjacent nonmalignant endometrium similar to the changes described in patients treated with either prolonged or unopposed estrogen. These changes include vascular thrombosis, focal stromal necrosis, focal glandular crowding, and hyperplasia of varying degrees. Tubal metaplasia is present in a third of cases. Mucin stains are negative. Most neoplasms are architecturally and cytologically well differentiated (i.e., grade 1). Most patients have surgical stage I disease.[101, 102] Myometrial invasion is present in approximately two-thirds of patients, varying from 5 to 70 percent of the myometrial thickness.[101,102]

The category of secretory adenocarcinoma may represent two clinical situations that have similar histopathologic appearances. One form occurs in premenopausal women, and here the adenocarcinoma is capable of responding to its hormonal environment. Usually a corpus luteum is present in the ovary, or the patient is taking exogenous progestogen therapy. However, a relationship to progesterone is not always demonstrable.[101] In this form, the secretory changes are cyclic and transient. If such a tumor is diagnosed on the basis of endometrial curettings, it sometimes has a nonsecretory histologic appearance on the hysterectomy

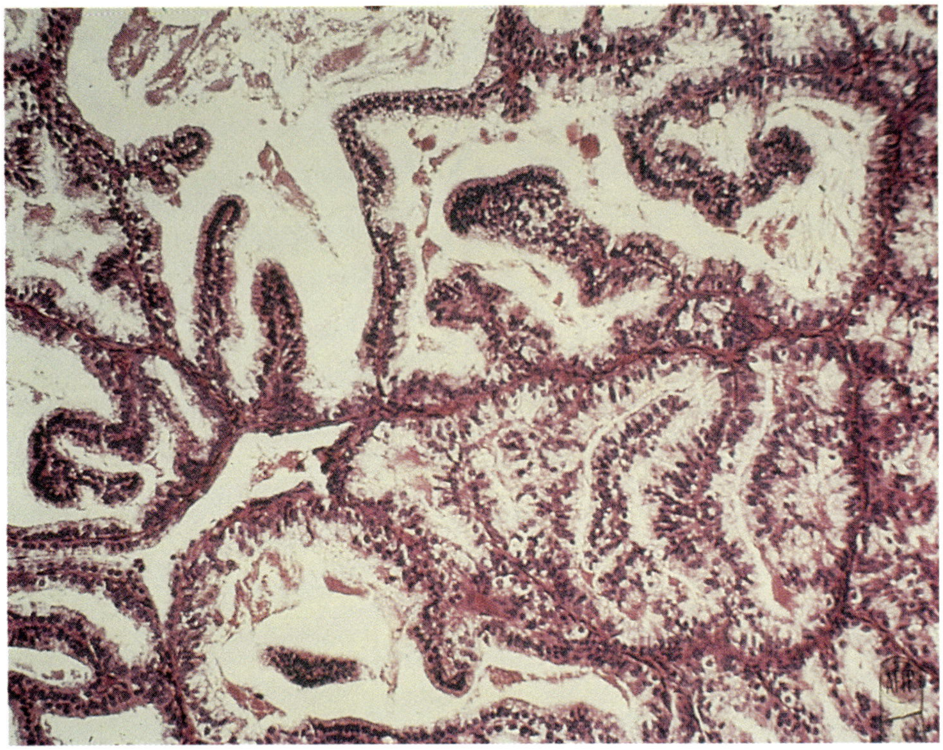

FIGURE 6-20
This is a secretory adenocarcinoma that shows back-to-back crowding. This neoplasm has no solid areas and minimal nuclear atypia (grade 1). The cells are tall columnar and contain secretory vacuoles in the cytoplasm. The secretory change resembles an early secretory endometrium. There are many sub- and supranuclear vacuoles.

specimen. The second form of secretory adenocarcinoma occurs in postmenopausal women who have a neoplasm that has become unregulated. These tumors exhibit secretion that is a normal cell function but is no longer under hormonal control.[101] Secretory activity in normal endometrium without exposure to estrogen and progesterone has been documented.[102a] There is one case report of secretory adenocarcinoma occurring in a woman with ovarian agenesis.[52] One neoplasm demonstrated positive immunocytochemical staining for carcinoembryonic antigen (CEA).[101]

The prognosis for patients with endometrial secretory adenocarcinoma is good owing to the fact that these tumors are usually early stage (i.e., stage I) and low grade (i.e., grade 1) at the time of the diagnosis.

Ciliated Cell Carcinoma

This is an extremely uncommon histopathologic variant of endometrial carcinoma. Only a few examples of this neoplasm exist in the literature. Microscopically, this neoplasm consists of glands lined in large part by cells containing cilia. Ciliated cell carcinoma has an association with exogenous estrogen administration.[103] These neoplasms are histopathologically low grade and seem to have a favorable prognosis.

Adenocarcinoma with Squamous Differentiation

Endometrial adenocarcinoma with squamous differentiation is a common histopathologic variant and continues to generate considerable controversy. Most endometrial carcinomas have foci of squamous differentiation. To be classified as an adenocarcinoma with squamous differentiation at least 5 percent of the neoplasm must demonstrate squamous change. This much squamous differentiation is present in approximately 25 percent of endometrial carcinomas.[82, 104] Recognition of the squamous elements in endometrial carcinoma is not difficult. The squamous differentiation varies from benign-appearing morule formation to malignant squamous differentiation. Considerable disagreement persists about its biologic significance. Beginning in 1968 an arbitrary division was made between two subtypes of endometrial adenocarcinoma with squamous differentiation. This division depended on whether the histopathologic appearance of the squamous differentiation was benign or malignant.[105] Adenoacanthoma (benign) and adenosquamous carcinoma (malignant) are the names of these two subtypes.[106] Adenoacanthoma was felt to represent a histopathologic subtype that had a favorable prognosis, whereas adenosquamous carcinoma was thought to confer an unfavorable prognosis. For a diagnosis of adenoacanthoma to be rendered, the nuclei of the squamous cells must be uniform, and nucleoli should be absent or small; bizarre giant cells must be absent. No mitotic figures should be present in the squamous cells.[104] The glandular component of an adenoacanthoma is also well differentiated. In contrast, the squamous cells in adenosquamous carcinoma have malignant features including pleomorphism, nuclear atypia, increased nuclear to cytoplasmic ratio, prominent nucleoli, and mitotic figures.[107] This neoplasm is a high-grade carcinoma. However, recent studies suggest that the distinction between adenoacanthoma and adenosquamous carcinoma is not of prognostic importance.[108] The poor differentiation of the glandular component in adenosquamous carcinoma accounts for the associated poor prognosis. Because the glandular component in adenoacanthoma is usually well differentiated (i.e., grade 1), this results in a more favorable prognosis. Currently, the term adenocarcinoma with squamous differentiation or change is used to denote the entire category of endometrial carcinoma and is the preferred terminology.[108]

It is recommended that squamous differentiation be diagnosed only when one or more of the following criteria are present: keratin pearl formation, distinct intercellular bridges, or the presence of three or more of the following: sheetlike growth without gland formation or palisading, sharp cell margins, eosinophilic, thick, or glassy cytoplasm, and a decreased nuclear to cytoplasmic ratio.[27,104]

Endometrial adenocarcinoma with squamous differentiation has epidemiologic features that are similar to those of endometrioid adenocarcinoma. The median age of women who have endometrial adenocarcinoma with squamous cell differentiation is 58 years. However, many are premenopausal. A high proportion have a history of exogenous estrogen use.[109–110] More than one-third of patients with this histopathologic variant are nulliparous.[104] Fifteen percent have diabetes mellitus. Almost half are obese, and almost half are hypertensive. The presenting complaint of most women with this neoplasm is abnormal uterine bleeding or postmenopausal bleeding.[104]

In endometrial adenocarcinoma with squamous differentiation the glandular component usually predominates and determines the architectural grade. Differentiation of the squamous component parallels that of the glandular components in more than 80 percent of cases. In the remaining cases they differ by only one grade.[104] Nuclear grading of endometrial adenocarcinoma with squamous differentiation is as important as it is in typical endometrial adenocarcinoma. Here also the nuclear grade of the glandular component (as previously described) determines the nuclear grade of the neoplasm. However, we believe that mention of the grade of the squamous component should also be made.

Morules—cells that have an oval to spindled appearance—are the most common feature of squamous change in endometrial carcinoma. When malignant, the squamous component varies in appearance from that of a well-differentiated keratinizing squamous cell carcinoma to that of a poorly differentiated nonkeratinizing type. The architectural grade of the squamous component is arbitrary. A proposed grading system defines three architectural grades. In grade 1, nests of squamous cells confined to the central or luminal aspects of the neoplastic glands (morule formation) are present. Architectural grade 2 consists of squamous nests in isolation from glands. They do not form part of the peripheral interface of the tumor with the myometrium or benign stroma. Architectural grade 3 consists of nests of squamous cells that form at least part of the peripheral interface between the tumor and the myometrium or stroma where there is a desmoplastic stromal response.[104]

At the time of surgery small 0.3- to 0.7-cm nodules may be seen on the surface of the ovary, fallopian tubes, omentum, or parietal peritoneum in patients with endometrial adenocarcinoma with squamous differentiation. These are keratin granulomas. They consist of laminated deposits of keratin surrounded by foam cells and foreign body giant cells.[111]

The prognosis of patients with adenocarcinoma with squamous differentiation correlates best with the histologic grade of the glandular component and is similar to the prognosis of patients with typical endometrial adenocarcinoma without squamous differentiation. However, some investigators suggest that patients with well-differentiated endometrial adenocarcinoma with squamous differentiation have a slightly better prognosis.[112–113] This is true despite a similar frequency of nodal metastases in patients with these two types of endometrial carcinoma. The reported 5-year survival rate of patients with high-grade endometrial adenocarcinoma with squamous differentiation is between 40 and 70 percent,[114] which is comparable to a 70 percent 5-year survival of patients with typical endometrial carcinoma.[114,115]

For each grading method (i.e., architectural, nuclear, or combined), both glandular differentiation and squamous differentiation correlate statistically with the frequency of pelvic and paraaortic lymph node metastases. The presence of deep myometrial invasion and poor histopathologic differentiation correlates with a more aggressive biologic behavior.[104] Deep myometrial invasion, vascular space involvement, and lymph node metastases are more common in high-grade tumors.[115] The frequency of lymph node metastases increases with increasing depth of invasion.[104]

Endometrial adenocarcinoma with squamous differentiation is at times difficult to distinguish from other histopathologic entities. To distinguish this adenocarcinoma with squamous differentiation from atypical hyperplasia with squamous differentiation, the identification of stromal invasion as outlined earlier is required.[22] The major diagnostic dilemma for the pathologist is distinguishing primary endometrial carcinoma with squamous differentiation from endocervical adenocarcinoma, which may be mixed adenocarcinoma and squamous carcinoma. As a general guideline, in endocervical mixed tumors the squamous epithelium predominates, whereas in the endometrium, the glandular component predominates. In addition, mucinous or signet ring–type cells are more characteristic of the endocervix.

Serous Adenocarcinoma (Uterine Papillary Serous Carcinoma)

Uterine papillary serous carcinoma (UPSC) comprises 1 to 9 percent of all endometrial carcinomas.[92, 116] This neoplasm occurs in older women at an average age of 70 years.[117] Unlike typical endometrial adenocarcinoma, nulliparity is not a prominent epidemiologic feature. This histopathologic variant is more frequent in African-American women than in white women. These patients also tend to be obese. As with the other histopathologic variants, there are no gross features that distinguish UPSC from other types of endometrial adenocarcinomas. This neoplasm grows in a papillary fashion with broad to fine fronds. These fronds contain a central fibrovascular core or stalk that supports the malignant cells. Secondary epithelial papillae that branch off the main stalk are common. These can appear as detached cell clusters or as individual detached cells, similar to those seen in ovarian serous tumors of low malignant potential[27, 100] (Fig. 6–21). Branching and refusion of the papillary processes is frequent. This may lead at times to a more solid-looking area that still has angular clefts and small glandular spaces. The surface of the papillae is characteristically uneven and ragged because the malignant epithelial cells are variable in size and shape. They arrange themselves in irregularly shaped stratified tufts. Foci of necrosis are common. Psammoma bodies are present in up to one-third of cases.[27] These are calcified, concentrically laminated bodies that form in the fibrovascular stalk. The central fibrovascular core may undergo hyaline change. Individual cells may appear small with larger nuclei than normal for the size of the cell, leading to a high nuclear to cytoplasmic ratio. These neoplasms are usually nuclear grade 2 or 3.[100] The nuclei are round to oval with marked pleomorphism and hyperchromasia. Large bizarre nuclei and macronuclei may be present. Solid areas of tumor may be present next to the papillary areas. Within each neoplasm solid areas usually have the same cyto-

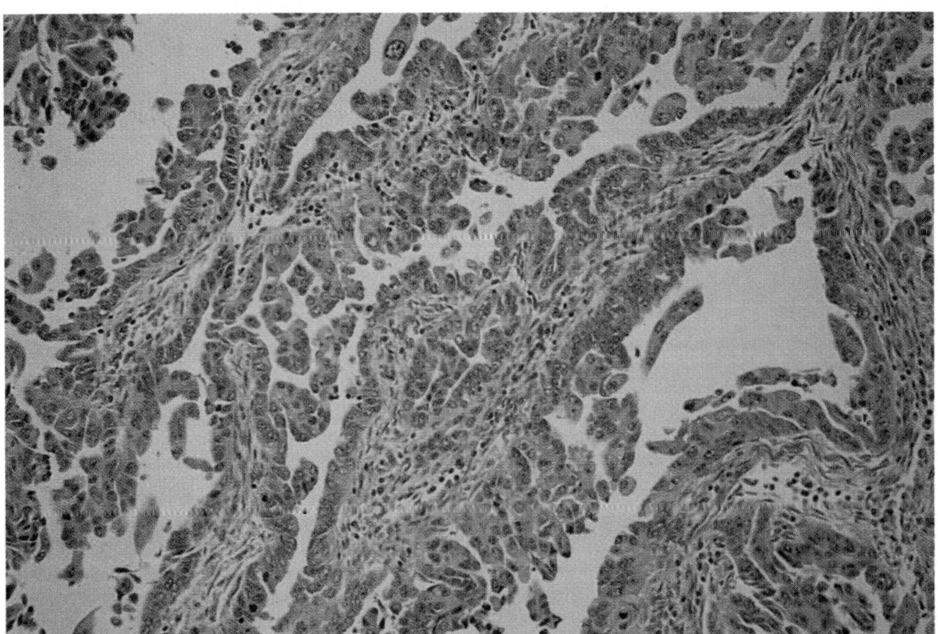

FIGURE 6–21
The uterine papillary serous carcinoma resembles its counterpart in the ovary. These papillae have thick connective tissue stalks. Individual cells and cell clusters are seen free in the glandular spaces.

pathologic features as the papillary areas. Mitotic figures are common and frequently abnormal (Table 6–5).

Deep myometrial invasion is common. It is present in approximately one-third of cases.[100, 116] In an additional third of cases the tumor invades only the inner half of the myometrium. Even in small uteri without gross myometrial invasion, the neoplasm may extensively invade endothelial lined spaces within the myometrium.[118] Surgical staging of patients with this histopathologic variant frequently reveals a more advanced stage than the apparent clinical stage. Thirty-three percent of patients have surgical stage I disease, 25 percent surgical stage II, 12 percent surgical stage III, and 30 percent surgical stage IV.[98, 116] Metastases to the lung and liver are common.[118]

The advanced surgical stage, high architectural grade, high nuclear grade, and deep myometrial invasion common with this neoplasm confer a poor prognosis for patients with this disease. The cornerstone of therapy is abdominal hysterectomy, bilateral salpingo-oophorectomy, and surgical staging. Staging should include sampling of the omentum and random peritoneal surfaces as done for epithelial tumors of the ovary. The 5-year survival rate for patients with this disease is only 26 to 35 percent.[97, 116–117] The 10-year survival rate is 14 percent.[116] UPSC is estrogen and progesterone receptor negative.

The morphologic and cytologic features of UPSC are similar to those of papillary serous carcinomas of ovarian and tubal origin. To distinguish primary UPSC from a primary serous adenocarcinoma of the ovary that has metastasized to the endometrium, the following criteria are used: the dominant disease is in the uterus and ovarian involvement consists of lymphatic involvement in the ovarian hilus or, if ovarian cortical involvement exists, it should be only microscopic and part of more widespread disease.[100]

Clear Cell Adenocarcinoma

Clear cell adenocarcinoma of the endometrium is less common than UPSC and constitutes 1.5 to 5 percent of all endometrial carcinomas. The first two cases reported in the English language appeared in 1957.[119] To date there have been over 140 reported cases.[120] It had been thought that this neoplasm was of mesonephric origin owing to its occurrence in the mesonephric remnants and its microscopic resemblance to renal cell carcinoma. Recent studies provide evidence favoring a müllerian origin.[121] Not only is this malignancy found in organs of müllerian origin (e.g., endometrium, vagina) but also its behavior and microscopic appearance are similar to those of other types of carcinoma that arise from the müllerian epithelium.[121] Additional evidence supporting a müllerian origin is the presence of squamous metaplasia in some cases as well as the coexistence of typical endometrial carcinoma in others.[120]

The age range of patients with clear cell adenocarcinoma of the endometrium is between 35 and 77 years, but most women are postmenopausal.[120] Twenty percent are nulliparous, and 20 percent have a documented history of current or past estrogen use. Twenty-five percent of patients are obese, 20 percent have diabetes mellitus, and approximately 50 percent are hypertensive.[120] Fifteen percent of women with this histopathologic variant of endometrial carcinoma have the triad of obesity, hypertension, and diabetes mellitus.[120] In 16 percent of cases there is a history of prior pelvic irradiation.[120]

Most patients complain of postmenopausal bleeding or abnormal uterine bleeding at presentation. Pelvic pain without bleeding or an asymptomatic pelvic mass are uncommon presentations. An occasional patient may present with cervical cytologic findings positive for adenocarcinoma.[120]

These neoplasms may be polypoid, granular, irregular, soft, fungating, grayish-tan or pink, hemorrhagic, and necrotic. The tumor mass tends to be larger than that of typical endometrial adenocarcinoma. It usually involves most of the endometrial surface.[121] In 25 percent of cases the tumor arises in an endometrial polyp.[120] Myometrial invasion is present in 60 percent of cases.

There are four histopathologic patterns including papillary, tubulocystic, glandular, and solid, and three cell types including clear, hobnail, and flattened or cuboidal.[120, 121] Most of these neoplasms contain more than one histopathologic pattern and more than one cell type, but usually one pattern predominates. The characteristic feature of the solid pattern is the presence of sheets of large polygonal tumor cells that have clear to slightly eosinophilic cytoplasm (Fig. 6–22). The nuclei are usually large, round to oval in shape, and often bizarre and hyperchromatic. Cell borders are distinct. The clear cytoplasm stains positive with periodic acid–Schiff and is partially resistant to diastase digestion. This indicates that both glycogen and mucin are present.[121] An occasional tumor contains lipid.[122] The tubulocystic pattern shows a combination of tubular and cystic spaces lined by the tumor cells. The tubular pattern may contain tumor, which varies from well to poorly differentiated. When cystic spaces are present they are frequently lined by flattened or

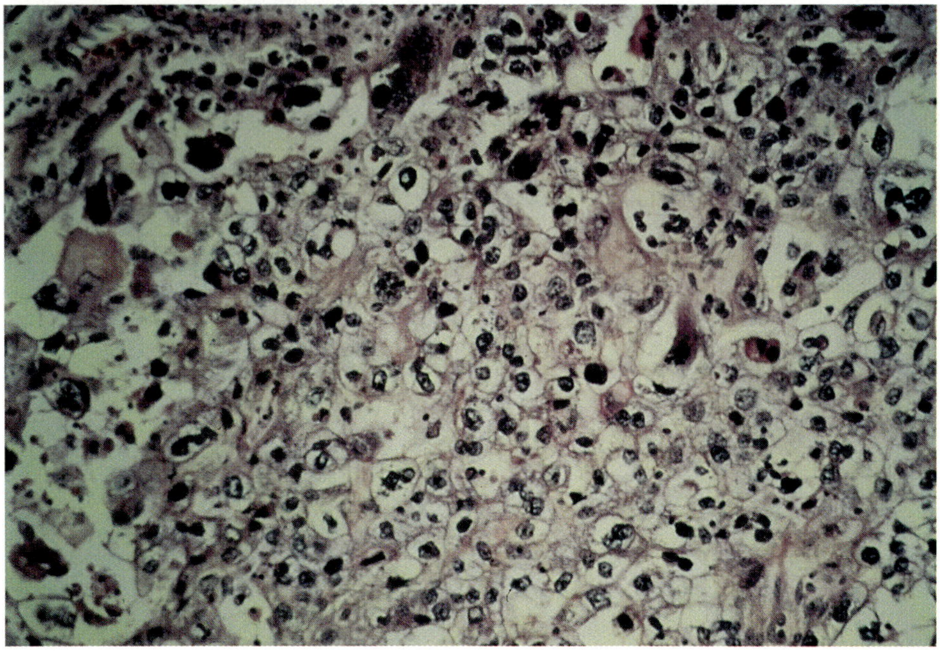

FIGURE 6-22
The solid pattern of clear cell endometrial adenocarcinoma is demonstrated. The cells have clear cytoplasm. The cell borders are distinct. There is marked nuclear pleomorphism.

cuboidal cells. Pink homogeneous or granular secretions are present within the gland lumens.[121] The papillary pattern demonstrates fronds of epithelial tumor cells that cover thin stalks of connective tissue. Hobnail cells are a prominent feature of this histopathologic pattern. The hobnail cells contain bulbous nuclei that project from the surface of the individual cell (Fig. 6–23). A typical hobnail cell nucleus is large with a sharp but often irregular margin. The chromatin tends to concentrate about the periphery of the nucleus.[120] Nucleoli are often large and conspicuous and may be multiple. Mitotic activity is usually brisk but may be variable.

The nuclear grade of clear cell carcinoma is usually high. A proposed nuclear grading system for clear cell carcinoma follows. Tumors that show the greatest uniformity of nuclei are grade 1. Tumors with little nuclear uniformity and large, irregular, and often multiple nucleoli are grade 3. Those with intermediate characteristics are grade 2.[120] A distinctive feature of clear cell adenocarcinoma is the presence of epithelial hyaline bodies in tumors with the papillary, tubulocystic, and glandular

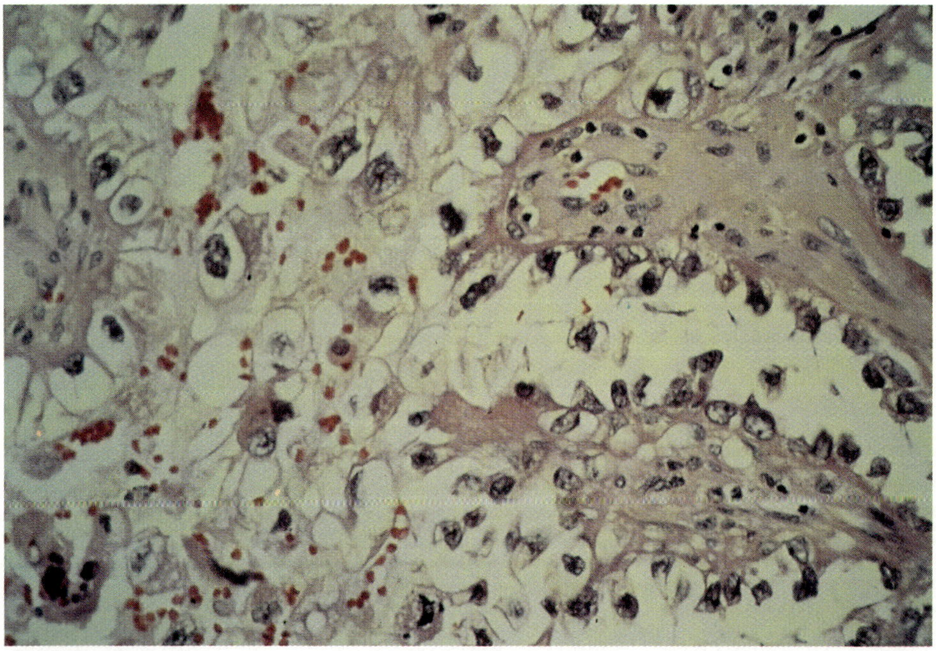

FIGURE 6-23
This clear cell endometrial carcinoma has both clear cells *(left)* and hobnail cells. The cytoplasm of the hobnail cells seems to have collapsed around the nucleus. The nuclei stick out toward the lumen.

patterns, they are present in two-thirds of these tumors.[120] Sometimes they stain lightly with eosin and resemble mucin-containing vacuoles. In tumors with the papillary pattern there may be a dense acellular hyalinization of the stalk of some of the fronds. This occurs around blood vessels or may be generalized. An inflammatory infiltrate may be present. Necrosis is present in half of the cases.

Myometrial invasion occurs in more than half of the cases and varies in depth from 5 to 100 percent of the myometrial thickness.[120, 121] Intravascular tumor invasion is uncommon and occurs in 5 percent of cases. The adjoining endometrium is hyperplastic in approximately one-third of cases and atrophic in the remainder. Peritoneal washings are positive in 5 to 15 percent of patients. Positive peritoneal cytologic findings show clusters of glandular-type cells with clear cytoplasm similar to those found in the endometrium. As in UPSC, pleomorphic and bizarre nuclei are common. The papillary pattern with hobnail cells is difficult at times to differentiate from UPSC. Sometimes these two histopathologic variants coexist.

Estrogen receptors and progesterone receptors are usually absent.[122] Patients with clear cell adenocarcinoma of the endometrium usually have advanced stage disease at diagnosis. This contributes to the poor prognosis associated with this histopathologic variant.

The cornerstone of therapy of endometrial clear cell adenocarcinoma is total abdominal hysterectomy and bilateral salpingo-oophorectomy plus surgical staging. Due to the high grade of most of these neoplasms and the frequent presence of deep myometrial invasion, most patients with this histopathologic variant of endometrial adenocarcinoma receive pelvic radiation. Tumor recurrence is common. The vagina is the most common site of recurrence. Long-term survival is similar to that of patients with UPSC. The 5-year survival rate of patients with this neoplasm has been reported to be between 35 and 60 percent.

Mucinous Adenocarcinoma

Mucinous adenocarcinoma is the least common type of endometrial adenocarcinoma. To make this diagnosis the adenocarcinoma must be predominantly mucinous and the mucin must be demonstrable in an intracytoplasmic location.[27] On gross examination this tumor appears similar to the typical endometrial adenocarcinoma. Polypoid lesions are common. Irregular crowded glands that contain one layer of columnar mucinous-type cells characterize this neoplasm. The cells are tall and have small regular nuclei at the base of the cell. These cells resemble the cells of normal endocervical epithelium. They frequently line papillary structures.[123] A prominent tufted appearance may be present in some areas. Pseudostratification to two or three cell layers may be present. Nuclear pleomorphism is minimal. Mitotic activity is scant. The stroma consists of spindle-shaped cells, thin-walled blood vessels, and scattered acute and chronic inflammatory cells. Foam cells are common. The stroma resembles endometrial-type stroma rather than the more fibrous endocervical stroma.

Mucicarmine stain is the easiest method of demonstrating intracytoplasmic mucin.[123] These cells also stain positive with periodic acid–Schiff and Alcian blue stains. Carcinoembryonic antigen (CEA) is also demonstrated in these cells with immunoperoxidase stains.[27]

Mucinous adenocarcinoma and endometrioid adenocarcinoma of the endometrium frequently occur together. A transition between the two cell types is usually observed when mucinous endometrial adenocarcinoma is admixed with typical endometrial adenocarcinoma. The areas with mucinous differentiation are usually on the endometrial surface. The adjacent uninvolved endometrium often contains varying degrees of endometrial hyperplasia.

Typical endometrial adenocarcinoma (i.e., endometrioid adenocarcinoma) frequently contains intraluminal mucin. The term mucin-rich adenocarcinoma serves to distinguish this neoplasm from a mucinous adenocarcinoma, which contains intracytoplasmic mucin. Minor foci of mucinous differentiation occur in 9 to 33 percent of typical endometrial adenocarcinomas.[123, 124]

Mucinous endometrial adenocarcinoma must be differentiated from endometrial extension of a primary endocervical adenocarcinoma. The following criteria help to establish the endometrial origin of the neoplasm: a transition between endometrioid adenocarcinoma and mucinous adenocarcinoma, areas of tufting, pseudostratification, atypical mucinous epithelium, and the identification of endometrial-type stroma within the mucinous adenocarcinoma.[124]

This histopathologic variant is usually low-grade and its prognosis is similar to that of other well-differentiated endometrial adenocarcinomas.

Rare Histopathologic Variants of Endometrial Carcinoma

Rare histopathologic variants of endometrial carcinoma include pure squamous cell carcinoma, verrucous squamous carcinoma, neuroendocrine carcinoma, and giant cell carcinoma. A review of the medical literature in English reveals over 30 reported cases of endometrial squamous cell carcinoma.[125] This histopathologic variant is associated with pyometra and cervical stenosis. The reported cases of pure squamous cell carcinoma of the endometrium have occurred in older women. Sheets of squamous epithelium replace the normal endometrium. The squamous epithelium may appear well differentiated and keratinized or poorly differentiated. The presence of intercellular bridges identifies the epithelium as squamous in a poorly differentiated tumor. An occasional endometrial gland may be seen trapped among the malignant squamous epithelium. Deep myometrial invasion and extrauterine extension are common findings. To render a diagnosis of pure squamous cell carcinoma of the endometrium the following criteria must be met: an adenocarcinoma is not present in the endometrium; the squamous carcinoma in the endometrium does not have a connection with the squamous epithelium of the cervix; and there is no squamous carcinoma of the cervix.[126] The differential diagnosis of squamous cell carcinoma of the endometrium includes poorly differentiated endometrial adenocarcinoma. However, intercellular bridges are not seen in an adenocarcinoma. Endometrial extension of a primary cervical neoplasm is another consideration. If a high-grade cervical intraepithelial lesion or invasive squamous cell carcinoma of the cervix with extension to the endometrium is present, by convention the neoplasm is considered primary in the cervix.

Verrucous carcinoma is a rare variant of squamous cell carcinoma that has unique clinical and pathologic characteristics. Its origin in the endometrium is extremely rare.[128] On gross examination the endometrium has a friable, pink or gray, papillary appearance. On microscopic examination replacement of the endometrium by superficial, well-differentiated sheets of squamous carcinoma is apparent; these sheets form wartlike papillary folds without fibrovascular cores. Superficial keratinization may occur. Focal superficial invasion into the myometrium may be seen. The tumor border is pushing rather than infiltrating. Some endometrial glands may show a transition from columnar epithelium to malignant squamous epithelium, possibly through subcylindric reserve cell hyperplasia.[128] Patients with this type of neoplasm seem to have a good prognosis.

A rare neoplasm that is more common in the cervix but may occur in the endometrium is the carcinoid tumor.[129] These neoplasms appear as a uniform population of small cells with oval to round nuclei and scant cytoplasm. Special stains identify the presence of neurosecretory granules in the cytoplasm.

Neoplasms that contain osteoclastic-type giant cells or syncytiotrophoblastic-type giant cells rarely occur in the endometrium. The former may exist together with a poorly differentiated adenocarcinoma. Immunocytochemical stains for human chorionic gonadotropin (hCG) may be helpful in identifying the latter.[129]

Mixed Carcinoma

Mixed carcinoma of the endometrium includes any histopathologic combination of the types discussed earlier. To qualify as a mixed carcinoma the second cell type must constitute at least 10 percent of the volume of the tumor as estimated from multiple tissue sections. The significance and prognosis of mixed endometrial carcinoma is unknown. Documentation in the medical literature of the clinical behavior of these neoplasms is lacking.

Adenocarcinoma Arising in the Lower Uterine Segment

Adenocarcinoma arising in the lower uterine segment deserves separate consideration because its clinical behavior is different from that of adenocarcinoma arising in the uterine fundus. Approximately 8 percent of endometrial neoplasms arise in the lower uterine segment.[93] Neoplasms that arise in this anatomic location have been called corpus et colli tumors. The mean age of patients with adenocarcinoma arising in the lower uterine segment is 49 years, with a range of 37 to 56 years. Most patients are premenopausal, and almost all have been pregnant.[130] Obesity, hypertension, nulliparity, and diabetes mellitus do not appear to be risk factors. These epidemiologic findings are different from those observed in patients with typical endometrial adenocarcinoma.[130] Almost all patients present with abnormal uterine bleeding. Seventy-five percent of women with endometrial adenocarcinoma in this anatomic location have an abnormal Papanicolaou smear, which in most cases has been interpreted as adenocarcinoma. In some patients the abnormal cervical cytology shows either atypical glandular cells or cells suggestive of a squamous lesion.

These tumors range in size between 1.8 cm and 7.7 cm, with a mean of 3.2 cm. Twenty-five percent appear as ulcers and 75 percent as nodules or polyps. Superficial necrosis is common. On microscopic examination one of several histopathologic patterns is observed. Over half appear as solid sheets of cells, one-third have tubules or glands, and approximately 10 percent are papillary. The majority are high grade. Only 16 percent are architectural grade 1. Squamous differentiation is present in 75 percent. In 75 percent of cases there is lymphatic space involvement.[130] The adjacent endometrium is usually hyperplastic or has atypical glands. Myometrial invasion is common. In 50 percent of cases the tumor invades to the outer half of the myometrium. Because of its anatomic location, the pattern of spread of this tumor has features in common with both cervical and fundal neoplasms. Metastases to lymph nodes at the time of initial surgery are present in one-third of patients.[93] Approximately one-third of these neoplasms recur.[130] Pelvic recurrence is less common than distant recurrence.

This tumor may be difficult to differentiate from a primary endocervical adenocarcinoma with extension to the lower uterine segment. In primary endocervical adenocarcinoma, adjacent adenocarcinoma in situ is usually seen.

The lower uterine segment location of an endometrial adenocarcinoma is seldom known preoperatively. After total abdominal hysterectomy, bilateral salpingo-oophorectomy, peritoneal lavage, and surgical staging most patients receive adjuvant postoperative radiation because of the presence of high-risk histopathologic findings. These include deep myometrial invasion, lymph node metastases, and poorly differentiated tumor. The overall 5-year survival rate for patients with endometrial adenocarcinoma in this location is 62 percent compared with over 70 percent for patients with typical endometrial adenocarcinoma.[130]

Adenocarcinoma Arising in Adenomyosis

Adenocarcinoma arising in adenomyosis without involvement of the surface endometrium is rare.[131] Adenocarcinoma arising in adenomyosis was found in 3 percent of patients who underwent hysterectomy for endometrial adenocarcinoma.[89a] A diagnosis of adenocarcinoma in adenomyosis is made if the adenomyotic foci are found more than one high-power microscope field below the basal endometrium and such foci are not connected to the endometrial adenocarcinoma. In the focus of adenomyosis a transition from benign to malignant is observed, and normal endometrial stroma accompanies the epithelium (Fig. 6–24). The prognosis of adenocarcinoma arising in adenomyosis depends on the surgical stage, histopathologic grade, and depth of invasion of the synchronous adenocarcinoma of the surface endometrium. However, patients with adenocarcinoma arising in adenomyosis tend to have stage I disease, well- to moderately differentiated tumors, and minimal invasion of the myometrium by the synchronous endometrial adenocarcinoma.[89a, 131a] The cases reported to date have had an excellent prognosis even when the adenocarcinoma arising in adenomyosis was deep in the myometrium.[89a, 131a]

Adenocarcinoma Arising in Endometrial Polyps

Adenocarcinoma occurs in approximately 1 in 200 endometrial polyps, and conversely, polyps are found in 12 to 34 percent of uteri that have endo-

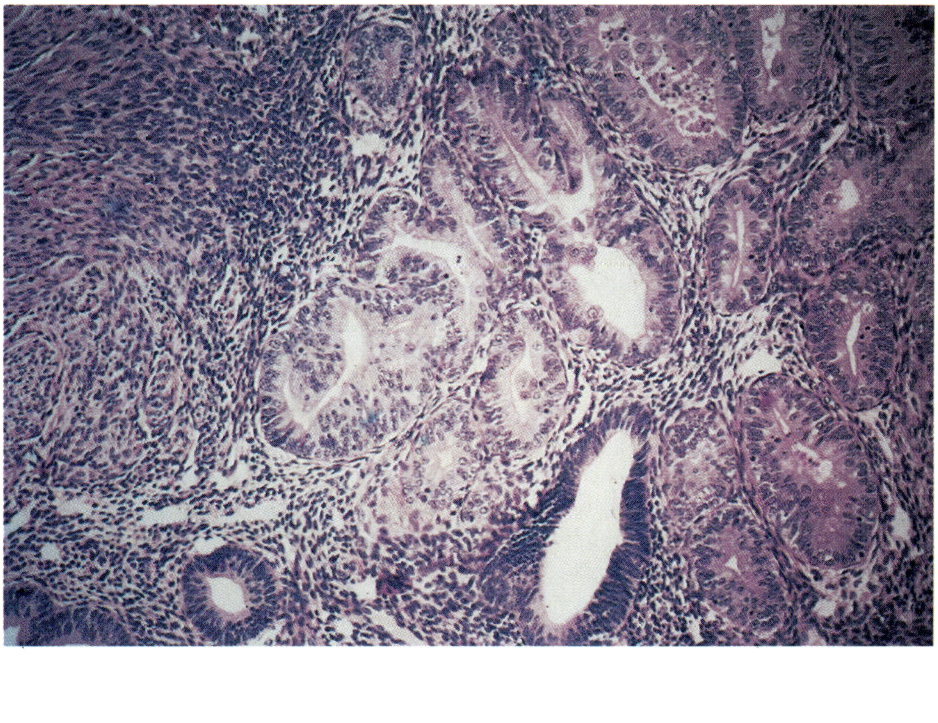

FIGURE 6–24
This is an adenocarcinoma arising in a focus of adenomyosis. Normal myometrium is seen *(top left)*. Normal endometrial glands and stroma are seen *(bottom left and center)*. The hyperplastic, complex, crowded glands within endometrial stroma are consistent with grade 1 endometrioid adenocarcinoma *(center)*. This area was found deep in the myometrium.

metrial carcinoma.[132, 133] Among women who had a previous diagnosis of endometrial polyps the risk that endometrial carcinoma will develop at a later time is 3.5 percent.[134] The histopathology of carcinoma arising in an endometrial polyp is variable. The surrounding endometrium may be atrophic, normal, or hyperplastic. Unless the neoplasm invades the stalk of the polyp or the myometrium, the prognosis is excellent.

The treatment for adenocarcinoma arising in and limited to an endometrial polyp is total abdominal hysterectomy, bilateral salpingo-oophorectomy, and surgical pathologic staging. In the young woman in whom preservation of reproductive function is strongly desired, one may opt to follow the patient closely after polypectomy, provided the neoplasm did not invade the stalk of the polyp and there is no involvement of the surrounding endometrium. This requires hysteroscopic and histopathologic evaluation of the entire endometrial cavity. There is one report of endometrial carcinoma arising in a large atypical polypoid uterine adenomyoma.[135] It was a poorly differentiated adenosquamous carcinoma associated with extensive adenomyosis. Metastases to paraaortic lymph nodes were present.

General Clinical Features

There appear to be two distinct clinical types of endometrial carcinoma. Type I has a good prognosis and arises in a background of hyperplasia in perimenopausal women. Type II has a poorer prognosis, occurs in older postmenopausal women, and is not associated with hyperplasia.[76, 136] The former has an association with endocrine and metabolic disturbances. Findings in this group include a history of anovulatory bleeding and infertility; a delayed onset of menopause; an estrogenic vaginal smear in the postmenopausal period; the presence of obesity, hyperlipidemia, diabetes, and hypertension; the existence of estrogen-producing lesions of the ovary; and the presence of endometrial hyperplasia, leiomyomas, and adenomyosis.[41, 76] Type I endometrial carcinomas are usually of low histopathologic grade and have less myometrial invasion, fewer lymph node metastases, lower surgical stage, and a better 5-year survival than those considered to be type II.[76] Type II neoplasms are unusual histopathologic variants, have a high nuclear grade with aneuploid DNA content, and deeply invade the myometrium.[137] There is a good correlation between nuclear grade 3 and aneuploidy.[138] Aneuploid tumors are more likely to recur, particularly outside the pelvis.[88]

Prognostic Variables in Endometrial Carcinoma

A number of variables have been identified as having prognostic significance in patients with endometrial carcinoma. These include a variety of clinical, surgical, and microscopic findings. Clinical indicators that have an association with prognosis include age at diagnosis[83, 105, 114, 139–141] and race.[76, 136] Although there is an epidemiologic association with obesity, hypertension, and diabetes mellitus these are not useful predictors of outcome. Surgical and pathologic findings of value in determining prognosis include the presence of extrauterine disease,[82, 85, 141] the depth of myometrial invasion,[86, 105, 114] tumor size,[142] lymph node metastases,[93, 94] gross cervical involvement,[142] histopathologic type,[97, 100, 116, 117, 119–121] histopathologic grade,[82, 86, 94] associated endometrial hyperplasia,[136, 143] peritoneal cytology,[144–151] vascular invasion,[83, 152] estrogen and progesterone receptor status of the neoplasm,[153–160] HER-2/*neu* expression,[83a] and flow cytometry and morphometric analysis.[96, 137, 161–163] The depth of the endometrial cavity[163] and the histopathologic findings on endocervical curettage[90, 91] may also be useful in predicting outcome in some cases. Neoplasms that involve the lower uterine segment tend to behave more aggressively, as discussed earlier.[130] We will consider the impact of each of these variables on prognosis, independently and in association.

Age

After exclusion of patients with clear cell and papillary serous tumors, age is a good predictor of biologic behavior in endometrial carcinoma.[164] In some studies, age at diagnosis is the single most important clinical determinant of survival.[82] This is true even after correcting for the fact that 10 to 15 percent of women with endometrial carcinoma die of unrelated causes. Endometrial carcinomas in younger women tend to be low-grade, stage I tumors with minimal myometrial invasion. These neoplasms typically develop in a background of endometrial hyperplasia. Postmenopausal women tend to have tumors with unfavorable histopathologic types and more advanced stage, and they have poorer survival rates.[76] Grade 3 endometrial carcinomas are uncommon in women under the age of 50 years.[165] In women under the age of 60, 91 percent of endometrial carcinomas are confined to the uterus and have only superficial myometrial invasion. These characteristics are found in 61 percent of women 60 years of age or older.[165]

Race

Race has never been considered a significant prognostic variable for endometrial carcinoma. However, African-American women tend to have tumors of higher grade and higher stage, and they have poorer survival rates than white women.[76] Also, a larger proportion of African-American women have unfavorable histopathologic types, particularly papillary serous neoplasms.[99a, 100] The survival rate for African-American women with endometrial endometrioid adenocarcinoma with or without squamous differentiation is 42 percent, which is considerably lower than the 80 percent survival rate for this tumor in white women.[82]

Uterine Depth

Two factors that are not part of the current surgical staging system but may have clinical importance are the depth of the endometrial cavity and the endocervical curettage findings. The depth of the uterine cavity correlates with nodal metastases. Approximately 45 percent of all endometrial carcinomas occur in uteri that sound to greater than 8 cm.[85] This corresponds to stage IB in the clinical classification system. For each histopathologic grade of disease, the probability of tumor spread to the pelvic and paraaortic lymph nodes increases as much as twofold when the uterus measures more than 8 cm in depth.

Endocervical Curettings

Before the current surgical staging system was used, endocervical curettage was the clinical tool that, in the absence of gross cervical involvement, differentiated clinical stage I from stage II disease. Positive findings on endocervical curettage frequently proved misleading because no endocervical tumor was found in many of these patients. At present we do not perform endocervical curettage during evaluation of the patient with endometrial carcinoma unless the patient is not a candidate for surgical staging. If the patient is not a surgical candidate, endocervical curettage is performed for clinical staging. If a gross lesion is seen on the cervix, a punch biopsy is obtained.

Surgical Staging

Disease stage is a well-known prognostic indicator. However, clinical staging has the disadvantage of assigning too low a stage in 10 to 20 percent of patients with endometrial carcinoma[85, 166, 166a, 167] (Table 6–6). Except in the recent literature, most published reports on endometrial carcinoma refer to the clinical stage. The reported 5-year survival rate of patients with clinical stage I endometrial carcinoma varies from 70 to 90 percent. This decreases to 50 to 77 percent for patients with stage II disease, 27 to 30 percent for stage III disease, and 0 to 10 percent for stage IV disease.[158–169] In a large study of 865 cases, there were no cancer-related deaths in patients with clinical stage I, grade 1 endometrial endometrioid adenocarcinoma with or without squamous differentiation.[82]

The current surgical staging system subdivides stage II endometrial adenocarcinoma into stage IIA (i.e., endocervical gland involvement only) and stage IIB (i.e., involvement of the cervical stroma). Approximately 10 percent of patients with endometrial carcinoma have surgical stage II disease.[166a, 170] In one study, 60 percent of patients with surgical stage II endometrial adenocarcinoma had involvement only of the glandular epithelium. None of these women developed recurrence. Of the remaining 40 percent who had surgical stage IIB disease, two thirds developed recurrence. All the recurrences were extrapelvic.[170] Although endocervical stromal invasion is associated with a poorer prognosis, involvement of only the endocervical glands by endometrial carcinoma is associated with a clinical behavior similar to that of surgical stage I disease.

The presence of gross cervical involvement is associated with a poorer prognosis.[142] When treated with external beam radiotherapy, intracavitary application of cesium followed by extrafascial hysterectomy, and bilateral salpingo-oophorectomy, the median survival time for women without gross cervical disease is 94.2 months compared to 29.1 months for women with gross cervical disease.[142]

TABLE 6–6.
Comparison of Clinical and Surgical Staging in Endometrial Carcinoma

		Surgical Stage			
Clinical Stage		*Stage I*	*Stage II*	*Stage III*	*Stage IV*
I	135	111	2	16	6
II	19	6	5	5	3
III	3			2	1
IV	12				12
Total	169	117	7	23	22

From Vardi JR, Tadros GH, Anselmo MT, Rafla S: The value of exploratory laparotomy in patients with endometrial carcinoma according to the new International Federation of Gynecology and Obstetrics staging. Obstet Gynecol 1992; 80: 204–208, with permission from The American College of Obstetricians and Gynecologists.

Gross cervical involvement commonly coexists with deep myometrial invasion, another indicator of worsened prognosis.[171] In the past, women with cervical extension of endometrial carcinoma received external and internal radiation followed by an extrafascial hysterectomy.[142] At present, we reserve this approach for patients who have gross cervical involvement by endometrial carcinoma.

The presence of residual tumor in the postradiation hysterectomy specimen does not seem to be associated with a worsened prognosis.[172] In one study, women undergoing a hysterectomy after radiation therapy for endometrial carcinoma who had no residual tumor had a recurrence rate of 25 percent, whereas patients with residual tumor who had had prior radiation therapy had a 21 percent recurrence rate.[172]

Extrauterine disease is an important predictor of clinical behavior in endometrial carcinoma. The presence or absence of extrauterine disease is an integral part of the surgical staging system. However, complete surgical staging is impossible to accomplish in some women due to age, obesity, or medical contraindications.[167] Frequent sites of extrauterine spread include pelvic and paraaortic lymph nodes, the uterine adnexae, and the peritoneum.[85] Metastases to these sites may be missed if surgical staging is not performed.[166, 167]

Uterine adnexal involvement with metastatic endometrial carcinoma can be a difficult histopathologic diagnosis. The pathologist must differentiate between metastatic disease and synchronous primaries (i.e., ovary and endometrium). Although the ovary is a frequent site of metastasis from endometrial carcinoma, the ovary and endometrium are the most frequent primary sites in patients with synchronous genital cancers.[173a] In more than 50 percent of cases both tumors are of the same histopathologic type, endometrioid adenocarcinoma.[173b, 173c] The presence of a large diffuse tumor mass in the ovary and a well-differentiated endometrioid adenocarcinoma in the endometrium without myometrial invasion suggests synchronous primaries. Other combinations are more difficult to diagnose. The 5-year survival rate of patients with synchronous stage I ovarian and stage I endometrial carcinomas is approximately 90 percent,[173b, 173c] whereas it is approximately 30 percent for aggressively managed patients with stage IIIA endometrial adenocarcinoma (i.e., metastasis to the uterine adnexa).[173a]

Depth of Myometrial Invasion

The depth of myometrial invasion is one of the most important variables in predicting the clinical behavior of endometrial carcinoma.[86, 105, 114, 164] The current surgical staging system recognizes the importance of this finding (see Table 6–3). Approximately 75 percent of patients with stage I endometrial adenocarcinoma have no myometrial invasion (stage Ia) or less than 50 percent myometrial invasion (stage IB).[166a]

Accurate preoperative evaluation of the depth of myometrial invasion has been elusive. Recently, the use of magnetic resonance imaging (MRI) to predict the depth of myometrial invasion has proved reliable. MRI accurately identified all but one of 18 cases with histopathologically proven deep myometrial invasion.[173] Hysterosalpingography (HSG) may be another useful tool in the preoperative evaluation of patients with endometrial carcinoma.[174] There is concern that HSG causes transtubal transport of cancer cells into the peritoneal cavity. However, there is no evidence that this has an impact on clinical outcome.[174]

With the current surgical staging system, gross examination of the specimen is important. Because the depth of myometrial invasion correlates with incidence of nodal metastases, an intraoperative estimate of the depth of myometrial invasion will help the gynecologic surgeon weigh the risks against the benefits of performing a paraaortic node dissection.[175] Visual examination of the cut uterus accurately identifies the depth of invasion in over 85 percent of patients.[175, 176] Gross examination of the uterine specimen becomes less reliable as the grade of adenocarcinoma increases. With grade 1 neoplasms, the depth of myometrial invasion as measured by gross examination is accurate in 87 to 91 percent of cases.[175, 176] In neoplasms that proved to be grade 3, the depth of invasion as estimated by gross examination correlated with microscopic examination in only 31 percent of cases in one study[176] and in 71 percent in another.[175]

Recurrences occur in 9 to 15 percent of patients with endometrial adenocarcinomas clinically confined to the uterus.[86, 164, 168] The depth of myometrial invasion correlates positively with the rate of recurrence (Fig. 6–25). In one study, less than 10 percent of patients with tumors that invaded the myometrium to less than half its thickness experienced a recurrence.[168] In contrast, recurrences occurred in 30 percent of patients with endometrial adenocarcinomas with more than 50 percent myometrial invasion. Sixty-five percent of endometrial adenocarcinomas that recur are poorly differentiated neoplasms with deep myometrial invasion.[86] Deep myometrial invasion is also a predictor of aortic node metastases.[87] Histopathologic tumor grade and depth of myometrial invasion appear to

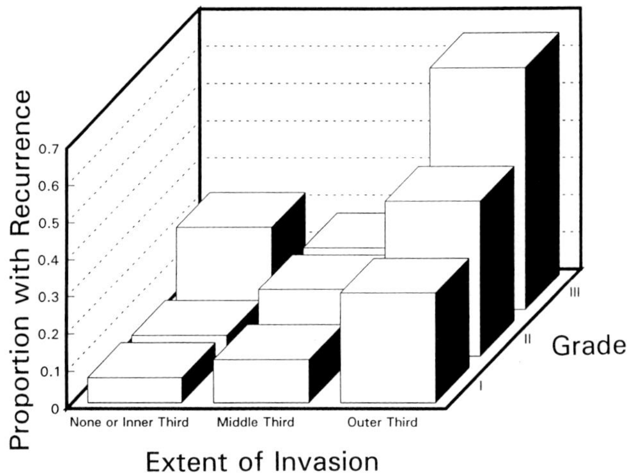

FIGURE 6-25
This graph compares tumor recurrence versus tumor grade and depth of myometrial invasion in patients with endometrial adenocarcinoma. (From Podczaski , Kaminski P, Gurski K, et al: Detection and patterns of treatment failure in 300 consecutive cases of "early" endometrial cancer after primary surgery. Gynecol Oncol 1992;47:323–327.)

be the most important factors in predicting recurrence from endometrial adenocarcinoma.[85]

Tumor Size

Tumor size has also been found to be an important prognostic factor in endometrial carcinoma.[141a] In a study of 142 patients with clinical stage I endometrial carcinoma, tumor size was found to correlate with survival and rate of metastasis.[141a] The most important clinical correlate is that seen in patients with grade 2 endometrial carcinomas with less than one-half myometrial invasion. No lymph node metastases were found if the tumor measured less than 2 cm; but 18 percent had nodal metastases when the tumor was larger than 2 cm.

Lymph Node Metastases

The patient with uterine cancer and pelvic or paraaortic lymph node metastases has at least stage IIIC disease (see Table 6–3). More than 10 percent of patients with endometrial carcinoma have occult lymph node metastases that will remain undetected unless lymph node dissection or lymph node sampling is an integral part of the surgical procedure.[166] The presence of lymph node metastasis in patients with endometrial carcinoma is associated with unfavorable histopathologic subtypes, high tumor grade, and deep myometrial invasion. Stage I, grade 1 endometrioid endometrial adenocarcinoma with myometrial invasion limited to the inner third of the myometrium has limited metastatic potential.[85, 86, 162, 164, 166] As any of these factors changes, the frequency of lymph node metastases increases. Surgical pathologic staging of endometrial cancer suggests the following as risk factors for lymph node metastases. In tumors confined to the corpus (i.e., stage I) there is a negligible risk of lymph node metastases (1) if the cancer is limited to the endometrium (i.e., no myometrial invasion) regardless of histopathologic grade; (2) if myometrial invasion is confined to the inner third in grade 1 or 2 tumors; and (3) if a grade 1 tumor invades to the middle third of the myometrium.[86, 93] Conversely, a substantial risk for lymph node metastases exists if examination of the uterine specimen identifies a grade 3 tumor with any depth of myometrial invasion, deep myometrial invasion by cancer of any grade, or vascular space involvement.[86, 93] Tumor extension to the cervical stroma or adnexa is also associated with an increased frequency of lymph node metastases. Although most studies have examined the presence of pelvic node metastasis, studies addressing the issue of paraaortic node metastasis have reached essentially the same conclusions. Patients who have well-differentiated tumors are at low risk for paraaortic node metastases. With grade 2 tumors the risk is 13.6 percent, and with grade 3 tumors the risk is 37.5 percent.[177] The paraaortic nodes are negative for metastasis when myometrial invasion is absent. They are positive in 4.5 percent of cases in which there is superficial myometrial invasion and in 45.5 percent of cases in which deep myometrial invasion exists.[177]

Histopathologic Cell Type

Endometrial carcinomas may be divided into favorable and unfavorable histopathologic cell types. Sixty-six to 77 percent of all endometrial carcinomas have the typical endometrioid appearance.[78, 177–179] Another 14 to 24 percent are well-differentiated endometrioid adenocarcinomas with squamous differentiation. The remainder include high-grade adenosquamous neoplasms, 6 to 11 percent; serous neoplasms, 4 to 9 percent; clear cell tumors, 1 to 3 percent, and secretory carcinomas, 0 to 2 percent.[78, 177–179] Histopathologic variants associated with poor prognosis include clear cell, papillary serous, and poorly differentiated neoplasms with or without squamous differentiation.[97, 100, 116, 117, 119–121, 165] In disease clinically confined to the uterus, the histopathologic cell type correlates with the frequency of recurrence.[169] Table 6–7 presents the frequency of various histopathologic cell types and 5-year survival rate for patients with stage I endometrial carcinoma.[78]

TABLE 6–7.
Frequency of Histopathologic Cell Types and 5-Year Survival Rate of Patients with Stage I Endometrial Carcinoma

Histopathologic Type	Frequency	Survival
Adenocarcinoma	66%	88%
Adenocarcinoma with squamous differentiation	16%	91%
Adenosquamous	5%	62%
Serous	8%	63%
Clear cell	3%	43%
Secretory	2%	89%

Modified from Fanning J, Evans MC, Peters AJ, et al: Endometrial adenocarcinoma histologic subtypes: Clinical and pathologic profiles. Gynecol Oncol 1989; 32: 288–291.

Histopathologic Grade

Histopathologic grade and depth of myometrial invasion (see Fig. 6–25) are strongly associated with prognosis in endometrial carcinoma.[22, 85, 86] Both high tumor grade and deep myometrial invasion increase the risk of tumor recurrence. After exclusion of patients with clear cell and papillary serous tumors, the worst survival rates for clinical stage I endometrial carcinoma occur in patients who have grade 3 tumor, myometrial invasion of more than one-third, vascular space involvement, or occult cervical stromal invasion.[165] Poorly differentiated neoplasms account for 57, 65, and 90 percent of endometrial carcinomas of surgical stage II, III, and IV, respectively.[167] A substantial risk of pelvic and paraaortic lymph node metastasis exists if the surgical pathologic study of the uterus identifies any myometrial invasion for grade 3 tumor, or deep myometrial invasion by cancer of any grade.[30, 93] Recurrences occur in 65 percent of patients who have grade 3 neoplasms that invade to the outer third of the myometrium.[86] Studies that specifically address paraaortic node metastasis suggest that patients who have well-differentiated endometrial carcinoma are at low risk for metastasis to this site. This risk increases to 37.5 percent in patients with poorly differentiated neoplasms.[180]

Associated Endometrial Hyperplasia

When hyperplasia is admixed with endometrial carcinoma in the biopsy, curettage, or hysterectomy specimen, the histopathologic features of the accompanying carcinoma are generally favorable. The surgical stage tends to be low, and survival rates are significantly better.[136] The carcinoma that develops in a background of endometrial hyperplasia is usually a well-differentiated endometrioid adenocarcinoma. These tumors tend to occur in younger women. Uterine papillary serous carcinoma and endometrial clear cell carcinoma rarely develop in a background of hyperplasia; they tend to occur in older women and frequently present in an advanced surgical stage with deep myometrial invasion.[76]

Peritoneal Cytology

Positive peritoneal cytology has an adverse effect on prognosis of endometrial cancer. Obtaining peritoneal fluid for cytologic examination is part of the surgical staging of endometrial carcinoma. The process by which the malignant cells gain access to the peritoneal cavity is unknown.[181] Valid postulates include tubal transportation enhanced by preoperative uterine manipulation or instrumentation, invasion to the uterine serosa, and lymphatic spread to peritoneal surfaces. The possibility of synchronous multifocal disease should also be entertained.

Peritoneal cytologic findings that are positive for endometrial adenocarcinoma are groups of obviously cytologically malignant cells. These cells are found in clusters and have large nuclei with prominent nucleoli and clumped chromatin (Fig. 6–26). They must be differentiated from reactive mesothelial cells, which may also have enlarged nuclei with some atypia and may occur in clusters and strips (Fig. 6–27). Comparison of the cells in the cytology specimen with those in the resected tumor is the best method of making this distinction. If radiation therapy has been given prior to hysterectomy the mesothelium will be even more reactive and atypical in appearance. Care should be taken never to make a diagnosis of malignancy on the basis of a peritoneal lavage specimen unless the tumor cells are the same as those seen in the uterus. There may be a few cases in which the peritoneal cytologic findings remain merely suspicious and are not definitely positive for adenocarcinoma.[181]

The prevalence of positive peritoneal cytologic findings in all stages of endometrial carcinoma ranges from 6 to 22 percent.[144, 145, 149–151] Approximately 5 percent of women who have clinical stage I endometrial adenocarcinoma have positive peritoneal cytologic findings,[144, 148] but this figure may be as high as 17 percent.[151] Forty-five percent of patients with a positive peritoneal cytologic examination have high-grade tumors and extrauterine disease.[144] In contrast, these are present in only 2 percent of patients with negative peritoneal cyto-

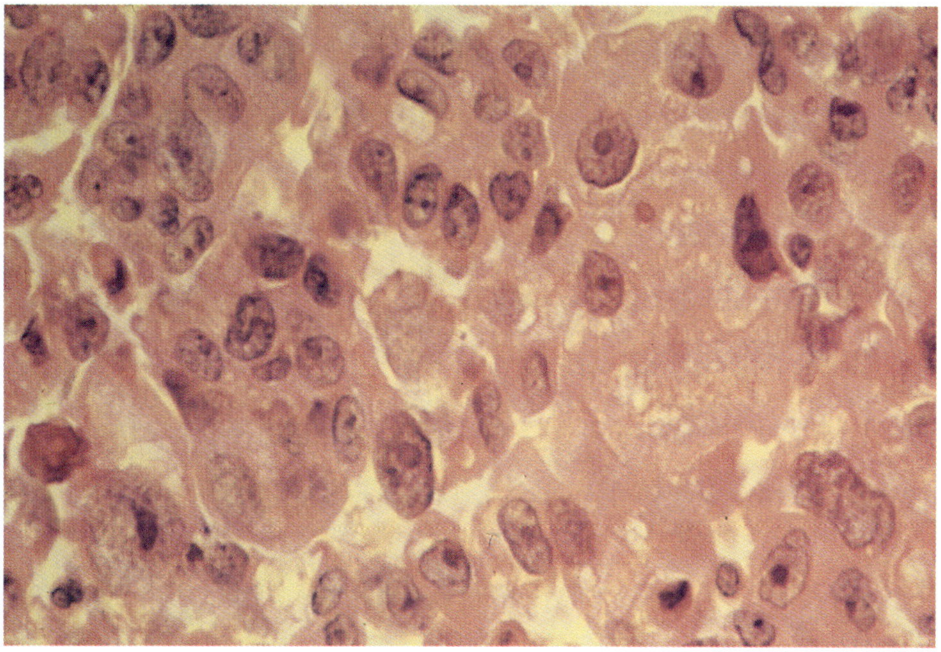

FIGURE 6-26
This is a cell block cytologic preparation of peritoneal washings obtained from a patient who had endometrial adenocarcinoma. The cells are large with pleomorphic nuclei. Macronucleoli are present. The chromatin pattern is variable, and the cellular groupings are disorganized. These features are diagnostic of malignancy.

logic findings. The clinical and surgical stage is likely to be greater than stage II in patients with positive peritoneal cytologic features. Positive peritoneal cytologic findings are present in 19.5 percent of patients with clinical stage II disease, 68.7 percent of those with stage III disease, and 85.7 percent of these in stage IV.[151] Nine to 13 percent of patients with a grade 1 tumor have positive peritoneal cytologic features, 17 to 21 percent of those with a grade 2 lesion, and 32 percent of those with a grade 3 tumor.[150–151] Positive peritoneal cytologic findings correlate with the depth of myometrial invasion in some studies. Peritoneal cytologic features were positive in 13 percent of cases with superficial or no myometrial invasion compared with 34 percent of cases with deep myometrial invasion in one study.[151]

Recurrence is seen in 17 to 50 percent of women who have endometrial carcinoma and positive peritoneal cytologic findings as the only indication of extrauterine disease.[148–151] The site of recurrence in patients with positive peritoneal cytologic

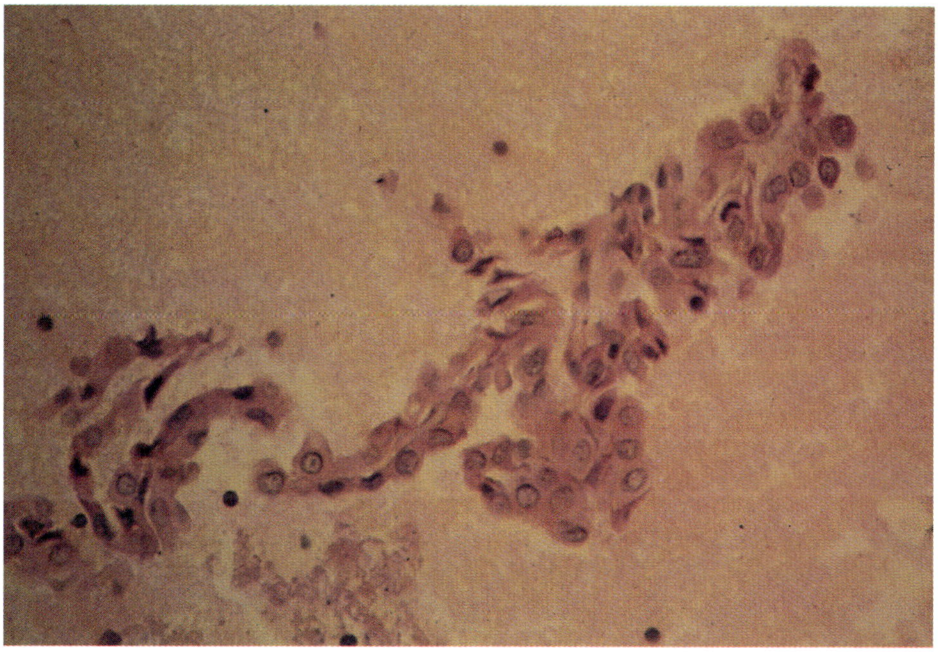

FIGURE 6-27
This cell block cytologic preparation shows strips of reactive mesothelium lifted from the peritoneum by peritoneal lavage. There is minimal nuclear variability. No macronucleoli are seen. There is an orderly arrangement of cells forming a structure that could be confused with a papillary fragment rather than a strip.

findings favors the upper abdomen (87.2 percent) rather than the pelvis (12.8 percent).[151] More than half of patients with positive peritoneal cytologic findings remain disease free.[151] Patients with uterine papillary serous carcinoma have an increased frequency of positive peritoneal cytologic features.[144] An analysis of poor prognostic factors in endometrial carcinoma, including grade 3, deep myometrial invasion, tumor size greater than 2 cm, lymph node metastasis, presence of extrauterine disease, and positive peritoneal cytologic examination, showed that the presence of positive peritoneal cytologic findings had no relation to the length of time to disease recurrence.[150] Other studies suggest that positive peritoneal cytologic findings, in the absence of other poor prognostic factors, are not associated with a worse prognosis.[87, 144] A negative peritoneal cytologic examination, however, is a good positive predictor of disease-free survival.[151] Nonetheless, 3 to 9 percent of patients with negative peritoneal cytologic examinations experience a recurrence of endometrial carcinoma.[148, 150, 151] In one study, positive peritoneal cytologic findings had no influence on survival when there was no extrauterine tumor.[83a] The 5-year survival rate for patients with extrauterine disease and negative peritoneal cytologic findings was 73 percent, but it was 13 percent if cytologic findings were positive. All the recurrences in the latter group occurred at distant sites, which suggests the need for systemic therapy.

Vascular Invasion

The identification of lymphatic or vascular space involvement by endometrial carcinoma is uncommon. Capillary-like space involvement is seen in 15 to 26 percent of these neoplasms.[85] Recurrence of endometrial carcinoma may reflect a failure to detect lymphatic space involvement at the time of original treatment.[83] When vascular invasion is present, the risk of pelvic lymph node metastasis increases fourfold, and the risk of paraaortic node metastasis doubles.[83, 85, 163] Vascular invasion-associated changes (VIAC) have been recently identified as an important prognostic variable in stage I endometrioid endometrial adenocarcinoma.[83, 83a] VIAC is defined as the presence of vascular invasion or perivascular lymphocytic infiltrates in the myometrium. The combination of VIAC and depth of myometrial invasion is a good predictor of survival in this group of patients. If neither VIAC nor myometrial invasion is present, the survival rate is 95 percent.[83] If VIAC and deep myometrial invasion are both present, the survival rate drops to 35 percent.[83] VIAC also correlates with tumor DNA ploidy.[163]

Estrogen and Progesterone Receptor Status

The quantity of estrogen and progesterone receptors in endometrial cancer varies; they are usually present in smaller concentrations than in normal cycling endometrium.[182] The presence of hormone receptors correlates with tumor grade. Receptors are present less frequently in poorly differentiated tumors.[153, 158] The literature on estrogen receptor (ER) and progesterone receptor (PR) in neoplastic endometrium is difficult to understand owing to different definitions of what constitutes the presence of receptors. For ER, 5 to 100 fmol/mg protein[154] and for PR, 10 to 50 fmol/mg protein defines the presence of receptors (i.e., receptor positive).[153, 154] Receptor status is independent of other factors known to be associated with prognosis. ER status does not correlate well with prognosis, but the absence of PR is associated with a poor prognosis.[153] Fifty-seven to 76 percent of endometrial carcinomas are both ER and PR positive.[153, 155] The majority of tumors that are ER and PR positive occur in obese women.[153] On the other hand, 17 to 24 percent of endometrial carcinomas are both ER and PR negative.[153, 155] There is a distinct survival difference between patients with receptor-positive tumors and those with receptor-negative tumors. Receptor status correlates with clinical stage and histopathologic grade but not with the depth of myometrial invasion. Sixty-eight percent of well-differentiated, 68 percent of moderately differentiated, and 25 percent of poorly differentiated neoplasms are ER and PR positive. The 5-year survival rate for patients with disease that is clinically confined to the uterus is better in tumors that are ER and PR positive (86 percent) than in tumors that are ER and PR negative (67 percent) or ER positive and PR negative (52 percent).[156, 160] Patients with tumors that are ER negative and PR positive had a 5-year survival rate of 88 percent.[156] Therefore, PR status is a significant prognostic factor. In some studies it is second in importance to clinical stage.[155] Fifty percent of patients with ER- and PR-negative endometrial carcinomas (all stages) die within 12 months.[153] Patients with endometrial carcinoma without lymph node metastasis who die within 12 months of the diagnosis have ER and PR negative tumors.[153] The presence of lymph node metastasis with ER- and PR-negative tumor identifies a group of patients who respond particularly poorly to treatment.[153]

Immunocytochemical analysis of sex steroid receptors is possible in paraffin-embedded, formalin-fixed tissue. Immunocytochemical and biochemical determination of ER and PR status in formalin-fixed tissue correlates positively with survival.[155] Scoring of the immunocytochemically stained tissue relies on two objective findings: the intensity of the nuclear stain and the percentage of stained cells.[155] The advantage of this technique is that the assay is determined directly on malignant cells only, whereas the chemical assay is performed on a weighed piece of tissue and the results may be skewed by nontumor tissue.

Oncogene Expression

The HER-2/*neu* oncogene codes for a specific cell-surface glycoprotein similar to the human growth factor receptor. Immunocytochemical staining for HER-2/*neu* correlates inversely with progression-free survival and overall survival.[83a] The 5-year progression-free survival rate is 56 percent for patients whose tumor stains strongly for HER-2/*neu* compared to 95 percent for patients whose tumors show minimal or no staining. For patients with surgical stage I disease, strong staining is associated with a 62 percent 5-year progression-free survival rate compared to 97 percent for those with minimal or no staining.[182a]

Flow Cytometry and Morphometric Analysis

DNA ploidy and nuclear morphometry do not seem to add additional prognostic information that is useful in distinguishing high-risk and low-risk endometrial carcinomas. The relationship between morphometry and clinical grading is very good. Pathologists can accurately estimate the proportion of endometrial tumors arranged in a solid or glandular pattern.[108, 161] Morphometric assessment of the proportion of undifferentiated cells lining the gland lumens has not been shown to improve the accuracy of prediction of clinical outcome beyond conventional architectural grading.[161]

Features of endometrial carcinoma cells suggestive of a poor prognosis include the mean shortest nuclear axis and the DNA index (the ratio of DNA content of cells being analyzed to DNA content of normal control cells; a diploid DNA index is 1 ± 0.1). These two features correlate positively with the depth of myometrial invasion and poor outcome.[88,96]

Measurement of DNA content by flow cytometry in endometrial cancer may be useful for supplementing traditional strong prognostic indicators such as age, tumor grade, and depth of myometrial invasion. Aneuploid tumors are those that have a DNA index of more than 1.1 or less than 0.9. Aneuploidy correlates positively with the presence of metastatic disease. Forty-six percent of surgical stage III and IV neoplasms are aneuploid, and 69 percent have an S-phase fraction of 9 percent or greater.[162] Within a given stage and tumor grade, the S-phase fraction is an objective measurement that is useful for the identification of prognostically different subgroups of patients.[183] Many poorly differentiated neoplasms are aneuploid, and aneuploid neoplasms tend to invade the myometrium deeply.[180] The proliferative fraction is defined as the percentage of cells in S-phase plus the percentage in G2 mitosis. A proliferative fraction of 14 percent or greater is present in 73 percent of tumors of patients who relapse and in 79 percent of tumors of patients who die.[162]

Multivariate analysis reveals that the triad consisting of depth of myometrial invasion, tumor DNA ploidy, and VIAC correlates strongly with survival.[163] The long-term survival rate is only 10 percent for patients with aneuploid neoplasms that have VIAC and deep myometrial invasion. Patients who have neoplasms with a peridiploid DNA content, no VIAC, and no myometrial invasion have a 93 percent long-term survival rate.[163] Determination of the DNA content of a particular endometrial adenocarcinoma may be useful when the surgical and pathologic findings are inconclusive in assigning a degree of risk. Thus, DNA content may prove especially helpful in cases of grade 2 endometrial adenocarcinomas, in which aneuploid neoplasms have twice the metastatic potential.[137] Most endometrial adenocarcinomas are histopathologic (i.e., architectural) grade 1, nuclear grade 1, and peridiploid. These neoplasms are unlikely to metastasize, whereas poorly differentiated, nuclear grade 3, aneuploid endometrial adenocarcinomas are associated with a high risk of metastases.[137]

Cervical Cytology and Endometrial Carcinoma

Cervical cytologic examination is a well-established screening test for cervical cancer. Endometrial cells, normal or abnormal, may also be present in cervical cytologic preparations. Approximately 25 to 36 percent of endometrial carcinomas shed cells that can be seen on a diagnostic cervical-vaginal smear.[183a] Sometimes it is difficult to tell whether these cells are of endocervical, endometrial, or ovarian origin. However, their specificity for malignancy is excellent. Because the sensitivity is low, cervical cytologic examination is not an adequate screening tool for endometrial cancer.

The need for routine cervical cytologic examinations in perimenopausal and postmenopausal women is controversial. Many of these women continue to have regular cervical cytologic smears despite being at low risk for cervical cancer. Walton et al[184] recommended discontinuing cervical cancer screening in patients older than 60 years. Nonetheless, many gynecologists continue to perform annual cervical cancer screening on older women because older women can develop cervical cancer, and other genital tract malignancies can be picked up on a Papanicolaou smear.[185]

Normal-appearing endometrial cells in women of reproductive age are seen during menses and up to day 10 to 14 of the normal menstrual cycle (Fig. 6–28). After this, the presence of endometrial cells is a matter of concern.[186, 187] The presence of normal endometrial cells in a cervical cytologic preparation obtained from a postmenopausal woman warrants further investigation because this is evidence of microscopic uterine bleeding. The causes of such bleeding include endometrial polyp, hyperplasia, or carcinoma. The presence of atypical endometrial cells at any age is of more concern. As the atypia progresses the nuclear size increases, the chromatin pattern alters, and micronuclei and macronucleoli appear. Cell size and pleomorphism also increase. These cytologic changes correspond to an increasing degree of atypical endometrial hyperplasia and grade of endometrial carcinoma.[187]

Mildly atypical endometrial cells show slight nuclear enlargement (i.e., greater than 40 μm^2) and an altered nuclear to cytoplasmic ratio. These changes suggest a benign process or endometrial hyperplasia.[188] Moderately atypical cells have moderate nuclear enlargement, hyperchromasia, and focal alterations in chromatin distribution. These alterations are seen as a change from an even distribution of chromatin to an irregular clumping pattern. These changes warrant further clinical evaluation.[188] Severely atypical cells show a further increase in nuclear size (i.e., 60 to 80 μm^2), irregular distribution of chromatin particles, and the presence of nucleoli (Fig. 6–29). These changes usually correlate with atypical hyperplasia or adenocarcinoma.[188] When atypical endometrial cells are present in a cervical cytologic specimen, endometrial sampling demonstrates abnormal findings in 42 percent of samples. Eleven percent show endometrial polyps, 11 percent show endometrial hyperplasia, and 20 percent are adenocarcinomas. Of the adenocarcinomas, 44 percent are endometrial grade 1, 37 percent endometrial grade 2, 11 percent endometrial grade 3, 4 percent carcinoma of the fallopian tube, and 4 percent ovarian serous tumor of low malignant potential.[188] Endometrial adenocarcinoma in these samples may or may not contain areas of squamous differentiation. The histopathologic findings and the frequency of these findings depend on the age of the patient being studied and the degree of cytologic atypia present.[186] In women over 59 years of age in whom atypical endometrial cells are detected on cervical cytologic examination, 57 per-

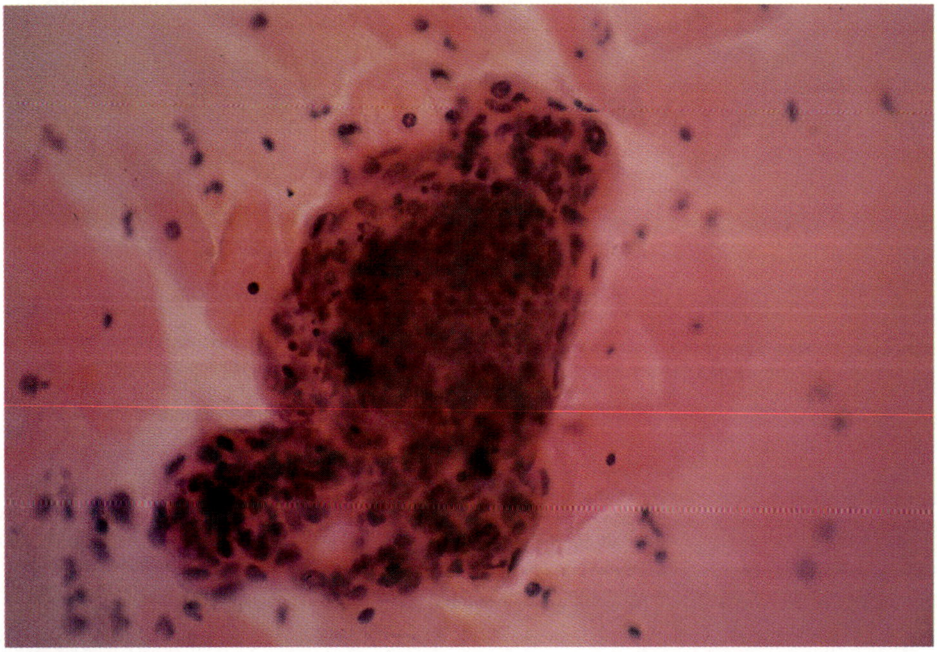

FIGURE 6–28
This Papanicolaou-stained smear was obtained from a woman who was on day 9 of her normal menstrual cycle. A background of normal superficial squamous cells is present. A ball of endometrial cells seen in the center is composed of endometrial stromal cells in the middle and epithelial cells on the outside. There is evidence of degeneration and infiltration by inflammatory cells. Such a cell ball is known as exodus. This is normal during the first half of the menstrual cycle but would be suspicious for endometrial cancer or hyperplasia if shed by a postmenopausal woman.

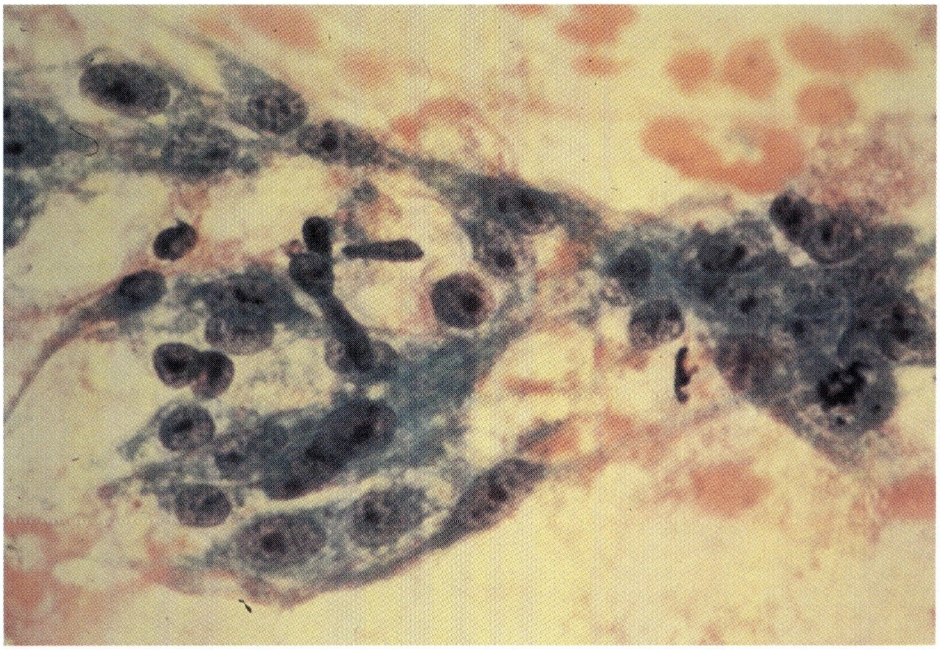

FIGURE 6-29
This Papanicolaou-stained smear shows a sheet of highly abnormal cells in a bloody background. The nuclei are enlarged, and the nucleoli are prominent and pleomorphic. Mitosis is present on the far right. This is suggestive of adenocarcinoma.

cent have adenocarcinoma. In contrast, 10 percent of women between 50 and 59 years of age in whom atypical endometrial cells are found in a cervical cytologic preparation have adenocarcinoma.[187] The more advanced the degree of atypia and the older the patient, the more likely it is that adenocarcinoma will be detected.

All women in whom a cervical smear unequivocally demonstrates adenocarcinoma are found to have some type of carcinoma on histopathologic evaluation. If there is no primary carcinoma of the cervix, 40 percent of the remainder have a primary endometrial adenocarcinoma.[189] Thus, although the prevalence of cervical cancer may decline in older women, cervical cytologic examination may retain its value as a screening tool for endometrial cancer. Cervical cytologic examination should be part of the evaluation of women with abnormal uterine bleeding, but if it is negative, more aggressive diagnostic modes such as endometrial biopsy or dilatation and curettage should be employed.

When endometrial stromal cells (also called endometrial histiocytes) are present on a routine cervical-vaginal smear obtained from a postmenopausal woman, it is possible that an endometrial lesion such as an endometrial polyp, hyperplasia, or carcinoma is present. The presence of both endometrial epithelial and stromal cells correlates even more closely with the presence of cancer or hyperplasia. Stromal cells are usually recognized as clusters and small groups of cells that have elongated nuclei and scant cytoplasm. When they are present only as single cells they may not be distinguishable from small macrophages.

Tumor Markers

Tumor markers in gynecologic cancers are undergoing active research. They may be detected in serum or in paraffin-fixed tissue. As a blood test, tumor markers may serve as a screening tool or may help in the follow-up of patients with a specific neoplasm.

CA 125 is a tumor-associated antigen that was originally identified in ovarian serous carcinomas, but it is also expressed in some endometrial carcinomas as well as in many other conditions. CA 125 expression is identifiable both in blood and in paraffin-fixed tissue. Serum CA 125 values greater than 35 U/ml are present in 12 percent of patients who have endometrial adenocarcinoma confined to the uterus and in 65 percent of patients with extrauterine disease.[190] Evaluation of CA 15-3 in endometrial carcinoma shows a serum level of greater than 30 U/ml in 17 percent of patients with localized disease and in 65 percent of those with advanced disease.[190] A serum level of tumor-associated glycoprotein 72 (TAG 72) of greater than 6 U/ml is found in 4 percent of patients with localized disease and in 30 percent of those with metastatic disease. The use of a combination of tumor markers (i.e., CA 125, TAG 72, or CA 15-3) does not improve the sensitivity and specificity for the detection of endometrial carcinoma compared with the use of CA 125 alone.[190] The tumor-associated antigens CA 125, TAG 72, and CA 15-3 are all accurate for the prediction of extrauterine disease (sensitivity 65 percent, specificity 88 percent). Eighty-two percent of women with advanced endometrial carcinoma have serum elevations of CA 125 and CA 15-3.[190] However, these tumor markers are not acceptable as a screening test for endometrial carcinoma because most patients with endometrial carcinoma have disease confined to the uterus and such cases will be missed. In the early stage of disease there is a low prevalence of elevated serum levels of any tumor marker. The use of tumor markers may be of value in the follow-up of patients at risk for recurrence.

Localization of CA 125 and CA 19-9 in formalin-fixed, paraffin-embedded tissue from patients with endometrial carcinoma is now possible. CA 125 is present in virtually all clear cell endometrial carcinomas, in 75 percent of uterine papillary serous carcinomas, and in 50 percent of endometrioid endometrial carcinomas, regardless of histopathologic grade.[9] CA 19-9 is a glycoprotein related to the Lewis A blood group. Its expression in paraffin-fixed tissue correlates with the prevalence of the Lewis A blood phenotype. In paraffin-fixed tissue CA 19-9 is present in 80 percent of clear cell endometrial carcinomas and in 40 percent of uterine papillary serous carcinomas. In endometrioid endometrial carcinoma, CA 19-9 is present in 88 percent of grade 1 tumors but in only 45 percent of grade 3 tumors.[9]

MSN-1 is a murine monoclonal antibody that recognizes the Lewis B carbohydrate moiety on glycolipids and possibly other carbohydrate moieties as well. When tested on a variety of normal and abnormal endometrial paraffin-embedded tissues, a positive reaction to MSN-1 was seen in 40 percent of patients with proliferative endometria, 100 percent of those with secretory endometria, 25 percent of those with simple hyperplasia, 100 percent of those with complex atypical hyperplasia, and 100 percent of those with typical endometrial adenocarcinomas grades 1 and 2. This antibody does not recognize tissue from individuals who are Lewis B negative.[191]

A variety of other tumor markers are currently under investigation. Twelve percent of endometrial adenocarcinomas of a variety of histopathologic cell types stain positive for intracytoplasmic amylase. This is considered a potential tumor marker for some endometrial adenocarcinomas.[192] Serum placental protein 4 (PP4) levels are high in 48 percent of patients with endometrial carcinoma. The frequency of elevated serum levels was 47 percent in patients with stage I uterine carcinoma.[193] In recurrent tumors, PP4 levels decreased to the normal range after treatment, and thus PP4 may prove useful as a marker of tumor activity.[193]

Clinical Correlations

Management

In the management of patients with endometrial carcinoma the physician must consider the risk of surgery and the disease stage. Because endometrial carcinoma frequently occurs in older and morbidly obese women, some patients are not candidates for surgery. Treatment of these patients consists primarily of radiation therapy. The staging of these patients is done using the clinical staging system (Table 6–8). In another group of women with endometrial carcinoma surgery is possible, but complete surgical staging is not feasible owing to complicating medical conditions or obesity.

In women who are surgical candidates, staging includes peritoneal lavage for cytologic evaluation, hysterectomy, bilateral salpingo-oophorectomy, surgical debulking if necessary, and selective pelvic and paraaortic lymphadenectomy. In women with UPSC, which has a pattern of spread similar to that of papillary serous carcinoma of the ovary, we recommend omental biopsy and sampling of the peritoneal surfaces. Postoperative radiation therapy is appropriate in patients who have stage I disease and poor prognostic indicators. These traditionally include deep myometrial invasion and grade 3 carcinomas. Approximately 20 percent of patients have tumors with these characteristics and are thus considered candidates for adjuvant radiation therapy.[194]

Visual examination of the sectioned uterus can accurately determine the depth of myometrial invasion in 85 percent of patients.[175] Frozen section, if necessary, can increase this accuracy to 96.5 percent. Likewise, frozen section accurately predicts histopathologic grade in 95 percent of instances as well as the presence of occult cervical

TABLE 6–8.

Clinical Staging of Endometrial Cancer To Be Used When Surgical Staging Is Not Possible. Use of Clinical Staging Should Be Noted

Stage I	Disease confined to the corpus
IA	Uterus sounds to 8 cm or less
IB	Uterus sounds to more than 8 cm
Stage II	Endometrial cancer extends to the cervix (positive endocervical curettings or ectocervical biopsy, with or without gross cervical involvement)
Stage III	Disease extends outside of the uterus but is still confined to the pelvis except for extension to bladder or rectal mucosa, which is stage IVA
Stage IVA	Tumor involves the bladder or rectal mucosa
Stage IVB	Extrapelvic metastasis

invasion.[83a] Careful gross examination of the uterus at the time of surgery, along with selective frozen section diagnosis, could eliminate the need for lymph node dissection in some patients.[83a,194,195]

The management of patients with grade 1 endometrial adenocarcinoma confined to the uterus with superficial or no myometrial invasion consists of peritoneal lavage for cytologic evaluation and careful exploration of the abdomen, followed by abdominal hysterectomy with bilateral salpingo-oophorectomy. The metastatic potential of these early, well-differentiated tumors is almost negligible, and the risks of extensive surgical staging outweigh its benefits, especially in obese or medically unstable patients. Complete surgical staging is appropriate in patients with more advanced tumors.

The management of patients with clinical stage II endometrial adenocarcinoma consists of initial surgical staging. Only 37 percent of women with clinically suspected but not proven cervical involvement will be found to have surgical stage II disease.[196] When cervical involvement is grossly evident or there is a biopsy-proven diagnosis of cervical involvement, radical abdominal hysterectomy, bilateral salpingo-oophorectomy, bilateral pelvic lymphadenectomy, and paraaortic lymph node sampling may be appropriate in selective cases. Preoperative radiation followed by an extrafascial hysterectomy is used in patients with bulky stage II endometrial carcinoma. The need for adjuvant postoperative therapy in patients with stage II endometrial carcinoma depends on the extent of cervical involvement, the depth of myometrial invasion, and the histopathologic tumor type and grade. Thirty percent of these women are at low risk for pelvic recurrence and will not benefit from adjuvant therapy.[196] Radiation therapy to the pelvis is used in patients with high-risk factors for nodal metastasis or pelvic recurrence regardless of whether or not the surgically removed nodes show carcinoma. Patients who have surgically confirmed pelvic or paraaortic lymph node metastasis require radiation therapy to the whole pelvis (5040 cGy) with extension of the radiation field to include the paraaortic nodes if they are involved.[197]

Patients with surgical stage III disease limited to the adnexa or pelvis require an attempt at surgical excision of all visible tumor. Postoperative radiation is given with good results.[173d] Patients with stage IVA disease benefit from radiation therapy to the pelvis. In patients with stage IVB disease, control of pelvic disease with radiation therapy or surgery is appropriate. Progestational agents can be used.[198] Patients who have well-differentiated neoplasms respond better to progestational agents than those who have poorly differentiated neoplasms. Eighty-seven percent of patients with well-differentiated endometrial adenocarcinoma respond to progestins, whereas only 14 percent of patients with poorly differentiated neoplasms demonstrate a clinical response.[198] Chemotherapy regimens that contain doxorubicin, cyclophosphamide, and cisplatin are associated with clinical response rates of approximately 45 percent in patients who have stage IVB endometrial adenocarcinoma.[198a,198b]

The 5-year survival rate of patients with surgical stage I endometrial carcinoma is between 83 and 97 percent.[164,166a,167] Patients with surgical stage II disease that is superficial and microscopic experience a 5-year survival rate of close to 90 percent. Patients with surgical stage II disease with high-risk factors for recurrence have a 5-year survival rate of 65 percent with adjuvant radiation.[196] Patients with paraaortic lymph node involvement or pelvic and paraaortic lymph node involvement who are treated with surgery and radiation have a 5-year survival rate of 47 and 43 percent, respectively.[197] Recurrence following radiation therapy is likely to occur outside the radiation fields.[197] The long-term survival of patients with stage IV disease is 10 percent or less.[198]

Detection of Recurrence

Recurrence occurs in up to 16 percent of women with endometrial carcinoma that is clinically confined to the uterus.[86,165,168] The average time from surgery to recurrence is 2.2 years.[165] Forty-seven percent of recurrences are detected within the first year of follow-up, and 70 percent are detected by the end of the second postoperative year.[86] Sixty-one percent of recurrences occur at distant sites, 34 percent are within the pelvis, and 6 percent are both local and distant.[86] Patients treated with radiation therapy to the pelvis after hysterectomy are more likely to experience recurrent tumors outside the pelvis. Only 5 percent of patients with disease confined to the uterus who receive postoperative radiation therapy have tumors that recur in the pelvis.[86] Approximately half of the recurrences occur in asymptomatic individuals. The combination of physical examination and chest radiograph is the most effective approach to detection of endometrial carcinoma recurrence in asymptomatic women. The combination of a careful medical history, physical examination, vaginal cytology, and chest radiograph is sufficient to detect all cases of recurrence.[86]

Estrogen Replacement Therapy

Endometrial adenocarcinoma is an estrogen-sensitive neoplasm. According to the package insert of every commercially available estrogen-containing preparation in the United States, endometrial adenocarcinoma is an absolute contraindication for estrogen replacement therapy. There is no consideration of the patient's age, menopausal status before the diagnosis of endometrial carcinoma, or estrogen and progesterone receptor status of the neoplasm. There is no question that the effects of menopause are physically and psychologically devastating in some women. Estrogen easily relieves vasomotor symptoms and prevents vaginal atrophy.[199] The Nurses Health Study demonstrated a 50 percent reduction in the incidence of heart disease in women who were on estrogen replacement.[200] The benefits of preventing, or at least severely retarding the progression of osteoporosis, may alone outweigh the theoretic risk of estrogen replacement in some women treated for endometrial carcinoma.[201, 202] Osteoporosis affects over 20 million women in the United States. Almost all are over 45 years of age. Oven 1 million fractures occur annually in women who have osteoporosis, leading to an estimated annual cost of 7 billion dollars.[201]

There is no good evidence that estrogen significantly increases the risk of recurrence of endometrial carcinoma.[203] Many women may benefit from estrogen replacement despite previous therapy for endometrial carcinoma. In a retrospective study of 268 women with stage I endometrial cancer, 47 patients received estrogen replacement therapy after surgery. There was only one recurrence (2.3 percent) in the estrogen-treated group compared to a 14.9 percent recurrence rate among women who did not receive estrogen therapy.[204] The groups were not statistically different in regard to tumor grade, depth of myometrial invasion, rate of nodal metastasis, rate of positive peritoneal cytologic findings, or tumor estrogen or progesterone receptor status. Thus, at least in patients without adverse prognostic indicators, a history of endometrial cancer does not seem to be a contraindication to estrogen replacement therapy.[204] Indeed, a survey of gynecologic oncologists indicates that 83 percent approved the use of estrogen replacement therapy for patients previously treated for stage I, grade 1 endometrial carcinoma. Fifty-six percent used it in patients with a history of stage I, grade 2 endometrial carcinoma, and 39 percent prescribed estrogen replacement for patients with a history of stage I, grade 3 tumors.[205] The patient should participate in the decision of whether or not to use estrogen replacement based on information about the risks and benefits. Although estrogen replacement in these women will not cause a recurrence, it may shorten the time to recurrence. In the United States, the Gynecologic Oncology Group is conducting a study that randomizes the choice of patients with surgical stage I or stage II endometrial carcinoma to receive or not to receive estrogen replacement therapy.

UTERINE SARCOMA

Classification

Uterine sarcomas are uncommon neoplasms. In the United States they account for less than 5 percent of all malignant uterine neoplasms. Most uterine sarcomas are classified as leiomyosarcoma, carcinosarcoma, or endometrial stromal sarcoma. Most reports in the literature include only a small number of patients with these rare neoplasms. Table 6–9 presents a detailed classification of uterine sarcomas based on that proposed by Ober.[206] A classification of mixed epithelial and nonepithelial tumors of the uterus modified from that of the International Society of Gynecologic Pathologists is shown in Table 6–10.[207] The relative frequency of uterine sarcomas, gathered from different sources, is presented in Table 6–11.[208–211] The Surveillance, Epidemiology, and End Results (SEER) study reports the annual incidence of uterine sarcomas as 17.1 per million women per year.[209] Most are carcinosarcomas (malignant mixed mesodermal tumors) and leiomyosarcomas.[209] The rate in African-American women is

TABLE 6–9.
Detailed Classification of Uterine Sarcomas

- I. Pure sarcoma
  - A. Pure homologous
    1. Leiomyosarcoma
    2. Low-grade stromal sarcoma
    3. High-grade stromal sarcoma
  - B. Pure heterologous
    1. Rhabdomyosarcoma (includes sarcoma botryoides)
    2. Chondrosarcoma
    3. Osteosarcoma
    4. Liposarcoma
- II. Mixed sarcoma (homologous or heterologous)
- III. Mixed epithelial-nonepithelial tumors (see Table 6–10)
- IV. Sarcoma unclassified
- V. Malignant lymphoma

Modified from Ober WB: Uterine sarcomas: Histogenesis and taxonomy. Ann NY Acad Sci 1959; 75: 568–585.

TABLE 6–10.

International Society of Gynecologic Pathologists Classification of Uterine Mixed Epithelial-Nonepithelial Tumors (1989)

Benign	Adenofibroma
	Adenomyoma (atypical polypoid adenomyoma)
Malignant	Adenosarcoma
	Homologous
	Heterologous
	Carcinosarcoma (malignant mixed mesodermal or müllerian tumor)
	Homologous
	Heterologous
	Carcinofibroma

Modified from Silverberg SG: Mixed müllerian tumors. *In* Sasano N (ed): Current Topics in Pathology, 85. Gynecological Tumors. New York, Springer Verlag, 1992, pp 36–56.

33.4 per million women per year, whereas in white women it is 16 per million per year. The report by Peters et al excluded leiomyosarcoma.[212] These authors reported that 77 percent of uterine sarcomas were carcinosarcomas (mixed mesodermal tumors), 20 percent were high-grade endometrial stromal sarcomas, and 3 percent were rhabdomyosarcomas.

The terms that describe uterine sarcomas are easy to understand. The prefix adeno- or carcino- identifies the epithelial component as benign or malignant, respectively. The suffix fibroma, myoma, or sarcoma describes the stromal component as benign for the first two or malignant for the last. The term homologous refers to mesenchymal tissue that is native to the müllerian system (i.e., smooth muscle, endometrial stroma, and blood vessels). The term heterologous refers to mesenchymal tissues not native to the uterus (i.e., striated muscle, cartilage, bone or fat).[207]

Adenosarcoma

Adenosarcoma accounts for approximately 8 percent of all uterine sarcomas (see Table 6–11). It is

TABLE 6–11.

Frequency of Specific Types of Sarcomas Relative to All Uterine Sarcomas[208–211]

Histopathologic Type	*Frequency*
Carcinosarcoma	22–48%
Leiomyosarcoma	27–50%
Endometrial stromal sarcoma	11–33%
Adenosarcoma	8%
Unclassified	4–6%
Angiosarcoma	3%
Miscellaneous	3%

characterized by an admixture of benign but sometimes atypical endometrial glands with a malignant stromal component.[213] This neoplasm was first described in 1974.[213] More than 200 cases of uterine adenosarcomas have now been reported in the literature.[213–219, 221–225] The largest series is that recently reported by Clement and Scully.[214]

Two theories are espoused to explain the origin of this neoplasm. One suggests a neoplastic process that simultaneously produces benign glands and malignant stroma.[214] The other proposes that benign normal endometrial glands are trapped within the malignant stroma.[215] These neoplasms, in contrast to other uterine sarcomas, have a low malignant potential. Recurrence tends to be local and occurs in approximately 25 percent of cases. Distant metastases occur in less than 5 percent of cases.[214] Adenosarcoma represents a type of mixed stromal-epithelial tumor that lies between the benign papillary adenofibroma and the highly malignant heterologous carcinosarcoma. Despite the number of reports in the literature, large gaps still exist in our knowledge of its epidemiology, histogenesis, and clinical and pathologic features.

By definition the stromal elements of adenosarcoma are malignant and the glands are benign. Heterologous nonepithelial elements such as striated muscle, cartilage, bone, and fat may be present. Criteria for the diagnosis of this neoplasm have not been clarified. Some authors require four mitotic figures per 10 high-power microscope fields (HPF) in the most active area of tumor to distinguish an adenosarcoma from a benign adenofibroma.[216] Others demand either one to two mitotic figures per 10 HPF in the most active areas, or a cytologically malignant-appearing stromal component.[214] Besides mitotic activity and pronounced stromal cellular atypia, the identification of myometrial invasion or the presence of malignant heterologous tissue also serves to identify the malignant nature of this neoplasm.[216]

The mean age of women with adenosarcoma is between 55 and 60 years, but it can occur in young women and even children.[214, 216, 217] The youngest patient reported to have developed adenosarcoma is an 11 year old girl[218]; the oldest is an 89-year-old woman.[214, 219] Sixty-two percent of women with adenosarcoma are older than 50 years. Eighty percent are white, and 30 percent are nulligravida.[214] In 5 percent of cases there is a history of prior pelvic irradiation. In another 5 percent there is an association with endogenous or exogenous estrogen.[214, 215] Adenosarcoma may arise in an otherwise unremarkable endometrial polyp.

Seventy-five percent of patients present with abnormal vaginal bleeding or postmenopausal bleeding. Pelvic pain is the presenting complaint in approximately 5 percent of patients.[214] Other uncommon findings at presentation include abnormal cervical cytologic findings, vaginal discharge, dysmenorrhea, dysuria, urinary tract infection, abdominal swelling due to ascites, and complaints referable to uterine prolapse.[214] The most common finding on pelvic examination is a mass protruding through the cervical os, which occurs in over 40 percent of cases.[214] It may resemble an endocervical polyp. In some patients the mass partially fills the vagina. Other findings include an enlarged uterus in one-third of patients. An occasional patient presents with a pelvic mass.[214]

Adenosarcoma is frequently confused with other conditions of the uterus. On retrospective review the initial histopathologic diagnosis was correct in 33 percent of cases, partially correct in 22 percent, and incorrect in the remainder.[214] Thus, in adenosarcoma, incorrect pathologic diagnoses are as common as correct ones. The most common incorrect benign diagnoses include benign endometrial or endocervical polyp, adenofibroma, and endometrial stromal hyperplasia. The most common incorrect malignant diagnoses include malignant endometrial stromal sarcoma, carcinosarcoma (malignant mixed mesodermal tumor), and sarcoma botryoides.[214]

This tumor is polypoid in appearance and frequently fills the entire endometrial cavity (Fig. 6–30). The tumor diameter averages 5 cm and ranges between 1 and 17 cm. The mass is almost always solitary. Usually the polyp is broad based, but on occasion it may be pedunculated. The tumor surface is generally smooth and shiny, but an occasional tumor has a papillary granular appearance. Most adenosarcoma originate in the fundal endometrium. However, 6 percent of these neoplasms originate in the cervix, and 4 percent originate within the myometrium. The cut surface has a spongy appearance. The color may be pink, white, gray, tan, or yellow, and there may be areas of hemorrhage and necrosis. The consistency is soft, fish flesh–like, or gelatinous; an occasional tumor is firm. Cystic spaces, up to 1 cm in diameter, are present on cut sections. Focal necrosis is present in 20 percent of cases and focal hemorrhage in 13 percent.[214] The tip of the polypoid mass may be necrotic, particularly if it extends through the cervical os. Myometrial invasion, when present, is readily apparent. Extrauterine extension is rare. When extrauterine spread is present it usually consists of ovarian involvement.[214]

This is a biphasic tumor composed of an admixture of benign or atypical glands within a sarcomatous stroma (Fig. 6–31). The growth pattern resembles that of cystosarcoma phylloides of the breast with the epithelial component growing in a broad leaflike pattern.[220] In three-fourths of cases the surface is smooth and is covered by glands. A minority of tumors have either a papillary appearance or stroma lined by glandular epithelium, resulting in a villoglandular or villous pattern.[214]

The glands in adenosarcoma are interspersed throughout a sarcomatous stroma. The glandular architecture is a mixture of the cytologically bland

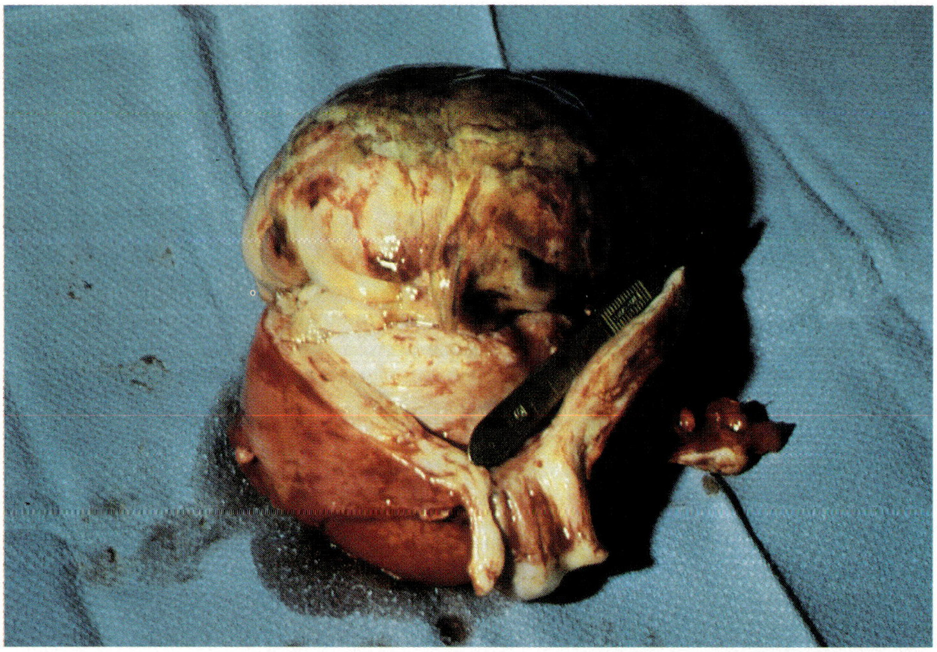

FIGURE 6–30
This large adenosarcoma fills the endometrial cavity. The tumor has a smooth, yellow, shiny surface with areas of hemorrhage. (Courtesy of Dr. John Wheelock.)

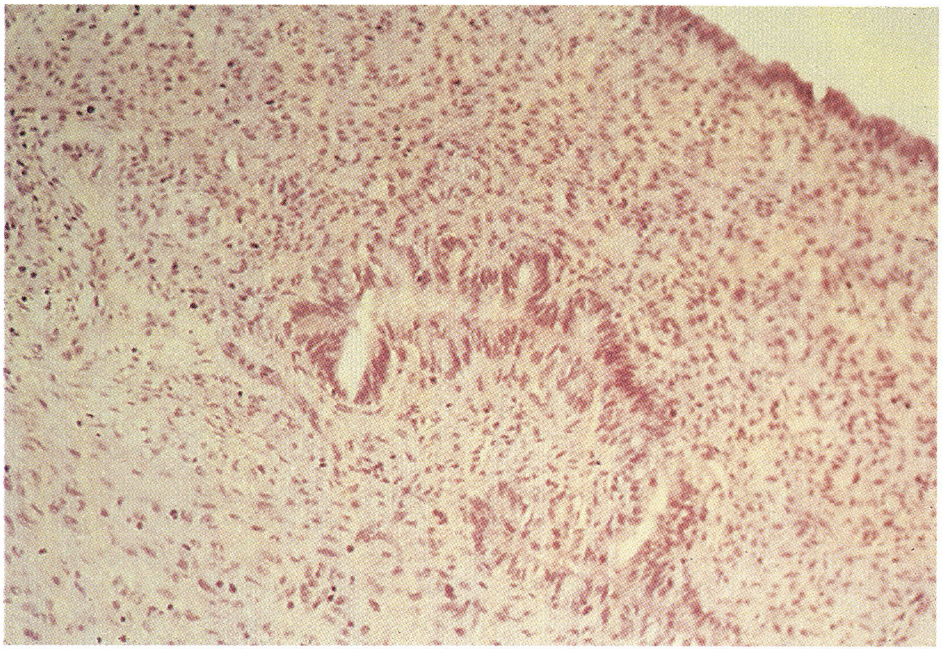

FIGURE 6-31
A sarcomatous stroma with benign endometrial glands that are an intrinsic part of the neoplasm is characteristic of adenosarcoma. The surface is covered by benign epithelium.

and atypical glandular epithelium. Individual glands vary in size. Small tubules with cuboidal or pseudostratified columnar epithelium resemble those of proliferative endometrium. Cystically dilated glands resemble those seen in simple hyperplasia. Compressed slitlike glands may form complex anastomoses. In these areas the glandular epithelium may appear flattened. The nuclei are basally oriented. Besides the typical endometrioid appearance of the epithelium, any of the previously described metaplastic processes of the endometrium may be present. Mucinous and tubal metaplasia are most common. Hobnail or clear cell metaplasia is the least common.[214, 222] A secretory glandular pattern is uncommon.[214] Cells with squamous differentiation may form solid nests,[213] typically on the surface of the tumor.[215]

Architectural atypia may be present but is usually focal. In rare cases the glandular crowding may approach that seen with well-differentiated adenocarcinoma. Cytologic atypia of the glandular epithelium is present in up to one-third of cases. It may be moderate to severe. Cytologic atypia consists of nuclear enlargement, pleomorphism, hyperchromasia, coarsening of chromatin, and prominent nucleoli.[214] If adenocarcinoma is present, the diagnosis is malignant mixed mesodermal tumor rather than adenosarcoma.

The stromal component of an adenosarcoma is by definition malignant. It is usually a low-grade sarcoma. The stromal cells are spindle shaped with mild to moderate nuclear polymorphism and hyperchromasia. The stroma tends to condense around the glands forming periglandular cuffs in over three-fourths of cases.[214] A cambium layer, an area of increased cellularity, may be present beneath the surface epithelium in some tumors.[214] Fibrosis may also be present in this area. The type of malignant component most commonly present is typical endometrial stromal sarcoma. In some cases the stromal component resembles smooth muscle cells.[213, 214, 222] A myxoid, spindle cell stroma with foci of hypercellular low-grade fibrosarcoma occurs in 12 to 54 percent of cases.[214, 222] Hyalinization may obliterate the sarcomatous stroma in some instances.[213, 221, 224] This may impart a deceptively benign appearance to the neoplasm.[214] The stroma in 20 percent of adenosarcomas contains areas with foamy macrophages.[213, 223] Mitotic activity is prominent in the stroma. The mean mitotic count is nine mitotic figures per 10 HPF. A mitotic count as high as 40 mitotic figures per 10 HPF is rarely seen.[213, 214, 221] Nuclei are hyperchromatic. An occasional tumor contains rare foci of mitotically inactive multinucleate giant cells, resembling those seen in vaginal polyps.[214]

Although the stroma in the majority of adenosarcomas is homologous, a heterologous sarcomatous component occurs in approximately one-fourth of cases.[214, 222] This takes the form of rhabdomyoblastic, chondroblastic, osteoblastic, and, rarely, liposarcomatous differentiation. The most common heterologous element is the rhabdomyoblast. Tumors that contain rhabdomyoblasts can resemble embryonal rhabdomyosarcoma. When this occurs, the stroma consists of packed primitive-appearing cells that have scanty cytoplasm and brisk mitotic activity. The nuclei of these cells are hyperchromatic and pleomorphic. Admixed with these cells are cells that are round and strap shaped or stellate. These cells contain abundant eosinophilic cytoplasm with easily recognizable cross striations. These tumor cells stain positive for myoglobin with immunoperoxidase stains.[214] Primitive cartilage is the second most common heterologous element, and this is followed by malignant bone and adipose tissue.

The adjacent uninvolved endometrium in cases of adenosarcoma may be proliferative, secretory, atrophic, or hyperplastic. In five cases a separate endometrial adenocarcinoma was present.[214] The uninvolved myometrium may contain adenomyosis or benign leiomyomas.

Approximately 15 to 20 percent of adenosarcomas invade the myometrium and rarely the myometrial vessels.[214] Myometrial invasion is usually superficial, and deep myometrial invasion occurs in less than 5 percent of cases. Invasion is usually infiltrative, but on occasion a pushing margin is seen.[214, 216] At the time of initial surgery 6 percent of patients have pelvic node metastasis, and 6 percent have positive peritoneal cytologic findings.[222]

Patients with adenosarcoma have a recurrence rate of 23 to 40 percent following hysterectomy.[214, 216, 222] Recurrence can occur as late as 10 years after surgery. In Clement and Scully's series of 100 cases, 60 percent of patients were alive 5 years after surgery with no evidence of recurrence, 13 percent died of other causes without tumor recurrence, and 26 percent had tumor at the time of death.[214]

Some patients with tumors that have as few as two mitotic figures per 10 HPF experience recurrence.[213, 214] The tumor usually recurs in the vagina, pelvis, or abdomen.[213, 214, 216, 222] At these sites recurrences are either pure sarcoma or adenosarcoma, whereas at sites outside the abdomen they tend to be pure sarcoma. Rarely, a recurrence may take the form of a carcinosarcoma (malignant mixed mesodermal tumor).[214] Vaginal recurrences appear as polypoid or papillary lesions arising from the vaginal apex. Their appearance may be similar to that of granulation tissue. Biopsy and microscopic examination are needed for diagnosis. Pelvic and abdominal recurrences involve the bowel, vagina, and bladder. Recurrences outside the pelvis also involve the omentum, mesentery, and retroperitoneal structures.[214] Metastasis outside the abdomen occurs in less than 5 percent of cases.

Deep myometrial invasion appears to be the most important factor in predicting recurrence.[214,216] Recurrence occurs in 35 to 46 percent of patients with adenosarcoma that invades deep into the myometrium. The mean mitotic rate of tumors that recur is 11 per 10 HPF compared to nine per 10 HPF in tumors that do not recur. Twenty percent of recurrent tumors, however, have mitotic counts of two to three mitoses per 10 HPF.[214] The triad of deep myometrial invasion, heterologous stromal elements, and mitotic activity of greater than ten mitotic figures per 10 HPF is associated with a poor prognosis.[216] Inclusion of patients with adenosarcoma who have these features in investigational protocols that study the effectiveness of adjuvant systemic chemotherapy is appropriate.

Although the therapy for adenosarcoma is hysterectomy, in a young woman polypectomy under hysteroscopic guidance may be appropriate if the adenosarcoma takes the form of a pedunculated endometrial polyp and the base of the polyp is not involved.[214] The treatment of recurrent tumor is excision followed by irradiation or chemotherapy. Half of patients with recurrence succumb to this malignancy.[214]

There are two distinct histopathologic variations of adenosarcoma that deserve attention in detail. These are the müllerian adenosarcoma with sex cord–like elements, also known by the acronym MASCE, and adenosarcoma with sarcomatous overgrowth.

Müllerian Adenosarcoma with Sex Cord–like Elements (MASCE)

Adenosarcoma may rarely contain sex cord–like elements within the stromal component. These have solid nests, trabeculae, or tubules that may be solid or hollow.[224] Clement and Scully documented eight cases of MASCE.[225] The age range of patients with this histopathologic variant is 22 to 85 years, with a median age of 41 years. The major complaint of these patients at presentation is abnormal uterine bleeding. The gross features are no different from those of adenosarcoma as described earlier. Myometrial invasion is present in most and is identified by gross examination in 37.5 percent of cases or by microscopic examination in another 37.5 percent.[225] In contrast to the typical adenosarcoma, the invasion of this tumor shows a pushing rather than an infiltrative border. The invasion is always confined to the inner half of the myometrium. The epithelial component has the appearance of proliferative endometrium, secretory endometrium with subnuclear vacuoles, or endocervical-type, tubal-type, or squamous-type epithelium.[225] As with typical adenosarcoma, some of the cystic glands have a flattened or low cuboidal epithelial lining. The nuclear features are bland, but occasionally atypical nuclei are present. The stromal component is always that of low-grade endometrial stromal sarcoma with a diffuse growth pattern.[225] The stroma contains periglandular condensation and forms polypoid or papillary projections into the gland lumens. This feature is also seen in over half of adenosarcomas without sex cord–like elements.[214] The malignant stroma exhibits only a mild degree of nuclear pleomorphism. The mitotic rate is between 1 and 15 mitotic figures per 10 HPF, but most tumors have less than three mitotic figures per 10 HPF.[225] Foci of stromal fibrosis and hyalinization may be present but are not prominent features. Sex cord–like elements, which account for 5 to 50 percent of the tumor, are interspersed within the adenosarcoma.[225] The presence of sex cord–like elements is multifocal in most cases. In some cases they form a discrete solitary mass at the base of the adenosarcoma. The individual cells are benign, round to oval epithelial-type cells. They often contain abundant eosinophilic or foamy lipid-rich cytoplasm. They arrange themselves in solid nests or trabeculae. Anastomosing or plexiform arrangements and solid or hollow tubules are also seen. The nuclei of sex cord–like element cells are round to oval, uniform or mildly atypical, and have fine chromatin with a vesicular appearance. Nucleoli may be either inapparent or prominent, depending on the degree of atypia. The nuclei may have grooves. These cells resemble granulosa cells or Sertoli cells, which also have a lipid-rich cytoplasm, or luteinized ovarian stromal cells.[225] Of the eight patients reported by Clement and Scully, six underwent a hysterectomy and have been followed for 3 to 11 years without recurrence.[225]

The differential diagnosis of MASCE includes endometrial stromal tumor with sex cord–like elements. Deep myometrial invasion is more common with endometrial stromal tumors, and the benign glandular component of adenosarcoma is not seen in endometrial stromal tumor.

Adenosarcoma with Sarcomatous Overgrowth

The other histopathologic variant of adenosarcoma is adenosarcoma with overgrowth by high-grade sarcoma. Sarcomatous overgrowth is seen in approximately 10 percent of adenosarcomas.[214, 222, 224] The definition of sarcomatous overgrowth is the presence of a pure sarcoma, usually but not necessarily of a higher grade and mitotic rate, that overgrows a typical adenosarcoma and accounts for at least 25 percent of the total tumor volume.[224] In some cases the sarcomatous overgrowth accounts for as much as 90 percent of the tumor volume.[224] These neoplasms are extremely aggressive, and their behavior is typically one of rapid progression and death.[222, 224] The age of women with sarcomatous overgrowth of an adenosarcoma is between 32 and 82 years. All cases reported were in white parous women. All had abnormal uterine bleeding as the presenting complaint, and all had an enlarged uterus on examination.[222,224]

The gross appearance of this variant of adenosarcoma is no different from that described earlier for adenosarcoma. The microscopic appearance is also similar; there are both benign glandular and sarcomatous components. Periglandular stromal condensation is also seen. However, sarcomatous areas without a glandular component occupy more than 25 percent of the tumor. The border between the adenosarcoma and the sarcomatous overgrowth is well demarcated in some neoplasms, but in others a gradual transition occurs.[222, 224] The areas of sarcomatous overgrowth are usually of a higher grade. In half of the cases the sarcomatous overgrowth appears poorly differentiated and has pleomorphic, nonspecific, oval to spindle-shaped cells separated by variable amounts of collagen (Fig. 6–32). An occasional tumor has tumor cells with bizarre, multiple, or multilobed nuclei and a moderate amount of eosinophilic cytoplasm suggestive of a rhabdomyoblast.[222, 224] The sarcomatous overgrowth appears as a high-grade endometrial stromal sarcoma in 20 percent of cases.[224] The individual cells exhibit moderate to marked nuclear pleomorphism. The mitotic count is usually more than ten mitotic figures per 10 HPF.

Myometrial invasion occurs in more than half of the patients. An infiltrative pattern of invasion is seen in most cases, but some have pushing borders. Unlike the other variants of adenosarcoma, deep invasion to the serosal surface is common. Heterologous elements are present in 16 to 59 percent of cases.[214, 222] If there is no sarcomatous overgrowth, striated muscle as a heterologous element is seldom seen. The presence of striated muscle cells should prompt a search for sarcomatous overgrowth.[222] Extrauterine spread to contiguous structures occurs in approximately 10 percent of cases. Metastases are uncommon but may be seen on the surface of the liver, diaphragm, and right lung.[224] Patients with adenosarcoma with sarcomatous overgrowth have an ominous prognosis.[222] The tumor recurs in 44 to 70 percent of cases. In contrast, neoplasms without sarcomatous overgrowth have a recurrence rate of 14 to 25 percent. Hematogenous metastases occur in approximately half of the patients who have adenosarcoma with sarcomatous overgrowth but in less

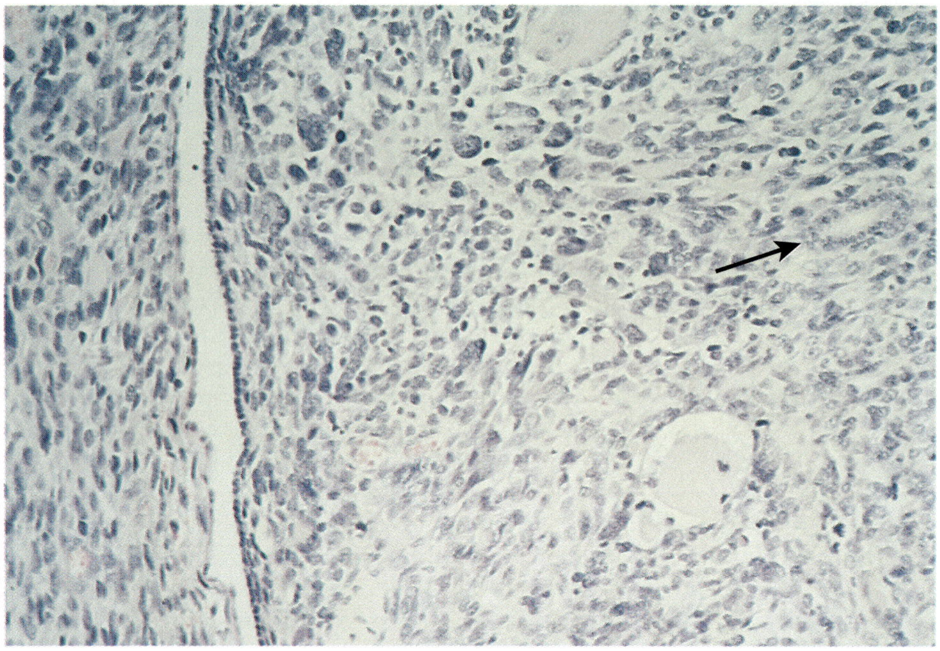

FIGURE 6–32
In this adenosarcoma the sarcomatous cells are markedly pleomorphic with severe nuclear atypia. A benign epithelium covers the adenosarcoma *(left)*. A benign gland is also seen *(arrow)*.

than 5 percent of those without it. Lymphatic space involvement is present in 29 percent of cases.[222] Sixty percent of patients whose neoplasm contains sarcomatous overgrowth die of this disease.[224] Rhabdomyosarcomatous differentiation and extrauterine spread are indicators of an extremely poor prognosis.

The origin of a poorly differentiated sarcoma from a well-differentiated sarcoma may occur in bone and soft tissue tumors as well as adenosarcoma. Stromal overgrowth, although uncommon, is also seen in cytosarcoma phylloides of the breast.[220] Cytosarcoma phylloides and müllerian adenosarcoma have many similar histopathologic features.

Carcinofibroma

Carcinofibroma is extremely rare. By definition the glandular epithelium is malignant, and the stroma is benign fibromatous tissue. Unlike a typical endometrial adenocarcinoma, which has an altered stroma or a desmoplastic stromal response, the carcinofibroma is truly biphasic, and the benign stromal component is an integral part of the neoplasm.

Endometrial Stromal Tumors

The category of endometrial stromal tumors consists of benign endometrial stromal nodules, discussed in the preceding chapter, and endometrial stromal sarcoma. Seven percent of endometrial stromal tumors are benign stromal nodules, and the remaining 93 percent are malignant.[226] The morphology differentiates the endometrial stromal nodule from endometrial stromal sarcoma. Whereas the endometrial stromal nodule has a well-circumscribed margin, the endometrial stromal sarcoma has an infiltrative invasive margin. The mitotic count divides endometrial stromal sarcoma into either low-grade or high-grade tumors.[227] High-grade endometrial stromal sarcoma has more than ten mitotic figures per 10 HPF in the areas of greatest mitotic activity. Endometrial stromal sarcoma accounts for 11 to 33 percent of all uterine sarcomas (see Table 6–11). Some authors consider low-grade and high-grade endometrial stromal sarcoma different expressions of the same entity.[227] Others hold that there are two distinct diseases, one that behaves as a neoplasm of low malignant potential and resembles normal proliferative endometrial stroma, and another with a clinical behavior similar to that of high-grade sarcoma.[228] The women who harbor this latter type of tumor tend to be older.[228] The second theory allows some neoplasms that show normal stromal differentiation but have mitotic counts of greater than ten mitotic figures per 10 HPF to be classified as low-grade endometrial stromal sarcoma.[228]

Low-Grade Endometrial Stromal Sarcoma (Endolymphatic Stromal Myosis or Stromatosis)

The main histopathologic difference between low-grade and high-grade endometrial stromal sarcoma is the number of mitotic figures per 10 HPF in the most active area. The biologic behavior of a low-grade endometrial stromal sarcoma differs dramatically from that of the high-grade neoplasm. Low-grade endometrial stromal sarcoma has a protracted clinical course with recurrences occurring many years after surgery.[229]

Low-grade endometrial stromal sarcoma was first described by Doran and Lockyer in 1909. In 1940 Goodall suggested the term stromal endometriosis for this neoplasm. Henderson coined the term endolymphatic stromal myosis in 1946.[230] This term continues to be used widely to designate this neoplasm. Other terms that make the literature on this entity confusing include stromatoid mural sarcoma, stromal myosis, uterine stromal endometriosis, interstitial endometriosis, benign stromal endometriosis, endometrial sarcoid, fibromyosis uteri of endometrial type, endometrioid sarcoma, grade 1 stromal sarcoma,[229] stromomyoma, uterine angiomatosis, and endometriosis interstitiale.[230]

Low-grade endometrial stromal sarcoma accounts for approximately 80 percent of all endometrial stromal tumors. The characteristics of low-grade endometrial stromal sarcoma lie between those of the endometrial stromal nodule and those of the high-grade endometrial stromal sarcoma.[231] The nondecidualized endometrial stromal cell is not particularly distinctive. Therefore, a universally acceptable morphologic definition of this entity has not been successful. The rarity, indolent course, and morphologic ambiguity of this neoplasm continue to defy efforts to identify statistically credible prognostic criteria.[226] Normal endometrial stroma during the proliferative phase is not particularly different from other stroma. The uniqueness of endometrial stroma does not become apparent until the luteal phase of the menstrual cycle, during pregnancy, or with the use of exogenous progestogen. Many authorities on the subject require that cells of low-grade endometrial stromal sarcoma be identical to, or closely resemble, those of endometrial stroma during the proliferative phase of the menstrual cycle[227] (Fig. 6–33). The only characteristic feature of endometrial stroma during the proliferative phase is its monotonous cytologic uniformity.

Women with low-grade endometrial stromal sarcoma are younger than women who have other uterine sarcomas. Fifty percent of low-grade endometrial stromal sarcomas occur in perimenopausal women.[230] Half are older than 45 years, and only 10 percent are older than 65 years.[226] However, 21 percent of patients are 30 years of age or younger, and this neoplasm occasionally occurs in women younger than 20.[226] The youngest reported patient with this neoplasm was 8 years old.[232] Ninety-two percent of patients who have this tumor are white. Ten percent have a history of prior estrogen use.[229]

The most common presenting complaint is abnormal vaginal bleeding.[226, 229, 230] Pelvic discomfort, usually associated with abnormal vaginal bleeding, also occurs. On rare occasions, the diagnosis is suspected on the basis of cervicovaginal cytology.[233] In 10 percent of cases the neoplasm is incidentally found in a hysterectomy specimen.[230] Endometrial sampling, the main clinical tool for evaluating abnormal uterine bleeding, is not sensitive enough to detect early-stage stromal sarcoma.[233] In only 10 percent of patients was the diagnosis of an endometrial stromal proliferation

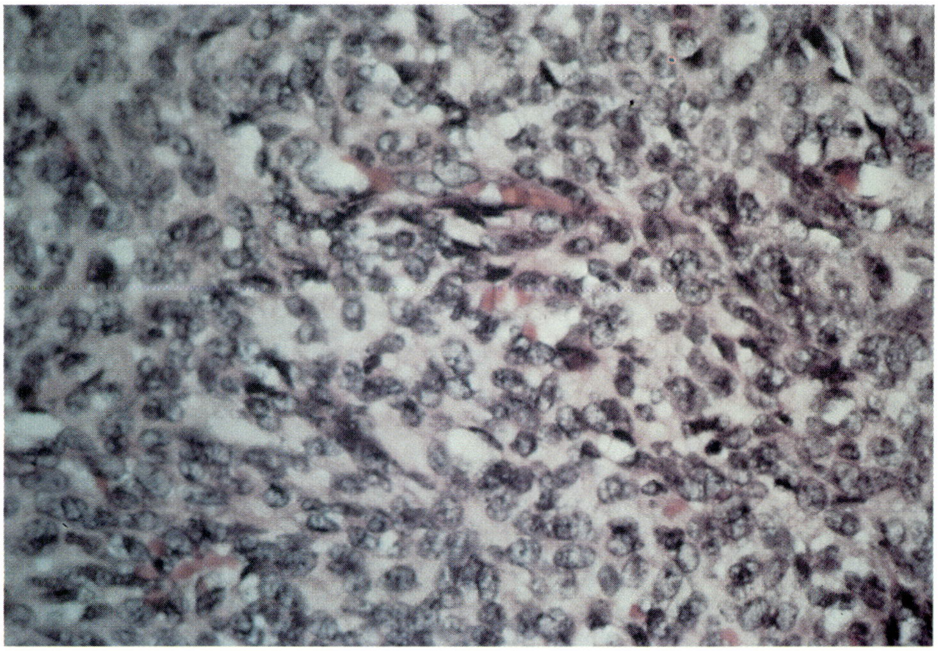

FIGURE 6–33
The endometrial stromal sarcoma cell lacks differentiation and resembles the endometrial stromal cell of the proliferative phase. There is little pleomorphism and minimal cytologic atypia. The nuclei are rounded to oval. The cells have scant cytoplasm.

correctly made on tissue removed with curettage.[226] The diagnosis of an endometrial stromal nodule versus low-grade endometrial stromal sarcoma cannot be made from uterine curettings. The finding of large fragments of endometrial stroma without endometrial glands in a curettage specimen obtained from a postmenopausal woman may warrant a hysterectomy to establish the correct diagnosis. Similar findings in a premenopausal woman who desires preservation of childbearing potential warrant careful follow-up with ultrasound, computed tomography,[226] and possibly hysteroscopy.

Most low-grade endometrial stromal sarcomas seem to be confined to the uterus at the time of initial surgery. Only a few cases demonstrate obvious spread beyond the uterus when the patient is first seen. Despite this seemingly favorable initial impression, a third or more of patients develop recurrences.[226] There is a significant discrepancy between clinical and surgical staging. Although 82 percent of neoplasms are clinical stage I, only 66 percent are surgical stage I. Likewise, only 8 percent are clinical stage III compared to 21 percent that are surgical stage III.[229]

Low-grade endometrial stromal sarcoma has three distinct appearances. It can present as a firm mass within the myometrium that resembles a leiomyoma. Neoplasms like this generally bulge into the endometrial cavity. In some other cases the uterus may appear normal or globular, similar to the uterus involved with adenomyosis. The least common presentation is that of a polypoid mass projecting into the endometrial cavity that replaces the endometrium and invades deeply into the myometrium. The low-grade endometrial stromal sarcoma is white to pale yellow. Areas of necrosis and hemorrhage are common. The cut surface is characteristically pale yellow in color and soft or rubbery in consistency. Wormlike bands may extend from the cut surface, in some cases penetrating deeply even beyond the myometrium.

This neoplasm grows in tongues and nests, and in islands of stromal tissue that replace the endometrium and invade the myometrium (Fig. 6–34). The histopathology is monotonous, consisting of small cells that have round to oval nuclei and a minimal amount of cytoplasm. Mitoses are infrequent (less than 10 mitoses per 10 HPF). Minimal to mild cytologic atypia may be present. Cytologic atypia includes nuclear hyperchromatism, enlarged nuclei, prominent nucleoli, and irregular nuclear membranes. Differentiation of the small, dark, endometrial stromal cells from pericytes and lymphocytes by light microscopy is at times difficult. On electron microscopy the low-grade endometrial sarcoma cells closely resemble those of the normal postmenstrual day 5 endometrium.

Myometrial invasion is seen as serpiginous tongues of neoplasm that diffusely infiltrate the myometrium. Typically there is an accompanying desmoplastic inflammatory reaction.[226] This tumor simulates adenomyosis, but there is no glandular component. Frequently there is a concentration of cells around small blood vessels.[230] Lymphovascular space involvement extending deep into the

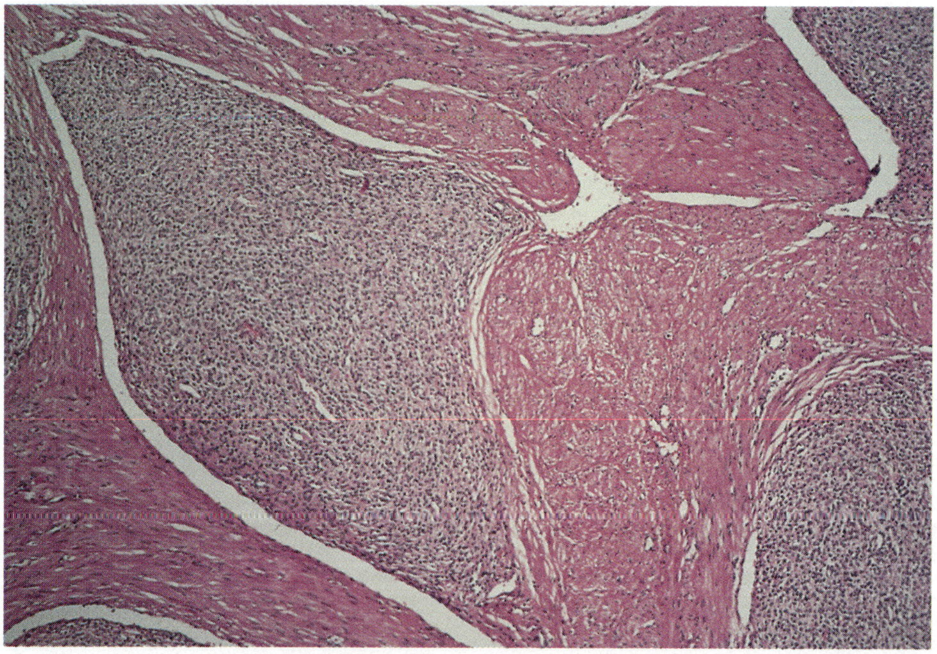

FIGURE 6–34
Seen here are islands of low-grade endometrial stromal sarcoma that penetrate the myometrium. The low-grade endometrial stromal sarcoma has a monotonous pattern of small cells with round to oval nuclei.

myometrial vessels and at times even beyond the confines of the uterus into the pelvic vessels is a common finding. On microscopic examination the neoplasm has the appearance of plugs within the vascular spaces. Intravascular growth occurs in over 50 percent of cases.[226]

Mitotic activity in low-grade endometrial stromal sarcoma is by definition less than ten mitoses per 10 HPF. Most of these tumors contain one to three mitotic figures per 10 HPF. If one adopts the theory presented previously that endometrial stromal sarcoma consists of two diseases, approximately 14 percent of neoplasms contain more than ten mitotic figures per 10 HPF but have normal stromal differentiation.[228] Forty-one percent contain only rare mitotic figures.[226] In performing a mitotic count one should include only definite mitotic figures and exclude lymphocytes, karyorrhectic nuclear fragments, and particles of hematoxylin, which can mimic mitotic figures.[234] Also, one should not gerrymander microscopic fields by low-power observations. It is necessary to count at least five sets of 10 MPF per slide.[226, 234] The DNA content of this tumor tends to be diploid.[235]

Occasionally individual glands may be present within islands of low-grade endometrial stromal sarcoma. These are usually endometrioid in type, sparse in distribution, and benign in appearance. Rarely atypical glandular proliferations, to the point of being back-to-back glandular structures, may be present.[236] These glands could represent focal epithelial differentiation within the tumor or entrapment of non-neoplastic endometrial or adenomytotic glands. The presence of occasional glands within the tumor does not change the diagnosis or alter the prognosis.

A prominent vascular pattern, which takes the form of a network of small arteries, is usually present. Chronic inflammation, characterized by plasma cells, is present in 70 percent of cases.[226] Foci of hyalinization are seen in 42 percent.[226] Thirty-eight percent of low-grade endometrial stromal sarcomas demonstrate microscopic hemorrhage, and 27 percent have foam cells not in areas of necrosis.[226] Most low-grade endometrial stromal sarcomas stain positive for cytokeratin, and all stain positive for vimentin using immunocytochemical techniques.[236]

Adenomyosis is present in adjacent normal myometrium in 27 percent of cases. Leiomyomas are also frequent. Nine percent of patients have an associated ovarian neoplasm.[230] Low-grade endometrial stromal sarcomas are characterized by frequent recurrences and occasional metastases, even after long intervals of time.[232] The interval between the initial treatment and the diagnosis of recurrence averages 5 years, but recurrences may occur as late as 25 years after surgery.[229] This has prompted many to use long-term oral progestogen as an adjuvant in the treatment of this condition.[229]

Endometrial Stromal Sarcoma Resembling Ovarian Sex Cord Tumor

This histopathologic variant of low-grade endometrial stromal sarcoma deserves detailed attention. This variant has sex cord or epithelioid differentiation within a low-grade endometrial stromal sarcoma. This differs from, and is more common than, glandular differentiation. The designation of uterine tumor resembling ovarian sex cord tumor is appropriate. When sex cord elements are a prominent feature of the neoplasm,[238] sex cordlike or epithelioid differentiation takes the form of cells arranged in small nests, cords, trabeculae, and solid or hollow tubules (Fig. 6–35). The cords, trabeculae, and solid tubules frequently have a plexiform arrangement.[238] The reported frequency of sex cordlike elements within a low-grade endometrial stromal sarcoma varies from 9 to 60 percent.[227, 230, 238, 239] The presence of sex cord differentiation has no effect on clinical outcome.[226]

The average age of women with low-grade endometrial stromal sarcoma with sex cord or epithelioid features is 49 years. The age range is between 35 and 71 years. The tumors range in size from 3.5 to 10 cm and average 6.9 cm. The gross features are similar to those of any other low-grade endometrial stromal sarcoma. The presence of epithelial-like or sex cord–like differentiation may be diffuse or focal. The cells grow in nests and rarely in well-developed glands, broad trabeculae, cords, or papillary structures.[238] Nests of cells with lipid-rich cytoplasm may be seen in some cases. The mitotic activity in this tumor is low to moderate and never exceeds ten mitotic figures per 10 HPF.[238]

The cells in areas of epithelioid differentiation express vimentin, muscle-specific actin, desmin, and cytokeratin using immunocytochemical techniques. They do not express epithelial membrane antigen. The epithelioid differentiation thus appears to be muscle in nature rather than epithelial, as in epithelioid smooth muscle uterine tumors. This differentiation toward smooth muscle is unusual. True myoepithelial neoplasms occur in organs such as the breast and salivary glands, which have myoepithelial cells. Myoepithelial cells are not present in the uterus. However, both endometrium and myometrium are derived from mes-

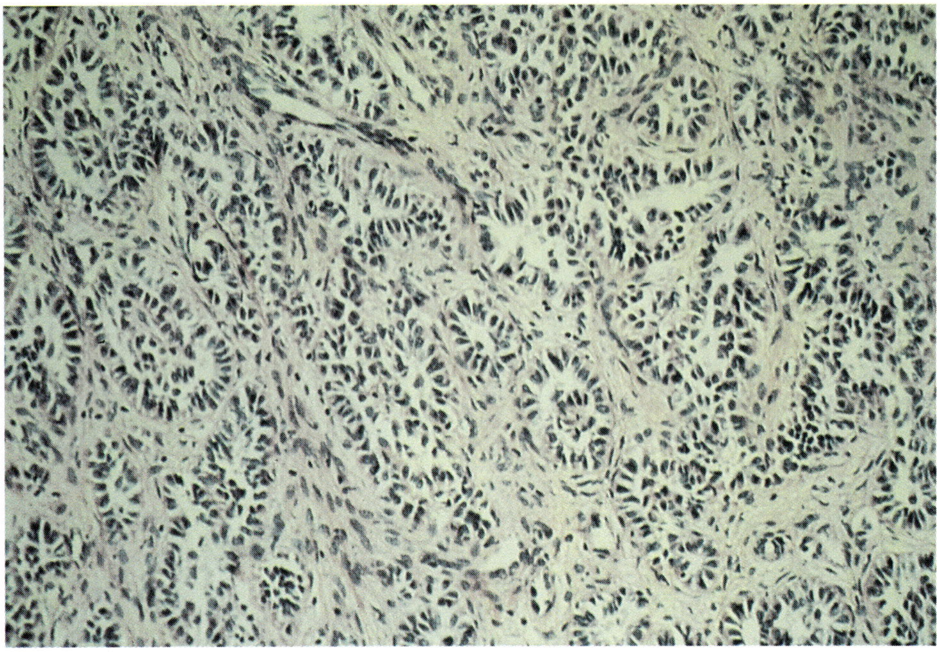

FIGURE 6–35
This is an endometrial stromal tumor with sex cord–like elements organized into a tubular pattern.

oderm, and endometrial stromal cells have the potential to differentiate toward smooth muscle.[240]

A rare low-grade endometrial stromal sarcoma may show smooth muscle differentiation or an admixture of distinct zones of unambiguous smooth muscle and endometrial stromal cells. These neoplasms tend to behave more like low-grade endometrial stromal sarcomas than mitotically active leiomyomas.[226] The term stromomyoma has been used to describe these cases.[241]

Differential Diagnosis

Low-grade endometrial stromal sarcomas must be differentiated from high-grade tumors. High-grade endometrial stromal sarcomas occur in older women, have a higher mitotic count, and are more anaplastic. The mitotic count usually exceeds 20 mitotic figures per 10 HPF. Smooth muscle uterine tumors with low mitotic activity may also be confused with low-grade endometrial stromal sarcoma. The cells in uterine smooth muscle tumors are different from those of endometrial stromal tumors. Smooth muscle cells have abundant eosinophilic cytoplasm and fusiform nuclei. Foam cells do not occur in uterine smooth muscle tumors but do occur in some low-grade endometrial stromal sarcomas. Carcinosarcoma may also be confused with a low-grade endometrial stromal sarcoma. The presence of a malignant epithelial component associated with the sarcoma defines the carcinosarcoma. Mitotic activity in carcinosarcoma is greater than in low-grade endometrial stromal sarcoma.

Clinical Management

The 5-year survival rate for patients with stage I disease is 88 percent, and for those who have stage II low-grade endometrial stromal sarcoma it is 66 percent. However, recurrences are frequent.[226] There is no association between the original tumor size and the risk of recurrence. Recurrences occur in 47 percent of patients whose tumors have minimal cytologic atypia and rare mitotic figures.[226] Of patients who have surgical stage I disease, 35 percent develop pelvic recurrence, 11.7 percent have pelvic and distant recurrence, and 9 percent have distant recurrence only. In stage III disease the recurrence rate is 72 percent. Seventy-five percent of women with stage III low-grade endometrial stromal sarcoma die of this disease. Of patients with surgical stage IV tumors, 86 percent develop recurrence, and 60 percent die of the disease.[226] Recurrent tumors are usually sensitive to hormonal therapy.[229] The most frequent sites of recurrence are the pelvis and abdomen. Forty-two percent of women who experience one recurrence will also have a second. Local excision of vaginal recurrence is successful in some patients.[226] The lung is an uncommon site of recurrence for this tumor. The time to recurrence ranges from 3 to 274 months. The interval without disease averages 34 months for patients with stage I disease and 4 months for those with stage IV disease.[226]

The treatment of low-grade stromal sarcoma is abdominal hysterectomy with bilateral salpingo-oophorectomy and surgical staging. There is evidence that many low-grade endometrial stromal sarcomas are hormone dependent or hormone responsive. The determination of tumor estrogen and progesterone content may prove useful in selecting patients for hormonal therapy.[242] Two-thirds of patients with low-grade endometrial stromal sarcoma respond to hormonal treatment. Of all the uterine sarcomas, low-grade endometrial stromal sarcoma has the highest median progesterone receptor content (113.9 fmol/mg cytosol protein).[243] Progesterone therapy appears to be more useful than cytotoxic agents in the treatment of patients with this neoplasm.[233] A variety of progestogens and antiestrogens have been used for treatment of patients with low-grade endometrial stromal sarcoma. These include megestrol acetate, medroxyprogesterone acetate, intramuscular hydroxyprogesterone caproate, and tamoxifen. Forty-six percent of patients experience a partial (23 percent) or complete (23 percent) response to hormonal therapy. Low-grade endometrial stromal sarcoma is also extremely radiosensitive. Radiation therapy may be used for local control. Although radiation therapy and progestational therapy are useful modalities for the treatment of patients with low-grade endometrial sarcoma, traditional chemotherapy is of limited value. Only 17 percent of patients respond to doxorubicin hydrochloride.[229]

Because of the high recurrence rate we recommend the indefinite use of a progestogen or antiestrogen after total abdominal hysterectomy and bilateral salpingo-oophorectomy. Radiation is used for the control of recurrences that fail to respond to hormonal therapy.

High-Grade Endometrial Stromal Sarcoma

High-grade endometrial stromal sarcoma differs from low-grade endometrial stromal sarcoma both in degree of mitotic activity and in biologic behavior. High-grade endometrial stromal sarcoma infiltrates the myometrium widely, has an aggressive clinical course with a high rate of metastases, and has a high mortality rate.[232] In one series only 13 percent of all endometrial stromal tumors were high grade.[226] There are few, if any, differences in the biologic behavior of high-grade endometrial stromal sarcomas and other uterine sarcomas such as leiomyosarcoma, pure heterologous sarcoma, undifferentiated sarcoma, and carcinosarcoma.[226]

The median age of patients with high-grade endometrial stromal sarcoma is 57 years. This tumor is found with almost equal frequency in white and African-American women.[209] Fourteen percent of patients are nulliparous, and 29 percent are premenopausal. Five percent have a history of previous pelvic irradiation. Eighty-six percent of patients present with abnormal uterine bleeding, 19 percent with vaginal discharge, 24 percent with abdominal pain, and 10 percent with gastrointestinal or genitourinary complaints.[212]

The diagnosis of high-grade endometrial stromal sarcoma requires a demonstration of mitotic activity of more than ten mitoses per 10 HPF and infiltrating tumor margins.[212] However, according to some investigators, a few of these neoplasms have fewer than ten mitotic figures per 10 HPF but behave biologically in an aggressive fashion similar to neoplasms that have a higher mitotic count.[228]

High-grade endometrial stromal sarcomas are soft, fleshy, polypoid tumors. They can be pink, tan, gray, or white. Areas of hemorrhage and necrosis are common. The tumor frequently fills the endometrial cavity. Gross evidence of myometrial invasion is usually readily apparent owing to the associated hemorrhage and necrosis. Growth beyond the uterus is common.[227]

The tumor cells resemble the stromal cells of proliferative endometrium but have considerable cytologic atypia. Sheets of monotonous cells with basophilic nuclei and indistinct cytoplasm characterize endometrial stromal neoplasms. Cellular pleomorphism is the hallmark of high-grade neoplasms. Stromal sarcoma grows as a well-demarcated layer of mass toward the uterine lumen.[211] Mitotic figures, by definition, must exceed ten per 10 HPF. The finding of over 20 mitotic figures per 10 HPF is frequent. Infiltration of the myometrium is wide and deep. Spread outside the uterus is common.[232] These tumors stain positive for vimentin and are negative for keratin and cytokeratin using immunocytochemical techniques.[236]

Sixty-one percent of patients have clinical stage I disease, 15 percent have stage II, and 23 percent have stage IV disease.[212, 226] The prognosis for these patients is poor. Survival rates for patients with high-grade endometrial stromal sarcoma are similar to those of patients with malignant mixed mesodermal tumor. The depth of myometrial invasion is strongly associated with the presence of extrauterine disease and determines the prognosis.[212,226]

Leiomyosarcoma

Leiomyosarcoma and carcinosarcoma are the most common malignant nonepithelial tumors of the uterus (see Table 6–11). Leiomyosarcoma accounts for 0.21 to 6 percent of all uterine smooth muscle tumors.[244] One estimate of its prevalence is 0.5 to 0.67 per 100,000 women who are 20 or more years of age.[245] The incidence is 6.4 per million women per year.[209] In reported series, leiomyosarcoma accounts for 16 to 50 percent of all uterine sarcomas and 1 to 6 percent of all malignant uterine tumors.[246, 247] It seems to occur more frequently in African-American than in white women.[244, 245] The frequency of leiomyosarcoma in white women is 6.1 per million women, and in African-American women it is 9.9 per million.[209]

Women who have a leiomyosarcoma tend to be younger than those who have other uterine sarcomas. Nonetheless, leiomyosarcoma is rare in women 40 years of age or less. The peak incidence is the fifth decade.[248] The patients' mean age is 52.5 years. The range is between 26 and 86 years.[233, 244, 249, 250] Fifty to 75 percent of women with a diagnosis of leiomyosarcoma are premenopausal,[244, 246, 249] and 15 to 20 percent are nulliparous.[244,249]

The most frequent presenting symptom is abnormal uterine bleeding, which occurs in two-thirds of cases.[244, 249, 251] Other signs and symptoms at presentation include pelvic pain, pelvic mass, dysmenorrhea, vaginal discharge, symptoms referable to anemia, and symptoms due to pressure on adjacent organs. Patients who have advanced disease may present with fever, weight loss, weakness, lethargy, and symptoms referable to neoplastic involvement of adjacent pelvic organs.[252] In 10 to 15 percent of cases the leiomyosarcoma is an incidental finding discovered on routine pelvic examination of an asymptomatic woman. In these cases the clinical impression is that of an enlarged uterus consistent with leiomyomas, but at surgery leiomyosarcoma is discovered. The duration of symptoms varies considerably. Some women report symptoms for less than 1 month, whereas others have had symptoms for more than a year.[244] When the leiomyosarcoma is in a submucus location, involves the cervix, or is bulky and projects into the endometrial cavity, fragments of neoplasm may be seen in curettage specimens. This occurs in up to 50 percent of cases.[246, 247] In less than 1 percent of patients with advanced disease, cells suspicious for malignancy may be seen on cervicovaginal cytologic examination.[233]

A major source of confusion is the inconsistent criteria for the diagnosis of leiomyosarcoma and the controversy regarding prognostic factors.[248] The distinction between benign and malignant uterine smooth muscle tumors depends on three factors: mitotic activity, cytologic atypia, and invasion.[232] Smooth muscle tumors that have invaded contiguous organs or blood vessels are by definition malignant.[232] In the absence of obvious invasion the diagnosis of malignancy rests on the other two criteria. These criteria were discussed in detail in Chapter 5, but, owing to their importance, they will be revisited here. A benign uterine smooth muscle tumor has fewer than five mitotic figures per 10 HPF in the most mitotically active area and lacks cytologic atypia. Uterine smooth muscle tumors that have greater than ten mitotic figures per 10 HPF in the most active areas and also show cytologic atypia are also clearly malignant. Smooth muscle tumors that contain five to nine mitotic figures per 10 HPF in the most active areas and have cytologic atypia are also considered leiomyosarcomas, but they have low metastatic potential.[232, 252, 253] An occasional uterine smooth muscle tumor lacks cytologic atypia but contains five to nine mitotic figures per 10 HPF in the most active area. Such a tumor is classified as mitotically active leiomyoma.[232, 252, 253] Only a few cases fall into this category.[232] In a critical appraisal of patients with mitotically active leiomyomas, aggressive clinical behavior was not seen if the tumor had been sampled adequately and examined carefully.[253]

Tumor sampling of a grossly atypical uterine smooth muscle tumor and mitotically active leiomyoma is important and requires one tissue block per centimeter of greatest tumor diameter.[250] Accurate mitotic counting in uterine smooth muscle tumors is essential. The mitotic count is performed in tissue from the most mitotically active area of the neoplasm. To aid in counting mitotic figures accurately, a 4- to 5-μm section of tissue is preferable. A light hematoxylin and eosin stain or a mucicarmine stain helps to distinguish mitotic figures from pyknotic, folded, bizarre, or hyperchromatic nuclei.[234, 246] The observer should count only clearly recognizable mitotic figures.[239, 246] To determine mitotic activity, the observer counts the number of mitotic figures in at least four or five sets of ten consecutive microscope high-power (400 ×) fields. The eyepieces should be 10 × wide field devices. The set with the highest count determines the mitotic count for the tumor. Lack of a systematic, compulsive, and careful approach to mitosis counting may account for reports of tumors with few mitotic figures that have recurred and metastasized.

Most malignant uterine smooth muscle tumors

show pleomorphism. Only rarely does a neoplasm with greater than ten mitotic figures per 10 HPF lack nuclear atypia. Uterine smooth muscle tumors without nuclear atypia and mitotic counts as high as 15 per 10 HPF have been reported to follow a benign course (see also Chapter 5).[83a] Nuclear atypia varies from none to marked and is classified based on the most abnormal area. An estimate of cellularity (low or high) is also appropriate. Comparison with adjacent normal uterine smooth muscle helps in determining the degree of tumor cellularity.[246] Also estimated is the proportion of tumor composed of spindle and round, epithelioid-type cells. Areas of necrosis are identified. A description of the tumor interface with normal tissue as either circumscribed or infiltrating is mandatory. Vascular invasion, whenever observed, requires documentation.[246]

The uterus containing a leiomyosarcoma is large, and the cervix to fundus length exceeds 10 cm in most cases. It has a nodular appearance. Benign leiomyomas are frequently also present. The frequency of benign leiomyomas coexisting with a leiomyosarcoma varies from 22 to 76 percent.[245, 252] The leiomyosarcoma is usually unifocal. Only 5 percent of leiomyosarcomas are multiple. In two-thirds of cases the leiomyosarcoma is confined to the uterus. In the remaining one-third there is spread beyond the uterus.[224, 249, 251] Leiomyosarcoma appears as a mass with a peculiar yellow hue and a soft brainlike or fish fleshlike consistency.[246] The cut surface is also soft or fleshy. Distinct zones consisting of gray-yellow, pink, or tan-colored tissue are apparent on cut sections. Unlike benign leiomyomas, which have a well-defined pseudocapsule, leiomyosarcoma has poorly defined borders. On occasion a leiomyosarcoma may be predominantly white in color and firm to hard in consistency. It may have a whirling fibrous pattern similar to that seen in a leiomyoma. Leiomyosarcoma, like the benign leiomyoma, often bulges above the plane of section. Necrotic and cavitated areas, cream and brown in color, are common (Fig. 6–36).

The gross appearance of malignant smooth muscle tumors is deceptive. A correct diagnosis of leiomyosarcoma occurs in only 30 percent of cases before microscopic examination. Deep myometrial invasion, when present, is usually obvious on inspection. The size of a leiomyosarcoma ranges from 0.5 to 40 cm.[245, 249, 250] The median size is approximately 9 cm. The majority of neoplasms arise intramurally, but some are submucosal and others arise in a subserosal location (Fig. 6–36). Uncommonly, it may arise in the cervix.[245] The location of uterine leiomyosarcoma is submucosal in 20 to 25 percent of cases, intramural in 50 to 65 percent, and subserosal in 15 to 16 percent.[245] The surrounding endometrial cavity may show compression by the tumor.

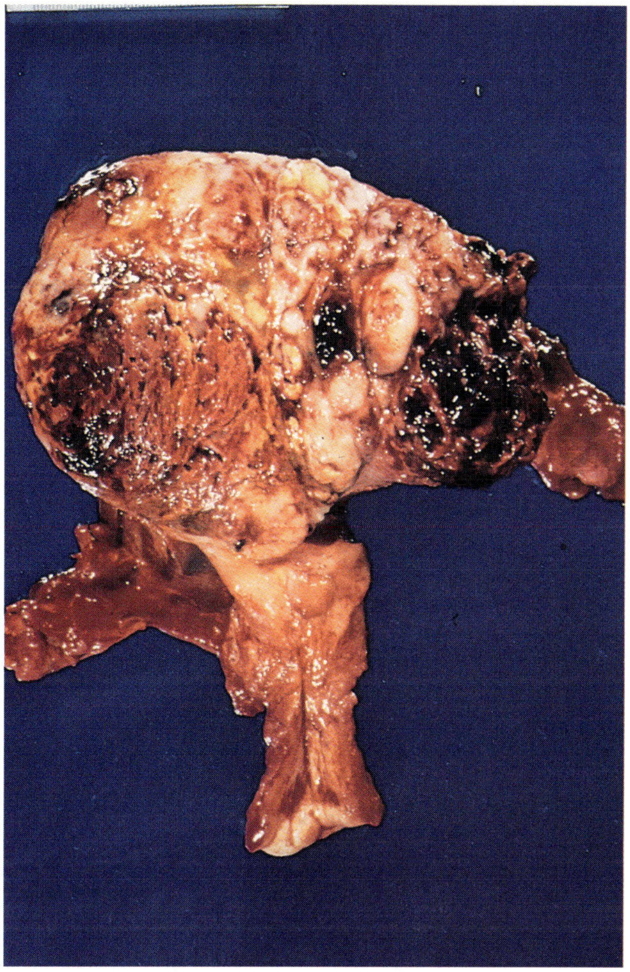

FIGURE 6–36
A large, fleshy leiomyosarcoma with hemorrhage and necrosis is seen arising subserosally from the uterine fundus. The uterus is of normal size. The normal cervix is seen at the bottom.

These neoplasms are densely cellular, have increased mitotic activity, and are cytologically atypical and pleomorphic[245] (Fig. 6–37). The degree of cytologic atypia, pleomorphism, and mitotic activity varies greatly from neoplasm to neoplasm. Spindle cells arranged in bundles intersecting at various angles are the hallmark of leiomyosarcoma. Individual cells appear fusiform and have abundant eosinophilic cytoplasm, which has a fibrillar appearance when stained with phosphotungstic acid hematoxylin (PTAH) stain. In some areas the tumor cells appear rounded or irregular and pleomorphic. The nuclei of these cells are blunt, and the cells possess copious eosinophilic cytoplasm. Cytoplasmic intranuclear inclusions,

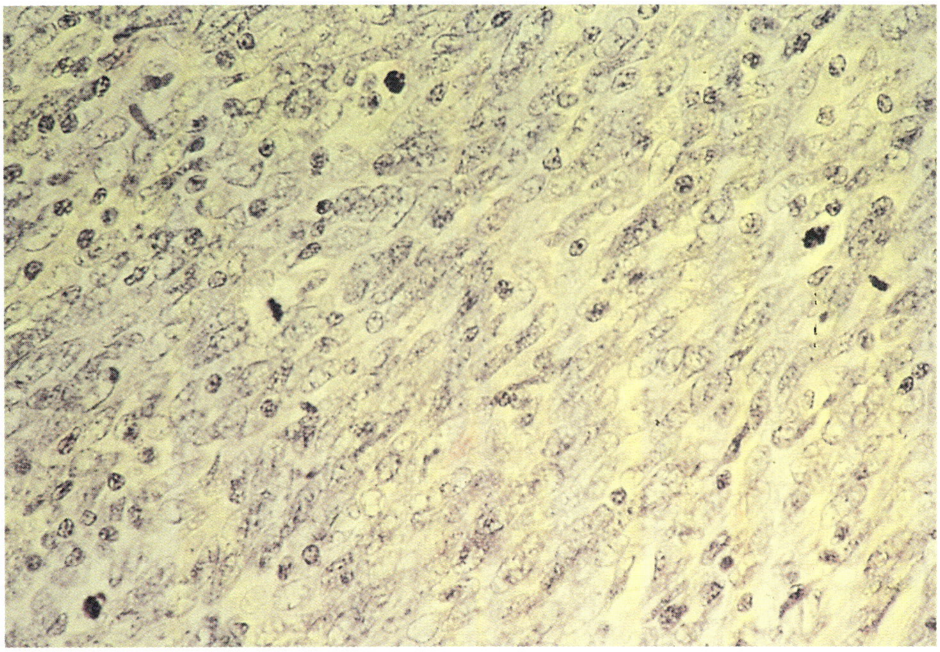

FIGURE 6-37
This leiomyosarcoma shows an increase in the number of fusiform cells as well as nuclear atypia and pleomorphism. Several mitotic figures are seen. A uterine smooth muscle tumor with cytologic atypia and five or more mitotic figures per ten HPF is considered a leiomyosarcoma.

which are actually invaginations of the cytoplasm into the nucleus, are common. They are present in 40 to 50 percent of tumors. The presence of intranuclear inclusions, however, is a poor predictor of malignancy. They are frequently present in leiomyosarcoma but are also present in 50 percent of bizarre leiomyomas.[250] Atypical mitotic figures are frequent. Multinucleate giant cells (symplastic giant cells) are common and occur in up to three-fourths of leiomyosarcomas. These multinucleate cells are the result of endonuclear reduplication. They appear as aggregates of smooth muscle nuclei that are clustered in an irregular fashion, and they have only minor degrees of nuclear hyperchromatism and pleomorphism.[250] They have no distinguishing cell boundaries. The other type of giant cell seen in leiomyosarcoma is the osteoclastic giant cell. The characteristic feature of this cell is the presence of densely staining, irregularly shaped masses of nuclear material that displays extreme pleomorphism. These cells contain up to 50 small round or oval nuclei with evenly dispersed chromatin. They have amphophilic, often foamy cytoplasm.[254] The only other sarcoma which contains similar giant cells is the malignant fibrous histiocytoma. The two types of giant cells frequently coexist.[254]

There is controversy about whether leiomyosarcoma arises de novo or arises in an otherwise benign leiomyoma. Leiomyosarcomas are usually single, and most do not suggest an origin from a leiomyoma, either typical or atypical. However, in 4 to 23 percent of cases, an origin from a leiomyoma is possible.[247,250]

The differential diagnosis of leiomyosarcoma includes cellular leiomyoma, endometrial stromal sarcoma, hemangiopericytoma, and rhabdomyosarcoma.[244] Mitotic activity and cellular atypia distinguish a benign from a malignant uterine smooth muscle tumor. The bland, monotonous, small cells of endometrial stromal sarcoma are different from the pleomorphic cells of leiomyosarcoma. The absence of cross striations excludes rhabdomyosarcoma. Hemangiopericytoma contains angular clefts and vascular-like spaces. Intravenous leiomyomatosis, leiomyomatosis peritonealis disseminata, and benign metastasizing leiomyoma could be confused with a leiomyosarcoma that has spread outside the uterus.[250] Mitotic activity in benign uterine smooth muscle neoplasms is low, but it exceeds 10 mitoses per ten HPF in most sarcomas.

Eighty-three percent of women with a leiomyosarcoma die of this disease 4 months to 14 years after the initial diagnosis and treatment.[248] At initial surgery 63 to 70 percent of leiomyosarcomas appear to be confined to the uterus (surgical stage I or II).[233, 247] The remaining tumors show extrauterine spread. The lung is the most common site of metastasis, followed by bone, liver, and other intraabdominal organs, particularly the small bowel.[249, 251] In one study, 74 percent of patients with disease confined to the uterus developed recurrence.[247] Of those with extrauterine disease, all developed recurrence within a median time of 3 months.

Prognostic factors associated with an unfavorable outcome include high mitotic rate, high histopathologic grade, infiltrating tumor border,[244] postmenopausal status, large uterine size, and extrauterine extension.[244, 245, 250] Vascular invasion is an indicator of an extremely poor prognosis. The frequency of vascular invasion varies from 10 to 67 percent.[244, 245, 250] Less than 25 percent of women with leiomyosarcoma with vascular invasion survive this disease.[250]

Two indicators of a favorable outcome are the menstrual status of the patient and the gross appearance of the tumor. Only 15 percent of premenopausal patients die of disease compared to 77 percent of postmenopausal patients.[250] However, premenopausal patients with tumor invasion of the vascular channels do poorly. Over half of these women succumb to the disease when the diagnosis of sarcoma is obvious on gross inspection.[250] Origin of a leiomyosarcoma in a leiomyoma confers a more favorable prognosis, but this is uncommon.[255, 257] Tumors with pushing margins are also associated with a better prognosis.[244] There also appears to be a correlation between an increase in mitotic activity and a decrease in survival.[244, 255]

Factors that do not appear to be of prognostic significance include the size of the uterus, the presence or absence of atypical mitotic figures, the presence of symplastic giant cells, and the presence or absence of nuclear inclusions.[244, 255]

Factors of questionable prognostic significance include duration of symptoms, race, and size of tumor. Women who have had a shorter duration of symptoms, less than 6 months, appear to do better than women who have had a longer duration of symptoms.[244] African-American women appear to have a lower survival rate than white women.[244] However, these findings may be a reflection of more advanced surgical stage.[233] In one study 67 percent of women with neoplasms less than 5 cm in diameter survived, whereas no patient with a tumor larger than 5 cm in greatest diameter survived.[248] Another study showed no association between tumor size and survival.[244]

The median survival of patients with leiomyosarcoma is 43 months. Fifty-one percent of patients develop local recurrence and 78 percent develop distant metastases. Adjuvant radiation or chemotherapy has no impact on disease-free survival or overall survival.[247, 257] Although the pelvis is the most common site of recurrence, it is often associated with concomitant extrapelvic disease.[233, 247, 251, 257] The reported long-term survival varies from virtually zero to 68 percent.[233, 244, 246] Most women develop recurrence and die of disease within 2 years. In one series the 10-year survival rate was 27 percent for patients with all stages of leiomyosarcoma and 48 percent for those with stage I disease.[233] The 5-year survival rate of patients with disease confined to the uterus (i.e., surgical stage I and II) is approximately 50 percent with or without adjuvant chemotherapy.[257] All patients with extrauterine disease at the time of surgery die within 2 years.[247]

Treatment of the patient with a leiomyosarcoma consists of hysterectomy, bilateral salpingo-oophorectomy, and an attempt at surgical debulking of any obvious tumor metastases. Because this neoplasm typically spreads by direct extension and hematogenous routes, the value of lymph node dissection is questionable. In the majority of cases the surgeon does not know the correct diagnosis until microscopic examination of the uterine specimen is performed.[244] Treatment after the initial surgery requires individual attention and depends on the presence or absence of extrauterine disease. Adjuvant chemotherapy has no impact on the survival rate of patients with surgical stage I or II disease.[257] An intravaginal radioactive implant may decrease the frequency of local recurrence in these patients.[257] Radiation therapy may be used in an attempt to achieve control of pelvic residual disease. However, objective responses to radiation therapy are few.[247] Leiomyosarcoma is the least radiosensitive sarcoma that occurs in the müllerian system.[247] Patients with advanced disease could be treated with chemotherapy. However, chemotherapy is also not very effective in this disease. Doxorubicin, the most active drug against sarcomas, produces only a 16 percent response rate in these cases.[247] The duration of response averages 4 months.[247] These patients should be encouraged to participate in investigational protocols. Solitary pulmonary metastases have been successfully resected surgically with long-term survival.[244, 257a] All patients who have obvious extrauterine disease at the time of surgery die within 2 years.

Carcinosarcoma—Malignant Mixed Mesodermal (Müllerian) Tumor

Carcinosarcoma accounts for 1 to 6 percent of all malignant neoplasms of the uterine corpus. Twenty-two to 48 percent of all uterine sarcomas fall into this category (see Table 6–11). The prevalence of carcinosarcoma is 8.2 cases per million women per year.[209] This makes malignant mixed mesodermal tumor (MMT) the most common of the uterine sarcomas. By definition this neoplasm is composed of malignant epithelial and stromal components. Carcinosarcoma is further subdivided into neoplasms that demonstrate only homologous stromal elements and those demonstrating heterologous stromal elements. Homologous elements include endometrial stroma, smooth muscle, and fibrous connective tissue. Heterologous elements include tissues not native to the müllerian system (e.g., striated muscle, cartilage, bone, and occasionally fat). This group of neoplasms has had a confusing variety of names. Some authors reserve the term carcinosarcoma for mixed mesodermal tumors with homologous elements and call tumors with heterologous elements mixed mesodermal tumors. Others use the term mixed mesodermal tumor with the adjective homologous or heterologous to denote the stromal component. The term mixed müllerian tumor is more general because these neoplasms may also occur in the fallopian tube, cervix, and ovary. The ovary is clearly not a müllerian duct derivative. Other names found in the literature that describe tumors that have the appearance of a carcinosarcoma include sarcoma botryoides, carcinosarcomatoides, and mesenchymal sarcoma.[258] In 1989 the International Society of Gynecologic Pathologists adopted the name carcinosarcoma with the adjective homologous or heterologous to denote this group of neoplasms.[207]

The pathogenesis of carcinosarcoma is of interest. There has been considerable speculation about whether this neoplasm represents a collision tumor (i.e., two independent tumors that meet) or a composition tumor. In cell culture carcinosarcoma cells can differentiate along the lines of both carcinoma and sarcoma.[259] This tumor appears to originate from totipotential mesodermal cells, which have the capacity to form both epithelium and stroma.[260]

Because this tumor is uncommon we do not have a good understanding of its epidemiologic features. Patients with a carcinosarcoma have the epidemiologic characteristics of patients who have typical endometrial carcinoma, i.e., nulliparity, obesity, and diabetes. In the past it was thought that carcinosarcoma was associated with prior pelvic irradiation, but this has not been a consistent feature in recent series.[212, 261, 262] A few cases of carcinosarcoma have developed on a background of functioning ovarian lesions and exogenous estrogen therapy.[263] They tend to occur later in life than other uterine sarcomas and confer the worst prognosis of all uterine sarcomas.[233] In older series homologous carcinosarcomas were more common than heterologous tumors. The arrival of immunocytochemical techniques has allowed easier detection of heterologous elements.[264, 265] This is particularly true of striated muscle with the use of myoglobin and actin antibodies. Although cartilage was formerly the most common heterologous element found in carcinosarcoma,[260] in recent studies striated muscle is the most common.[210] Rhabdomyosarcoma is found in approximately 60 percent of heterologous carcinosarcomas, and chondrosarcoma is found in most of the remainder.

Carcinosarcoma occurs almost exclusively in postmenopausal women. The patients' mean age is 61 years,[260] and the median age is 62 years. The age range is 44 to 88 years.[258, 260, 262] Only a few patients are premenopausal.[242, 244, 246] There is an isolated case report of a carcinosarcoma in a 4-year-old girl.[266] Although 80 to 85 percent of patients with carcinosarcomas are white,[260, 267] the incidence in African-American women is three times higher than that in white women. The incidence of carcinosarcoma is 20.3 cases per million African-American women per year, whereas it is 7.5 per million white women per year.[209] African-American women are most likely to have heterologous elements. Seventy percent of carcinosarcomas in African-American women contain heterologous elements, but only one-third of the neoplasms in white women have heterologous elements.[267] Approximately 20 percent of patients are nulliparous,[258, 260, 267] and 16 to 47 percent are obese.[260, 267] Sixty-one percent are hypertensive, and 21 percent are diabetics.[267] Six to 14 percent of women with carcinosarcoma have a history of previous pelvic radiation therapy.[262, 267] There appears to be an increase in the incidence of carcinosarcoma in recent years, but the reason for this increase is unknown.[267]

By far the most common presenting complaint is postmenopausal vaginal bleeding.[233, 267] The occasional premenopausal patient typically presents with abnormal uterine bleeding. A watery or blood-tinged vaginal discharge may be the only clinical sign in some postmenopausal women.[260] An uncommon presentation is "tumor abortus." This refers to spontaneous passage of the polypoid neoplasm in part or in its entirety. Rare patients present with symptoms of advanced disease. These symptoms include weight loss and complaints referable to the intestinal or urinary systems. Carcinosarcoma is a rapidly growing neoplasm, and the median duration of symptoms is 2.8 months.[233, 267]

On physical examination uterine enlargement is present in two-thirds of patients. More than 20 percent have tumor protruding through the cervical os (Fig. 6–38). Rarely, the diagnosis is suggested by cervicovaginal cytologic examination.[268] Thirty-five to 46 percent of women with carcinosarcoma have cervicovaginal cytologic findings that are suspicious for malignancy or frankly malignant.[233, 258, 267] Typically it is the epithelial component that is present in the cytology smear. Curettage establishes a diagnosis of cancer in more

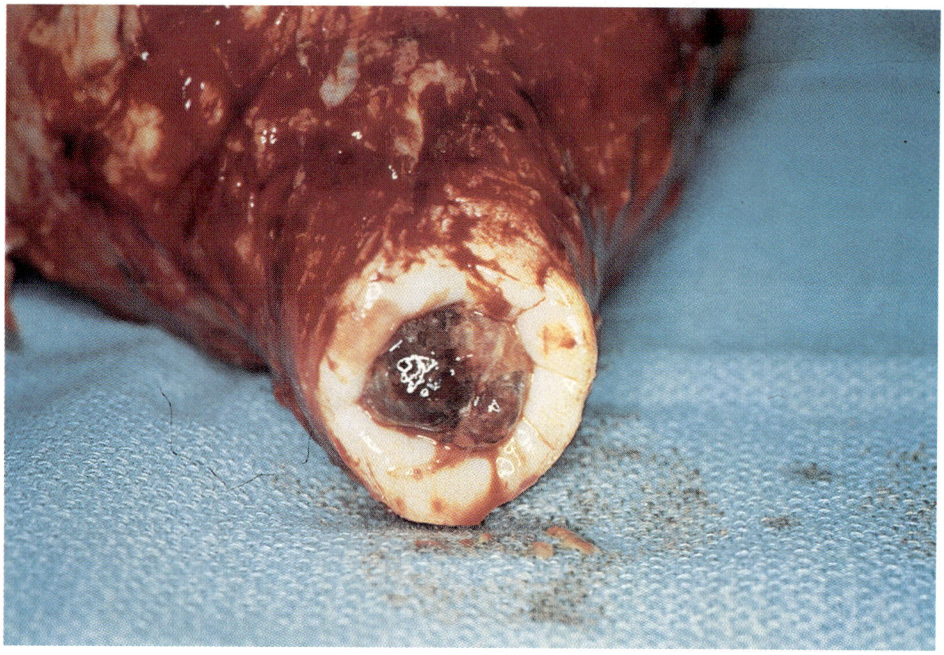

FIGURE 6-38
This is a carcinosarcoma presenting as a polypoid mass protruding through the cervical os. This is a hysterectomy specimen. Normal cervical tissue is seen around the hemorrhagic, variegated polypoid mass.

than 80 percent of cases. In 68 percent of these cases the multiphasic nature of the neoplasm is apparent on the curettage specimen, whereas in the remainder only adenocarcinoma or only sarcoma is present. In some cases the diagnosis is made on cervical biopsy or vaginal vault biopsy. In some patients the correct diagnosis is not made until the hysterectomy specimen has been carefully reviewed.[267]

Carcinosarcoma is usually polypoid. Pedunculated exophytic growth also occurs. The tumor is usually solitary, soft, friable, and tan or gray in appearance (Fig. 6-39). Focal hemorrhage, which can be extensive, is present in one-third of cases, and necrosis is present in one-half.[260, 269] The maximum tumor diameter ranges from 1.4 cm to 20 cm; the average diameter is 7.8 cm.[260] In 9 percent of tumors the diameter is less than 2 cm; in 43 percent it is 2 to 5 cm; in 39 percent it is 5 to 10 cm; and in 9 percent it exceeds 10 cm.[270] The tumor mass is usually larger than that seen with endometrial adenocarcinoma. The tumor surface is typically smooth, but the cut surface is usually fleshy and variegated. Two thirds of polypoid neo-

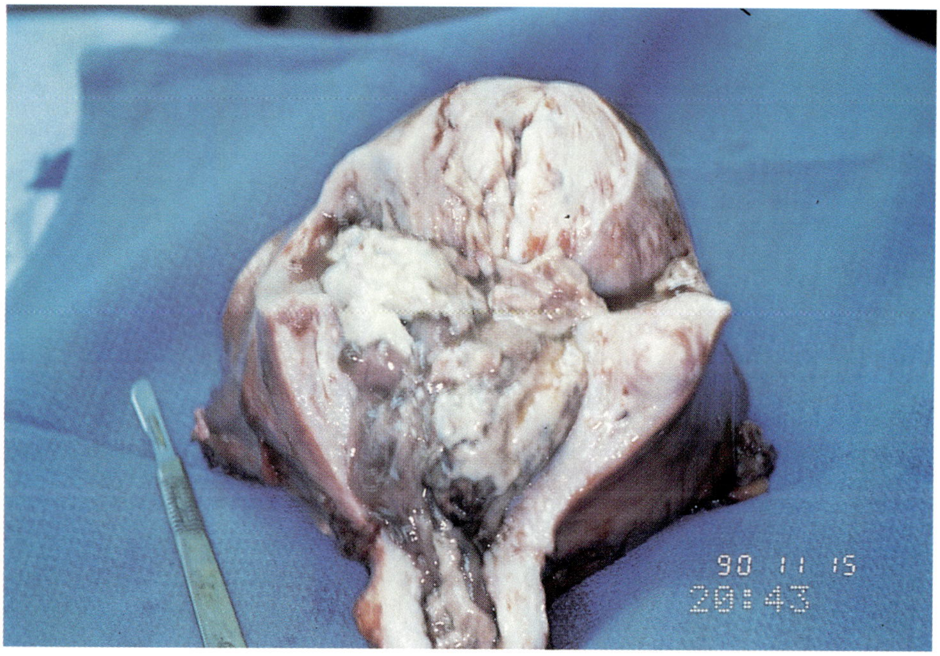

FIGURE 6-39
This uterus has been opened anteriorly, with the incision extended toward each uterine cornu. A pinkish gray, fleshy mass fills the endometrial cavity. Areas of necrosis are apparent. A polypoid portion of the tumor extends into the endocervical canal. The tumor involves the fundal myometrium. A 1.5 cm intramural leiomyoma is seen on the anterior myometrium *(right)*.

plasms have a single attachment to the uterus. The width of this attachment varies from 1 to 2.5 cm. The remaining tumors are sessile polypoid lesions with a broad base or tumors that have multiple sites of attachment to the uterus.[261] A few carcinosarcomas appear as diffuse plaques. The location of carcinosarcoma within the uterus involves the fundus in 19 percent of cases. Approximately one fourth demonstrate cervical extension.[270] Deep myometrial invasion, when present, is usually grossly apparent (see Fig. 6–39).

Carcinosarcoma contains both a malignant epithelial component (i.e., carcinoma) and a malignant stromal component (i.e., sarcoma). One of the tumor elements, either the glandular or the stromal, predominates. In most cases the stromal component accounts for more than half of the tumor volume.[269] The epithelial component may have the appearance of any of the cell types of müllerian origin. Endometrioid-type epithelium is found in most cases, but serous, mucinous, and clear cell carcinoma are not uncommon. (Fig. 6–40). Squamous differentiation in endometrioid-type epithelium, as in endometrial adenocarcinoma, occurs frequently. Rarely, pure squamous carcinoma may be the epithelial component. A mix of cell types occurs in many carcinosarcomas. The predominant epithelial cell type is endometrioid in 58 percent of cases, adenosquamous in 26 percent, papillary serous in 10 percent, and clear cell in 2 percent.[269]

The stromal component is usually an undifferentiated high-grade sarcoma, but occasionally it is well differentiated. The stromal component in homologous carcinosarcoma may show areas of differentiation that include endometrial stromal sarcoma, leiomyosarcoma, and fibrosarcoma. The endometrial stromal sarcoma component is usually high grade and shows a preponderance of small, pleomorphic, oval to spindle-shaped cells that have a high nuclear to cytoplasmic ratio. The cytoplasm is usually scant. The nuclei are hyperchromatic, oval or round, and have prominent nucleoli. Some amount of endometrial stromal sarcoma is present in over half of carcinosarcomas. Mitotic activity is usually brisk.[269] The mitotic count exceeds 20 mitoses per 10 HPF in 57 percent of cases, 10 to 20 mitotic figures per 10 HPF in 23 percent, and five to nine per 10 HPF in 14 percent; the remainder have fewer than five mitotic figures per 10 HPF.[270]

Heterologous elements, tissues that are not native to the müllerian system, are present in half to two-thirds of carcinosarcomas[261, 267, 270] (Fig. 6–41). These elements include rhabdomyosarcoma, chondrosarcoma, osteosarcoma, and, uncommonly, liposarcoma.[269, 270] A rare carcinosarcoma may exhibit neuroectodermal differentiation.[217] In approximately 25 percent of heterologous carcinosarcomas more than one heterologous element is present. The proportion of carcinosarcomas with heterologous elements is increasing in recent series, probably owing to improved diagnosis as a result of immunocytochemical techniques.[26]

Due to advances in immunocytochemistry, rhabdomyosarcoma is now the most common heterologous element found in carcinosarcoma. In most cases, the rhabdomyoblasts involve many micro-

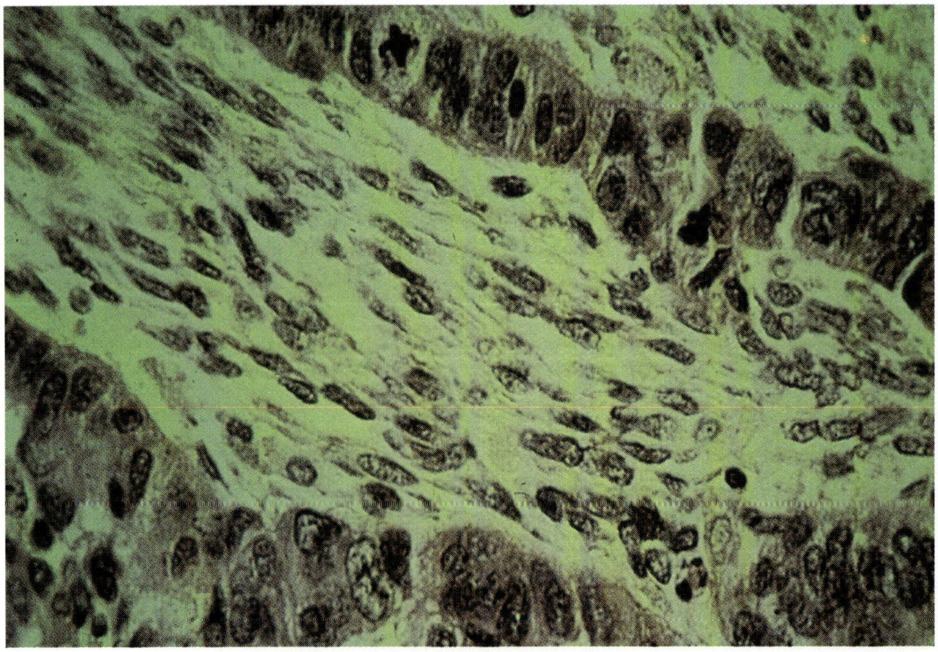

FIGURE 6–40
A malignant epithelium with marked nuclear atypia and pleomorphism is set in a background of a stromal sarcoma. An abnormal mitosis is seen in the epithelium *(top)*. Some of the epithelial cells have cilia.

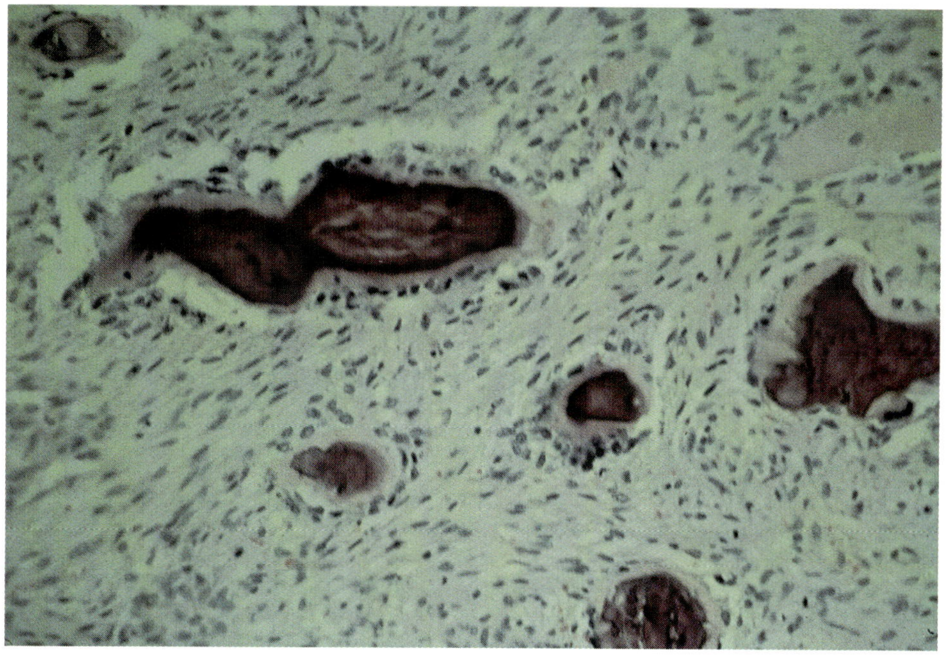

F I G U R E 6 – 4 1
A sarcomatous stroma with neoplastic, partially calcified osteoid tissue is seen. A malignant epithelial component was visible in other areas. A diagnosis of carcinosarcoma with heterologous elements was rendered.

scopic areas. Large pleomorphic cells, some of which demonstrate cross striations, are present throughout the neoplasm (Fig. 6–42). Both racquet-shaped cells and strap cells with cross striations are seen. To qualify as rhabdomyosarcoma two or more cells with unequivocal cross striations as well as large, nonstriated, deeply eosinophilic cells with granular cytoplasm should be identified. These cells sometimes contain large vesicular nuclei. Phosphotungstic acid hematoxylin (PTAH) stain may prove helpful in identifying cross striations, but this is rarely done anymore because immunocytochemical staining for myoglobin is simple and specific for striated muscle. Its sensitivity is 80 to 90 percent.[264] Immunocytochemical staining for actin is even more helpful than myoglobin in identifying rhabdomyoblasts. In six cases in which cross striations were present on light microscopy, immunocytochemical staining was positive in three cases with antimyoglobin, in five using anti-desmin antibodies, and in all six with anti-actin antibodies.[264] In three cases thought to be homologous tumors on light microscopy, the presence of actin showed the neoplasms to be heterologous.[269]

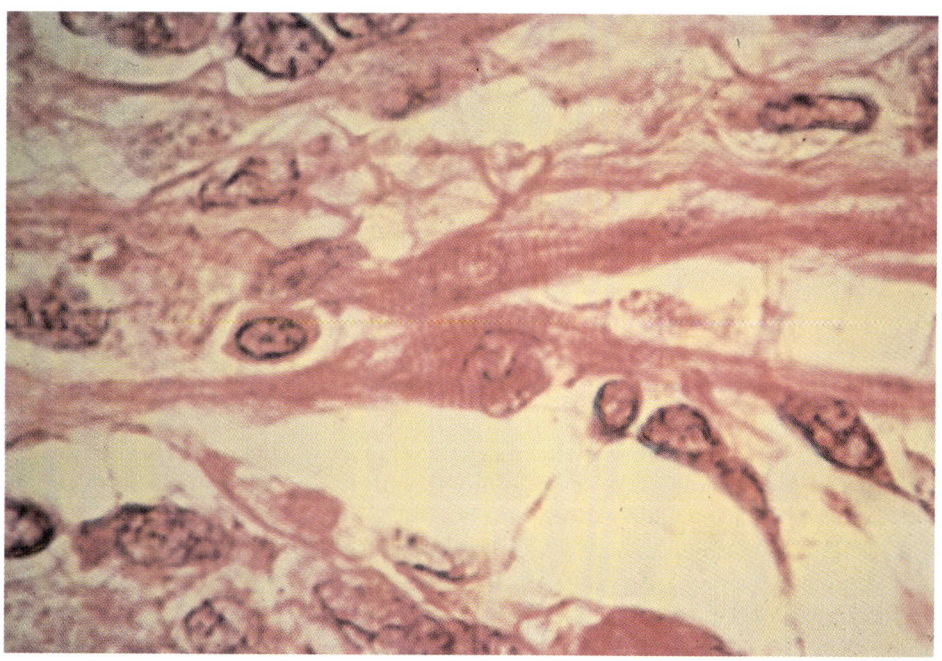

F I G U R E 6 – 4 2
Two malignant rhabdomyoblasts are seen *(center)*. Cross striations are easily observed.

Actin is present in 45 percent of carcinosarcomas.[264] Vimentin is present focally in glandular epithelium but is typical of all mesodermal cells. Immunologic markers for the stromal component include vimentin, desmin, actin, myoglobin, and α_1-antichymotrypsin.[265, 269, 270] Staining for epithelial membrane antigen or cytokeratin may be useful in identifying an epithelial component in some poorly differentiated neoplasms.[265] In as many as 25 percent of carcinosarcomas diagnosed as homologous, immunocytochemical staining identifies rhabdomyoblasts.[265] Some carcinosarcoma cells have eosinophilic cytoplasm that contains hyaline droplets. These droplets stain positive for α^1-antitrypsin.[272]

Neural tissue, when present in a carcinosarcoma, appears as large confluent tongues of glial tissue. Smaller nests of neural tissue may be present within the myometrium.[271] Other heterologous elements, unlike neural tissue, generally occur in small microscopic foci. The rare tumor with neural tissue stains positive with immunocytochemical staining methods against glial fibrillary acidic protein (GFAP) and S-100.[271]

Histopathologic grading of carcinosarcomas involves grading both the epithelial and stromal components. The histopathologic grade of carcinosarcoma does not seem to relate to prognosis and is not used to guide subsequent therapy. However, attempts to correlate carcinosarcoma grade with other clinical and pathologic findings continue to be made. There is no standard grading system for these neoplasms. The most commonly employed grading system for the epithelial component is similar to that previously described for endometrial carcinoma. Briefly, the epithelial component is called grade 1 if 5 percent or less of the tumor exhibits solid sheets of cells, grade 2 if 6 to 50 percent of the neoplasm has solid areas, and grade 3 if more than 50 percent has solid, sheetlike growth.[270] Some authors suggest that if the epithelial component of a carcinosarcoma is less than 25 percent solid it should be given a grade of 1, whereas the presence of 26 to 50 percent solid areas constitutes a grade 2.[253] Significant nuclear atypia increases the grade by one.[269]

Fourteen to 29 percent of carcinosarcomas have a well-differentiated epithelial component.[233, 261, 269, 270] The majority, therefore, are grade 2 or 3. The adjacent uninvolved endometrium is atrophic in most carcinosarcomas, but occasionally proliferative or hyperplastic endometrium is seen.[258]

A proposed histopathologic grading of the stromal component is as follows.[269, 270] A grade 1 stromal component contains relatively bland, polygonal to spindle-shaped cells, and there is a large amount of collagen separating the stromal cells. The nuclei show minor degrees of pleomorphism. Nucleoli are inconspicuous. A grade 2 stromal component is more cellular and pleomorphic than grade 1. Some intervening collagen is present. The nuclei are irregular, and an occasional pink nucleolus is seen. A grade 3 stromal component is very cellular, and the cells are anaplastic and pleomorphic. Nuclei vary greatly in size and shape. Occasional bizarre nuclei are present, and large red nucleoli are common. Necrosis may be present; fibrosis is absent. Using this grading of the malignant stroma of carcinosarcoma, 16 percent are identified as grade 1, 41 percent as grade 2, and 43 percent as grade 3.[269]

The strongest prognostic indicator in patients with carcinosarcoma is the depth of myometrial invasion.[212, 273] Myometrial invasion with or without lymphatic space involvement is present in 78 to 93 percent of carcinosarcomas.[260, 269, 270] Myometrial invasion is superficial in only 25 to 35 percent of instances.[269, 270] More than half of carcinosarcomas demonstrate lymphatic or vascular space involvement.[270]

Microscopic examination of metastases of carcinosarcoma shows carcinoma in 75 percent of cases, sarcoma in 10 percent, and both in 15 percent.[269, 270] The sarcomatous metastases contain heterologous elements in 50 percent of cases. Histopathologic findings in the heterologous elements in the metastases usually mirror those of the primary tumor. The heterologous elements found in metastases, in order of frequency, are rhabdomyosarcoma, chondrosarcoma, and osteosarcoma.[269]

Making the diagnosis of carcinosarcoma is usually not difficult, but differentiation from adenosarcoma is occasionally a problem. This is important because adenosarcoma is associated with a much better prognosis. Adenosarcoma generally occurs in younger women, and the epithelial component is clearly benign. Any focus of a malignant epithelial component establishes the correct diagnosis as carcinosarcoma. Endometrial stromal tumors may at times differentiate into tubular, glandlike, or sex cord structures. In these neoplasms the glandlike differentiation is always benign or of low-grade malignancy. Leiomyosarcoma and endometrial stromal sarcoma tend to spread hematogenously, whereas carcinosarcoma spreads first to the pelvic nodes.[269] Immunocytochemical techniques may prove useful in the differentiation of carcinosarcoma from undifferentiated sarcoma. Distinguishing carcinosarcoma from undifferentiated carcinoma may also be difficult. Immunocytochemical techniques sometimes can establish the correct diagnosis.

The treatment of patients with carcinosarcoma consists of hysterectomy, bilateral salpingo-oophorectomy, and surgical staging and debulking if necessary. Preoperative radiation therapy may be used in selected patients, particularly if there is bulky cervical involvement.[261] Postoperative chemotherapy is used in patients with advanced disease (i.e., stages III and IV). Ifosfamide is the most active cytotoxic agent available for the treatment of carcinosarcoma.[274] The combination of cisplatin and ifosfamide is currently being evaluated. Radiation therapy may be used for local control of recurrent or residual disease. Patients with stage I or II disease may be treated with chemotherapy or radiation. Radiation directed to the pelvis prevents local recurrences. The use of adjuvant cisplatin and ifosfamide in patients with totally resected stage I or II uterine carcinosarcoma is being studied by the Gynecologic Oncology Group.

There is no difference in the surgical stage distribution of homologous and heterologous carcinosarcomas. Sixty to 70 percent appear grossly to be confined to the uterus.[212] However, the surgical stage is higher in 15 to 20 percent of patients.[267]

In approximately one-third of patients extrauterine disease is present at the time of initial surgery.[260, 261] Sites of extrauterine disease include the ovary (40 percent), fallopian tube (33 percent), omentum (33 percent), lymph nodes (33 percent), peritoneum (13 percent), and occasionally the intestines, liver, and other sites.[269] In patients with disease clinically confined to the uterus, microscopic extrauterine disease is found in 19 percent, usually in positive pelvic or paraaortic lymph nodes. When the presence of extrauterine disease is obvious clinically, 85 percent of patients have positive pelvic or paraaortic lymph nodes. The majority of patients with metastasis to lymph nodes have tumors in which lymphatic space involvement has been identified.[270] Sixty-two percent of women with nodal metastasis have deep myometrial invasion. However, 10 percent of women with tumor clinically limited to the endometrium also have positive lymph nodes.

The prognosis of women with carcinosarcoma is poor. The reported overall 5-year survival rate is between 18 and 42 percent.[260, 261, 269, 270, 273, 275] Factors associated with survival include stage, cytology of peritoneal washings, depth of myometrial invasion, lymphatic space involvement, race, previous irradiation, and mode of therapy.[267] Age is not an important factor. Surgical stage and depth of myometrial invasion appear to be the most important prognostic indicators.[212, 273] Of these two factors, surgical stage appears to be most closely related to survival.[267, 273, 276, 277] The presence of malignant cells in peritoneal lavage fluid indicates an extremely poor prognosis. All patients reported to have carcinosarcoma apparently confined to the uterus but with positive peritoneal washings have died of the disease.[277a] Fifty-two percent of patients have superficial myometrial invasion or no invasion, 18 percent have invasion to the middle third, and 30 percent have myometrial invasion to the outer third. When considered as an independent variable, the depth of myometrial invasion does not appear to be related to survival. Even with superficial invasion, more than half of the patients eventually die of the disease.[267] With deep myometrial invasion the 5-year survival rate is 15 to 30 percent.[261, 267] Deep myometrial invasion does correlate with an increased risk of metastatic disease.[270] Lymphatic or vascular space involvement conveys a poorer prognosis.[270] With lymphatic space involvement the survival rate is 18 percent, but it is 53 percent in women without lymphatic space involvement. Involvement of the uterine isthmus or cervix also conveys a poorer prognosis.[270]

The grade of the carcinomatous element does not predict survival. The survival rate is 25 percent for patients in whom the epithelial component of the carcinosarcoma is grade 1, 55 percent if it is grade 2, and 43 percent if it is grade 3.[261]

In the past, the presence of heterologous elements was thought to be associated with a poorer prognosis, but this opinion has not been confirmed by larger and more recent studies.[270, 273] The type of heterologous element was also thought to have an impact on survival. The presence of rhabdomyoblasts was thought to be associated with a poorer prognosis, whereas the presence of cartilage was associated with a better prognosis.[212, 260] Again, a larger prospective study has not confirmed these findings.[270] The presence or absence of stromal heterologous elements, the type of such elements when present, the grade of the stromal component, and the mitotic count of the stromal component do not correlate with survival.[270]

The origin of a carcinosarcoma and its confinement entirely within an endometrial polyp occur uncommonly. Without evidence of extension through the stalk, the outlook for survival is excellent.[267, 278] The type of attachment of a polypoid tumor also appears to correlate with prognosis. Patients whose neoplasm has a pedunculated attachment to the uterus have a 5-year survival rate that exceeds 50 percent, whereas more than 25 percent of patients whose neoplasm has a broad-based attachment die within 12 months. The size of the neoplasm may affect survival. Women with small tumors, defined as measuring less than 5 to

7 cm, have a 5-year survival of 69 percent. Women with tumors larger than 7 cm have a 5-year survival of less than 10 percent.[260, 261] In early disease, (i.e., stage I) the patient with a small carcinosarcoma attached through a stalk rather than a broad base has the best prognosis.[260]

Estrogen and progesterone receptors are found in 25 to 56 percent of uterine sarcomas.[156, 243] The reported median estrogen receptor concentration is 10.7 fmol/mg cytosol protein and that of progesterone receptor is 15.8 fmol/mg cytosol protein. This is lower than the median concentration of these receptors in both endometrial and breast carcinomas.[243] Disease stage, tumor grade, and mitotic count do not appear to be associated with estrogen and progesterone receptor levels. Patients less than 50 years of age have higher progesterone receptor levels. There is no apparent age difference for estrogen receptor levels.[263]

The tumor-associated antigens CA 125 and CA 19-9 are readily demonstrable in the epithelial component of carcinosarcoma. CA 125 is present in 60 percent of neoplasms at least focally, and CA 19-9 is present in 51 percent.[279] The degree of expression correlates with the cell type and histopathologic grade of the epithelial component. Papillary serous, clear cell, and well-differentiated neoplasms are more likely to stain positive for CA 125 and CA 19-9.[279] Because recurrences of carcinosarcoma contain an epithelial component in 90 percent of cases, measurement of CA 125 and CA 19-9 in the serum may be useful in the follow-up of these patients.[279]

Pure Heterologous Uterine Sarcomas

Pure heterologous uterine sarcomas are extremely rare. They include rhabdomyosarcoma and chondrosarcoma. Although osteosarcoma and liposarcoma might occur in the uterus, we know of no reported cases of these neoplasms occurring as pure heterologous uterine sarcomas.

Pure rhabdomyosarcoma arising anywhere in the female genital tract is uncommon. Primary pure heterologous rhabdomyosarcoma arising in the uterus is extremely rare. Rhabdomyosarcoma usually occurs in childhood, when the term embryonal rhabdomyosarcoma or sarcoma botryoides is used. Genital rhabdomyosarcoma usually arises in the vagina. Fewer than 60 reported cases of pure uterine rhabdomyosarcomas are found in the literature.[280] Most rhabdomyosarcomas found in the uterus are part of a mixed epithelial-stromal neoplasm, usually a carcinosarcoma.[281] The incidence of pure rhabdomyosarcoma in a population is difficult to ascertain. In one large institution only one case of pure rhabdomyosarcoma was accessioned in the pathology laboratory during a 25-year period During that time there were over 5 million people at risk.[282] These tumors compose 2.9 to 5.7 percent of all uterine sarcomas.[210, 212]

Pure uterine rhabdomyosarcoma occurs in older women, usually in the seventh decade of life.[212, 281] Occurrence of this neoplasm in a 22-year-old and in a 42-year-old woman has been reported.[281] The chief complaint at presentation is abnormal or postmenopausal uterine bleeding.[212]

On physical examination a soft friable mass that protrudes through the cervix is commonly seen. It may resemble a prolapsed fibroid or an endometrial polyp. The mass may fill the upper vagina. Spontaneous passage (i.e., abortion) of all or part of the neoplasm may occur with this rapidly growing malignancy. The tip of the lesion frequently has areas of ulceration and hemorrhage. At initial surgery many uterine rhabdomyosarcomas seem to be confined to the uterus.[280–282] In the endometrium the neoplasm appears as reddish, tan, or gray solitary nodules. The tumor diameter varies from 2 to 14 cm. Hemorrhage and necrosis are common findings on the cut surface.

There seem to be two distinct histopathologic variants, one occurring in younger women and the other in older women. Although there are only a few reports of this neoplasm in younger women, in these women the neoplastic nodules closely resemble the embryonal rhabdomyosarcoma that arises in the vagina. Primitive small sarcoma cells encircle normal non-neoplastic endometrial glands. There is a condensation of cells forming a cambium layer beneath the surface epithelium. The cytoplasm of the rhabdomyoblast is brightly eosinophilic and fibrillar, and cross striations are easily recognizable (see Fig. 6–42). Cells with easily recognizable cross striations are usually plentiful. Other areas are highly cellular and show compact sheets of spindle-shaped cells. No other heterologous elements are present.

The second histopathologic variant occurs in older women. Numerous pleomorphic spindle-shaped cells, numerous epithelioid rhabdomyoblasts that have abundant eosinophilic cytoplasm and easily identifiable cross striations, and occasional strap cells that have cytoplasmic cross striations are present.[280, 281] Mitotic activity is brisk and usually exceeds 20 mitotic figures per 10 HPF. Areas of necrosis and hemorrhage may be extensive. Immunocytochemical staining for muscle-specific actin is positive in all instances. No malignant epithelial component or other heterologous elements are present. Deep myometrial invasion is common.[280]

Rhabdomyosarcoma of the uterus is a biologically aggressive neoplasm. Patients with pure uterine rhabdomyosarcoma generally have advanced disease at the time of diagnosis. The usual course is rapid progression, with death occurring within months despite aggressive adjuvant radiation therapy and chemotherapy.[212, 280, 281] Pelvic radiation therapy may control local disease. In many patients the disease, if not widespread at the time of diagnosis, spreads rapidly, and only palliative treatment and supportive care are appropriate. However, there is one reported case of a patient who had a solitary lung lesion. Resection of the lung lesion and multiagent chemotherapy resulted in a disease-free survival of more than 2 years at the time of the report.[281]

Chondrosarcoma is the second most common pure heterologous sarcoma occurring in the uterus. In one series there was one case among 70 uterine sarcomas.[212] However, in other large series of uterine sarcomas there were no primary uterine heterologous sarcomas other than rhabdomyosarcoma.[270, 277] Areas of chondrosarcoma appear highly differentiated.[210] The plump cells contain large double nuclei. Chondroblastic areas merge almost imperceptibly with the adjacent undifferentiated spindle cell sarcoma.

Angiosarcoma (Malignant Hemangioendothelioma)

Angiosarcoma is a tumor of blood vessels. In 1943 Stout characterized these neoplasms as being composed of vascular channels that had a tendency to anastomose and were lined by an excess of atypical endothelial cells.[283] Two criteria must be met to diagnose a primary vascular neoplasm in the uterus: the tumor cells are of vascular origin, and the tumor is not one of the more common endometrial tumors with an extensive vascular pattern. The prominent vascularity of many uterine neoplasms, especially vascular leiomyomas, can easily lead to an erroneous diagnosis of a primary vascular tumor.[284] There are only approximately ten well-documented examples of uterine angiosarcoma in the medical literature.[284]

The presenting complaint of patients with uterine angiosarcoma is abnormal vaginal bleeding. Curettage may increase bleeding instead of controlling it. Hysterectomy may become a medical emergency.

On gross examination, the myometrium appears diffusely thickened. The vascular tumor is brownish-red in color and firm in consistency.

These neoplasms consist of nests of cells that frequently form anastomosing vascular channels of varying caliber (Fig. 6–43). Papillary projections into the lumens are present. The individual cells have large vesicular nuclei, prominent nucleoli, and a moderate amount of amphophilic cytoplasm. Mitotic figures are abundant. With immunocytochemical staining techniques, stain factor VIII stains positively.[284]

The treatment of uterine angiosarcoma is abdominal hysterectomy and bilateral salpingo-oophorectomy. Because there are so few cases in the literature, the prognosis for patients with this tumor is difficult to ascertain, but it appears to be poor.

Miscellaneous Rare Uterine Sarcomas

Primitive neuroectodermal neoplasms, arising as a primary neoplasm in the uterus, are extremely uncommon.[285] They are soft polypoid tumors that

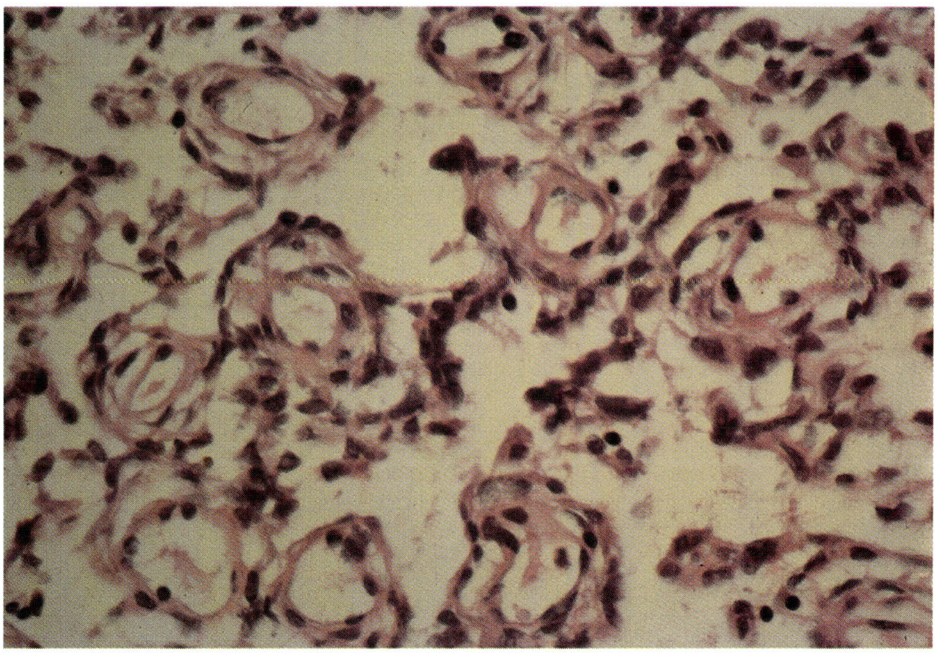

FIGURE 6–43
This angiosarcoma shows a proliferation of vascular channels lined by atypical cells. Atypical cells that have pyknotic and pleomorphic nuclei are seen in between the vessels.

fill and expand the endometrial cavity. Transmural infiltration of the myometrium may occur. Necrosis is common. On microscopic examination a malignant proliferation with a heterogeneous appearance replaces the endometrium. Malignant oval to spindle-shaped cells with a high nuclear to cytoplasmic ratio are present. Nucleoli are not a prominent feature.[285] Unlike teratomas, there are no mesodermal or endodermal elements in a neuroectodermal neoplasm. These tumor cells resemble those seen in medulloblastoma, retinoblastoma, neuroblastoma, and Ewing sarcoma. Chromogranin, S-100, and neuron-specific enolase can be used to identify the neuroendocrine cells. Primitive neuroepithelial cells form rosettes. Variably differentiated neuroblasts, occasional ganglion cells, oligodendrocytes, and bipolar and multipolar astrocytes are seen. Choroid plexus–like areas may be present. All these elements are present in variable amounts. Primitive neuroectodermal tumors exhibit an extremely aggressive biologic behavior.[285]

There is a case report of a malignant rhabdoid tumor arising as a primary neoplasm in the uterus of a 46-year-old woman.[286] The patient presented with metrorrhagia. Physical examination revealed an enlarged uterus consistent with uterine fibroids. The uterus contained a 9-cm, circumscribed, soft mass in the myometrium. The tumor showed areas of hemorrhage, necrosis, and cystic degeneration. Both the diffuse and the alveolar growth patterns of a rhabdoid tumor were identified on microscopic examination. The tumor cells were uniform and had large nuclei with prominent "owl eye" nucleoli, abundant eosinophilic cytoplasm, and large cytoplasmic globules that were PAS positive and diastase resistant.[286] Mitotic figures were infrequent. The histogenesis of this neoplasm is uncertain.

Tumors Metastatic to the Uterus

Malignant tumors may spread to either the endometrium or the myometrium by direct extension or by hematogenous metastasis. Extension to the endometrium occurs from primary or secondary cancers of the fallopian tube or the cervix. Extension to the uterine serosa or myometrium may occur from primary or secondary cancer of the ovary, fallopian tube, colon, or appendix. Tumors that are metastatic to the uterus maintain the histopathologic appearance of the primary neoplasm. The ovary requires special comment. When endometrioid adenocarcinoma is present in both the uterus and the ovary, it is more often the result of synchronous primary neoplasms than of metastasis from one to the other. Ovarian carcinoma metastasizes to the endometrium infrequently, whereas endometrial carcinoma spreads to the ovary more commonly.[287]

The presence of endometrial metastasis causes abnormal or postmenopausal uterine bleeding. Myometrial or serosal involvement may result in a pelvic mass. With a cancer that originates outside the pelvis, uterine involvement is usually part of a widespread disease process. On rare occasions, endometrial sampling for abnormal uterine bleeding may be diagnostic of breast, stomach, colon, or other nongynecologic neoplasms (Fig. 6–44).[288] Rarely, a cervical cytologic smear that reveals frankly malignant cells may be the initial clue to a cancer metastatic to the uterus.[189]

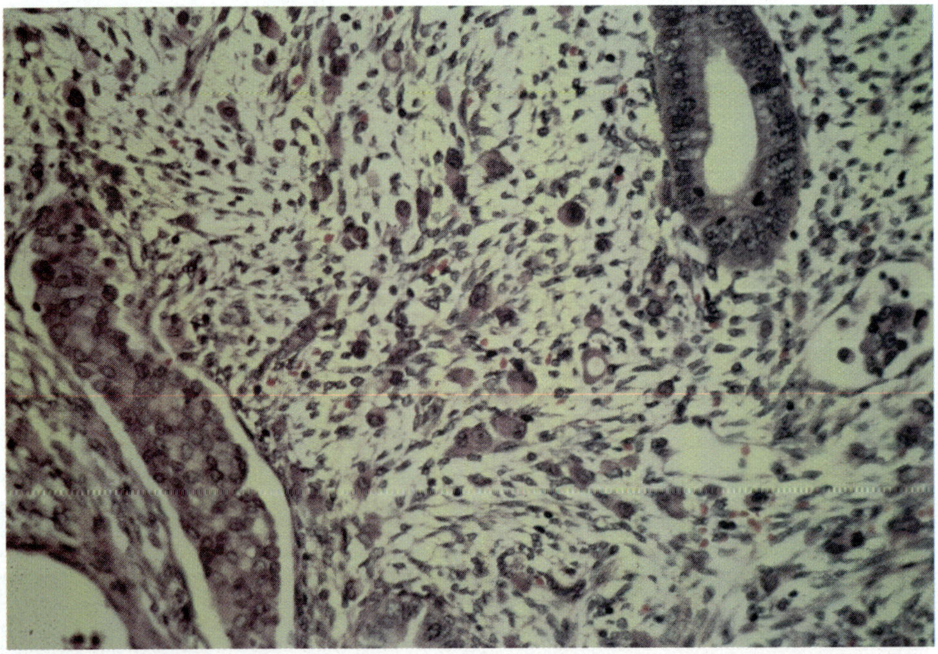

FIGURE 6–44
Single malignant cells are seen infiltrating the endometrial stroma. These cells differ in appearance from the cells lining the normal endometrial gland *(right)*. A nest of malignant cells is seen in a lymphovascular space *(left)*; some of the cells have vacuoles. This proved to be metastatic gastric adenocarcinoma.

REFERENCES

1. Vellios F: Endometrial hyperplasia and carcinoma in situ. Gynecol Oncol 1974;2:152–161.
2. Campbell PE, Barter RA: The significance of atypical hyperplasia. J Obstet Gynaecol Br Commonw 1961;68:668–672.
3. Hertig AT, Sommers SC, Bengloff H: Genesis of endometrial carcinoma: III. Carcinoma in situ. Cancer 1949;2: 946–971.
4. Gusberg SB, Kaplan AL: Precursors of corpus cancer: IV. Adenomatous hyperplasia as stage 0 carcinoma of the endometrium. Am J Obstet Gynecol 1963;87: 662–678.
5. Gusberg SB, Moore DB, Martin F: Precursors of corpus cancer: II. A clinical and pathological study of adenomatous hyperplasia. Am J Obstet Gynecol 1954;68:1472–1481.
6. Beutler HH, Dockerty MB, Randall LM: Precancerous lesions of the endometrium. Am J Obstet Gynecol 1963;86:433–443.
7. Kurman RJ, Kaminski PF, Norris NJ: The behavior of endometrial hyperplasia: A long term study of "untreated" hyperplasia in 170 patients. Cancer 1985;56:403–412.
8. Katayama KP, Jones HW: Chromosomes of atypical (adenomatous) hyperplasia and carcinoma of the endometrium. Am J Obstet Gynecol 1967;97:978–983.
9. Podczaski E, Kaminski PF, Zaino R: CA 125 and CA 19-9 immunolocalization in normal, hyperplastic, and carcinomatous endometrium. Cancer 1993;71:2551–2556.
10. Ausems EWMA, van der Kamp J-K, Baak JPA: Nuclear morphometry in the determination of the prognosis of marked atypical endometrial hyperplasia. Int J Gynecol Pathol 1985;4:180–185.
11. Colgan TJ, Norris JH, Foster W, Kurman RJ, Fox CH: Predicting the outcome of endometrial hyperplasia by quantitative analysis of nuclear features using a linear discriminant function. Int J Gynecol Pathol 1983;1:347–352.
12. Norris HJ, Becker RL, Mikel UV: A comparative morphometric and cytophotometric study of endometrial hyperplasia, atypical hyperplasia and endometrial carcinoma. Hum Pathol 1989;20:219–223.
13. Ferenczy A: Cytodynamics of endometrial hyperplasia and neoplasia: Part II. In vitro DNA histoautoradiography. Hum Pathol 1983;14:77–82.
14. Winkler B, Alvarez S, Richart RM, Crum CP: Pitfalls in the diagnosis of endometrial neoplasia. Obstet Gynecol 1984;64:184–194.
15. Gambrell RD, Bagnell CA, Greenblatt RB: Role of estrogens and progesterone in the etiology and prevention of endometrial cancer. Am J Obstet Gynecol 1983;146:696–707.
16. Gusberg SB, Kardon P: Proliferative endometrial response to theca-granulosa tumors. Am J Obstet Gynecol 1971;111:633–643.
17. Mishell DR: Menopause. *In* Droegemmueller W, Herbst AL, Mishell DR, Stenchever MA (eds): Comprehensive Gynecology, 2nd ed. St. Louis, Mosby–Year Book, 1992, pp 1083–1084.
18. Carlson JA Jr, Arger P, Thompson S, Carlson EJ: Clinical and pathologic correlation of endometrial cavity fluid detected by ultrasound in the postmenopausal patient. Obstet Gynecol 1991;77:119–123.
19. Kaminski PF, Stevens CW Jr: The value of endometrial sampling in abnormal uterine bleeding. Am J Gynecol Health 1988;2:130–133.
20. Garner WL, Wheelock JB, Kaminski PF: Postmenopausal bleeding: An outpatient approach. Am J Gynecol Health 1989;3:165–168.
21. Hendrickson MR, Kempson RL: Endometrial epithelial metaplasias: Proliferations frequently misdiagnosed as adenocarcinoma: Report of 89 cases and proposed classification. Am J Surg Pathol 1980;4:525–542.
22. Kurman RJ, Norris HJ: Evaluation of criteria for distinguishing atypical endometrial hyperplasia from well-differentiated carcinoma. Cancer 1982;49:2547–2559.
23. Ferenczy A, Gelfand M: The biologic significance of cytologic atypia in progestogen-treated endometrial hyperplasia. Am J Obstet Gynecol 1989;160:126–133.
24. Lee KR, Scully RE: Complex endometrial hyperplasia and carcinoma in adolescents and young women 15–20 years of age: A report of 10 cases. J Obstet Gynecol Pathol 1989;8:201–213.
25. Daniell JF, Kurtz BR, Ke RW: Hysteroscopic endometrial ablation using the rollerball electrode. Obstet Gynecol 1992;80:329–332.
26. Lauchlan SC: Conceptual unity of the müllerian tumor group. Cancer 1968;22:601–610.
27. Sidawy MK, Silverberg SG: Endometrial carcinoma: Pathologic factors of therapeutic and prognostic significance. Pathol Annu 1992;27(Pt. 2):153–185.
28. Boring CC, Squires TS, Tong T: Cancer Statistics 1993. CA Cancer J Clin 1993;43:7–26.
29. Koss L, Schreiber K, Oberlander S, Moussoris H, Lesser M: Detection of endometrial carcinoma and hyperplasia in asymptomatic women. Obstet Gynecol 1984;64:1–11.
30. Gusberg SB: Current concepts in cancer: The changing nature of endometrial cancer. N Engl J Med 1980;302:729–731.
31. Baron JA, LaVecchia C, Levi F: The antiestrogenic effect of cigarette smoking in women. Am J Obstet Gynecol 1990;162:502–514.
32. Brinton LA, Hoover RN: The endometrial cancer collaborative group: Estrogen replacement therapy and endometrial cancer risk: unresolved issues. Obstet Gynecol 1993;81:265–271.
33. Brinton LA, Barrett RJ, Berman ML, Mortel R, Twiggs LB, Wilbanks GD: Cigarette smoking and the risk of endometrial cancer. Am J Epidemiol 1993;137:281–291.
34. Gambrell RD, Bagnell CA, Greenblatt RB: Role of estrogens and progesterone in the etiology and prevention of endometrial cancer: Review. Am J Obstet Gynecol 1983;146:696–707.
35. Davies JL, Rosenshein NB, Antunes CMF, Stolley PD: A review of the risk factors for endometrial cancer. Obstet Gynecol Surv 1981;36:107–116.
37. Schenker JG, Weinstein D, Okon E: Estradiol and testosterone levels in the peripheral and ovarian circulation in patients with endometrial cancer. Cancer 1979;44:1809–1812.
38. Kessler II: Cancer and diabetes mellitus: A review of the literature. J Chronic Dis 1971;23:579–600.
39. Lynch HT, Krush AH, Larsen AL: Hereditary and endometrial carcinoma. South Med J 1967;60:231–235.
40. Rodriquez J, Hart WR: Endometrial cancers occurring 10 or more years after pelvic irradiation for carcinoma. Int J Gynecol Pathol 1982;1:135–144.
41. Ziel HK: Estrogen's role in endometrial cancer. Obstet Gynecol 1982;60:509–515.
42. Greene JW: Feminizing mesenchymomas (granulosa-cell and theca-cell tumors) with associated endometrial carcinoma: Review of the literature, and a study of the material of the Ovarian Tumor Registry. Am J Obstet Gynecol 1951;61:147–153.
43. Docekrty MB, Mussey E: Malignant lesions of the uterus associated with estrogen-producing ovarian tumors. Am J Obstet Gynecol 1951;61:147–153.
44. Gray LA, Christopherson WM, Hoover RN: Estrogens and endometrial carcinoma. Obstet Gynecol 1977;49; 385–389.
45. Sommers SC, Hertig AT, Bengloff H: Genesis of endometrial carcinoma: II. Cases 19 to 35 years old. Cancer 1949;2:957–963.
46. Judd HL, Lucas WE, Yen SSC: Serum 17 β-estradiol and estrone levels in postmenopausal women with and without endometrial cancer. J Clin Endocrinol Metab 1976; 43:272–278.
47. Rizkallah TH, Tovell HMM, Kelly WG: Production of es-

trone and fractional conversion of circulating androstenedione to estrone in women with endometrial carcinoma. J Clin Endocrinol Metab 1975;40:1045–1056.

48. Benjamin I, Block RE: Endometrial response to estrogen and progesterone therapy in patients with gonadal dysgenesis. Obstet Gynecol 1977;50;136–138.
49. Dewhurst J, DeKoos EB, Haines RM: Replacement hormone therapy in gonadal dysgenesis. Br J Obstet Gynaecol 1975;82:412–416.
50. Sirota DK, Marinoff SC: Endometrial carcinoma in Turner's syndrome following prolonged treatment with diethylstilbestrol. Mt Sinai J Med 1975;42:586–590.
51. Cutler BS, Forbes AP, Ingersol RM, Scully RE: Endometrial carcinoma after stilbestrol therapy in gonadal dysgenesis. N Engl J Med 1972;287:628–631.
52. Gray PH, Anderson CT Jr, Munnell EW: Endometrial adenocarcinoma and ovarian agenesis: Report of a case. Obstet Gynecol 1970;35:513–518.
53. Dowsett JH: Corpus carcinoma developing in a patient with Turner's syndrome treated with estrogen. Am J Obstet Gynecol 1963;86:622–625.
54. Krishnamurthy S, Adcock LL, Okagaki T: Endometrial carcinoma following estrogen-progesterone therapy in Turner's syndrome: A case report and review of the literature. Gynecol Oncol 1977;5:291–298.
55. Louka MH, Ross RD, Lee JH Jr, Lewis GC Jr: Endometrial carcinoma in Turner's syndrome. Gynecol Oncol 1978;6:294–304.
56. McCarroll AM, Montgomery DAD, Harley JMcG, McKown EF, MacHenry JC: Endometrial carcinoma after cyclical oestrogen-progestogen therapy for Turner's syndrome. Br J Obstet Gynaecol 1975;82:421–423.
57. Roberts G, Wells AL: Oestrogen-induced endometrial carcinoma in a patient with gonadal dysgenesis. Br J Obstet Gynaecol 1975;82:417–420.
58. Lyon FA: The development of adenocarcinoma of the endometrium in young women receiving long-term sequential oral contraception: Report of 4 cases. Am J Obstet Gynecol 1975;123:299–301.
59. Silverberg SG, Makowski EL: Endometrial carcinoma in younger women taking oral contraceptive agents. Obstet Gynecol 1975;46:503–506.
60. Kelly HW, Miles PA, Buster JE, Schragg WH: Adenocarcinoma of the endometrium in women taking sequential oral contraceptives. Obstet Gynecol 1976;47:200–202.
61. Kauffman RH, Reeves KO, Dougherty CM: Severe atypical endometrial changes and sequential contraceptive use. JAMA 1976;236:923–926.
62. Mack TM, Pike MC, Henderson BE, Pfefer RI, Gerkins VR, Arthur M, Brown SE: Estrogens and endometrial cancer in a retirement community. N Engl J Med 1976;294:1262–1267.
63. Hoogerland DL, Buchler DA, Crowley JJ, Carr WF: Estrogen use—risk of endometrial carcinoma. Gynecol Oncol 1978;6:451–458.
64. Antunes CMF, Stolley PD, Rosenshein NB, Davies JL, Tonascia JA, Brown C, Burnett L, Rutledge A, Pokempner M, Garcia R: Endometrial cancer and estrogen use: Report of a large case-control study. N Engl J Med 1979;300:9–13.
65. Jick H, Watkins RN, Hunter JR, Dinan BJ, Madsen S, Rothman KJ, Walker AM: Replacement estrogens and endometrial cancer. N Engl J Med 1979;300:218–222.
66. Hulka BS, Fowler WC Jr, Kaufman DG, Grimson RC, Greenberg BG, Hogue JR, Berger GS, Pulliam CG: Estrogen and endometrial cancer: Cases and two control groups from North Carolina. Am J Obstet Gynecol 1980;137:92–101.
67. Jelovsek FR, Hammond CB, Woodard BH, Draffin R, Lee KL, Creasman WT, Parker RT: Risk of exogenous estrogen therapy and endometrial cancer. Am J Obstet Gynecol 1990;137:85–91.
68. Gordon J, Reagan JW, Finkle WD, Ziel HK: Estrogen and endometrial carcinoma: An independent pathology review supporting original estimate. N Engl J Med 1977; 297:570–571.
69. Hammond CB, Jelovsek FR, Lee KL, Creasman WT, Parker RT: Effects of long-term estrogen replacement therapy: II. Neoplasm. Am J Obstet Gynecol 1979; 133:537–547.
70. Shapiro S, Kaufman SW, Slone D, Rosenberg L, Miettinen OS, Stolley PD, Rosenshein NB, Watring WE, Levitt T Jr, Knapp RC: Recent and past use of conjugated estrogens in relation to adenocarcinoma of the endometrium. N Engl J Med 1980;303:485–489.
71. Cook JW, Doods EC: Sex hormones and cancer-producing compounds. Nature 1933;131:205–206.
72. Horowitz RI, Feinstein AR: Alternative analytic methods for case-control studies of estrogens and endometrial cancer. N Engl J Med 1978;299:1091–1094.
73. Horowitz RI, Feinstein AR, Horowitz SM, Robboy SJ: Necropsy diagnosis of endometrial cancer and detection bias in case control studies. Lancet 1981;2:66–88.
74. Shapiro S, Kelly JP, Rosenberg L, Kaufman DW, Helmrich SP, Rosenshein NB, Lewis JL, Knapp RC, Stolley PD, Schottenfeld D: Risk of localized and widespread endometrial cancer in relation to recent and discontinued use of conjugated estrogens. N Engl J Med 1985;313:969–972.
75. Stubblefield PG: Oral contraceptives and neoplasia. J Reprod Med 1984;29(7S):524–529.
76. Bokham JV: Two pathogenetic types of endometrial carcinoma. Gynecol Oncol 1983;15:10–17.
77. FIGO stages—1988 revision. Gynecol Oncol 1989;35:125–126.
78. Fanning J, Evans MC, Peters AJ, Samuel M, Harmon ER, Bates JS: Endometrial adenocarcinoma histologic subtypes: Clinical and pathologic profiles. Gynecol Oncol 1989;32:288–291.
79. Oakley G, Nahas WA: Endometrial adenocarcinoma: Therapeutic impact of preoperative histopathologic examination of endometrial tissue. Eur J Gynaec Oncol 1989;10:255–260.
80. Soothill PW, Alcock CJ, Mackenzie IZ: Discrepancy between curettage and hysterectomy histology in patients with stage I uterine malignancy. Br J Obstet Gynecol 1989;96:478–481.
81. Anderson WA, Taylor PT, Fechner RE, Pinkerton JAV: Endometrial metaplasia associated with endometrial carcinoma. Am J Obstet Gynecol 1987;157:597–604.
82. Connelly PJ, Alberhasky RC, Christopherson WM: Carcinoma of the endometrium: III. An analysis of 865 cases of adenocarcinoma and adenoacanthoma. Obstet Gynecol 1982;59:569–575.
83. Ambros RA, Kurman RJ: Combined assessment of vascular and myometrial invasion as a model to predict prognosis in stage I endometrial adenocarcinoma of the uterine corpus. Cancer 1992;69:1424–1430.
83a. Hernandez E: Pathological findings and prognosis from uterine malignancy. Curr Opinion Obstet Gynecol 1993;5:480–485.
84. Eifel P, Ross J, Hendrickson M, Cox RS, Kempson R, Martinez AA: Adenocarcinoma of the endometrium: Analysis of 256 cases with disease limited to the uterine corpus: Treatment comparisons. Cancer 1983;52:1026–1031.
85. Creasman WT, Morrow CP, Bundy BN, Homesley HD, Graham JE, Heller PB: Surgical pathologic spread patterns of endometrial cancer: A Gynecologic Oncology Group study. Cancer 1987;60:2035–2041.
86. Podczaski E, Kaminski P, Gurski K, MacNeill C, Stryker JA, Singapuri K, Hackett TE, Sorosky J, Zaino R: Detection and patterns of treatment failure in 300 consecutive cases of "early" endometrial cancer after primary surgery. Gynecol Oncol 1992;47:323–327.
87. Morrow CP, Bundy BN, Kurman RJ, Creasman WT, Heller P, Homesley HD, Graham JE: Relationship between surgical-pathological risk factors and outcome in

clinical stage I and stage II carcinoma of the endometrium: A Gynecologic Oncology Group study. Gynecol Oncol 1991;40:55–65.
88. Sorbe B, Risberg B, Frankendal B: DNA ploidy, morphometry, and nuclear grade as prognostic factors in endometrial carcinoma. Gynecol Oncol 1990;38:22–27.
89. Mittal KR, Barwick KW: Diffusely infiltrating adenocarcinoma of the endometrium: A subtype with poor prognosis. Am J Surg Pathol 1988;12:754–758.
89a. Hernandez E, Woodruff JD: Adenocarcinoma in adenomyosis. Am J Obstet Gynecol 1980;138:829–832.
90. Kadar NRD, Kohorn EI, LiVolsi VA, Kapp DS: Histologic variants of cervical involvement by endometrial carcinoma. Obstet Gynecol 1982;59:85–92.
91. Frauenhoffer EE, Zaino RJ, Wolff TV, Whitney CW: Value of endocervical curettage in the staging of endometrial carcinoma. Int J Gynecol Pathol 1987;6:195–202.
92. Bigelow B, Vekshtein V, Demopoulos R: Endometrial carcinoma, stage II: Route and extent of spread to the cervix. Obstet Gynecol 1983;62:363–366.
93. Boronow RC, Morrow CP, Creasman WT, DiSaia PJ, Silverberg SG, Miller A, Blessing JA: Surgical staging in endometrial cancer: Clinical-pathologic findings of a prospective study. Obstet Gynecol 1984;63:825–832.
94. Morrow CP, Bundy BN, Kurman RJ, Creasman WT, Heller P, Homesley HD, Graham JE: Relationship between surgical-pathological risk factors in clinical stage I and II carcinoma of the endometrium: A Gynecologic Oncology Group study. Obstet Gynecol 1970;35:437–443.
95. Ng ABP, Reagan JW: Incidence and prognosis of endometrial carcinoma by histologic grade and extent. Obstet Gynecol 1970;35:437–443.
96. Van der Putter HWHM, Baak JPA, Koenders TJM, Kurver PHJ, Stolk HG, Stolte LAM: Prognostic value of quantitative pathologic features and DNA content in individual patients with stage I endometrial carcinoma. Cancer 1989;63:1378–1387.
97. Christopherson WM, Alberhasky RC, Connelly PJ: Carcinoma of the endometrium: II. Papillary adenocarcinoma: A clinical pathology study of 46 cases. Am J Clin Pathol 1982;77:534–540.
98. Chen JL, Trost DC, Wilkinson EJ: Endometrial papillary adenocarcinomas: Two clinicopathological types. Int J Gynecol Pathol 1985;4:279–288.
99. O'Hanlan KA, Levine PA, Harbatkin D, Feiner C, Goldberg GL, Jones JG, Rodriguez-Rodriguez L: Virulence of papillary endometrial carcinoma. Gynecol Oncol 1990; 37:112–119.
99a. Dunton C, Balsara G, McFarland M, Hernandez E: Uterine papillary serous carcinoma: A review. Obstet Gynecol Surv 1991;46:97–102.
100. Hendrickson M, Ross J, Eifel P, Martinez A, Kempson R: Uterine papillary serous carcinoma, a highly malignant form of endometrial adenocarcinoma. Am J Surg Pathol 1982;6:93–108.
101. Christopherson WM, Alberhasky RC, Connelly PJ: Carcinoma of the endometrium: I. A clinicopathologic study of clear-cell and secretory carcinoma. Cancer 1982;49:1511–1523.
102. Tobon H, Watkins GJ: Secretory adenocarcinoma of the endometrium. Int J Gynecol Pathol 1985;4:328–335.
102a. Erhmann RL, McKelvey HA, Hertig AT: Secretory behavior of endometrium in tissue culture. Obstet Gynecol 1961;17:416–433.
103. Hendrickson MR, Kempson R: Ciliated carcinoma: A variant of endometrial carcinoma: A report of 10 cases. Int J Gynecol Pathol 1983;2:1–12.
104. Zaino RJ, Kurman R, Herbold D, Gliedman J, Bundy BN, Voet R, Advani H: The significance of squamous differentiation in endometrial carcinoma. Cancer 1991;68:2293–2302.
105. Ng ABP: Mixed carcinoma of the endometrium. Am J Obstet Gynecol 1968;102:506–515.
106. Ng ABP, Reagan JW, Storalski JP, Wentz WB: Mixed adenosquamous carcinoma of the endometrium. Am J Clin Pathol 1973;59:765–781.
107. Silverberg SG: New aspects of endometrial carcinoma. Clin Obstet Gynecol 1984;11:189–208.
108. Zaino RJ, Kurman RJ: Squamous differentiation in carcinoma of the endometrium: A critical appraisal of adenoacanthoma and adenosquamous carcinoma. Semin Diagn Pathol 1988;5:154–171.
109. Silverberg SG, Mullen D, Faraci JA, Makowski EL, Miller A, Finch JL, Sutherland JV: Endometrial carcinoma: Clinical pathologic comparison of cases in postmenopausal women receiving and not receiving estrogens. Cancer 1980;45:3018–3026.
110. Robboy SJ, Miller AW III, Kurman RJ: The pathologic features and behavior of endometrial carcinoma associated with exogenous estrogen administration. Pathol Res Pract 1982;174:237–256.
111. Kim K-R, Scully RE: Peritoneal keratin granulomas with carcinomas of endometrium and ovary and atypical polypoid adenomyoma of endometrium: A clinicopathological analysis of 22 cases. Am J Surg Pathol 1990;14:925–932.
112. Liu CT: A study of endometrial carcinoma with emphasis on morphologically variant types. Am J Clin Pathol 1972;57:562–573.
113. Nahhas WA, Lund CJ, Rudolph JH: Carcinoma of the corpus uteri: A ten year review of 225 patients. Obstet Gynecol 1971;38:564–570.
114. Silverberg SG, Bolin WG, De Giorgi LS: Adenoacanthoma and mixed adenosquamous carcinoma of the endometrium: A clinicopathologic study. Cancer 1972;30:1307–1314.
115. Alberhasky RC, Connelly PJ, Christopherson WM: Carcinoma of the endometrium: IV. Mixed adenosquamous carcinoma: A clinical-pathological study of 68 cases with long-term follow-up. Am J Clin Pathol 1982;7:655–664.
116. Abeler VM, Kjørstad KE: Serous papillary carcinoma of the endometrium: A histopathological study of 22 cases. Gynecol Oncol 1990;39:266–271.
117. Jeffrey JF, Krepart GV, Lotocki RJ: Papillary serous adenocarcinoma of the endometrium. Obstet Gynecol 1986;67:670–674.
118. Gallion HH, Van Nagell JR, Powell DF, Donaldson ES, Higgins RV, Kryscio RJ, Pavlik EJ, Nelson K: Stage I serous papillary carcinoma of the endometrium. Cancer 1989;63:2224–2228.
119. Kay S: Clear cell carcinoma of the endometrium. Cancer 1957;10:124–130.
120. Kanbour-Shakir A, Tobon H: Primary clear cell carcinoma of the endometrium: A clinicopathologic study of 20 cases. Int J Gynecol Pathol 1991;10:67–78.
121. Kurman RJ, Scully RE: Clear cell carcinoma of the endometrium: An analysis of 21 cases. Cancer 1976;37:872–882.
122. Yorishima M, Hirura M, Moriwaki S, Nakanishi Y, Yokoyama T, Tanaka M, Chiba T: Clear cell carcinoma of the endometrium with lipid-producing activity. Int J Gynecol Pathol 1989;8:286–295.
123. Ross JC, Eifel PJ, Cox RS, Kempson RL, Hendrickson MR: Primary mucinous adenocarcinoma of the endometrium: A clinicopathologic and histochemical study. Am J Surg Path 1983;7:715–729.
124. Czernoblisky B, Katz Z, Lancet M, Gaton E: Endocervical-type epithelium in endometrial carcinoma. Am J Surg Pathol 1980;4:481–489.
125. Pritzker J, Anselmo MT, Veridiano NP, Tancer ML: Squamous cell carcinoma of the endometrium: A case report. J Reprod Med 1992;37:194–198.
126. Fluhman CF: Squamous epithelium in the endometrium in benign and malignant conditions. Surg Gynecol Obstet 1928;46:309–316.
127. Kanbour AI, Stock RJ: Squamous cell carcinoma in situ of the endometrium and fallopian tube as superficial extension of invasive cervical carcinoma. Cancer 1978;42:570–580.

128. Ryder DE: Verrucous carcinoma of the endometrium: A unique neoplasm with long survival. Obstet Gynecol 1982;59:78S–80S.
129. Ueda G, Sato Y, Yamasaki M, Inoque M, Hiramatsu K, Tanaka Y: Argyrophil cell adenocarcinoma of the endometrium. Gynecol Oncol 1978;6:467–473.
129a. Pesce C, Merino MJ, Chambers JT, Nogales F: Endometrial carcinoma with trophoblastic differentiation: An aggressive form of uterine cancer. Cancer 1991;68:1799–1802.
130. Hachisuga T, Kaku T, Enjoji M: Carcinoma of the lower uterine segment: Clinicopathologic analysis of 12 cases. Int J Gynecol Pathol 1989;8:26–35.
131. Coleman HI, Rosenthal AH: Carcinoma developing in areas of adenomyosis. Obstet Gynecol 1959;14:342–348.
131a. Mittal KR, Barwick KW: Endometrial adenocarcinoma involving adenomyosis without true myometrial invasion is characterized by frequent preceding estrogen therapy, low histologic grades, and excellent prognosis. Gynecol Oncol 1993;49:197–201.
132. Peterson WF, Novak ER: Endometrial polyps. Obstet Gynecol 1956;8:40–49.
133. Salm R: The incidence and significance of early carcinomas in endometrial polyps. J Pathol 1972;108:47–53.
134. Armenia CC: Sequential relationship between endometrial polyps and carcinoma of the endometrium. Obstet Gynecol 1967;30:524–529.
135. Kay S, Frable WJ, Goplerud DR: Endometrial carcinoma arising in a large polypoid adenomyoma of the uterus. Int J Gynecol Pathol 1988;7:391–398.
136. Beckner ME, Mori T, Silberberg SG: Endometrial carcinoma: Nontumor factors in prognosis. Int J Pathol 1985;4:131–145.
137. Symonds DA: Prognostic value of pathologic features and DNA analysis in endometrial carcinoma. Gynecol Oncol 1990;39:272–276.
138. Mittal KR, Schwartz PE, Barwick KW: Architectural (FIGO) grading, nuclear grading, and other prognostic indicators in stage I endometrial adenocarcinoma with identification of high-risk and low-risk groups. Cancer 1988;61:538–545.
139. Salazar OM, DePapp EW, Bonfioglio TA, Feldstein ML, Rubin P, Rudolph JH: Adenosquamous carcinoma of the endometrium. Cancer 1977;40:119–130.
140. Pokoly T: A comparison of the clinical behavior of uterine adenocarcinomas and adenoacanthoma. Am J Obstet Gynecol 1970;108:1080–1084.
141. Demopoulos RI, Dubin N, Noumoff J, Blaustein A, Sommers G: Prognostic significance of squamous differentiation in stage I endometrial adenocarcinoma. Obstet Gynecol 1980;68:45–50.
141a. Schink JC, Rademaker AW, Miller DS, Lurain JR: Tumor size in endometrial cancer. Cancer 1991;67:2791–2794.
142. Podczaski ES, Kaminski P, Manetta A, Louk D, Andrews C, Larson J, DeGeest K, Mortel R: Stage II endometrial carcinoma treated with external beam radiotherapy, intracavitary application of cesium, and surgery. Gynecol Oncol 1989;35:251–254.
143. Deligdisch L, Cohen CJ: Histologic correlates and virulence implications of endometrial carcinoma associated with adenomatous hyperplasia. Cancer 1895;56:1452–1455.
144. Grimshaw RN, Tupper WC, Fraser RC, Tompkins MG, Jeffrey JF: Prognostic value of peritoneal cytology in endometrial carcinoma. Gynecol Oncol 1990;36:97–100.
145. Creasman WT, DiSaia MD, Blessing J, Wilkinson RH, Johnston W, Weed JC: Prognostic significance of peritoneal cytology in patients with endometrial cancer and preliminary data concerning therapy with intraperitoneal radiopharmaceuticals. Am J Obstet Gynecol 1981;141:921–927.
146. Soper JT, Creasman WT, Clarke-Pearson DT, Sullivan DC, Vergadoro F, Johnston WW: Intraperitoneal chromic phosphate P32 suspension therapy of malignant peritoneal cytology in endometrial carcinoma. Am J Obstet Gynecol 1985;151:191–196.
147. Yazigi R, Piver MS, Blumenson L: Malignant peritoneal cytology as prognostic indicator in Stage I endometrial cancer. Obstet Gynecol 1983;62:359–361.
148. Turner DA, Gershenson DM, Atkinson N, Sneige ZN, Wharton AT: The prognostic significance of peritoneal cytology for stage I endometrial cancer. Obstet Gynecol 1989;74:775–780.
149. Szpak CA, Creasman WT, Clarke-Pearson DL, Sullivan JC, Vergadoro F, Johnson WW: Prognostic value of cytologic examination of peritoneal washings in patients with endometrial carcinoma. Acta Cytol 1981;256:640–646.
150. Lurain JR, Rumsey NK, Schink JC, Wallenmark CB, Chmiel JS: Prognostic significance of positive peritoneal cytology in clinical stage I adenocarcinoma of the endometrium. Obstet Gynecol 1989;74:175–179.
151. Harouny VR, Sutton GP, Clark SA, Geisler HE, Stehman FB, Ehrlich CE: The importance of peritoneal cytology in endometrial carcinoma. Obstet Gynecol 1988;72:394–398.
152. Sivridis E, Buckley CH, Fox H: The prognostic significance of lymphatic vascular space invasion in endometrial carcinoma. Br J Obstet Gynecol 1981;94:991–994.
153. Liao BS, Twiggs LB, Leung BS, Yu WCY, Potish RA, Prem KA: Cytoplasmic estrogen and progesterone receptors as prognostic parameters in primary endometrial carcinoma. Obstet Gynecol 1986;67:463–467.
154. Chambers JT, MacLusky N, Eisenfield A, Kohorn E, Lawrence R, Schwartz PE: Estrogen and progestin receptor levels as prognosticators for survival in endometrial cancer. Gynecol Oncol 1988;31:65–77.
155. Chambers JT, Carcangiu ML, Voynick IM, Schwartz PE: Immunohistochemical evaluation of estrogen and progesterone receptor content in 183 patients with endometrial carcinoma: Part II. Correlation between biochemical and immunohistochemical methods and survival. Am J Clin Pathol 1990;94:55–60.
156. Kleine W, Maier T, Geyer H, Pfleiderer A: Estrogen and progesterone receptors in endometrial cancer and their prognostic relevance. Gynecol Oncol 1990;38:59–65.
157. Spona J, Giysch E, Kubista E, Salzer H, Korler B: Enzyme immunoassay and scatchard plot estimation of estrogen receptor in gynecological tumors. Cancer Res 1986;46:4310S–4312S.
158. Soper JT, Segreti EM, Novotny DB, Mutch D, Creasman WT, McCarthy KS Jr: Estrogen and progesterone receptor content of endometrial carcinomas: Comparison of total issue versus cancer component analysis. Gynecol Oncol 1990;36:363–368.
159. Segreti EM, Novotomy DB, Soper JT, Mutch DG, Creasman WT, McCarthy KS: Endometrial cancer: Histologic correlates of immunohistochemical localization of progesterone receptor and estrogen receptor. Obstet Gynecol 1989;73:780–785.
160. Creasman WT: Prognostic significance of hormone receptors in endometrial cancer. Cancer 1993;71:1467–1470.
161. Zaino RJ, Laskaris A, Whitney C, Sharkey FE: Morphometric analysis of endometrial adenocarcinoma: 2. A comparison of architectural differentiation determined morphometrically with subjective grading. Int J Gynecol Pathol 1987;6:620–628.
162. Podratz KC, Wilson TO, Gaffey TA, Cha SS, Katzmann JA: Deoxyribonucleic acid analysis facilitates the pretreatment identification of high-risk endometrial cancer patients. Am J Obstet Gynecol 1993;168:1206–1215.
163. Ambros RA, Kurman RJ: Identification of patients with stage I uterine endometrioid adenocarcinoma at high risk of recurrence by DNA ploidy, myometrial invasion, and vascular invasion. Gynecol Oncol 1992;45:235–239.
164. Kadar N, Malfetano JH, Homesley HD: Determinants of survival of surgically staged patients with endometrial cancer histologically confined to the uterus: Implications for therapy. Obstet Gynecol 1992;80:655–659.

165. Schultz MJ, Shen JT: Treatment of stage I endometrial carcinoma. J Reprod Med 1989;34:167–172.
166. Cowles TA, Magrina JF, Masterson BJ, Capen CV: Comparison of clinical and surgical staging in patients with endometrial carcinoma. Obstet Gynecol 1985;66:413–416.
166a. Abeler VM, Kjørstad KE: Endometrial adenocarcinoma in Norway. Cancer 1991;67:3093–3103.
167. Vardi JR, Tadros GH, Anselmo MT, Rafla S: The value of exploratory laparotomy in patients with endometrial carcinoma according to the new International Federation of Gynecology and Obstetrics staging. Obstet Gynecol 1992;80:204–208.
168. Lurain JR, Rice BL, Rademaker AW, Poggensee LE, Schick JC, Miller DS: Prognostic factors associated with recurrence in clinical stage I adenocarcinoma of the endometrium. Obstet Gynecol 1991;78:63–69.
169. Burke TW, Heller PB, Woodward JE, Davidson SA, Hoskins WJ, Park RC: Treatment failure in endometrial carcinoma. Obstet Gynecol 1990;75:96–101.
170. Fanning J, Alvarez PM, Tsikada Y, Piver MS: Prognostic significance of the extent of cervical involvement by endometrial cancer. Gynecol Oncol 1991;40:46–47.
171. Trimble EWL, Jones HW III: Management of stage II endometrial adenocarcinoma. Obstet Gynecol 1988;71: 323–326.
172. Larson DM, Copeland LJ, Gallager S, Wharton JT, Gershenson DM, Rutledge FN: The significance of residual tumor after preoperative pelvic irradiation for stage II endometrial cancer. Obstet Gynecol 1987;70:916–919.
173. Chen SS, Rumancik WM, Spiegel G: Magnetic resonance imaging in stage I endometrial carcinoma. Obstet Gynecol 1990;75:274–277.
173a. Eisner RF, Neiberg RK, Berek JS: Synchronous primary neoplasms of the female reproductive tract. Gynecol Oncol 1989;33:335–339.
173b. Choo YA, Naylor B: Multiple primary neoplasms of the ovary and uterus. Int J Gynaecol Obstet 1982;20:327–334.
173c. Eifel P, Hendrickson M, Ross J, Ballon S, Martinez A, Kempson R: Simultaneous presentation of carcinoma involving the ovary and the uterine corpus. Cancer 1992;50:163–170.
173d. Greven KM, Lanciano RM, Corn B, Case D, Randall ME: Pathologic Stage III endometrial carcinoma: Prognostic factors and patterns of recurrence. Cancer 1993;71:3697–3702.
174. Stock RJ, Gallup DG: Hysterography in patients with suspected uterine cancer: Radiographic and histologic correlations and clinical implications. Obstet Gynecol 1987; 69:872–878.
175. Doering DL, Barnhill DB, Weiser EB, Burke TW, Woodward JE, Park RC: Intraoperative evaluation of depth of invasion in stage I endometrial carcinoma. Obstet Gynecol 1989;74:930–933.
176. Goff BA, Rice LW: Assessment of depth of myometrial invasion in endometrial adenocarcinoma. Gynecol Oncol 1990;38:46–48.
177. Piver MS, Lele SB, Barlow JJ, Blumenson L: Para-aortic lymph node evaluation in stage I endometrial carcinoma. Obstet Gynecol 1982;59:97–100.
178. Underwood PB, Lutz MM, Kruetner A, Miller MC III, Johnson RD: Carcinoma of the endometrium: Radiation followed immediately by operation. Am J Obstet Gynecol 1977;128:86–98.
179. Burrell MO, Franklin EW, Powell JL: Endometrial cancer: Evaluation of spread and follow-up in one hundred eighty-nine patients with stage I and stage II disease. Am J Obstet Gynecol 1982;144:181–185.
180. Christopherson WM, Connelly PJ, Alberhasky RC: Carcinoma of the endometrium: V. An analysis of prognosticators in patients with favorable subtype and stage I disease. Cancer 1983;51:1705–1709.
181. Hernandez E, Rosenhein NB, Dillon MB, Villar J: Peritoneal cytology in Stage I endometrial adenocarcinoma. J Nat Med Assoc 1985;77:799–803.
182. Janne O, Kauppila A, Kontula K, Syrjala P, Vihko R: Female sex steroid receptors in normal, hyperplastic and carcinomatous endometrium: The relationship to serum steroid hormones and gonadotropins and changes during medroxyprogesterone acetate administration. Int J Cancer 1979;24:545–554.
182a. Hetzel DJ, Wilson TD, Keeney GL, Roche PC, Cha SS, Podratz KC: HER-2/neu expression: A major prognostic factor in endometrial cancer. Gynecol Oncol 1992:45:179–185.
183. Stendahl U, Strang P, Wagenius G, Bergstrom R, Tribukait B: Prognostic variables of proliferation in endometrial adenocarcinomas: A multivariate analysis of clinical and flow cytometric variables. Int J Gynecol Pathol 1991;10:271–284.
183a. Anderson GH: Cytologic screening programs. *In* Bibbo M (ed): Comprehensive Cytopathology. Philadelphia, WB Saunders, 1991, pp 53–54.
184. Walton RJ, Blanchet M, Boyes DA, Carmichael J, Marshall KG, Miller AB, Thompson DW: Detection of cancer of the cervix uteri. Union Medicale Du Canada 1976; 105:997–1047.
185. Kaminski PF, Sorosky JI, Wheelock JB, Stevens CW Jr: The significance of atypical cervical cytology in an older population. Obstet Gynecol 1989;73:13–15.
186. Gondos B, King EB: Significance of endometrial cells in cervico-vaginal smears. Ann Clin Lab Sci 1977;7:486–490.
187. Ng AB, Regan JW, Hawliczek S, Wentz BW: Significance of endometrial cells in the detection of endometrial carcinoma and its precursors. Acta Cytol 1974;18:356–361.
188. Cherkis RC, Patten SF, Dickinson JC, Dekanich AS: Significance of atypical endometrial cells detected by cervical cytology. Obstet Gynecol 1987;69:786–789.
189. Lyon DS, Kaminski PF, Wheelock JB: Significance of a positive Papanicolaou smear in a well-screened population. South Med J 1989;82:190–192.
190. Soper JT, Berchuk A, Olt GJ, Soisson AP, Clarke-Pearson DL, Bast RC Jr: Preoperative evaluation of serum CA 125, TAG 72, and CA 15-3 in patients with endometrial carcinoma. Am J Obstet Gynecol 1990;163:1204–1209.
191. Propatich C, Nozawa S, Rojas M, Chapman WB, Silverberg SG: MSN-1 antibody in the evaluation of female genital tract adenocarcinomas. Int J Gynecol Pathol 1990; 9:73–79.
192. Ueda G, Yamasaki M, Inoue M, Tanaka Y, Inoue Y, Nishino T, Ogawa M: Immunohistochemical demonstrations of amylase in endometrial carcinomas. Int J Gynecol Pathol 1986;5:47–51.
193. Ota Y, Inaban N, Shirotake S, Fukazawa I, Takamizawa H, Bohn H: Enzyme immunoassay for placental protein (PP4) and its possible diagnostic significance in patients with genital tract cancer. Arch Gynecol Obstet 1990; 247:139–147.
194. Paterson E, Spratt D, Tomkiewicz Z, Lewis C, Rathbun P: Management of Stage I carcinoma of the uterus. Obstet Gynecol 1982;59:755–758.
195. Malviya VK, Deppe G, Malone JM, Sundareson AS, Lawrence WD: Reliability of frozen section examination in identifying poor prognostic indicators in stage I endometrial adenocarcinoma. Gynecol Oncol 1989;34:299–304.
196. Mannel RS, Berman ML, Walker JL, Manetta A, DiSaia PJ: Management of endometrial cancer with suspected cervical involvement. Obstet Gynecol 1990;75:1016–1022.
197. Potish RA, Twiggs LB, Adcock LL, Savage JE, Levitt SH, Prem KA: Paraaortic lymph node radiotherapy in cancer of the uterine corpus. Obstet Gynecol 1985;65:251–256.
198. Aalders JG, Abeler V, Kolstad P: Stage IV endometrial carcinoma: A clinical and pathological study of 83 patients. Gynecol Oncol 1984;17:75–84.
198a. Dunton CJ, Pfeifer SM, Braitman LE, Morgan MA, Carlson JA, Mikuta JJ: Treatment of advanced and recurrent endometrial cancer with cisplatin, doxorubicin, and cyclophosphamide. Gynecol Oncol 1991;41:113–116.

198b. Burke TW, Stringer CA, Morris M, Freedman RS, Gershenson DM, Kavanagh JJ, Edwards CL: Prospective treatment of advanced or recurrent endometrial carcinoma with cisplatin, doxorubicin, and cyclophosphamide. Gynecol Oncol 1991;40:264–267.
199. Leiblum S, Bachmann G, Kemmann E, Colburn D, Swartzman L: Vaginal atrophy in the postmenopausal woman: The importance of sexual activity and hormones. JAMA 1983;249:2195–2198.
200. Stampfer MJ, Golditz GA, Willett WC, Manson JE, Rosner B, Speizer FE, Hennekens CH: Postmenopausal estrogen therapy and cardiovascular disease: Ten year follow-up from the Nurses Health Study. N Engl J Med 1991;325:756–762.
201. Riffee JM: Osteoporosis: Prevention and management. Am Pharm 1992;NS32:665–676.
202. Cummings SR, Black DM, Rubin SM: Lifetime risk of hip, Colles' or vertebral fracture and coronary disease among white postmenopausal women. Arch Intern Med 1989; 149:2445–2448.
203. Cresman WT: Recommendations regarding estrogen replacement therapy after treatment of endometrial cancer. Oncol 1992;6:23–26.
204. Creasman WT, Henderson D, Hinshaw W, Clarke-Pearson DL: Estrogen replacement therapy in the patient treated for endometrial cancer. Obstet Gynecol 1986;67: 326–330.
205. Committee on Gynecologic Practice: Estrogen replacement therapy and endometrial cancer. ACOG Committee Opinion. August 1993, p 126.
206. Ober WB: Uterine sarcomas: Histogenesis and taxonomy. Ann NY Acad Sci 1959;75:568–585.
207. Silverberg SG: Mixed müllerian tumors. *In* Sasano N (ed): Current Topics in Pathology, 85. Gynecological Tumors. New York, Springer Verlag, 1992, pp 36–56.
208. Zaloudek C, Norris HJ: Mesenchymal tumors of the uterus. *In* Kurman RJ (ed): Blaustein's Pathology of the Female Genital Tract, 3rd ed. New York, Springer Verlag, 1987, p 374.
209. Harlow BL, Weiss NS, Lofton S: The epidemiology of sarcomas of the uterus. JNCI 1986;76:399–402.
210. Bocker W, Stegner HE: A light and electron microscopic study of endometrial sarcomas of the uterus. Virchows Arch [A] 1975;368:141–156.
211. Saksela E, Lampinen V, Procope B-J: Malignant mesenchymal tumors of the uterine corpus. Am J Ostet Gynecol 1974;120:452–460.
212. Peters WA, Kumar NB, Fleming WP, Morley GW: Prognostic features of sarcomas and mixed tumors of the endometrium. Obstet Gynecol 1984;63:550–556.
213. Clement PB, Scully RE: Müllerian adenosarcoma of the uterus: A clinicopathologic analysis of ten cases of a distinctive type of müllerian mixed tumor. Cancer 1974; 34:1138–1149.
214. Clement PB, Scully RE: Müllerian adenosarcoma of the uterus: A clinicopathologic analysis of 100 cases with a review of the literature. Hum Pathol 1990;21:363–381.
215. Katzenstein A-LA, Askin FB, Feldman PF: Müllerian adenosarcoma of the uterus: An ultrastructural study of four cases. Cancer 1977;40:2233–2242.
216. Zaloudek CJ, Norris HJ: Adenofibroma and adenosarcoma of the uterus: A clinicopathologic study of 35 cases. Cancer 1981;48:354–366.
217. Vellios F: Papillary adenofibroma-adenosarcoma: The uterine cystosarcoma phylloides. Prog Surg Pathol 1980;1:205–219.
218. Chen KTK: Rhabdomyosarcomatous uterine adenosarcoma. Int J Gynecol Pathol 1985;4:146–152.
219. Hariri J: Müllerian adenosarcoma of the endometrium: Review of the literature and report of two cases. Int J Gynecol Pathol 1983;2:182–191.
220. Ward RM, Evans HL: Cystosarcoma phyllodes: A clinicopathological study of 26 cases. Cancer 1986;58:2282–2289.
221. Baker TR, Piver MS, Lele SB, Tsukada Y: Stage I uterine adenosarcoma: A report of six cases. J Surg Oncol 1988;37;128–132.
222. Kaku T, Silverberg SG, Major FJ, Miller A, Fetter B, Brady MF: Adenosarcoma of the uterus: A Gynecologic Oncology Group clinicopathologic study of 31 cases. Int J Gynecol Pathol 1991;11:75–88.
223. Gloor E: Müllerian adenosarcoma of the uterus: Clinicopathologic report of five cases. Am J Surg Pathol 1979;3:203–209.
224. Clement PB: Müllerian adenosarcomas of the uterus with sarcomatous overgrowth: A clinicopathological analysis of 10 cases. Am J Surg Pathol 1989;13:28–38.
225. Clement PB, Scully RE: Müllerian adenosarcoma of the uterus with sex cord like elements: A clinicopathologic analysis of eight cases. Am J Clin Pathol 1989;91:664–772.
226. Chang KL, Grabtree GS, Liam-Tan SK, Kempson RL, Hendrickson MR: Primary uterine endometrial stromal neoplasms: A clinicopathologic study of 117 cases. Am J Surg Pathol 1990;14:415–438.
227. Norris HJ, Taylor HB: Mesenchymal tumor of the uterus. I: A clinical and pathological study of 53 endometrial stromal tumors. Cancer 1966;19:755–766.
228. Evans HL: Endometrial stromal sarcoma and poorly differentiated endometrial sarcoma. Cancer 1982;50:2170–2182.
229. Piver MS, Rutledge FN, Copeland L, Webster K, Blumenson L, Suh O: Uterine endolymphatic stromal myosis: A collaborative study. Obstet Gynecol 1984;64:173–178.
230. Thatcher SS, Woodruff JD: Uterine stromatosis: A report of 33 cases. Obstet Gynecol 1984;59:428–434.
231. Lillemore TJ, Perrone T, Norris HJ, Dehner LP: Myogenous phenotype of epithelial-like areas in endometrial stromal sarcomas. Arch Pathol Lab Med 1991;115:215–219.
232. Kempson RL, Bari W: Uterine sarcomas: Classification, diagnosis, and prognosis. Hum Pathol 1970;1:331–349.
233. Kahanpaa KV, Wahlstrom T, Grohn P, Heinonen E, Nieminen U, Widholm O: Sarcoma of the uterus: A clinicopathologic study of 119 patients. Obstet Gynecol 1986;67:417–424.
234. Scully RG, Kempson RL, Norris NJ: Mitosis counting I–III. Hum Pathol 1976;7:481–484.
235. Goldfarb S, Richart RM, Okagaki T: Nuclear DNA content in endolymphatic stromal myosis. Am J Obstet Gynecol 1970;106:525–529.
236. Clement PB, Scully RE: Endometrial stromal sarcomas of the uterus with extensive endometrioid glandular differentiation: A report of three cases that caused problems in differential diagnosis. Int J Gynecol Pathol 1992;11:163–173.
237. Binder SW, Nieberg RK, Cheng L, Al-Jitawai A: Histologic and immunohistochemical analysis of nine endometrial stromal tumors: An unexpected high frequency of keratin protein positivity. Int J Gynecol Pathol 1991;10:191–197.
238. Clement PB, Scully RE: Uterine tumors resembling ovarian sex cord tumors: A clinicopathologic analysis of fourteen cases. Am J Clin Pathol 1976;66:512–525.
239. Fekete PS, Vellios F: The clinical and histologic spectrum of endometrial stromal neoplasma: A report of 41 cases. Int J Gynecol Pathol 1984;3:198–212.
240. Bird CC, Willis RA: The production of smooth muscle by the endometrial stroma of the adult human uterus. J Pathol Bacteriol 1965;90:75–81.
241. Tang CK, Toker C, Ances IG: Stromomyoma of the uterus. Cancer 1979;43:308–316.
242. Dunton C, Kelsten ML, Brooks SE, Viglione MJ, Carlson JA, Mikuta JJ: Low-grade stromal sarcoma: DNA flow cytometric analysis and estrogen/progesterone receptor data. Gynecol Oncol 1990;37:268–275.
243. Sutton GP, Stehman FB, Michael H, Young PCM, Ehrlich CE: Estrogen and progesterone receptors in uterine sarcomas. Obstet Gynecol 1986;68:709–714.
244. Silverberg SG: Leiomyosarcoma of the uterus. Obstet Gynecol 1971;38:613–628.
245. Christopherson WM, Williamson EO, Gray LA: Leiomyosarcoma of the uterus. Cancer 1971;29:1512–1517.

246. Gallup DG, Cordray DR: Leiomyosarcoma of the uterus: Case reports and a review. Obstet Gynecol Surv 1979;34:300–312.
247. Berchuk A, Rubin SC, Hoskins WJ, Saigo PE, Pierce VK, Lewis JL Jr: Treatment of uterine leiomyosarcoma. Obstet Gynecol 1988;71:845–850.
248. Evans HL, Chawla SP, Simpson C, Finn KP: Smooth muscle neoplasm of the uterus other than ordinary leiomyoma: A study of 46 cases, with emphasis on diagnostic criteria and prognostic factors. Cancer 1988;62:2239–2247.
249. Hannigan EV, Gomez LG: Uterine leiomyosarcoma: A review of prognostic clinical and pathologic features. Am J Obstet Gynecol 1979;134:557–564.
250. Burns B, Curry RH, Bell MEA: Morphologic features of prognostic significance in uterine smooth muscle tumors: A review of 84 cases. Am J Obstet Gynecol 1979;135:109–114.
251. Hart WR, Billman JK Jr: A reassessment of uterine neoplasms originally diagnosed as leiomyosarcomas. Cancer 1978;41:1902–1910.
252. Taylor HB, Norris NJ: Mesenchymal tumors of the uterus: IV. Diagnosis and prognosis of leiomyosarcoma. Arch Pathol 1966;82:40–44.
253. O'Connor DM, Norris HJ: Mitotically active leiomyomas of the uterus. Hum Pathol 1986;5:260–268.
254. Marshall RJ, Braye SG, Jones DB: Leiomyosarcoma of the uterus with giant cells resembling osteoclasts. Int J Gynecol Pathol 1986;5:260–268.
255. Dinh TV, Woodruff JD: Leiomyosarcoma of the uterus. Am J Obstet Gynecol 1982;144:817–823.
256. Stearns HC, Sneedon VD: Leiomyosarcoma of the uterus. Am J Obstet Gynecol 1966;26:374–380.
257. Omura GA, Blessing JA, Major F, Lifshitz S, Ehrlich CL, Mangan C, Beecham J, Park R, Silverberg S: A randomized trial of adjuvant Adriamycin in uterine sarcomas: A Gynecologic Oncology Group study. J Clin Oncol 1985;3:1240–1245.
257a. Levenback C, Rubin SC, McCormack PM, Hoskins WJ, Atkinson ED, Lewis JL Jr: Resection of pulmonary metastases from uterine sarcomas. Gynecol Oncol 1992;45:202–205.
258. Shaw RW: Müllerian mixed tumour of the uterine corpus: A clinical histopathological review of 28 patients. Br J Obstet Gynecol 1983;90:562–569.
259. Ishiwata I, Ono I, Ishiwata C, Nakaguchi T, Soma M, Mukai M, Ishikawa H: Heterotransplantation of mixed mesodermal tumor cells in nude mouse: Histology of metastatic foci. Gynecol Oncol 1987;27:189–196.
260. Norris HJ, Roth E, Taylor HB: Mesenchymal tumors of the uterus: II. A clinical and pathologic study of 31 mixed mesodermal tumors. Obstet Gynecol 1966;28:57–63.
261. Schweizer W, Demopoulos R, Beller U, Dubin N: Prognostic factors for malignant mixed müllerian tumors of the uterus. Int J Gynecol Pathol 1990;9:129–136.
262. Clement PB, Scully RE: Uterine tumors with mixed epithelial and mesenchymal elements. Semin Diagn Pathol 1988;5:199–222.
263. Press MF, Scully RE: Endometrial "sarcomas" complicating ovarian thecoma, polycystic ovarian disease and estrogen therapy. Gynecol Oncol 1985;21:135–154.
264. Meis JM, Lawrence D: The immunohistochemical profile of malignant mixed müllerian tumor: Overlap with endometrial adenocarcinoma. Am J Clin Pathol 1990;94:1–7.
265. Auerbach HE, LiVolsi VA, Merino MJ: Malignant mixed müllerian tumors of the uterus: An immunohistochemical study. Int J Gynecol Pathol 1988;7:123–131.
266. Amr SS, Tavassoli FA, Hassan AA, Issa AA, Madanat FF: Mixed mesodermal tumor of the uterus in a 4-year old girl. Int J Gynecol Pathol 1986;5:371–378.
267. Dinh TV, Slavin RE, Bhagavan BS, Hannigan EV, Tiamson EM, Yandell RB: Mixed müllerian tumors of the uterus: A clinicopathological study. Obstet Gynecol 1989;74:388–392.
268. Tenti P, Babilonti L, LaFianza A, Zampatti C, Carneval L, Sonnino P, Franchi M: Cytology of malignant mixed mesodermal tumor of the uterus: Experience of 10 cases. Eur J Gynaecol Oncol 1989;10;125–128.
269. Bitterman P, Chun B, Kurman RJ: The significance of epithelial differentiation in mixed mesodermal tumors of the uterus. Am J Surg Pathol 1990;14:317–328.
270. Silverberg SG, Major FJ, Blessing JA, Fetter B, Askin FB, Lioa S-Y, Miller A: Carcinosarcoma (malignant mixed müllerian tumor) of the uterus: A Gynecologic Oncology Group pathologic study of 203 cases. Int J Gynecol Pathol 1990;9:1–19.
271. Gersell DJ, Duncan DA, Fulling KH: Malignant mixed müllerian tumor of the uterus with neuroectodermal differentiation. Int J Gynecol Pathol 1989;8:169–178.
272. Dictor M: Ovarian malignant mixed mesodermal tumor: The occurrence of hyaline droplets containing α-1-antitrypsin. Hum Pathol 1982;13:930–933.
273. Lotocki R, Rosenshein NB, Grumbine F, Dillon M, Parmley T, Woodruff JD: Mixed müllerian tumors of the uterus: Clinical and pathologic correlations. Int J Gynaecol Obstet 1982;20:237–243.
274. Sutton GP, Blessing JA, Rosenshein NB, Photopulos G, DiSaia PJ: Phase II trial of ifosfamide and mesna in mixed mesodermal tumors of the uterus (a Gynecologic Oncology Group study). Am J Obstet Gynecol 1989;161:309–312.
275. Podczaski ES, Woomert CA, Stevens CH Jr, Manetta A, Larson JE, Zaino RJ, Mortel R: Management of malignant mixed mesodermal tumors of the uterus. Gynecol Oncol 1989;32:240–244.
276. Spanos WJ Jr, Wharton JT, Gomez L, Fletcher GH, Oswald MJ: Malignant mixed müllerian tumors of the uterus. Cancer 1984;53:311–316.
277. Wheelock JB, Krebs H-B, Schneider V, Goplerud DR: Uterine sarcoma: Analysis of prognostic variables in 71 cases. Am J Obstet Gynecol 1985;151:1016–1022.
277a. Kanbour AI, Buchsbaum HJ, Hall A, Kanbour AI: Peritoneal cytology in malignant mixed müllerian tumors of the uterus. Gynecol Oncol 1989;33:91–95.
278. Kahner S, Ferenczy A, Richart RM: Homologous mixed müllerian tumors (carcinosarcoma) confined to endometrial polyps. Am J Obstet Gynecol 1975;121:278–279.
279. Podczaski E, Kaminski P, Hackett TE, Olt GJ, Zaino R: Tissue CA 125 and CA 19-9 in malignant, mixed mesodermal tumors of the uterus. Gynecol Oncol 1993;49:56–60.
280. Podczaski E, Sees J, Kaminski P, Sorosky J, Larson JE, DeGeest K, Ziano RJ, Mortel R: Rhabdomyosarcoma of the uterus in a postmenopausal patient. Gynecol Oncol 1990;37:439–442.
281. Hart WR, Craig JR: Rhabdomyosarcoma of the uterus. Am J Clin Pathol 1978;70:217–223.
282. Christopherson WM, Richard M: Uterine mesenchymal tumors. Pathol Annu 1981;16:215–246.
283. Stout AP: Hemangio-endothelioma: A tumor of blood vessels featuring vascular endothelial cells. Ann Surg 1943;118:445–464.
284. Witkin GB, Askin FB, Geratz D, Reddick RL: Angiosarcoma of the uterus: A light microscopic, immunohistochemical, and ultrastructural study. Int J Gynecol Pathol 1987;6:176–184.
285. Hendrickson MR, Scheithauer BW: Primitive neuroectodermal tumor of the endometrium: Report of two cases, one with electron microscopic observations. Int J Gynecol Pathol 1986;5:249–259.
286. Cho KR, Rosenshein NB, Epstein JI: Malignant rhabdoid tumor of the uterus. Int J Gynecol Pathol 1989;8:381–387.
287. Ulbright TM, Roth LM: Metastatic and independent cancers of the endometrium and ovary: A clinicopathologic study of 34 cases. Hum Pathol 1985;16:28–34.
288. Kumar NB, Hart WR: Metastases to the uterine corpus from extragenital cancers: A clinicopathologic study of 63 cases. Cancer 1982;50:2163–2169.

7

The Fallopian Tubes

Richard J. Stock

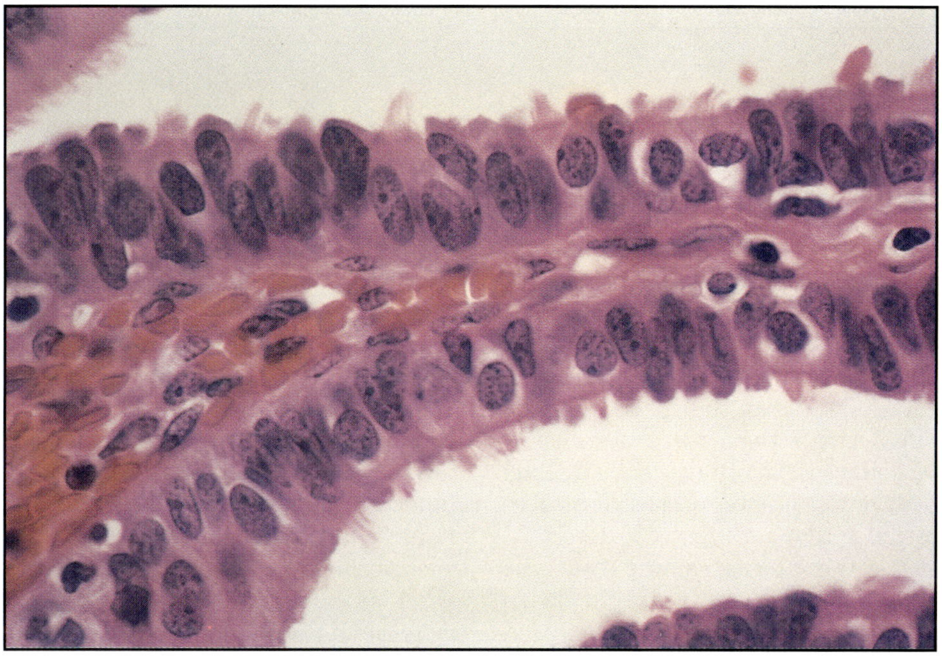

The uterine tubes were mentioned in the Hindu medical writings as early as 1000 to 800 B.C., but their attachments and functions were not suggested until the observations of Fallopius (1561) and deGraaf (1672). Up to the time of Fallopius, the tubes were believed to be conduits of female semen, somewhat analogous to the function of the vas deferens. Tubal connections were not clearly delineated; some believed that they were attached to the bladder, whereas others proposed attachment to the uterus. Fallopius correctly described the attachments to the uterus, noting that the shape of the tube is comparable to that of a classical musical instrument and therefore naming it the "tuba uteri." deGraaf was the first to suggest that the tubes function by transporting eggs to the uterus. Blundell (1819) commented upon the muscular movements of the tube, while Bischoff (1842) suggested that transport of eggs through the tube is secondary to both contractions of the tube and ciliary activity of the tubal epithelium.[1] Today we view the fallopian tubes as active, but not indispensable, in facilitating fertilization and transport of the zygote.

Most of the clinical and pathologic problems of the fallopian tubes concern either infection or fertility. A challenging area for evaluation is documentation of damage and the effects of the healing processes subsequent to infections and surgical interventions. There are major pathophysiologic consequences of this healing. To understand these processes better, evaluation of the tubal specimens by the pathologist might include imaginative and innovative techniques, such as the use of combinations of radiographic injectable materials with histopathologic markers for confirming tubal patency, the use of serial longitudinal sections, and clearing methods.[2, 3]

THE NORMAL FALLOPIAN TUBE

Embryology

Early in embryogenesis, the mesonephric system forms from the mesoderm. The mesonephric tubules enlarge, creating a ventral bulge in the coelomic cavity. This is developed by 30 days from conception. The ridge divides longitudinally into what is referred to as the lateral mesonephric ridge and the medial genital ridge. Together they form the urogenital ridge, which contains the mesonephric (wolffian) duct, the undifferentiated gonad, and the developing adrenal gland. In all embryos by about the fourth to fifth week post conception a groove develops on the lateral side of the mesonephric ridge that closes to form a tube that is parallel and medial to the wolffian duct. The cranial portion remains open. This duct, which is lined by coelomic epithelium, constitutes the paramesonephric, or müllerian, duct. The müllerian ducts fuse in the midline as they extend caudally, forming the genital cord. In the absence of testicular determining factor, embryonic testes, and testosterone, the müllerian ducts develop as the internal female genitalia while the wolffian ducts become vestigial.[4] The cranial portion of the müllerian duct forms the fallopian tube, and the fused portion constitutes the uterus. The cranial end of the müllerian duct remains open, forming the tubal fimbriae. Vestigial remnants of the wolffian duct exist within the mesosalpinx and are incorporated into the superficial muscularis of the lateral aspect of the uterus. The fallopian tube develops quite rapidly with early coiling followed by the formation of luminal crypts that later turn into luminal folds. These folds extend the length of the fallopian tube. Ciliated cells appear by the fourth month of gestation. By birth, ciliated and secretory cells are well developed, as are the plicae.[5]

The most common anomalies involving the fallopian tube are caused by the failure of the müllerian duct to develop on one or both sides. Complete failure of development of the müllerian duct is usually associated with an abnormality in the development of the urogenital ridge, which results in the absence of the ipsilateral kidney and collecting ducts. Most of the anomalies are associated with incomplete development or failure of fusion of the caudal aspects of the müllerian duct. Failure of fusion results in various forms of duplication of the internal female genitalia from the vaginal canal to the uterus. The fallopian tubes are rarely affected by the anomalies associated with fusion, except with respect to the angle of entrance of the tube into the fundal portion of the uterine horn. Rare instances of hypoplasia have also been reported.[6]

Fallopian tube anomalies can be divided into three groups: (1) absence, which could be complete, partial, or segmental; (2) duplication, which could be complete, partial, or accessory; and (3) multiple lumens and accessory fimbriae. The most common anomaly is accessory fimbriae (Fig. 7–1). This is believed to result from incomplete folding of the cephalic portion of the müllerian duct or local differentiation of cells that creates pedunculated foci with a fimbriated end. The reported incidence of accessory fimbriae occurring in the ampullary and infundibular portion of the fallopian tube ranges from 2 to 6 percent. Beyth et al. suggested that such accessory fimbriae may be a contributing factor to infertility.[7] An association with ectopic pregnancy and endometriosis has also been proposed. In our own studies on patients undergoing elective sterilization, the incidence of accessory fimbria is 3 percent; in patients with ectopic pregnancy, the incidence is also 3 percent.

One of the rarest anomalies of the fallopian tube is duplication or other multiples of the fallopian tube on one or both sides. Embryologically this can be explained by the development of two or more grooves on the mesonephric ridge. In the few reported cases of the occurrence of multiples of the fallopian tube on one side, each has terminated in the body of the uterus. In our own series of 440 elective laparoscopic sterilizations, we have seen one case of a partial unilateral duplication (lateral third only) of the fallopian tube.

Anatomy

The fallopian tube begins at the junction of the tube with the uterine cavity and extends through the muscular portion of the uterus, to end at its attachment to the ovary. The tube is attached to the ovary by the *fimbria ovarica,* which attaches to the lateral surface of the cranial portion of the

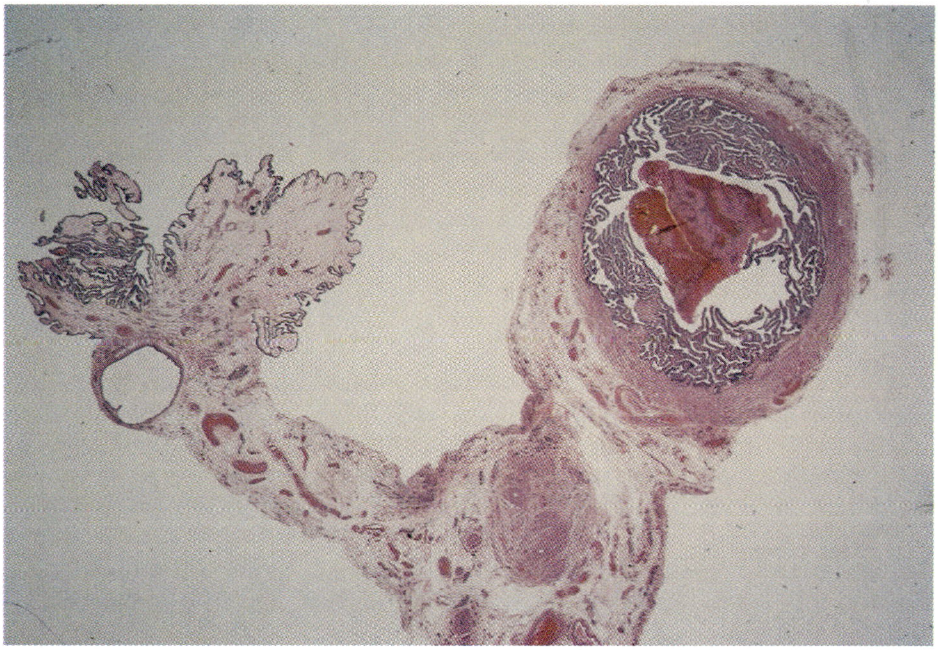

FIGURE 7–1
This is a cross section of a fallopian tube in which there was an ectopic pregnancy. An accessory fimbria, attached on the left, does not have a lumen and does not communicate with the tube. The stalk has a fibrovascular core.

ovary. The length of the fallopian tube is measured from the cornu (i.e., junction of the tube with the body of the uterus) to the fimbriae. A normal fallopian tube length averages 8 to 11 cm. The fallopian tube is covered by the broad ligament, which drapes over the round ligament and then over the tube flowing posteriorly to the lateral portion of the uterus and down to the level of the uterosacral ligaments, where it extends laterally to the pelvic side wall. The fallopian tube is usually divided into four segments. The first is the interstitial or intramural portion, which extends from the junction with the endometrium to the uterine serosa; the second is the isthmic portion, extending from the uterotubal junction to the ampulla; the third is the ampulla; and the fourth is the infundibulum. The infundibulum incorporates both the opening of the tube to the peritoneal cavity (or ostium) and the finger-like projections (fimbriae) that protrude from it.

In the past, the interstitial portion of the fallopian tube was studied because of an earlier suggestion of the presence of a sphincter or valve in this area. No anatomic valve has been found, although Rocker noted that the tube angles acutely just before its entrance into the uterine cavity.[8] The interstitial portion of the tube varies from 1 to 3.5 cm in length; it has been described as taking one of several courses through the myometrium. Sweeney noted that of 100 tubes studied, 8 followed a curved course, 23 followed a straight course, and 67 followed a tortuous route of 2 cm to 3.5 cm through the myometrium.[9]

On cross section the interstitial portion of the tube demonstrates four primary folds within a well-defined longitudinal muscle layer. The isthmus varies from 2 to 3 cm in length and constitutes the most muscular segment of the fallopian tube. It has three distinct muscular layers. The mid-isthmus also is the narrowest segment of the tubal lumen. The ampullary-isthmic junction can be defined by a palpable difference secondary to the change in the muscular configuration of the wall. The ampulla varies from 5 to 8 cm in length. On cross section the longitudinal folds appear much more complex than those seen in the isthmus. The well-defined inner longitudinal muscularis of the isthmic portion of the tube is lost in the ampullary portion. The muscular configuration of the ampullary portion is primarily circular with interdigitating longitudinal fibers. The infundibulum varies from 1 to 2 cm. The luminal diameter decreases from nearly 2 cm in the ampullary portion to only about 1 to 2 mm at the ostium. The makeup of the muscular wall is the same as the ampullary portion of the tube.

The blood supply to the fallopian tube arises from both the uterine and the ovarian arteries. Borell and Fernstrom demonstrated by arteriography that the uterine artery usually supplies the isthmic and proximal ampullary portion of the tube, while the ovarian artery supplies the infundibulum and the distal portion of the ampulla.[10] However, they also noted that the distribution was not uniform; in some instances it was the ovarian artery that supplied all of the fallopian tube, whereas in other instances it was the uterine artery. The arterial blood supply to the tubes arises from a rich anastomosis of arcading vessels in the mesosalpinx that connect to linearly running arterial channels coursing along the antimesenteric border of the tube. The venous drainage follows the course of the arterial supply. The lymphatic drainage of the tube was originally demonstrated by Pauerstein. It consists of three distinct lymphatic networks draining the mucosa, the muscularis, and the serosa, respectively.[11] Pauerstein also noted that the configuration of lymphatic drainage changes during the course of reproductive life. All three intrinsic lymphatic networks combine to enter into the mesosalpinx and from there follow the broad ligament lymphatics, finally to enter the paraaortic lymph nodes.

Histology

The outer serosal surface of the fallopian tube is a continuation of the broad ligament. The broad ligament has a lining of mesothelial cells, underlying connective tissue, and a thin layer of circular and longitudinal smooth muscle cells that converge at the antimesenteric portion of tube.

The inner mucosal layer is surrounded by tubal muscularis except in the interstitial segment. There is a scant amount of connective tissue that contains vessels and a scant number of stromal cells. Beginning in the interstitial portion of the fallopian tube, the mucosa forms four to six folds, or plicae, that extend out into the isthmic portion (Fig. 7–2). In the ampullary portion, these folds become much more complex with extensive branching (Fig. 7–3). The epithelial cell layer of the mucosa is composed of three histologic cell types: secretory, ciliated, and intercalary (or peg) cells (Fig. 7–4). The distribution and proportion of the ciliated cells vary with the age of the patient, the location within the tube, and the hormonal milieu.[12] Ciliated cells are more prevalent in the ampullary portion of the tube and tend to be located at the apical portions of the plicae. The ciliated cell is a glandular columnar cell. Transmis-

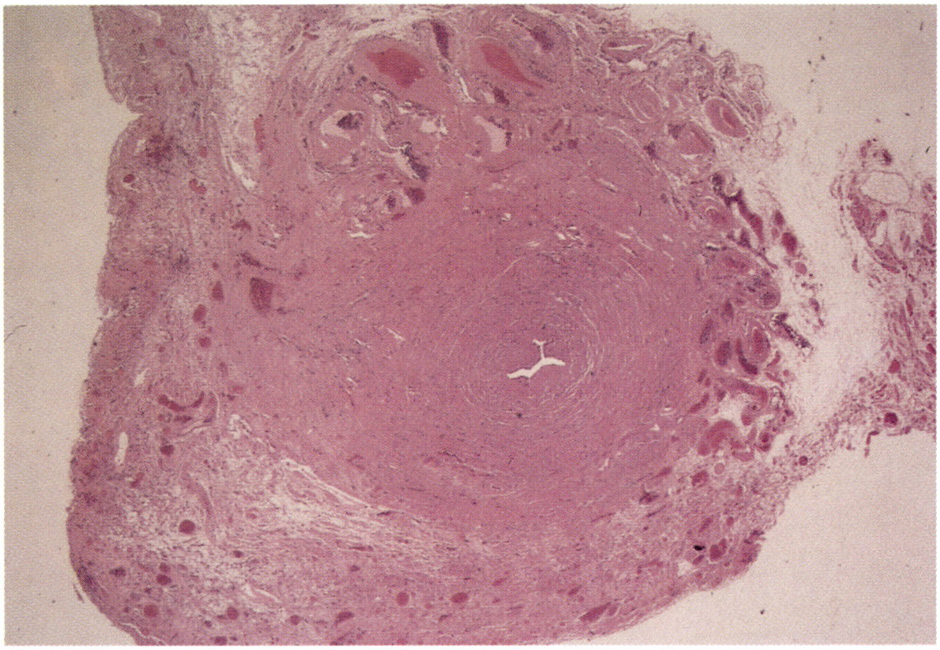

FIGURE 7–2
The isthmic portion of fallopian tube has several primary folds, and the muscle is thick. The inner circular layer of muscle is easily identified.

sion electron microscopy reveals the typical ultrastructural appearance of cilia, with basal bodies and rootlets.[13] The ciliated cells are viewed as necessary for sperm transport, although fertility has been observed in patients with nonfunctional ciliated cells (Kartagener syndrome).[14] The secretory cell is columnar and approximately the same size as the ciliated cell. It has an oval to elongated nucleus that has a denser chromatin pattern than that of the ciliated cell. Both ciliated and secretory cells have a small but distinct nucleolus. The intercalary columnar (peg) cell has a thin, dark-staining nucleus. This cell is believed to be a morphologic variant of the secretory cell. In addition to these three columnar cell types, a smaller, distinct cell with a rounded, dark nucleus may be seen. Because it is located in the basal portion of the epithelium it was originally thought to be a reserve cell for the tubal mucosa. However, electron microscopic studies have shown that this cell is of lymphocytic origin.[15]

The stroma is sparse in most areas around the tube but somewhat more prominent in the ampullary and infundibular portions. In these areas the

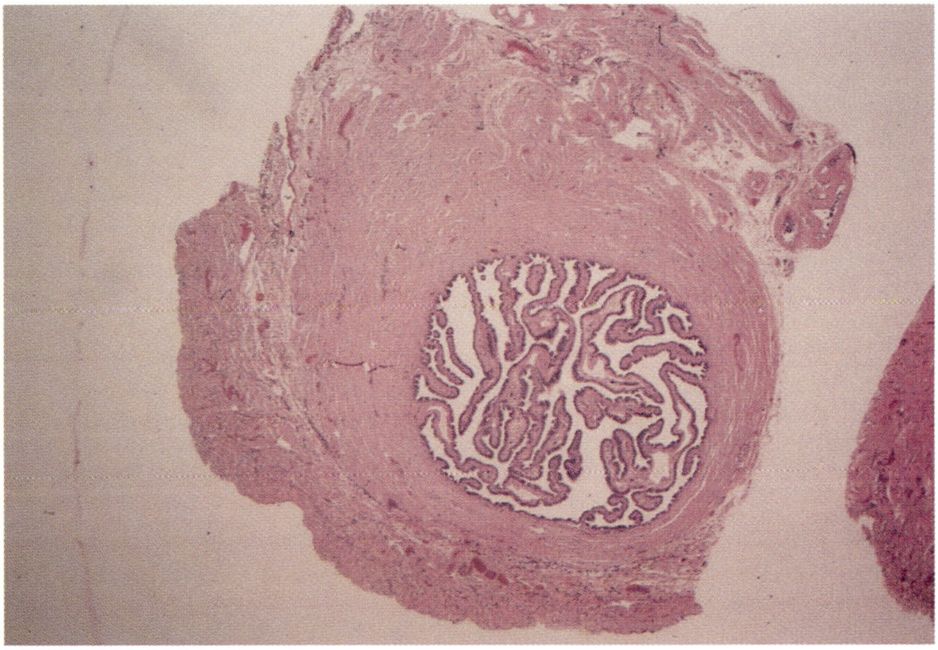

FIGURE 7–3
An ampullary segment of fallopian tube shows that the primary folds arborized to form a complex pattern. The muscularis is less prominent.

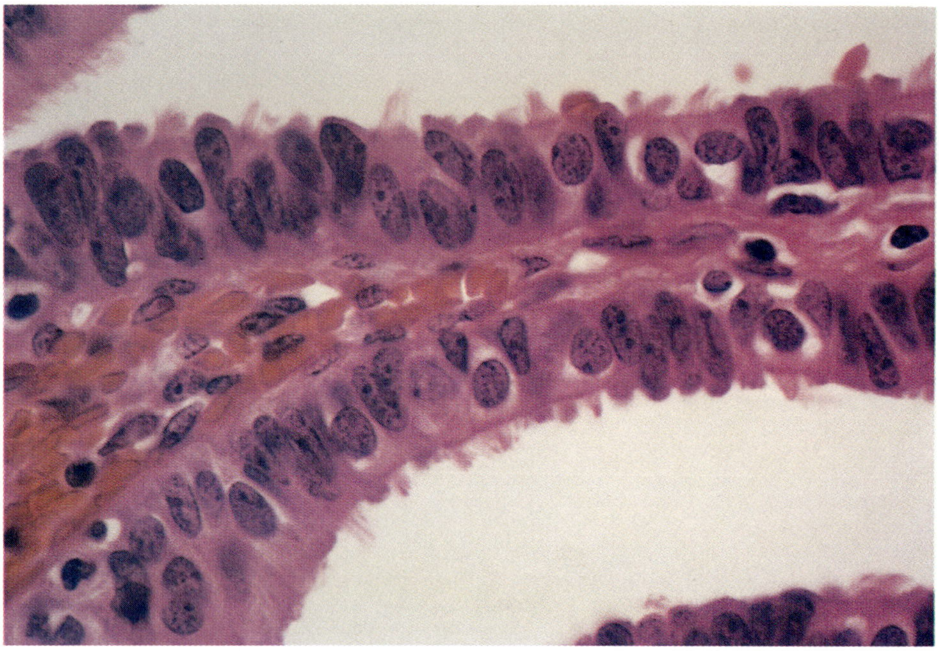

FIGURE 7-4
The tubal epithelium consists of columnar ciliated cells, peg cells, and nonciliated cells. Also seen is a small, dark lymphocytic cell located at the base of the epithelium (*upper left*). The stroma is sparse. The ciliated cells have a round, centrally located nucleus and a terminal bar. The secretory cells have an elongated nucleus with a dense chromatin pattern. Both cells have distinct small nucleoli.

loose-textured connective tissue contains fine reticulum and collagen fibers. Fibroblasts and mast cells may be identified in these areas. From our own studies of segments of tubes removed during interval or postpartum sterilization, we have seen plasma cells in the stroma in 30 percent of cases. Fibroblast proliferation may occur with infection, aging, or vascular injury. This results in plical fibrosis.

The mesosalpinx is covered anteriorly and posteriorly by the leaves of the broad ligament. It contains the arteries, veins, and lymphatics. Also contained in the mesosalpinx and in close approximation with the tube are remnants of the mesonephric (wolffian) duct. These remnants consist of small, rounded lumens surrounded by two layers of smooth muscle, the inner being longitudinal (Fig. 7–5). The epithelium consists of cuboidal to low columnar nonciliated cells that are separated from the muscular layer by a well-defined basal lamina. Other more convoluted tubules with a low columnar epithelium that may be stratified and contain ciliated cells may be identified in the mesovarium. Their muscular coat disappears as the

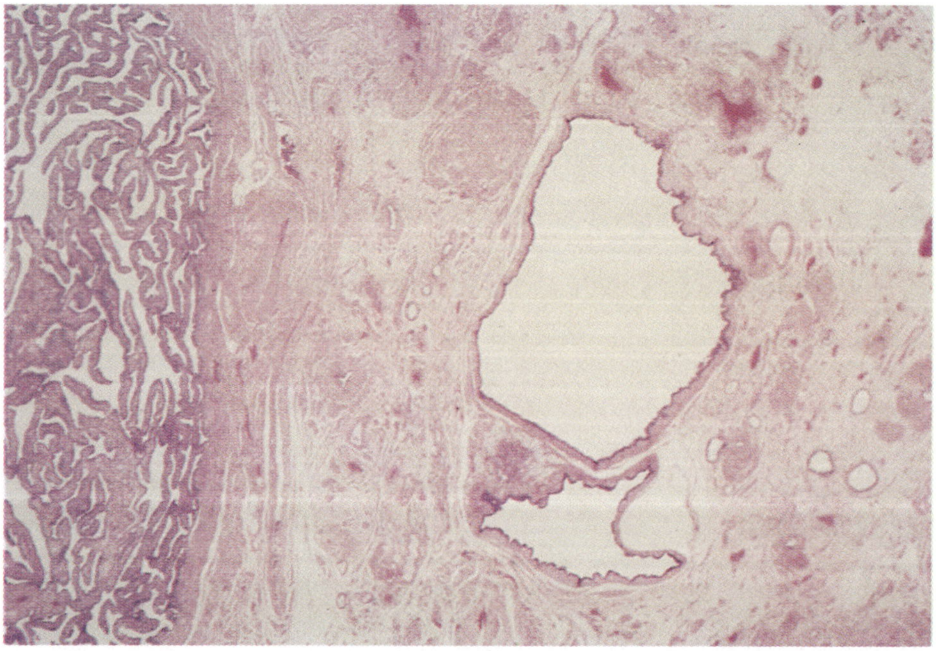

FIGURE 7-5
This is a cross section through the tube (*left*) and mesosalpinx. Two dilated vestigial mesonephric ducts are seen. These wolffian duct remnants are lined by low cuboidal, nonciliated cells. Muscle is seen to surround each duct remnant.

remnants are found closer to the hilum of the ovary. In this region, adrenal rests may occasionally be identified.[16]

Small cystic structures, referred to as hydatids of Morgagni, are frequently found attached to the tube along the ampulla and infundibulum. Morgagni was the first author to describe these structures and ascribe a clinical significance to them. The structures are of paramesonephric (müllerian) origin. They contain occasional plicae and are lined by ciliated and nonciliated cells. The wall contains smooth muscle. Rarely, torsion of a hydatid of Morgagni may result in a clinical picture similar to that of appendicitis. Some authors have suggested that the origin of the hydatids may be mesonephric rather than paramesonephric; however, in a study by Genadry et al. in 1977, none was found to be of mesonephric origin.[17]

METAPLASIA AND RELATED CHANGES

Metaplasia is a process wherein a fully differentiated tissue of one kind differentiates into a fully differentiated tissue of another kind. Metaplasia in the fallopian tube occurs in three areas—the serosa, the stroma, and the mucosa.

Serosal

Walthard Cyst

Walthard cysts (i.e., Walthard rests or nests) are a very common finding at surgery. They consist of solitary or scattered 1 to 3 mm, white to yellowish cystic nodules found on the serosal surface of the fallopian tube. They often have prominent vessels overlying the unilocular cyst. The cystic structures are lined by epithelium that is histologically similar to squamous metaplasia or urothelium (Fig. 7–6). The basal cells are polygonal, while the surface cells are flattened. Rarely, mucinous cells may be identified. The histologic characteristics are similar to those seen in Brenner tumors of the ovary.[18] Although Walthard cysts are frequently encountered at the time of surgery, the occurrence of a Brenner tumor of the fallopian tube has not been reported. Walthard cysts are a frequent observation but are of no clinical significance.

Stromal

Decidual Change

Decidual change in the fallopian tube is a hormonally stimulated transformation of the stromal cells. This type of change is usually identified in stromal cells underneath the tubal epithelium, although patches may occur anywhere in association with mesothelial surfaces. Earlier works describe decidual change at the site of implantation of an ectopic pregnancy. However, what had been called decidua is now recognized as actually being proliferating intermediate trophoblasts. Other authors have identified decidual changes not in the area of the eccyesis (i.e., extrauterine pregnancy) but rather in other portions of the fallopian tube. The occurrence of decidual changes at other than the

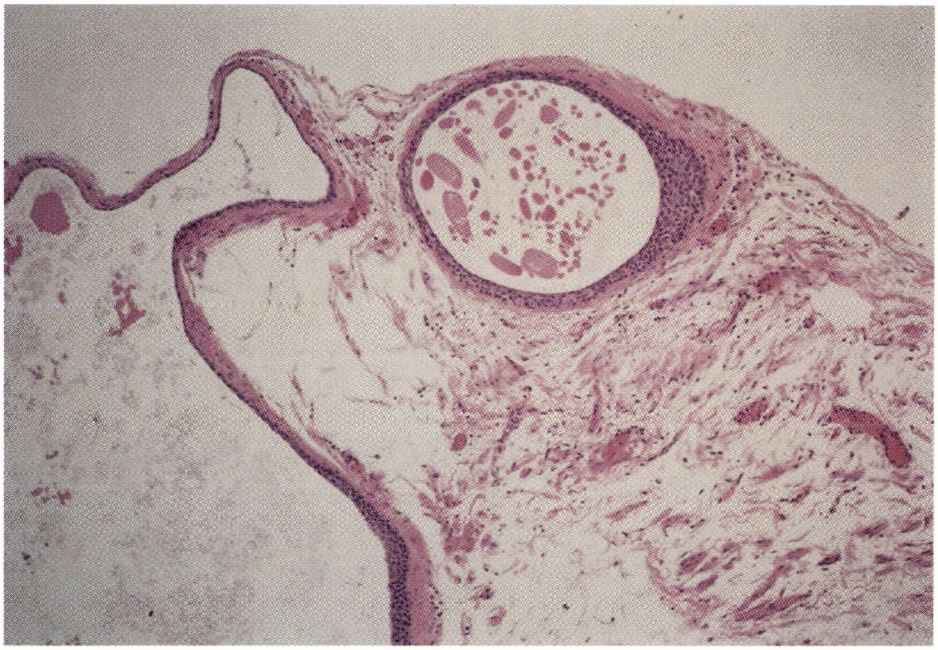

FIGURE 7–6
Two Walthard inclusion cysts are seen under the serosa of the fallopian tube. There is cellular debris in the lumina. The epithelium lining the cyst is stratified and recapitulates squamous metaplasia of the cervix. The larger cyst has areas lined by low cuboidal to flat epithelium.

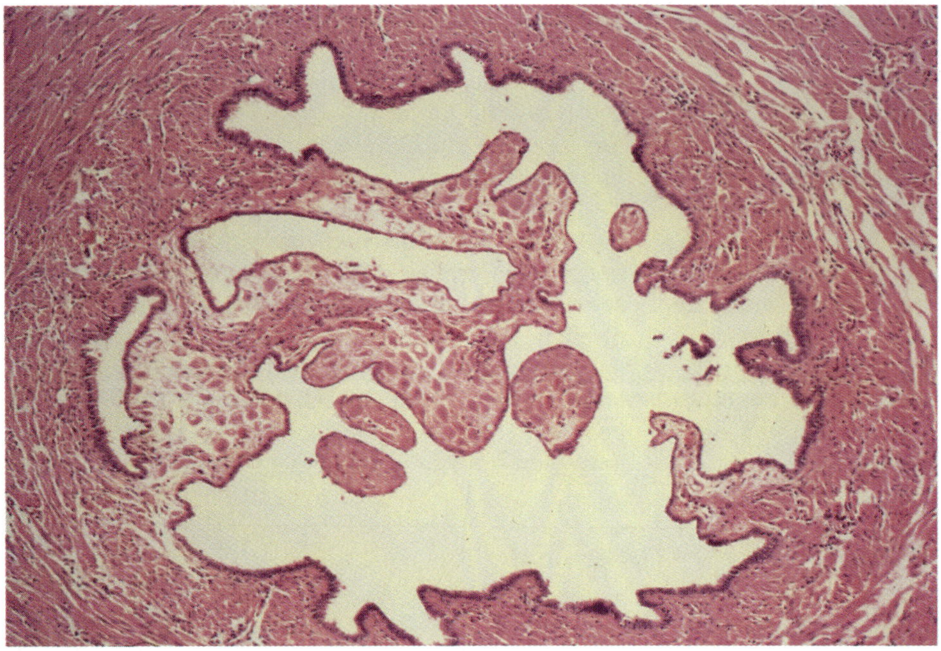

FIGURE 7-7
This cross section of the isthmic portion of a fallopian tube was taken from a postpartum tubal sterilization. Agglutination of plicae secondary to previous salpingitis is seen (*left and center*). The stromal cells of these agglutinated plicae show decidual change. They are plump, with abundant eosinophilic cytoplasm.

site of implantation has been reported in 21 percent of tubes with ectopic pregnancy.[19] After examining postpartum tubal sterilization specimens, Tilden and Winstedt reported a 12 percent incidence of decidual change.[19] After examining 195 postpartum tubal sterilization specimens, decidual change was noted in only 5 percent of cases (unpublished data, Richard J. Stock). However in 45 percent of those with decidua present, there was concurrent evidence of chronic salpingitis identified by plical agglutination (Fig. 7–7) and/or salpingitis isthmica nodosa. In a series of 37 cases of ectopic pregnancy, 14 percent had decidual changes in a site distant from the implantation sites (unpublished data, Richard J. Stock). In this series, 40 percent were directly associated with evidence of chronic salpingitis or salpingitis isthmica nodosa. In the examination of tubes from patients who became pregnant following a sterilization procedure, decidual change is quite common at the site of the prior surgical procedure. In our experience, decidual transformation is most often seen in association with areas of prior tubal injury.

Fibrosis

Fibrosis or hyalinization of the fallopian tube is associated with aging.[20] In the postmenopausal woman, there is an increase in hyalinized and fibrotic tissue within the plicae. This change also occurs in patients who undergo sterilization procedures with division of the tube. The amount of fibrosis is related to the time from sterilization to examination of the segments of tube and is confined to the lateral portion of disrupted tube. The same changes are seen in patients who have a previous history of salpingitis, especially those who have had recurrent episodes.

Ovarian Stromal Metaplasia

Stromal metaplastic changes that resemble ovarian stroma have also been identified.[21] Honoré[21] reports that the condition is very uncommon and that it is seen mostly in the stroma of the fimbriae. The change is apparently seen mostly in perimenopausal women. It has no clinical significance.

Psammoma Bodies

Psammoma bodies are seen in the serosa, submucosa, or lumen of the fallopian tube. A psammoma body is a small, round, concentrically laminated, calcified structure. Psammoma bodies are associated with many neoplastic and non-neoplastic conditions (e.g., pelvic inflammatory disease, ectopic pregnancy, ovarian carcinoma).

Psammoma bodies and dystrophic calcifications are often found in the subepithelial portions of the tube. The psammoma body could then be extruded into the tubal lumen. Psammoma bodies may travel through the fallopian tubes and be identified in cytologic smears taken from the cervix. The importance of this is that psammoma body formation need not be associated with a malignant process. A malignancy is likely, however, when a psammoma body is found in association with malignant-appearing epithelial cells.

Mucosal

Squamous Metaplasia

Squamous epithelial changes in the tubal mucosa can rarely be identified as areas of squamous morula formation. Immature squamous metaplasia is more often identified in the area of the uterotubal junction. As such it may be associated with the same factors that are associated with endometrial squamous metaplasia.[21]

Mucinous Metaplasia

Foci of mucinous metaplasia are rarely seen. This has been associated with the Peutz-Jeghers syndrome.[22] Mucinous metaplasia has also been reported in an instance of coexistent endocervical and ovarian mucinous adenocarcinomas. This illustrates the potential for similar neoplastic transformation of tissues of similar embryologic origin.[22A]

Papillary Eosinophilic Metaplasia

Papillary eosinophilic metaplasia can be a histopathologic pitfall, especially when associated with a papillary change (Fig. 7–8). Most lesions have been identified incidentally in postpartum tubal sterilization specimens and have occasionally been mistakenly reported as malignant.[23] Saffos et al. noted that even though this is a benign process it may have some disturbing cellular features.[24] These lesions involve only part of the circumference of the tubal mucosa. The papillary appearance is partly due to their origin from the tubal plicae. The papillary curves are thin. A light lymphocytic infiltrate is seen in the loose fibrovascular tissue. The metaplastic epithelium is confined to the surface. The cells are columnar, nonciliated, and arranged as a single layer or pseudostratified. Most of the cells have abundant eosinophilic cytoplasm; some contain mucin. The nuclei are round to oval with occasional prominent nucleoli. The nuclei are located at the base when there is a single cellular layer or at various levels within the cell when there is pseudostratification. Epithelial budding, similar to that seen with ovarian serous tumors of low malignant potential, is common. Mitotic activity is absent or rare. The few cases reported have had no malignant sequelae.[24]

Endometriosis and Endosalpingiosis

Although endometriosis has been considered by some to be a metaplastic process, others feel that it represents implantation from retrograde menstruation.[25–28] The luminal foci are most frequently found in association with prior tubal occlusive procedures and are located in the medial (i.e., proximal) portion of the fallopian tube (Fig. 7–9). The site of endometriosis is almost always in the immediate area of the prior surgical procedure. Foci of endometriosis are also identified in patients with tubal obstructive disease. Sampson

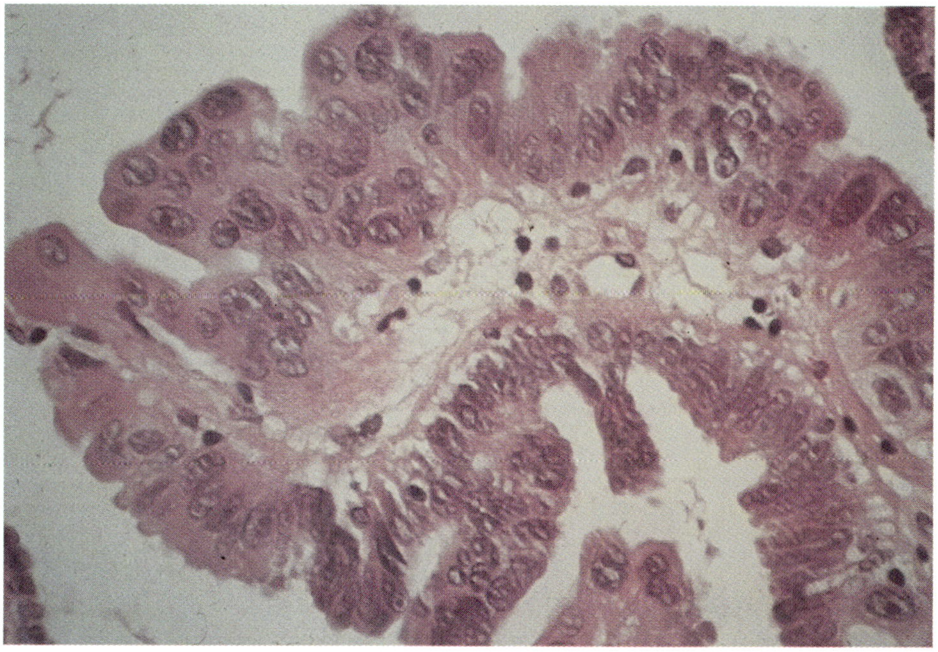

FIGURE 7–8
This is a free-floating papillary tissue fragment that was identified within the lumen of the tube in a patient who underwent a postpartum tubal sterilization procedure. It was mistakenly diagnosed as carcinoma. This is eosinophilic or oncocytic metaplasia. The fibrovascular core is thin and edematous and contains a few lymphocytes. The surface epithelial changes are focal. There is pseudostratification, pleomorphism, loss of polarity, nuclear atypia, and prominent nucleoli. However, there are no mitoses.

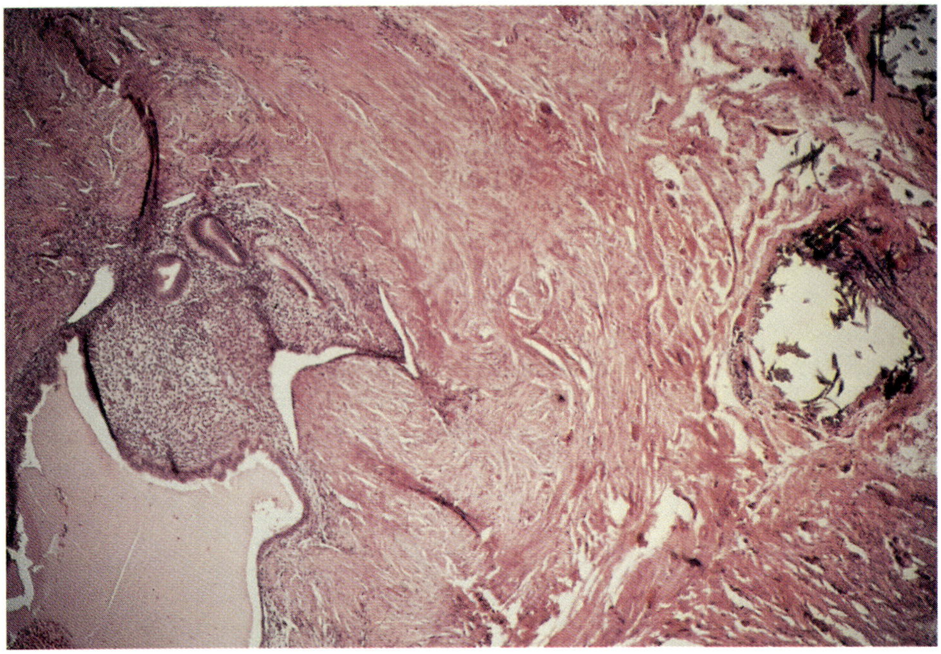

FIGURE 7-9
This histologic section is from the terminal aspect of the medial remaining tube following a postpartum sterilization. Remnants of suture material can still be identified along the right margin. A focus of endometriosis with normal endometrial glands and stroma is identified next to the tubal lumen. This is believed to represent retrograde implantation.

coined the term endosalpingiosis to describe a local proliferative nest of tubal mucosa found outside the tubal lumen following surgical intervention.[25] In his view, the endosalpingiosis could either retain its normal characteristics or undergo a metaplastic process, recapitulating the endometrium. Most of his cases were instances in which the tube and/or adnexa were removed because of acute or recurrent salpingitis. Novak challenged Sampson's data, since some of Sampson's illustrations are consistent with what is known as salpingitis isthmica nodosa.[29] In a second publication, Sampson compared his patients with 100 controls and concluded that the repair of salpingectomy wounds is one of the exceptions to the law of normal healing of hollow viscera. "In a very large percentage of these cases the growth of the tubal epithelium not only invades the tubal scar . . . but may continue to grow after healing has occurred."[30] The epithelium may be either of tubal type or of a metaplastic endometrial type. Sampson's concept was later taken to mean that the tubal epithelium has unique characteristics that may, in fact, be the cause of tubal ligation failures.[26]

Over the years the term endosalpingiosis has

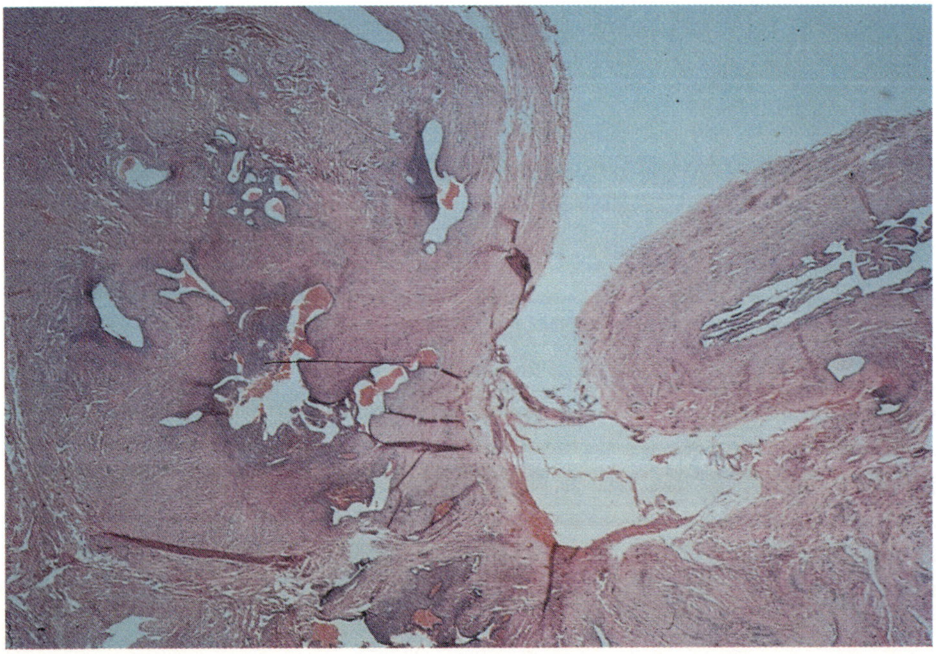

FIGURE 7-10
This is a longitudinal section through the area of a prior tubal sterilization procedure that was done utilizing unipolar electrocoagulation with high-frequency current. The area of tubal separation can be readily identified (*center*). The lateral (i.e., distal) segment of tube is on the right, and the medial segment is on the left. Multiple foci of endometriosis, with blood present in the gland lumen, are seen in the medial fallopian tube segment.

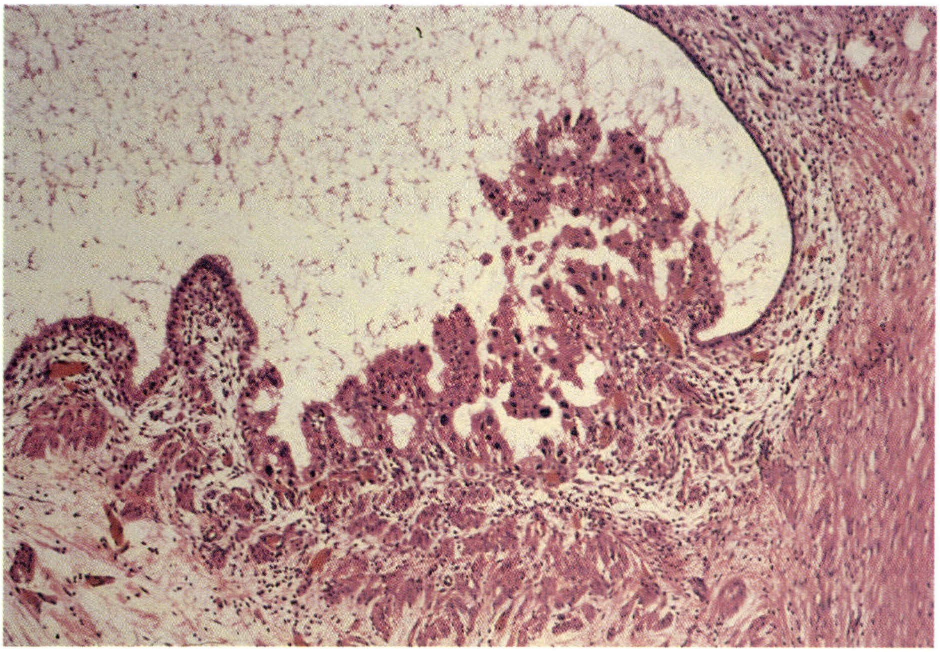

FIGURE 7-11
This is a section of fallopian tube from a patient who underwent a previous sterilization procedure and subsequently became pregnant. A focus of endometriosis located in the immediate area of the sterilization site in the medial remaining tubal segment is seen. An Arias-Stella change is present. The cells have large, bizarre, hyperchromatic nuclei.

been expanded to include foci in any site where ectopic tubal epithelium can be identified. It is common in retroperitoneal lymph nodes and should not be mistaken for metastatic adenocarcinoma. McCausland in 1982 suggested "endosalpingoblastosis" as a better term to apply to the dynamic activation of tubal epithelium after injury, especially that associated with electrocoagulation.[27] A series of tubes from 54 women who had undergone a segmental destructive procedure for sterilization were examined.[28] Both the medial and the lateral tubal segments were studied. The changes described by both Sampson and McCausland (i.e., endometriosis and endosalpingiosis) were identified only at the medial surgical site and could be explained by the nature of the injury and by retrograde menstruation (Fig. 7–10). The Arias-Stella changes seen with pregnancy (see Chapter 5) can also be seen in tubal endometriosis (Fig. 7–11).

ANATOMIC DISORDERS

Torsion

Torsion of the fallopian tube may occur as an isolated condition but most commonly also involves the ovary. Morgagni described a case of "lost" adnexa in 1748. Rokitansky in 1850 presented a major discussion on torsion of the adnexa along with a selected series of 18 cases of torsion of the tube, the ovary, or both. Reports in the first part of this century mostly focused on torsion of the fallopian tube rather than the adnexa.[31] In most of these cases, however, the ovary was also involved. Torsion of the adnexa has been classified in many ways: (1) the adnexal structure involved, (2) the age or condition of the patient, (3) the associated pathologic conditions of the tube or ovary, and (4) the mechanisms involved in torsion and the direction of the torsion. A thorough review of the clinical manifestations of torsion of the adnexa was presented by Merritt in 1991.[32] As was pointed out by Rokitansky, the importance of torsion is in its early clinical recognition. Most patients are in the reproductive age group, and salvage of the adnexa is therefore important. The pathologic findings associated with torsion can range from early focal tubal congestion and edema to migration or loss of a part of, or all, the adnexa.[31]

The patient with torsion of the adnexa presents with colicky, unilateral pelvic pain. She may develop a low-grade fever and mild leukocytosis. On pelvic examination, a tender, unilateral pelvic mass is felt. In some cases this mass appears to enlarge rapidly. This occurs if the torsion occludes venous return but only partially blocks arterial flow. This situation allows for vascular congestion and edema.

There has been much conjecture as to whether a normal fallopian tube can undergo torsion, but a review of the literature suggests that this is not the case.[31] For the uterine adnexa to undergo torsion there must be some alteration resulting in an unbalanced structure that is predisposed to torsion. The most common underlying causes are the large functional cysts and ovarian neoplasms. When the fallopian tube undergoes independent

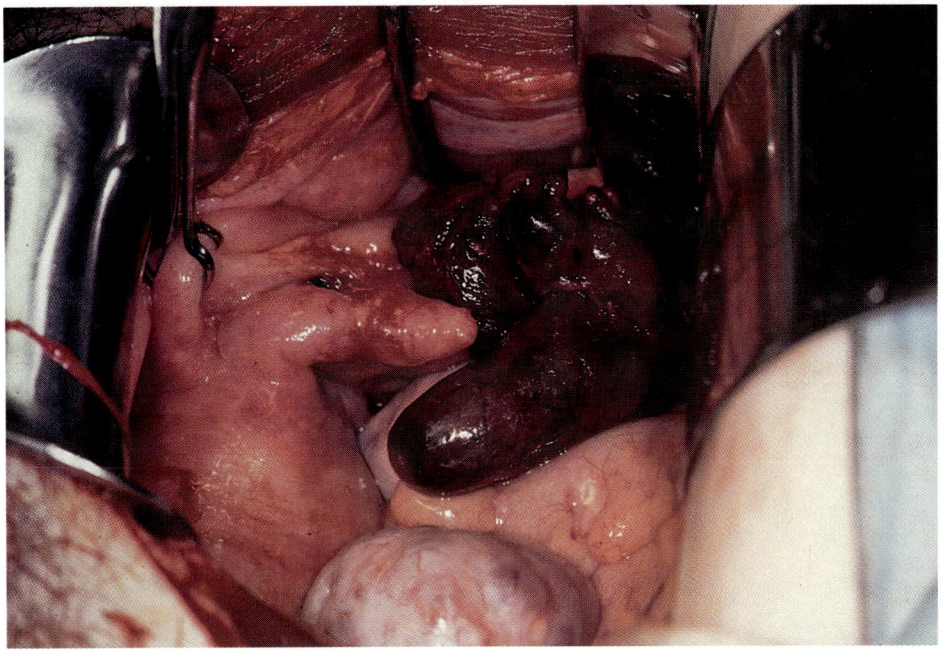

FIGURE 7–12
This patient had a previous Pomeroy tubal ligation and presented with acute onset of right lower quadrant pain. The medial aspect of the tube is identified attached to the uterus. The lateral remaining segment of tube is twisted on its own pedicle, resulting in hemorrhagic congestion and infarction. The surgical (Babcock) clamp is holding the round ligament, which attaches to the uterus anterior to the fallopian tube. A normal ovary is seen (*bottom center*).

torsion there almost always is prior distortion of the tube secondary to sterilization, ectopic pregnancy, or a hydrosalpinx (Fig. 7–12). Prior sterilization procedures or segmental resections leave a segment of tube on a pedicle, which may twist. Hemorrhagic congestion and edema are found in the tissue distal to the site of torsion (Fig. 7–13). There are differences in the degree of tissue edema and vascular congestion identified on either side of the point of constriction. In the area of constriction, vascular thrombosis may be seen. This leads to the clinical decision of whether to untwist the adnexa to assess viability, possibly risking a thromboembolic event. However, there have been no reported cases of thromboembolism secondary to untwisting congested, and possibly infarcted, adnexa. If the adnexa is obviously infarcted or if the patient is beyond her reproductive years (see Fig. 7–13), removal is accomplished without untwisting. If there appears to be no infarction, untwisting and observation for return of normal blood flow are recommended. Intraoperative Doppler flow ultrasound may be used to assess the adequacy of the blood flow.

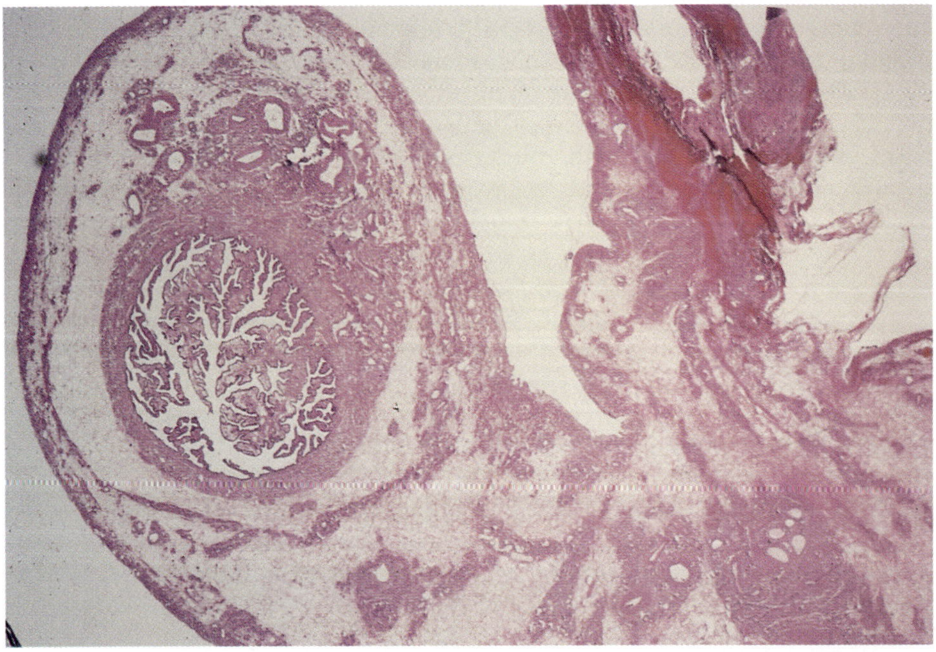

FIGURE 7–13
This is a cross section through the ampulla of a tube and its mesosalpinx in a case of adnexal torsion. There is marked edema and vascular dilatation. The presence of a paratubal cyst of paramesonephric origin predisposed this tube to torsion. The wall of the paratubal cyst, with hemorrhagic congestion can be seen in the upper right corner.

Prolapse

There are fewer than 100 cases of fallopian tube prolapse reported in the literature, and most of these have followed vaginal hysterectomy. The paucity of reported cases does not reflect the true incidence of this problem. The first case of tubal prolapse was described by Pozzi in 1902. Sapan and Solberg suggested that postoperative infection, hematoma, abscess formation, or the use of transvaginal drains were common factors associated with prolapse.[33] The diagnosis of prolapse is most frequently made early in the postoperative period, but reports have listed intervals of up to 20 years following surgery. When prolapse occurs in the early postoperative period, frequent complaints include bloody or watery discharge, postcoital spotting, and dyspareunia. The clinician may easily confuse the prolapsed fimbriated end with granulation tissue (Fig. 7–14). Biopsy specimens are likewise frequently mistakenly interpreted as granulation tissue. Symmonds et al. have pointed out an important clinical distinction—the fimbriated end of the tube is tender when manipulated or biopsied, and granulation tissue is not.[33a]

Some authors have commented on the value of cytology in suggesting the diagnosis of fallopian tube prolapse.[34] Glandular cells are easily recognized and should not be present in the posthysterectomy vagina. Since these cells may have features similar to endometrial cells, it is important to recognize the ciliated cells to distinguish prolapse from endometriosis. Unfortunately, most of the ciliated cells disappear because of the isolated acute and chronic inflammation. In terms of the biopsy material, the possibility of prolapse must be kept in mind. The pathologist needs to be informed of the site of the biopsy (i.e., vaginal apex) and the history of a previous hysterectomy. The true nature of the lesion can be identified by low-power microscopic examination, which shows distended and inflamed plicae or fimbriae; on higher power, surface cuboidal or columnar epithelial cells are identified.

The presence of a prolapsed fimbriated end of a fallopian tube into the vaginal vault is one explanation for the rarely reported instances of pregnancy occurring more than 7 months following hysterectomy.[35] It has also been related to cases of acute salpingitis and postcoital pneumoperitoneum. Prolapse identified years after surgery could be confused with well-differentiated adenocarcinoma.[36] Removal of the prolapsed fallopian tube may be accomplished by either a transvaginal surgical approach with the patient under anesthesia or by a combined laparoscopic and transvaginal approach.

Intussusception

Adams has reported the only case of intussusception in which a hydatid cyst of Morgagni was engulfed into the fallopian tube. A portion of the fimbriated end was pulled into the ampullary portion of the tube.[37]

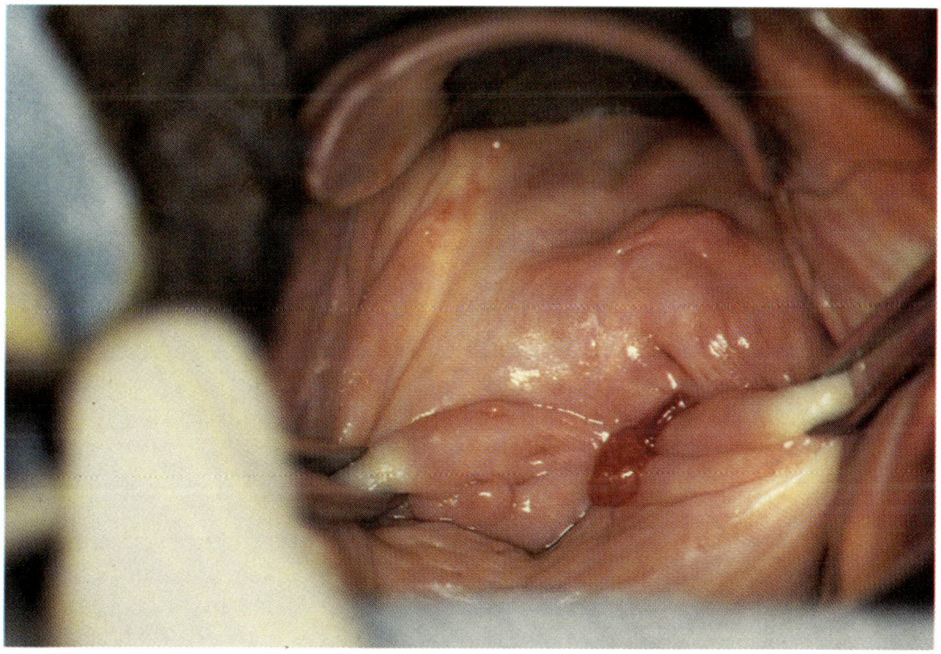

FIGURE 7–14
A speculum vaginal examination of a patient who previously underwent a vaginal hysterectomy and presented some months later with postcoital spotting is shown. At the apex of the vagina there is a reddened, pedunculated tissue mass that was tender on manipulation. This represents prolapse of the fimbriated end of the fallopian tube. It is frequently confused with granulation tissue. Granulation tissue is not tender.

TUBAL STERILIZATION

James Blundell in 1823 first suggested tubal obstruction as a mechanism for female sterilization. It was Samuel Lungren in 1880 who performed the first tubal ligation procedure by utilizing a silk ligature at the time of a cesarean section. German physicians in the later part of the nineteenth century conducted many experimental tubal sterilization procedures on animals. They experimented with different methods including excision, use of different suture materials, steam, galvanic current, and destructive chemicals. The failure rates, however, were too high.[38] Modern sterilization procedures became popular with the advent of laparoscopy in the 1960s.

The pathologist has three concerns when dealing with tubal sterilization specimens. The first is to confirm that an appropriate sterilization procedure has been performed when a segment of tube has been removed. The second is to recognize the long-term pathophysiologic changes after surgical sterilization, and the third is to try to identify the cause for a sterilization failure.

In the more traditional "tubal ligation" procedures a segment of fallopian tube is removed and submitted for pathologic examination in order to confirm that a complete segment of tube has been removed. The importance of identifying the intactness of the lumen of the removed segment was illustrated by a series of failures of the Uchida sterilization procedure in which only partial segments of the tubal lumen were removed.[39] The Uchida procedure removes an ampullary-isthmic segment of fallopian tube and buries the ligated proximal segment in the mesosalpinx.

Early in the 1970s, when laparoscopy was first used for sterilization procedures, high-frequency electrical current was employed to destroy segments of the tube; this was followed by resection of the intervening segment. Under these conditions, the pathologist had difficulty confirming the presence of a lumen, or even identifying an intact segment of tube, because of the coagulation injury. Orientation of the tube in order to identify the presence of a tubal lumen was frequently not possible.

The pathologic changes that are encountered subsequent to a tubal sterilization procedure often reflect the type of sterilization that was performed. For that reason the pathologist should be aware of the most frequently performed sterilization procedures.

Most postpartum period tubal ligations are performed by the so-called Pomeroy or "modified" Pomeroy procedure using a small laparotomy incision (minilaparotomy). During the Pomeroy procedure the middle segment of tube is elevated and doubly ligated using 1-0 chromic suture. The top of the tubal loop is then excised. Most of the "modifications" involve the use of other sizes or types of suture. The success of the procedure was attributed to the use of absorbable suture material, which leads to the eventual separation of the two tubal ends. Histopathologic examination of the tubal segment at the time of sterilization should identify a complete cross section of the lumen. A dissecting microscope may be helpful in some cases to determine proper orientation of the specimen in the tissue block. Examination of a tube removed after a previous Pomeroy procedure must focus on the changes that occur both at the point of ligature application and at the point of tubal excision. The success of the procedure is influenced by the degree of compression and necrosis at the ligature site and the healing process at the excision site. Separation of the severed ends of the tubes after suture breakdown is the most common occurrence. Compression injury at the ligature sites leads to luminal occlusion. The tubal segment that existed between the ligature and the excision site usually becomes a cystic remnant attached to the tubal end (Fig. 7–15). In unusual instances the two ends of the fallopian tube may stay in immediate proximity and undergo a spontaneous anastomosis at the excision site. If the static constriction of the ligature was either insufficient to initially occlude the lumen or to inflict sufficient injury to result in obstruction during the healing process, pregnancy could occur. The most common cause for sterilization failure is patency at the ligature site together with open communication between the peritoneal cavity and the tube at the excision site (Fig. 7–16). The plicae partially extrude, creating pseudofimbriae.[41] The occurrence of these tuboperitoneal fistulae is, probably, not related to the size or type of suture utilized.

Another type of sterilization procedure used until recently is the Kroner procedure. The distal tube, to include the fimbriated end, is excised after ligature placement. The failure rate for this procedure is relatively high; examination of these cases revealed the formation of a tuboperitoneal fistula at the proximal ligature site, rather than at the excision site as seen with the Pomeroy procedure.[41, 42] This may be a consequence of the ligature being placed on the ampulla, where the muscularis is very thin, but the plicae fill the lumen of the tube by creating a spongelike effect. Most of the damage is to the muscularis which results in fistulization. The pseudofimbriae that form are very well developed (Fig. 7–17).

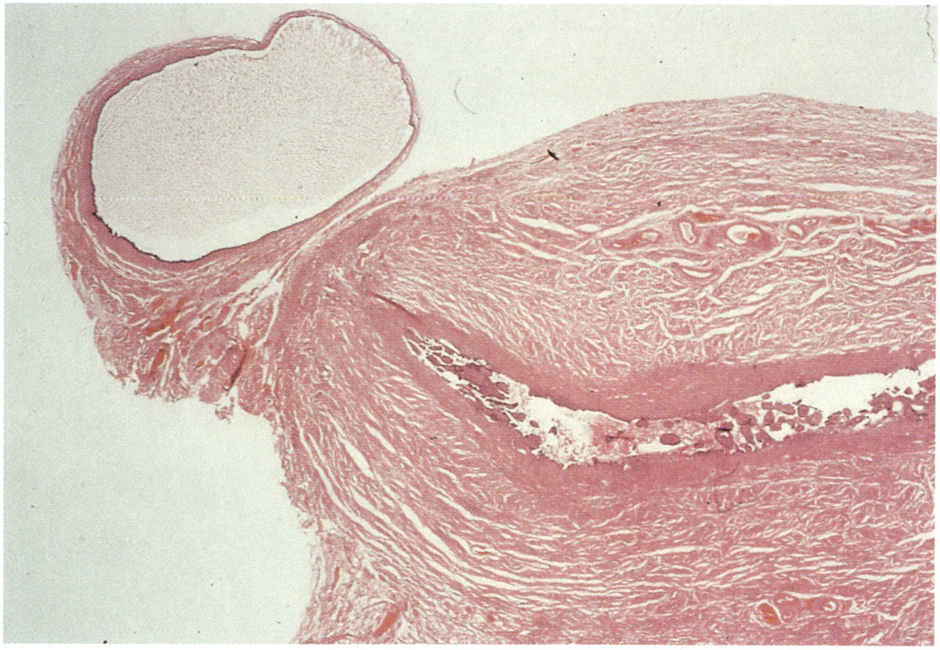

FIGURE 7–15
This is a longitudinal section taken from the medial portion of the fallopian tube in a patient who had previously undergone a Pomeroy sterilization procedure. The lumen is dilated and contains blood with pseudopolyp formation. The segment that represents the area between the placement of the ligature and the excision site remains attached to the distal aspect as a cystic remnant.

With the advent of laparoscopy, three basic methods have been utilized to achieve tubal occlusion. The first is electrocoagulation by the use of electrical energy usually delivered by bipolar equipment. This causes tissue desiccation and coagulation. The long-term effect is coagulative necrosis and fibrosis. The tubes used to be transected following electrocoagulation. However, higher failure rates were seen than without transection. Transection of the tube is usually not performed today. Monopolar electrical delivery systems utilized high-frequency electrosurgical generators; the end-point for tubal destruction is the observation of tissue swelling, explosion, and collapse. These end-point observations are not applicable when bipolar systems are used. With bipolar electrosurgical units the end-point is determined by the current flow between the two poles of the paddles that compress the fallopian tube. This is assessed by an ammeter that is attached to the electrosurgical generator and is a reflection of the increasing degree of tissue dehydration. Unfortu-

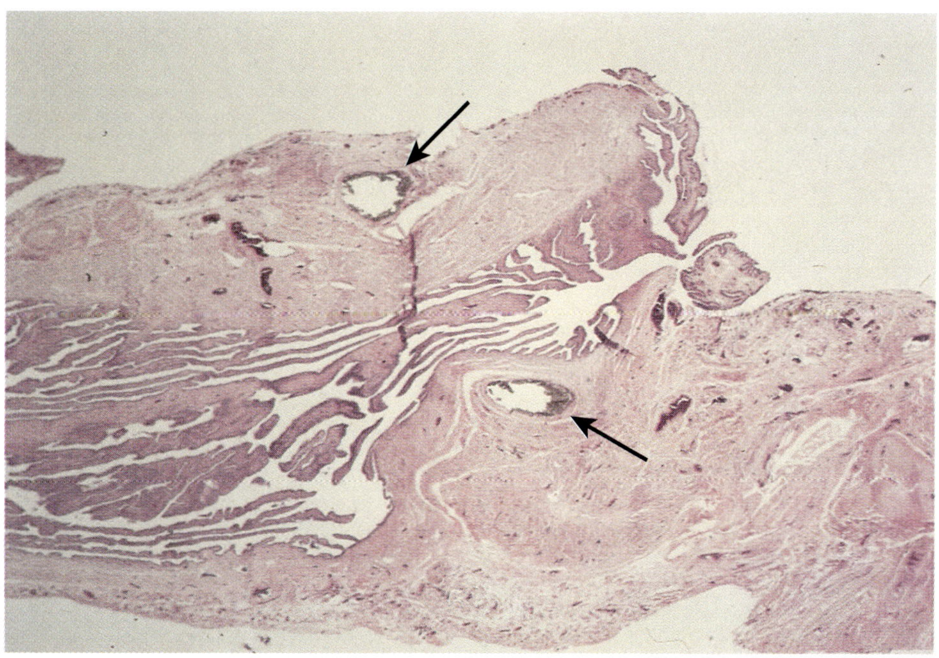

FIGURE 7–16
This is a longitudinal section through the tubal segment lateral to the sterilization site. The suture placement site can be readily identified by residual suture material seen in the muscle on either side of the lumen (*arrows*). The lumen remains open both at the point of ligature placement and the excision site (*top right*).

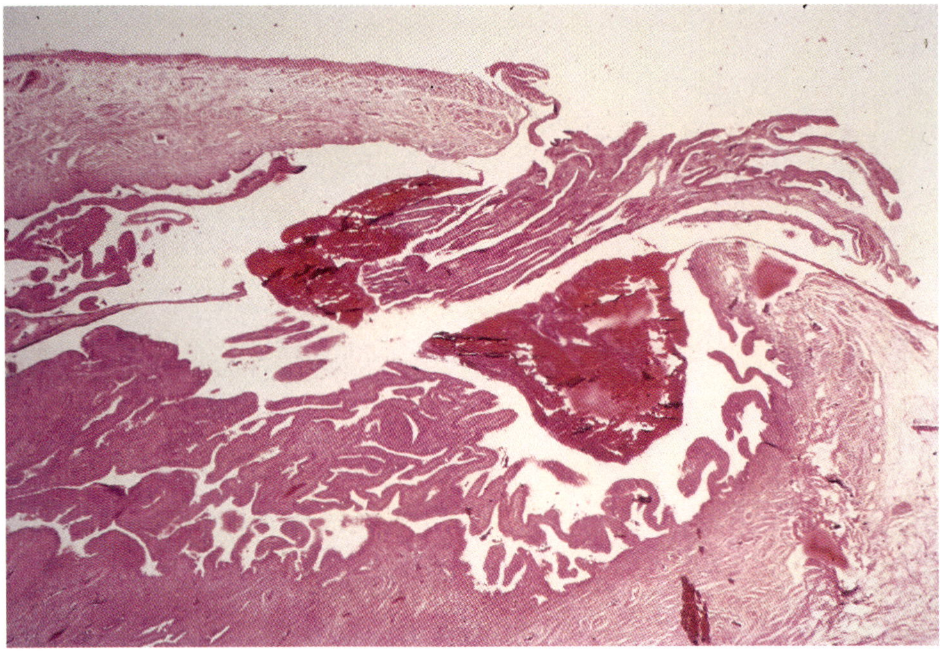

FIGURE 7-17
This is a longitudinal section through the terminal portion of the remaining fallopian tube following a Kroner sterilization procedure. A tuboperitoneal fistula has arisen at the point of ligature placement. The plicae in the ampulla readily protrude through the fistula forming pseudofimbria.

nately, bipolar sterilization procedures are frequently performed with electrosurgical units for which the end-point has not been accurately established.[43, 44] Most pregnancies following bipolar sterilization procedures are a reflection of this problem. By histopathology, marked changes in the muscularis are seen; there is diminished cross-sectional tubal size and evidence of coagulation necrosis involving both the blood vessels and the muscularis (Fig. 7–18).

Two mechanical obstructive techniques are also used for laparoscopic sterilization. One utilizes a Silastic band (Falope ring) that is placed around the base of a loop of fallopian tube. The other uses a clip (Hulka or Filshie) that is placed across the tube. The instrumentation for applying the Silastic band draws a 2.4 to 2.8 cm loop of fallopian tube into the instrument and then releases a band around the base of the loop. Continued compression of the tube at the point of application causes eventual loss of the muscularis, which leads to focal fibrosis. In about 40 percent of patients who are subsequently operated on, the proximal and distal ends of tube are visibly separated, with the

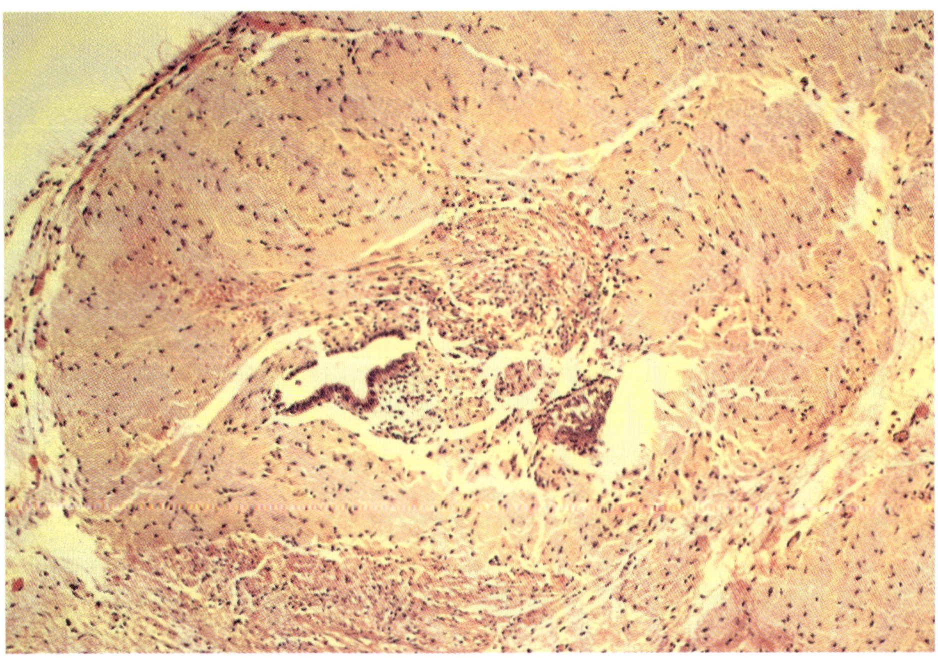

FIGURE 7-18
This is a cross section through the patent isthmic tubal remnant in a patient who previously underwent unipolar electrocoagulative sterilization with a subsequent intrauterine pregnancy. The lumen with a partial epithelial lining is visible within an area of hyalinized tissue. There is marked diminution of the cross-sectional size and little recognizable muscularis.

band or ring found in a variety of locations within the pelvis. The ring is usually attached to a fragment of tissue that on examination has the characteristics of the remaining segment of tube distal to the ligation site after a Pomeroy procedure. Failures associated with the silastic band sterilization are mostly secondary to misapplication of the band.[41, 43] Once the band is placed around the base of an intact loop of tube, it is not spontaneously ejected by muscular contractions. However, if the ring is placed over a portion of the tube without completely encircling the base of the loop, then subsequent muscular contractions of the tube may displace or eject it.[45] Pregnancy very rarely occurs following an adequately placed Falope ring. If pregnancy does ensue, it is a consequence of tubal separation and formation of a tuboperitoneal fistula.

The third technique for laparoscopic tubal obstruction is the use of clips. Although several clips have been marketed in the past, currently the Hulka and Filshie are the principal ones used. The Hulka clip is the only one approved for use in the United States. The Hulka spring clip consists of hinged straight plastic jaws with teeth. The clip is placed at a right angle across the isthmic portion of the fallopian tube. The teeth secure the tube so that it does not roll out during closure of the jaws. A continuous compression is achieved by a gold-coated stainless steel spring that slides over the clip, locks in place into preformed grooves, and compresses the tube. This maintains functional obstruction until the compressed segment is collapsed and fibrosed. Tubal separation at the point of application is rarely encountered following Hulka clip applications. The usual gross finding is a thin tissue envelope covering the clip and seemingly binding the tube in its original position. Pregnancies that occur subsequent to Hulka clip applications are almost always related to misapplication of the clip.[41, 43] The design of the clip is such that it will fit appropriately across the isthmic segment of most fallopian tubes when placed perpendicular to the tube. If the clip is placed at an angle to the tube, a portion may roll out upon closure of the clip, and interruption of the lumen is not achieved (Fig. 7–19).

The Filshie clip is widely used throughout the world. It is made of titanium and silicone rubber. In its application, a curved upper jaw latches under a hooked end, thus securing the tube in place. The silicone rubber bed provides a continuous compressive force that is almost 15 times that achieved by the Hulka clip. Like the Hulka clip, it is designed to be placed across the isthmus at a right angle. The compressive force results in focal necrosis, and tubal separation is encountered with a frequency similar to that seen with the Falope ring. Failures are usually related to misapplication. The few instances of other failures are a result of tuboperitoneal fistula formation at the site of tubal separation.

Other than the changes encountered at the site of the sterilization procedure, there are histopathologic changes identified in the tubes both medial and lateral to the site of obstruction. The most frequent finding in the segment of tube medial to the site of obstruction is luminal dilatation. Lu-

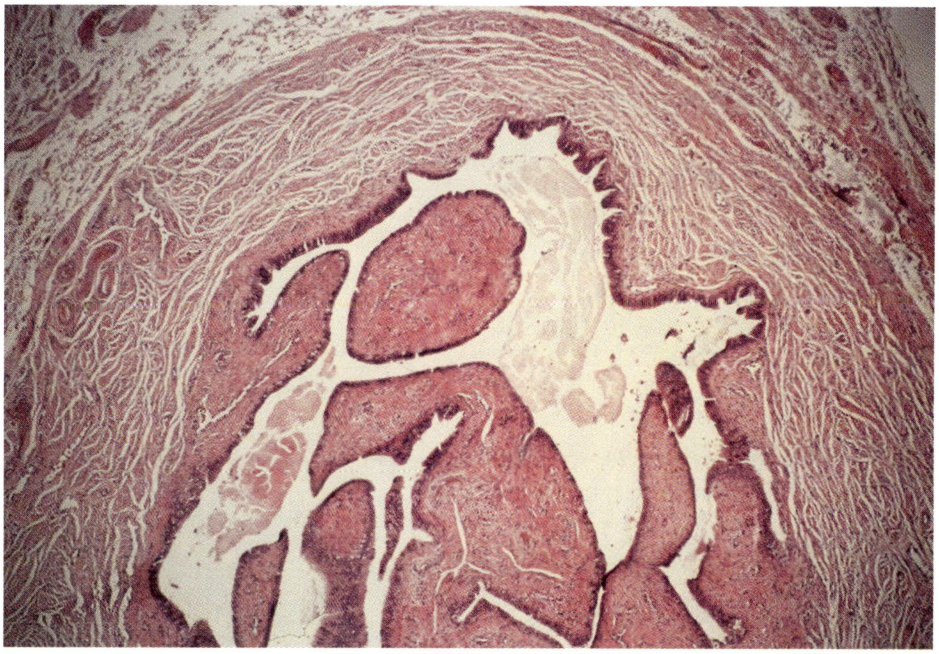

FIGURE 7–19
This is a cross section of the lateral aspect of a remaining tubal segment following a Pomeroy tubal sterilization. Hyalinized debris is contained within the lumen and plicae stromal fibrosis is evident.

minal dilatation is dependent upon the site of obstruction and the interval from the obstructive procedure to the time of examination. The Kroner procedure, which involves the more distensible ampulla, results more often in a grossly apparent hydrosalpinx. With the more proximal obstructive procedures, luminal dilatation is seen on microscopic examination but is seldom clinically obvious. This is explained by the thicker muscularis of the isthmic portion of the tube. The frequency and degree of dilatation increase with time regardless of its location. These changes are not identified in the presence of a tuboperitoneal fistula.[41] In addition to the dilatation, which is identified on low-power examination, there is separation of plicae and at times a polypoid appearance to them. The luminal contents frequently consist of menstrual blood and occasional menstrual debris. The stroma of the plicae contains chronic inflammatory cells and, in the presence of blood or shortly after the menstrual period, may contain multiple hemosiderin-laden macrophages. As mentioned previously, foci of endometriosis are usually encountered in the area immediately adjacent to the surgical site but only in the medial remnant of the tube (see Figs. 7–9 and 7–10).

In the lateral or distal remaining tubal segment, chronic inflammatory cell infiltrates are not identified, but they are seen in the medial remaining segment. Nor is endometriosis or pseudopolyp formation seen. Frequently encountered, however, are foci of intraluminal debris that represent products of plical degeneration in the immediate area of the surgical site. Hyalinization, calcification, and occasional psammoma bodies are present in varying degrees. Plical fibrosis, similar to that seen in a tube from a postmenopausal woman is encountered in the lateral segment following the more destructive midsegment sterilization procedures (see Fig. 7–19). Loss of cilia has also been identified by scanning electron microscopic studies.[46]

The success of sterilization reversal procedures has been found to be dependent upon the length of the reconstructed tube and the time lapse between sterilization and the anastomotic procedure. The importance of this interval is probably related to the increase in plical fibrosis, loss of ciliae, inflammatory changes, and hydrosalpinx formation as time passes.[46]

When the fallopian tubes are submitted for examination after a case of pregnancy that followed a sterilization procedure, it is important for the pathologist to determine the cause of the failure. In a patient with an ectopic pregnancy who has had removal of the involved tube, it is important to confirm whether the cause for the failure was on the side where the ectopic pregnancy occurred. There are many cases of ectopic pregnancy that have occurred contralateral to the side of tubal patency (Fig. 7–20). If that is the case, the patient remains at risk for a subsequent pregnancy. Gross examination at the time of surgery is important, since if the possibility of contralateral tubal patency exists, a repeat sterilization procedure should be performed. Pregnancy occurring subsequent to a sterilization procedure may well result in a medicolegal claim. The pathologist has a responsibil-

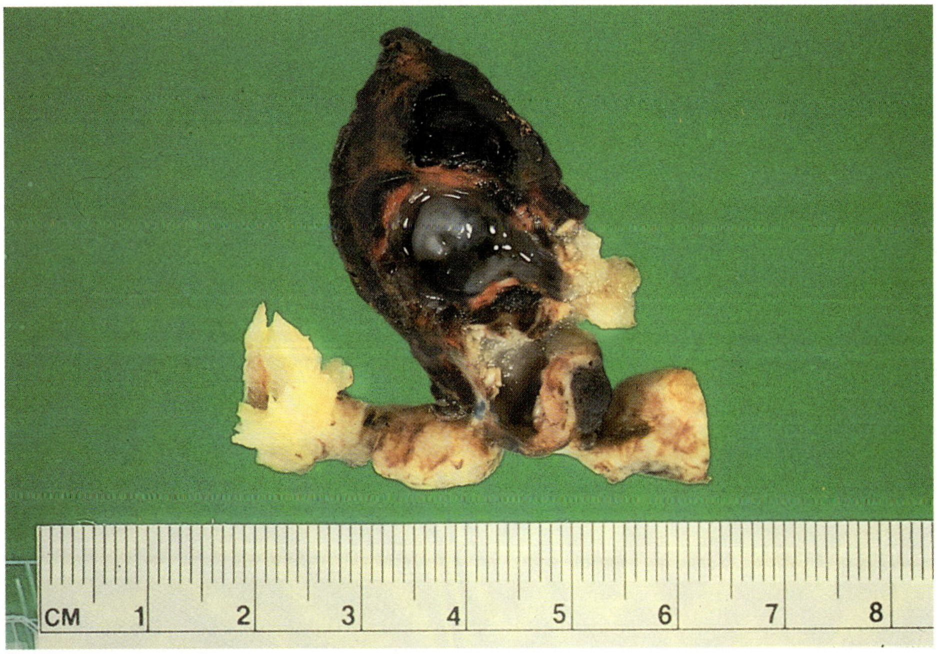

FIGURE 7–20
This shows a tubal pregnancy in the lateral segment of the tube following a Pomeroy sterilization procedure. The fimbriated end is seen on the left; the isthmus is on the right. The proximal tubal segment lumen was closed. The implantation is in the residual tube above the suture (blue suture remnants are seen). A tuboperitoneal fistula was present in the contralateral fallopian tube. A fetus surrounded by blood clots is evident.

ity to try to identify the etiology of the failure, since this may settle the legal issues. It is not only important to identify those cases in which an appropriate sterilization procedure had been carried out, but it is also critical to identify those cases in which a surgical error may have occurred. Working with a fresh, unfixed specimen facilitates the examination. The first step is to identify the prior surgical site, which is usually grossly apparent. The easiest way to determine whether there is a communication or fistula is to use a mixture of aqueous radiopaque dye with India ink and inject it with a flexible small-bore venous catheter that has been threaded into the isthmic lumen of the tubal specimen. A radiograph will delineate the status of the sterilization site. The India ink remains intraluminally and is seen on histologic sections.

INFLAMMATION

Pelvic inflammatory disease (PID) is a consequence of sexually transmitted infections and was noted to have dramatically increased in the 1960s and 1970s. Currently, PID is estimated to account for approximately 1 million physician visits per year and an annual cost of 4 billion dollars. The enormity of the problem is complicated by the long-term sequelae of chronic pelvic pain, infertility, and ectopic pregnancy.[47, 48] The term PID is used synonymously with acute salpingitis. The roles of laparoscopy, pelvic fluid analysis, and endometrial biopsy have become more important in the primary assessment of PID.[49]

In the past, most PID or salpingitis cases were attributed to *Neisseria gonorrhoeae*. However, more recently it is recognized that PID is often polymicrobial, and *Chlamydia trachomatis* is one of the most prevalent primary infective organisms. Granulomatous disease of the tube has become less frequent in the United States but still exists as a problem in third world countries.

Salpingitis can be divided into three groups: physiologic, granulomatous, and nongranulomatous.

Physiologic Salpingitis

It was noted by Black-Schaffer in 1944 that 38 percent of fallopian tube segments removed at the time of postpartum sterilization showed evidence of acute salpingitis.[50] The inflammatory infiltrate consisted principally of polymorphonuclear leukocytes and mononuclear cells that occupied the lumen and the mucosal surfaces. This was often accompanied by edema. Hellman subsequently reported the same observation but found only a 20 percent incidence of salpingitis. This declined as the time interval between delivery and sterilization increased.[51] These were asymptomatic patients. Subsequently, Nassberg et al. observed a similar pattern of acute inflammatory infiltrates in the tubes of women undergoing hysterectomy near the time of menstruation.[52] Menstrual debris is frequently identified with the inflammatory infiltrate, and no bacteria were isolated. It was noted that a similar reaction had been found by Smith when human menstrual blood was injected into a rabbit uterine horn, utilizing the opposite horn as a control.[51] It was believed that the menstrual blood or blood-associated products flowed back through the fallopian tubes and thus elicited a sterile inflammatory response. This was most likely to occur immediately post partum or during menstruation.

A more aggressive inflammatory response, which is likewise not accompanied by evidence of infection, is seen in the immediate postoperative period in patients who have undergone a sterilization procedure, salpingostomy, or repair of an aborted ectopic implantation site.

Granulomatous Salpingitis

Granulomatous reactions in the fallopian tube can be due to a host of etiologic agents, including *Mycobacterium tuberculosis*, *M. leprae*, actinomycosis, *Enterobius vermicularis*, schistosomiasis, and *Echinococcus granulosus*. They are also seen in patients who have Crohn disease, foreign body reaction, or sarcoidosis.

Tuberculous Salpingitis

Tuberculous salpingitis used to be a major cause of infertility in the United States but now is seen in less than 1 percent of cases. Tubal involvement occurs mostly by hematogenous spread from the pulmonary lesion. Autopsy studies of women who died of pulmonary tuberculosis reveal the presence of active tubal infection in approximately 8 percent of the cases.[36]

The presenting complaint of women with pelvic tuberculosis is infertility in 45 to 55 percent of instances, and pelvic pain and irregular bleeding in fewer cases.[54] The past medical history reveals a childhood contact in 20 percent of cases, and frequently a history of tuberculosis contracted around the time of menarche is elicited. Many of the cases that are diagnosed during infertility evaluations are discovered or suggested by the

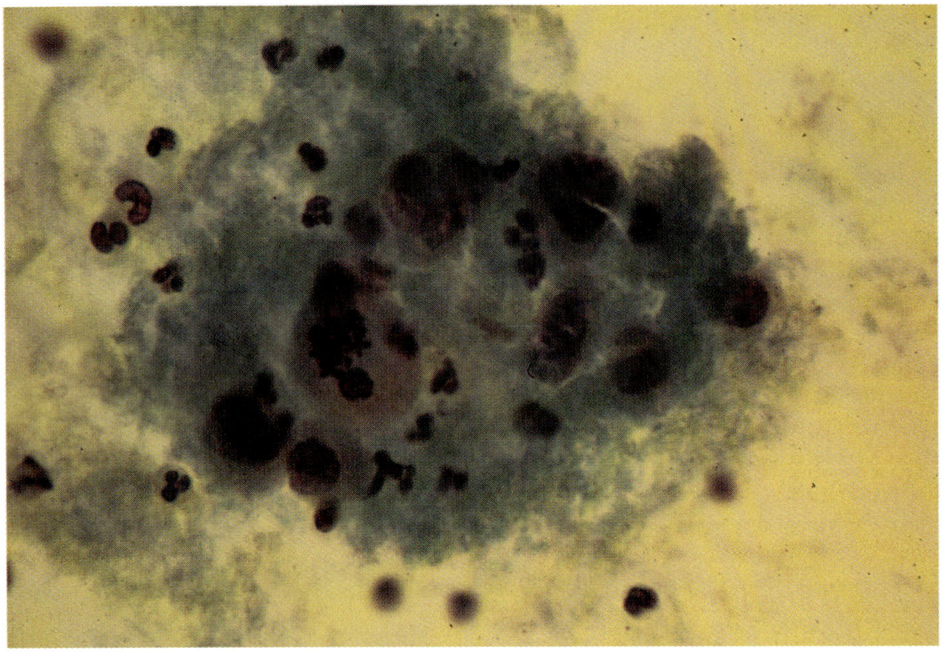

FIGURE 7-21
This cytologic preparation of a peritoneal lavage specimen shows markedly atypical epithelioid cells, a mitosis, and necrotic material in the shape of a granuloma. These cytologic findings and the multiple peritoneal nodules found at the time of laparoscopy were suggestive of carcinoma. A diagnosis of tuberculosis was made when caseating granulomas with acid-fast organisms were seen on histopathology. A definitive diagnosis of malignancy in a peritoneal lavage specimen should not be made in a patient without a known malignancy.

hysterosalpingographic finding of a pipe stem or drumstick appearance of the tubes.[55] The diagnosis is confirmed by histology or by culture of mycobacteria from endometrial biopsies. The gross appearance of tuberculous salpingitis is not very different from that of acute bacterial salpingitis, and the diagnosis is seldom made at the time of surgery. The granulomatous involvement of the omentum and peritoneum may be mistakenly interpreted as a metastatic process, especially when it is accompanied by ascites. A cytologic preparation of the ascitic fluid or peritoneal lavage can be mistaken for carcinoma owing to the atypia of the epithelioid cells (Fig. 7–21). On microscopy the tubal lesions involve mucosa and serosa. There is a typical granulomatous reaction composed of epithelioid cells and lymphocytes arranged in nodular aggregates. Caseation may be present, and giant cells, usually of the Langhans type, may be readily identified (Fig. 7–22). When there is an associated prominent epithelial cell proliferation, cellular pleomorphism, and mitotic activity, this could be mistaken for a primary fallopian tube carcinoma. A definitive diagnosis of tuberculosis is established

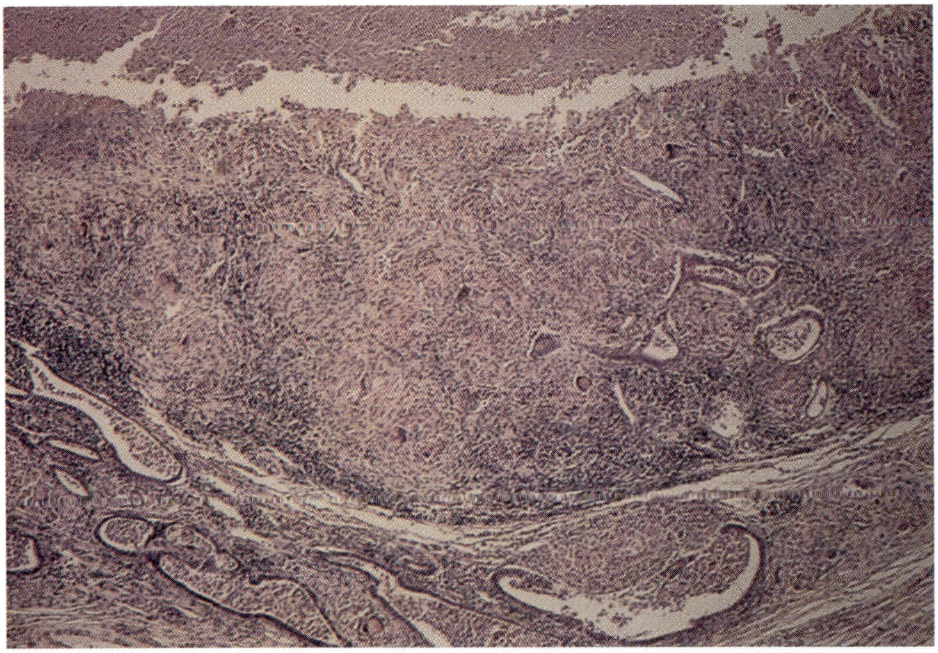

FIGURE 7-22
This fallopian tube is infected with *Mycobacterium* tuberculosis. The fallopian tube and residual epithelium are seen (*bottom*). Necrotic material fills the tubal lumen (*top*). The tuberculous granuloma (*center*) is characterized by multinucleated giant cells in a background of granulomatous inflammation. The granulomas are composed of epithelioid cells, giant cells, and connective tissue components. Small lymphocytes surround the granulomas, and these are seen as the more basophilic areas in this low power view.

by culture. Immunofluorescence and acid-fast stains can be utilized. However, those techniques cannot differentiate tuberculosis from the much rarer case of leprosy. They can identify neither atypical tuberculosis nor the sensitivity to antibiotics.

Foreign Body Reaction

Foreign material in the fallopian tube may elicit a foreign body giant cell reaction. The most common localized foreign body giant cell reactions are those seen secondary to prior surgical procedures that utilized high-frequency electrical current, laser, or suture. Focal scarring, a chronic inflammatory infiltrate, and foreign body giant cells with ingested material may be present.

A disseminated foreign body giant cell reaction was frequently seen in the fallopian tubes of women who underwent hysterosalpingography with an oil-based radiopaque dye. This oil-based material is no longer used owing to complications caused by intravasation and oil embolization.

Actinomycosis

Actinomyces as a cause of PID was unusual prior to the mid-1960s. After the introduction of the intrauterine contraceptive device (IUD) in the 1960s, reports of pelvic infections and abscesses caused by *Actinomyces* became more frequent.[56] Currently, it is believed that women who are at low risk for acquiring a sexually transmitted disease have little risk of PID while using an IUD.[57] It has also been suggested that the infections and abscesses in women wearing an IUD were not primary actinomycosis but rather of other bacterial origin, the *Actinomyces* being an opportunistic organism. The surgical findings in cases of actinomycosis are of acute salpingitis. In the gross specimen, "sulfur" bodies may be seen within the abscess. Microscopically there is an intense inflammatory infiltrate throughout the muscularis. In the mucosa there is a predominance of histiocytes, plasma cells, and lymphocytes. Giant cells and granulomatous lesions may be identified.

Actinomyces is a pleomorphic gram-positive rod with forms varying from bacilli to long, branching filaments. In an anaerobic environment, the organisms produce a polysaccharide protein that cements the filaments together, creating the "sulfur" granule (Fig. 7–23). These clumps consist of filamentous structures in which the filaments radiate outward from the center. *Actinomyces*-like organisms can be easily identified by cervical/vaginal Papanicolaou smear. Definitive diagnosis is established by culture. If *Actinomyces*-like organisms are seen on a Papanicolaou smear from a patient who is using an IUD and who has symptoms, the IUD should be removed and the patient treated with an appropriate antibiotic (e.g., ampicillin 250 mg four times a day for 14 days). If the patient has no symptoms and wishes to continue using the IUD, the Papanicolaou smear is repeated after a 14-day course of an appropriate antibiotic. The IUD is removed if the smear continues to show *Actinomyces*-like organisms or if the patient develops symptoms.

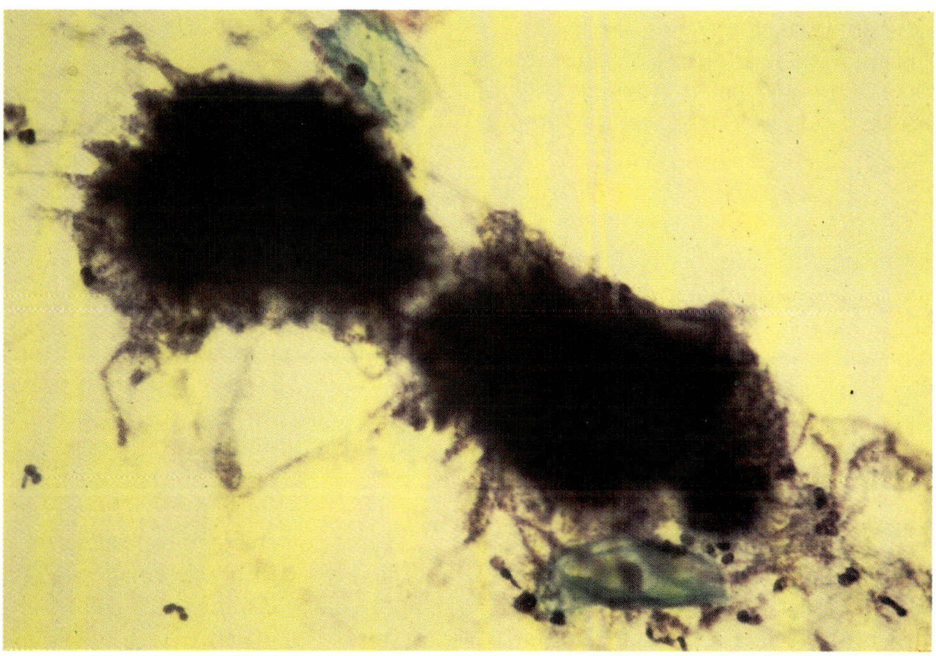

FIGURE 7–23
This cervical Papanicolaou smear shows two squamous cells and two "sulfur granules." The "sulfur granules" are colonies of *Actinomyces*. The bacteria form filaments that are seen radiating from the periphery. This Papanicolaou smear is from an asymptomatic woman with an intrauterine contraceptive device (IUD).

Parasitic Salpingitis

Parasites are a rare cause of salpingitis in the United States. The pinworm-related salpingitis *(Enterobius vermicularis)* results from the migration of the pinworm up through the genital tract to subsequently embed in the wall of the tube. There is an acute and chronic inflammatory response with eosinophils and Charcot-Leyden crystals (i.e., rhomboid eosinophilic crystals). The ova are identified by their size ($25\mu \times 50\mu$). However, they may be obscured by calcification in the granulomas.

Schistosomiasis is probably the most common form of granulomatous disease in the world, but it is rare in the United States. The diagnosis is made by identifying the ova of the schistosome. These are usually located in areas of fibrosis, which produces a nodular or fibrotic fallopian tube. On surgical exploration some patients are found to have extensive pelvic adhesions. The species that usually infects the tube is *Schistosoma haematobium*. This infection does not seem to affect fertility rates or to increase the incidence of ectopic pregnancy.[58]

Hydatid disease is the consequence of infection with *Echinococcus granulosus,* which may involve the female genital tract and, rarely, the fallopian tube.

Crohn Disease

Crohn disease originating in the ileum or colon can sometimes involve the tube and ovary, and then it produces a granulomatous salpingo-oophoritis. The lesions consist of a noncaseating granuloma that involve the entire thickness of the tubal muscularis. In cases of Crohn disease involving the fallopian tube, there may be epithelial proliferation and associated cellular atypia.[59]

Sarcoid

Sarcoidosis is commonly listed in the differential diagnosis of granulomatous disease of the fallopian tubes but has rarely been reported.[60] The histologic pattern is that of noncaseating granulomas. The diagnosis is one of exclusion.

Nongranulomatous Salpingitis

Acute Salpingitis

The patient with acute salpingitis typically presents with pelvic pain that starts approximately 1 week after menstruation. Sexual intercourse is painful. The pain progressively worsens and can involve the upper abdomen if pus escapes the fallopian tubes and moves up the right parasitic gutter to the upper abdomen. On physical examination the patient does not stand up straight. The body temperature is elevated. There is tenderness of the lower abdomen. Guarding and rebound tenderness are sometimes present. These findings may involve the entire abdomen if diffuse peritonitis has occurred. Pelvic examination may reveal a purulent discharge from the cervix. Gram stain preparation of this discharge may show gram-negative intracellular diplococci if the infection is caused by *N. gonorrhoeae*. Pelvic pain is elicited upon moving the cervix. Palpation of the adnexa reveals tenderness, and a mass may be felt if an abscess is present. However, palpation is compromised by the tenderness. The presence of an abscess may be confirmed by ultrasonography. Laboratory studies should include a hemogram, urinalysis, pregnancy test, and liver enzyme assay. The white blood cell count is elevated. The liver enzymes may be slightly elevated in the presence of perihepatitis. This occurs when pus accumulates between the liver and right hemidiaphragm. Filmy adhesions (i.e., violin string adhesions) between the liver and diaphragm may form in these cases. This complex is known as the Fitz-Hugh–Curtis syndrome.

Acute salpingitis is clinically diagnosed as PID when the foregoing constellation of signs and symptoms is present. The severity of the symptoms and findings is variable. Less severe symptoms are seen in patients infected with *C. trachomatis*.

After a presumptive clinical diagnosis of PID is made the patient is started on antibiotics. At present, ceftriaxone and doxycycline are recommended for uncomplicated cases. We prefer intravenous ampicillin, gentamicin, and clindamycin if a tuboovarian abscess is present. This combination of antibiotics recognizes the polymicrobial nature of the tuboovarian abscess with a significant anaerobic component. Although *N. gonorrhoeae* or *Chlamydia* may have been the initial offending organism, other pathogens soon proliferate in this fertile ground. If after 48 hours of antibiotics there is no clinical improvement, a laparoscopy is performed to confirm the diagnosis. The differential diagnosis includes appendicitis, ectopic pregnancy, adnexal torsion, diverticulitis, and infarcted uterine fibroid. Pelvic endometriosis and cancer are sometimes confused with acute PID, but a carefully obtained medical history should reveal the chronic nature of the symptoms in the former conditions.

The most common cause of acute salpingitis recognized in the past was infection with *N. gonorrhoeae* (gonococcus, GC). One of the largest studies conducted regarding the histologic findings correlated with bacteriologic confirmation was that of Curtis in 1921.[61] When there is a positive culture for GC, there is always grossly recognizable involvement of the tube. A history of recurrent episodes leads to thickening of the tubal wall and development of a pyosalpinx. Thickening and induration of the wall are seen. Glandlike nests of tubal epithelium that extend deep into the wall and lead to the development of diverticula may also be present. The inflammatory cellular infiltrate involves all layers of the tube but is most intense in the mucosa. The predominant inflammatory cell type is the polymorphonuclear leukocyte, but large numbers of lymphocytes and plasma cells are also present.[61]

Streptococcus-related infections have also been recognized. In these cases there is more of a perisalpingitis with less inflammation of the epithelium, and plasma cells are noted less often than in gonococcus-associated salpingitis.[61] The mechanism for tubal infection has been assumed to be passive transport from the endocervix through the endometrium into the tube itself for gonococci and lymphatic spread for streptococci. Falk examined cornual resection as therapy for patients with recurrent episodes of salpingitis. He found no recurrences in a group of 1000 women followed over a period of 8 years.[62] It was concluded that polymicrobial and gonococcal salpingitis were ascending infections. They occur either by passive transport or by the organisms attaching themselves to sperm or trichomonads. Falk's findings were reaffirmed by Hajj, who in 1978 reported on a series of 3500 laparoscopically performed sterilizations.[63] However, Vermesh et al. reported that 4 (8 percent) of 48 patients who had laparoscopically confirmed salpingitis had had a prior sterilization procedure.[64] In these cases, salpingitis of the lateral tubal segment was laparoscopically evident. *N. gonorrhoeae* was cultured from the cervix of one patient and *C. trachomatis* was cultured from the peritoneal fluid in another. The lateral segment involvement could be explained either by the presence of a tuboperitoneal communication or by lymphatic spread.

The pathophysiology of fallopian tube infection by *N. gonorrhoeae* is as follows. The gonococcus adheres to the nonciliated tubal epithelial cells with subsequent penetration, cell lysis, and sloughing. Adjacent ciliated cells are also destroyed in the process. The bacterium also penetrates the subepithelial connective tissue. This accounts for the edema, vascular engorgement, and infiltration by acute inflammatory cells throughout the layers of the tubal wall.

Although the inflammation is evident throughout the length of the tube, the degree of tissue response may be focally different (Fig. 7–24). In the face of untreated or resistant infection, microabscesses will form (Fig. 7–25). This eventually results in a tuboovarian complex or abscess.

In recent years *C. trachomatis* has attracted attention as a major etiologic agent in PID.[65] Both gonococcal and chlamydial tubal infections have been associated with the menstrual cycle. However, many questions remain regarding the association of cervical and tubal infection and the mechanisms for upper genital tract involvement.[66] Only about 8 percent of untreated cervical chlamydial infections progress to salpingitis.[67] The identification of *C. trachomatis* in culture is difficult. There have been a host of nonculture diagnostic tests made available for *Chlamydia* detection, but there are major problems with their specificity.[68] Chlamydial tubal infections are often subclinical, and lack of timely treatment could result in more tubal damage. The mechanism for tubal injury is not well known. It is speculated that it may be immune-mediated. The incubation period for *Chlamydia* is 1 to 3 weeks. The onset of symptoms for chlamydial and gonococcal tubal infections is similar. Approximately 80 percent of patients with either gonorrheal or chlamydial salpingitis have onset of symptoms within 7 days of menstruation.[66] In the case of gonorrhea this is believed to be related to the availability of iron in the menstrual blood, which facilitates the growth of the gonococcus. In the case of *Chlamydia*, it is believed that the increase in estrogen and progesterone late in the menstrual cycle may facilitate the growth of the organism. The histopathology of chlamydial infection is that of loss of cilia plus epithelial cell degeneration. Cytoplasmic inclusions may be found in the tubal epithelial cells, but this is not frequent or specific.

In the past, cells in cervical/vaginal Papanicolaou smears that had certain characteristics were considered to be "diagnostic" of chlamydial infection. These were metaplastic squamous or endocervical cells with cytoplasmic vacuoles containing basophilic or eosinophilic "dots" thought to represent coccoid bodies of *Chlamydia*. Comparison studies with culture and direct immunofluorescence using monoclonal antibodies to *Chlamydia* show that this cytologic finding is not specific or sensitive. Current cytopathologic classification (i.e., the Bethesda System) no longer supports basing this diagnosis on cervical/vaginal cy-

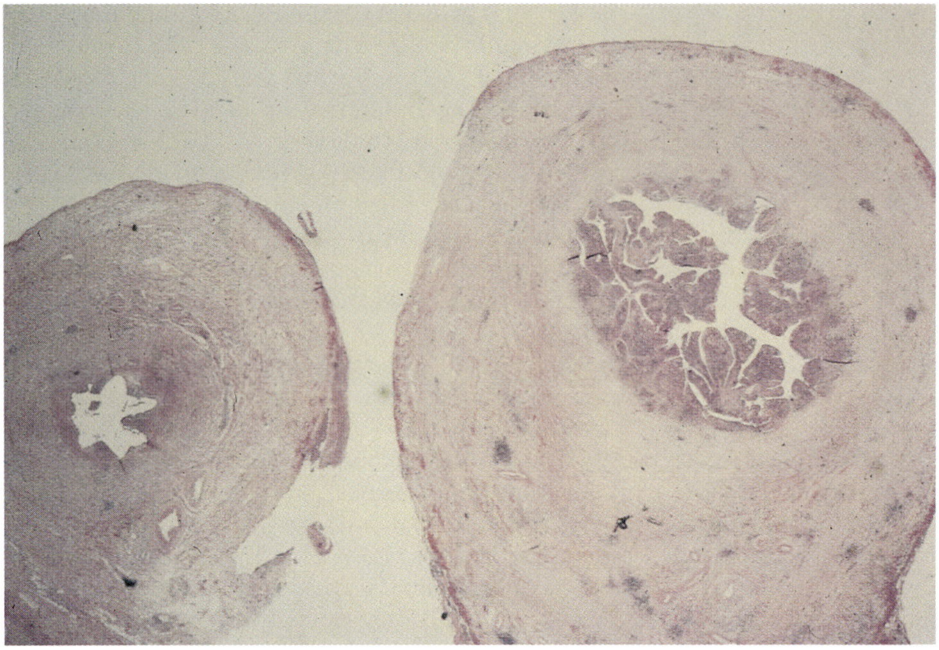

FIGURE 7-24
Cross sections of the isthmus (*left*) and ampulla of a tube that was removed from a woman with acute salpingitis. The mucosal inflammatory infiltrate (seen as blue cells) is more intense in the ampulla. Edema of the wall is very prominent. There is agglutination of the ampullary plicae. In the isthmus there is loss of epithelium and blunting of the plicae.

tology specimens. The long-term sequelae of chlamydial salpingitis are recurrent PID, chronic pelvic pain, infertility, and ectopic pregnancy.[48]

An associated infection of the surface of the ovary (perioophoritis) may occur in patients with salpingitis. Infections of the ovarian substance are extremely rare. When an ovarian abscess occurs, it is usually in association with a pyosalpinx. Ovarian abscess without pyosalpinx could occur after vaginal hysterectomy. This does not seem to be related to the phase of the menstrual cycle in which the hysterectomy was performed.

Chronic Salpingitis

The term chronic salpingitis does not mean a diagnosis of continuing infection or inflammation; rather, it indicates histopathologic alterations that have been interpreted as the consequences of prior infection. These include plical fibrosis and aggluti-

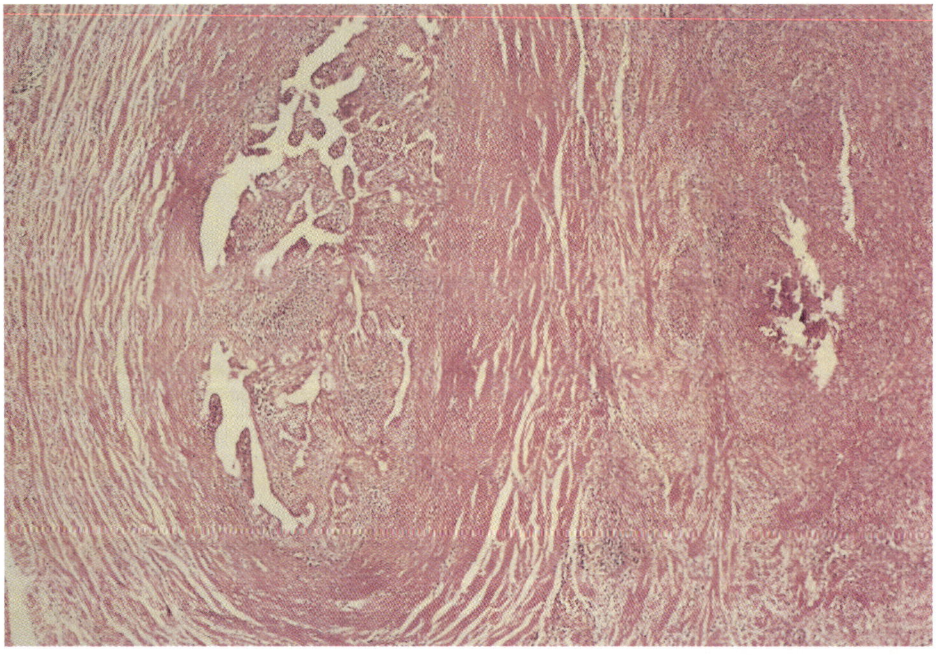

FIGURE 7-25
This cross section of a tube (*left*) and mesosalpinx was removed from a patient with PID unresponsive to antibiotics. Microabscess formation is evident in the mesosalpinx. The ampullary segment of tube shows fusion of its plicae. The stroma of the tubal plicae have an intense inflammatory infiltrate that focally extends to the muscularis.

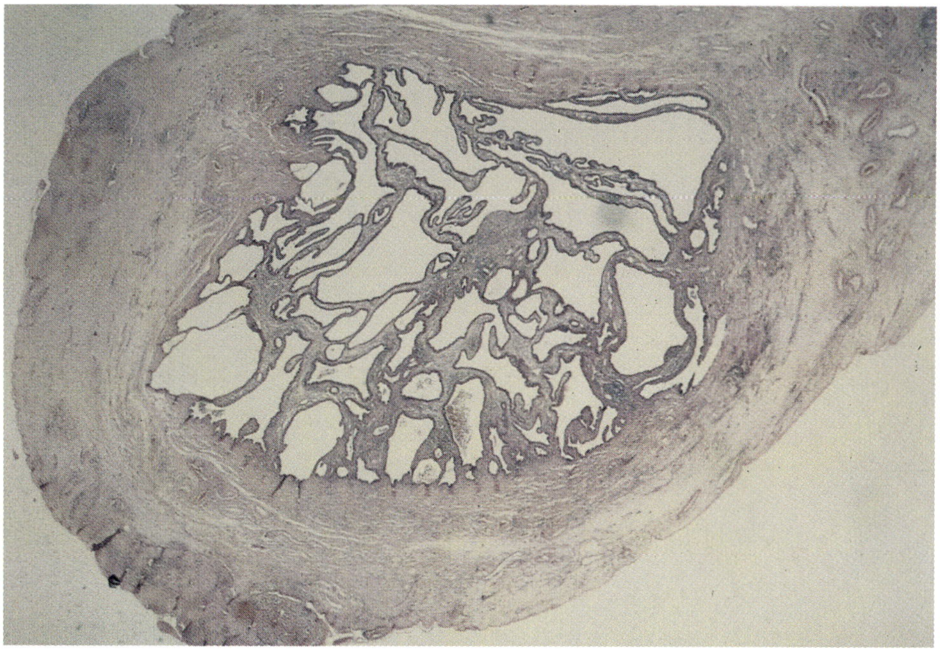

FIGURE 7-26
This cross section of the ampulla demonstrates plical agglutination with fluid accumulation, resulting in a pattern known as follicular salpingitis (named for its resemblance to ovarian follicles).

nation, fimbrial occlusion, and hydrosalpinx. Of less clear etiology is focal uterotubal obstruction with fibrosis and epithelial loss, and salpingitis isthmica nodosa (SIN).

The tube differs from the endometrium in that the presence of occasional plasma cells does not reflect a current or previous inflammatory process. Among the histopathologic alterations interpreted as chronic salpingitis, plical agglutination is the most common (see Fig. 7-7). This is seen more commonly in the ampulla (Fig. 7-26). In the mildest form only a few plicae may be involved. Extensive involvement of plicae leading to occlusion of the tube then results in an accumulation of fluid. This is referred to as follicular salpingitis (see Fig. 7-26). With continued fluid accumulation, the clinical appearance becomes that of an elongated, dilated sac, which constitutes a hydrosalpinx. Histologically there is separation of the plicae, and there may be varying degrees of luminal dilatation.

Another characteristic formerly attributed to prior inflammatory disease is plical fibrosis. This is a very subjective finding and one that may be present as a consequence of vascular interference, particularly after tubal occlusive procedures.

When obstruction of the uterotubal junction is found, one of several histopathologic diagnoses is present. The most common finding is obliterative luminal fibrosis (Fig. 7-27), followed by salpingitis isthmica nodosa (Fig. 7-28).[69] In addition, Sulak et al. have reported clinical obstruction secondary to "plugs" of amorphous hyalinized material.[70]

Salpingitis Isthmica Nodosa

Nodular lesions of the tube were described as early as 1818 by Meckel, but most people attribute the diagnosis of SIN to the description by Chiari in 1887, of tubal diverticula with focal muscular hypertrophy. It was Schauta in 1888 who coined the term "salpingitis isthmica nodosa." Although Chiari described this lesion in association with infection of the tube, von Recklinghausen in 1896 suggested that the etiology was congenital. Ries suggested that the lesion was akin to endometriosis and adenomyosis.[71, 72] Although this latter association has been postulated throughout the last 60 years, there have been no published studies relating the two entities.

The term salpingitis isthmica nodosa implies that the lesion is seen in the isthmic portion of the fallopian tube, whereas it is found scattered throughout the length of the tube. In detailed studies by Wrork and Broders the lesion was found to be unilateral in only 17 percent of the cases.[73] In recent years an association of SIN with ectopic pregnancy has been described. Majmudar et al., in a retrospective review of ectopic pregnancies identified 57 percent as being associated with SIN.[74] The SIN was confined to the isthmus in 63.2 percent, and in 26.8 percent it was located primarily within the ampulla. Dubuisson et al. noted that isthmic SIN was almost always associated with other histopathologic evidence of previous tubal infection.[75] As described above, SIN may cause tubal obstruction.

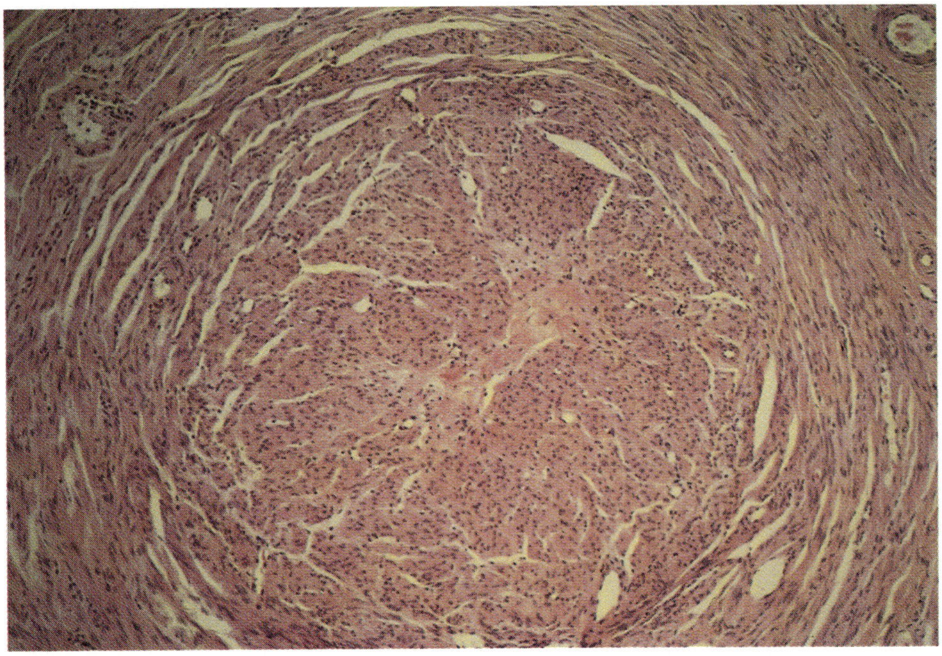

FIGURE 7-27
This is a cross section of the fallopian tube isthmus from an infertility patient who had uterotubal obstruction as demonstrated by hysterosalpingogram. There is no residual epithelium, and the lumen is replaced by fibrosis. Loose granulation tissue surrounds the dense collagen (*center*).

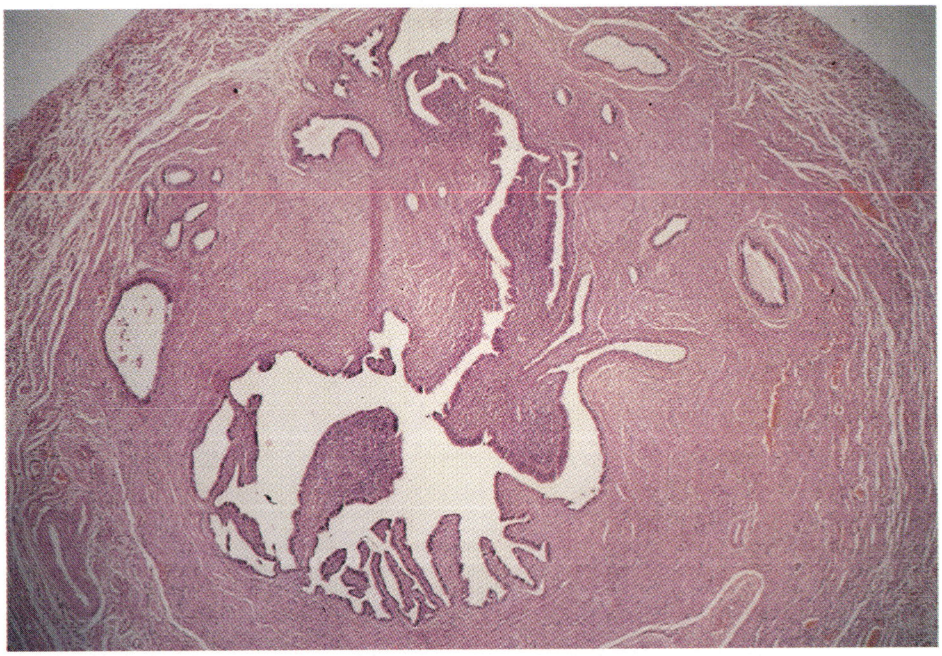

FIGURE 7-28
This is a cross section of the fallopian tube isthmus that demonstrates the diverticular nature of salpingitis isthmica nodosa (SIN). Invagination of tubal epithelium into the muscularis is seen (*top center*). Multiple glandlike structures lined by tubal epithelium and surrounded by muscle are seen in the muscularis. A dense inflammatory infiltrate is present in some of the tubal plicae and the diverticulum.

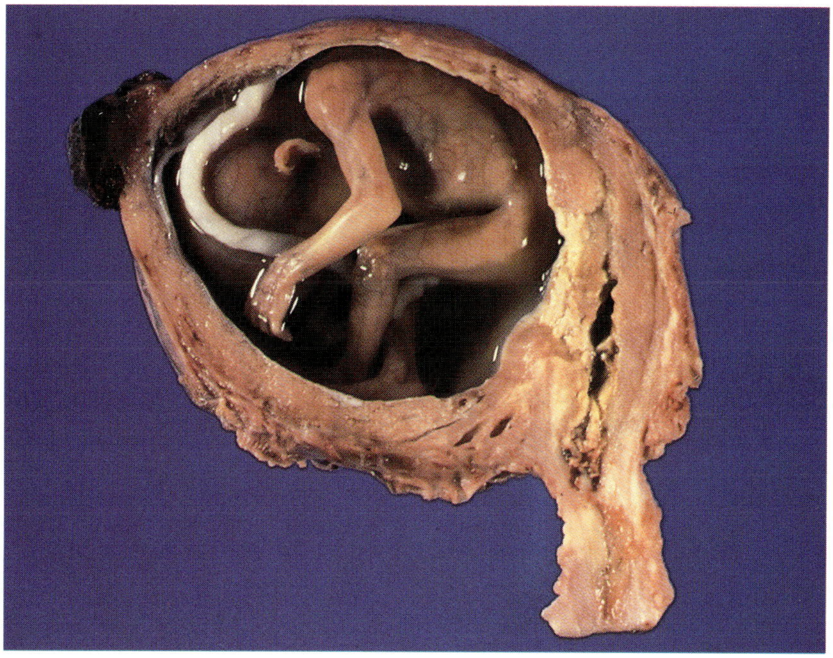

FIGURE 7–29
A twenty-week interstitial pregnancy with early myometrial disruption and well-defined placental disk formation is seen here. The endocervical and endometrial cavities are seen on the right. The decidualized endometrium appears yellow and shaggy. Most of the placenta is seen implanted on the upper portion of the tube. Interstitial pregnancies tend to be asymptomatic until the second trimester. Rupture can be catastrophic owing to sudden profuse hemorrhage. (From Stock RJ: Tubal pregnancy: associated histopathology. Obstet Gynecol Clin North Am 1991;18:73–93.)

The classic finding in SIN is diverticula that extend from the lumen of the fallopian tube into the muscularis with a surrounding muscular hypertrophy (see Fig. 7–28). Retrograde bleeding into the diverticula may result in an erroneous clinical diagnosis of ectopic pregnancy. In some instances the epithelium may have foci that recapitulate the endometrium. In rare instances there may be extensive muscular hypertrophy that may give the appearance of an adenomyoma. Accumulation of fluid within a diverticulum may result in a cystic mass that may become clinically palpable. Rarely, a pregnancy may implant in a diverticulum, creating a clinical picture similar to that of an interstitial pregnancy. However, rupture occurs much earlier than with a true interstitial pregnancy (Fig. 7–29).

TUBAL ECTOPIC PREGNANCY

Most ectopic pregnancies (95 to 97 percent) are located in the fallopian tube. Approximately 70 percent implant in the ampulla and 27 percent in the isthmus.[76] Less commonly, ectopic gestations can implant at the site of a tuboperitoneal fistula that has followed a sterilization procedure or, rarely, in a diverticulum of SIN as described above.

Ectopic pregnancy has been historically associated with primary and secondary infertility. Risk factors for tubal ectopic pregnancy include prior PID, IUD use, therapeutic abortions, prior tubal surgery, tubal sterilization, prior tubal pregnancy, and the use of modern reproductive technologies. However, only about 40 percent of patients with an ectopic pregnancy have any of these risk factors.[77] Histopathologic evidence of prior tubal infection has been reported to range from 19 to 95 percent. The issue of whether the fertilized oocyte may contribute to the ectopic implantation has been raised. Cytogenetic studies have not identified any karyotypic differences. However, a viable embryo with an appropriately developing gestation is seldom identified in a tubal pregnancy. Transvaginal ultrasound identifies an embryo in about 20 percent of tubal gestations. Prior to the use of ultrasound, embryos were identified histopathologically in about 5 percent of ectopic pregnancies.

The clinical diagnosis of a patient who presents with an acutely ruptured tubal ectopic pregnancy is simple. The patient complains of acute-onset abdominal pain, sometimes after coitus. The pain starts in the lower abdomen and later becomes generalized. Irritation of the diaphragm by the hemoperitoneum causes right shoulder pain. A history of amenorrhea and/or irregular vaginal bleeding is elicited. The physical examination is remarkable for tachycardia. Decreased pulse pressure or hypotension may be present. There are direct and rebound abdominal tenderness and guarding. Pelvic examination is difficult owing to exquisite tenderness to displacement of the cervix and uterus. The urine pregnancy test is positive, and the hemoglobin level may be low. If the blood loss is significant, the individual may lose consciousness. This patient needs to be resuscitated with crystalloids and possibly packed red blood cells and taken to the operating room for an exploratory laparotomy. Upon entering the abdomen, the uterus is elevated, the site of the ectopic gestation identified, and immediate hemostasis achieved by clamping the mesosalpinx. A salpingostomy or partial salpingectomy is performed.

Currently the clinical goal is to diagnose an ectopic pregnancy before it ruptures. The patient with amenorrhea, a positive urine pregnancy test, mild unilateral lower abdominal pain, and unilateral adnexal tenderness is evaluated with serial serum β-hCG determinations and transvaginal ultrasound. If the serum β-hCG titer fails to increase by 66 percent within 48 hours, an abnormal gestation is usually present (i.e., ectopic pregnancy or missed abortion).[77a] If the transvaginal ultrasound fails to demonstrate an intrauterine pregnancy when the serum β-hCG titer is ≥2000 mIu/ml (First International Reference Preparation), an ectopic pregnancy must be excluded.

In the presence of laparoscopic confirmation of an ectopic tubal pregnancy, either a conservative surgical procedure (e.g., salpingostomy) or tubal excision (partial or complete) may be performed. Alternatively, when a clinical diagnosis of early unruptured tubal ectopic pregnancy is made, the patient could be treated with intramuscularly administered methotrexate.[77b]

Whether a developing tubal gestation is interstitial, isthmic, or ampullary, the maternal-fetal interface presents a grossly expansive, rather than an infiltrative, process as described by some authors.[78] The implantation is superficial and replaces the tubal epithelium. Maternal tissue penetration by the intermediate trophoblast occurs just as it does in normal intrauterine pregnancy (see also Chapter 12). However, in the unruptured tubal pregnancy the villi and villus-associated trophoblast remain within the confines of the tubal muscularis.[76]

The clinical and histopathologic picture of an ectopic pregnancy varies depending upon its location in the tube and the extent of collapse of the implantation site. The distensibility of the ampullary portion of the tube usually allows for a partial retention of the plical pattern and luminal space. The placentation interrupts only the epithelial surface (Figs. 7–30 and 7–31). There is no identifiable epithelium with eccyeses located in the isthmic portion. The distended lumen impinges on the muscularis of the tube. The occurrence of rupture of the tube is not related to the point of implantation. The point of disruption usually is the result of vascular compromise secondary to a progressively distending lumen. Histopathologic specimens obtained at surgery in cases in which rupture is imminent show hemorrhagic necrosis and disruption of the muscularis without evidence of "invasive" trophoblastic material (see Fig. 7–31). When the tubal pregnancy is surgically removed or the tube spontaneously ruptures and the gestation is aborted, the tube collapses, leaving distorted architecture. The developing gestation distends the tube at the point of implantation and may override the tube medial and lateral to the site of implantation. With collapse and the production of an irregular contour, random cross sections of the tube may be misinterpreted as repre-

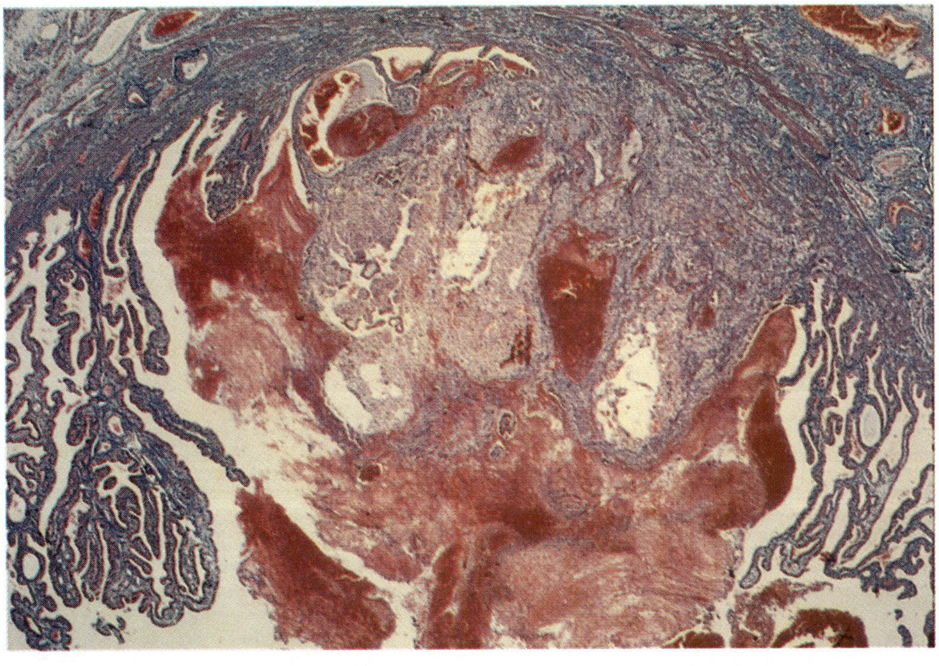

FIGURE 7–30
This is a cross section of the ampulla at the site of an aborting tubal pregnancy that demonstrates a mural implantation. The superficial nature of the implantation should be appreciated. This is a trichrome stain that shows the muscle and blood in red and the connective tissue in blue. Blood, trophoblasts, and a few villi are seen in the tubal lumen. The tubal plicae lateral to the implantation site are intact.

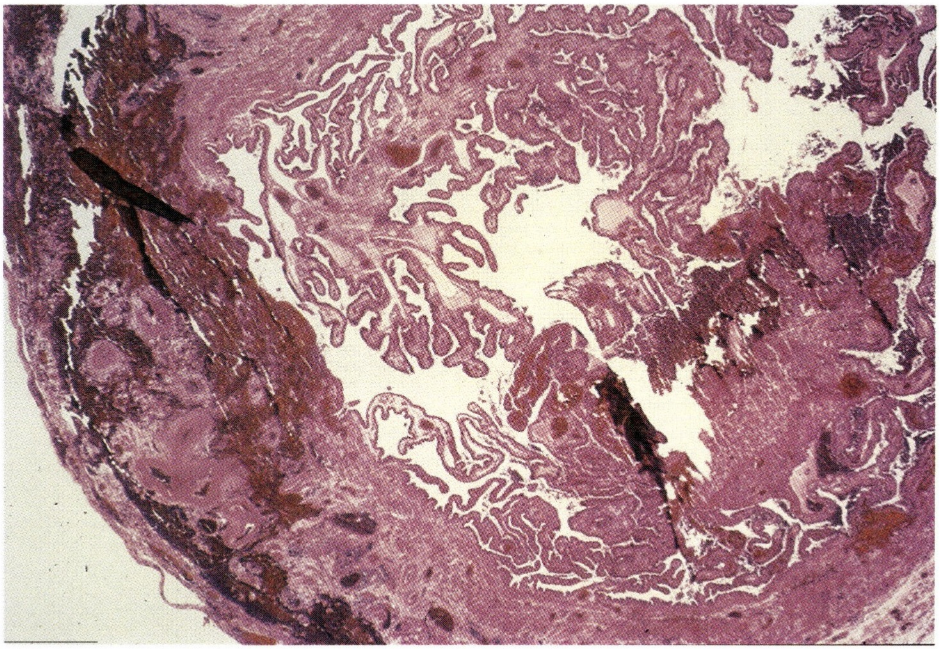

FIGURE 7-31
This is a cross section of the ampulla with an aborted plical implantation (*lower right*). Away from the implantation, the tubal wall demonstrates disruption of the muscularis with interstitial hemorrhage. Tubal rupture with an ectopic pregnancy is not necessarily related to the point of implantation but to vascular compromise secondary to a progressively distending lumen.

senting muscular invasion. Salpingographic studies of tubal segments removed with an intact gestation, as well as histopathologic studies of aborting tubal pregnancies, reflect the intraluminal location of the growing gestation.[76] Some authors argue that the early tubal gestations are intraluminal, while invasion of the muscularis is seen with more advanced gestations.[3]

When there is spontaneous disruption of the tube and partial extrusion of the products of conception, continuous bleeding occurs into the peritoneal cavity; this may result in the clinical picture of shock. The site of spontaneous disruption heals in the same way as a salpingostomy.[76]

It is important to realize that much of the distention of the tube associated with an ectopic pregnancy reflects the intermittent bleeding and the accumulation of blood clots within the more distensible lateral or distal portion. This tubal distention and the ooze of blood through the fimbria are responsible for the pain and adnexal tenderness experienced by the patient while the tube is intact. When the ectopic pregnancy is evacuated through a salpingostomy, too often the incision is made over the most distended portion of the tube, which represents the blood clot and not the implantation site. In such an instance the patient may return with acute symptoms secondary to continued bleeding or to the expansion of the implantation site that was not removed, i.e., persistent pregnancy.[76]

The question of recurrent ectopic pregnancy arises when conservative surgical procedures are performed. The incidence of recurrence is between 15 and 20 percent. Fifty percent of the recurrences are ipsilateral. In a study of tubes removed from 16 patients with recurrent ipsilateral ectopic pregnancies, the previous implantation site could be identified only in a third. However, the previous incision site could be identified in all.[2] Except for the occurrence of an ectopic pregnancy on the pseudofimbriae at the site of a tuboperitoneal fistula, recurrent eccyesis was not seen at the prior implantation site or at the previous surgical site. One of the cases revealed a pregnancy that implanted at a point of luminal obstruction created by a suture that had been placed to achieve hemostasis at the time of the original surgery. In this case the tubal incision had been made not over the implantation site but in proximity to it, damaging the medial normal segment of tube.

Conservative management of tubal eccyesis has gone beyond surgical procedures to that of chemical destruction of the gestation by either systemic or local injection techniques. The injected chemicals, methotrexate and hyperosmolar glucose solutions, have not resulted in microscopic damage in the few tubes that have been studied.[79, 80] It is possible that long-term absorption of the products of conception could result in focal obstruction or segmental tubal loss.[81]

Chronic Ectopic Pregnancy

The term chronic ectopic pregnancy is used to identify an unsuspected ectopic pregnancy of long standing that is already undergoing resorption. The term was used in the past to characterize an

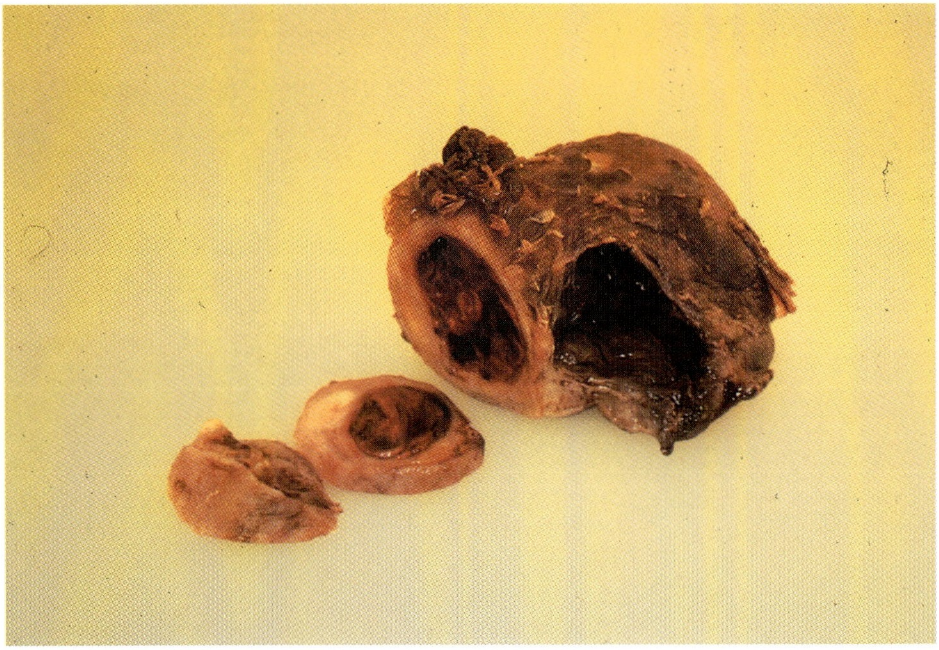

FIGURE 7-32
This fallopian tube was removed because of an asymptomatic pelvic mass identified on routine examination. The tube wall is thickened. The lumen is filled with blood clot. The tube has been sliced in cross section. Tubal fimbriae are seen on the top left. Rare "ghost" villi were identified on microscopic examination.

ectopic pregnancy associated with symptoms of pelvic pain but without acute abdominal symptoms or vascular instability. More recently the term has been applied to patients who have long-standing chronic pelvic pain and/or a pelvic mass but have a negative pregnancy test. A mass is identified in approximately 80 percent of cases. It consists of a resolving tubal pregnancy associated with a slow but continuous ooze of blood that has resulted in marked expansion of the tube, marked stromal edema, and muscular hypertrophy (Fig. 7–32).[82] Routine pregnancy tests in the past were invariably negative, whereas the more sensitive pregnancy tests in use today may be positive. A low titer β-hCG level is seen on quantitative measurement. By ultrasound the mass may be interpreted as solid and cystic. These ultrasound findings along with low hCG titers may be misinterpreted as a possible ovarian germ cell tumor; however, the diagnosis is quite evident at surgery.

Persistent Tubal Pregnancy

The term persistent tubal pregnancy is used to identify the patient with persistence of signs or symptoms of pregnancy after conservative management. The term originated in 1979, when Kelly et al. reported a patient who had to undergo a second operative procedure because of pain following the conservative removal of an ectopic pregnancy.[83] This is usually the result of failure to fully remove the implantation site. A second definition of persistent tubal pregnancy is persistence of an elevated hCG titer following a conservative procedure. These patients are asymptomatic, and the titers may reflect the presence of either viable trophoblastic tissue at the implantation site that was not completely removed or chorionic villi transplanted onto a peritoneal surface.[84] In either case, the titers usually disappear spontaneously in about 45 to 60 days. The hCG persistence can be seen after laparoscopic salpingostomy or salpingectomy if chorionic villi are spilled as the specimen is squeezed through the laparoscope trocar or laparoscopy incision.[84] This may be avoided by placing the specimen in a laparoscopic specimen bag prior to its removal from the peritoneal cavity.

Pregnancy After Sterilization

McCausland called attention to the inordinately high percentage of tubal gestations following sterilization by unipolar electrofulguration of the tube.[27] The incidence of ectopic pregnancy associated with other methods of tubal sterilization is not as high. Most pregnancies following a sterilization procedure using Hulka clips or Falope rings are intrauterine and are the result of misapplication of the clips or rings with a fairly intact and minimally damaged tubal lumen. Among the sterilization procedures that involve excision of a tubal segment, those pregnancies following a Kroner procedure are almost always intrauterine, whereas those following a Pomeroy procedure are frequently extrauterine. In the evaluation of a fallopian tube removed for an ectopic pregnancy in a patient who has had a prior sterilization, as discussed earlier, it is imperative to try to identify the mechanism of failure.[85]

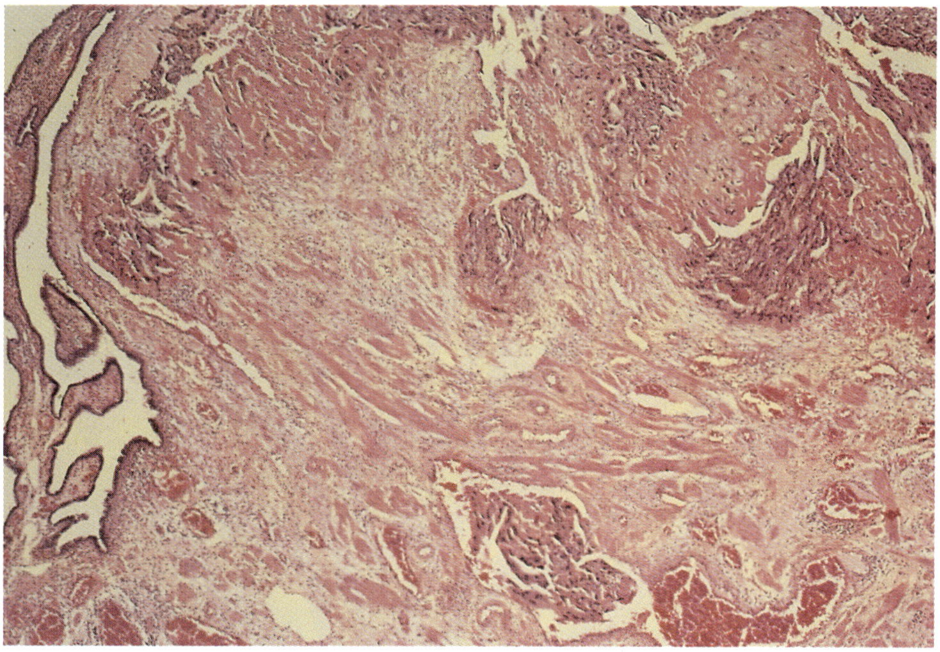

FIGURE 7-33
This cross section of a tube from a 19-year-old woman demonstrates the invasive and destructive pattern of growth seen with an early primary choriocarcinoma of the fallopian tube. Sheets of trophoblasts are seen at the top invading the muscularis of the tube. Trophoblasts are present in a vascular space *(bottom center)*. Intact tubal epithelium is seen on the left. (Courtesy of Dr. Henry J. Norris, Armed Forces Institute of Pathology, Washington, DC.)

GESTATIONAL TROPHOBLASTIC DISEASE

Gestational trophoblastic disease (GTD) is a term used to denote a spectrum of trophoblastic neoplasms that originate from a fertilized egg (see Chapter 12). The pathologic diagnoses include hydatidiform mole, invasive mole, placental site trophoblastic tumor, and choriocarcinoma. It has been estimated that gestational tubal choriocarcinoma has an incidence of 1 per 5333 tubal pregnancies or 1 per 1.6 million normal intrauterine pregnancies. In a review of the literature in 1981, 93 cases of primary choriocarcinoma of the fallopian tube were collected.[86] Ober and Maier considered only 58 as acceptable.[86] To these the authors added 18 cases from the files of the Armed Forces Institute of Pathology (AFIP). An estimate of the occurrence rate is obtained from the experience reported by regional trophoblastic treatment centers. In 1986 tubal choriocarcinoma accounted for 4 percent of 197 patients treated for choriocarcinoma and 1.7 percent of 459 patients treated for gestational trophoblastic disease at the John I. Brewer Trophoblastic Disease Center in Chicago, Illinois.[87] Of the 197 cases of known choriocarcinoma, 42.6 percent followed a hydatidiform mole, 28.9 percent followed a term pregnancy, 24.4 percent followed an abortion, and only 4.1 percent followed an ectopic pregnancy.

Most cases of GTD are persistent hydatidiform mole identified by plateauing or rising serum β-hCG titers. In the case of the fallopian tube, this is an extremely rare phenomenon. Ober and Maier identified only 22 cases of tubal hydatidiform mole in their review of the literature.[86]

The median age of patients with tubal choriocarcinoma is 33 years, and the majority present with symptoms consistent with an ectopic pregnancy, i.e., amenorrhea, abnormal vaginal bleeding, positive pregnancy test and vascular instability. Of the reported patients, few had hCG titers drawn preoperatively. The few who did had very high titers similar to these seen with intrauterine hydatidiform mole and choriocarcinoma. In the AFIP series of 18 cases, the size of the lesions varied from 2 mm to 18 cm (Fig. 7–33).[86] The incidence of metastases at the time of diagnosis is similar to that seen with uterine choriocarcinoma, and the therapeutic outcomes are equivalent. The histopathologic features are the same as those described in Chapter 12.

ATYPICAL EPITHELIAL PROLIFERATIONS

Atypical proliferations of the tubal epithelium have been described, in association with endometrial hyperplasia and carcinoma, as well as with benign and malignant ovarian neoplasms.[87a] These proliferations show epithelial stratification, intraepithelial glandlike spaces, and epithelial papillae. The presence of mitotic figures in these proliferations is thought to represent tubal carcinoma in situ (Fig. 7–34). However, this entity is not well defined. Progression of these atypical epithelial proliferations to cancer has not been documented.

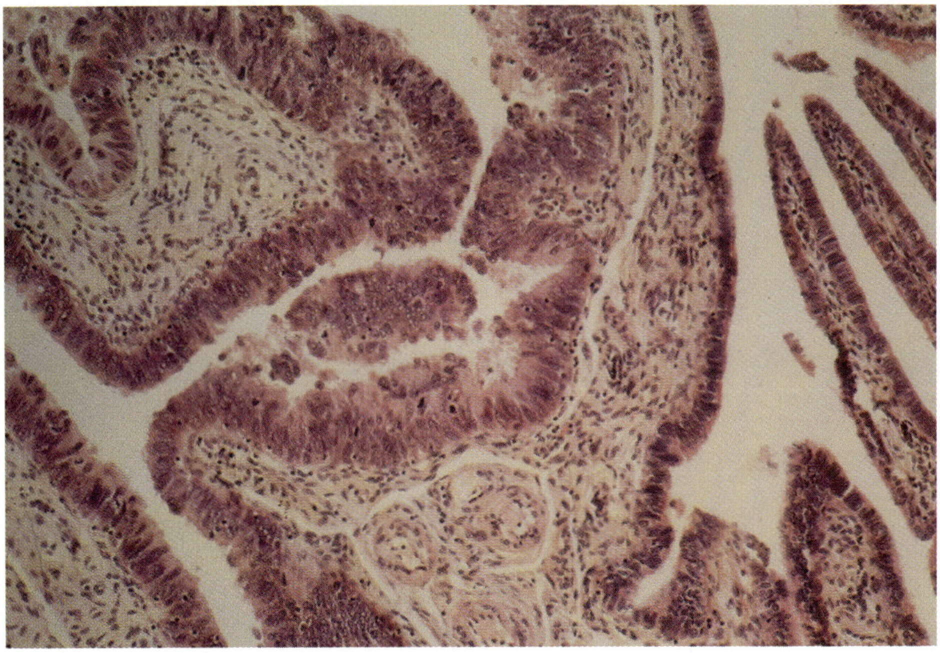

FIGURE 7–34
Normal fallopian tube epithelium is seen on the right. A single layer of columnar cells line the tubal folds. Adenocarcinoma in situ is seen on the left. This is characterized by cellular stratification, mitotic activity, and nuclear atypia.

NEOPLASMS

Neoplastic lesions of the fallopian tube can be divided into those originating within the tube itself, those originating within the mesosalpinx, and those that are metastatic.

Benign

Adenomatoid Tumor

Although rare, this is the most common of the benign neoplastic processes of the fallopian tube. The histogenesis of these lesions has been the cause of controversy. Adenomatoid tumors are found more frequently in men (epididymis) than in women. In women they occur with almost equal frequency in the tube and the uterine fundus.[88] In general, they are located adjacent to the mesothelial surface and are rather discrete, rarely exceeding 3 cm in diameter. In the fallopian tube, the lesions may occupy the space between the muscularis and the mesothelial surface or may involve the muscularis (Fig. 7–35). They are firm and have a white to yellowish appearance. By microscopic examination they consist of tightly packed tubular spaces lined by a flattened or cuboidal epithelium. This lesion has been referred to as adenoma, fibromyoma, lymphangioma, mesothelioma, and mesonephroma, which reflects the confusion regarding its histogenesis. Golden and Ash suggested the term adenomatoid because they believed that it was "morphologically correct and genetically neutral."[89] The tubular and cleftlike spaces contain no stainable material and no red blood cells. Masson et al. believed that the origin was mesothelial, and this has been confirmed by both ultrastructural and histochemical studies.[90]

On gross examination the lesion can occasionally be mistaken for an ectopic pregnancy. By frozen section it may be misinterpreted as an adenocarcinoma.[91]

Polyps

Interstitial luminal polyps can be identified by hysterosalpingography in infertility patients. However, most of the time these hysterosalpingographic findings represent foci of ectopic endometrium rather than true polyps. True polyps are rarely identified in other areas of the tube. These consist of papillomas, adenomatous polyps, and adenofibromas. The simplest form, the papilloma, is usually an incidental finding in a postpartum tubal segment removed for sterilization.[92] As mentioned previously, when the associated epithelium manifests eosinophilic metaplasia a mistaken diagnosis of adenocarcinoma might be made.

Adenofibroma is a rare tumor that may grow to a size that becomes clinically evident. The histology is the same as when this lesion is seen in other areas of the reproductive tract.[93]

Teratomas

The first case of a fallopian tube teratoma was reported in 1865. Mazzarella et al. reviewed a series of 44 cases reported up to 1972.[94] The ma-

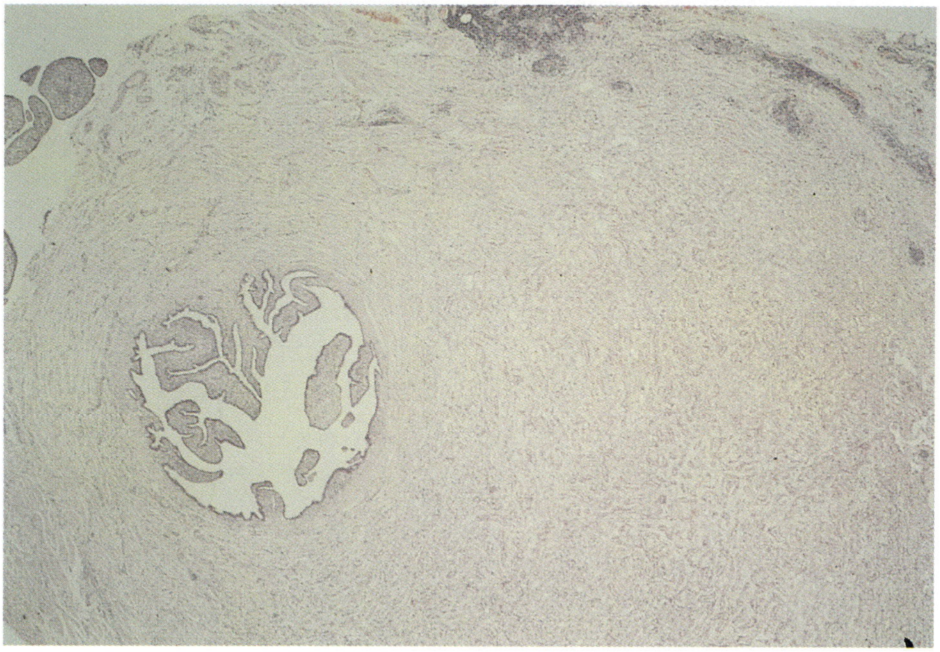

FIGURE 7-35
This is a cross section of a fallopian tube nodule that was identified incidentally at surgery. An adenomatoid tumor is seen (*right*) involving the muscularis and extending into the mesosalpinx. The tubular and cleftlike spaces are surrounded by a loose stroma. The adenomatoid tumors are benign and of mesothelial origin.

jority of lesions have been located intramurally and in the isthmic or ampullary portion of the fallopian tube. The age of the patients with these lesions varies from 21 to 60 years, with a mean of approximately 38 years. Forty percent of the women are nulliparous. There have been at least six cases reported in association with ectopic pregnancy.[95] In only two of the six cases was the teratoma on the ipsilateral side, and it therefore appears to be an incidental finding rather than a cause for ectopic pregnancy.

There have been rare cases of immature teratoma of the fallopian tube reported.[96] This lesion is considerably larger and presents as a pelvic mass. The histopathologic appearance of tubal teratomas is identical to that of teratomas of the ovary.

Leiomyomas

There are only about 60 cases of leiomyoma of the fallopian tube reported in the world literature. Most of these neoplasms are small and are associated with leiomyomas of the uterus. The finding of a leiomyoma of the fallopian tube is usually incidental, although rarely it may present as a pelvic mass. When a leiomyoma occurs in the interstitial portion of the fallopian tube it may cause infertility. When a leiomyoma is within the muscular portion of the fallopian tube it may be mistaken for an ectopic pregnancy.[97]

Other Mesodermal Tumors

Other tumors such as lipomas, hemangiomas, and neural tumors are rare in the fallopian tube.

Malignant

Primary Tubal Malignancies

Primary malignancies of the fallopian tube are almost always adenocarcinoma. It is the least frequent of the primary malignancies of the female genital tract. In multiple series, the incidence of fallopian tube adenocarcinoma varies from 0.1 to 0.5 percent of all gynecologic malignancies. The first case of fallopian tube malignancy was reported by Raynaud in 1847. The first pathologic description was made by Rokitansky in 1861, while Orthmann reviewed 13 cases by 1866. He described the pathology of primary fallopian tube malignancy and specifically excluded metastatic disease.[98] This was important, since nine out of ten malignancies found in the fallopian tube are metastatic.

Up to the present time there are about 1000 reported cases of primary tubal carcinoma. The age range of these patients at presentation varies from 18 to 94 years, with the median age in the late sixth decade of life. These neoplasms have been found in almost equal numbers in the right and left fallopian tubes. The rate of bilaterality is 17 to 33 percent.

The main presenting symptom of primary tubal carcinoma is vaginal discharge, which occurs approximately in 60 percent of patients. It may be watery, serosanguineous, bloody, or creamy. Lower abdominal cramping occurs in 28 percent of patients and a palpable pelvic mass in 85 percent. Martzloff in 1940 divided the patients with fallopian tube carcinoma into two categories according to the clinical presentation—those with an abnormal vaginal discharge and those without.[99] Pa-

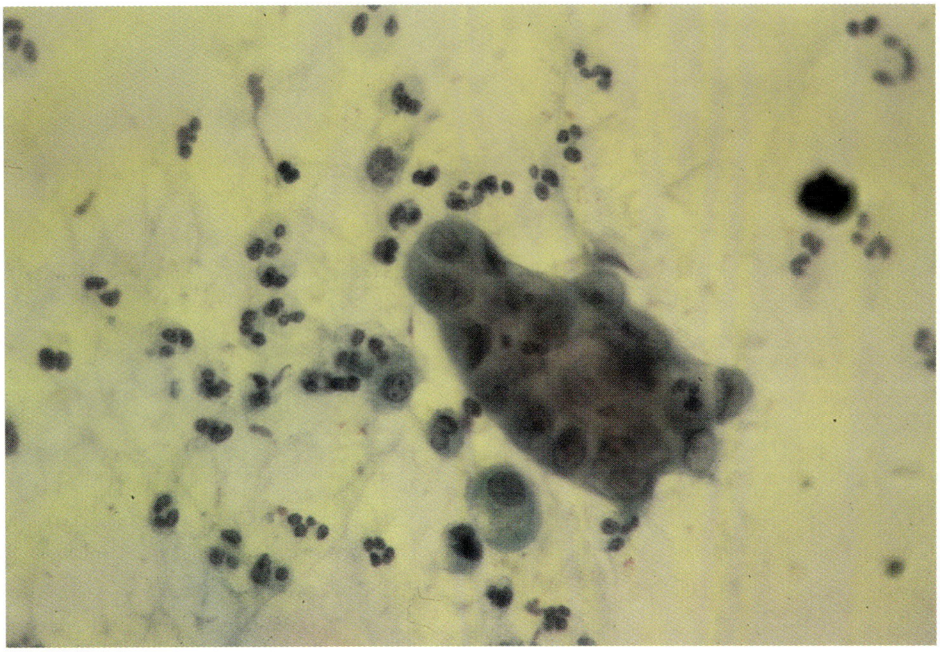

FIGURE 7-36
This cervical cytology specimen reveals a papillary cluster of malignant epithelial cells. The nucleoli are prominent. A cell with a vacuole containing a neutrophil is seen at the left of the cluster. These cytologic findings are consistent with a papillary adenocarcinoma of endometrial, fallopian tube, or ovarian origin. An endometrial curettage yielded two small detached fragments of adenocarcinoma in a patient without palpable adnexal masses who was subsequently found to have a small tubal adenocarcinoma (see Fig. 7-37).

tients without an abnormal vaginal discharge have signs and symptoms similar to those of patients with ovarian malignancies, i.e., abdominal distention and a pelvic mass. In patients with a vaginal discharge, Martzloff reported that 20 percent have the typical "hydrops tubae profluens" or "hydrorrhea tubae intermittens."[99] Latzko in 1915 was the first to call attention to this symptomatology, which consists of lower abdominal or pelvic colicky pain, with relief following a gush of fluid. Subsequent authors have rarely noted this particular symptom complex. The diagnosis of tubal carcinoma is seldom made preoperatively. Although extensively discussed in the past, the association of salpingitis and fallopian tube carcinoma has not been substantiated. The rate of involuntary infertility has been reported to be between 27 and 70 percent in patients with fallopian tube carcinoma.

Recently, attention has been directed to the presence of cervical cytology positive for an adenocarcinoma in the absence of a documented endometrial cancer or adnexal mass. The first case of fallopian tube carcinoma associated with a positive

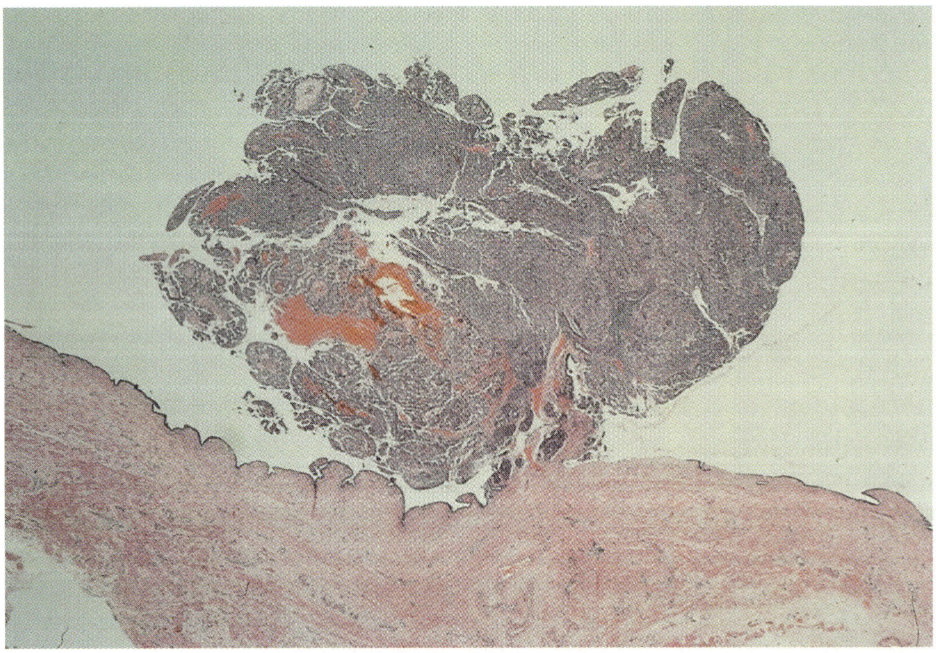

FIGURE 7-37
This is the small fallopian tube adenocarcinoma found in a patient with positive cervical cytology shown in Figure 7-36. Upon exploratory laparotomy and hysterectomy with bilateral salpingo-oophorectomy no gross lesions were identified within the uterine cavity or the ovaries. A 3 mm papillary adenosquamous carcinoma is identified arising from the fallopian tube epithelium.

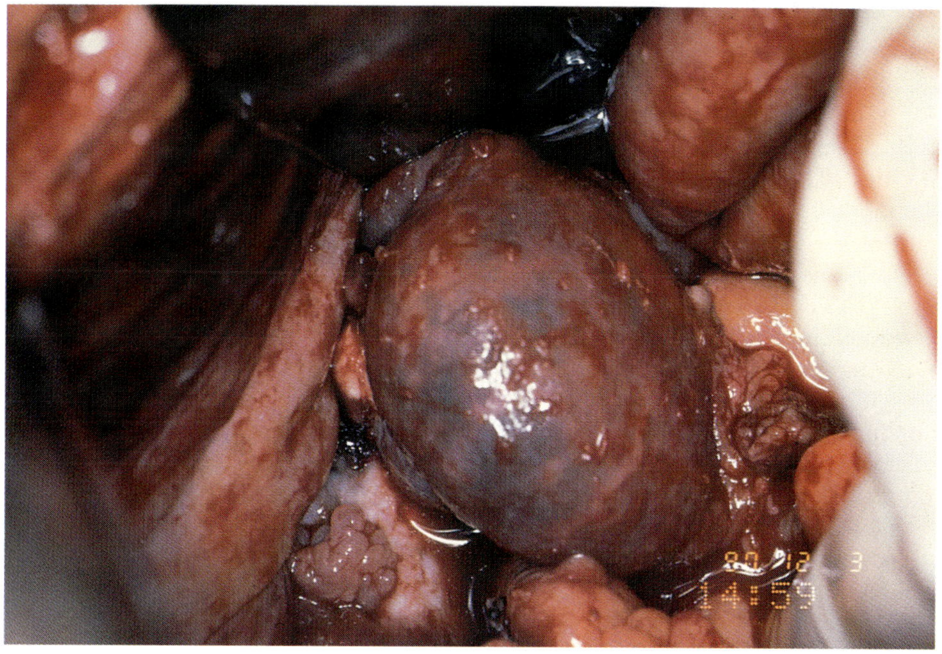

FIGURE 7-38
This is an intraoperative photograph of a right fallopian tube carcinoma. Portion of a normal left ovary and fallopian tube fimbria are seen (*bottom left*). The cancer distends the ampullary and infundibular portions of the tube and produces a bluish discoloration of the tubal serosa. The fimbria of the right fallopian tube is seen (*right center*). There are vascular adhesions on the serosa of the right fallopian tube.

cervical cytology was noted in 1950. The tubal location may be confirmed by hysterosalpingography. In a review of 128 cases of primary fallopian tube carcinoma collected between 1917 and 1982, 61 patients had preoperative cytology, with positive cytology in 45.9 percent of them.[101] The cytology preparations included cervical and endometrial aspiration samples. Positive cytology was present in 37.9 percent of the cervical smears, whereas the endometrial cytology was positive in 80 percent of the cases. The cytologic findings are not distinctive for tubal carcinoma. The findings are very similar to those of endometrial adenocarcinoma, but in cases of fallopian tube carcinoma there is a clean background on the cytology smear, only a few groupings of malignant cells are present, and the groupings are often papillary or globular (Figs. 7–36 and 7–37). The likelihood of obtaining a positive smear from either a cervical cytology or an endometrial aspiration increases if there is a bloody discharge or a discharge consistent with hydrops tubae profluens.[104] In the presence of a positive cytology, the diagnosis of tubal carcinoma should be suspected if no pelvic mass is

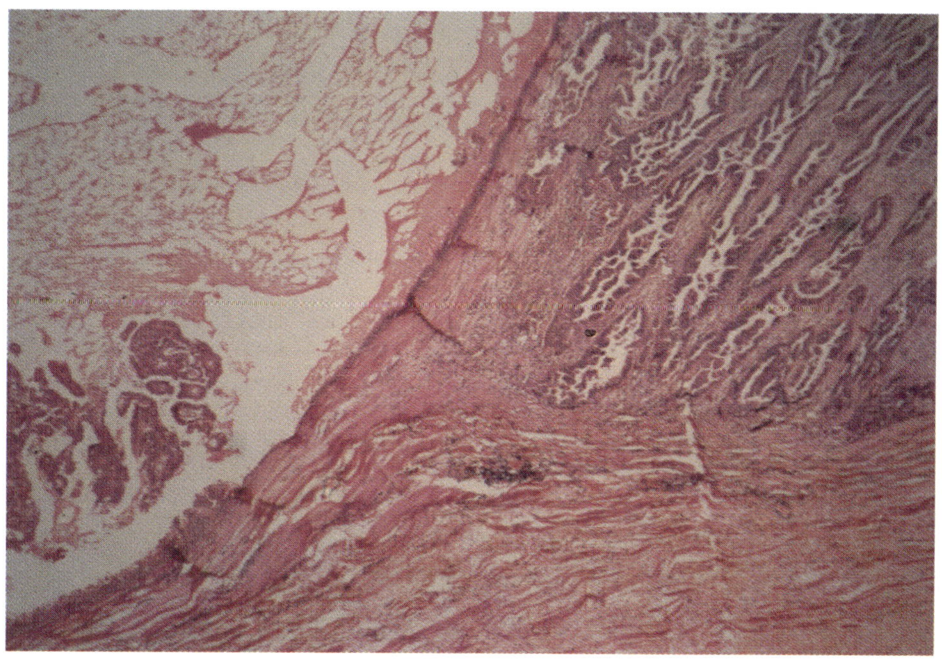

FIGURE 7-39
This fallopian tube adenocarcinoma has a papillary-alveolar pattern. The papillary component is seen on the left in the tubal lumen. The alveolar component is seen on the right invading the tubal muscularis, which is best seen at the bottom. The tumor has a pushing border. Transition from normal to malignant epithelium is seen on the luminal surface.

felt and an endometrial curettage yields either no malignancy or a few fragments of adenocarcinoma not referable to endometrial stroma. On exploration, the tumors are usually located in the ampulla. The lesions are grossly evident in approximately 70 percent of the cases, and are usually confined to the pelvis (Fig. 7–38).

In order to establish a diagnosis of primary fallopian tube carcinoma, three criteria need to be met: (1) The tumor is grossly within the tube; (2) there are no malignant lesions in the ovary, endometrium, or other pelvic structures, or, if tumor is present in adjacent structures, the bulk of the tumor is greatest in the tube; and (3) tubal mucosal involvement and epithelial transition from benign to malignant should be identified (see Fig. 7–37).[102]

The histopathologic description of tubal adenocarcinomas has varied over time. Three types have been described: papillary, alveolar, and medullary (or solid) (Fig. 7–39). In recent years, other types of tubal carcinomas have been reported, including 33 cases of mixed malignant müllerian tumors, 6 cases of endometrioid carcinomas, and a case of glassy cell carcinoma identified in a patient who was 10 weeks post partum.[102–105] Since the tube is of the same embryologic origin as the rest of the upper genital tract, neoplasms similar to those found in the ovaries and uterus (e.g., sarcoma) are also seen in the fallopian tube.

Like ovarian epithelial malignancies, fallopian tube adenocarcinomas are often associated with elevated serum CA 125.[106] The use of CA 125 with vaginal ultrasound as a screening tool has been reported to be useful in identifying at least two patients who had early fallopian tube carcinoma.[107] Although the pattern of metastatic spread of fallopian tube adenocarcinoma is similar to that of ovarian carcinoma, the reported 5-year survival rate after platinum-based chemotherapy (e.g., cisplatin, doxorubicin, cyclophosphamide) is as good as or better than that of patients with ovarian cancer.[108–110]

The actuarial 5-year survival rate for patients with fallopian tube adenocarcinoma (all stages) is 51 percent.[108] The staging of fallopian tube adenocarcinoma is similar to that of ovarian cancer (Table 7–1).

TABLE 7–1.
Fallopian Tube Tumor Staging According to the International Federation of Gynecology and Obstetrics (FIGO)

Stage	Description
Stage 0	Carcinoma in situ (limited to tubal mucosa)
Stage I	Growth limited to fallopian tubes
Stage IA	Growth limited to one tube with extension into submucosa and/or muscularis but not penetrating serosal surface; no ascites
Stage IB	Growth limited to both tubes with extension into submucosa and/or muscularis but not penetrating serosal surface; no ascites
Stage IC	Tumor either stage IA or stage IB but with extension through or onto tubal serosa or with ascites containing malignant cells or with positive peritoneal washings
Stage II	Growth involving one or both fallopian tubes with pelvic extension
Stage IIA	Extension and/or metastasis to uterus and/or ovaries
Stage IIB	Extension to other pelvic tissue
Stage IIC	Tumor either stage IIA or stage IIB and with ascites containing malignant cells or with positive peritoneal washings
Stage III	Tumor involving one or both fallopian tubes with peritoneal implants outside pelvis and/or positive retroperitoneal or inguinal nodes. Superficial liver metastasis equals stage III. Tumor appears limited to true pelvis but with histologically proven malignant extension to small bowel or omentum
Stage IIIA	Tumor grossly limited to true pelvis with negative nodes but with histologically confirmed microscopic seeding of abdominal peritoneal surfaces
Stage IIIB	Tumor involving one or both tubes with histologically confirmed implants of abdominal peritoneal surfaces, none exceeding 2 cm in diameter. Lymph nodes are negative.
Stage IIIC	Abdominal implant >2 cm in diameter and/or positive retroperitoneal or inguinal nodes
Stage IV	Growth involving one or both fallopian tubes with distant metastases. If pleural effusion is present, cytologic fluid must be positive for malignant cells to be stage IV. Parenchymal liver metastasis equals stage IV.

Note: Staging for fallopian tube carcinoma is by the surgical pathologic system. Operative findings designating stage are determined before tumor debulking.

(From Creasman WT: Revision in classification by International Federation of Gynecology and Obstetrics (letter). Am J Obstet Gynecol 1992;167:857–858.)

Metastatic Lesions

Eighty to ninety percent of all malignancies identified within the fallopian tube are metastatic from other sites. Of these, 60 percent originate in the ovary (Fig. 7–40). Other tumors that metastasize to the fallopian tube include tumors of the endometrium, cervix, breast, gastrointestinal tract, and lung as well as uterine choriocarcinoma and occasionally lymphomas.

The degree of involvement can be categorized as (1) intraluminal or intraepithelial, or (2) stromal or mural. In the first instance, free-floating fragments of tumor can be identified in fallopian tube sections of patients with primary endometrial or ovarian carcinomas. On occasion, superficial epithelial implantation may occur as a consequence of the transit of tumor fragments either from the

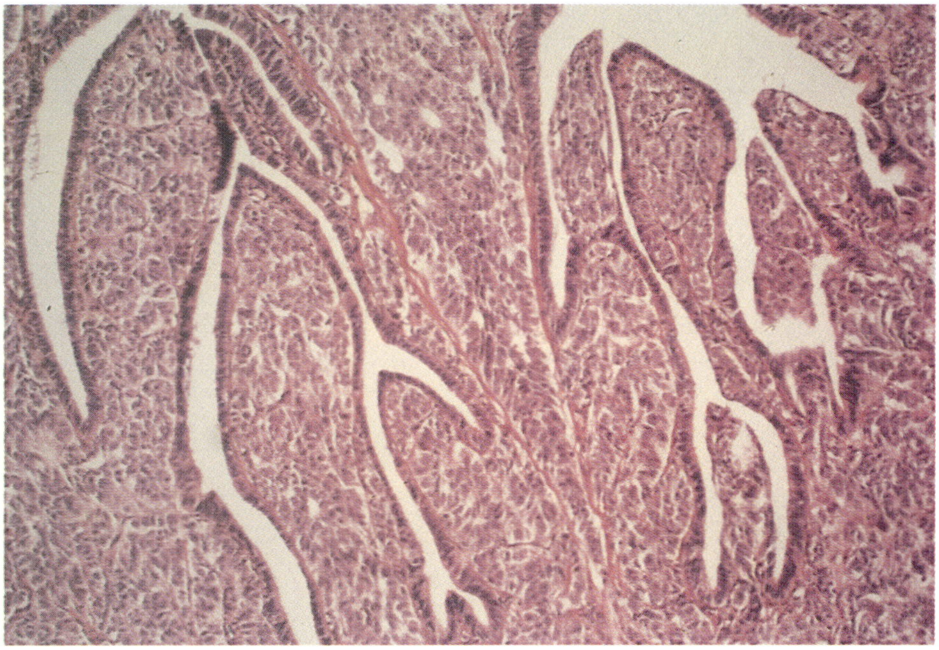

FIGURE 7-40
This is a section of tubal plicae in a case of a metastatic, poorly differentiated ovarian adenocarcinoma. The tumor completely replaces the plical stroma but leaves the overlying normal tubal epithelium intact.

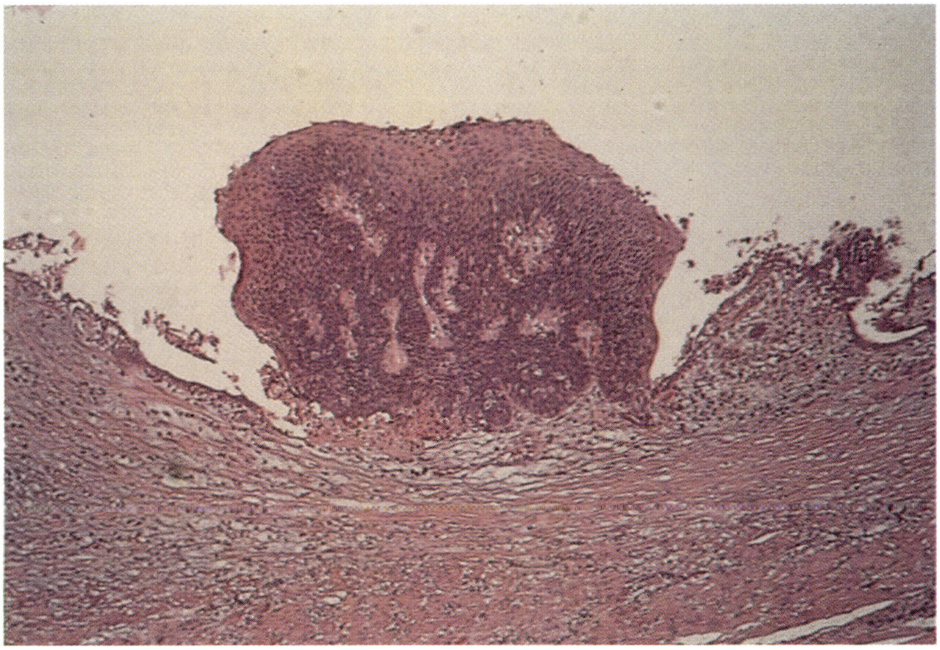

FIGURE 7-41
This cervical squamous cell carcinoma involved the fallopian tube. Residual normal fallopian tube epithelium is seen flanking the squamous carcinoma. The fallopian tube muscle bundles are at the bottom.

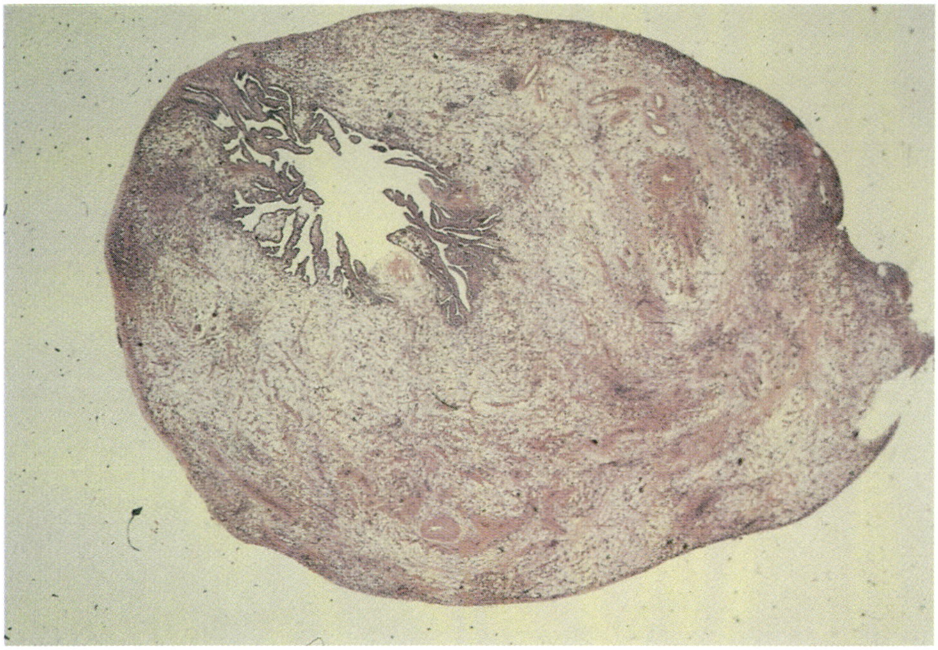

FIGURE 7-42
This is a cross section of a tube removed from a patient with a pelvic mass. The tumor infiltrates the tubal muscularis and the stroma of some of the luminal folds, giving it a myxoid appearance on lower magnification. This myxoid appearance was seen to be caused by the presence of mucin-containing signet ring cells. The tubal epithelium is normal. This patient was found to have a gastric carcinoma.

uterus to the peritoneal cavity or from the peritoneal cavity to the uterus. Another instance in which the epithelium of the fallopian tube may be involved is by horizontal spread of a squamous cell carcinoma of the cervix (Fig. 7–41). This is known as the zuckerguss (from the German "icing on the cake") pattern of spread. This is a very rare occurrence.[111]

The stromal or mural metastatic pattern is the most frequent (Fig. 7–42). The metastatic tumor will at times completely replace the connective tissue of the fallopian tube, giving the appearance of a "cast." This type of pattern, which replaces the stroma and particularly the plicae of the tube, must be distinguished from that of a primary carcinoma. In metastatic disease, epithelial atypia or transition from benign to malignant is not identified.

PARATUBAL LESIONS

The fallopian tube develops from the müllerian (paramesonephric) duct. This runs parallel to the wolffian (mesonephric) duct. Cystic lesions that arise within the broad ligament in the paratubal area may be of mesonephric, paramesonephric, or mesothelial origin. Gardner subdivided the cystic lesions that involve the broad ligament into intraligamentous and pedunculated. He believed that 36 percent of grossly visible intraligamentous cysts are paramesonephric in origin, whereas 43 percent are mesonephric.[16] More recently, Genadry and colleagues contended that the intraligamentous cysts (paraovarian cysts), 5 cm or greater in size are of a mesothelial origin.[17] There exists a great deal of controversy regarding the histogenesis of these cysts, albeit the lesions are contained between the leaves of the broad ligament. In cysts of paramesonephric origin, ciliated and secretory cells can be seen as well as occasional plicae. Cysts of mesonephric origin differ in that they have a well-defined basement membrane that can best be demonstrated utilizing an iron-hematoxylin or a periodic acid–Schiff stain.[111] The intraligamentous cysts are almost always benign. The clinical presentation is either that of an adnexal mass in an asymptomatic patient or that of pain associated with torsion of the adnexa. They occur predominantly in women of reproductive age and should be managed conservatively, sparing the adnexa.[111A] (Fig. 7–43)

The hydatids of Morgagni are considered a paramesonephric remnant and in the Gardner classification would be designated a pedunculated lesion.[111] Hydatids of Morgagni are quite common. Torsion is rare. The clinical picture resembles that of appendicitis when the lesion is on the right side. On occasion, epithelial proliferation may occur, which results in a serous epithelial lesion. A few rare cases of serous cystadenocarcinoma in a hydatid of Morgagni have been reported.[112]

Occasionally, adrenal rests are found in the mesosalpinx. The adrenal rest contains cells consistent with the zona fasciculata and the zona reticularis of the adult adrenal (Fig. 7–44).

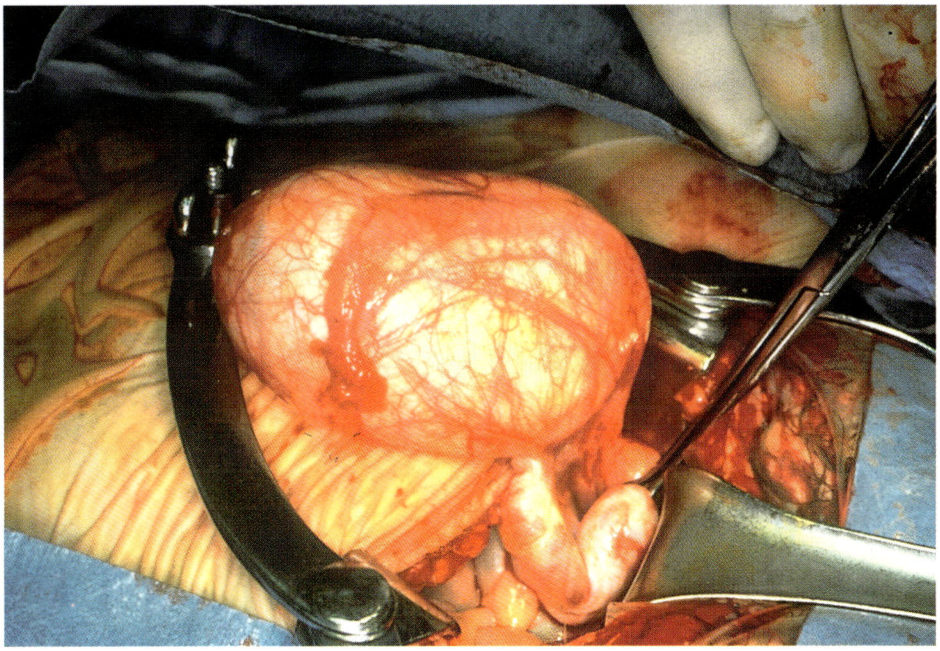

FIGURE 7-43
Intraligamentous paratubal cyst of paramesonephric origin is seen. The fallopian tube is stretched over the cyst. The bright red fimbriae which are seen on the cyst are sometimes mistaken for external excresences by ultrasound. The utero-ovarian ligament is not seen but is being held by a surgical clamp. The ovary in front of the clamp appears normal. The vessels of the mesosalpinx are stretched over the paratubal cyst.

The female adnexal tumor of probable wolffian origin can be found within the broad ligament or hanging from it or from the fallopian tube.[113–115] Its average size is 8 cm in diameter. These are firm to rubbery, yellow, lobulated tumors. Internally they are solid or solid and cystic and of gray-white or yellow-tan color. On microscopic examination the tumor may form tubules, cystic spaces, or a sievelike pattern. The tubules may be solid. They are lined by cuboidal to columnar cells that have round to oval uniform nuclei and scant cytoplasm. A few cells may have abundant pale cytoplasm. The cysts are usually lined by flattened cells. Electron microscopic studies favor a wolffian origin.[116] Of all reported cases, two tumors behaved in a malignant fashion.[117, 118] These two patients had late recurrences (i.e., more than 6 years after removal). One case proved fatal.[118]

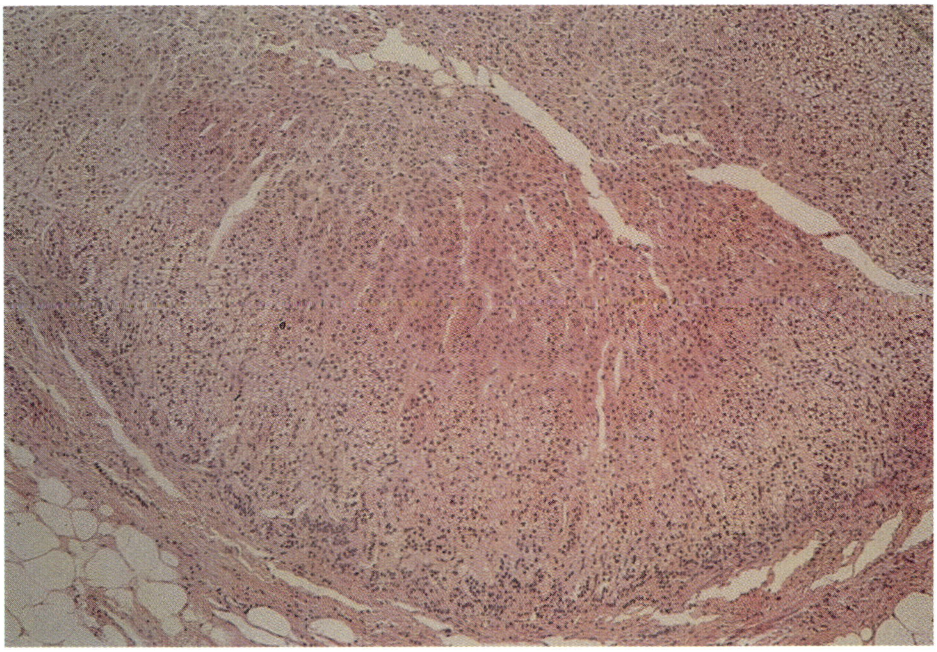

FIGURE 7-44
This adrenal rest in the mesosalpinx consists of two cell layers. The outer cells contain abundant, clear, vacuolated cytoplasm and are consistent with the cells found in the zona fasciculata of the adrenal gland. The inner cells have abundant eosinophilic cytoplasm and are consistent with the cells of the zona reticularis.

REFERENCES

1. Hunter RHF: The Fallopian Tubes: Their Role in Fertility and Infertility. New York, Springer-Verlag, 1988, pp 1–11.
2. Stock RJ: Histopathology of fallopian tubes with recurrent tubal pregnancy. Obstet Gynecol 1990;75:9–14.
3. Pauerstein CJ, Croxatto HB, Eddy CA, et al: Anatomy and pathology of tubal pregnancy. Obstet Gynecol 1986;67:301–308.
4. Berta P, Hawkins JR, Sinclair AH, et al: Genetic evidence equating SRY and the testis-determining factor. Nature 1990;348:448–450.
5. Woodruff JD, Pauerstein CJ: The Fallopian Tube—Structure, Function, Pathology and Management. Baltimore, Williams & Wilkins, 1969, pp 9–21.
6. Knab DR, Blanco LJ: Müllerian duct agenesis with a unilateral functioning segment of the rudimentary uterine horn. Am J Obstet Gynecol 1978;132:222–224.
7. Beyth Y, Kopolovic J: Accessory tubes: A possible contributing factor in infertility. Fertil Steril 1982;38:382–383.
8. Rocker I: The anatomy of the utero-tubal junction area. Proc R Soc Med 1964;57:707–709.
9. Sweeney WJ: The interstitial portion of the uterine tube: Its gross anatomy, course and length. Obstet Gynecol 1962;19:3–8.
10. Borell U, Fernstrom I: The adnexal branches of the uterine artery. Acta Radiol 1953;40:561–582.
11. Woodruff JD, Pauerstein CJ: The Fallopian Tube—Structure, Function, Pathology and Management. Baltimore, Williams & Wilkins, 1969, pp 34–37.
12. Ludwig H, Metzger H: The Human Female Reproductive Tract. New York, Springer-Verlag, 1976, pp 79–105.
13. Ferenczy A, Richart RM: Female Reproductive System: Dynamics of Scan and Transmission Electron Microscopy. New York, Wiley & Sons, 1974, pp 212–253.
14. Jean Y, Langlais J, Roberts KD, et al: Fertility of a woman with nonfunctional ciliated cells in the fallopian tubes. Fertil Steril 1979;31:349–350.
15. Odor DL: The question of "basal" cells in oviductal and endocervical epithelium. Fertil Steril 1974;25:1047–1062.
16. Gardner GH, Greene RR, Peckham BM: Normal and cystic structures of the broad ligament. Am J Obstet Gynecol 1948;55:917–939.
17. Genadry R, Parmley T, Woodruff JD: The origin and clinical behavior of the paraovarian tumor. Am J Obstet Gynecol 1977;129:873–879.
18. Roth LM: The Brenner tumor and the Walthard cell rest. An electron microscopic study. Lab Invest 1974;31:15–23.
19. Tilden IL, Winstedt R: Decidual reactions in fallopian tubes. Am J Pathol 1943;19:1043–1055.
20. Pinero DA Jr, Foraker AG: Aging in the fallopian tube. Am J Obstet Gynecol 1963;86:397–400.
21. Honore LH: Pathology of the fallopian tube. *In* Fox H (ed): Haines and Taylor's Obstetrical and Gynecological Pathology. Edinburgh, Churchill Livingstone, 1987, pp 484–485.
22. Fetissof F, Berger G, Bubois MP, et al: Female genital tract and Peutz-Jeghers syndrome: An immunohistochemical study. Int J Gynecol Pathol 1985;4:219–229.

22a. LiVolsi VA, Merino MJ, Schwartz PE: Coexistent endocervical adenocarcinoma and mucinous adenocarcinoma of ovary: a clinicopathologic study of four cases. Int J Gynecol Pathol 1983;1:391–402.

23. Starr AJ, Ruffolo EH, Shenoy BV, Marston BR: Primary carcinoma of the fallopian tube: A surprise finding in a postpartum tubal ligation. Am J Obstet Gynecol 1978;132:344–345.
24. Saffos RO, Rhatigan RM, Scully RE: Metaplastic papillary tumor of the fallopian tube: A distinctive lesion of pregnancy. Am J Clin Pathol 1980;74:232–236.
25. Sampson JA: Endometriosis following salpingectomy. Am J Obstet Gynecol 1928;16:461–499.
26. Rock JA, Parmley TH, King TM, et al: Endometriosis and the development of tuboperitoneal fistulas after tubal ligation. Fertil Steril 1981;35:16–20.
27. McCausland A: Endosalpingosis ("endosalpingoblastosis") following laparoscopic tubal coagulation as an etiologic factor of ectopic pregnancy. Am J Obstet Gynecol 1982;143:12–22.
28. Stock RJ: Postsalpingectomy endometriosis: A reassessment. Obstet Gynecol 1982;60:560–570.
29. Novak E: Comment on Dr. Sampson's paper 1928. Am J Obstet Gynecol 1928;16:742.
30. Sampson JA: Postsalpingectomy endometriosis (endosalpingiosis). Am J Obstet Gynecol 1930;20:443–480.
31. Stock RJ: Clinicopathologic changes resulting from adnexal torsion. J Reprod Med 1987;32:201–207.
32. Merritt DF: Torsion of the uterine adnexa: A review. Adolesc Pediatr Gynecol 1991;4:3–13.
33. Sapan IP, Solberg NS: Prolapse of the uterine tube after abdominal hysterectomy. Obstet Gynecol 1973;42:26–31.

33a. Symmonds RE, Counseller US, Pratt JH: Prolapse of a fallopian tube as a complication of hysterectomy. Am J Obstet Gynecol 1957;74:214–217.

34. Wolfendale M: Exfoliative cytology in a case of prolapsed fallopian tube. Acta Cytol 1980;24:545–548.
35. Reese WA, O'Connor R, Bouzoukis JF, Sutherland SF: Tubal pregnancy after total vaginal hysterectomy. Ann Emerg Med 1989;18:1107–1110.
36. Wheelock JB, Schneider V, Goplerud DR: Prolapsed fallopian tube masquerading as adenocarcinoma of the vagina in a postmenopausal woman. Gynecol Oncol 1985;21:369–375.
37. Adams BE: Intussusception of a fallopian tube. Am J Surg 1969;118:591–592.
38. Littig LW: The technique of tubal sterilization. Surg Gynecol Obstet 1912;15:514–520.
39. Stock RJ: Tubal patency following "Uchida" tubal ligation. Obstet Gynecol 1980;56:521–525.
40. Bishop E, Nelms WF: A simple method of tubal sterilization. NY State J Med 1930;30:214–216.
41. Stock RJ: Histopathologic changes in fallopian tubes subsequent to sterilization procedures. Int J Gynecol Pathol 1983;2:13–27.
42. Metz KGP: Failures following fimbriectomy: A further report. Fertil Steril 1978;30:269–273.
43. Soderstrom RM: Sterilization failures and their causes. Am J Obstet Gynecol 1985;152:395–403.
44. Soderstrom RM, Levy BS: Bipolar systems: Do they perform? Obstet Gynecol 1987;69:425–426.
45. Yoon IB, Poliakoff SR: Laparoscopic tubal ligation. J Reprod Med 1979;23:76–80.
46. Vasquez G, Winston RML, Boeckx W, Brosens I: Tubal lesions subsequent to sterilization and their relation to fertility after attempts at reversal. Am J Obstet Gynecol 1980;138:86–92.
47. Peterson HB, Walker CK, Kahn JG, et al: Pelvic inflammatory disease. JAMA 1991;1266:2605–2611.
48. Safrin S, Schachter J, Dahrouge D, Sweet RL: Long-term sequelae of acute pelvic inflammatory disease. Am J Obstet Gynecol 1992;166:1300–1305.
49. Kahn JG, Walker CK, Washington AE, et al: Diagnosing pelvic inflammatory disease. JAMA 1991;266:2594–2604.
50. Black-Schaffer B: Subclinical post-partum salpingitis and one-child sterility: A pathologic study. Am J Obstet Gynecol 1944;48:374–378.
51. Hellman LM: The morphology of the human fallopian tube in the early puerperium. Am J Obstet Gynecol 1949;57:154–163.
52. Nassberg S, McKay DG, Hertig AT: Physiologic salpingitis. Am J Obstet Gynecol 1954;67:130–137.
53. Schaefer G: Tuberculosis of the female genital tract. Clin Obstet Gynecol 1970;13:965–998.
54. Nogales-Ortiz F, Taracon I, Nogales-Ortiz F Jr: The pathology of female genital tuberculosis. Obstet Gynecol 1979;53:422–428.

55. White MM: The diagnosis of tubal tuberculosis. *In* World Congress on Fertility and Sterility Proceedings, 1st–2nd. Naples,1953–1956 NLM: W3 W0538E.
56. Dische EE, Burt JM, Davidson NJH, Puntambekar S: Tubo-ovarian actinomycosis associated with intrauterine contraceptive devices. J Obstet Gynaecol Br Commonw 1974;81:724–729.
57. Lee NC, Rubin GL, Borucki R: The intrauterine device and pelvic inflammatory disease revisited: New results from the women's health study. Obstet Gynecol 1988; 72:1–6.
58. Bland KG, Gelfand M: The effects of schistosomiasis on the fallopian tube in the African female. J Obstet Gynaecol Br Commonw 1970;77:1024–1027.
59. Brooks JJ, Wheeler JE: Granulomatous salpingitis secondary to Crohn's disease. Obstet Gynecol 1977;49:31s–33s.
60. Kay S: Sarcoidosis of the fallopian tubes. J Obstet Gynecol Br Emp 1956;63:871–874.
61. Curtis AH: Bacteriology and pathology of fallopian tubes removed at operation. Surg Gynecol Obstet 1921;33:621–631.
62. Falk HC: Interpretation of the pathogenesis of pelvic infection as determined by cornual resection. Am J Obstet Gynecol 1946;52:66–72.
63. Hajj SN: Does sterilization prevent pelvic infection? J Reprod Med 1978;20:289–290.
64. Vermesh M, Confino E, Boler LR, et al: Acute salpingitis in sterilized women. Obstet Gynecol 1987;69:265–267.
65. Cates W Jr, Wasserheit JN: Genital chlamydial infections: Epidemiology and reproductive sequelae. Am J Obstet Gynecol 1991;164:1771–1781.
66. Sweet RL, Blankfort-Doyle M, Robbie MO, Schachter J: The occurrence of chlamydial and gonococcal salpingitis during the menstrual cycle. JAMA 1986;255:2062–2064.
67. Rice PA, Schachter J: Pathogenesis of pelvic inflammatory disease: what are the questions? JAMA 1991;266:2587–2593.
68. Schachter J, Stamm WE, Chernesky MA, et al: Nonculture tests for genital tract chlamydial infection: What does the package insert mean, and will it mean the same thing tomorrow? (editorial). Sex Transm Dis 1992;19:243–244.
69. Fortier KJ, Haney AF: The pathologic specimen of uterotubal junction obstruction. Obstet Gynecol 1985;65:93–98.
70. Sulak PJ, Hayslip CC, Letterie GS, et al: Histology of proximal tubal occlusion. Fertil Steril 1987;48:437–440.
71. Ries E: Nodular forms of tubal disease. J Exp Med 1897;2:347–389.
72. Rabinovitz M: The pathogenesis of adenomyosalpingitis (salpingitis nodosa). Am J Obstet 1913;38:711–752.
73. Wrork DH, Broders AC: Adenomyosis of the fallopian tube. Am J Obstet Gynecol 1942;44:412–432.
74. Majmudar B, Henderson PH III, Semple E: Salpingitis isthmica nodosa: a high-risk factor for tubal pregnancy. Obstet Gynecol 1983;62:73–78.
75. Dubuisson JB, Aubriot FX, Cardone V, Vacher-Lavenu MC: Tubal causes of ectopic pregnancy. Fertil Steril 1986;46:970–972.
76. Stock RJ: Tubal pregnancy: associated histopathology. Obstet Gynecol Clin North Am 1991;18:73–93.
77. Stock RJ: The changing spectrum of ectopic pregnancy. Obstet Gynecol 1988;71:885–888.
77a. Kadar N, Caldwell BV, Romero R: A method of screening for ectopic pregnancy. Obstet Gynecol 1981;58:162–165.
77b. Stovall TG, Ling FW, Gray LA: Single-dose methotrexate for treatment of ectopic pregnancy and its indications. Obstet Gynecol 1991;77:754–757.
78. Budowich M, Johnson TRB, Genadry R, et al: The histopathology of the developing tubal ectopic pregnancy. Fertil Steril 1980;34:169–171.
79. Klinkert J, van Geldorp HJ, Chadha-Ajwani S, Huikeshoven FJM: Tubal damage after intratubal methotrexate treatment. Fertil Steril 1993;59:926–927.
80. Hönigl W, Pickel H, Tamussino K, Lang PF: Histopathology of the fallopian tube after local instillation of hyperosmolar glucose solution for unruptured tubal pregnancy. Fertil Steril 1993;59:1316–1318.
81. Haney AF: Bilateral tubal occlusion secondary to asymptomatic ectopic pregnancies. Obstet Gynecol 1986;67:52S–53S.
82. Cole T, Corlett RC Jr: Chronic ectopic pregnancy. Obstet Gynecol 1982;59:63–68.
83. Kelly RW, Martin SA, Strickler RC: Delayed hemorrhage in conservative surgery for ectopic pregnancy. Am J Obstet Gynecol 1979;133:225–226.
84. Reich H, Wilkie WL, DeCaprio J, et al: Peritoneal trophoblastic tissue implants after laparoscopic treatment of tubal ectopic pregnancy. Fertil Steril 1989;52:337–339.
85. Stock RJ, Nelson KJ: Ectopic pregnancy subsequent to sterilization: histologic evaluation and clinical implications. Fertil Steril 1984;42:211–215.
86. Ober WB, Maier RC: Gestational choriocarcinoma of the fallopian tube. Diagn Gynecol Obstet 1981;3:213–231.
87. Lurain JR, Sand PK, Brewer JI: Choriocarcinoma associated with ectopic pregnancy. Obstet Gynecol 1986; 68:286–287.
87a. Stern J, Buscema J, Parmley T, et al: Atypical epithelial proliferations in the fallopian tube. Am J Obstet Gynecol 1981;140:309–312.
88. Teel P: Adenomatoid tumors of the genital tract. Am J Obstet Gynecol 1958;75:1347–1353.
89. Golden A, Ash JE: Adenomatoid tumors of the genital tract. Am J Pathol 1945;21:63–73.
90. Taxy JB, Battifora H, Oyasu R: Adenomatoid tumors: A light microscopy, histochemical and ultrastructural study. Cancer 1974;34:306–316.
91. Grunebaum AN, Sedlis A: Adenomatoid tumor of the uterus simulating interstitial pregnancy. Obstet Gynecol 1982;59:87s–88s.
92. Gisser SD: Obstructing fallopian tube papilloma. Int J Gynecol Pathol 1986;5:179–182.
93. Kanbour AI, Burgess F, Salazar H: Intramural adenofibroma of the fallopian tube: light and electron microscopy. Cancer 1973;31:1433–1439.
94. Mazzarella P, Takashi O, Richart RM: Teratoma of the uterine tube. Obstet Gynecol 1972;39:381–388.
95. Kutteh WH, Albert T: Mature cystic teratoma of the fallopian tube associated with an ectopic pregnancy. Obstet Gynecol 1991;78:984–986.
96. Frost RG, Roongpisuthipong A, Cheek BH, Majmudar BN: Immature teratoma of the fallopian tube. J Reprod Med 1989;34:62–64.
97. Schust D, Stovall DW: Leiomyomas of the fallopian tube. J Reprod Med 1993;38:741–742.
98. Mitchell RM, Mohler RW: Primary carcinoma of the fallopian tube. Am J Obstet Gynecol 1945;50:283–292.
99. Martzloff KH: Primary cancer of the fallopian tube. Am J Obstet Gynecol 1940;40:804–817.
100. Sinha AC: Hydrops tubae profluens as a presenting symptom in primary carcinoma of the fallopian tube. Br Med J 1959;2:996–1001.
101. Takashina T, Ito E, Kudo R: Cytologic diagnosis of primary tubal cancer. Acta Cytol 1985;29:367–372.
102. Finn WF, Javert CJ: Primary and metastatic cancer of the fallopian tube. Cancer 1949;2:803–814.
103. Buchino JJ, Buchino JJ: Malignant mixed müllerian tumor of the fallopian tube. Arch Pathol Lab Med 1987;111:386–387.
104. Daya D, Young RH, Scully RE: Endometrioid carcinoma of the fallopian tube resembling an adnexal tumor of probable wolffian origin: a report of six cases. Int J Gynecol Pathol 1992;11:122–130.
105. Herbold DR, Axelrod JH, Bobowski ST, Freel JH: Glassy cell carcinoma of the fallopian tube. Int J Gynecol Pathol 1988;7:384–390.
106. Tokunaga T, Miyazaki K, Matsuyama S, Okamura H: Se-

rial measurement of CA 125 in patients with primary carcinoma of the fallopian tube. Gynecol Oncol 1990; 36:335–337.
107. Davies AP, Fish A, Woolas R, Oram D: Raised serum CA 125 preceding the diagnosis of carcinoma of the fallopian tube: Two case reports. Br J Obstet Gynaecol 1991; 98:602–603.
108. Barakat RR, Rubin SC, Saigo PE, et al: Cisplatin-based combination chemotherapy in carcinoma of the fallopian tube. Gynecol Oncol 1991;42:156–160.
109. Barakat RR, Rugin SC, Saigo PE, et al: Second-look laparotomy in carcinoma of the fallopian tube. Obstet Gynecol 1993;82:748–751.
110. Morris M, Gershenson DM, Burke TW, et al: Treatment of fallopian tube carcinoma with cisplatin, doxorubicin, and cyclophosphamide. Obstet Gynecol 1990;76:1020–1024.
111. Kanbour AI, Stock RJ: Squamous cell carcinoma in situ of the endometrium and fallopian tube as superficial extension of invasive cervical carcinoma. Cancer 1978;42:570–580.
111a. Stock RJ: Large intraligamentous cysts: technique of surgical removal and correlation of surgical observations and histologic findings pertaining to origin. J Reprod Med 1987;32:347–352.
112. Rojansky N, Ophir E, Sharony A, et al: Broad ligament adenocarcinoma—its origin and clinical behavior: A literature review and report of a case. Obstet Gynecol Surv 1985;40:665–671.
113. Kariminejad MH, Scully RE: Female adnexal tumor of probable wolffian origin: A distinctive pathologic entity. Cancer 1973;31:671–677.
114. Sivathondan Y, Salm R, Hughesdon PE, Faccini JM: Female adnexal tumour of probable wolffian origin. J Clin Pathol 1979;32:616–624.
115. Kao GF, Norris HJ: Juxtaovarian adnexal tumor: A clinical and pathologic study of 19 cases (abstract). Lab Invest 1978;38:350–351.
116. Demopoulos RI, Sitelman A, Flotte T, Bigelow B: Ultrastructural study of a female adnexal tumor of probable wolffian origin. Cancer 1980;46:2273–2280.
117. Taxy JB, Battifora H: Female adnexal tumor of probable wolffian origin: evidence for a low grade malignancy. Cancer 1976;37:2349–2354.
118. Abbot RL, Barlogie B, Schmidt WA: Metastasizing malignant juxtaovarian tumor with terminal hypercalcemia: A case report. Cancer 1981;48:860–865.

8

The Ovary: Normal, Physiologic Changes, Endometriosis, and Metastatic Tumors

Gulnar Balsara/Enrique Hernandez

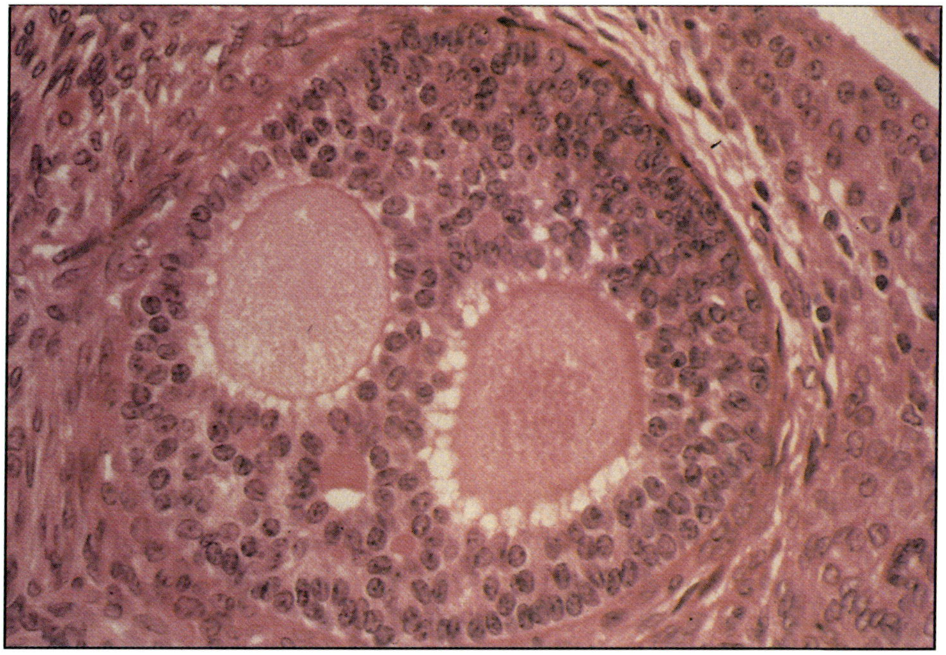

NORMAL ANATOMY

The ovaries are paired organs that lie within the pelvic peritoneal cavity. They are normally found behind the uterus and against the lateral pelvic sidewall. They are attached to the posterior aspect of the broad ligament by a double fold of peritoneum known as the mesovarium. The mesovarium attaches to the anterior surface of the ovary but does not enclose it. The mesovarium becomes the mesosalpinx as it approaches the fallopian tubes, which lie anterior and superior to the ovaries. The lateral pole of the ovary is attached to the pelvic sidewall by the infundibulopelvic or suspensory ligament. This is not a true ligament but a neurovascular bundle that lies within a connective tissue matrix. The medial pole of the ovary is attached by the utero-ovarian ligament to the uterus just inferior to the uterotubal junction.

The adult ovary is ovoid, measures approximately 3 cm in length, and weighs an average of 6.5 gm (Fig. 8–1). During a normal menstrual cycle a dominant follicle reaches a diameter of 2 to 2.5 cm, resulting in an ovarian diameter of approximately 5 cm. In the early reproductive years the ovarian surface is smooth and tan-white. Occasionally, translucent follicular cysts or yellow-orange corpora lutea are visible on the external surface (Fig. 8–2). On cut section three poorly defined zones are identified—the cortex, the medulla, and the hilum. As aging occurs, the ovarian surface develops irregular scars and appears more convoluted. After menopause the size of the ovaries gradually decreases to about 1 to 2 cm.

The ovaries receive their blood supply from the abdominal aorta through the ovarian artery, which runs within the infundibulopelvic ligament. It reaches the mesovarium, where it anastomoses with the ovarian branch of the uterine artery. Branches of these vessels enter the ovary through the hilum and course through the medulla to reach the corticomedullary junction. From this area straight arterioles radiate outward to supply the ovarian surface. The ovarian veins form the pampiniform plexus in the mesovarium and then traverse the infundibulopelvic ligament to join the inferior vena cava on the right and the renal vein on the left. The lymphatics of the ovary drain into the paraaortic lymph nodes at the level of the second lumbar vertebra. Lymphatics also run along the ovarian ligament and the round ligament to drain into the lingual lymph nodes.[1, 2] The nerve supply of the ovary is derived predominantly from the aortic plexus, which has both sympathetic and parasympathetic components. The sympathetic fibers provide vasomotor control. They are also believed to play a role in follicular maturation and ovarian hormone production.[3] The role of the parasympathetic nerves is unknown.

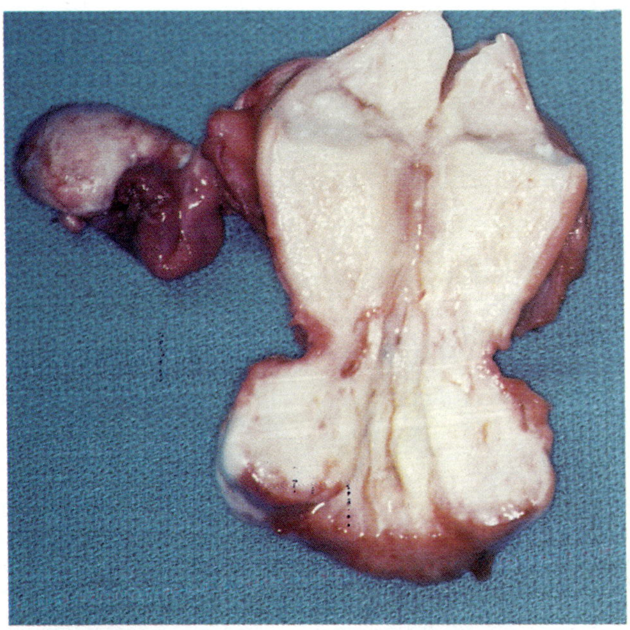

FIGURE 8–1
A normal ovary is shown still attached to the right side of the uterus. The fallopian tube lies below the ovary. Its normal anatomic position is superior and anterior to the ovary.

NORMAL HISTOLOGY

The surface epithelium of the ovary is composed of a single layer of low cuboidal to flattened cells that are separated from the underlying stroma by a well-defined basement membrane. This epithelium follows the external contour of the ovary, dipping down into crevices created by the convolutions (Fig. 8–3). If in one of these areas the epithelium loses its connection with the surface it may result in an epithelial inclusion cyst. The surface epithelial cells show positive immunoreactivity using antibodies to cytokeratin, vimentin,[4] estrogen, progesterone, and CA 125.[5] The ovarian stroma is composed of densely packed stromal cells. These cells are spindle shaped, have scant cytoplasm, and are arranged in cellular whorls within a dense reticulin framework. Collagen is present between the stromal cells and is particularly prominent in the superficial cortex. Stromal cells show positive immunoreactivity using antibodies to vimentin, actin, desmin, estrogen, and progesterone. With aging there is a decrease in stromal cellularity and an increased amount of collagen. Stromal cells also contain lipid, a feature

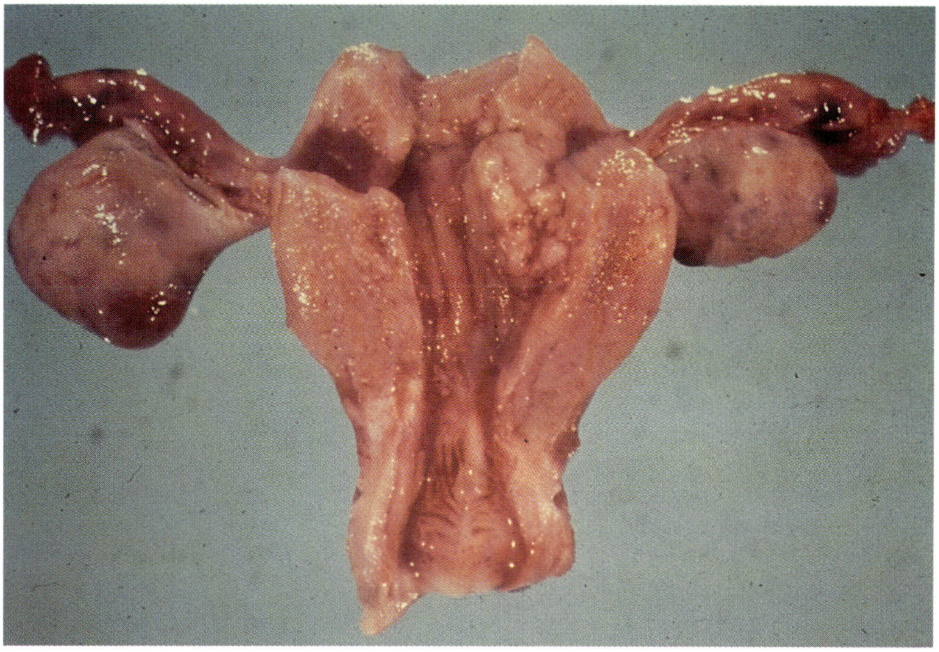

FIGURE 8-2
The ovary on the left shows a corpus luteum (reddish area). The fallopian tubes are stretched above the ovaries. The uterus has been opened anteriorly. A polypoid tumor is seen in the left cornu. (Courtesy of Dr. J. Donald Woodruff, The Johns Hopkins Hospital, Baltimore, MD.)

that is more prominent in postmenopausal ovaries and that may give them a yellowish color. A variety of other cell types are encountered in the ovary, all of which are believed to arise from ovarian stromal cells. The most prominent other cell type is luteinized stromal cells. These are most commonly scattered within the medulla. They may be single or small clusters. They are polyhedral cells with a central round nucleus, prominent nucleoli, and cytoplasm that is either clear or eosinophilic. These cells contain lipid and show positive immunoreactivity to testosterone. Luteinized stromal cells are believed to be influenced by gonadotropins and thus are found in increased numbers during pregnancy and the menopause.[6] Occasionally, excessive stromal luteinization may be associated with virilization (see also Chapter 11). Stromal cells can also differentiate into Leydig cells, fat cells, smooth muscle cells, endometrial stromal cells, or decidualized cells.[7] These latter cells are

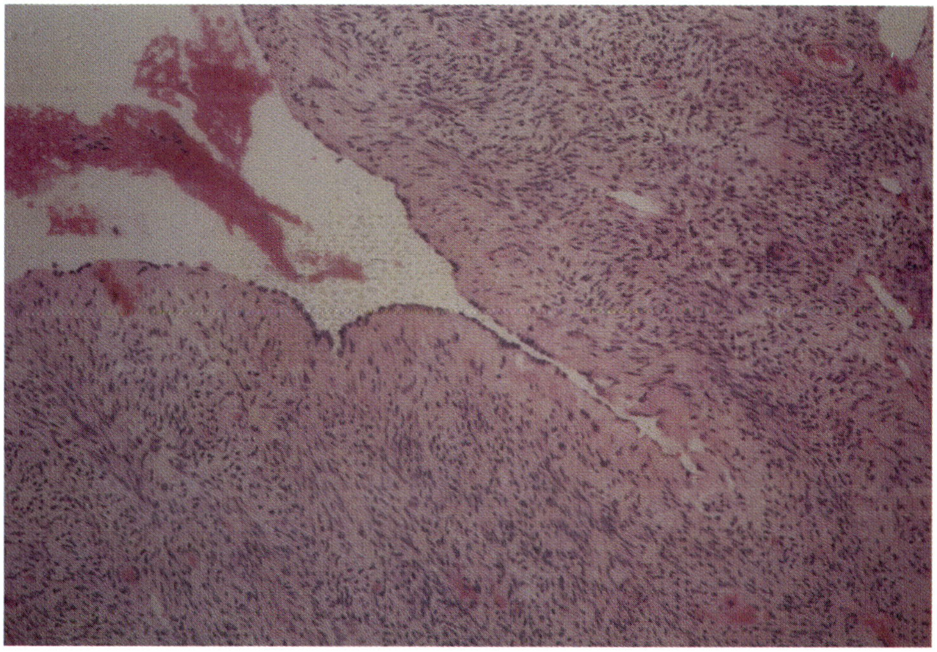

FIGURE 8-3
The surface of the ovary is lined by a single layer of cells that vary from low cuboidal to flattened. The dark nuclei of these cells are all that is visible at this magnification.

fairly consistently found during pregnancy. Rarely, stromal cells can also demonstrate neuroendocrine differentiation.

Ovaries of women who are of reproductive age have primordial follicles that are scattered as groups in a band within the superficial cortex. An average of 400,000 primordial follicles are found in each ovary at birth. This number progressively decreases during the reproductive years until none are found at menopause. At the center of the primordial follicle is the primary oocyte, which is a spherical cell of approximately 20 μm in diameter. The nucleus of the oocyte has finely dispersed chromatin and a thread-like nucleoli. The cytoplasm of the oocyte contains crescent-shaped eosinophilic structures called Balbiani's vitelline bodies.[8] The oocyte is surrounded by a single layer of inactive flattened granulosa cells. Beginning with the fifth to sixth month of intrauterine life and continuing until the menopause, the flattened granulosa cells surrounding the primary oocyte become cuboidal at the same time that the oocyte is enlarging, and this results in a primary follicle (Fig. 8–4). The granulosa cells secrete a glycosaminoglycan that gives rise to a translucent halo around the oocyte that is called the zona pellucida. Follicles in many different stages of development are present in ovaries of women of reproductive age (Fig. 8–5). The preantral (or secondary) follicle consists of several layers of granulosa cells surrounding an enlarged oocyte. Mitotic activity is seen within the granulosa cells. Preantral follicles are 50 to 400 μm in diameter. The antral (or tertiary) follicle consists of an eccentrically located oocyte that is surrounded by a large cavity called the antrum, which is filled with glycosaminoglycan-rich fluid. At this stage, the differentiation of the surrounding ovarian stromal cells into the theca interna and the theca externa becomes evident. The granulosa cells proliferate around the oocyte of the mature antral follicle (i.e., graafian follicle) to form the cumulus oophorus (Fig. 8–6). Normally during each menstrual cycle one mature follicle becomes the preovulatory (dominant) follicle. The preovulatory follicle measures an average of 20 mm in diameter. At this stage the oocyte and the cumulus become detached from the granulosa cells and float free within the antral fluid. The preovulatory follicle reaches the superficial cortex to protrude under the ovarian surface, where it initiates local tissue necrosis as a prelude to its rupture and the liberation of the oocyte-cumulus complex into the peritoneal cavity.[9] The point of rupture in the ovarian surface then heals and is ultimately converted to scar tissue.

Granulosa cells are typically 5 to 6 μm in diameter and polyhedral in shape. They have ill-defined borders, pale cytoplasm, and a round to oval nucleus that has a vesicular chromatin pattern. They rarely contain cytoplasmic lipid. When the antral follicle reaches 200 to 400 μm in diameter the formation of lacunae among the granulosa cells becomes apparent. These lacunae are round and contain eosinophilic, periodic acid–Schiff (PAS)-positive material that is separated from the granulosa cells by a basal lamina. These structures are

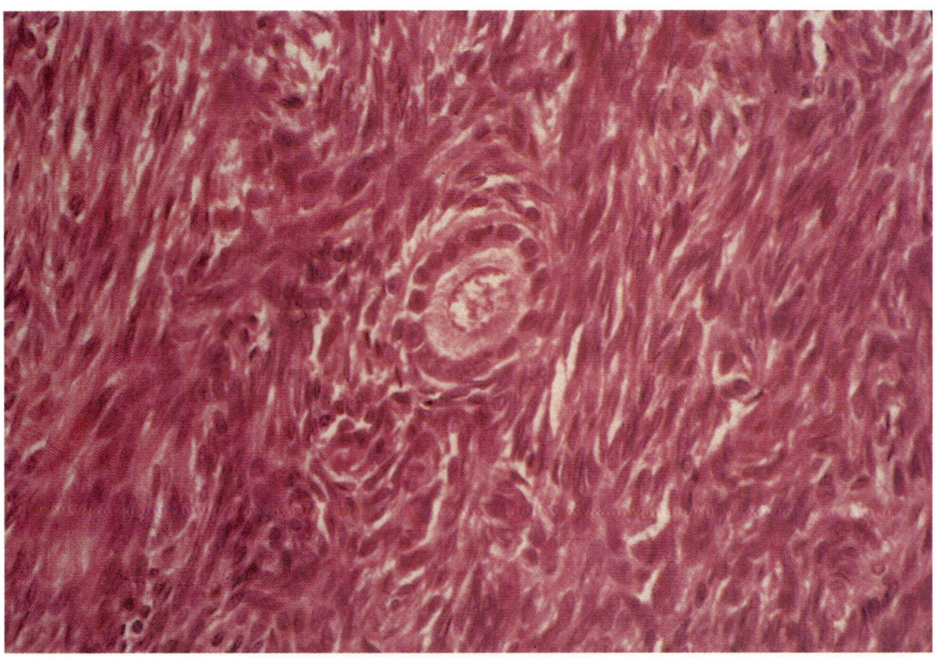

FIGURE 8–4
A primary follicle is shown within dense ovarian stroma. The oocyte is surrounded by a single layer of granulosa cells.

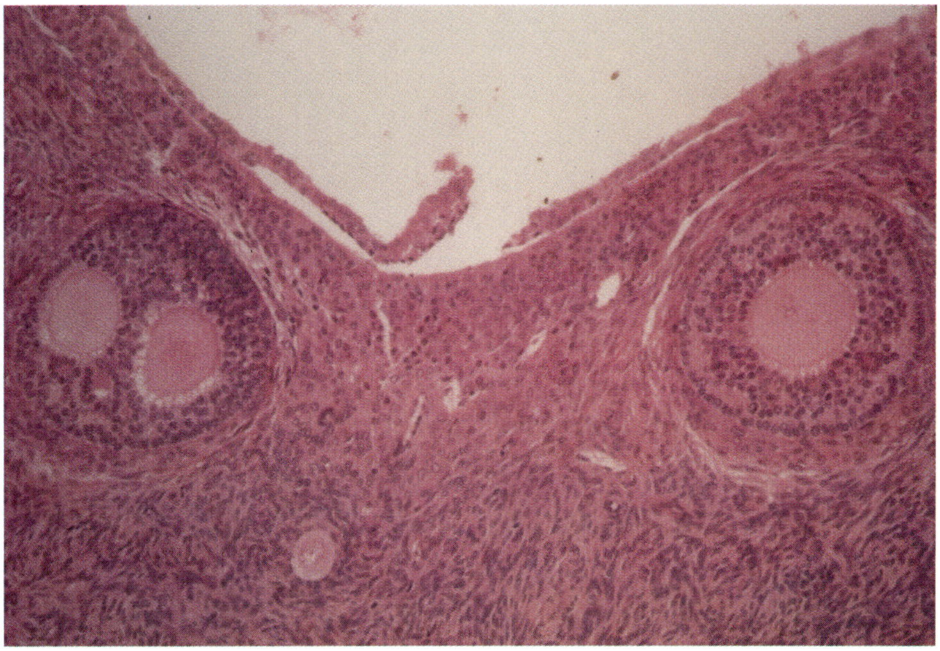

FIGURE 8–5
This histologic section of an ovary of a young woman shows follicles in multiple stages of development. The cavity of a large follicle is seen at the top. A primary follicle is seen at the bottom center. It is flanked by a preantral follicle on the right and an antral follicle on the left. The zona pellucida can be seen in the preantral and antral follicles.

known as Call-Exner bodies (Fig. 8–7). The theca cells are derived from the ovarian stromal cells that surround the developing follicle. The theca interna is well defined and is composed of three to four layers of cells separated from the granulosa cells by a well-defined basement membrane (Fig. 8–8). The cells of the theca interna are polygonal and have abundant eosinophilic cytoplasm and a rounded, central nucleus that has a vesicular chromatin pattern and a prominent nucleolus. They have variable amounts of intracytoplasmic lipid, and there is a dense reticulin framework surrounding each cell. The theca externa is poorly defined and its cells are intermediate in appearance between the cells of the theca interna and the nonspecialized ovarian stromal cells.

Following ovulation, if fertilization of the ovum has not occurred, the ruptured ovulatory follicle changes into the corpus luteum or yellow body of menstruation. This structure is yellowish-orange, convoluted and folded, and is approximately 2 cm in diameter. Central hemorrhage is present. Dur-

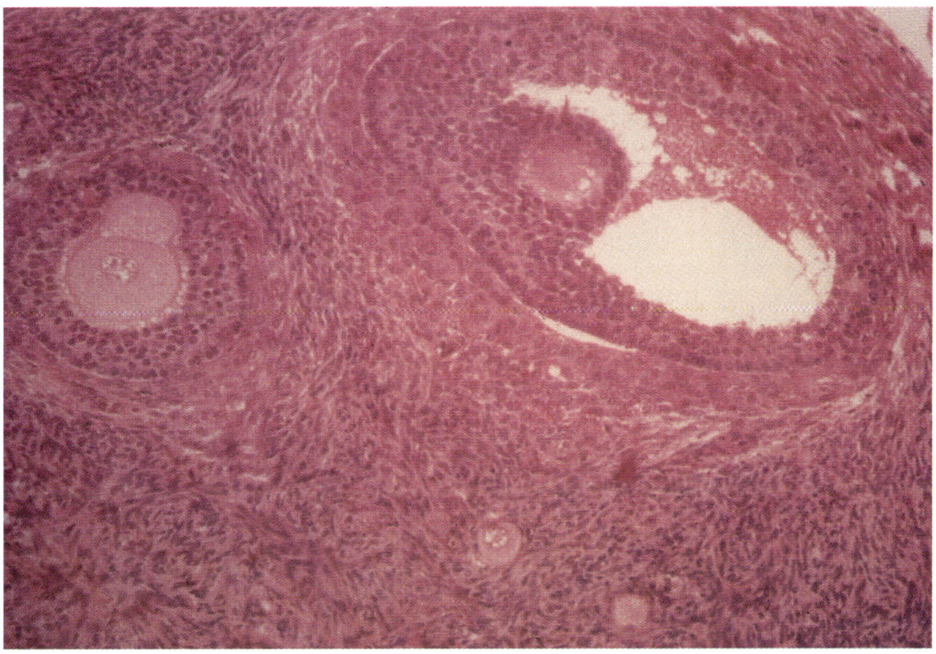

FIGURE 8–6
The antral follicle (*top right*) shows an eccentrically placed oocyte surrounded by granulosa cells, which is known as the cumulus oophorus. A cavity or antrum is seen. The theca interna under the granulosa cells is prominent. The theca externa is beginning to suggest itself. The follicle on the left is beginning to form the antrum. Its theca interna layer is not as prominent.

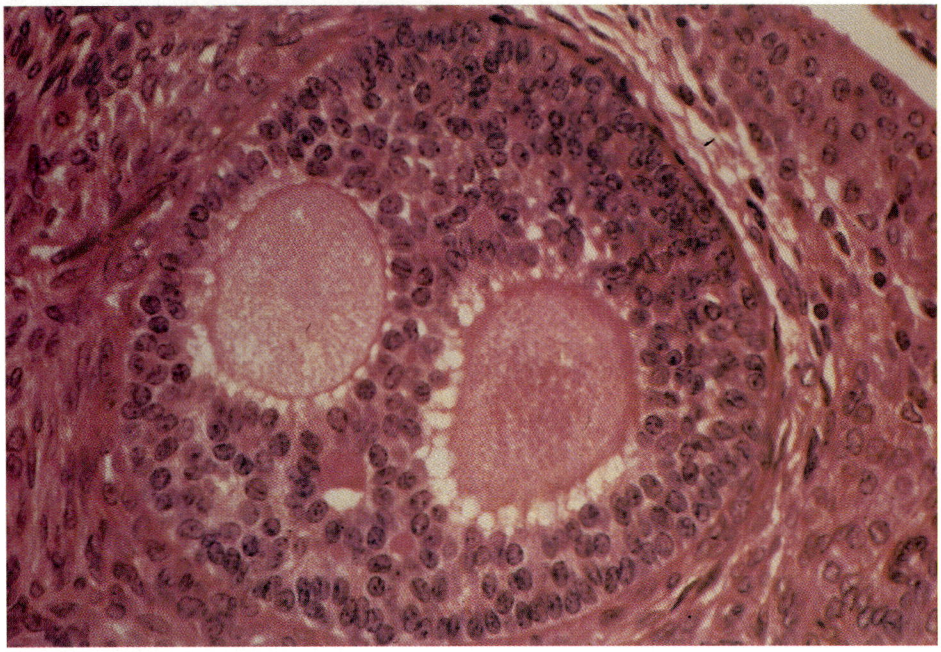

FIGURE 8–7
Call-Exner bodies are seen within an antral follicle and are best identified at the lower center. They are characterized by densely eosinophilic globules surrounded by a circle of granulosa cells.

ing the secretory phase of the menstrual cycle after rupture of the follicle the corpus luteum undergoes a series of changes. The granulosa cells become luteinized, which means that they become larger and have increased intracytoplasmic lipid. The theca interna cells form a thick layer that surrounds the granulosa cells (Fig. 8–9). The cells of the theca interna are generally smaller than the granulosa cells but contain a greater amount of lipid. Scattered among the granulosa cells and theca cells are the K cells, which are stellate in shape and have a deeply eosinophilic cytoplasm (Fig. 8–10). The nuclei sometimes are pyknotic. These are believed to be either degenerated granulosa or theca cells[10, 11] or possibly macrophages.[12] As the corpus luteum of menstruation matures, capillaries and fibroblasts from the theca interna extend into the central hemorrhagic cavity and form a fibrous lining layer (Fig. 8–11). Involutionary changes follow and become evident as shrinkage and pyknosis of the luteinized granulosa cells. These cells are ultimately phagocytized. Increasing

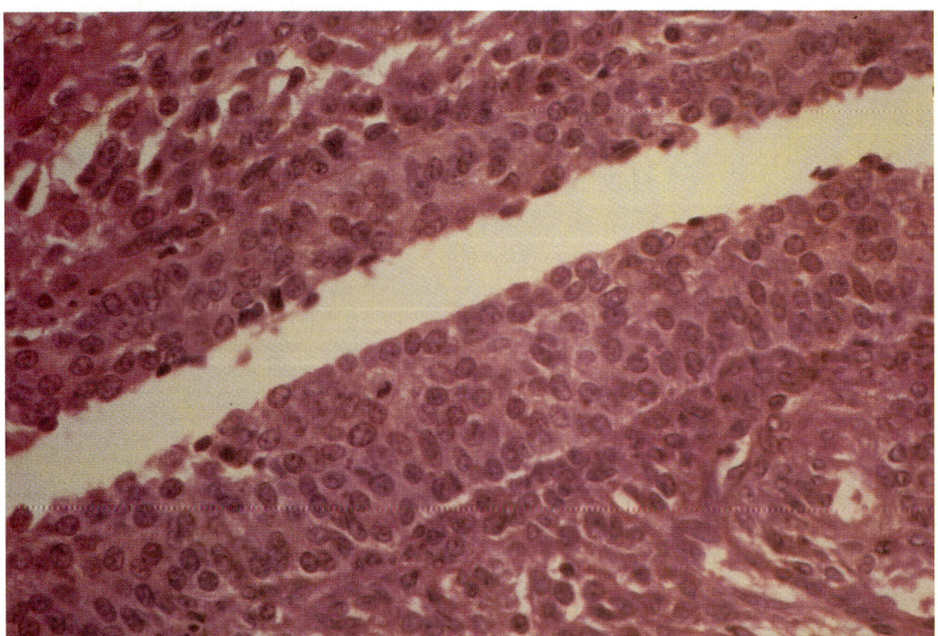

FIGURE 8–8
The granulosa cells (*center*) surround a flattened cavity. The theca interna layer is separated from the granulosa by a basement membrane, seen best at the top. The nuclei of the theca cells are more hyperchromatic than those of the granulosa cells. A reticulin stain of this would show a reticulin fiber framework around the theca cells.

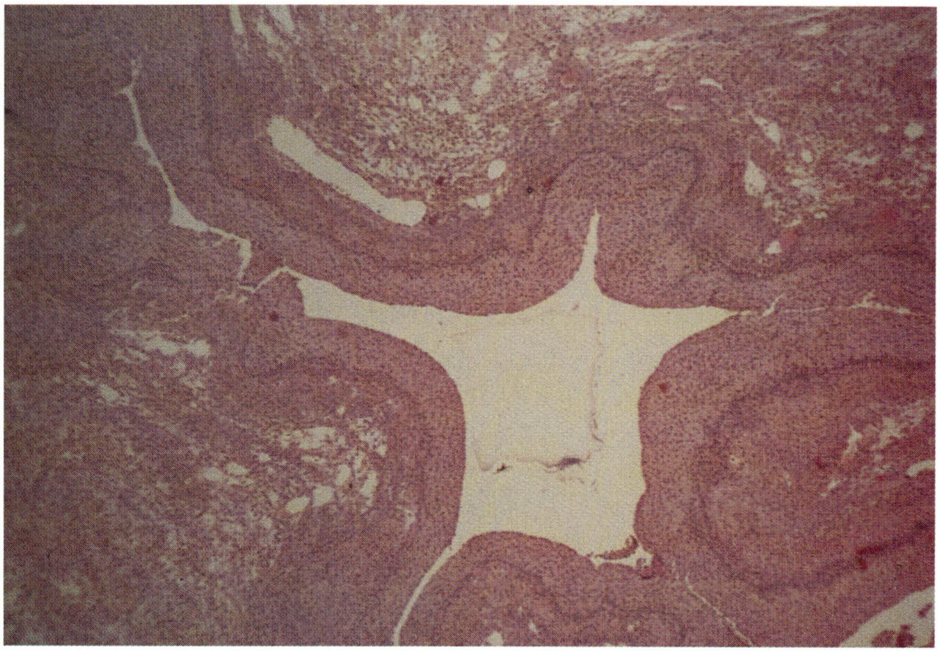

FIGURE 8–9
In this corpus luteum there is convolution of the granulosa and theca cell layers. A band of theca cells with hyperchromatic nuclei separates the granulosa cells from the thickened theca interna layer. Both the granulosa and the theca cells have increased cytoplasm from lipid accumulation. This appears as a yellow color on gross examination and is known as luteinization.

fibrosis of the central cavity occurs over several months, and this leads to the corpus albicans (i.e., white body). A mature corpora albicans is a dense collagenous structure that has a well-defined but convoluted border (Fig. 8–12). The process of aging of the corpus luteum has been described in detail by Corner.[13] Because there is great variability in the timing of the histologic appearance of the various stages of the corpus luteum, the histologic appearance cannot be used to indicate the ovulation date.

The postmenopausal ovary is small and shrunken and has a firm consistency. The cut surface is white. There is stromal atrophy and a decrease in the stromal cellularity associated with an increase in intercellular collagen. Primordial follicles are absent, and scattered corpora albicantia are present. In addition, the medullary blood vessels

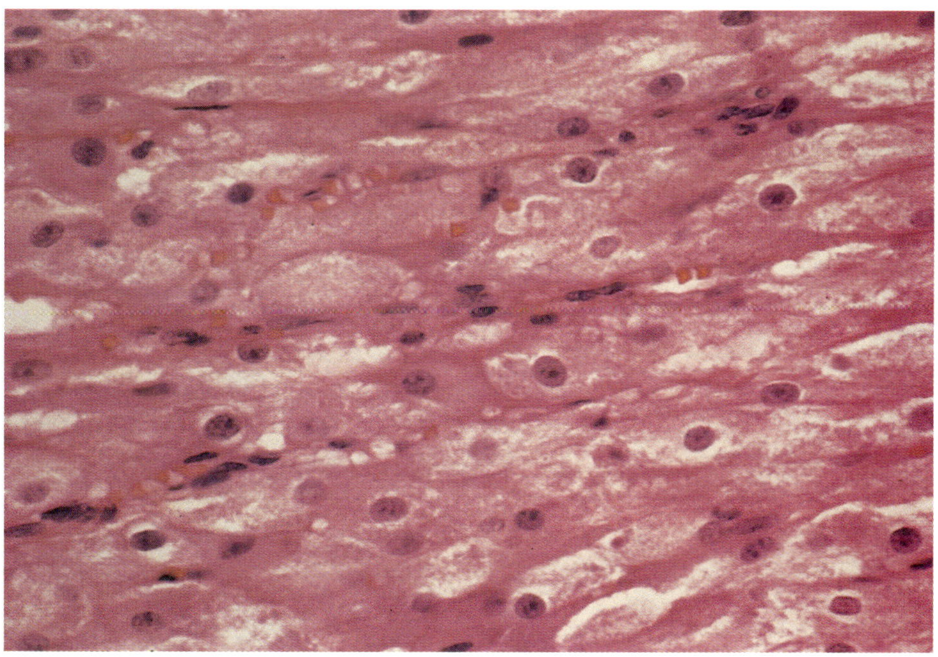

FIGURE 8–10
The "K" cells are interspersed among the luteinized theca cells. The theca cells have abundant cytoplasm with lipid accumulation. The "K" cells have dense eosinophilic cytoplasm and are stellate.

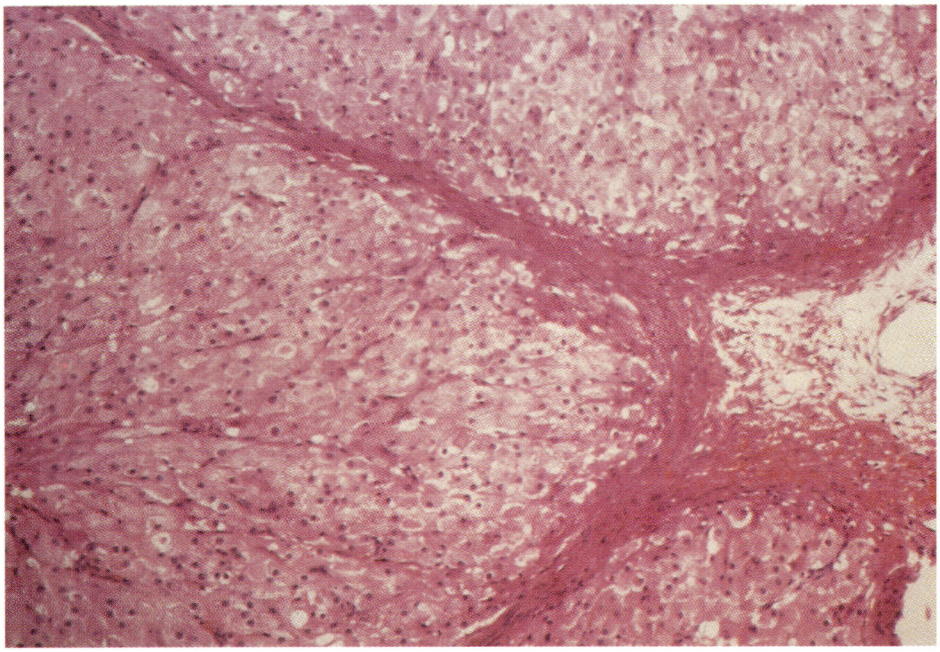

FIGURE 8-11
A maturing corpus luteum is seen. The granulosa cells are luteinized. Fibroblasts and capillaries are seen in the granulosa cell layer. The cavity seen at the far right is lined by loose fibrous connective tissue.

become more prominent. They have thick walls and increase in tortuosity, which may mimick a hemangioma. Other aging processes in the ovary include surface papillary proliferations, luteinization of stromal cells, and dense fibrosis.

FOLLICLE CYST

A follicle cyst is a non-neoplastic condition of the ovary. This cyst may attain a large size and may mimic a tumor. It arises from an ovarian follicle. Follicle cysts are usually solitary and most commonly occur in women of reproductive age, but they can be present during childhood or, rarely, after menopause.[14] They are generally discovered as an incidental finding at laparotomy or on pelvic ultrasound examination. Occasionally, a patient may present with either an adnexal mass or changes secondary to increased estrogen production (e.g., sexual precocity, endometrial hyperplasia).[14–16] The pathogenesis of the follicle cyst is

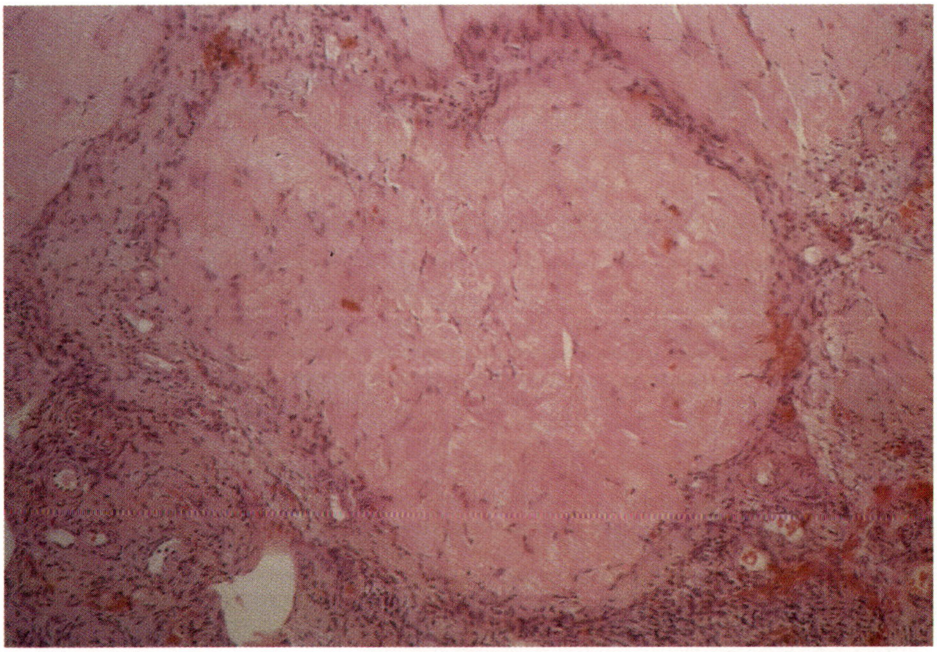

FIGURE 8-12
The convoluted shape of the corpus luteum is still apparent in this corpus albicans. However, the cells have been replaced by dense connective tissue.

believed to result from abnormal serum gonadotropin levels. Some cysts appear to be independent of gonadotropin control; these generally do not recur after removal. Rarely, a follicle cyst may rupture, causing a hemoperitoneum. This requires immediate surgical intervention.[17]

Solitary follicle cysts average 5 cm in diameter, have a thin wall, and are unilocular. They are lined by an inner granulosa cell layer and an outer theca interna layer (Fig. 8–13). Most follicle cysts regress spontaneously within 6 to 8 weeks and require no treatment. Follicle cysts can be distinguished both from follicles, which are typically less than 2 cm in diameter, and from surface epithelial inclusion cysts, which are lined by only a single layer of epithelial cells. Rarely, follicle cysts must be differentiated from unilocular granulosa cell tumors. The latter tend to be larger and demonstrate characteristic Call-Exner bodies. The microscopic appearance of both unilocular endometriotic cysts and cystic teratomas is sufficiently distinctive to pose no problem in differentiating them from follicle cysts.

Rarely, a specialized type of solitary follicle cyst can arise during pregnancy. It is similar to the classic follicle cyst described earlier except that it is larger and is lined by luteinized granulosa and theca cells that demonstrate nuclear atypia that is not associated with neoplasia. These changes are due to the high level of circulating human chorionic gonadotropin (hCG) associated with pregnancy.[18]

FOLLICLE HEMATOMA

A follicle hematoma is produced when there has been hemorrhage into the cavity of a cystic atretic follicle. The vessels of the theca layer are the source of the bleeding. Although these hematomas are generally small, they may occasionally reach a considerable size. Because of the hemorrhagic content, they can be confused with endometriotic cysts on gross examination. The lining of the follicle hematoma is composed of scattered granulosa and theca cells, fibrosis, and hyaline tissue (Fig. 8–14).

LUTEIN CYST

Both granulosa and theca cells are capable of undergoing luteinization under the influence of gonadotropins. Thus, lutein cysts of the ovary are divided into granulosa and theca lutein cysts depending on the cell of origin.

Corpus luteum cysts are the most common type of granulosa lutein cysts. They are solitary cysts of follicular origin that occur more commonly in women of reproductive age. Their clinical presentation, pathogenesis, behavior, and treatment are similar to those of follicle cysts. However, corpus luteum cysts are yellowish-orange in color, have a convoluted border, and contain serosanguineous or hemorrhagic fluid. A corpus luteum cyst is lined by granulosa and theca interna cells that show

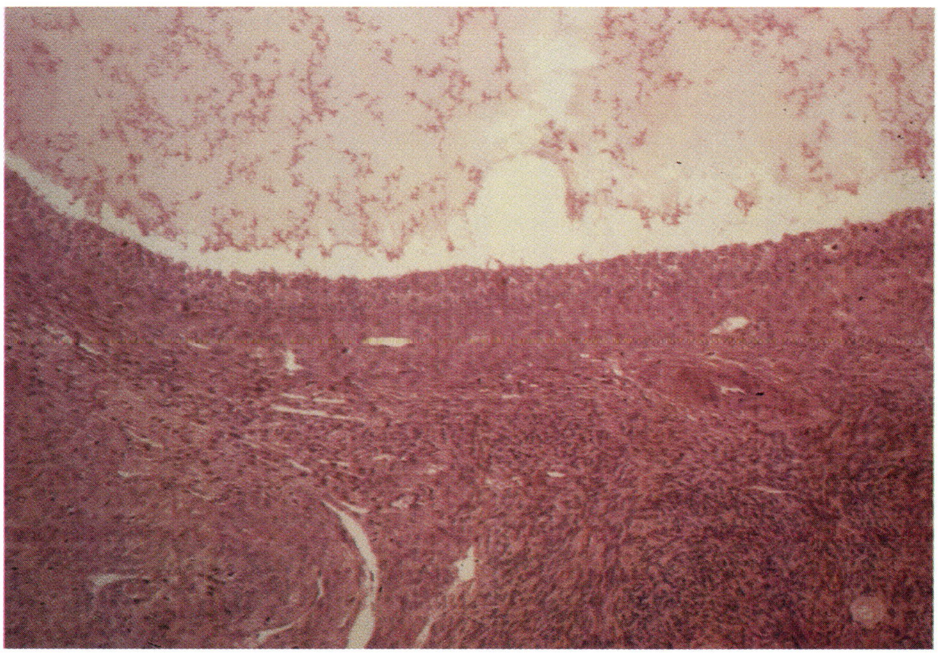

FIGURE 8-13
The large cavity is lined by an inner granulosa cell layer and an outer theca interna layer. A basement membrane separates these two layers.

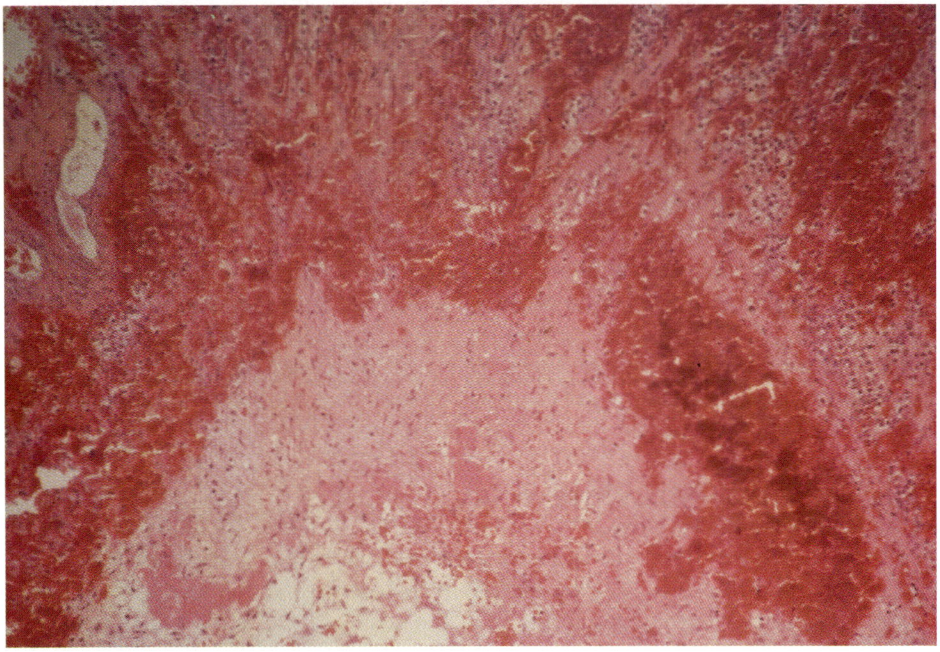

FIGURE 8-14
This follicle hematoma shows marked hemorrhage within the granulosa and theca cell layers. The center of the follicle is beginning to organize into dense fibrosis.

prominent luteinization. Involutional fibrosis of a corpus luteum cyst will result in a solid corpora albicans.

A theca lutein cyst is composed of luteinized theca cells. The granulosa cell layer is present, but it is narrow and the cells lack luteinization (Fig. 8–15). These cysts are generally very large, bilateral, and multiple (see also Chapter 12). They are filled with serous or hemorrhagic fluid. The nonspecialized stroma adjacent to the cysts may show edema and luteinization. Theca lutein cysts are also referred to as hyperreactio luteinalis. They are commonly associated with conditions in which there is a high level of circulating hCG (e.g., hydatidiform mole, choriocarcinoma, twin pregnancy).[19] These lutein cysts can be discovered by pelvic examination, ultrasound examination, or at the time of cesarean section. Complications associated with the presence of a theca lutein cyst include torsion, rupture with hemoperitoneum, and occasionally virilization. Rarely such a cyst will regress before delivery.[20] In gestational trophoblastic disease re-

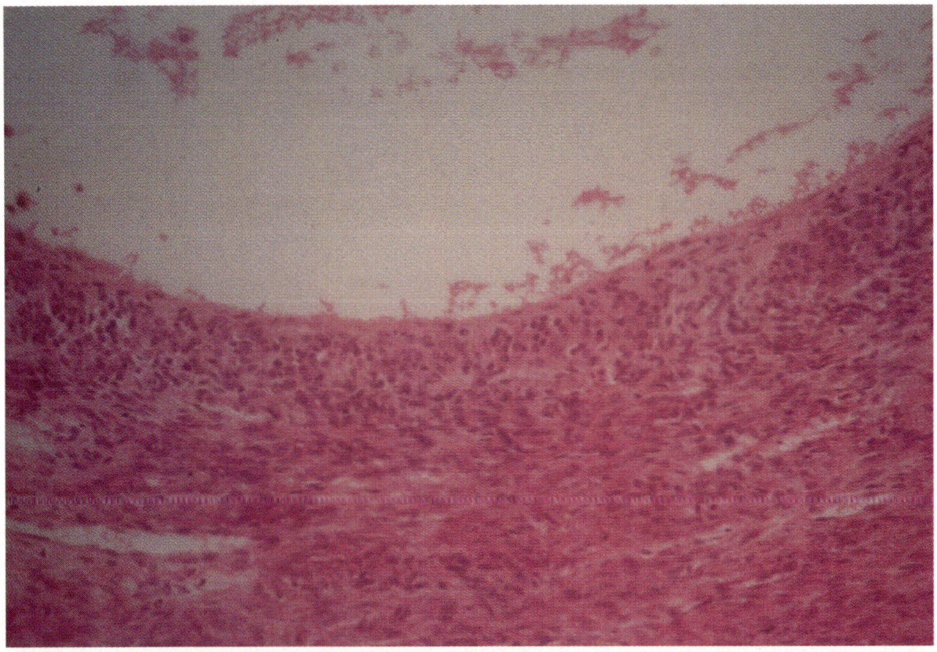

FIGURE 8-15
This theca lutein cyst is lined by luteinized theca cells. A separate granulosa cell layer is not evident on this photograph.

gression occurs within 3 months of the time of evacuation of the uterus. Surgery is required only when there has been a rupture or an infarction of the cyst.

LUTEOMA OF PREGNANCY

Luteoma of pregnancy, as the name implies, is a physiologic ovarian change associated with pregnancy. It typically occurs in black women in their third or fourth decade of life. It rarely produces a palpable pelvic mass. More often it is discovered incidentally at the time of cesarean section. It is believed to be the result of increased levels of hCG during pregnancy. The hCG induces a marked proliferation of luteinized ovarian stromal cells (Fig. 8–16). This in turn causes an elevation of plasma testosterone, which is responsible for the virilization of mother or fetus in a small proportion of cases.[21,22]

A luteoma of pregnancy may produce an ovary that is enlarged to approximately 7 cm (range, 5 to 25 cm) by either single or multiple, well-circumscribed, soft, yellowish-brown nodules. Both ovaries are involved in over one-third of cases. The nodules are composed of sheets, nests, or cords of polygonal cells that have abundant eosinophilic, lacy cytoplasm and a round, moderately hyperchromatic nucleus that has a prominent nucleolus (Fig. 8–17). Mitoses are usually not present, but in some cases up to seven mitoses per 10 high-power microscopic fields have been identified.[23]

Generally, luteoma of pregnancy is sufficiently characteristic in both its clinical presentation and its appearance to cause little difficulty in differentiating it from conditions such as corpus luteum of pregnancy and theca lutein cyst. Luteinized granulosa cell tumor and other steroid cell neoplasms must also be considered in the differential diagnosis (also see Chapter 11). These latter lesions are generally unilateral and present as a single enlarging nodule in the ovary. Multiple histologic sections reveal the characteristic patterns of these lesions, making it relatively easy to arrive at the correct diagnosis.

If the pregnancy has been terminated, the luteoma undergoes regression. This involves hemorrhage, necrosis, and finally scar formation. Concomitant with regression, plasma testosterone levels decrease to reach normal levels 2 weeks postpartum. Because this is a self-limited entity no treatment is necessary. However, if a solid adnexal mass is discovered (usually by ultrasound examination) during pregnancy or at the time of cesarean section it may not be possible to make the correct diagnosis unless a biopsy is obtained. To avoid contamination of the peritoneal cavity if the mass turns out to be a malignant neoplasm, biopsy is performed with the mass outside of the laparotomy incision after packing has been placed around the mass. The presence of bilateral solid ovarian tumors found during pregnancy in association with increased circulating testosterone levels favors the diagnosis of luteoma of pregnancy.

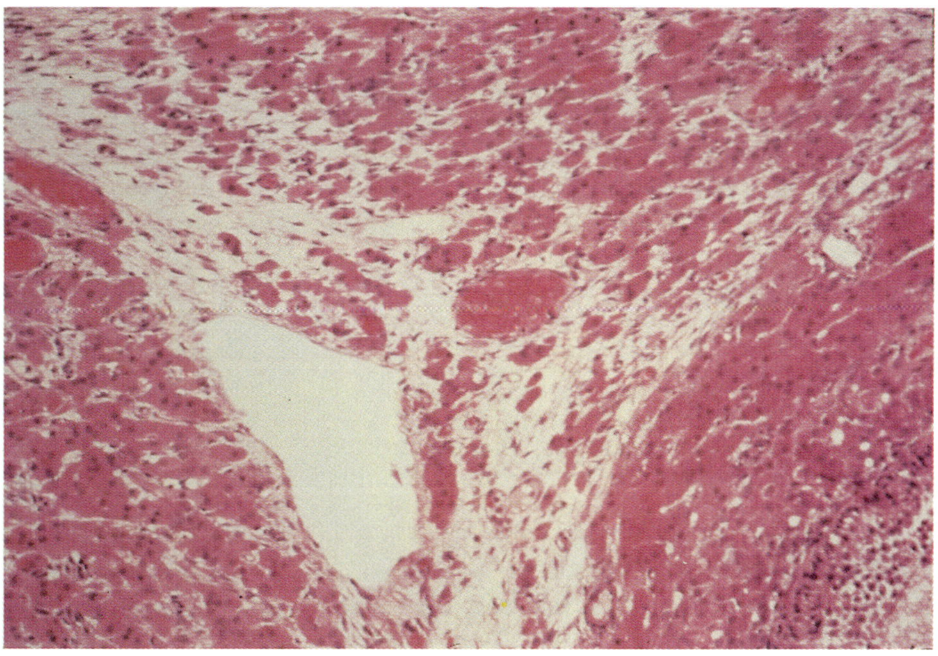

FIGURE 8–16
This luteoma of pregnancy has an increased vascularity. The ovarian stromal cells have uniform nuclei and abundant, deeply eosinophilic cytoplasm. (Courtesy of Dr. J. Donald Woodruff, The Johns Hopkins Hospital, Baltimore, MD.)

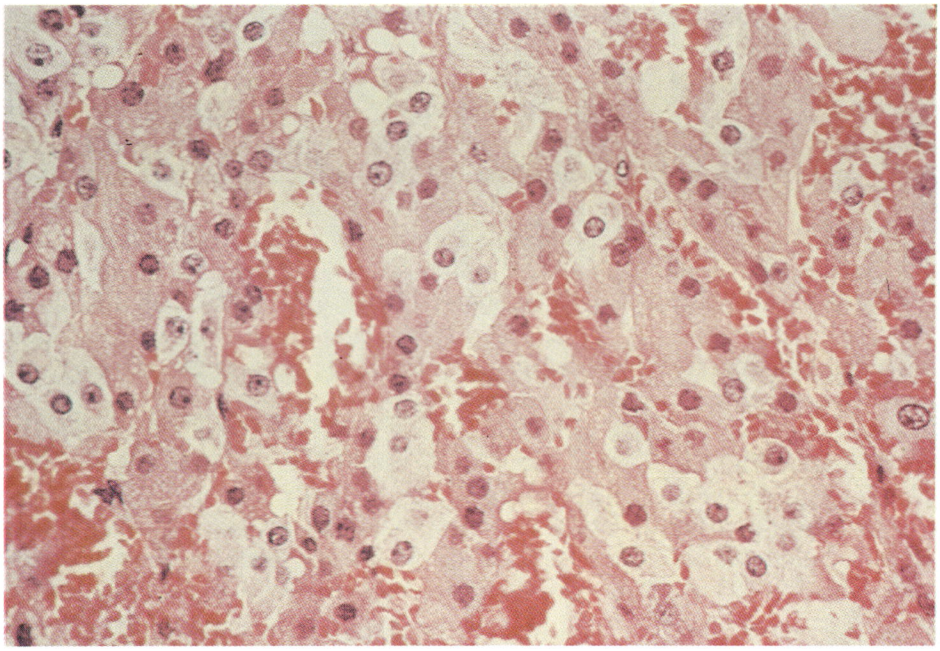

FIGURE 8-17
A high-power view of a luteoma of pregnancy is seen. The cytoplasm of the ovarian stromal cells is very abundant and varies from eosinophilic to pale. It has a lacy appearance. The nuclei are round and regular and have prominent nucleoli. (Courtesy of Dr. J. Donald Woodruff, The Johns Hopkins Hospital, Baltimore, MD.)

POLYCYSTIC OVARIES

The syndrome of polycystic ovaries (PCO) was first described in 1935 by Stein and Leventhal. It is a disorder characterized by slightly enlarged, sclerocystic ovaries associated with anovulation. It is usually identified in women in their third decade of life. Rarely, it may present as a palpable adnexal mass. Typically, the patient with PCO syndrome is obese, infertile, and hirsute. The patient experiences menstrual irregularities, which range from oligomenorrhea to menometrorrhagia.[24, 25] Rarely, the patient with PCO is normal in appearance or has frank virilization.[25a] Although studies have not documented a definite mode of inheritance, some cases of PCO syndrome have been familial.[25]

The pathogenesis of PCO syndrome is not completely understood, but a hypothalamic disturbance that causes an increased production of luteinizing hormone-releasing factor (LHRF) is central to the pathophysiology of the condition.[25,25b] This excess LHRF leads to erratic elevations of luteinizing hormone (LH), which, although not conducive to ovulation, stimulate the production of androgens (primarily androstenedione) by the theca interna cells.[26] Androstenedione is converted to estrone in peripheral adipose tissue, resulting in a reversal of the estradiol-estrone ratio and leading to an increased LHRF output. This in turn results in a tonic elevation of LH and selective inhibition of follicle-stimulating hormone (FSH) release. As a consequence of these hormonal changes, estrogen production by the follicle is diminished and an increased androgen environment occurs in the ovary. This, along with the elevated LH level, is responsible for the interruption in follicle growth and anovulation. Obesity associated with enhanced androstenedione conversion to estrone helps to maintain the increased LH production, and the subsequent chain of events leads to hyperandrogenism and anovulation.[27] The effect of unopposed estrogen is predominantly seen in the endometrium, which often shows the entire spectrum of hyperplastic changes (see Chapter 6). A small number of patients with PCO may go on to develop endometrial adenocarcinoma. If this happens, the tumor is almost always of low grade and is associated with minimal myometrial invasion.[28,29] Hyperprolactinemia is present in approximately one-fourth of the patients.[25] Although some patients with PCO have a coexisting pituitary adenoma, in the majority of cases a disturbance in the dopaminergic inhibition of prolactin secretion by the pituitary is believed to be responsible for the hyperprolactinemia.

On gross examination both ovaries typically are enlarged and round. On cut section the superficial cortex is thickened, white, and fibrotic. Situated below the cortex are multiple small cysts, usually of equal size, which average less than 1 cm in diameter. On microscopic examination the outer cortex is hypocellular and there is an increase in collagen, producing the appearance of a true capsule (Fig. 8-18). There is also an increased number of thick-walled vessels. The cysts are generally

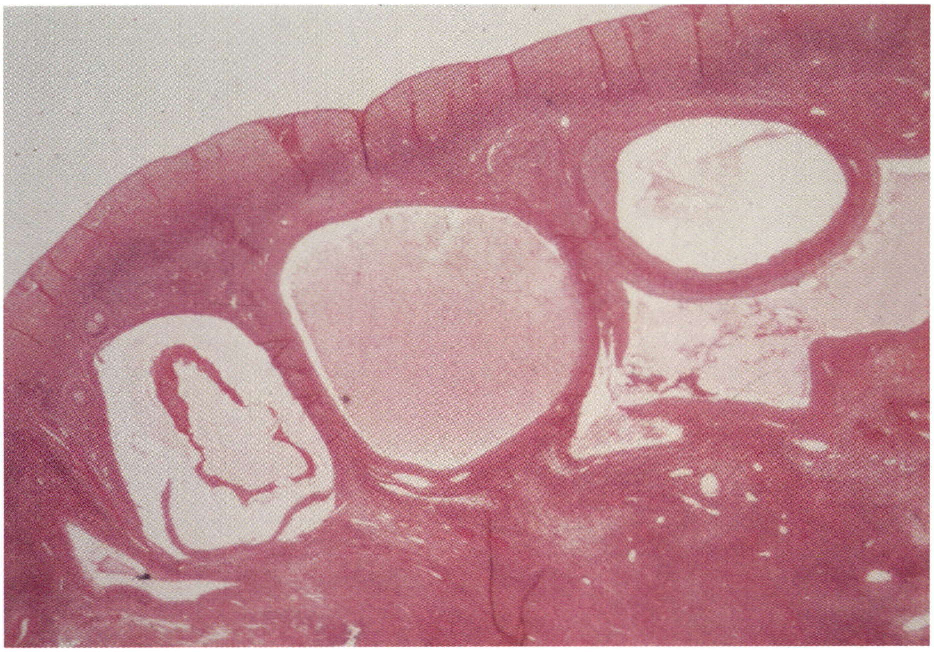

FIGURE 8-18
A low-power view of a polycystic ovary shows that the ovarian cortex near the surface is slightly fibrotic, giving the appearance of a thickened capsule. Several cystic follicles are seen.

lined by nonluteinized granulosa cells surrounded by an outer layer of hyperplastic, luteinized theca interna cells (follicular hyperthecosis). This hyperplasia is due to the high tonic LH levels. Although a normal number of primordial follicles are present, the follicles that demonstrate a midantral stage of development are more common than normal. Corpora lutea and corpora albicantia are generally absent, but their presence does not exclude the diagnosis of PCO in an otherwise typical case. The deeper cortex and medulla show stromal hyperplasia, and focally cells with luteinization are present. Classic PCO must be distinguished from other conditions that cause PCO and anovulation. These are often secondary to other abnormalities of gonadotropin release such as virilizing adrenal tumors, Cushing syndrome, and estrogen- and androgen-secreting ovarian tumors.

Polycystic ovaries can be seen in children or in young girls during the first year after the onset of puberty. PCO has been reported in patients who are taking long-term oral contraceptive treatment[30] and in patients with some non-neoplastic conditions such as stromal hyperthecosis[31] and Leydig cell hyperplasia.

The treatment of PCO is tailored to the patient's wishes. If the patient does not desire a pregnancy, oral contraceptives can be used to cause cyclic and controlled withdrawal uterine bleeding. These will protect the endometrium from the unopposed estrogen characteristic of this syndrome and will reduce androgen levels in the circulation. Alternatively, a progestin (e.g., 10 mg medroxyprogesterone acetate) is given for the first 12 to 14 days of every month. If the patient desires pregnancy, clomiphene citrate is used. Clomiphene blocks the effect of estrogen on the hypothalamus, resulting in increased FSH and LH output. This in turn initiates the events that occur in the normal ovulatory cycle including follicle recruitment, increased circulatory estradiol levels with a concomitant gradual decrease in the secretion of gonadotropins, and eventual triggering of an endogenous LH surge, resulting in ovulation.

OVARIAN EDEMA

Ovarian edema is characterized by enematous enlargement of one or both ovaries. The condition is typically seen in women who are in their twenties. They generally present with pelvic pain and irregular menstrual cycles. A small percentage of these patients may exhibit hirsutism or virilization.[32] Serum testosterone levels are elevated in some but not in all cases. The condition is bilateral in approximately 25 percent of cases. An enlarged adnexal mass can be palpated on pelvic examination. The condition is believed to follow periodic episodes of torsion of an ovary that previously was enlarged by fibromatosis or stromal hyperplasia.[32] The resulting vascular congestion and lymphatic dilatation induces an accumulation of edematous fluid within the ovarian stroma. The ovary is enlarged, ranging in size from 5 to 35 cm. It is soft to palpation and has a smooth, tan-white external surface (Fig. 8-19). Cross section reveals a white, fibrotic cortical layer below the capsule and tan-

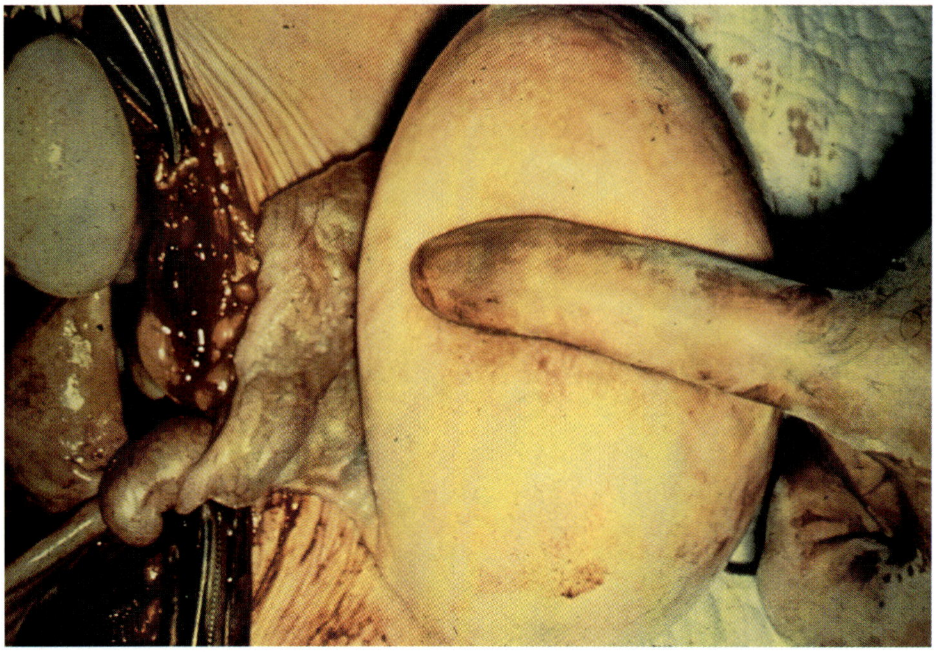

FIGURE 8-19
An enlarged edematous ovary is being held by the surgeon. The surface is smooth and tan-white. Its vascular pedicle (*left*) is twisted. (Courtesy of Dr. J. Donald Woodruff, The Johns Hopkins Hospital, Baltimore, MD.)

white, gelatinous interior that oozes edematous fluid when pressure is applied. On microscopic examination the ovarian stromal cells are widely separated by pale pink edematous fluid. The superficial cortex is uninvolved in the edematous process and appears fibrotic. In more than one-third of cases foci of luteinized cells are present, accounting for the androgenic manifestations (Fig. 8–20). Ovarian edema must be distinguished from fibrosis and from a sclerosing stromal tumor that may occasionally show myxoid degeneration.

ENDOMETRIOSIS

Endometriosis is the presence of normal endometrial glands and stroma at a site other than the endometrium. Endometriosis is most commonly found in mesothelium-covered surfaces (e.g., peritoneum, pleura), and the ovary is one of the sites most frequently involved.[33] Several theories have been advanced to explain the origin of endometriosis. These include metaplastic transformation of the mesothelium, implantation of endometrium

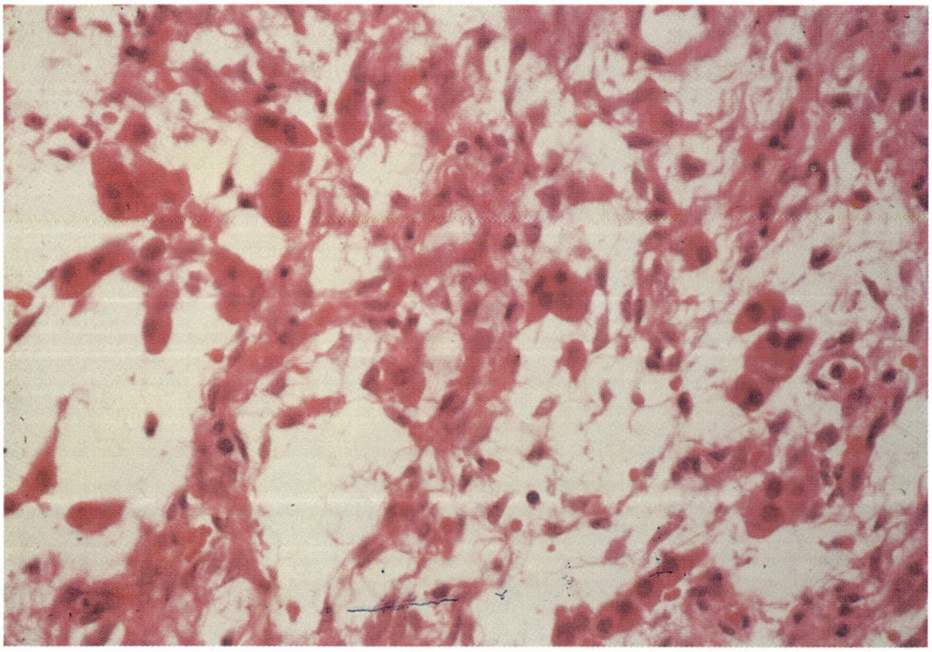

FIGURE 8-20
The ovarian stromal cells are separated by extracellular edema fluid. Some of the cells have abundant, deeply eosinophilic cytoplasm diagnostic of luteinization. (Courtesy of Dr. J. Donald Woodruff, The Johns Hopkins Hospital, Baltimore, MD.)

from retrograde menstruation, and hematogenous or lymphatic embolization.[34] These theories are used to explain endometriosis that occurs at various distant sites (e.g., pelvis, pleura, postsurgical abdominal skin scar).

Women who have endometriosis may experience pain and infertility. Infertility associated with endometriosis can occur even in the presence of minimal disease, and the explanation for this is not clear. Paradoxically, some patients who have minimal endometriosis experience severe pain, whereas others who have severe endometriosis have no symptoms.

The typical endometriotic implant is described as "powder burn–like." This is a puckered, blue-black lesion (Fig. 8–21). However, areas of scarring, telangiectasia, redness, and small clear vesicles as well as apparently normal peritoneum have been found to contain endometriosis.[35, 36] Endometriotic implants may contain only endometrial glands or endometrial stroma, or both. In many cases, scarring and the presence of hemosiderin-laden macrophages are the only evidence of previous endometriosis. Implants of endometriosis respond to sex hormones. During the menstrual cycle the glands and stroma of endometriosis may undergo changes similar to those seen in the normal endometrium. During menstruation they can bleed. In the ovary, chronic cyclic bleeding from endometriosis may result in an endometrioma, the so-called chocolate cyst (Fig. 8–22).

Modern surgical management of endometriosis involves laparoscopic identification of endometriotic implants and their ablation using laser or electrocautery techniques.[37, 38] Modern medical management involves prescription of danocrine or gonadotropin-releasing hormone analogs.[36, 38a] Progestogens may also be used for medical management.[39]

TUMORS METASTATIC TO THE OVARIES

Metastasis to the ovaries occurs in only 5 percent of women who have cancer.[40] However, 5 to 10 percent of all malignant ovarian tumors are secondary neoplasms that have presented as possible primary ovarian tumors.[41] Those cancers that most frequently spread to the ovaries (excluding those that spread by direct extension) include metastases from the breast, colon or rectum, endometrium, and cervix.[42, 43] Although autopsy series of patients who died from leukemia or lymphoma have found that the ovaries are the site of metastatic spread in 25 percent of cases, premortem ovarian enlargement as an initial manifestation of disease occurs in less than 1 percent of patients.[44] Metastatic malignant tumors to the ovaries are bilateral in approximately 60 percent of cases.[40] When metastatic disease to the ovaries presents as a solid tumor, the microscopic appearance is usually distinctive enough to allow an accurate diagnosis. However, cystic metastases, especially metastatic colon adenocarcinoma, are frequently misdiagnosed as a primary ovarian carcinoma. This subject will be further discussed in the chap-

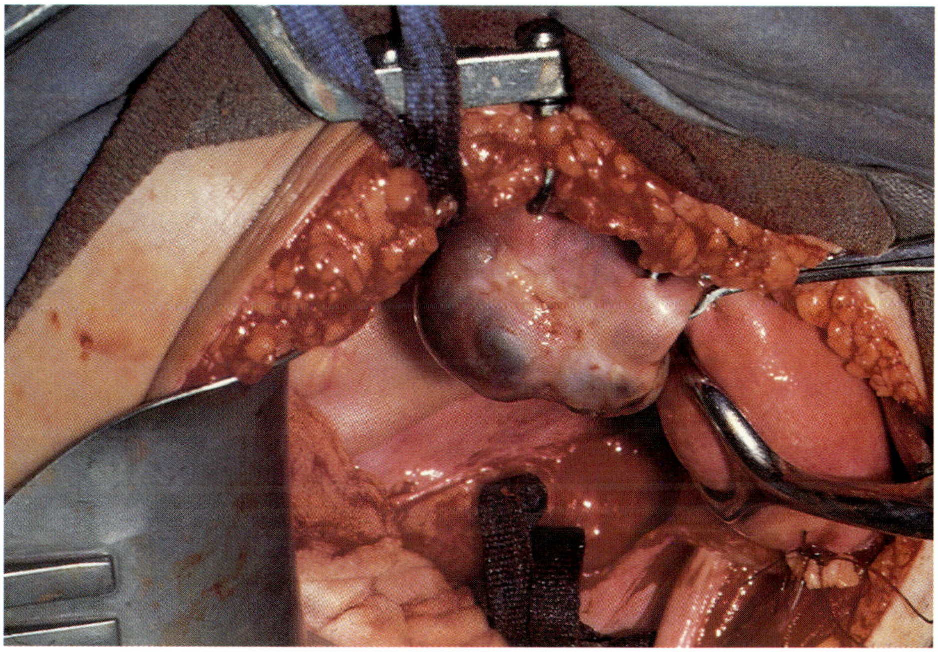

FIGURE 8-21
A slightly enlarged left ovary is shown. Several bluish cysts are present under the ovarian surface. The irregular bluish-brown areas on the ovarian surface closer to the uterus suggest endometriosis. By microscopic examination, all these changes proved to be endometriosis.

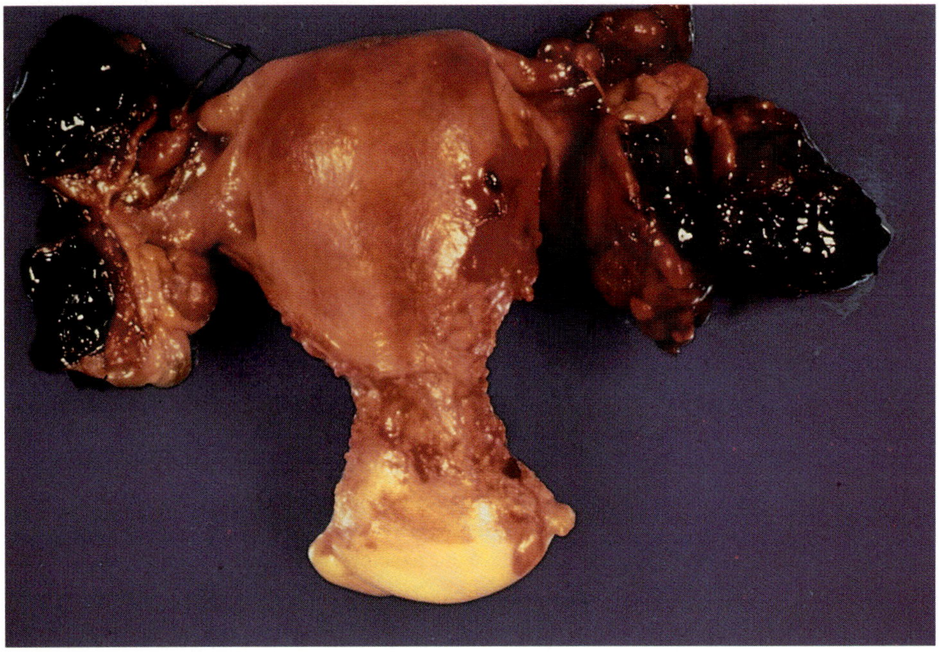

FIGURE 8-22
This hysterectomy specimen shows bilateral endometriomas flanking a normal uterus. The cysts have been opened, and their content consists of old blood that often is dark brown and thick, giving the nickname of chocolate cyst. A dark brown spot of endometriosis is seen on the serosal surface of the uterine fundus. (Courtesy of Dr. Deborah Powell, University of Kentucky, Lexington, KY.)

ter on epithelial ovarian tumors (Chapter 9). Two situations not covered in other chapters, breast cancer metastatic to the ovaries and the Krukenberg tumor, will be discussed here.

Breast Cancer Metastatic to the Ovary

Metastasis to the ovary from breast cancer occurs in the presence of recurrent or advanced disease. The presence of tumor in the ovary is not grossly recognized in half of the cases.[41] In a third of cases the metastases are microscopic (less than 1 mm). The ovary is enlarged to more than 5 cm in only 15 percent of cases. Bilateral ovarian involvement is present in one-half of cascs. In three-fourths of cases the microscopic appearance is described as a single file or ductal-type arrangement. These are infiltrating rows of cells that show nuclear mold-

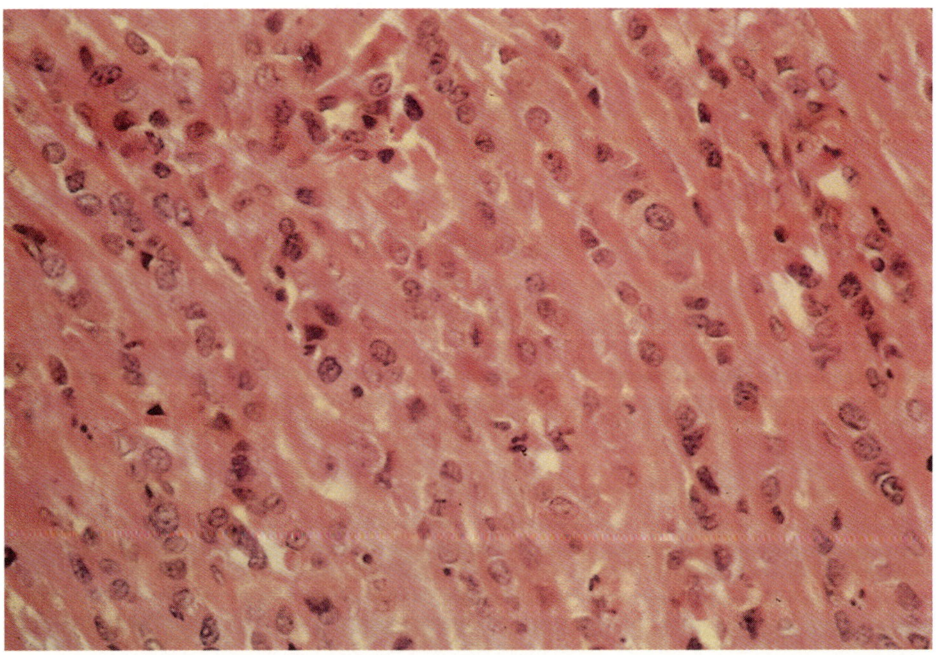

FIGURE 8-23
Rows of single-file cells from a breast cancer infiltrate the ovarian stroma. The cells have scant cytoplasm, and there is nuclear pleomorphism.

ing. These patterns are usually easily recognized as metastases of breast cancer (Fig. 8–23). Other cases present various histopathologic features that may mimic either a primary ovarian tumor or tumor-like conditions such as luteoma, hyperthecosis, dysgerminoma, granulosa cell tumor, or carcinoid tumor.[41, 43] All women who have an ovarian carcinoma should have a careful breast examination and bilateral mammograms to exclude the presence of metastatic disease or a second primary. If synchronous ovarian and breast cancer occurs, the histopathology of both lesions should be compared to exclude the presence of metastatic disease.

Krukenberg Tumor

This tumor was originally believed by Krukenberg in 1896 to be an unusual type of mucin-producing, primary fibrosarcoma of the ovary. The tumor now recognized as a Krukenberg tumor is a signet ring cell carcinoma that infiltrates a very cellular but nonmalignant stroma.[45] Although most Krukenberg tumors represent metastatic carcinomas to the ovaries, primary ovarian Krukenberg tumors have been reported. These are thought to arise from an ovarian teratoma.[46]

In one series of 27 Krukenberg tumors the age range of patients was between 20 and 70 years.[45] Almost half of the patients were 40 years of age or younger. Review of a series of 48 cases of Krukenberg tumor from the Emil Novak Ovarian Tumor Registry revealed that the patients' average age was 40 years.[46]

The presenting signs and symptoms of patients with a Krukenberg tumor are related to the presence of a pelvic or abdominal mass or other metastases. Abdominal swelling and pain are the most common symptoms. Abnormal vaginal bleeding occurs in a few patients.

Gastric carcinoma is the most frequent primary tumor that metastasizes to the ovary to produce Krukenberg tumor. Colonic carcinoma is the next most frequent primary site. The presence of a primary gastrointestinal carcinoma is found before the ovarian tumor is discovered in only 25 percent of cases. In 50 percent of cases the ovarian and gastrointestinal tumors are diagnosed synchronously.[45]

Most Krukenberg tumors present as bilateral, solid ovarian masses with a maximum diameter of between 2.5 and 15 cm. Usually the ovaries are asymmetrically enlarged, and they are lobulated and firm (Fig. 8–24). On cut section they are yellowish-tan, pink, or gray-white in color. The entire ovary is replaced by ill-defined nodules. Edematous, gelatinous, or myxoid areas may also be present.[45]

The histopathologic appearance of Krukenberg tumor is that of diffuse infiltration of the cellular but benign stroma by mucin-secreting cells, many of which have a signet ring appearance (Fig. 8–

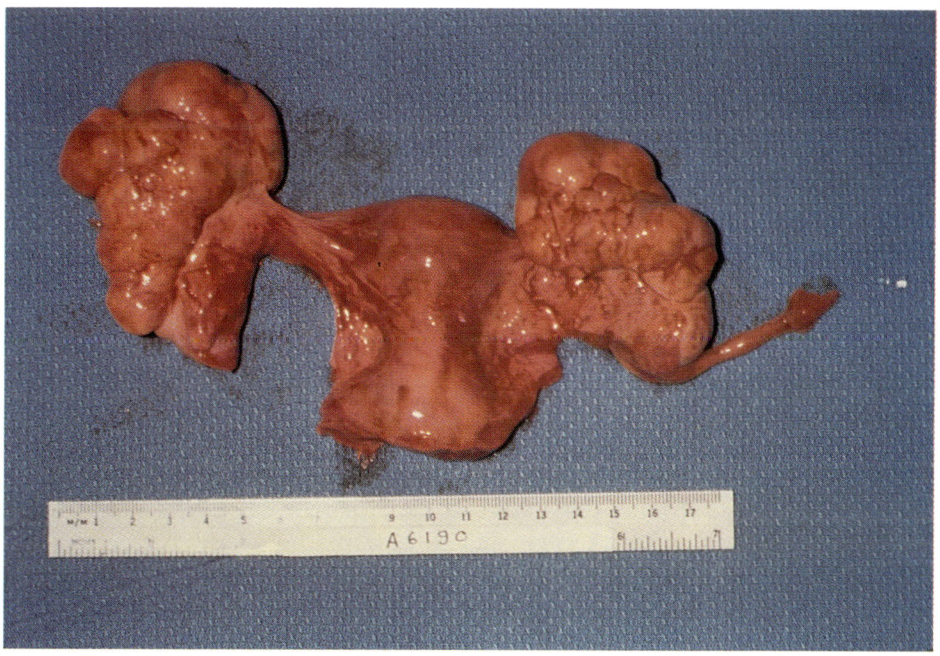

FIGURE 8–24
This autopsy specimen was removed from a 24-year-old woman who had a small gastric carcinoma. Both ovaries are enlarged, lobulated, and yellowish orange. They felt firm. By microscopic examination, metastasis from the gastric carcinoma was confirmed.

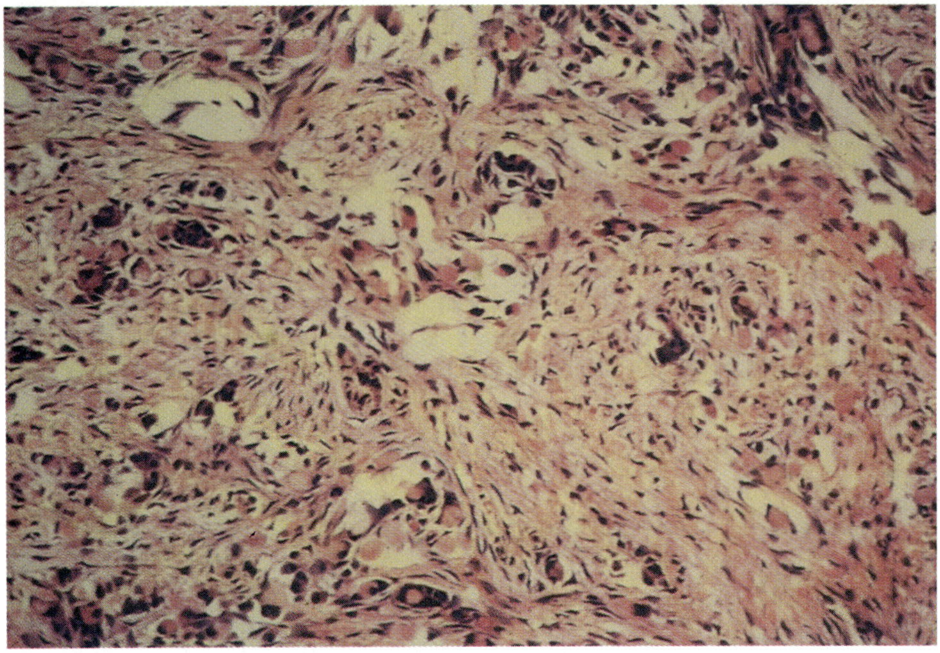

FIGURE 8–25
The histopathologic appearance of a Krukenberg tumor is seen. There is infiltration of a fibrotic stroma by malignant cells. Some of these cells have a signet-ring appearance. These are the ones with the abundant pale pink cytoplasm and the nucleus pushed to the side. (Courtesy of Dr. J. Donald Woodruff, The Johns Hopkins Hospital, Baltimore, MD.)

25). These cells have large intracytoplasmic vacuoles that push the nucleus to an eccentric position against the cytoplasmic membrane. The vacuoles indent and distort the nuclear shape. Some of the carcinoma cells are not vacuolated but contain a granular cytoplasm. Single malignant cells are found within the stroma, but they may also form linear cords, trabeculae, and clusters. Acini are found in the majority of cases, but these may be focal. Scattered small glands or tubules may be seen. In some instances solid sheets of signet ring carcinoma cells are found. The accompanying ovarian stroma is cellular and may assume a storiform or whorled pattern associated with dense collagen formation. When the malignant cells are relatively dispersed within a hyperplastic stroma the tumor may be misdiagnosed as a fibroma or fibrous histiocytoma. The presence of mucin-secreting carinoma cells in these cases can be identified using a mucicarmine stain or periodic acid–Schiff (PAS) stain. The presence of PAS-positive material indicates the presence of glycogen, which is found in a variety of benign and malignant cells. If a duplicate histologic section is pretreated with diastase and then stained by the PAS technique, all of the positive staining reaction will disappear if it is due to the presence of glycogen. No reduction in positive staining indicates the presence of mucin. It has been recommended that this PAS with diastase digestion technique be used before any ovarian tumor is diagnosed as a primary stromal neoplasm.[45] This PAS stain may disclose the presence of carcinomatous cells in areas where they are not otherwise easily visualized.

Areas of edema are also frequently present in Krukenberg tumors, especially near the medulla. Carcinomatous cells in lymphovascular spaces are found in more than half of cases when a careful search is made. These are more frequent in the hilum, mesovarium, and mesosalpinx regions.

CLASSIFICATION OF OVARIAN NEOPLASMS

The following chapters cover the neoplasms that arise in the ovaries. WHO classifies benign and malignant ovarian neoplasms into nine major groups (Table 8–1).[47] We have divided ovarian

TABLE 8–1.

Major Histopathologic Groups of Ovarian Neoplasms According to the WHO Classification

1. Common epithelial tumors
2. Sex-cord stroma (specialized stroma) tumors
3. Lipid (lipoid) cell tumors
4. Germ cell tumors
5. Gonadoblastoma
6. Soft tissue tumors not specific to the ovary
7. Unclassified tumors
8. Secondary (metastatic) tumors
9. Tumor-like conditions

tumors into those of epithelial, germ cell, and stromal (specialized stroma and nonspecific mesenchyme) origin. These will be discussed in Chapters 9, 10, and 11, respectively.

REFERENCES

1. Way S: The lymphatics of the pelvis. *In* Scientific Foundation of Obstetrics and Gynecology. Phillips EE, Barnes J, Newton M (eds): London, Heinemann, 1977, pp 118–126.
2. Plentl AA, Friedman EA: Lymphatic System of the Female Genitalia. Philadelphia, WB Saunders, 1971.
3. Jacobowitz D, Wallach EE: Histochemical and chemical studies of the autonomic innervation of the ovary. Endocrinology 1967;81:1132–1139.
4. Miettinen M, Lento V, Virtanen I: Expression of intermediate filaments in normal ovaries and ovarian epithelial, sex-cord stromal, and germinal tumors. Int J Gynecol Pathol 1983;2:64–71.
5. Kabawat SE, Bast RC Jr, Bhan AK, Welch WR, Knapp RC, Colvin RB: Tissue distribution of coelomic-epithelium-related antigen recognized by the monoclonal antibody OC 125. Int J Gynecol Pathol 1983;2:275–285.
6. Boss JH, Scully RE, Wagner KH, Cohen RB: Structural variations in the adult ovary: Clinical significance. Obstet Gynecol 1965;25:747–763.
7. Israel SL, Rubenstone A, Meranze DR: The ovary at term: I. Decidua-like reaction of surface cell proliferation. Obstet Gynecol 1954;3:399–407.
8. Hertig AT: The primary human oocyte: Some observations on the fine structure of Balbiani's vitelline body and the origin of the annulate lamellae. Am J Anat 1968;122:107–138.
9. Balboni GC: Structural changes: Ovulation and luteal phase. *In* Serra GB (ed): The Ovary. New York, Raven Press, 1983.
10. Nelson WW, Greene RR: Some observations on the histology of the human ovary during pregnancy. Am J Obstet Gynecol 1958;76:66–89.
11. White RF, Hertig AT, Rock J, Adams E: Histological and histochemical observations of the corpus luteum of human pregnancy with special reference to corpora lutea associated with early normal and abnormal ovaries. Contrib Embryol 1951;34:55–74.
12. Gillim SW, Christensen AK, McLennan CE: Fine structure of the human menstrual corpus luteum at its stage of maximum secretory activity. Am J Anat 1969;126:409–428.
13. Corner GW Jr: The histological dating of the human corpus luteum of menstruation. Am J Anat 1956;98:377–401.
14. Strickler RC, Kelley RW, Askin FB: Post-menopausal ovarian follicle cyst: An unusual case of estrogen excess. Int J Gynecol Pathol 1984;3:318–322.
15. Muechler EK, Florack AT, Cary D, Kapakis M: Isosexual precocious puberty with luteinized follicular cyst. NY State J Med 1982;82:1353–1356.
16. Monteleone JA, Monteleone PL, Danis RK: Pseudo-precocious puberty associated with isolated follicle cyst of the ovary. J Pediatr Surg 1973;8:949–950.
17. Hallat JG, Steele CH Jr, Snyder M: Ruptured corpus luteum with hemoperitoneum: A study of 173 surgical cases. Am J Obstet Gynecol 1984;149:5–9.
18. Clement PB, Scully RE: Large solitary luteinized follicle cyst of pregnancy and puerperium. Am J Surg Pathol 1980;4:431–438.
19. Caspi E, Schreyer P, Bukovsky J: Ovarian cysts in pregnancy. Obstet Gynecol 1973;42:388–398.
20. Levine SC, Huffaker J, Jacobsen JB, Brodey PA, Fisch AE: Second trimester spontaneous regression of theca lutein cysts. Obstet Gynecol 1982;6:125–126.
21. Wolff E, Glasser M, Gordon GG, Olivo J, Southren AL: Virilizing luteoma of pregnancy. Am J Med 1973;54:229–233.
22. Garcia-Bunuel R, Berek JS, Woodruff JD: Luteoma of pregnancy. Obstet Gynecol 1975;45:407–414.
23. Sternberg WH, Barclay DL: Luteoma of pregnancy. Am J Obstet Gynecol 1966;95:165–181.
24. Yen SSC: The polycystic ovary syndrome. Clin Endocrinol 1980;12:177–203.
25. Futterweit W: Polycystic ovarian disease. Clinical Perspectives in Obstetrics and Gynecology. New York, Springer-Verlag, 1985.

25a. Young RH, Scully RE: Ovarian pathology in infertility. *In* Krans FT (ed): Pathology of Reproductive Failure. Baltimore, Williams & Wilkins, 1991, pp 104–139.

25b. McKenna TJ: Pathogenesis and treatment of polycystic ovary syndrome. N Engl J Med 1988;318:558–562.

26. Biggs JSG: Polycystic ovarian disease: Current concepts. Aust NZ J Obstet Gynecol 1981;21:26–36.
27. Bates GW, Whitworth NS: Effect of body weight reduction on plasma androgens in obese, infertile women. Fertil Steril 1982;38:406–409.
28. McDonald TW, Malkasian GD, Gaffey TA: Endometrial cancer associated with feminizing ovarian tumors and polycystic ovarian disease. Obstet Gynecol 1977;49:654–658.
29. Jafari K, Javaheri G, Ruiz G: Endometrial adenocarcinoma and the Stein-Leventhal syndrome. Obstet Gynecol 1978;51:97–100.
30. Plate WP: Ovarian changes after long-term oral contraceptives. Acta Endocrinol 1967;55:71–77.
31. Castleman B, Scully RE, McNeely BU (eds): Case records of the Massachusetts General Hospital: Weekly clinicopathologic exercises, case 49-1972 (hyperthecosis of ovaries). N Engl J Med 1972;287:1192–1195.
32. Young RH, Scully Re: Fibromatosis and massive edema of the ovary, possibly related entities: A report of 14 cases of fibromatosis and 11 cases of massive edema. Int J Gynecol Pathol 1984;3:153–178.
33. Williams TJ, Pratt JH: Endometriosis in 1,000 consecutive celiotomies: Incidence and management. Am J Obstet Gynecol 1977;129:245–250.
34. Glass RH: Infertility. *In* Yen SSC, Jaffe RB (eds): Reproductive Endocrinology, 3rd ed. Philadelphia, WB Saunders, 1991, pp 698–701.
35. Murphy AA, Green WR, Bobbie D, de la Cruz Z, Rock JA: Unsuspected endometriosis documented by scanning electron microscopy in visually normal peritoneum. Fertil Steril 1986;46:522–524.
36. Strauss JF III, Guroide E: The endometrium: Regulation and dysfunction. *In* Yen SSC, Jaffe RB (eds): Reproductive Endocrinology, 3rd ed. Philadelphia, WB Saunders, 1991, 341–344.
37. Seiler JC, Gidwani G, Ballard L: Laparoscopic cauterization of endometriosis for fertility: A controlled study. Fertil Steril 1986;46:1098–1100.
38. Rock JA: Infertility: Surgical aspects. *In* Yen SSC, Jaffe RB (eds): Reproductive Endocrinology, 3rd ed. Philadelphia, WB Saunders, 1991, pp 724–726.

38a. Emmi AM: The use of GnRH agonists in the medical therapy of endometriosis in the woman with pain. Semin Reprod Endocrinol 1993;11:119–126.

39. Luciano AA, Turksoy N, Carleo J: Evaluation of oral medroxyprogesterone acetate in the treatment of endometriosis. Obstet Gynecol 1988;72:323–327.
40. Ulbright TM, Roth LM, Stehman FB: Secondary ovarian neoplasia: A clinicopathologic study of 35 cases. Cancer 1984;53:1164–1174.
41. Gagnon Y, Têtu B: Ovarian metastases of breast carcinoma: A clinicopathologic study of 59 cases. Cancer 1989;64:892–898.
42. Mazur MT, Hsueh S, Gersell DJ: Metatstases to the female genital tract: Analysis of 325 cases. Cancer 1984;53:1978–1984.

43. Woodruff JD, Murthy YS, Bhaskar TN, Bordbar F, Tseng S-S: Metastatic ovarian tumors. Am J Obstet Gynecol 1970;107:202–209.
44. Osborne BM, Robboy SJ: Lymphomas or leukemia presenting as ovarian tumors: An analysis of 42 cases. Cancer 1983;52:1933–1944.
45. Holtz F, Hart WR: Krukenberg tumors of the ovary: A clinicopathologic analysis of 27 cases. Cancer 1982;50:2438–2447.
46. Woodruff JD, Novak ER: The Krukenberg tumor: Study of 48 cases from the Ovarian Tumor Registry. Obstet Gynecol 1960;15:351–360.
47. Serov SF, Scully RE: Histological Typing of Ovarian Tumors. Geneva, World Health Organization, 1973.

9

Epithelial Tumors of the Ovary

Deborah E. Powell

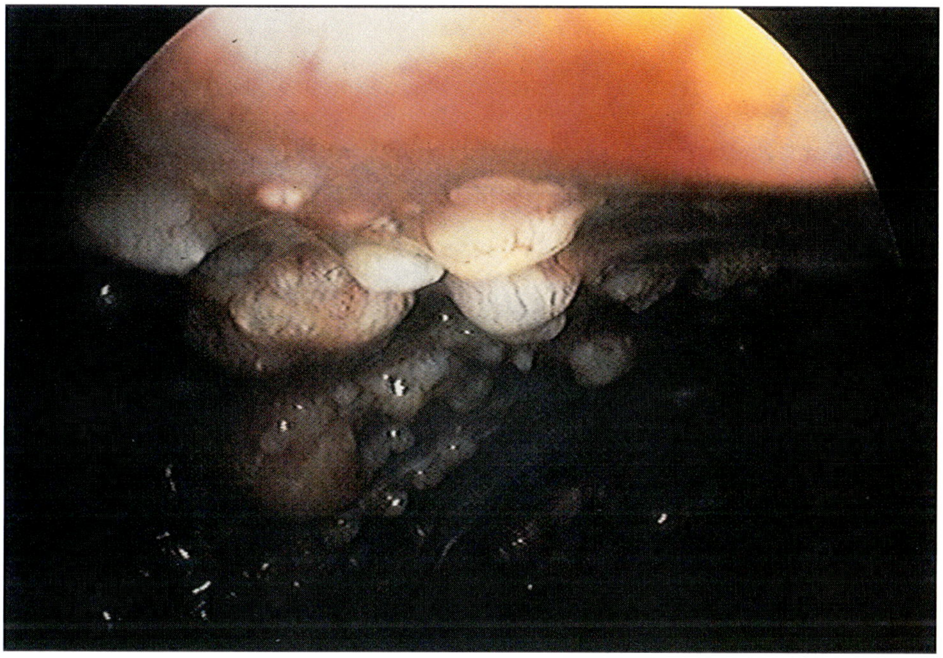

Epithelial ovarian neoplasms constitute the most common tumors of the human ovary. Epithelial neoplasms exist in three major biologic categories: benign, borderline or low malignant potential tumors (LMP), and carcinomas. Epithelial neoplasms of the ovary are generally considered tumors of adult women, the peak age incidence of the malignant tumors being the sixth and seventh decades of life. However, it should be noted that malignant epithelial ovarian neoplasms can be seen in very young women as well. Epithelial ovarian cancer is responsible for 80 to 90 percent of all malignant ovarian tumors. Benign and LMP tumors are more commonly found in younger women, the peak incidence of LMP tumors occurring about a decade earlier than that of carcinomas. Epithelial neoplasms are uncommon in children.[3] Patients who have malignant epithelial neoplasms have a high mortality in general. This is usually the result of late diagnosis, and there is presently great interest in the development of screening modalities for the early detection of epithelial ovarian cancer. This chapter presents the presumed histogenesis and epidemiology of these tumors, the biology of the three different subtypes, and a discussion of the histopathologic appearance and behavior of the five major categories of epithelial tumors: serous, mucinous, endometrioid, clear cell, and Brenner tumors of the ovary. Small cell tumors and transitional carcinomas of the ovary are also discussed briefly.

EPIDEMIOLOGY OF OVARIAN TUMORS

A number of risk factors have been associated with an increased incidence of malignant epithelial neoplasms of the ovary.[4] These are Caucasian race, age, low parity, infertility, a family history of ovarian cancer, a personal history of breast or endometrial cancer, and radiation exposure. Numerous epidemiologic studies have considered these as well as other potential risk factors for ovarian cancer. For example, several studies have shown a decreased risk of development of invasive ovarian cancer in patients who have used oral contraceptive pills (OCPs),[4–7] and some have shown that risk is further decreased by increased duration of use of OCPs.[6, 7] Although nulliparity has been shown in several studies[4–6] to be associated with an increased risk of ovarian cancer, at least one study has shown a slight increase in risk in women who have had multiple pregnancies when the woman's age at the time of the first pregnancy was 35 years or older.[6] However, the same authors showed that the relative risk of ovarian cancer decreased with each successive pregnancy. This study also showed, as have others, an increased risk with infertility.[4, 6] Whether lactation confers a protective effect is still controversial. No protective effect was found in studies by Booth et al[6] and Hildreth et al[5], but a slight protective effect was found in the study by Hartge et al.[4] Several studies have suggested an increased risk for women who have a late onset of menopause,[5, 6, 8] but there has been little evidence to suggest increased risk with early menarche. Some studies have shown a decreased risk with prior sterilization or hysterectomy.[6, 9] Environmental factors such as alcohol, cigarette smoking, and particularly talc exposure have been of considerable interest. One study has shown a weak increase in risk of ovarian cancer with alcohol use but no increased risk in users of cigarettes.[4] Booth et al[6] found a slight increase in risk of ovarian cancer among women who frequently (daily or weekly) used talc in the genital area compared to women who never or infrequently used it.

Familial ovarian cancer accounts for approximately 5 percent of all epithelial ovarian cancers and exists in three forms: the hereditary breast-ovarian cancer syndrome, the Lynch syndrome II (a familial syndrome of predisposition to endometrial, breast, ovarian, and colonic cancers), and the less common site-specific familial ovarian cancer in which ovarian cancer is the only tumor found in affected families.[10] These syndromes show an autosomal dominant inheritance pattern.[11] Some studies have found that familial ovarian cancer tends to occur at a younger age than sporadic tumors.[12] However, other studies[10] have not found significant age differences among patients who have familial versus sporadic ovarian cancer. Recent genetic studies have shown a linkage with one or more genes on the long arm of chromosome 17 (17q12-q23). This locus is referred to as BRCA-1 when found in breast-ovarian cancer syndrome patients.[13] This gene is currently under active investigation and this chromosomal region may prove to be important in other familial cancer syndromes. The BRCA-1 gene has recently been identified and cloned, and a number of different mutations are being identified.[13A] This is an important step in what will be a long process of unraveling the genetic alterations in familial and ultimately in sporadic ovarian cancer.

A few epidemiologic studies have examined benign and LMP (borderline) ovarian tumors.[14–17] Two studies have suggested that a family history of ovarian cancer is associated with an increased risk of ovarian cancer but not of LMP tumors.[15, 18] In one study[17] a slightly increased risk of developing an LMP ovarian tumor was associated with older age at the time of the first birth. A slightly decreased risk was found with the use of OCPs. No association of LMP and ovarian tumors has been found with lifelong menstrual pattern or age at menarche or menopause. For benign ovarian epithelial tumors some association was found with earlier menarche and as for carcinomas, with a longer interval between marriage and first birth. Some differences were noted between benign serous and mucinous tumors, and endometrioid tumors.[16]

To summarize, the risk of ovarian cancer is greatest in nulliparous or infertile women, in women with a positive family history of ovarian cancer, and in women who themselves have a breast or endometrial cancer.[19] Risk increases with age. There may be a decreased risk among long-term users of OCPs. The role of talc exposure in histogenesis is undetermined at the present time. Some studies indicate that risk factors for LMP tumors may differ from those for carcinoma.

HISTOGENESIS, PATHOGENESIS, AND BIOLOGIC BEHAVIOR

The ovary is covered by a single layer of epithelial cells, which are rarely seen in routine histologic sections (Fig. 9–1). This epithelium is a mesothelium similar to that investing other pelvic organs. Embryologically it is derived from the lateral plate mesoderm, as is the peritoneum. A number of other sites in the female genital tract have the same embryologic origin from the lateral plate mesoderm: the fallopian tubes, uterus, cervix, and upper portion of the vagina. The similar embryologic origin is the basis for a unifying theory of histogenesis that encompasses ovarian epithelial tumors of different histologic composition. The undifferentiated ovarian mesothelium is considered capable of differentiation along several different cell lines, giving rise to, for example, tumors bearing a resemblance to fallopian tube epithelium, endocervix, and endometrium.

Although epithelial ovarian tumors are believed to arise from the ovarian surface epithelium, the agents responsible for neoplastic transformation are unknown. Some epithelial tumors arise on the surface of the ovaries, whereas others develop within the ovary itself. The latter tumors are believed to develop from small inclusion cysts of surface epithelium that become trapped within the cortical stroma (Fig. 9–2). These epithelial inclusion cysts presumably develop during ovulation when repair of the defect caused by rupture of the follicle may lead to trapping of epithelial cells within the ovary itself. These microscopic inclusion cysts are very common and are usually lined by a layer of single epithelial cells. However, in appropriate circumstances, neoplastic transformation may occur. During this process the epithelium lining the cysts, like that covering the ovary, may proliferate and differentiate in a number of müllerian patterns to form the different types of epithelial tumors.

It has been standard teaching that benign, borderline, and malignant tumors of the ovary arise

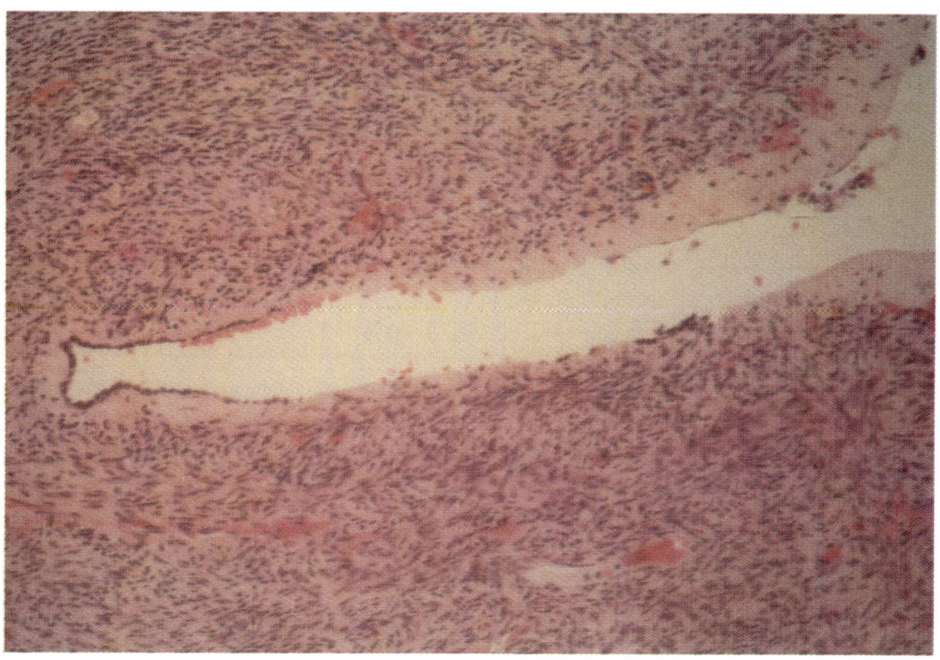

FIGURE 9–1
This is a section through the surface of an ovary showing an invagination lined by mesothelium. This mesothelium is well preserved at the tip of the invagination. The cells are rounded to cuboidal and have scant cytoplasm.

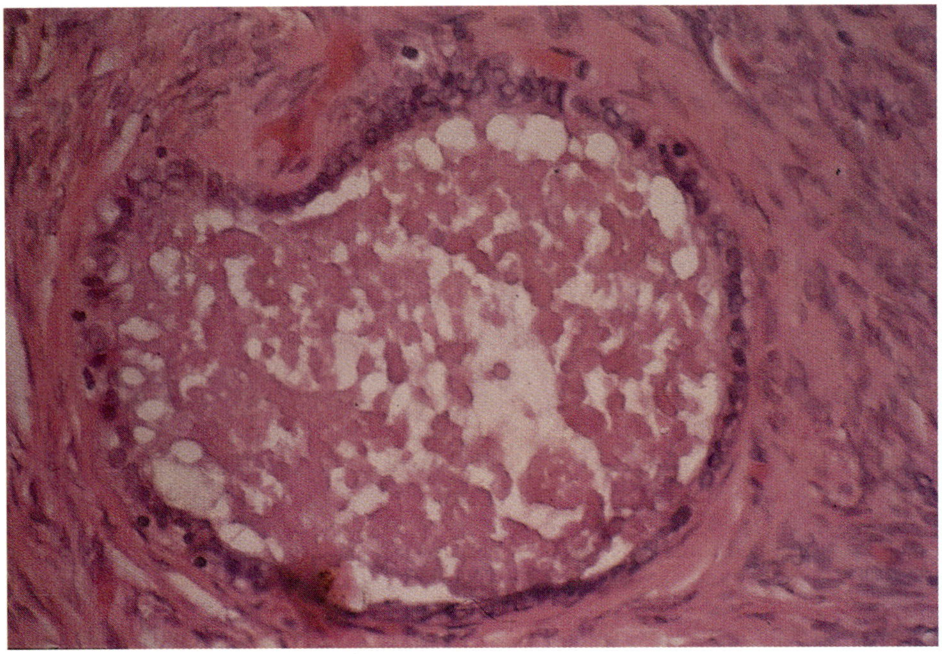

FIGURE 9-2
An ovarian epithelial inclusion cyst is seen. Most of the cyst is lined by a single layer of cuboidal cells. The nuclei are prominent, and the cytoplasm is scant. There is trapped debris in the cyst.

separately and do not form a continuum of malignant progression, unlike the progression that occurs with other human neoplasms, for example, the adenoma to carcinoma sequence of colonic tumors. However, it has been observed for some time that borderline and even malignant mucinous tumors may contain areas of histologically benign epithelium.[20] Recently, some authors have suggested that in some circumstances serous as well as mucinous malignant and LMP tumors may arise from preexisting benign neoplasms.[21, 22] Several types of studies support this concept. Histologic studies show areas of benign epithelium in borderline and malignant serous and mucinous tumors. In addition, areas of transition from benign to malignant epithelium can be identified in some tumors.[22, 23] Epidemiologic studies from England have shown a fivefold increased incidence of benign ovarian tumors in first- and second-degree relatives of patients with ovarian cancer. Finally, electron microscopic studies from Sweden demonstrate a benign to malignant epithelial transition in ovarian tumors.[22]

If certain benign tumors can undergo malignant transformation, the development of screening procedures to detect and remove benign epithelial tumors before such a transformation has occurred becomes important. It is certain, however, that many, if not most, benign epithelial ovarian tumors do not undergo malignant change. It is important to develop ways to differentiate benign from potentially or unequivocally malignant tumors before surgery. Ongoing research in many laboratories is attempting to unravel the molecular genetic events that occur during the pathogenesis of these tumors. It is entirely possible and even likely that a cascade of gene alterations will be identified that are similar to those already shown to be important in the pathogenesis of carcinoma of the colon. It is not at all impossible to believe that in the future samples of the epithelial lining or of the fluid obtained from a cystic ovarian tumor may be subjected to genetic analysis, allowing assessment of the malignant potential of the neoplasm.

LOW MALIGNANT POTENTIAL OVARIAN TUMORS

The terms low malignant potential (LMP) and borderline ovarian epithelial tumors are synonyms for a group of tumors that are usually associated with highly favorable prognosis. This category of tumors has been adopted both by the World Health Organization (WHO) Histological Classification of Ovarian Tumors and by the International Federation of Gynecologists and Obstetricians (FIGO). Currently, LMP is the preferred term because, although uncommon, some of these tumors do spread to involve distant sites and ultimately prove fatal for patients. They should not be confused with grade 1 carcinomas. The category of LMP tumors is most applicable to the serous and mucinous tumors; nevertheless, LMP forms of endometrioid and clear cell carcinomas have been identified, and proliferative or LMP Brenner tumors are also reported with some frequency.

LMP ovarian tumors constitute between 14 and 16 percent of all epithelial ovarian neoplasms.[23a] They are more frequent in women who are in their fourth or fifth decade of life. This age is lower than the age of patients who have epithelial ovarian cancer.[23a, 24] Despite the generally favorable survival of patients with LMP tumors (81 to 95 percent 5-year survival rate and 68 to 90 percent 10-year survival rate),[25] some women will die from LMP ovarian tumors. Some studies suggest that 15 to 20 percent of patients will eventually die from this disease, and death may occur many years to decades after the original diagnosis.[26] Attempts to identify patients in this poor prognosis category by histopathologic grading of the epithelial atypia have been unrewarding. The prognosis is related in general to the stage of disease, but stage in itself is not a uniform predictor of survival.[27] Some studies have shown a positive predictive value of morphometric analysis of LMP serous and mucinous tumors. Tumors that have a high mitotic activity index and a high epithelium to stroma ratio have been reported to be strongly associated with poor patient survival.[25]

Recently, increased attention has been paid to the characterization of peritoneal and other extraovarian implants of LMP tumors.[28–31] Thirty to 40 percent of patients with LMP ovarian tumors have extraovarian implants.[28] These may be found either within the pelvis (stage II) or at extrapelvic sites (stage III). The rare case of an LMP ovarian tumor implant on the abdominal skin has been reported.[31a] It should be noted that endosalpingiosis (the presence of benign endocervical, tubal, or endometrial type glands) is frequently found in patients who have epithelial ovarian tumors (Fig. 9–3). Endosalpingiosis must be differentiated by histopathologic examination from the diagnosis of tumor implants. Some studies have suggested that implants are more common with exophytic than with intraovarian LMP tumors.[32]

Tumor implants may be classified as invasive or noninvasive. Criteria for invasive implants have been defined as infiltration into the underlying tissue in a destructive and irregular pattern.[28] In most instances the invading tumor shows a distinct glandular pattern with atypical cells resembling low-grade carcinomas (Fig. 9–4). A stromal response is often seen in the presence of invasive implants. However, noninvasive implants of a desmoplastic type may also show a marked stromal reaction.[28] Within these noninvasive desmoplastic implants, the tumor shows a lack of destructive extension into the underlying tissue. The desmoplastic implants may be present as plaquelike areas on the pelvic peritoneum and are often infiltrated by a large number of both mononuclear and acute inflammatory cells and occasionally by hemorrhage and fibrin. These implants may show nests, papillae, or small clusters of tumor cells, but, most important, a destructive growth pattern is absent (Fig. 9–5). In noninvasive, nondesmoplastic implants there is a lack of associated fibrosis and inflammation, and the tumor exists as epithelial islands and papillae. Psammoma bodies are frequently found with all types of implants (Fig. 9–6). In a large study investigating the prognostic significance of different patterns of implants in

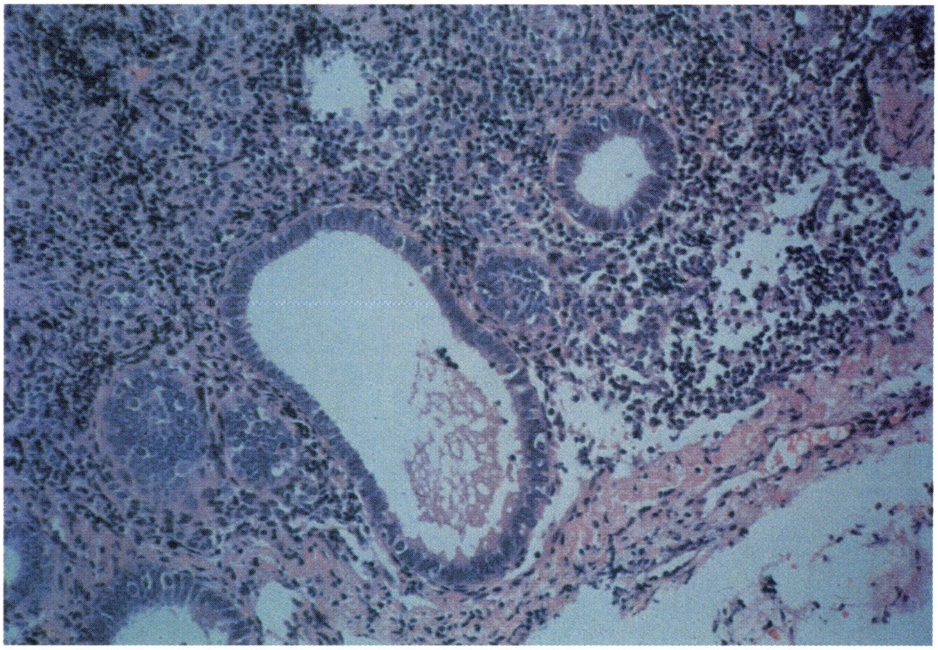

FIGURE 9–3
Glands in the subcortical area of a lymph node are lined by a single layer of columnar cells similar to the cells of the fallopian tube epithelium. This is endosalpingiosis and should not be confused with metastases from an adenocarcinoma.

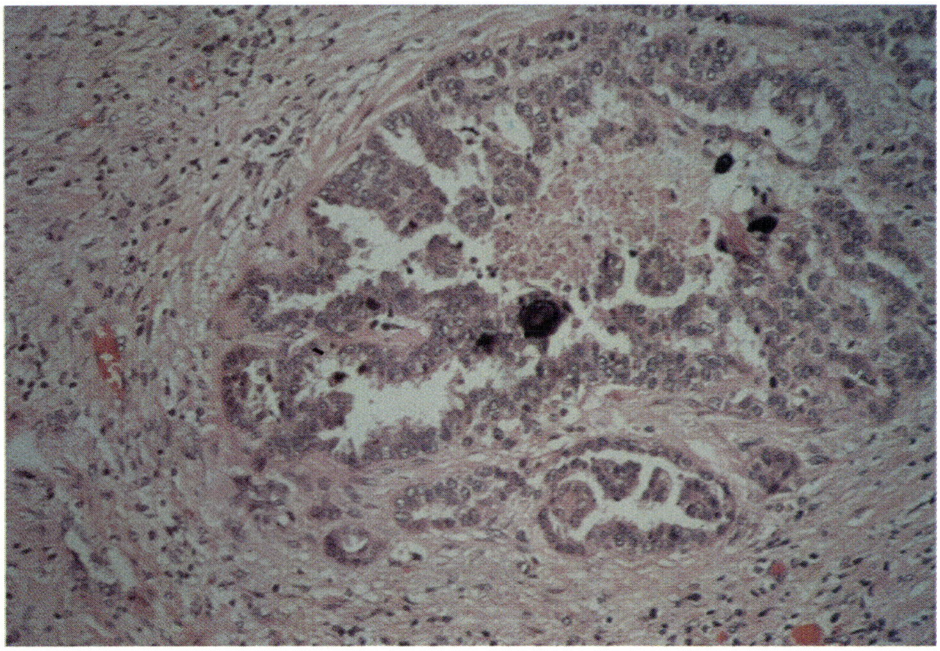

FIGURE 9-4
This extraovarian tumor implant in a patient who had an ovarian serous LMP tumor is consistent with a grade 1 serous adenocarcinoma. There is a complex papillary glandular pattern, cellular stratification, and mild pleomorphism. A psammoma body is seen in the center.

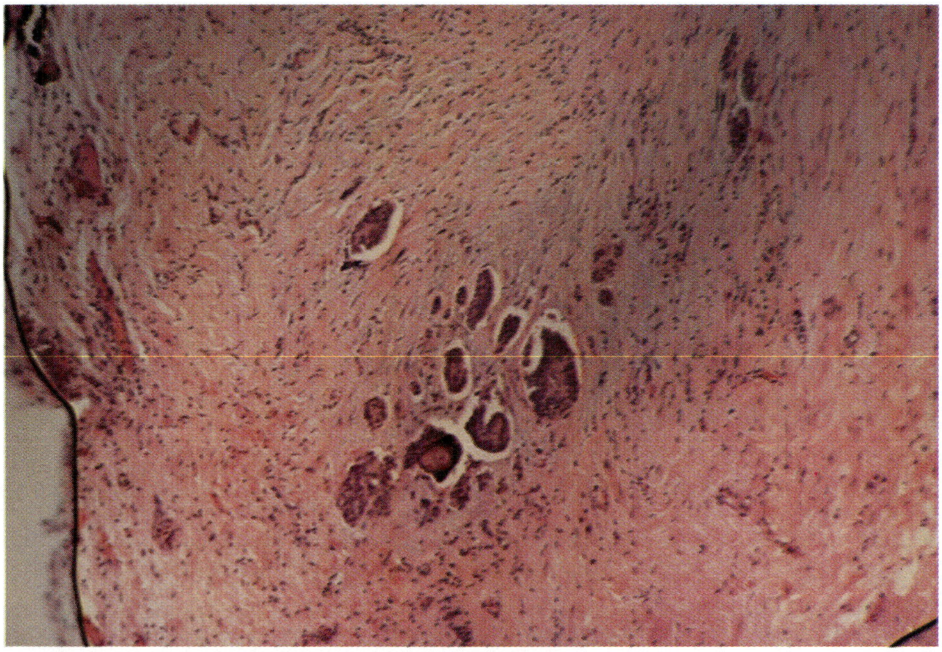

FIGURE 9-5
In this noninvasive implant, clusters and nests of tumor cells are found in fibrotic stroma. The stroma around the tumor cell nests has a purplish, wavy appearance. This type of fibrotic response is known as desmoplasia. There is no tissue destruction by the tumor, and on higher power (see Fig. 9-6) there is little cytologic atypia.

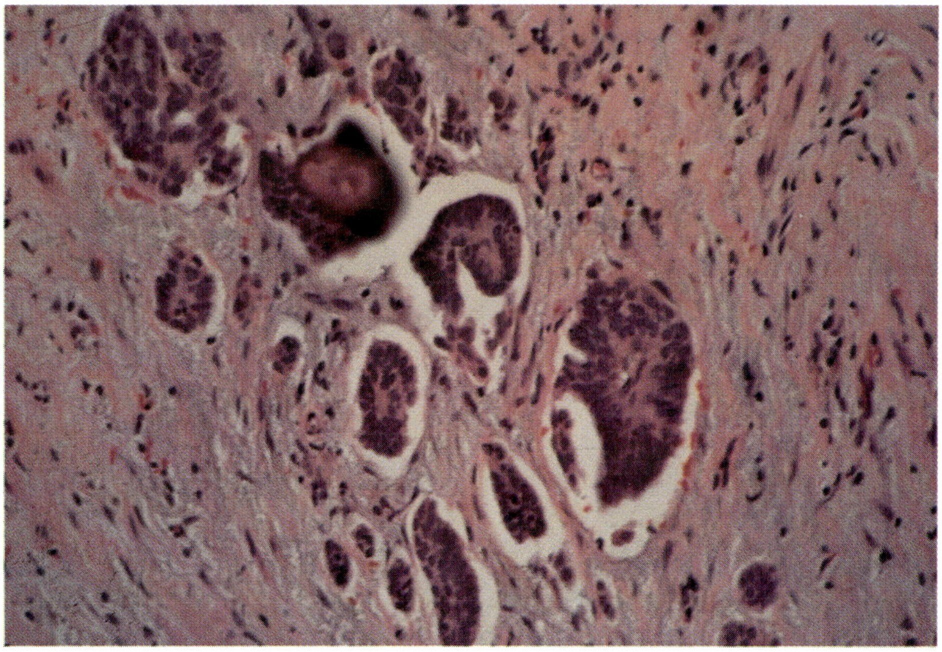

FIGURE 9-6
This is a high-power view of Figure 9–5. The cell clusters have a papillary configuration. There is little cytologic atypia and no mitotic activity. The dense purple structure in one of the cell clusters is a psammoma body.

LMP epithelial tumors, it was found that the most significant prognostic factors were the presence of true invasive implants and the presence of marked cytologic atypia in both invasive and noninvasive implants.[28] Both of these factors were highly statistically significant. In addition, the presence of mitotic activity in both invasive and noninvasive implants and the presence of residual tumor, as grossly determined by the operating surgeon, were also considered to be associated with a poor prognosis. The authors of this study suggested that patients who have either invasive implants or implants (whether invasive or noninvasive) that have marked cytologic atypia might benefit from adjuvant or adjunctive therapy. Patients lacking the features mentioned in this section are thought to have a very good prognosis. Other studies[33, 34] have suggested that the histopathologic features of the implant, including an invasive phenotype, are not related to prognosis. It is possible that different criteria for the diagnosis of invasiveness account for the disparate results. It is important to remember that the presence of desmoplastic fibrosis alone is not a criteria for invasiveness, and the finding of a desmoplastic stromal response without epithelial invasion or marked cytologic atypia does not affect prognosis.[28] Likewise, the presence of necrosis in the implants and the presence or number of psammoma bodies are not of prognostic significance. Other investigators[30] have found results similar to those of Bell et al.[28]

Other methodologies used for establishing the prognosis of LMP tumors include cytogenetic analysis and flow cytometry. The large majority of LMP ovarian tumors are diploid, but a few cases of aneuploid neoplasms have been reported. Larger studies must be done to assess whether aneuploid DNA patterns in LMP tumors are associated with poor prognosis.[35] Histopathologic criteria for the diagnosis of LMP tumors differs significantly for the different histopathologic subtypes. These criteria will be discussed in the subsequent sections of this chapter.

As noted earlier, endosalpingiosis is frequently associated with LMP ovarian tumors as well as ovarian adenocarcinoma. This may present a problem in differential diagnosis both histopathologically and cytopathologically.[36] Psammoma bodies may also be associated with endosalpingiosis, which may further complicate pathologic interpretation. Endosalpingiosis usually shows isolated cystic structures lined by a single layer of cuboidal or columnar epithelial cells that may or may not be ciliated and may or may not be associated with psammoma bodies (see Fig. 9–3).

Papillary mesothelial hyperplasia that occasionally is florid has been associated with both LMP ovarian tumors and carcinomas. These mesothelial proliferations are occasionally mistaken for metastatic tumors or tumor implants[37] (Figs. 9–7 and 9–8). Potential causative factors of papillary mesothelial hyperplasia include mechanical irritation by a large tumor, ascites, tumor rupture, and endometriosis. Papillary mesothelial hyperplasia may also be associated with psammoma bodies. Histochemical or immunocytochemical studies may in some rare instances be required to differentiate mesothelial from epithelial cells. Adenocarcinoma

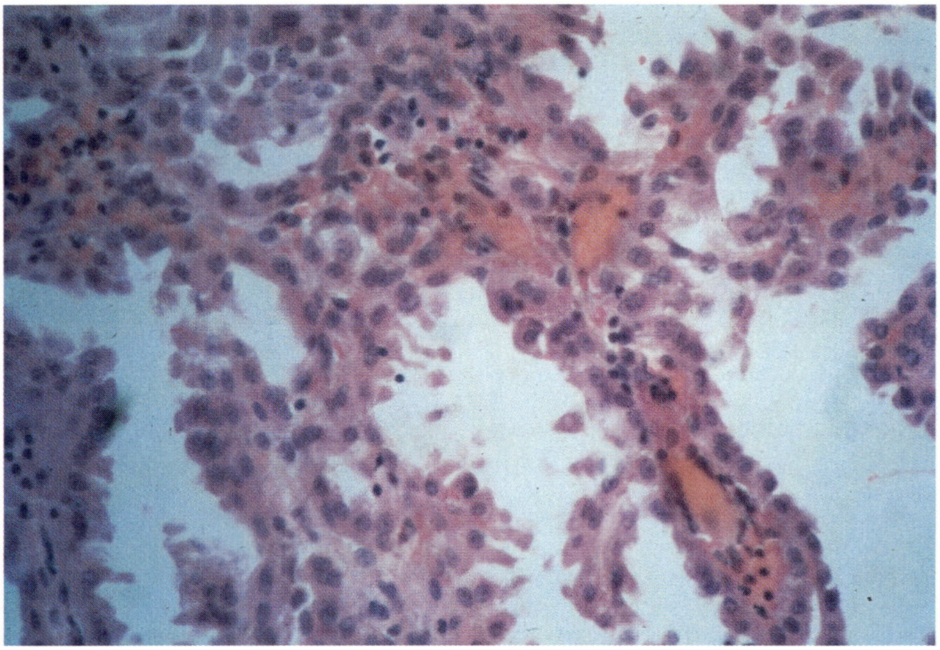

FIGURE 9–7
This high-power view shows a focus of papillary mesothelial hyperplasia. Reactive mesothelial cells that are round or cuboidal line structures in a papillary configuration. The cells have abundant pink cytoplasm. The nuclei are oval and have prominent nucleoli. There is no pleomorphism. This pattern is sometimes difficult to distinguish from a serous LMP ovarian tumor.

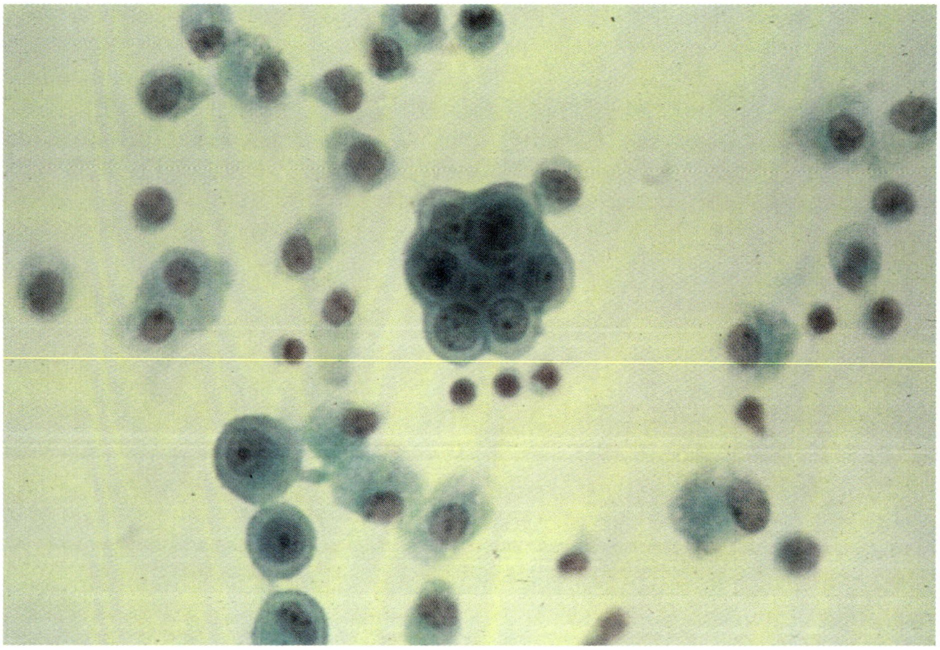

FIGURE 9–8
This cytologic preparation of peritoneal fluid from a patient without tumor shows a cluster of reactive mesothelial cells in a papillary configuration. The cells have round, uniform nuclei and prominent nucleoli. There is abundant cytoplasm with a clear zone surrounding the nucleus. This is typical of reactive mesothelial cells. The nuclear to cytoplasmic ratio seen is also typical of mesothelial cells.

cells may stain for milk fat globule-related antigen (MFGRA), whereas reactive mesothelial cells do not.[38]

HISTOPATHOLOGIC SUBTYPES OF EPITHELIAL OVARIAN TUMORS

Serous Tumors

Serous tumors are the most common epithelial ovarian neoplasms. Although the majority of ovarian serous tumors are either benign or LMP, the majority of malignant ovarian epithelial tumors are also of the serous type.[20, 27, 39] Serous adenocarcinoma accounts for approximately 50 percent of all epithelial ovarian cancers.[2] Serous tumors are tumors of adult women with a median age in the sixth decade of life. As mentioned previously, both benign and LMP tumors tend to occur more frequently than do carcinomas in younger patients, but there is considerable overlap. Serous tumors are more commonly bilateral (10 to 30 percent of cases) than any of the other epithelial ovarian tumors.

Because there are multiple forms of benign serous tumors the appearance on gross examination is variable. The tumor may present as a solitary large cyst or as a multicystic tumor that completely replaces the ovarian parenchyma (Fig. 9–9). It may also present as a firm mass composed of variably sized cystic spaces with an intervening fibrous stroma. Contents of the cysts may be clear, straw-colored, or occasionally more mucinous in character.

The lining epithelium of benign serous tumors (e.g., serous cystadenoma) is a single layer of columnar epithelial cells, some of which are ciliated (Fig. 9–10). These cells resemble those lining the fallopian tubes. Mild epithelial proliferation or hyperplasia may be seen in some cases, but this is never a major component.

A serous tumor may be either a papillary tumor arising on the surface of the ovary or a cystic mass within the ovarian parenchyma. When the tumor is formed from a proliferation of both the epithelium and the fibrous stroma, it is referred to as an adenofibroma.

Histopathologic criteria for LMP serous tumors, whether of the exophytic (surface) or intraovarian (cystic) type, include epithelial hyperplasia and proliferation, often in micropapillary or tufting patterns or in a papillary hyperplastic epithelial configuration (Fig. 9–11). Characteristically, intraovarian LMP tumors have cystic spaces within which there is a grossly nodular or granular pattern that corresponds to papillary projections of the tumor seen microscopically (Fig. 9–12). Stratification of epithelial cells may be marked. Stratification to more than 10 to 12 cell layers is not uncommon. Mitotic activity is present (usually less than one mitosis per high-power microscopic field), although abnormal mitotic figures are not usually seen. Cytologic atypia may be present and may be marked in some cases[40] (Fig. 9–13). In particular, cytoplasmic eosinophilia associated with markedly atypical nuclei may be noted. The single criterion

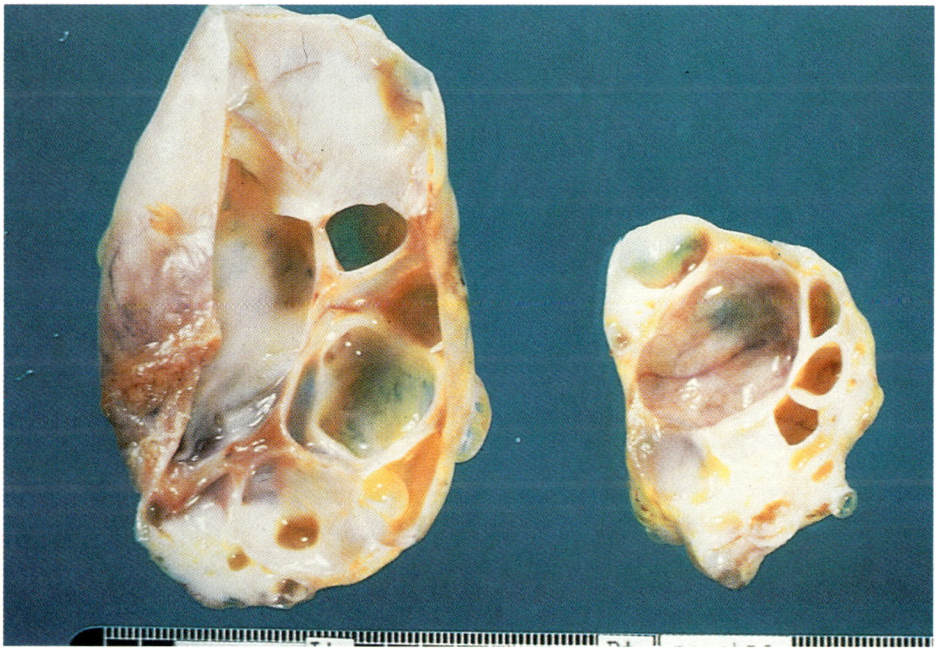

FIGURE 9–9
A benign multicystic serous ovarian tumor has different-sized cystic spaces with smooth walls. There are no papillary excrescences.

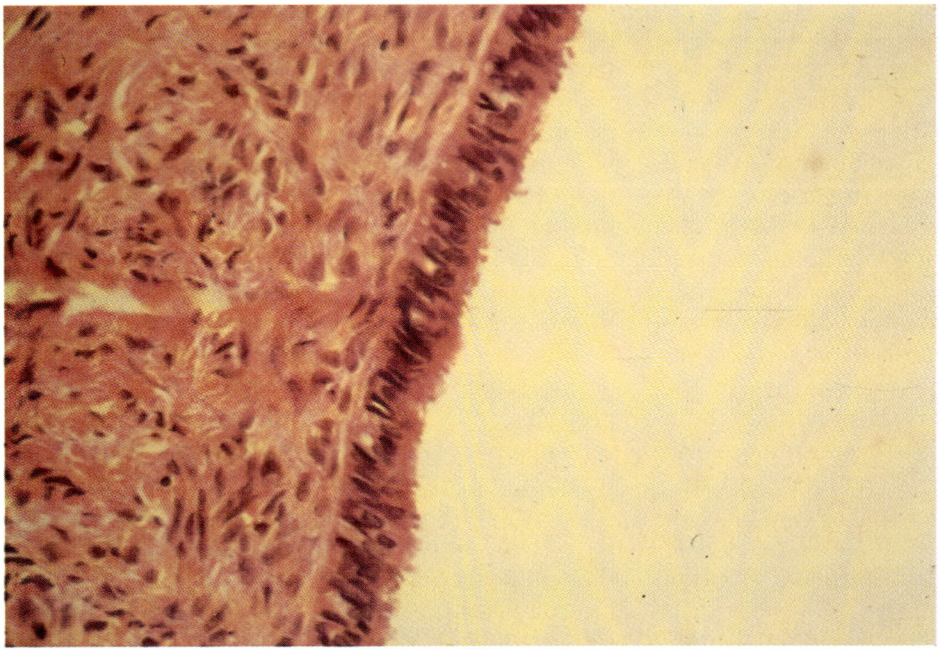

FIGURE 9-10
The lining of this serous cystadenoma consists of a single layer of columnar cells, many of which are ciliated. It resembles the cells of the fallopian tube epithelium.

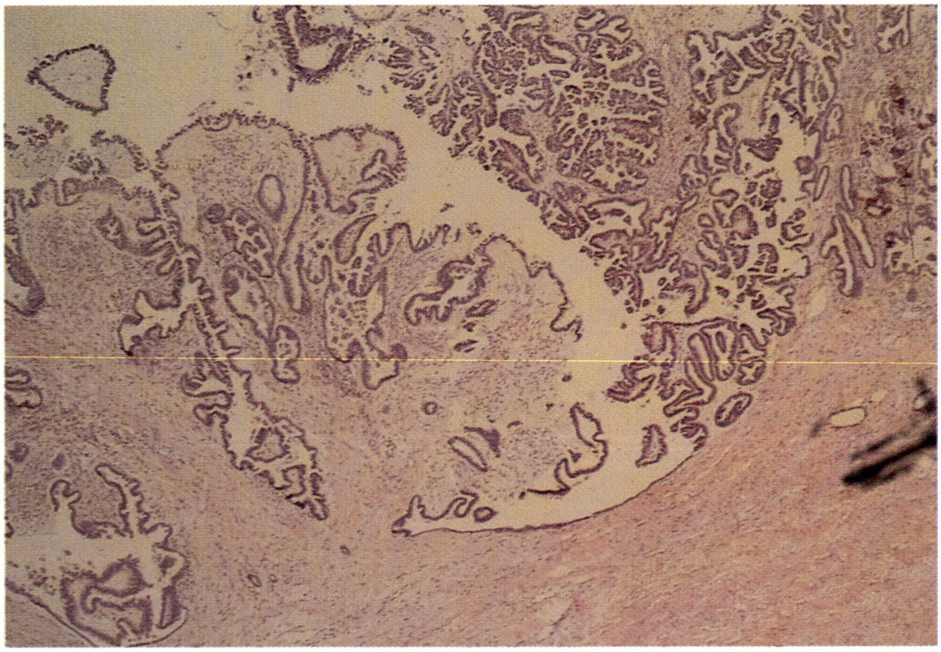

FIGURE 9-11
This is a low-power view of a serous LMP ovarian tumor. Wide fibrovascular papillae are seen *(left)*, and there is a complex papillary pattern *(right)*. Only the surface is involved. There is no stromal invasion.

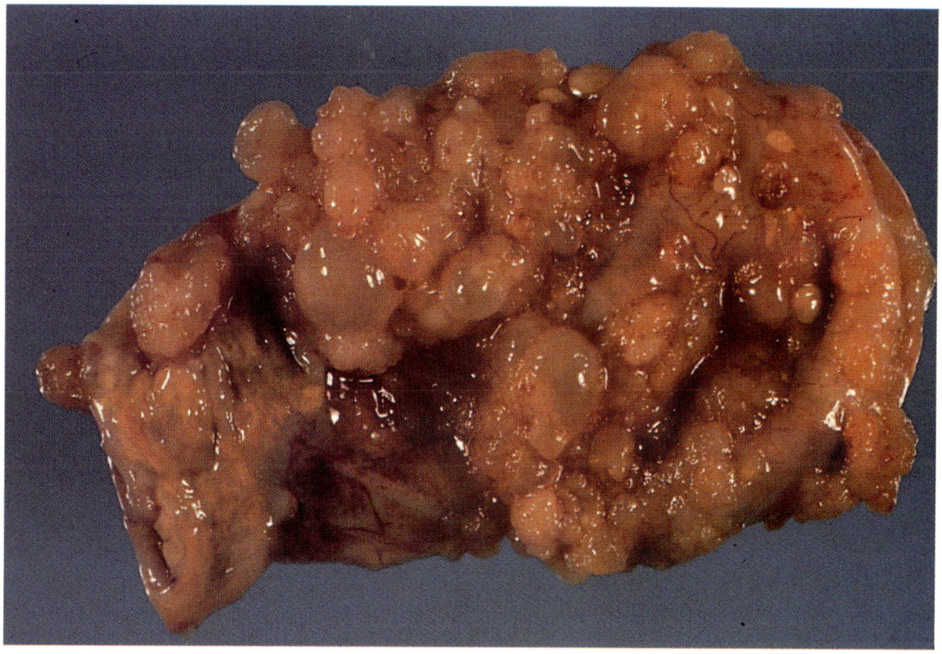

FIGURE 9-12
Although the outer surface of this ovarian cystic tumor was smooth, the inside wall had multiple small cysts and yellow papillary nodules. The microscopic examination showed a serous LMP tumor.

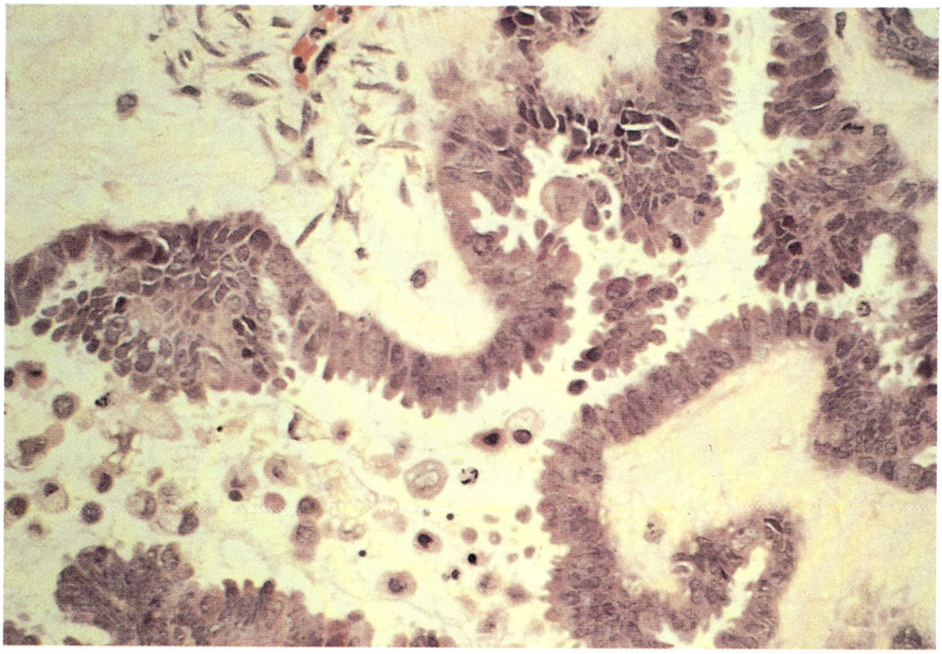

FIGURE 9-13
This serous LMP tumor shows columnar cells lining fibrovascular papillae. There is cytologic atypia and some cellular stratification. One mitotic figure is seen *(right upper corner)*. Individual tumor cells and clusters of cells are seen in the cystic space. This microscopic picture is very characteristic of this tumor.

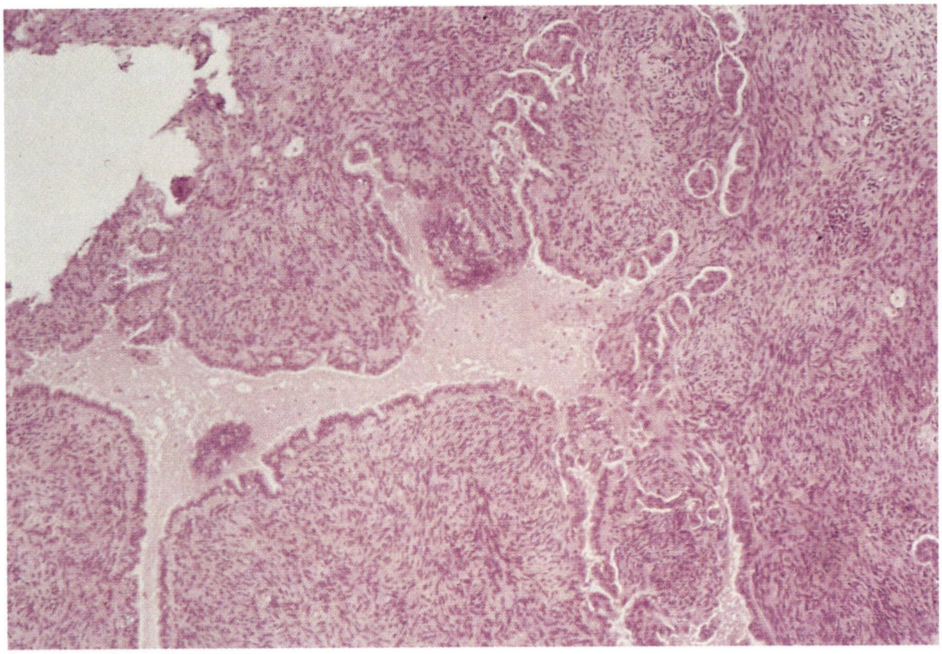

FIGURE 9–14
A serous LMP tumor has cells that line papillae. Clusters of tumor cells are seen to extend into the stroma *(right upper corner)*. This suggests microinvasion.

differentiating LMP tumors from true carcinomas of serous type is the absence of demonstrable ovarian stromal invasion in LMP tumors.

The question of the significance of the so-called microinvasion[41] has been raised, but at the present time there is no convincing evidence of a worse prognosis with microinvasion. Most reported cases of microinvasive LMP serous tumors have been found in patients who had stage I disease and were expected to do well even if the tumor was actually a grade 1 adenocarcinoma. Thus the exact significance or definitional criteria for microinvasion in serous carcinomas of the ovary is unclear. Microinvasion is usually suggested by a few nests of epithelial cells that are clearly seen to extend into the stroma immediately adjacent to the cyst wall (Fig. 9–14). Occasionally a desmoplastic stromal response may be identified as well.

Serous ovarian carcinomas can arise within the ovary as well as from the surface (Fig. 9–15). Invasion must be documented for a diagnosis of carcinoma to be made. The invasive tumor frequently shows papillary formations of epithelial cells (Fig. 9–16). Psammoma bodies are frequently present.

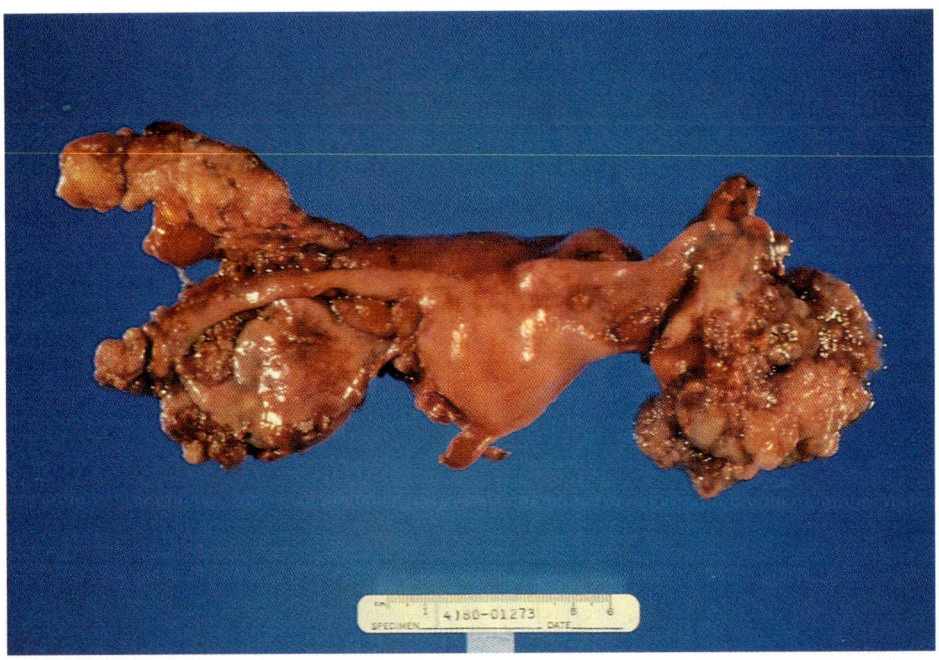

FIGURE 9–15
The uterine fundus is seen flanked by solid tumor masses that replaced the normal ovaries. Papillary nodules or excrescences are present on the surface of the tumor. The fallopian tubes are stretched over the tumor masses. This appearance is typical of an ovarian serous carcinoma.

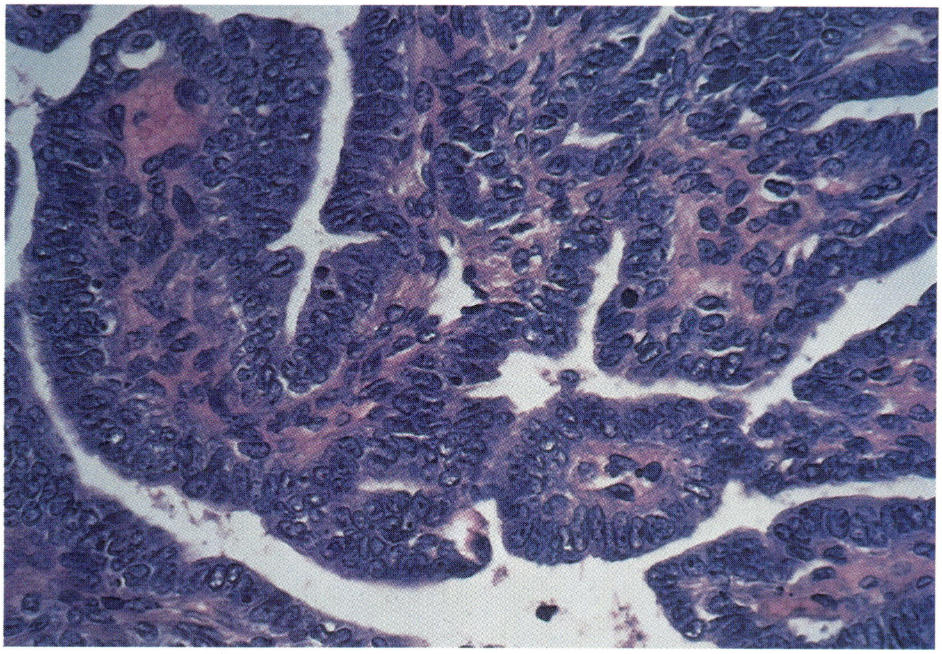

FIGURE 9-16
This grade 2 serous ovarian carcinoma has a papillary configuration, but acinar structures are also seen *(upper right corner)*. Many of the cells are columnar. There is stratification. Several mitoses are seen. Pleomorphism is more prominent in the acinar structures.

These spherical masses of laminated calcium are characteristic of papillary tumors in the ovary as well as other sites (Fig. 9–17). Some tumors may exhibit a more glandular than papillary pattern of invasive growth. High-grade tumors frequently are present as sheets of cells showing considerable anaplasia and numerous, often atypical, mitotic figures. Only rare papillary or glandular foci and a distant resemblance of the cells to those of the fallopian tube permit the diagnosis of a serous neoplasm; otherwise, a diagnosis of undifferentiated or poorly differentiated adenocarcinoma is made (Fig. 9–18). Grading of epithelial tumors will be discussed in detail in a subsequent section.

Papillary serous tumors may arise primarily from the peritoneal surfaces.[43, 44] Primary peritoneal papillary carcinoma accounts for approximately 7 percent of neoplasms originally diagnosed as ovarian serous adenocarcinoma.[45] Primary peritoneal papillary carcinoma is identical to papillary serous carcinoma in the ovary and frequently contains psammoma bodies. This tumor is believed to arise from extraovarian mesothelium, which, as mentioned previously, is embryologically

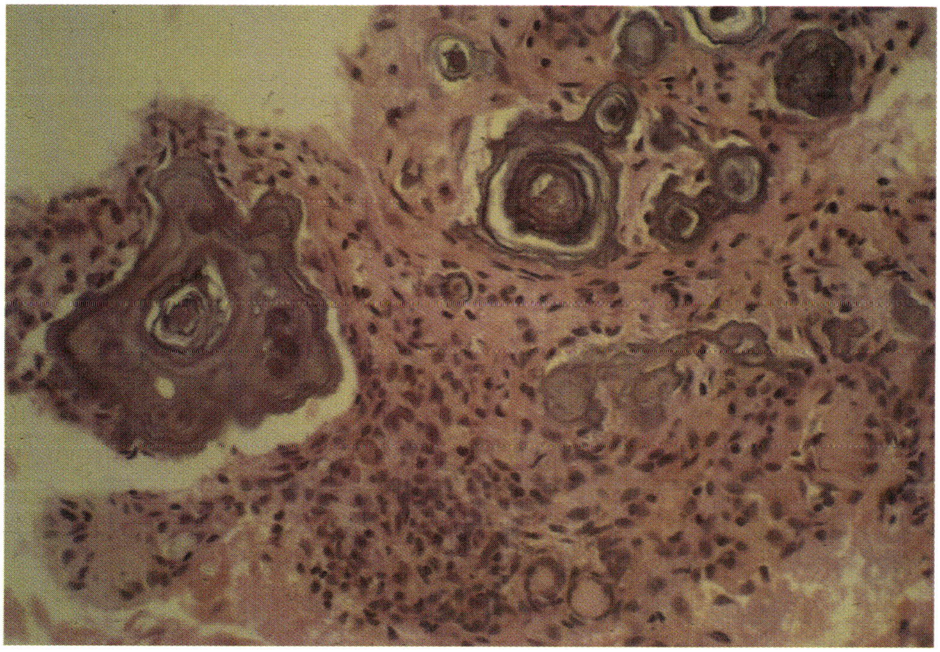

FIGURE 9-17
This cell block of a peritoneal lavage specimen shows multiple psammoma bodies. Concentric annular rings are characteristic of this structure. The purplish color indicates calcification. No malignant cells are seen in this preparation; the presence of psammoma bodies does not necessarily indicate malignancy. The patient from whom this peritoneal lavage was obtained had chronic pelvic inflammatory disease.

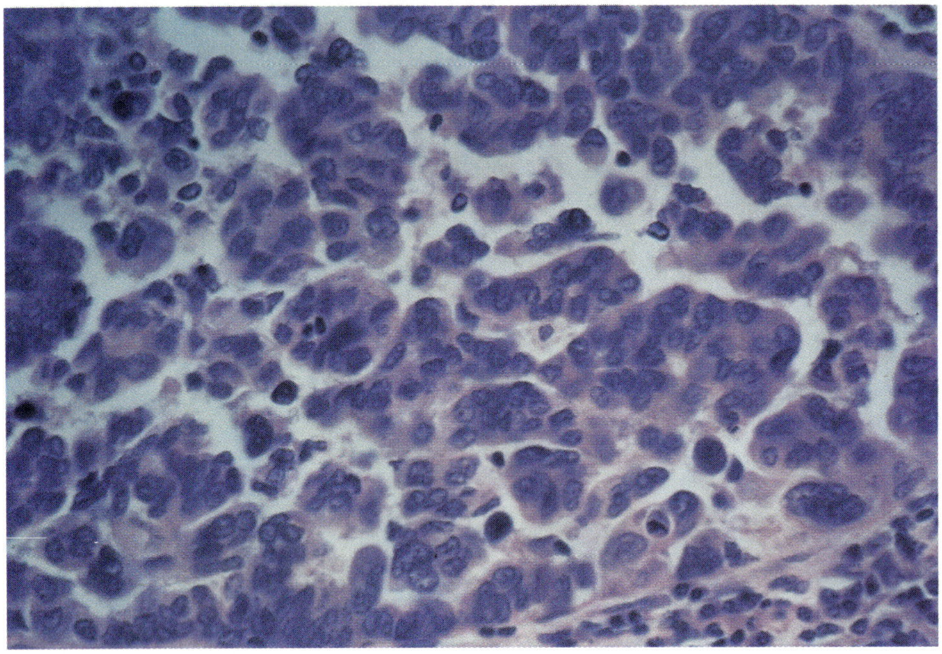

FIGURE 9–18
This is a poorly differentiated adenocarcinoma that retains some papillary configuration. There is marked pleomorphism and nuclear atypia.

derived from the lateral plate mesoderm, as is the ovarian surface epithelium and müllerian ducts. Because of its embryologic origin, this mesothelium is believed to have a potential for müllerian differentiation. The usual clinical presentation is ascites with widespread studding of the peritoneal surfaces with tumor. Minimal involvement of the ovarian surface may be present. The clinical behavior of primary peritoneal papillary carcinoma is similar to that of ovarian papillary serous adenocarcinoma.

Peritoneal papillary serous tumors must be differentiated from malignant mesothelioma of the peritoneal cavity. The latter is uncommon in women unless they have been exposed to asbestos.[43] Mesotheliomas rarely contain numerous psammoma bodies or intracytoplasmic mucin. The cells of mesothelioma are round or plump and cuboidal and not columnar as are the cells of peritoneal papillary serous carcinoma[46] (Fig. 9–19).

Other differences between ovarian adenocarcinoma and malignant mesothelioma have been studied.[38] Ovarian adenocarcinomas stain for MFGRP by immunocytochemistry. In contrast, the

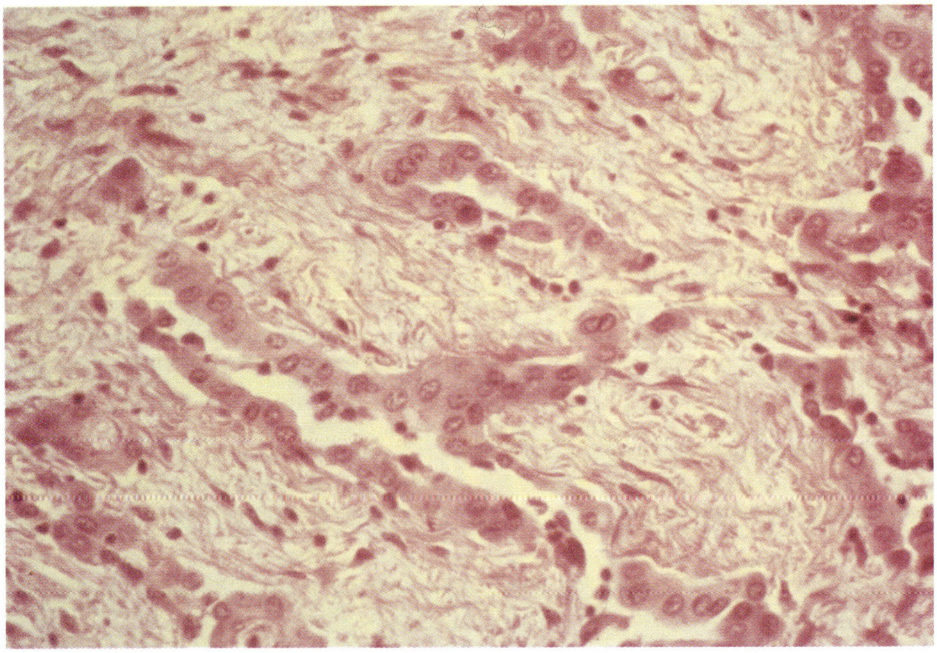

FIGURE 9–19
This is a high-power view of an epithelial malignant mesothelioma. The malignant mesothelial cells line slit-like spaces. There is a fibrotic connective tissue background. The cells are relatively uniform and have the abundant pink cytoplasm and oval nucleus typical of reactive mesothelial cells. It is necessary to see this specimen at lower magnification to be sure that there is a tumor mass here, in order to make a definitive diagnosis of malignancy.

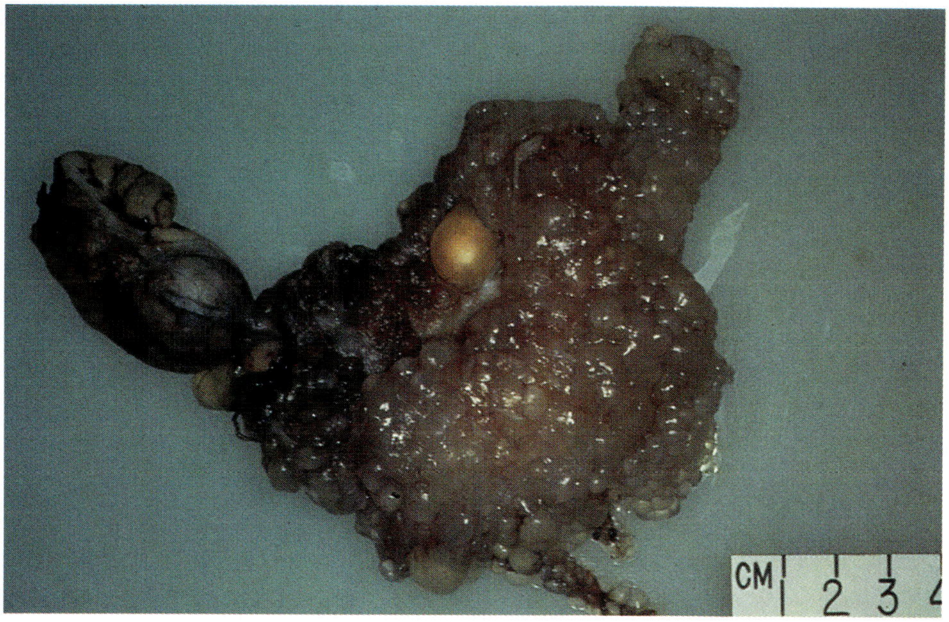

FIGURE 9-20
This multicystic structure replaced the normal omentum. The cysts contained clear to straw-colored fluid. The cyst walls are thin. At the time of surgery this lesion was thought to represent a malignancy; by microscopic examination, however, it was a benign multicystic mesothelioma.

normal, reactive, or neoplastic mesothelial cells do not.[38] This is paradoxical because both ovarian adenocarcinomas and malignant mesotheliomas are thought to arise from the same epithelium (mesothelium).[47] Electron microscopic studies have also documented differences between ovarian adenocarcinoma and malignant mesothelioma. Ovarian adenocarcinoma usually has only a few, short, thick, stubby microvilli, which are usually limited to the apical portion of the cells.[38] Mesothelioma typically has abundant long, thin, sinuous microvilli that are distributed over most of the cell surface.

Mesothelial neoplasms, however, represent a spectrum of disease that includes the adenomatoid tumor, the localized fibrous mesothelioma, multicystic mesothelioma (Figs. 9–20 and 9–21), well-differentiated papillary mesothelioma of the peritoneum, and diffuse malignant mesothelioma.[48–50] Adenomatoid tumor is benign, and the localized fibrous mesothelioma is also benign in most cases.[48] The multicystic mesothelioma[49, 50] and the well-differentiated papillary mesothelioma are of LMP, whereas the diffuse malignant mesothelioma is a highly aggressive neoplasm.

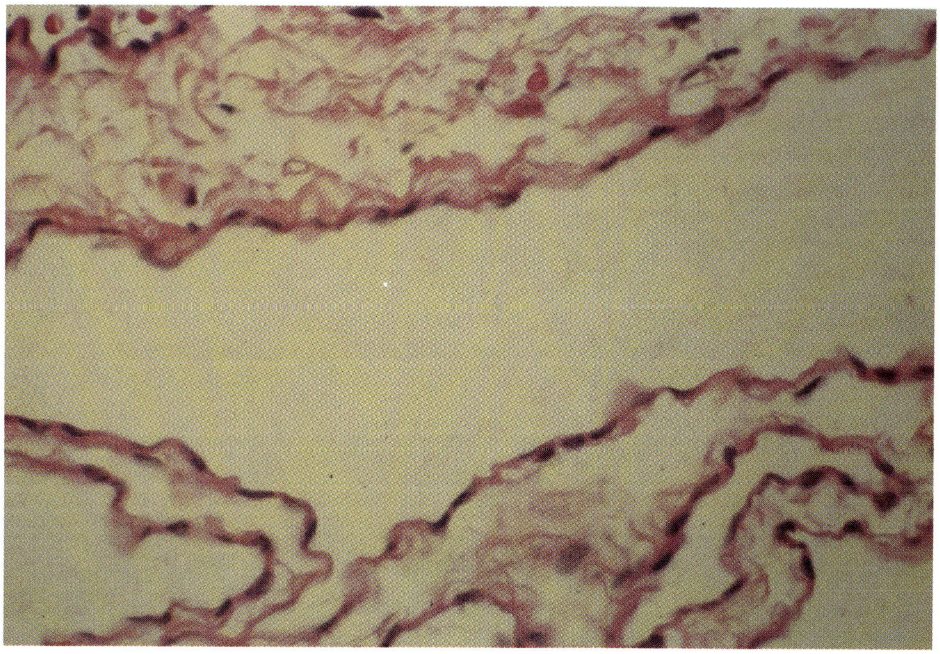

FIGURE 9-21
This is the microscopic appearance of the lesion shown in Figure 9–20. Multiple cystic spaces are lined by a single layer of flattened mesothelial cells. The variable-sized cysts are embedded in a delicate fibrovascular stroma.

It is the epithelial type of malignant mesothelioma that resembles a serous ovarian tumor. Mesotheliomas may also be of the sarcomatous type or may be mixed epithelial and sarcomatous. The sarcomatous pattern is recognizable from the sheets of spindle-shaped cells that do not have distinct cell borders and do not have epithelial-type growth patterns such as papillary groups or lining of slitlike spaces. The importance of recognizing this sarcomatous pattern is that if it is found, the tumor can be correctly classified as a malignant mesothelioma, either of sarcomatous type or mixed epithelial and sarcomatous type, and not as an epithelial ovarian tumor.

Because epithelial ovarian tumors are thought to arise from the surface epithelium (a mesothelium) and because they usually present with spread to other peritoneal (mesothelial) surfaces, the concept of these neoplasms as mesotheliomas has been advocated, particularly by Woodruff and Parmley.[47] These authors have also suggested that advanced-stage disease may in fact represent a multifocal tumor origin or "field effect" in a tissue (mesothelium) at risk rather than metastatic disease. This compelling theory is further advanced by the finding of advanced-stage LMP tumors without invasive metastases,[31] and by the frequent (over 30 percent) synchronous bilaterality of the serous epithelial tumors.

Recent studies attempting to validate this theory have focused on molecular genetic techniques to study the clonality of the ovarian tumor and peritoneal implants in patients with advanced-stage ovarian cancer. Using analysis of specific allelic deletions and methylation patterns of the hypoxanthine phosphoribosyl transferase (HPRT) gene on active and inactive X chromosomes, Tsao et al[51] showed the presence of similar patterns in both the ovarian tumors and the extraovarian implants, suggesting a monoclonal origin. They analyzed high-grade serous tumors, and the molecular evidence points to the ovarian tumor as primary and the extraovarian sites as metastatic. However, the possibility exists that this may not be the case for low-grade carcinomas and LMP tumors. Further studies of these tumors are needed. A recent report investigated the clonality of papillary peritoneal serous carcinoma.[52] Using analysis of patterns of allelic loss and differing P53 gene mutations, it was demonstrated that in contrast to stage III high-grade ovarian serous carcinomas, primary peritoneal papillary serous carcinomas are polyclonal and thus may truly represent multifocal rather than metastatic disease.

Mucinous Tumors

Mucinous tumors of the ovary are the second most common type of epithelial ovarian neoplasms. Like their serous counterparts, they exist in benign, LMP, and malignant forms. Ovarian mucinous adenocarcinoma accounts for approximately 10 percent of all ovarian epithelial cancer.[2] They are more frequently intracystic than exophytic. Two histopathologic subtypes are recognized, intestinal and müllerian. Compared with serous tumors, a higher percentage of mucinous tumors occurs as benign neoplasms. They are seldom bilateral. These tumors are found in adult women in the third to seventh decades of life, with benign and LMP tumors seen more commonly at the lower end of this spectrum. Mucinous tumors frequently display a variety of epithelial patterns within a single tumor.[20] This fact, coupled with the large size of these tumors, mandates extensive sampling to avoid missing focal areas of LMP or cancer in a neoplasm in which the major portion of the epithelium appears benign. One tissue section for each centimeter of maximum tumor diameter is suggested for histopathologic sampling. There appears to be an association of mucinous tumors with Peutz-Jeghers syndrome[53] and with mucinous adenocarcinoma of the endocervix.[54]

Most benign mucinous tumors are cystic lesions (i.e., mucinous cystadenoma) that often reach a very large size (up to several kilograms) and are frequently multilocular (Figs. 9–22 and 9–23). Very large mucinous cystadenomas may show areas of necrosis due to outgrowth of the blood supply. In general, the cysts of a mucinous cystadenoma are thin-walled and have no nodularity or papillae, whereas those that are malignant may have these features (Fig. 9–24). Intestinal-type mucinous tumors are more common. The müllerian or endocervical type has been recognized relatively recently. Both tumor types may produce mucin. The classic intestinal type of benign mucinous tumor shows cysts lined primarily by goblet cells with abundant apical cytoplasmic mucin and basally placed small nuclei (Fig. 9–25). Occasionally other cell types such as Paneth cells and argyrophil or argentaffin cells may be present.[55, 56] The müllerian type of benign tumor is lined by columnar epithelial cells that have mucin-rich cytoplasm. Classic goblet cells are less often seen.

Some mucinous tumors may have a predominant benign proliferative stromal or fibrous component. Mucinous adenofibromas are quite rare.[57] When mucinous adenofibromas occur they are similar to the more common serous or endometrioid adenofi-

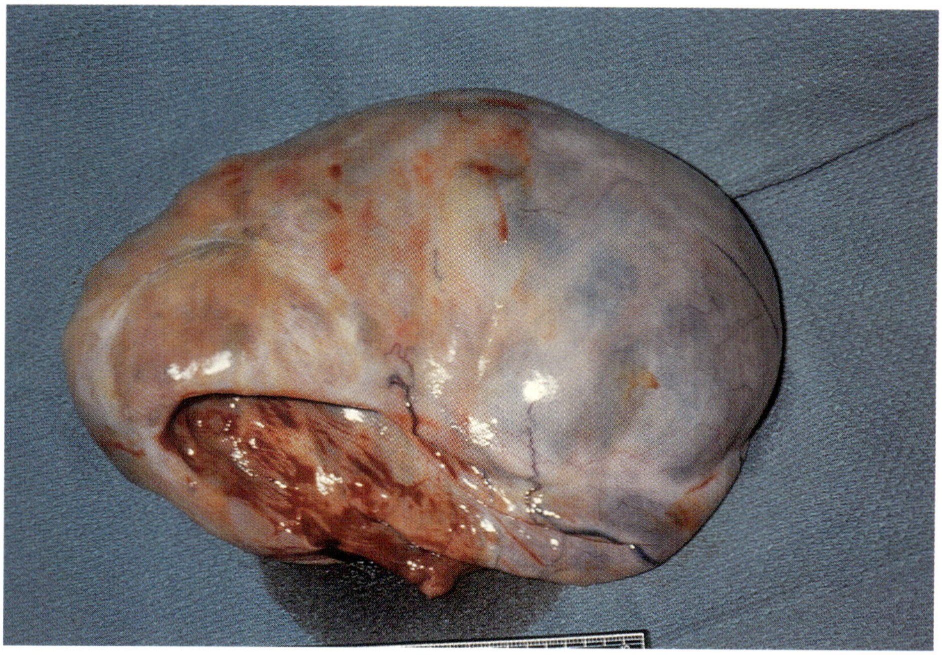

FIGURE 9-22
This large mucinous ovarian tumor has a smooth capsule with a lobulated appearance secondary to the multicystic nature of the neoplasm. This is a mucinous cystadenoma.

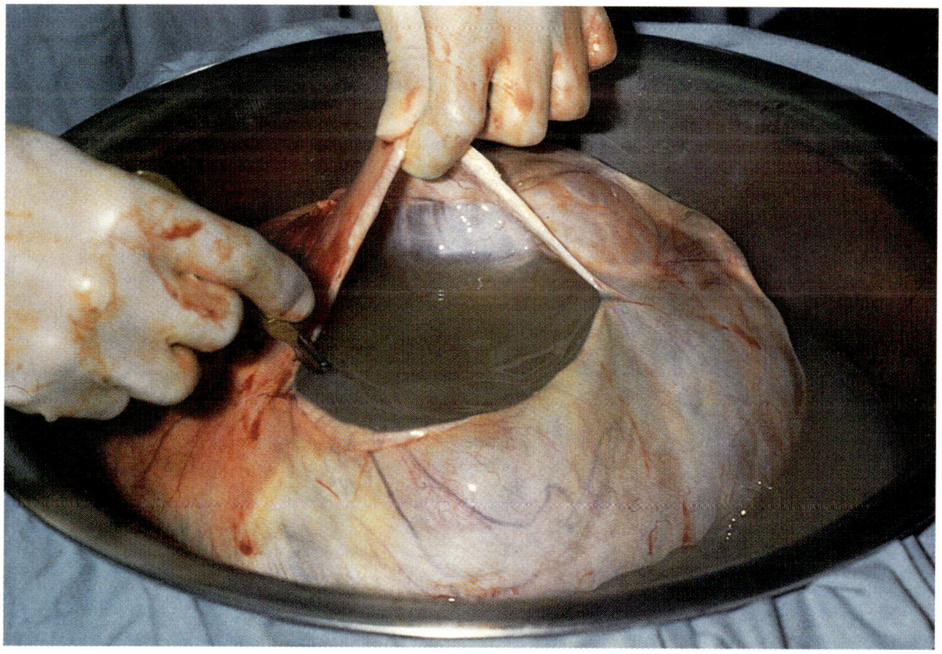

FIGURE 9-23
One of the multiple cysts that form the ovarian mucinous tumor shown in Figure 9–22 is being opened. The cyst is filled with thick, green-brown, mucoid fluid.

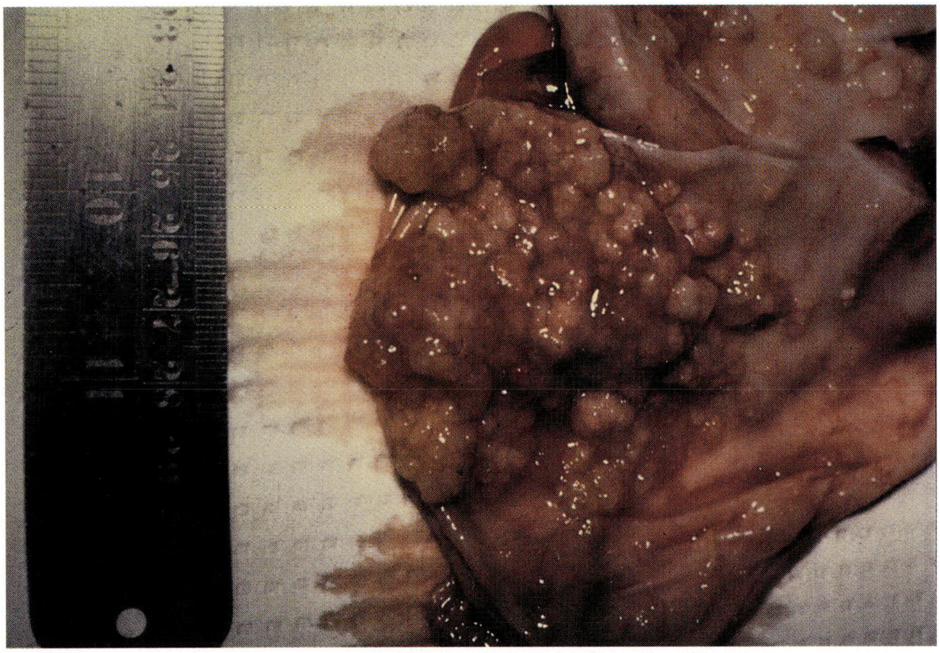

FIGURE 9-24
This is the inside wall of a mucinous cystadenocarcinoma. Multiple papillary nodules that resemble those of serous carcinoma are seen.

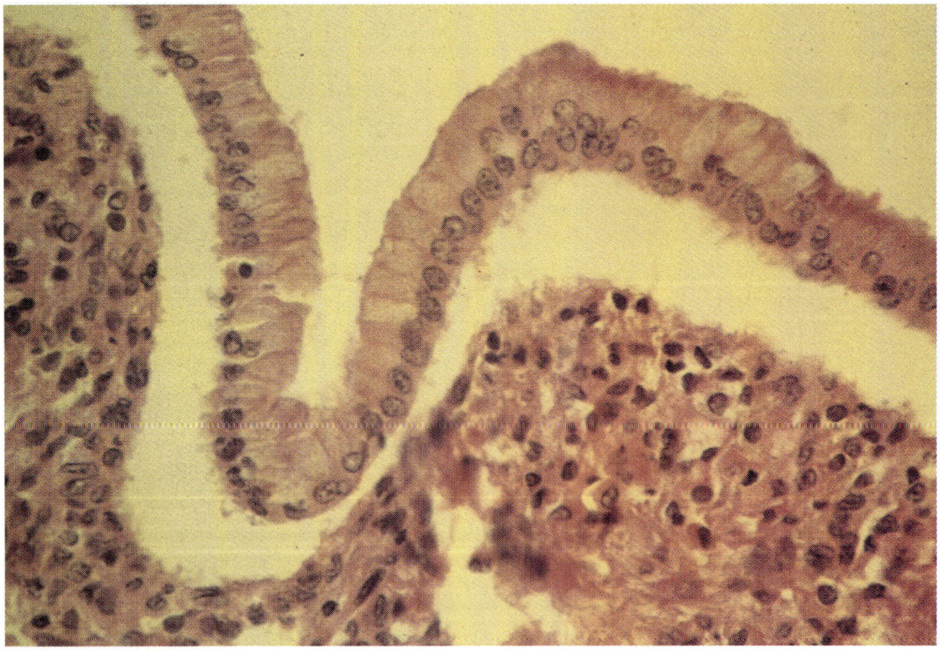

FIGURE 9-25
This is a high-power view of an ovarian mucinous cystadenoma. The cyst is lined by a single layer of columnar cells. The nuclei are basally oriented. Abundant apical cytoplasmic mucin is present.

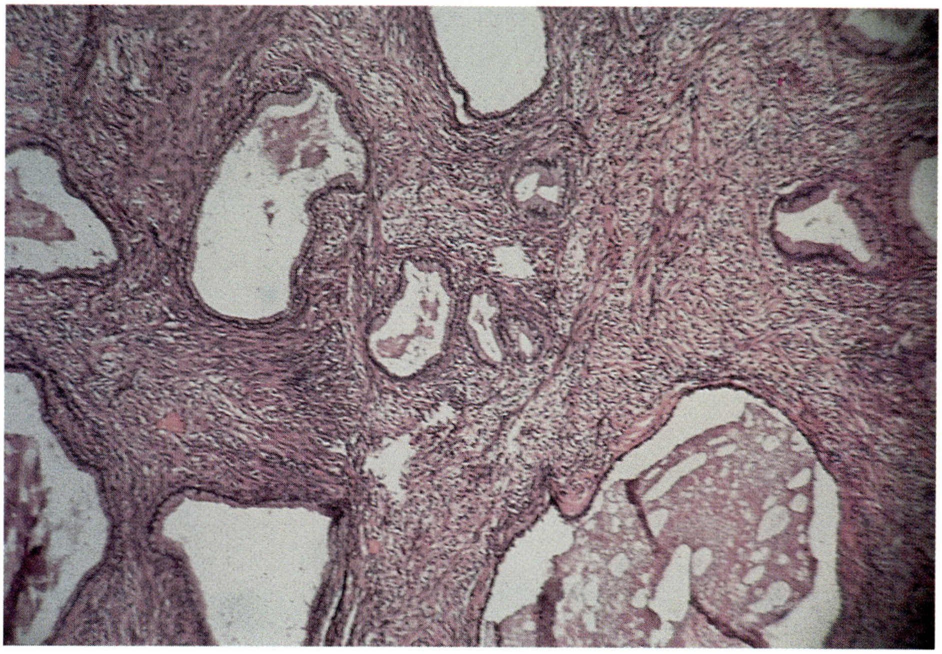

FIGURE 9-26
Multiple simple glands are seen within a benign proliferative stroma. The glands are lined by a single layer of mucin-secreting cells. This is a mucinous cystadenofibroma.

bromas consisting of a mixture of stromal elements and cysts lined by glandular epithelium (Fig. 9-26). Most of the epithelium is bland, but a few mucinous adenofibromas have been identified that show varying degrees of epithelial atypia. Even the lesions that have epithelial atypia are classified as benign. The recognition of mucinous adenofibroma as an unusual but distinct category is important, however, since it is necessary to differentiate these neoplasms from metastatic mucinous adenocarcinoma of the ovary, which will be discussed later in this section.

Mucinous LMP lesions have much less histopathologic variability than serous LMP tumors. Like serous LMP tumors, mucinous LMP tumors show evidence of epithelial proliferation. The epithelial cells retain evidence of intracytoplasmic mucin. Minimal (0-1 mitosis per high-power microscopic field) mitotic activity consisting of normal mitotic figures and a moderate degree of epithelial atypia may be present. There is a limit to the degree of cellular stratification that may be present in mucinous LMP tumors (Fig. 9-27). According to the criteria of Hart and Norris,[58] muci-

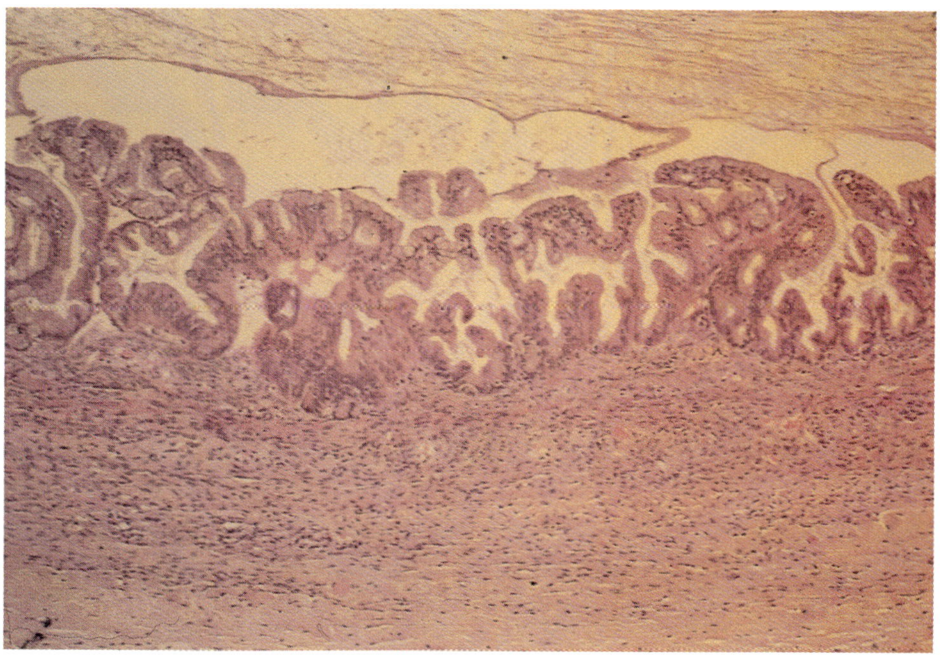

FIGURE 9-27
This mucinous LMP tumor has a more complex architecture than a mucinous cystadenoma. There is cellular stratification. Intracytoplasmic mucin and goblet cells are still prominent, especially at the surface. There is no stromal invasion. Mucinous material is seen within the cyst cavity *(top)*.

nous neoplasms with epithelial stratification of four or more cell layers should be classified as malignant. Other authors have not totally accepted this criterion. It is useful to recognize that the distinction between LMP and grade 1 mucinous carcinomas is difficult. This is especially true because the diagnosis of stromal invasion in mucinous tumors is very tenuous owing to the propensity of these neoplasms to form small epithelial lined cysts that may be mistaken for malignant glands invading the stroma of the ovary.

Some biologic as well as histopathologic differences exist between the more common mucinous LMP tumors of intestinal type and the less common mucinous LMP müllerian tumors.[59] The latter tumors have a papillary architecture that is more reminiscent of serous LMP tumors. The tumor is lined by endocervical-type cells and may have areas of larger polygonal cells with marked nuclear atypia. Frequent inflammatory reactions and focal necrosis are also common. Endometriosis was present in 30 percent of mucinous LMP müllerian-type tumors in one study.[59] In contrast, intestinal-type mucinous LMP tumors are larger and are much less often bilateral. Their lining epithelium contains goblet cells and often silver-positive argyrophil cells. Papillary formations are infrequent, and there is no associated endometriosis. Pseudomyxoma peritonei can occur with the intestinal type but usually does not occur with the müllerian-type mucinous LMP tumors. If mucinous LMP tumors are confined to the ovary, their prognosis is excellent.[33,60]

Marked epithelial atypia in mucinous neoplasms in addition to loss of cytoplasmic mucin and increased mitotic activity usually warrant a diagnosis of low-grade carcinoma rather than mucinous LMP tumor. Likewise, a cribriform pattern is rarely seen in LMP neoplasms but is usually a feature of mucinous carcinoma.[61] Frankly malignant mucinous tumors of the intestinal type often resemble colonic carcinomas. They show palisading or stratification of hyperchromatic nuclei with pleomorphism and increased mitotic activity (Fig. 9–28). Some cells show mucin secretion, and others show preservation of mucin within the cytoplasm. The endocervical or müllerian-type tumors do not resemble colonic carcinomas. The latter may be more likely to be confused with endocervical or even endometrioid carcinomas of the ovary.

Pseudomyxoma peritonei is a finding associated with mucinous tumors and frequently presents a difficult diagnostic problem.[62] Pseudomyxoma peritonei presents clinically with massive intraperitoneal mucin due to deposits of tumor on serosal surfaces that produce abundant mucin. In many instances, the tumor implants may appear benign or of LMP. It can be difficult if not impossible to identify epithelium within the pools of mucin despite numerous histologic sections. The synchronous occurrence of mucinous tumors of the ovary and appendix in cases of pseudomyxoma peritonei has long been recognized.[63] This situation results in several questions: (1) Are the two tumors simultaneous primary lesions or does one represent a metastasis from the other? (2) Which lesion is responsible for the peritoneal implants? (3) Are

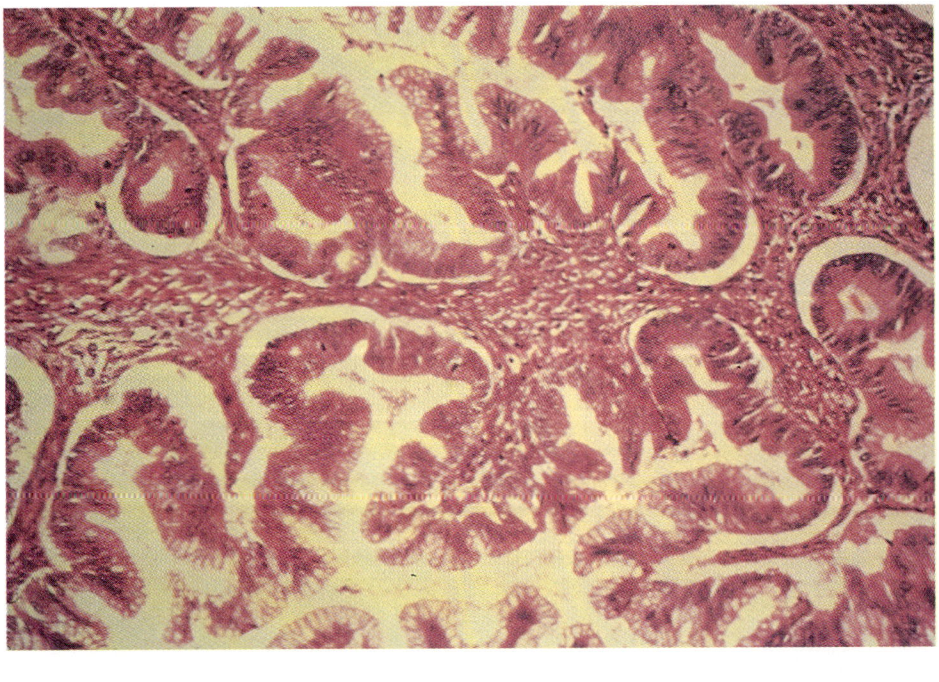

FIGURE 9–28
This ovarian mucinous carcinoma has papillary, acinar, and cribriform patterns. The papillary tumor *(lower area)* shows intracytoplasmic mucin, while the acinar groups *(upper right and left)* are formed by more poorly differentiated cells. There is brisk mitotic activity. (Courtesy of Dr. J. Donald Woodruff, The Johns Hopkins Hospital, Baltimore, MD.)

the peritoneal implants themselves primary lesions representing a transformation of the peritoneum in a manner analogous to that described for peritoneal papillary serous carcinoma? Two recent papers have addressed this issue and reached different conclusions.[64, 65] One study of 22 cases of appendiceal and ovarian neoplasms, of which 21 were synchronous, concluded that in most instances the ovarian tumor represented metastasis from the appendix.[65] These authors recommended that patients with pseudomyxoma peritonei and an ovarian tumor have the appendix removed even if it is grossly normal. They also concluded that when tumor cells were identified within the implants of pseudomyxoma peritonei the patient had a poorer prognosis. They recommend that when a diagnosis of pseudomyxoma peritonei is made the report should read, "pseudomyxoma peritonei, tumor cells identified" or "no tumor cells identified" because of the difference in prognosis. In contrast, in an analysis of 25 cases of ovarian and appendiceal mucinous lesions, 23 of which were synchronous lesions, Seidman et al[64] concluded that the tumors of the appendix and ovary probably represented separate, independent primaries. They also suggested that the peritoneal implants themselves might represent additional primary sites and not metastasis from either ovary or appendix. Part of this interpretation was based on immunoperoxidase studies in 15 of their cases using four epithelial antigens that revealed concordance for all four of the antigens in only one-third of the cases. It is apparent that the findings of these two studies do not conclusively answer the question, which will need to be approached by other methodologies. Clonality studies, as have been done with serous epithelial tumors, represent the best available approach to defining an answer to this problem.[51]

Mucinous tumors, whether benign, LMP, or frankly malignant, are occasionally associated with varying sized mural nodules that are found within the wall of a cystic tumor. These mural nodules show varying histologies, often with marked atypia. Sarcomas, (including one rhabdomyosarcoma), anaplastic carcinomas, and sarcomatous-like lesions have been described in them.[66–70] Even more rarely, carcinoid tumors have been associated with mucinous LMP tumors or adenocarcinomas.[71] Although in general carcinoid tumors are considered teratomas belonging to the category of germ cell tumors, it appears that rarely they can arise from argentaffin cells within the mucinous tumor. It should be noted also that some pathologists believe that mucinous tumors of intestinal type are themselves teratomas and that only müllerian-type mucinous tumors are epithelial in origin. This interpretation is not universally accepted.

Metastatic Mucinous Tumors

Occasionally metastatic tumors to the ovary, in particular those from the gastrointestinal tract, pancreas, or biliary tract, may mimic primary ovarian mucinous tumors.[72] This is particularly true of metastatic tumors that are predominantly cystic.[73] However, solid metastatic tumors with considerable stromal fibrosis may occasionally be confused with atypical mucinous adenofibromas. Within the predominantly cystic tumors, transition from histologically benign to malignant epithelium has been used as an indicator of a primary ovarian tumor because such transition areas are seen frequently in ovarian mucinous tumors.[20, 22] However, it should be noted that in some cases metastatic tumors show similar transition areas.[72] Studies of the clonality of the neoplasm, like those described in the section on serous tumors, may be required to answer this question, particularly in tumors that are synchronous in the ovary and some other site such as the gastrointestinal tract. Because of this situation, the gynecologic surgeon, when removing an ovarian neoplasm, should always carefully explore the entire abdomen. This exploration should include palpating the stomach and pancreas. Inspection and palpation of the liver, gallbladder, appendix, and small and large intestines is routinely performed.

Endometrioid Tumors

Endometrioid tumors of the ovary are much less common than the serous or mucinous types. However, in some series malignant endometrioid carcinomas are more common than mucinous carcinomas. They account for less than 10 to 24 percent of all epithelial ovarian cancers.[74] Benign and LMP endometrioid tumors are unusual. They usually occur as adenofibromas that contain glandular structures associated with fibrous stroma. In 10 to 28 percent of endometrioid tumors endometriosis can be identified either in the ovaries or elsewhere in the pelvis.[75] In a distinctly smaller number (approximately 5 to 10 percent) of cases, the origin of the endometrioid carcinoma can be demonstrated within an endometriotic cyst, often with an adjacent area of hyperplasia.[20] The patient in whom it can be demonstrated that the origin of the endometrioid carcinoma is from a site of endometriosis tends to be younger (by a decade on average) than the patient in whom no such origin can be demonstrated.[75]

As mentioned, benign endometrioid tumors are relatively uncommon and are usually found as adenofibromas or cystadenofibromas. These benign tumors show abundant fibrous stroma and widely spaced glands lined by a nonproliferating endometrial-type epithelium, often with squamous metaplasia but without evidence of atypia. These tumors usually are found at a slightly younger age than are endometrioid carcinomas. Several reports have described intermediate forms of endometrioid tumors, varyingly categorized as atypical, proliferative, and LMP.[76–79] The terms proliferative and LMP tumor describe different degrees of epithelial proliferation and atypia both quantitatively and qualitatively.[77] Proliferative endometrioid adenofibromas show less atypia and less epithelial proliferation than do LMP tumors, but, unlike the adenofibromas, they may show papillary or cribriform growth patterns.

Fewer studies have been done to elucidate criteria for endometrioid LMP tumors than for serous or mucinous types, possibly because endometrioid LMP tumors are less frequently identified. In most of these studies endometrioid LMP tumors are a combination of epithelial and fibrous elements (endometrioid adenofibromas). Less commonly, atypical epithelium that resembles atypical or complex hyperplasia of the endometrium is identified in foci of cystic ovarian endometriosis. These areas may represent intermediate differentiation between endometriosis and endometrial adenocarcinoma but are not classically included in descriptions of endometrioid LMP tumors. One study distinguished proliferating endometrioid tumors from LMP endometrioid tumors using quantitative criteria.[79] In proliferative endometrioid tumors, epithelial proliferation with multiple cell layering is seen, and occasionally cytologic atypia may be identified, but there should be no solid areas of epithelium exceeding 5 mm uninterrupted by stroma. In contrast, endometrioid LMP tumors show one or more areas of glandular proliferation that exceed 5 mm without intervening stroma. Papillary patterns are also identified in endometrioid LMP tumors lined by epithelial cells that exhibit nuclear stratification and epithelial atypia, analogous to the changes seen in complex hyperplasia of the endometrium (see Chapter 6). In general, stromal invasion is not present; however, microscopic foci of stromal invasion can be seen in a few of these tumors but have not been associated with an adverse prognosis.[79]

Coexisting endometriosis can be seen both within the same ovary as LMP endometrioid tumors and at extraovarian sites within the pelvis. This coexistence has been confirmed by several studies. The origin of these LMP lesions from endometriosis has been difficult to confirm. Some studies of LMP endometrioid tumors[76, 78, 79] have also found evidence of coexisting intrauterine endometrial hyperplasia or carcinoma, similar to the situation with ovarian endometrioid carcinomas, which are associated with synchronous endometrial carcinoma in approximately 25 percent of cases. The biologic behavior of the proliferative and LMP endometrioid tumors in all of the reported studies has been benign. This is also the case for LMP tumors with rare foci of microinva-

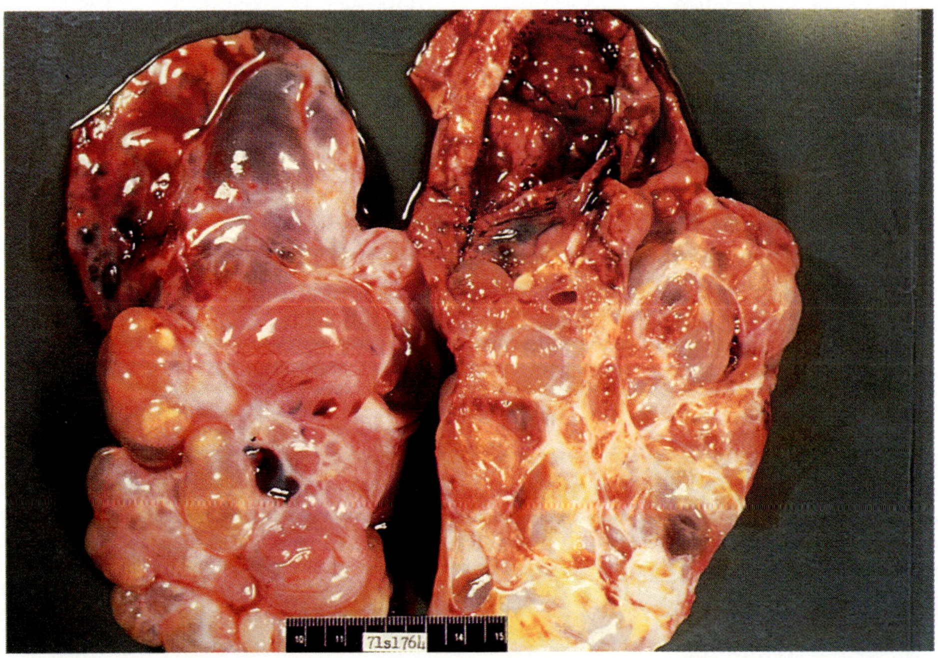

FIGURE 9–29
This ovarian endometrioid carcinoma is both solid and cystic. A large hemorrhagic area is seen *(top).*

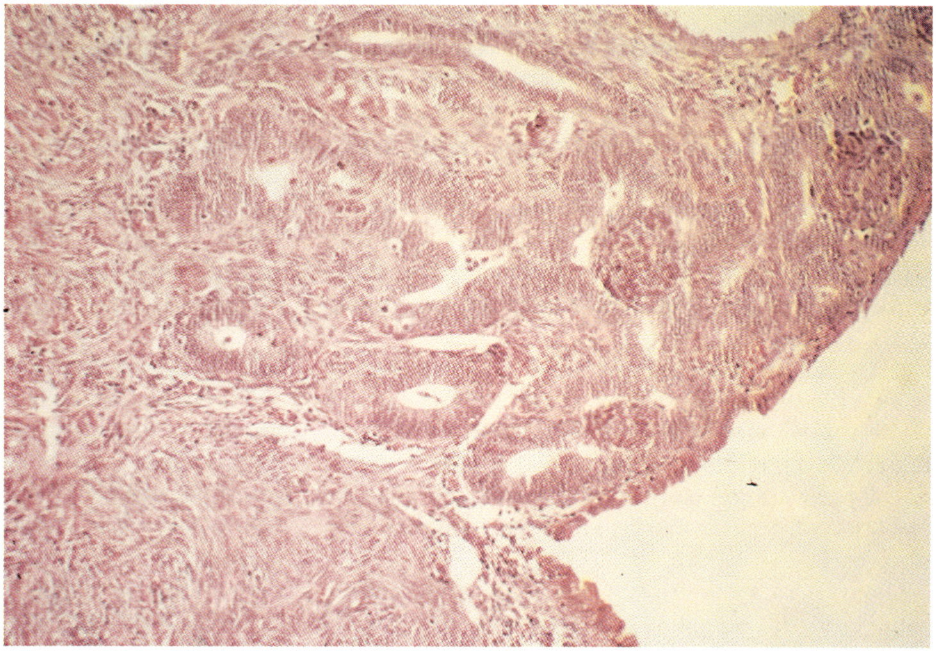

FIGURE 9-30
A focus of endometrioid adenocarcinoma is seen just under the ovarian mesothelium. Three endometrial stromal clusters (balls of small dark cells) seem to be present within the tumor glands. Two simple glands *(top, right)* are lined by a single layer of cells and are consistent with endometriosis.

sion. However, tumors with extensive foci of microinvasion in several low-power fields should probably be considered malignant.[77] The endometrioid LMP and proliferative tumors are usually confined to one ovary and do not show extraovarian spread, unlike serous LMP tumors.

Endometrioid carcinomas account for approximately 20 percent of all primary ovarian epithelial cancers[24] (Fig. 9–29). As mentioned previously, in approximately 5 to 10 percent of cases they are identified arising within areas of endometriosis (Fig. 9–30). Even when this origin is not seen, there is associated endometriosis in approximately 28 percent of cases.[80] Ovarian endometrioid carcinomas frequently exhibit cystic as well as papillary, cribriform, and solid growth patterns. In well-differentiated tumors the epithelium is a pseudostratified columnar form and resembles endometrial epithelium. Like endometrial adenocarcinoma, ovarian endometrioid carcinoma may contain areas of benign or malignant squamous epithelium (Fig. 9–31). Prognosis is related to histopathologic grade and to stage. In general, the prognosis for stage I tumors is good.[81] However, as

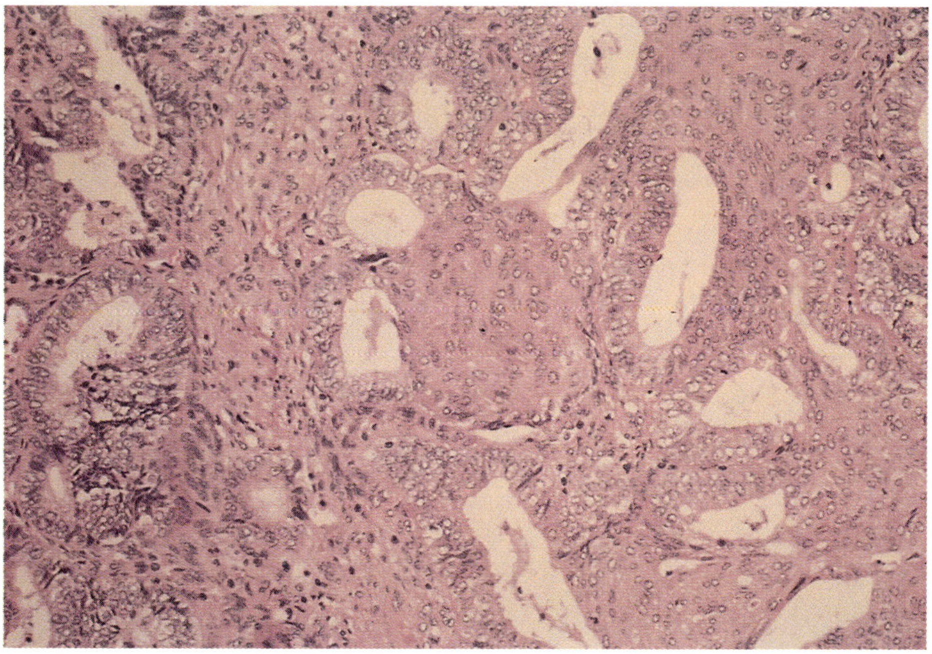

FIGURE 9-31
This is a well-differentiated ovarian endometrioid adenocarcinoma with areas of squamous differentiation *(center, right)*.

with all epithelial carcinomas, the prognosis for advanced-stage tumors is poor. In one study the 5-year survival rate was 87 percent for patients with stage I disease, 48 percent for stage II, 41 percent for stage III, and 20 percent for stage IV.[74] Tumor grade and amount of postsurgical residual disease are also significant prognostic factors.

In approximately 25 percent of cases of ovarian endometrioid carcinomas, synchronous endometrial carcinomas are present. Often the two tumors are histologically similar. In most of these cases the two tumors appear to arise as synchronous primary neoplasms. In one study the 5-year survival rate of patients with endometrioid carcinomas with or without endometrial cancers was similar for all stages, supporting the theory that the two tumors represent synchronous primary neoplasms.[82]

Ovarian mixed mesodermal tumors (carcinosarcoma and adenosarcoma) can be included in the category of endometrioid tumors because the epithelial component resembles endometrial adenocarcinoma. Rarely, they have been reported to arise within endometriosis.[83] The presence of stromal elements also allows them to be classified under ovarian stromal tumors (see Chapter 11). Adenosarcomas are characterized by malignant cellular stroma and benign epithelium. They are frequently large and may have a somewhat more favorable prognosis than carcinosarcoma in which both epithelial and stromal components are malignant[84, 85] (Fig. 9–32). Ovarian carcinosarcoma is an aggressive tumor that usually presents with disease outside of the pelvis and kills most patients within 6 months of diagnosis.[86] In most cases the tumor is confined to the abdominal cavity.[87] Although the mixture of malignant stromal and epithelial tissues may suggest a diagnosis of malignant teratoma, the differentiation between teratoma and carcinosarcoma should not be difficult. First, malignant teratoma is a tumor of children and young adults, whereas carcinosarcoma is found in menopausal and postmenopausal patients. Second, the tumor elements of malignant teratoma are immature fetal-type tissues (see Chapter 10), whereas those of carcinosarcoma are of the adult type. Third, neuroectoderm is common in teratoma but quite rare in carcinosarcoma.

Endometrial stromal sarcomas of the ovary are rare tumors that may be misdiagnosed as carcinosarcoma or as adenosarcoma. They are also frequently misclassified as some other type of ovarian sarcoma or as a tumor of the specialized ovarian stroma.[88] They are often bilateral and are commonly associated with endometriosis. They may also be associated with intrauterine endometrial stromal sarcomas, either synchronously or metachronously. In some of these cases clinical evidence suggests to separate primary tumors.[88] A histopathologic distinction of high- and low-grade tumors on the basis of mitotic counts and cytologic atypia has important prognostic implications.

Ovarian endometrioid carcinomas are occasionally misdiagnosed as other tumor types. This occurs most commonly if the endometrioid tumor has a prominent fibrous stromal component or if much of the tumor is composed of squamous epithelium. In the latter case, the tumor may be mis-

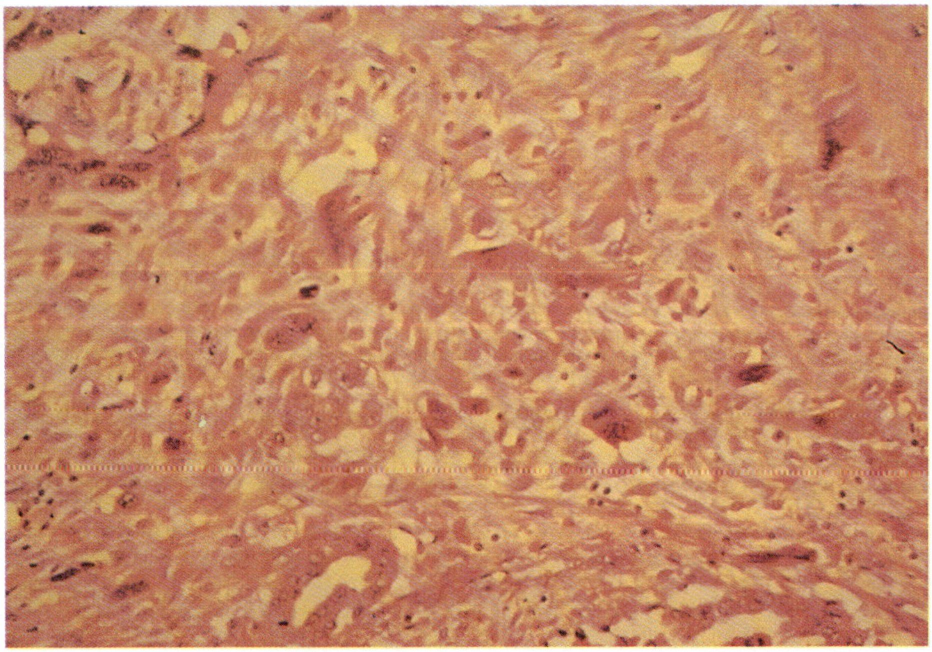

FIGURE 9–32
This ovarian carcinosarcoma shows malignant glandular structures *(bottom)*. Most of the rest of the field is composed of a poorly differentiated sarcomatous component. Many of the cells are spindle-shaped; others are large and bizarre.

diagnosed as a Brenner tumor. As will be discussed later, Brenner tumors may contain areas of glandular and squamous epithelium, but the glandular epithelium is mucinous, not endometrioid.

Another problem in the differential diagnosis is the endometrioid carcinomas that resemble Sertoli-Leydig or granulosa cell tumors.[89] These endometrioid carcinomas show prominent areas of small or elongated tubal structures within a fibrous stroma that may occasionally contain luteinized cells. If multiple sections are taken from these areas of atypical endometrioid carcinoma, squamous epithelium or a benign endometrioid adenofibroma can be identified. The glandular elements in the endometrioid carcinoma may stain for mucin. Immunostaining for epithelial membrane antigen may be helpful because in one series it was positive in all cases of ovarian endometrioid carcinoma but present in only one Sertoli-Leydig cell tumor.[90]

Clear Cell Tumors

Clear cell carcinoma of the ovary has been recognized as a neoplasm of müllerian derivation ever since the association of this tumor with endometriosis and endometrioid tumors was noted by Scully and Barlow in 1967.[91] Prior to that time the tumor had been described as mesonephric in origin (ovarian mesonephroma of Schiller). Clear cell tumors, like endometrioid tumors of the ovary, most commonly are found as malignant neoplasms.

In both their benign and malignant forms clear cell tumors are characterized by two distinctive cell types, clear cell and hobnail cell. The clear cells, as the name implies, have a large amount of pale to clear cytoplasm that can be demonstrated to contain glycogen (Fig. 9–33). The nuclei of these cells are somewhat vesicular and in the LMP and malignant varieties show nuclear enlargement, coarse chromatin, and nucleoli as well as pleomorphism. The hobnail cells have a more eosinophilic but scant cytoplasm with a large nucleus, which in some cells sticks out toward the gland lumen (Fig. 9–34). Less commonly, flattened or eosinophilic cells are recognized. Occasionally these comprise the dominant cell type.[92] These cells are more commonly found in the carcinomas.[93] These varying cell types frequently line tubules or cysts in both the benign and malignant tumors and form solid sheets or papillary structures in the carcinomas.

Several studies have demonstrated an increased incidence of coexisting endometriosis in the involved ovary or in the pelvis of patients who have a clear cell carcinoma. In fact, the association of endometriosis with clear cell carcinoma is higher than that of any other ovarian tumor and is present in approximately half of the cases.[27, 82, 93] This observation has prompted some authors to suggest that, as is true for endometrioid carcinomas, clear cell carcinomas may also arise in some instances from endometriosis. This origin cannot be demonstrated as often for clear cell tumors as for endometrioid carcinomas, but the frequent association with endometriosis is difficult to ignore, as is the fact that clear cell tumors also may arise from the endometrium.

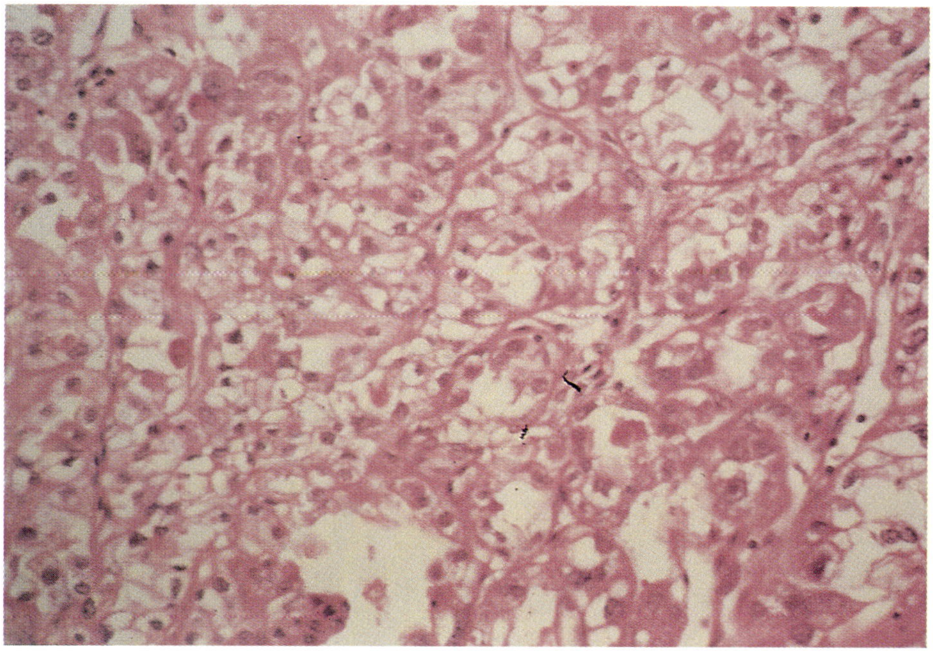

FIGURE 9–33
An ovarian clear cell carcinoma is composed of sheets of cells that contain clear vacuolated cytoplasm. Some vesicular nuclei with prominent nucleoli are seen.

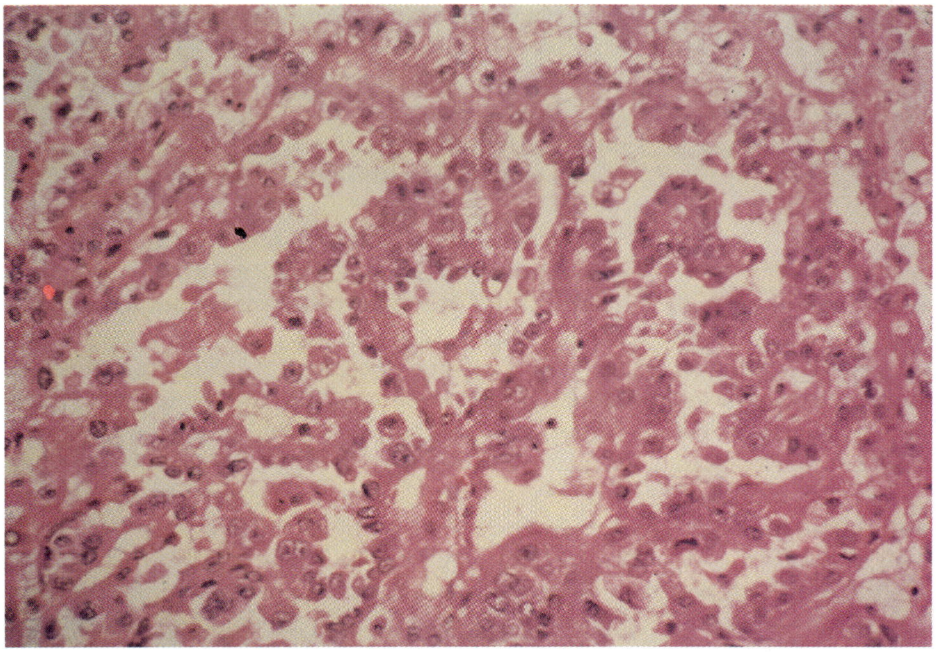

FIGURE 9-34
This area of an ovarian clear cell carcinoma shows hobnail cells rather than clear cells. The cells have scant eosinophilic cytoplasm. They line thin fibrovascular papillary stalks. There are many vesicular nuclei that have prominent nucleoli. Some of the nuclei protrude toward the spaces.

Benign and LMP forms of clear cell tumors are rare and usually exist as adenofibromatous neoplasms with a marked stromal component. The benign tumors generally show small cystic or tubular structures lined by clear or hobnail cells without evidence of significant atypia or proliferation. These tubules are widely spaced within a fibrous stromal component. The tumors designated as LMP show a similar pattern of small cysts or tubules arrayed within a stroma composed of spindle-shaped cells. However, the epithelium lining the cysts and tubules shows evidence of proliferation, epithelial tufting, and nuclear atypia but no significant mitotic activity.[94, 95] Occasionally a solid group of cells can be recognized.[95] Usually the LMP tumors also show areas of benign clear cell adenofibroma. In some cases, small areas of invasive carcinoma can be observed within these LMP neoplasms.[94, 95] These areas are characterized by stromal invasion, often with accompanying desmoplasia. The area of microinvasive tumor shows varying patterns of solid, cystic, and even papillary growth.[94] Occasionally more extensive carcinomatous growth can be observed.[95] The frequent coexistence of LMP and benign patterns within a single tumor, occasionally with identifiable microinvasion, has prompted speculation of progressive neoplastic transformation from benign through atypical to malignant in some of these tumors.[94] Notably, all tumors with only benign or LMP patterns have behaved in a clinically benign fashion, whereas those with microinvasive foci occasionally show recurrence or metastasis.[94] Therefore, a clear cell tumor with evidence of invasion, even if it is focal, should be given a diagnosis of carcinoma.[24] As with clear cell carcinomas, an association between clear cell adenofibroma and endometriosis exists.[94]

Clear cell carcinoma is also known to coexist with adenofibroma, and large tumors require careful sampling for this reason. Clear cell carcinomas are less common than serous, mucinous, and endometrioid cancers. They account for approximately 6 percent of all epithelial ovarian cancers.[96] The age of the patient is similar or slightly younger than that of patients who have other types of epithelial ovarian cancer. The median age was 50.6 years in one series.[93] As previously mentioned, there is a high frequency of associated endometriosis. The frequency of coexisting endometriosis either in the involved ovary or in the pelvis was 47 percent in cases of clear cell carcinoma and 28 percent in cases of endometrioid carcinomas but was less than 6 percent in patients who had mucinous tumors and 3 percent in patients with serous carcinomas.[80]

Clear cell carcinoma exhibits not only a variety of cell types but also a number of architectural patterns. The most common architectural patterns are tubulocystic and papillary patterns (see Fig. 9-34), but solid patterns of invasive growth are also seen (see Fig. 9-33). One study reported a more favorable prognosis for tumors exhibiting a predominantly tubulocystic pattern,[93] although other studies have not confirmed this.[82, 96] Unlike data for other ovarian epithelial cancers, histopathologic grading of clear cell carcinomas does not correlate with prognosis.[93,96,97]

Some studies have indicated a poorer survival rate for patients with clear cell carcinoma than for patients with other types of epithelial ovarian cancer.[98] A 5-year survival rate for patients with stage I clear cell carcinoma of approximately 50 percent, as reported in some series,[93, 99] is significantly worse than that of patients with stage I serous or endometrioid cancers.[98] A large number of stage I clear cell carcinomas appear to be stage IC. Rupture of the tumor capsule at the time of surgery may be due to a high frequency of adhesions, perhaps related to associated endometriosis. Stage IC clear cell carcinoma is associated with a poorer prognosis despite aggressive chemotherapy.[96] Clear cell carcinoma has a propensity to be found in lymph nodes when it recurs. The occurrence of nodal metastases is significantly greater for clear cell than for serous carcinoma.[98]

Clear cell carcinoma is frequently mixed with endometrioid carcinoma. If each tumor element is present in more than 10 percent of the tumor, the neoplasm should be classified as mixed epithelial carcinoma. Clear cell carcinomas may also be confused with other tumor types. The most common problems in the differential diagnosis include endodermal sinus tumor, hepatoid carcinoma, lipid cell tumor, and other tumors of the specialized ovarian stroma. The differential diagnosis also includes metastatic renal clear cell carcinoma. Although renal clear cell carcinoma rarely metastasizes to the ovary, it may present as an ovarian mass in the absence of a known renal primary. Helpful histopathologic features in differentiating metastatic renal carcinoma include a lack of hobnail cells and the absence of the variety of histopathologic patterns characteristic of ovarian clear cell carcinomas.[100]

Undifferentiated Carcinoma

Undifferentiated carcinoma accounts for a varying percentage of ovarian carcinomas depending on the study cited. By definition, these are anaplastic tumors that do not exhibit features of differentiation sufficient to classify them as one of the subtypes of epithelial ovarian cancers. Because serous and endometrioid carcinomas are the most common ovarian carcinomas, it is likely that an undifferentiated carcinoma is of one of these two types. Nevertheless, for accuracy, if histopathologic features that allow a tumor to be classified into one of the major categories are not present, it is preferable to designate it as undifferentiated. This is particularly important because recent molecular studies appear to suggest that the molecular genetics of the different histopathologic types may not be similar.[101, 102] Undifferentiated carcinoma often exhibits a sheetlike growth pattern with marked cellular anaplasia (Fig. 9–35). It is often widely disseminated at the time of diagnosis.[39]

Mixed Epithelial Tumors

Mixtures of different histopathologic patterns are frequently found in epithelial ovarian tumors.[103] For example, combinations of endometrioid and clear cell carcinomas are very common. In general, if a tumor is composed of different histopathologic

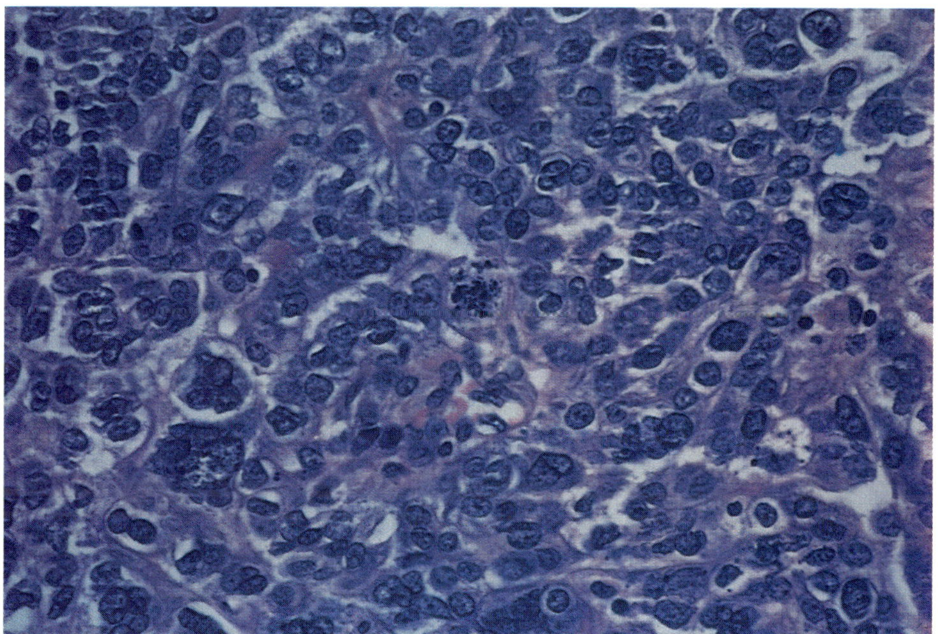

FIGURE 9–35
This tumor demonstrates marked cellular atypia and lack of architectural differentiation. However, the presence of vague slit-like areas suggests an adenocarcinoma. Several tumor giant cells and an abnormal mitosis *(center)* are seen. This is an undifferentiated carcinoma.

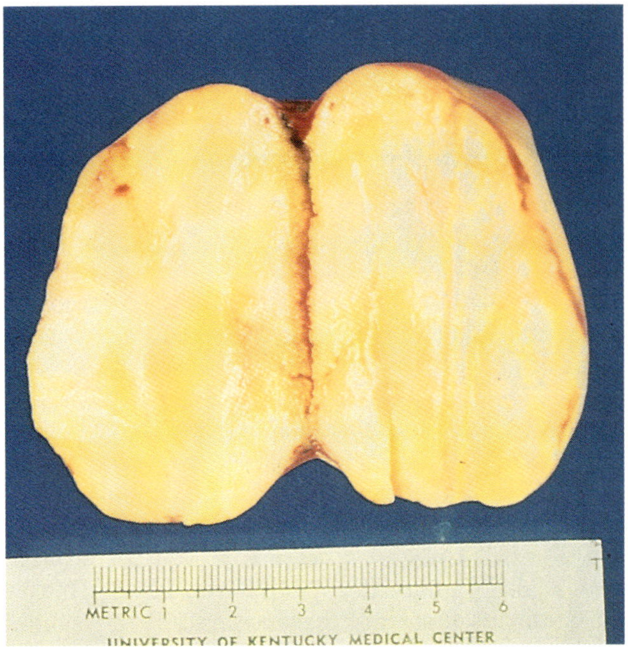

FIGURE 9-36
This solid, yellowish tumor replaced the normal ovary. Microscopic examination showed a benign Brenner tumor.

types and two or more types each compose more than 10 percent of the tumor, it should be classified as mixed and the specific histopathologic types should be mentioned.[80]

Brenner Tumors and Transitional Cell Carcinomas

The ovarian Brenner tumor most commonly is found as an incidental small tumor within an ovary removed for other reasons. Occasionally a Brenner tumor is large and presents as a pelvic mass (Fig. 9–36). The typical benign Brenner tumor is composed of fibrous stroma in which there are small nests of epithelial cells. These epithelial cell nests resemble transitional epithelium (Fig. 9–37). The cells have regular nuclei with small nucleoli and are characterized by very prominent, easily recognized nuclear grooves, a feature found also in cells of granulosa tumors and referred to as coffee bean nuclei (Fig. 9–38). The cytoplasm is palely eosinophilic. Often, cystic spaces containing an eosinophilic material are present within the clusters of cells, which resemble the Call-Exner bodies of granulosa cell tumors.

Classically, this benign tumor is small, usually less than 2 cm. Its histogenesis is controversial, but it is probably the result of a neoplastic change and metaplasia of ovarian surface epithelium inclusions. The occurrence of Walthard inclusions (i.e., Walthard rest, Walthard cyst) has been described on the ovaries, fallopian tubes, and uterine serosa (Fig. 9–39), all covered by mesothelium. The variety of epithelia that can be found in these inclusions are similar to those described for the Brenner tumor.

Malignant and intermediate forms of the Brenner tumor are recognized.[24, 103a] Both malignant and intermediate Brenner tumors are characterized by an overgrowth of the epithelial component of the tumor. The intermediate varieties have been characterized most recently by Roth et al[104] as metaplastic, proliferating, and LMP forms. In their definition, metaplastic tumors are benign Brenner tumors that frequently show admixtures of other types of epithelium, which often lines the

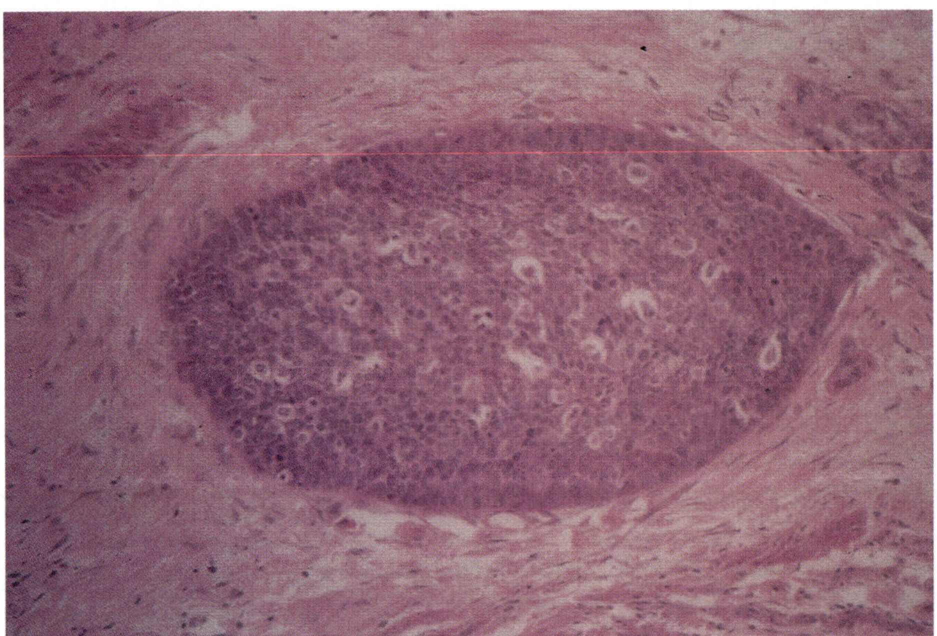

FIGURE 9-37
A nest of transitional cells surrounded by a fibrous stroma is seen in this benign Brenner tumor.

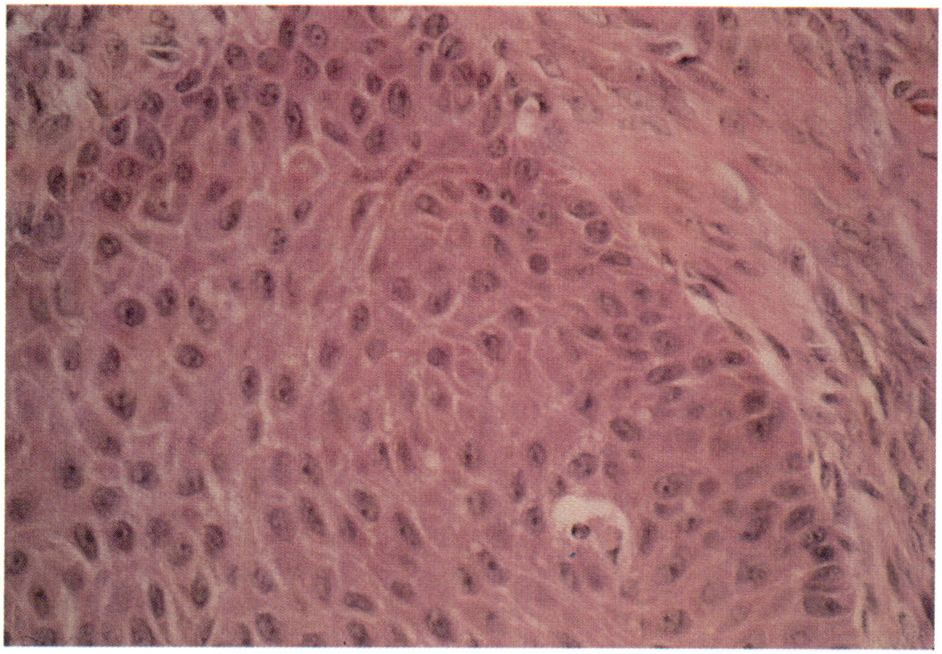

FIGURE 9-38
The Brenner tumor shown is composed of a very uniform population of cells. The nucleoli are prominent, and nuclear grooves are seen in some of the cells. The intercellular spaces are prominent; some intercellular bridges are seen, which suggests squamous differentiation.

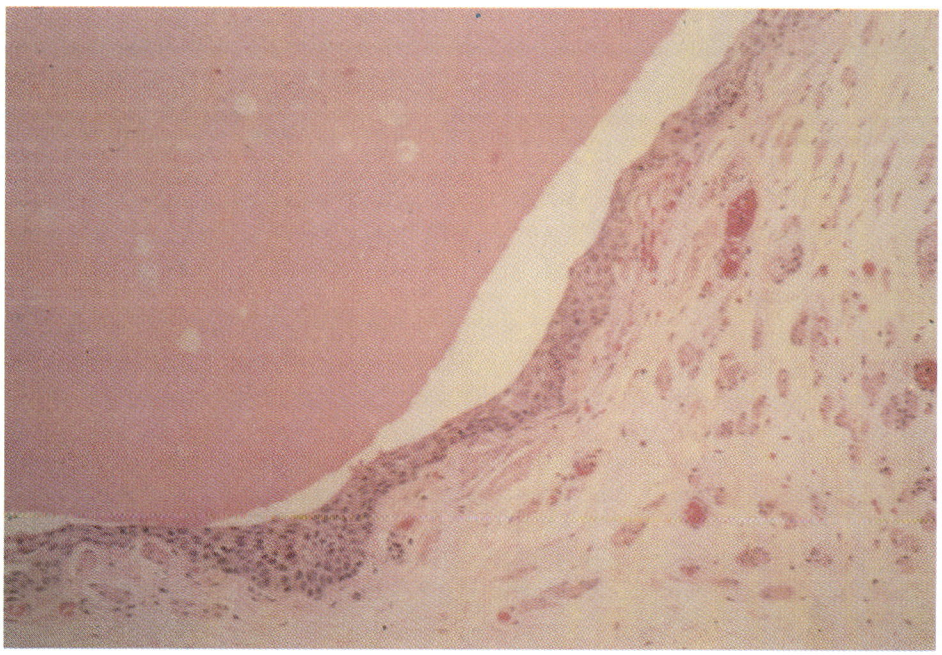

FIGURE 9-39
This Walthard inclusion was found on the surface of a fallopian tube. The inclusion wall is lined by epithelium that resembles immature squamous metaplasia as seen in the transformation zone of the cervix. The inclusion contents consist of fluid and cellular debris.

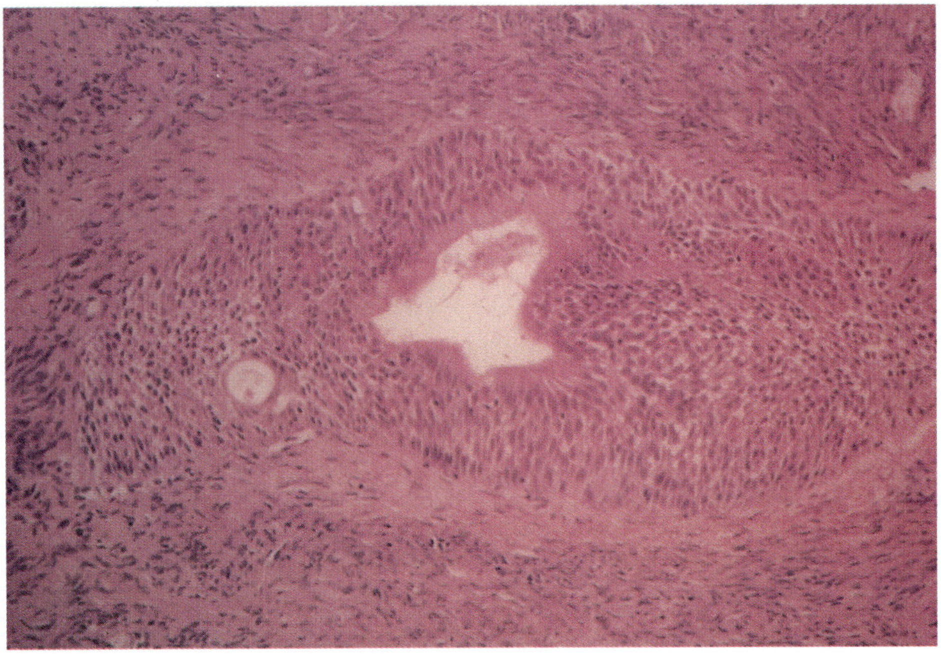

FIGURE 9–40
This nest of Brenner tumor cells has a central cystic space lined by glandular metaplastic cells that resemble those of the endocervix.

cystic spaces. Most commonly, this epithelium is a mucinous epithelium, but squamous epithelium is also often present (Fig. 9–40). Proliferating Brenner tumors resemble low-grade transitional cell carcinomas of the urinary bladder. These tumors are often cystic, the cystic structures being lined by bands of proliferating multilayered transitional-type epithelium that is often arrayed in papillary formations. Mild to moderate cytologic atypia and mitotic activity may be present, but stromal invasion is notably absent.[23a] To date, no proliferative Brenner tumor has been associated with a patient death. This suggests that these are benign neoplasms.

A lack of stromal invasion also characterizes the rare LMP Brenner tumor. Like the proliferating tumors, LMP Brenner tumors are also often cystic with a proliferating undulating urothelial pattern but also show significant nuclear atypia and mitotic activity. Thus, these tumors look like in situ or papillary grade 3 transitional cell carcinomas of the bladder. Not infrequently, squamous differentiation can be seen in these LMP tumors; when present, it resembles squamous cell carcinoma in situ. Both proliferating and LMP Brenner tumors should be accompanied by identifiable areas of benign Brenner tumor to make a correct diagnosis. Not infrequently, a transition between benign and proliferating neoplasm may be present. Flow cytometric studies have demonstrated that LMP and proliferating Brenner tumors are most commonly diploid.[105] One proliferating Brenner tumor was tetraploid.[105] Progressively increasing S phase fractions are noted in benign, proliferating, and LMP Brenner tumors. Malignant Brenner tumors are characterized by the presence of stromal invasion, which is occasionally difficult to recognize.[106] It is now generally accepted that to make a diagnosis of malignant Brenner tumor, areas of benign or proliferating Brenner tumor must be present within the ovary. In addition, there must be a papillary and invasive tumor that resembles transitional cell carcinoma with varying degrees of nuclear atypia and pleomorphism. Malignant Brenner tumor may also be characterized by areas of squamous cell carcinoma (Fig. 9–41) and, less commonly, by areas of glandular differentiation within the transitional tumor cell nests. Flow cytometric studies have described most malignant Brenner tumors as aneuploid with elevated S phase fractions.

Brenner tumor, of either the benign or malignant type, may be associated with mucinous tumors of the ovary and may represent two separate primary neoplasms. More recently, the entity of transitional cell carcinoma of the ovary has been described.[107–109] Transitional cell carcinoma is a malignant tumor of the ovary that resembles transitional cell carcinoma of the urinary bladder (Fig. 9–42). This tumor can be differentiated from a malignant Brenner tumor by the absence of any identifiable areas of benign or proliferating Brenner neoplasm. Transitional cell carcinoma of the ovary must show evidence of stromal invasion. Histopathologically it is graded similarly to transitional carcinomas of the urinary bladder. Like malignant Brenner tumor, transitional cell carcinoma of the ovary may have some components of squa-

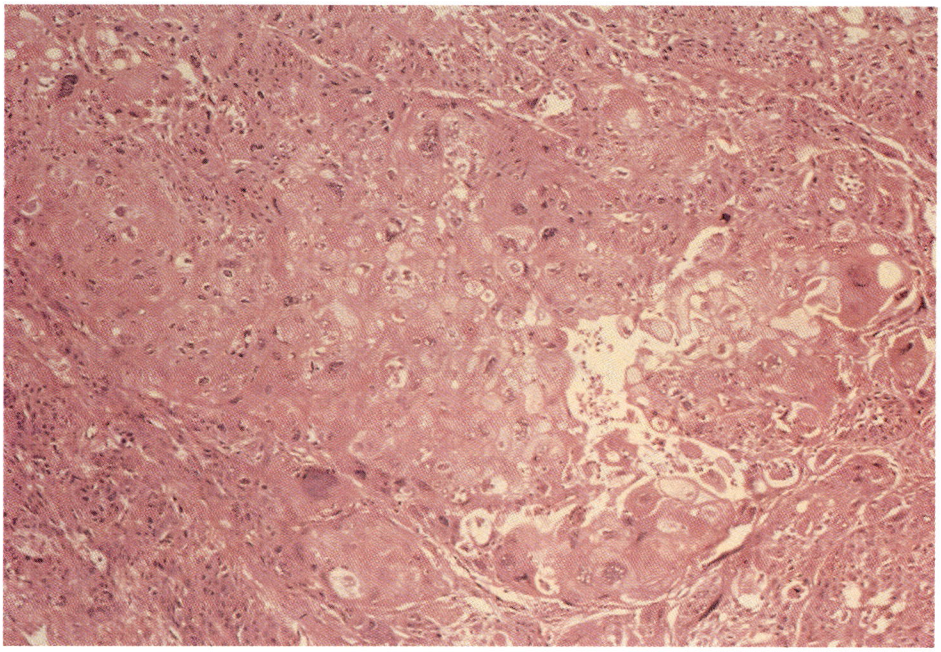

FIGURE 9-41
This is an area of poorly differentiated, keratinizing squamous cell carcinoma within a Brenner tumor. At the periphery of this area the cells appear transitional. This is a malignant Brenner tumor.

mous carcinoma or adenocarcinoma, but these are usually relatively minor portions of the neoplasm. The few flow cytometric studies of these tumors have indicated that most if not all transitional cell carcinomas are aneuploid.[105, 108] Compared with malignant Brenner tumor, transitional cell carcinomas appear to be more aggressive neoplasms.[107] They more commonly present as advanced-stage disease. When stage IA transitional cell carcinoma is compared with stage IA malignant Brenner tumor, there is a decreased survival for patients with transitional cell carcinoma. It has been suggested that transitional cell carcinomas of the ovary arise directly from the ovarian surface epithelium in a fashion analogous to serous or mucinous tumors rather than from existing benign or proliferating Brenner tumors. In contrast, the malignant Brenner tumor is thought to arise from a preexisting benign or proliferating Brenner neoplasm.

Some studies have suggested that transitional cell carcinoma may be a fairly common element in high-grade ovarian carcinomas admixed with other elements.[110] In a review of ovarian carcinomas at the M.D. Anderson Cancer Center from 1979 to

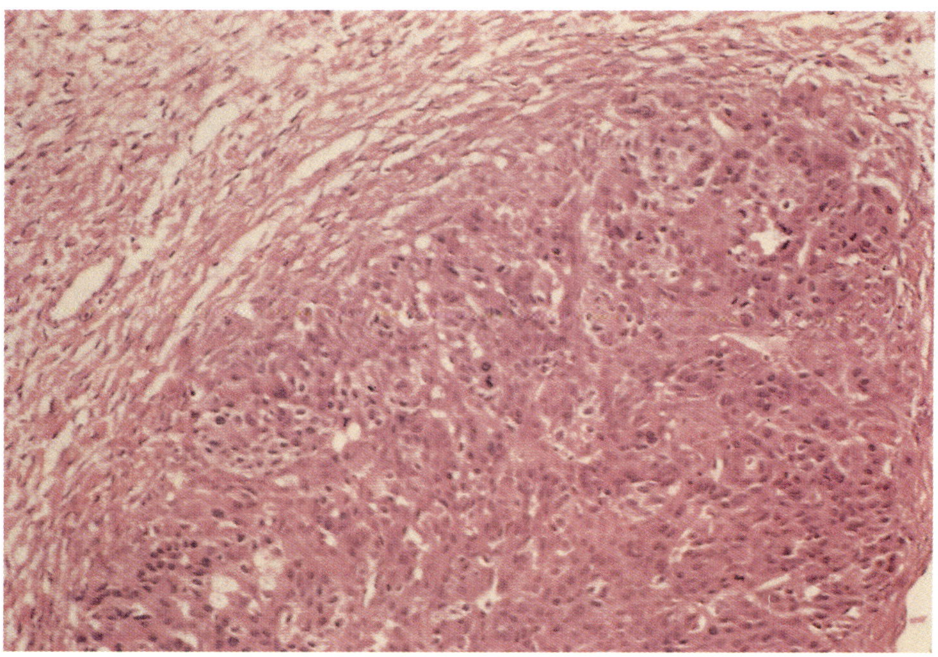

FIGURE 9-42
This malignant ovarian tumor forms a nodule, from which cells are invading the stroma. The cells are small and transitional in appearance. The cytoplasm is abundant. There is moderate nuclear pleomorphism and brisk mitotic activity. This is an ovarian transitional cell carcinoma.

1983, 9.4 percent of the tumors were found to have areas of transitional cell carcinoma.[110]

Small Cell Carcinomas

Although small cell carcinoma of the ovary is not typically included with epithelial tumors, evidence suggests that it is epithelial in origin. Therefore, it is included in this chapter for completeness. Recent reports suggest that small cell carcinoma of the ovary should be subclassified into at least two distinct histopathologic types.[111, 112] The most commonly recognized entity, ovarian small cell carcinoma of the hypercalcemic type, has been described in a large number of reports beginning with the initial descriptions by Dickersin et al.[113] More recently, ovarian small cell carcinoma of pulmonary type has also been described.[111]

Ovarian small cell carcinoma of hypercalcemic type is a tumor primarily of children and young adults. The patients' average age is 23 years.[112] This tumor is characteristically unilateral, and in over half of the patients it presents at an advanced stage. It is associated with high mortality rates. In a significant percentage (over 60 percent) of cases there is an association with hypercalcemia. The serum levels of calcium fall into the normal range after complete tumor removal. The hypercalcemia associated with small cell carcinoma of the ovary is rarely symptomatic. The mechanism for production of hypercalcemia is unknown, although one tumor has been shown to contain a parathyroid hormone–like polypeptide.[114] On gross inspection, these tumors resemble ovarian dysgerminoma or lymphoma. They are solid, yellow to white in color, and have frequent areas of hemorrhage or necrosis. Although much of the neoplasm is composed of small cells arranged diffusely or in small cords or clusters, large cells with abundant eosinophilic cytoplasm, large vesicular nuclei, and prominent nucleoli may be seen (Fig. 9–43). In addition, rounded cystic structures containing eosinophilic material resembling follicles are a frequent finding in small cell carcinomas of hypercalcemic type (Fig. 9–44). These tumors usually have a high mitotic count, but flow cytometric studies show that most are diploid.[115] Ultrastructurally, dense core granules have been described infrequently, and the cells appear to be epithelial with intercellular junctions, basal laminae, and rare microvilli. Immunocytochemical staining is positive for cytokeratin and occasionally for epithelial membrane antigen. Some tumors are positive for neuron-specific enolase and chromogranin.[116]

It has been difficult to include the hypercalcemic type of small cell carcinoma of the ovary in the traditional histogenetic classification of ovarian neoplasms. The patients' age suggests that this tumor should fit better in the categories of germ cell tumor or tumors of the specialized ovarian stroma. However, electron microscopic and immunocytochemical data suggest that the tumor is of epithelial origin. As mentioned previously, these tumors are highly malignant. They are usually unilateral, and tumor in the contralateral ovary has been described only rarely. For stage IA tumors, there is little experience with adjuvant radiation or chemotherapy. In patients with more

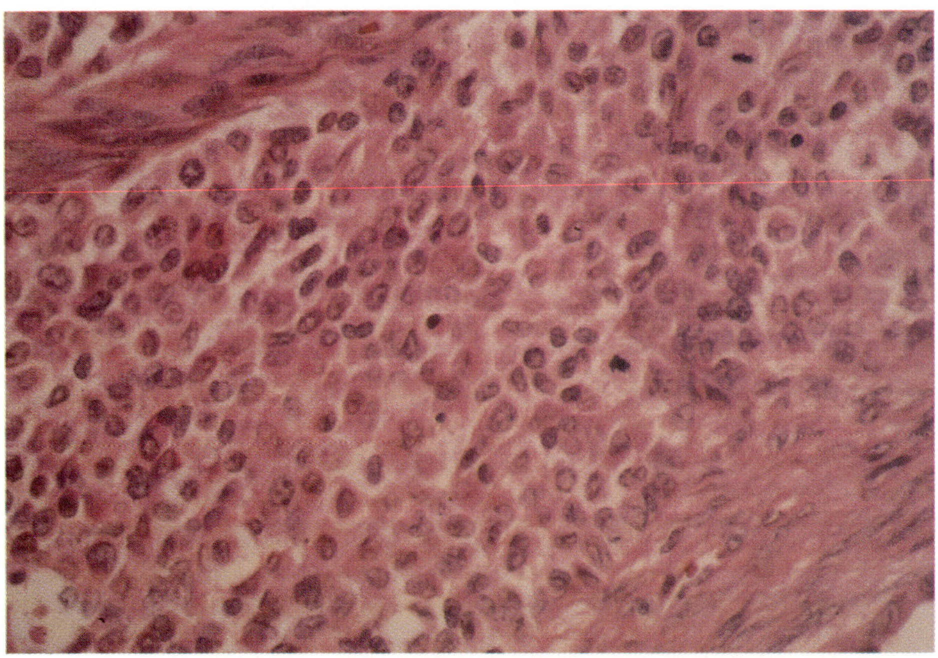

FIGURE 9–43
High-power view of an ovarian small cell carcinoma of hypercalcemic type. Most of the nuclei are large and have a vesicular chromatin pattern. Many cells have abundant eosinophilic cytoplasm. Mitoses are seen. (Courtesy of Department of Pathology, Frankford Hospital, Philadelphia, PA.)

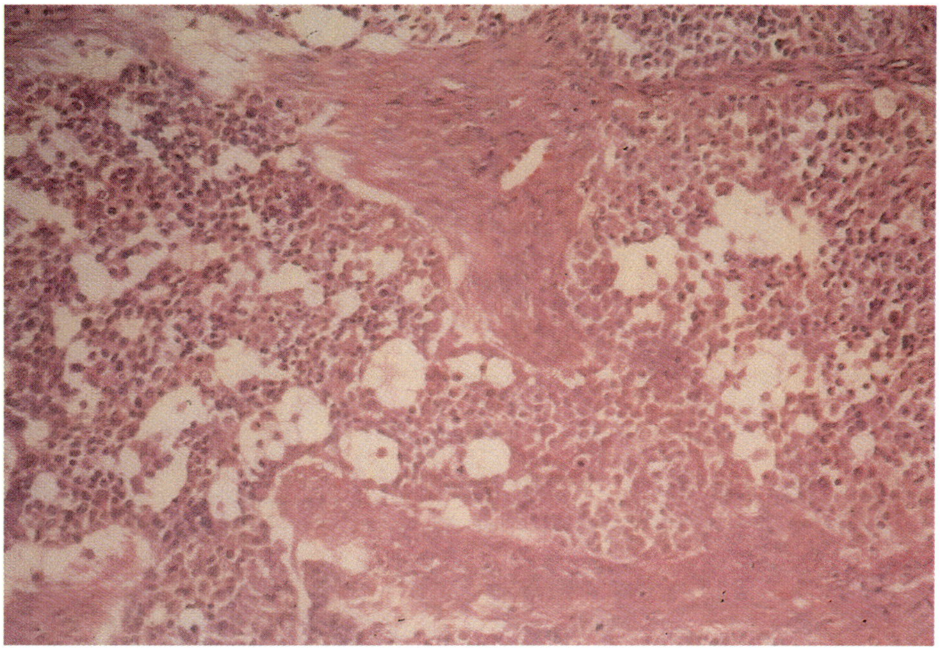

FIGURE 9-44
In this low-power view of the tumor seen in Figure 9–43 it is apparent that the cells are forming spaces and that the pattern is reminiscent of granulosa cell tumor. (Courtesy of Department of Pathology, Frankford Hospital, Philadelphia, PA.)

advanced disease the response to radiation and chemotherapy has been disappointing. At present, however, these modalities appear to provide the only hope of survival for patients with higher than stage IA disease.[117]

Ovarian small cell carcinoma of pulmonary type is a recently described entity that differs significantly from the relatively more common small cell carcinoma of hypercalcemic type. Small cell carcinoma of pulmonary type resembles other small cell carcinomas that occur in a number of organs including the lung. When they arise as primary tumors in the ovary, they occur in adult women who have a mean age of 59 years. There is almost an equal distribution of unilateral and bilateral tumors. Small cell carcinoma of pulmonary type is a predominantly solid neoplasm composed of small cells that have scant cytoplasm, hyperchromatic nuclei, and inconspicuous small nucleoli. This tumor shows a diffuse to focally trabecular growth pattern and in general lacks the folliclelike spaces and characteristic large cells seen in the hypercalcemic type of small cell carcinoma of the ovary. Some but not all tumor cells stain for cytokeratin or epithelial membrane antigen. In addition, some tumors stain for neuron-specific enolase, and a smaller percentage are positive for chromogranin. Unlike the ovarian small cell carcinoma of hypercalcemic type, flow cytometry in several cases has revealed that more than 50 percent of the tumors are aneuploid. Several tumors have been associated with other types of epithelial neoplasia, including Brenner and endometrioid tumors. Argyrophil granules have been identified in some neoplasms. Clinical evidence of hypercalcemia is not present. Like the ovarian small cell carcinomas of hypercalcemic type, this tumor is highly malignant. Five of seven patients in one reported series that had adequate follow-up died of disease within 13 months.[111] Interestingly, one patient developed a syndrome of inappropriate antidiuretic hormone secretion.

STAGING AND HISTOPATHOLOGIC GRADING OF MALIGNANT EPITHELIAL NEOPLASMS

Epithelial ovarian cancer is staged according to the FIGO system outlined in Table 9–1. As mentioned previously, most patients (two-thirds) who have epithelial ovarian cancer present with advanced-stage disease (stage III or IV) because the tumor is usually asymptomatic while still confined to the ovary, and no screening modalities are currently of proven usefulness.

Histopathologic grading systems for epithelial ovarian cancer use both architectural and nuclear features.[39, 97] In general, for all histopathologic types, grade 1 tumors show evidence of stromal invasion but maintain a well-defined papillary or glandular growth pattern, and cytologic features show some preservation of the morphologic features of their benign counterparts but there is definite nuclear atypia and pleomorphism. In contrast, grade 3 tumors show a more solid or sheetlike growth pattern, and there are only infrequent foci of glandular or papillary differentiation. There is marked nuclear pleomorphism and fre-

TABLE 9–1.
FIGO Staging of Malignant Ovarian Neoplasms

Stage I	Tumor confined to the ovaries
IA	One ovary, no ascites, intact capsule
IB	Both ovaries, no ascites, intact capsule
IC	Ruptured capsule; capsular involvement; positive peritoneal washings; or malignant ascites
Stage II	Ovarian tumor with pelvic extension
IIA	Pelvic extension to uterus or tubes
IIB	Pelvic extension to other pelvic organs (e.g., bladder, rectum, or vagina)
IIC	Pelvic extension and findings similar to those noted under IC
Stage III	Tumor outside the pelvis or positive retroperitoneal or inguinal lymph nodes
IIIA	Microscopic seeding outside the true pelvis
IIIB	Grossly visible tumor nodules. None measuring more than 2 cm
IIIC	Tumor nodules greater than 2 cm or positive lymph nodes
Stage IV	Distant organ involvement, including liver parenchyma or pleural space
	(Pleural effusion must be proved to contain malignant cells by cytopathology. Surface liver involvement in stage III)

quent mitotic activity. Newer grading systems have also added patterns of invasion, capsular penetration, and vascular invasion.[118] The fact that there can be significant interobserver variability in the grading of ovarian carcinoma should be recognized. In one study, two gynecologic pathologists disagreed in 33 percent of cases when evaluating 68 ovarian carcinomas.[119]

CLINICAL FEATURES OF EPITHELIAL OVARIAN TUMORS

As mentioned previously, epithelial ovarian cancer is a tumor of adult women. The peak incidence is in the sixth decade of life.[11] It is the fifth most common malignant tumor of women in the United States and has the highest mortality of any of the tumors of the female genital tract. When these tumors are detected as stage I disease, usually as an incidental finding on pelvic examination in an asymptomatic patient, treatment consists of total abdominal hysterectomy, bilateral salpingo-oophorectomy, and surgical staging. No additional therapy is needed if the tumor is stage IA or IB and grade I or of LMP.[120] In a nulliparous woman who wishes to preserve fertility and who has a stage IA tumor of either grade 1 or LMP, removal of the involved ovary with preservation of the uterus and contralateral adnexa could be considered.

Careful surgical staging is necessary in the evaluation of every case of ovarian neoplasm. This consists of adequate exploration of the entire abdomen. This is best done through an ample vertical midline incision. Peritoneal lavage for cytology is performed immediately on entering the peritoneal cavity. At least 200 ml of normal saline is poured into the pelvis, and a similar amount is used in each paracolic gutter. The peritoneal cavity is rinsed with the fluid, which is subsequently retrieved and submitted for cytopathologic evaluation. The peritoneal washings are placed in containers containing Saccomano's carbowax solution or, alternatively, 1000 units of heparin are added for each 100 ml of fluid retrieved. If ascites is present, a sample is obtained and submitted in a similar fashion (Fig. 9–45). Scrapings of the diaphragm are obtained with a wooden spatula and smeared onto a glass slide, which is immediately fixed and submitted for cytopathologic evaluation. This procedure has been found to be more sensitive than obtaining random samples for biopsy.[127] However, if adhesions or irregularities of the diaphragm are identified, samples of these should be taken for biopsy (Fig. 9–46). Any adhesions or areas of irregularity of the peritoneal surfaces are also submitted for biopsy. If none are present, random biopsy samples are obtained of both paracolic gutters, cul-de-sac, pelvic sidewalls, and bladder peritoneum. At least a partial omentectomy is performed. Samples of pelvic and paraaortic nodes are obtained. Metastases to the pelvic lymph nodes can occur without para-aortic node involvement and vice versa.[122] The appendix should also be removed, since it is frequently involved with tumor, and appendicitis could be confused with chemotherapy-induced typhlitis or with intestinal obstruction secondary to tumor.[123] About 20 to 25 percent of patients who on initial inspection seem to have an epithelial carcinoma confined to the ovary are found after careful surgical staging to have extrapelvic or retroperitoneal lymph node involvement.[122,124]

The 5-year survival rate is 94 percent for patients with adequate staging who have stage IA or IB, grade 1 epithelial ovarian cancer treated by surgery only.[120] There are not enough data to assess whether patients with grade 2 tumors need adjuvant chemotherapy. Patients with stage IA or IB, grade 3 tumors and those with tumors that are stage IC or above should receive adjuvant chemotherapy.[125] At present, cisplatin, carboplatin, and Taxol are considered the most cytotoxic agents active against this disease.[126] The use of high-dose chemotherapy with bone marrow or peripheral stem cell transplantation is being investigated.[127]

More than two-thirds of patients with epithelial

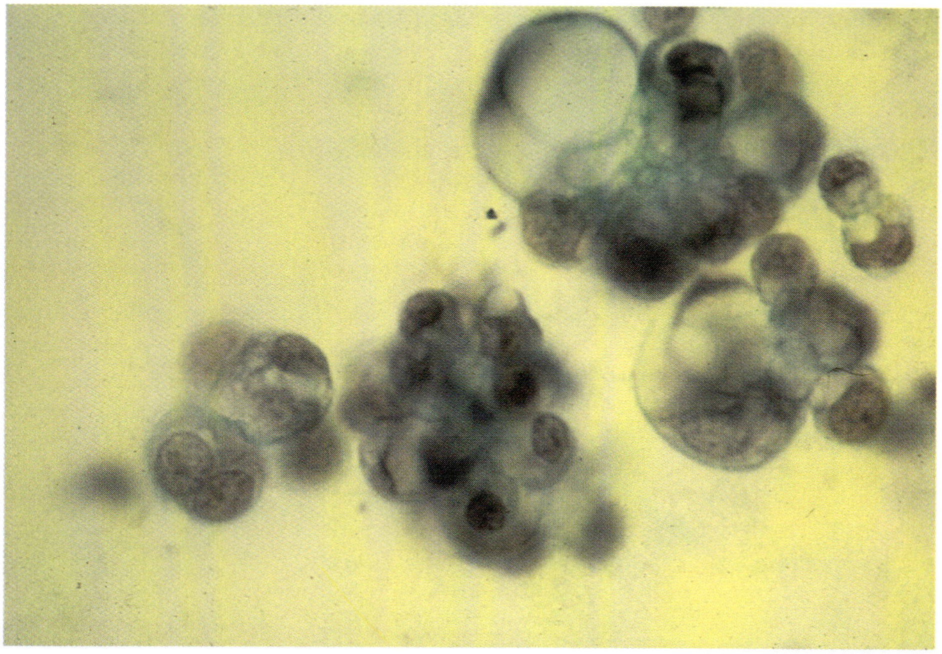

FIGURE 9-45
This is a cytologic preparation of ascitic fluid from a woman who had serous ovarian carcinoma. There are groups of cells arranged in a papillary configuration. There are variable-sized vacuoles in the cytoplasm. These round vacuoles are common in cytologic preparations of serous tumors and these cells should not be misdiagnosed as mucinous. The presence of large papillary groups of pleomorphic cells in peritoneal fluid is diagnostic of malignancy.

ovarian cancer have stage III or IV disease at diagnosis. Most have stage III disease. Although no prospective studies have been performed, retrospective studies consistently show that maximal tumor reduction (i.e., cytoreduction or tumor debulking) is associated with a better prognosis.[128]

A recent survey of the American College of Surgeons collected long-term survival data on 5156 patients who were diagnosed in the United States with ovarian carcinoma in 1983.[129] The 5-year survival rates for stages I, II, III, and IV were 89 percent, 57 percent, 24 percent, and 12 percent, respectively; when the data were stratified further to substages, the 5-year survival rates were: IA, 92 percent; IB, 85 percent; IC, 82 percent; IIA, 69 percent; IIB, 56 percent; IIC, 51 percent; IIIA, 39 percent; IIIB, 26 percent; IIIC, 17 percent; and IV, 12 percent.

In an effort to change these statistics research into the early detection of ovarian cancer is being performed at many centers.[130, 131] Most are using a combination of serum tumor markers and ultrasonography. Results at this time are preliminary and are somewhat disappointing.[132]

Elevated serum levels of CA-125 antigen (more than 200 units/ml) in the presence of a pelvic mass

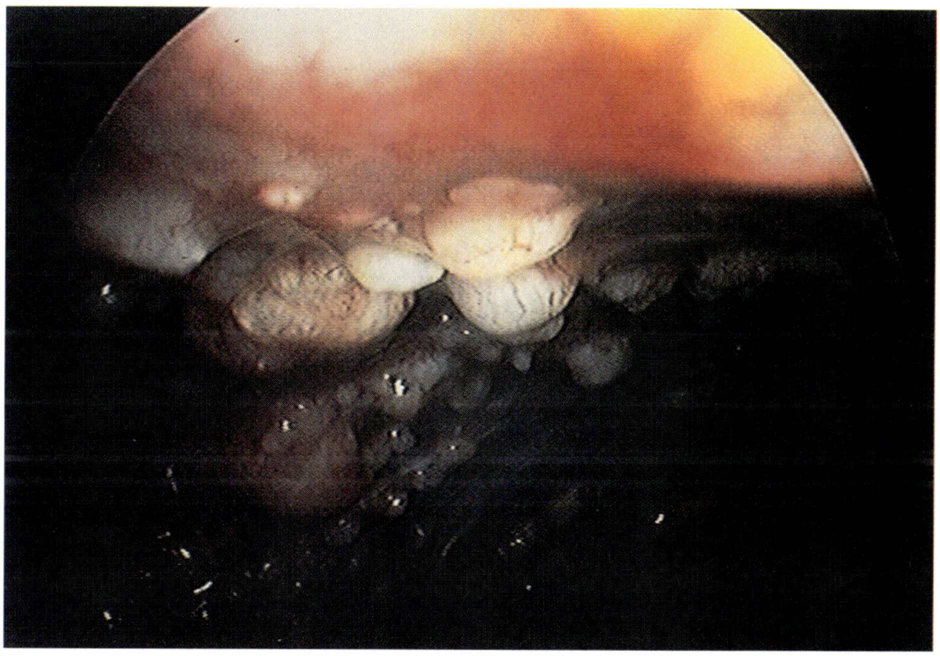

FIGURE 9-46
Photograph of the right hemidiaphragm obtained through a laparoscope. The light shines brighter on the diaphragm closer to the scope *(top)*. Multiple variable-sized tumor nodules stud the diaphragm. This patient had stage IIIC ovarian serous carcinoma. The above findings were documented at second-look laparoscopy.

is strongly predictive of ovarian cancer.[133] This antigen is not specific for ovarian cancer, however, and may be elevated in a variety of benign conditions including endometriosis and pregnancy as well as with other malignant tumors.[11] Because of its relatively low sensitivity and specificity it is not recommended as a screening modality at this time but may be used with other modalities to lend weight to a suspected diagnosis or, more commonly, to follow patients with ovarian cancer postoperatively. It should be noted that patients with mucinous tumors are unlikely to have elevated CA-125 levels but may have elevated CA 19-9 levels.[134]

In addition to stage, histopathologic grade and amount of residual tumor are other factors that have been used to predict prognosis. Several studies have shown that amplification of HER-2/*neu* oncogene in tumor cells is associated with poor prognosis in epithelial ovarian cancer.[135, 136] Flow cytometry of ovarian carcinoma has shown that tumor ploidy is an important prognostic factor for both early and advanced-stage disease.[35, 137–140] In addition, S phase fraction provides additional prognostic information in diploid tumors.[137] Even patients with stage III diploid ovarian carcinomas have a significantly longer survival than those with aneuploid tumors.[138] In one study, when multiple prognostic factors were evaluated statistically, only tumor ploidy and the presence of ascites were significant factors in predicting survival.[140] A recent study suggested that aneuploid tumors with a high DNA index may represent a high-risk subgroup of patients with well-differentiated early-stage epithelial ovarian cancer.[141] It should be noted that ovarian carcinomas are heterogeneous, and differences in DNA ploidy pattern are identified when multiple sites are assayed.[142] Therefore, when performing flow cytometry studies multiple samples should be analyzed.

Prognosis is also related to tumor type. Patients who have mucinous stage I tumors have an excellent prognosis, better than that of patients with stage I tumors of other histopathologic types.[143] In advanced-stage tumors, however, the prognosis for mucinous neoplasms approximates that of serous and clear cell carcinomas. Patients who have endometrioid carcinomas of stage II and above have a somewhat better overall 5-year survival (60 percent) than those with tumors of other histopathologic types. As mentioned previously, the survival for patients with small cell carcinoma is extremely poor. The prognosis for LMP tumors is excellent, with most studies reporting that over 90 percent of patients survive more than 10 years.[28] Factors associated with poor prognosis for LMP tumors include advanced stage and the presence of invasive tumor implants or tumor implants with marked cytologic atypia.[27]

REFERENCES

1. Yanik R: Ovarian cancer: Age contrast in incidence, histology, disease stage at diagnosis, and mortality. Cancer 1993;71:517–523.
2. Rosenshein NB, Hernandez E, Rosenblatt K: Risk factors for ovarian cancer. *In* Gold E (ed): The Changing Risk of Disease in Women: An Epidemiologic Approach. Lexington, KY, DC Heath and Co, 1984, pp 221–231.
3. Hernandez E, Rosenshein NB, Parmley NB: Mucinous cystadenocarcinoma in a premenarchal girl. South Med J 1982;75:1265–1267.
4. Hartge P, Schiffman MH, Hoover R, McGowan L, Lesher L, Norris HJ: A case-control study of epithelial ovarian cancer. Am J Obstet Gynecol 1989;161:10–16.
5. Hildreth NG, Kelsey JL, LiVolsi VA, Fischer DB, Holford TR, Mostow ED, Schwartz PE, White C: An epidemiologic study of epithelial carcinoma of the ovary. Am J Epidemiol 1981;114:398–405.
6. Booth M, Beral V, Smith P: Risk factors for ovarian cancer: A case-control study. Br J Cancer 1989;60:592–598.
7. LaVecchia C, Decarli A, Fasoli M, Franceschi S, Gentile A, Negri E, Parazzni F, Tognoni G: Oral contraceptives and cancers of the breast and of the female genital tract: Interim results from a case-control study. Br J Cancer 1986;54:311–317.
8. Parazzini F, La Vecchia C, Negri E, Gentile A: Menstrual factors and the risk of epithelial ovarian cancer. J Clin Epidemiol 1989;42:443–448.
9. Hankinson SE, Hunter DJ, Colditz GA, Willet WC, Stampfer MJ, Rosner B, Hennekensch CH, Speizer FE: Tubal ligation, hysterectomy, and risk of ovarian cancer: A prospective study. JAMA 1993;270:2813–2818.
10. Buller RE, Anderson B, Connor JP, Robinson R: Familial ovarian cancer. Gynecol Oncol 1993;51:160–166.
11. Canuistra SA: Cancer of the ovary. N Engl J Med 1993;329:1550–1559.
12. Lynch HT, Lynch JF: Hereditary ovarian cancer. Hematol Oncol Clin North Am 1992;6:783–811.
13. Narod SA, Feunteun J, Lynch HT, Watson P, Conway T, Lynch J, Lenoir GM: Familial breast-ovarian cancer locus on chromosome 17q12-q23. Lancet 1991;338:82–83.

13a. Miki Y, Swensen J, Shattuck-Eidens D, et al: A strong candidate for the breast and ovarian cancer susceptibility gene BRCA 1. Science 1994;266:66–71.

14. Harlow BL, Weiss NS, Lofton S: Epidemiology of borderline ovarian tumors. J Nat Cancer Inst 1987;78:71–74.
15. Harlow BL, Weiss NS, Roth GJ, Chu J, Daling JR: Case-control study of borderline ovarian tumors: Reproductive history and exposure to exogenous female hormones. Cancer Res 1988;48:5849–5852.
16. Parazzini F, La Vecchia C, Franceschi S, Negri E, Cecchetti G: Risk factors for endometrioid, mucinous and serous benign ovarian cysts. Int J Epidemiol 1989;18:108–112.
17. Parazzini F, Restelli C, La Vecchia C, Negri E, Chiari S, Maggi R, Mangioni C: Risk factors for epithelial ovarian tumors of borderline malignancy. Int J Epidemiol 1991; 20:871–877.
18. Schildkraut JM, Thompson WD: Familial ovarian cancer: A population-based case-control study. Am J Epidemiol 1988;128:456–466.
19. McGowan L, Parent L, Lednar W, Norris HJ: The woman at risk for developing ovarian cancer. Gynecol Oncol 1979;7:325–344.
20. Scully RE: Tumors of the ovary and maldeveloped gonads.

In Armed Forces Institute of Pathology: Atlas of Tumor Pathology, Second Series, Fascicle 16. Washington, D.C., Armed Forces Institute of Pathology, 1979.
21. Powell DE, Puls LE, van Nagell JR Jr, et al: Current concepts in epithelial ovarian tumors: Does benign to malignant transformation occur? Hum Pathol 1992;23:846–847.
22. Puls LE, Powell D, DePriest PD, Gallion HH, Hunter JE, Kryscio RJ, van Nagell JR Jr: Transition from benign to malignant epithelium in mucinous and serous ovarian cystadenocarcinoma. Gynecol Oncol 1992;47:53–57.
23. Fox H: Pathology of early malignant change in the ovary. Int J Gynecol Pathol 1993;12:153–155.
23a. Colgan TJ, Norris HJ: Ovarian epithelial tumors of low malignant potential: a review. Int J Gynecol Pathol 1983; 1:367–382.
24. Russell P: The pathological assessment of ovarian neoplasms: II. The proliferating "epithelial" tumors. Surgical Pathology of the Ovaries. London, Churchill-Livingstone, 1989.
25. Baak JPA, Fox H, Langley FA, Buckley CH: The prognostic value of morphometry in ovarian epithelial tumors of borderline malignancy. Int J Gynecol Pathol 1985;4:186–191.
26. Aure JC, Hoeg K, Kolstad P: Clinical and histologic studies of ovarian carcinoma: Long-term follow-up of 990 cases. Obstet Gynecol 1971;37:1–9.
27. Leake JF, Currie JL, Rosenshein NB, Woodruff JD: Long-term follow-up of serous ovarian tumors of low malignant potential. Gynecol Oncol 1992;47:150–158.
28. Bell DA, Weinstock MA, Scully RE: Peritoneal implants of ovarian serous borderline tumors: Histologic features and prognosis. Cancer 1988;62:2212–2222.
29. Kurman RJ, Trimble CL: The behavior of serous tumors of low malignant potential: Are they ever malignant? Int J Gynecol Pathol 1993;12:120–127.
30. McCaughery WTE, Kirk ME, Lester W, Dardick I: Peritoneal epithelial lesions associated with proliferative serous tumors of ovary. Histopathology 1984;8:195–208.
31. Shiraki M, Otis CN, Donovan JT, Powell JL: Ovarian serous borderline epithelial tumors with multiple retroperitoneal nodal involvement: Metastasis or malignant transformation of epithelial glandular inclusions: Gynecol Oncol 1992;46:255–258.
32. Segal GH, Hart WR: Ovarian serous tumors of low malignant potential (serous borderline tumors): The relationship of exophytic surface tumor to peritoneal "implants". Am J Surg Pathol 1992;16:577–583.
33. Bostwick DG, Tazelaar HD, Ballon SC, Hendrickson MR, Kempson RL: Ovarian epithelial tumors of the borderline malignancy: A clinical and pathologic study of 109 cases. Cancer 1986;58:2052–2065.
34. Michael H, Roth LM: Invasive and non-invasive implants in ovarian serous tumors of low malignant potential. Cancer 1986;57:1240–1247.
35. Friedlander ML, Hedley DW, Swanson C, Russel P: Prediction of long-term survival by flow cytometric analysis of cellular DNA content in patients with advanced ovarian cancer. J Clin Oncol 1988;6:282–290.
36. Sidawy MK, Silverberg SG: Endosalpingiosis in female peritoneal washings: A diagnostic pitfall. Int J Gynecol Pathol 1987;6:340–346.
37. Clement PB, Young RH: Florid mesothelial hyperplasia associated with ovarian tumors: A potential source of error in tumor diagnosis and staging. Int J Gynecol Pathol 1993;12:51–58.
38. Battifora H, Kopinski MI: Distinction of mesothelioma from adenocarcinoma: An immunohistochemical approach. Cancer 1985;55:1679–1685.
39. Russell P, Bannatyne P: Surgical Pathology of the Ovaries. London, Churchill-Livingstone, 1989.
40. Katzenstein AA, Mazur MT, Morgan TE, Kao M-S: Proliferating serous tumors of the ovary: Histologic features and prognosis. Am J Surg Pathol 1990;39:284–288.
41. Tavassoli FA: Serous tumor of low malignant potential with early stromal invasion (serous LMP with microinvasion). Mod Pathol 1988;1:407–414.
42. Hanselaar AGJM, Vooijs GP, Mayall B, Ras-Zeijlmans GJ, Chadha-Ajwani S: Epithelial markers to detect occult microinvasion in serous ovarian tumors. Int J Gynecol Pathol 1993;12:20–27.
43. Folyle A, Al-Jabi M, McCaughey WTE: Papillary peritoneal tumors in women. Am J Surg Pathol 1981;5:241–250.
44. Killackey MA, Davis AR: Papillary serous carcinoma of the peritoneal surface: Matched case comparison with papillary serous ovarian carcinoma. Gynecol Oncol 1993; 51:171–174.
45. Lele SB, Piver MS, Matharu J, Tsukada Y: Peritoneal papillary carcinoma. Gynecol Oncol 1988;31:315–320.
46. Fronum G-L, Gershenson DM, Silva EG: Papillary serous carcinoma of the peritoneum. Obstet Gynecol 1990;75:89–95.
47. Parmley TH, Woodruff JD: The ovarian mesothelioma. Am J Obstet Gynecol 1974;120:234–241.
48. Daya D, McCaughey TE: Well-differentiated papillary mesothelioma of the peritoneum: A clinicopathologic study of 22 cases. Cancer 1990;65:292–296.
49. Schneider V, Partridge JR, Gutierrez F, Hurt WG, Maizels MS, Demay RM: Benign cystic mesothelioma involving the female genital tract: Report of four cases. Am J Obstet Gynecol 1983;145:355–359.
50. Weiss SW, Tavassoli FA: Multicystic mesothelioma: An analysis of pathologic findings and biologic behavior in 37 cases. Am J Surg Pathol 1988;12:737–746.
51. Tsao SW, Mok CH, Knapp RC, Oike K, Muto MG, Welch WR, Goodman HM, Sheets EE, Berkowitz RS, Lau CC: Molecular genetic evidence of a unifocal origin for human serous ovarian carcinoma. Gynecol Oncol 1993;48:5–10.
52. Muto MG, Welch WR, Mok SC, Fishbaugh PM, Lau CC, Goodman HM, Sheets EE, Knapp RC, Berkowitz RS: Evidence for a multifocal origin of papillary serous carcinoma of the peritoneum. Gynecol Oncol 1994;52:127.
53. Young RH, Clement PB, Scully RE: The ovary. *In* Sternberg SS (ed): Diagnostic Surgical Pathology. New York, Raven Press, 1989.
54. LiVolsi VA, Merino MJ, Schwartz PE: Coexistent endocervical adenocarcinoma and mucinous adenocarcinoma of the ovary: A clinicopathologic study of 4 cases. Int J Gynecol Pathol 1983;1:391–401.
55. Aguirre P, Dayal Y, Scully RE, DeLellis RE: Mucinous tumors of the ovary with argyrophil cells: An immunohistochemical analysis. Am J Surg Pathol 1984;8:345–356.
56. Sasaki E, Sasano N, Kimura N, Andoh N, Yajima A: Demonstration of neuroendocrine cells in ovarian mucinous tumors. Int J Gynecol Pathol 1989;8:189–200.
57. Bell DA: Mucinous adenofibromas of the ovary: A report of 10 cases. Am J Surg Pathol 1991;15:227–232.
58. Hart WR, Norris HJ: Borderline and malignant mucinous tumors of the ovary: Histologic criteria and clinical behavior. Cancer 1973;3:1031–1045.
59. Rutgers JL, Scully RE: Ovarian müllerian mucinous papillary cystadenomas of borderline malignancy: A clinicopathologic analysis. Cancer 1988;61:340–348.
60. Chaitin BA, Gershenson DM, Evans HL: Mucinous tumors of the ovary: A clinicopathologic study of 70 cases. Cancer 1985;55:1958–1962.
61. Hart WR: Ovarian epithelial tumors of borderline malignancy (carcinomas of low malignant potential). Hum Pathol 1977;8:541–549.
62. Kahn MA, Demopoulos RI: Mucinous ovarian tumors with pseudomyxoma peritonei: A clinicopathological study. Int J Gynecol Pathol 1992;11:15–23.
63. Michael H, Sutton G, Roth LM: Ovarian carcinoma with extracellular mucin production: Reassessment of "pseudomyxoma ovarii et peritonei." Int J Gynecol Pathol 1987;6:298–312.
64. Seidman JD, Elsayed AM, Sobin LH, Tavassoli FA: Asso-

ciation of mucinous tumors of the ovary and appendix: A clinicopathologic study of 25 cases. Am J Surg Pathol 1993;17:22–34.
65. Young RH, Gilks CB, Scully RE: Mucinous tumors of the appendix associated with mucinous tumors of the ovary and pseudomyxoma peritonei: A clinicopathological analysis of 22 cases supporting an origin in the appendix. Am J Surg Pathol 1991;15:415–429.
66. Czernobilsky B, Dgani R, Roth LM: Ovarian mucinous cystadenocarcinoma with mural nodule of carcinomatous derivation: A light and electron microscopic study. Cancer 1983;51:141–148.
67. Prat J, Scully RE: Ovarian mucinous tumors with sarcoma like mural nodules: A report of seven cases. Cancer 1979;44:1333–1344.
68. Prat J, Scully RE: Sarcomas in ovarian mucinous tumors: A report of two cases. Cancer 1979;44:1327–1331.
69. Prat J, Young RH, Scully RE: Ovarian mucinous tumors with foci of anaplastic carcinoma. Cancer 1981;50:300–304.
70. Tsujimura T, Kawano K: Rhabdomyosarcoma coexistent with ovarian mucinous cystadenocarcinoma: A case report. Int J Gynecol Pathol 1992;11:58–62.
71. Robboy SJ: Insular carcinoid of ovary associated with malignant mucinous tumors. Cancer 1984;54:2273–2276.
72. Young RH, Hart WR: Metastases from carcinoma of the pancreas simulating primary mucinous tumors of the ovary. Am J Surg Pathol 1989;13:748–756.
73. Ulbright TM, Roth LM, Stehman FB: Secondary ovarian neoplasia: A clinicopathologic study of 35 cases. Cancer 1984;53:1164–1174.
74. Kline RC, Wharton JT, Atkinson EN, Burke TN, Gershenson DM, Edwards CL: Endometrioid carcinoma of the ovary: Retrospective review of 145 cases. Gynecol Oncol 1990;39:337–346.
75. Mostoufigadeh GHM, Scully RE: Malignant tumors arising in endometriosis. Clin Obstet Gynecol 1980;23:951–963.
76. Bell DA, Scully RE: Atypical and borderline endometrioid adenofibromas of the ovary: A report of 27 cases. Am J Surg Path 1985;9:205–214.
77. Norris HJ: Proliferative endometrioid tumors and endometrioid tumors of low malignant potential of the ovary. Int J Gynecol Pathol 1983;12:134–140.
78. Roth LM, Czernobilsky B, Langley FA: Ovarian endometrioid adenofibromatous and cystadenofibromatous tumors: Benign, proliferating and malignant. Cancer 1981;48:1838–1845.
79. Snyder RR, Norris HJ, Tavassoli F: Endometrioid proliferative and low malignant potential tumors of the ovary: A clinicopathologic study of 46 cases. Am J Surg Pathol 1987;12:661–671.
80. Russell P: The pathological assessment of ovarian neoplasms: I. Introduction to the common epithelial tumors and analysis of benign "epithelial" tumors. Pathology 1979;11:5–26.
81. Czernobilsky B, Silverman BB, Mikuta JJ: Endometrioid carcinoma of the ovary: A clinical pathologic study of 75 cases. Cancer 1970;26:1141–1152.
82. Brescia RJ, Dubin N, Demopoulos RI: Endometrioid and clear cell carcinomas of the ovary: Factors affecting survival. Int J Gynecol Pathol 1989;8:132–138.
83. Marchevsky AM, Kaneko M: Bilateral ovarian endometriosis associated with carcinosarcoma of the right ovary and endometrioid carcinoma of the left ovary. Am J Clin Pathol 1978;70:709.
84. Clement PB, Scully RE: Extrauterine mesodermal (müllerian) adenosarcomas: A clinicopathologic analysis of five cases. Am J Clin Pathol 1978;69:276–283.
85. Kao GF, Norris HJ: Benign and low grade variants of mixed mesodermal tumor (adenosarcoma) of the ovary and adnexal region. Cancer 1978;42:1314–1324.
86. Hernandez W, DiSaia PJ, Morrow CP, Townsend DE: Mixed mesodermal sarcoma of the ovary. Obstet Gynecol 1977;49:595–635.
87. Deligdisch L, Plate S, Cohen CJ: Extrauterine pelvic malignant mixed mesodermal tumors: A study of 10 cases with immunohistochemistry. Int J Gynecol Pathol 1988; 7:361–372.
88. Young RH, Prat J, Scully RE: Endometrioid stromal sarcomas of the ovary: A clinicopathologic analysis of 23 cases. Cancer 1984;52:1143–1155.
89. Young RH, Prat J, Scully RE: Ovarian endometrioid carcinomas resembling sex cord-stromal tumors: A clinicopathological analysis of 13 cases. Am J Surg Pathol 1982; 6:513–522.
90. Aguirre P, Thor AD, Scully RE: Ovarian endometrioid carcinomas resembling sex cord-stromal tumors: An immunohistochemical study. Int J Gynecol Pathol 1989; 8:364–373.
91. Scully RE, Barlow JF: "Mesonephroma" of the ovary: Tumor of müllerian nature related to endometrioid carcinoma. Cancer 1967;20:1405–1417.
92. Young RH, Scully RE: Oxyphilic clear cell carcinoma of the ovary: A report of nine cases. Am J Surg Pathol 1987;11:661–667.
93. Montag AG, Jenison EL, Griffiths CT, Welch WR, Lavin PT, Knapp RC: Ovarian clear cell carcinoma: A clinicopathologic analysis of 44 cases. Int J Gynecol Pathol 1989;8:83–96.
94. Bell DA, Scully RE: Benign and borderline clear cell adenofibromas of the ovary. Cancer 1985;56:2922–2931.
95. Roth LM, Langley FA, Fox H, Wheeler JE, Czernobilsky B: Ovarian clear cell adenofibromatous tumors: Benign, of low malignant potential, and associated with invasive clear cell carcinoma. Cancer 1984;53:1156–1163.
96. Kennedy AW, Biscotti CV, Hart WR, Thason LJ: Histologic correlates of progression-free interval and survival in ovarian clear cell adenocarcinoma. Gynecol Oncol 1993; 50:334–338.
97. Sorbe B, Frankendal B, Veress B: Importance of histologic grading in the prognosis of epithelial ovarian carcinoma. Obstet Gynecol 1982;59:576–582.
98. Jenison EL, Montag AG, Griffiths CT, Welch WR, Lavin PT, Greer J, Knapp RC: Clear cell adenocarcinoma of the ovary: A clinical analysis and comparison with serous carcinoma. Gynecol Oncol 1989;32:65–71.
99. Czernobilsky B, Silverman BB, Enterline HT: Clear cell carcinoma of the ovary: A clinicopathologic analysis of pure and mixed forms and comparison with endometrioid carcinoma. Cancer 1970;25:762–772.
100. Young RH, Hart WR: Renal cell carcinoma metastatic to the ovary: A report of three cases emphasizing possible confusion with ovarian clear cell adenocarcinoma. Int J Gynecol Pathol 1992;11:96–1104.
101. Eccles DM, Russell SEH, Haites NE, Atkinson R, Bell DW, Gruber L, Hickey I, Kelly K, Kitchener H, Leonard R: Early loss of heterozygosity on 17q in ovarian cancer. Oncogene 1992;7:1069–2072.
102. Pieretti M, Powell DE, Gallion HH, et al: Genetic alterations on chromosome 17 distinguish different types of epithelial ovarian tumors. Hum Pathol. In press.
103. Hernandez E, Rosenshein NB, Bhagavan BS, Parmley TH: Tumor heterogenity and histopathology in epithelial ovarian cancer. Obstet Gynecol 1984;63:330–334.
103a. Woodruff JD, Dietrich D, Genadry R, Parmley TH: Proliferative and malignant Brenner tumors. Am J Obstet Gynecol 1981;141:118–125.
104. Roth LM, Dallenbach-Hellweg G, Czernobilsky B: Ovarian Brenner tumors: I. Metaplastic, proliferating and of low malignant potential. Cancer 1985;56:582–591.
105. Martin AR, Kotylo PK, Kennedy JC, Fineberg NS, Roth LM: Flow cytometric DNA analysis of ovarian Brenner tumors and transitional cell carcinomas. Int J Gynecol Pathol 1992;11:188–196.
106. Roth LM, Czernobilsky B: Ovarian Brenner tumors: II. Malignant. Cancer 1985;56:592–601.
107. Austin RM, Norris HJ: Malignant Brenner tumor and transitional cell carcinoma of the ovary: A comparison. Int J Gynecol Pathol 1987;6:29–39.

108. Robey SS, Silva EG, Gershenson DM, McLemore D, el-Naggar A, Ordonez NG: Transitional cell carcinoma in high-grade, high-stage ovarian carcinoma: An indicator of favorable response to chemotherapy. Cancer 1989;63:839–847.
109. Young RH, Scully RE: Urothelial and ovarian carcinomas of identical cell types: problems in interpretation. Int J Gynecol Pathol 1988;7:197–211.
110. Silva EG, Robey-Cafferty SS, Smith TL, Gershenson DM: Ovarian carcinomas with transitional cell carcinoma pattern. Am J Clin Pathol 1990;93:457–465.
111. Eichhorn JH, Young RH, Scully RE: Primary ovarian small cell carcinoma of pulmonary type: a clinicopathologic, immunohistologic and flow cytometric analysis of 11 cases. Am J Surg Pathol 1992;16:926–938.
112. Scully RE: Small cell carcinoma of hypercalcemic type. Int J Gynecol Pathol 1993;12:148–152.
113. Dickersin GR, Kline IW, Scully RE: Small cell carcinoma of the ovary with hypercalcemia: A report of eleven cases. Cancer 1982;49:188–197.
114. Burton PBJ, Knight DE, Quirks P, et al: Parathyroid hormone related peptide in ovarian carcinoma (letter). J Clin Pathol 1990;43:784.
115. Eichhorn JH, Bell DA, Young RH, Swymer CM, Flotte TJ, Preffer RI, Scully RE: DNA content and proliferative activity in ovarian small cell carcinomas of the hypercalcemic type: implications for diagnosis, prognosis and histogenesis. Am J Clin Pathol 1992;98:579–586.
116. Aguirre P, Thor AD, Scully RE: Ovarian small cell carcinoma: Histogenetic considerations based on immunohistochemical and other findings. Am J Clin Pathol 1989; 92:140–149.
117. Benrubi G, Rosen B, Pitel P, Fyles A, DePetrillo A: The response of the small cell cancer of the ovary with hypercalcemia to sequencing chemotherapy (abstract). Gynecol Oncol 1991;40:178.
118. Bichel P, Jakobsen A: A new histologic grading index in ovarian carcinoma. Int J Gynecol Pathol 1989;8:147–155.
119. Hernandez E, Bhagavan BS, Parmley TH, Rosenshein NB: Interobserver variability in the interpretation of epithelial ovarian cancer. Gynecol Oncol 1984;17:117–123.
120. Young RC, Walton LA, Ellenberg SS, Homesley HD, Wilbanks GD, Decker DG, Miller A, Park R, Major F Jr: Adjuvant therapy in stage I and stage II epithelial ovarian cancer: Results of two prospective randomized trials. N Engl J Med 1990;322:1021–1027.
121. Jahdon ME, Morgan MA, Kelstein ML, Carlson JA Jr, Mikuta JJ: Cytologic smears of peritoneal surfaces as a sampling technique in epithelial ovarian carcinoma. Cancer 1990;75:102–105.
122. Burghardt E, Girardi F, Lanhousen M, Tamussino K, Stettner H: Patterns of pelvic and paraaortic lymph node involvement in ovarian cancer. Gynecol Oncol 1991; 40:103–106.
123. Malfetano JH: The appendix and its metastatic potential in epithelial ovarian cancer. Obstet Gynecol 1987;69:396–398.
124. Young RC, Decker DG, Wharton JT, Piver S, Sindelar WF, Edwards BK, Smith JP: Staging laparotomy in early ovarian cancer. JAMA 1983;250:3072–3076.
125. Piver MS, Malfetano J, Baker TR, Hempling RE: Five-year survival for stage IC or stage I grade 3 epithelial ovarian cancer treated with cisplatin-based chemotherapy. Gynecol Oncol 1992;46:357–360.
126. McGuire WP, Hoskins WJ, Brady MF, Kucera PR, Look KY, Partridge EE, Davidson M: A phase III trial comparing cisplatin/cytoxan (PC) and cisplatin/taxol (PT) in advanced ovarian cancer (AOC). Proc Am Soc Clin Oncol 1993;12:255.
127. Stiff PJ, McKenzie RS, Alberts DS, Sosman JA, Dolan JR, Rad N, McCloskey T: Phase I clinical and pharmacokinetic study of high-dose mitoxantrone combined with carboplatin, cyclophosphamide, and autologous bone marrow rescue: High response rate for refractory ovarian carcinoma. J Clin Oncol 1994;12:176–183.
128. Bertelsen K: Tumor reduction surgery and long-term survival in advanced ovarian cancer: A DACOVA study. Gynecol Oncol 1990;38:203–209.
129. Nguyen HN, Averette HE, Hoskins W, Sevin B-U, Penalver M, Steren A: National survey of ovarian carcinoma VI: Critical assessment of current International Federation of Gynecology and Obstetrics staging system. Cancer 1993;72:3007–3011.
130. DePriest PD, van Nagell JR Jr, Gallion HH, Shenson D, Hunter JE, Andrews SJ, Powell DE, Pavlik EJ: Ovarian cancer screening in asymptomatic post menopausal women. Gynecol Oncol 1993;51:205–209.
131. Bourne TH, Campbell S, Reynolds K, Hampson J, Blatt L, Crayford TJB, Whitehead MI, Collins WP: The potential role of serum CA-125 in an ultrasound-based screening program for familial ovarian cancer. Gynecol Oncol 1994;52:372–385.
132. Averette HE, Steren A, Nguyen HN: Screening in gynecologic cancers. Cancer 1993;72:1043–1049.
133. Di Xia C, Schwartz PE, Xinguo L, Zhan Y: Evaluation of CA-125 levels in differentiating malignant from benign tumors in patients with pelvic masses. Obstet Gynecol 1988;72:23–27.
134. Gadducci A, Ferdeghini M, Prontera C, Moretti L, Mariani G, Bianchi R, Fioretti P: The concomitant determination of different tumor markers in patients with epithelial ovarian cancer and benign ovarian masses: Relevance for differential diagnosis. Gynecol Oncol 1992;44:147–154.
135. Berchuck A, Kamel A, Whitaker R, Kerns B, Olt G, Kinney R, Soper JT, Dodge R, Clarke-Pearson DL, Marks P: Overexpression of HER-2/neu is associated with poor survival in advanced epithelial ovarian cancer. Cancer Res 1990;50:4087–4091.
136. Slamon DJ, Godolphen W, Jones LA, Holt JA, Wong SG, Keith DE, Levin WJ, Stuart SG, Udove J, Ullrich A: Studies of HER-2-neu proto-oncogene in human breast and ovarian cancer. Science 1989;244:707–712.
137. Kallioniemi O-P, Punnonen R, Mattila J, Lehtinen M, Koivula T: Prognostic significance of DNA index, multiploidy, and S-phase fraction in ovarian cancer. Cancer 1988;61:334–339.
138. Khoo SK, Hurst T, Kearsley J, Dickie G, Free K, Parsons PG, Whitaker S, Ward B: Prognostic significance of tumor ploidy in patients with advanced ovarian carcinoma. Gynecol Oncol 1990;39:284–288.
139. Merkel DE, McGuire WL: Ploidy, proliferative activity and prognosis: DNA flow cytometry of solid tumors. Cancer 1990;65:1194–1205.
140. Rodenburg CJ, Cornelisse CJ, Heintz PAM, Hermans J, Fleuren GJ: Tumor ploidy as a major prognostic factor in advanced ovarian cancer. Cancer 1987;59:317–323.
141. Schueler JA, Cornelisse EJ, Hermans J, Trimbos JB, van der Burg ME, Fleuren GJ: Prognostic factors in well-differentiated early-stage epithelial ovarian cancer. Cancer 1993;71:787–795.
142. Zangwill BC, Balsara G, Dunton C, Varello M, Rebane BA, Hernandez E, Atkinson BF: Ovarian carcinoma heterogeneity as demonstrated by DNA ploidy. Cancer 1993; 71:2261–2267.
143. Hogberg T, Carstensen J, Simonsen E: Treatment results and prognostic factors in a population-based study of epithelial ovarian cancer. Gynecol Oncol 1993;48:38–49.

10

Ovary—Germ Cell Tumors

Dennis M. O'Connor

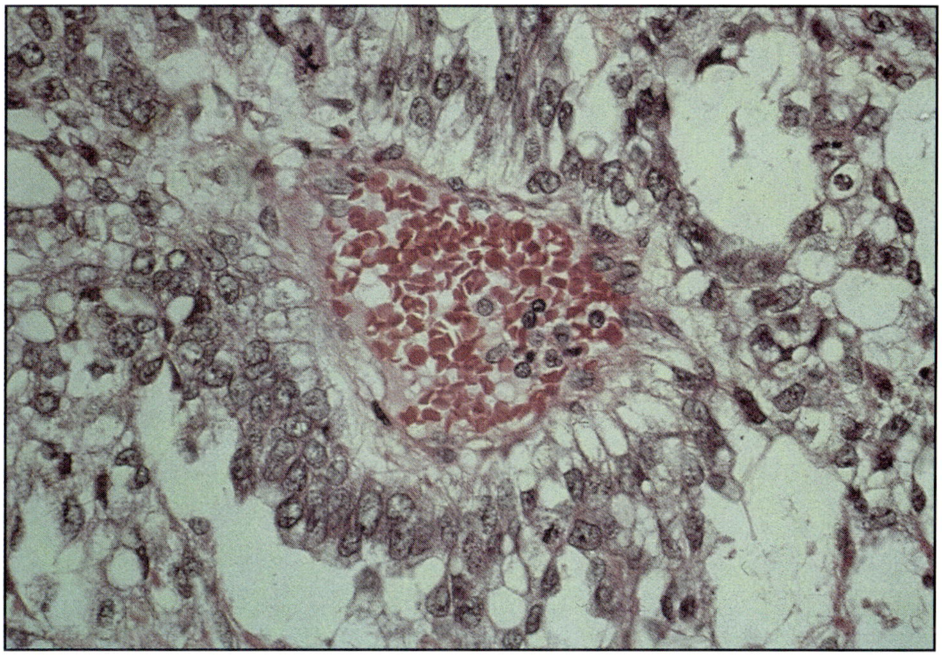

Germ cell tumors are the second most common group of ovarian neoplasms. In the Western hemisphere, germ cell neoplasms account for 20 to 25 percent of ovarian tumors.[1, 2] For multiple reasons the germ cell tumors have often been difficult to conceptualize. Owing to the rarity of individual tumor types, initial descriptions of these lesions were drawn from either case reports or extremely small series. For many years the terminology was imprecise, and confusion often arose over the appropriate wording to indicate metastatic potential. Histopathologic criteria were inadequately described and not easily reproducible. The occurrence of tumors with different germ cell types compounded the difficulty of establishing histopathologic patterns. Prognostic features were not well delineated, since the majority of patients with malignant neoplasms did not survive despite different treatment modalities.

More recently a uniform understanding of the pathogenesis of germ cell tumors has evolved. New biologic markers have been identified and used to follow the clinical behavior of malignant tumors. New chemotherapy regimens that are highly effective in reducing mortality have helped improve our understanding of the behavior of these unusual neoplasms.

Of the ovarian germ cell tumors, the vast majority are mature cystic teratomas (dermoid cysts). Only 2 to 3 percent of all ovarian germ cell tumors are malignant.[2] Germ cell tumors are more common in younger women; two thirds to three fourths of all benign ovarian tumors in patients under the age of 40 years are mature cystic teratomas.[2, 3] The younger the patient, the greater the likelihood of a malignant tumor type. Twenty-five percent of germ cell tumors in patients under the age of 15 years are malignant.[3, 4] Likewise, 80 percent of malignant ovarian neoplasms in patients under the age of 20 years are of germ cell origin.[3]

PATHOGENESIS

The first person to propose a germ cell origin for this category of tumors was Askanazy, who believed that the types of tissue differentiation seen in a teratoma represent development of displaced totipotential germinal cells into multiple mature layers.[5] The presence of homologous germ cell tumors in the male and the occurrence of these tumors at sites along the path of germ cell migration supported this theory. Origin from primordial germ cells has become the accepted theory of histogenesis. The interrelationship between the different germ cell tumors and their potential cells of origin was summarized by Teilum.[6, 7] Figure 10–1 outlines the Teilum classification. Tumors that arise from primordial germ cells without potential for differentiation are classified as dysgerminomas. Further differentiation along germ cell lines results in the totipotential cells that lead to embryonal carcinomas. Embryonal carcinoma cells have the inherent ability to differentiate into either embryonal or extraembryonic elements. The

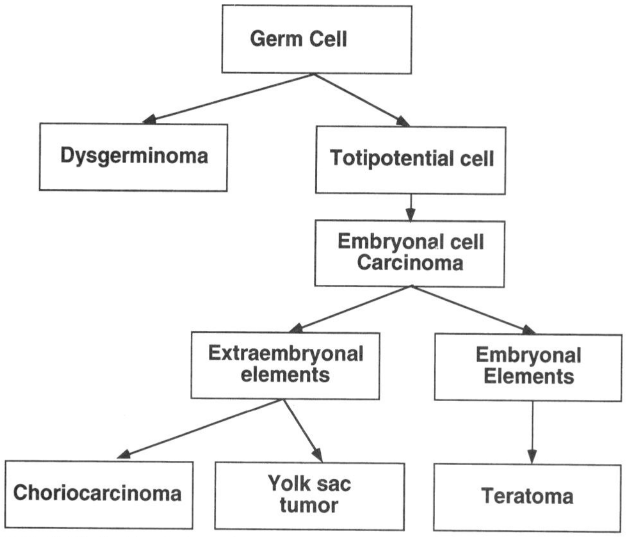

FIGURE 10–1
The pathogenesis of ovarian germ cell tumors as described by Telium is outlined.

embryonal elements may further differentiate in tumors that have cells similar to those seen in the embryo proper (i.e., teratomas). The extraembryonic elements lead to tumors similar to cells found in extraembryonic tissues (i.e., choriocarcinoma from trophoblastic type cells and yolk sac tumors from endodermal type cells). Various degrees of differentiation may occur within the same tumor, which explains the occurrence of mixed germ cell tumors. These tumors also arise from the germ cells in the testis. The different frequency of tumor types found in the testis versus the ovary may reflect the difference in organizational proteins produced by the ovum or spermatozoon.[8] What causes the malignant transformation of primordial germ cells is unknown. However, lack of expression of the ovarian tumor gene (OUT) has been shown to result in abnormal development of primordial germ cells.[9]

Figure 10–2 is a graphic representation of germ cell differentiation during embryogenesis and of the tumors that can arise from the associated theoretical parent cell. In this theoretical schema, the dysgerminoma represents a tumor composed of undifferentiated germ cells. Cells corresponding to the 4- to 32-cell morula give rise to the embryonal carcinoma. Further differentiation results in a blastular stage, which contains cells with the potential to develop into extraembryonic tissues. The trophoblastic precursor cell is the parent cell of the choriocarcinoma; the endoderm lining the yolk sac gives rise to the yolk sac tumor. The blastular stage also contains the inner cell mass, or embryoblast. These cells are the parent cells of teratomas and embryoid bodies, depending on the ultimate degree of differentiation. This schema, we believe, helps to better conceptualize the various differentiation patterns of all the germ cell tumors.

CLASSIFICATION

The most commonly accepted classification for ovarian germ cell tumors is that proposed by the World Health Organization (WHO).[10] There are eight categories of tumor. The three most common types are dysgerminoma, yolk sac tumor, and teratoma. The yolk sac tumor and teratoma are divided into various subcategories according to gross appearance and histopathologic features. Table 10–1 summarizes this classification with minor modifications.

FIGURE 10–2
A graphic representation of the postulated pathogenesis of ovarian germ cell tumors is presented.

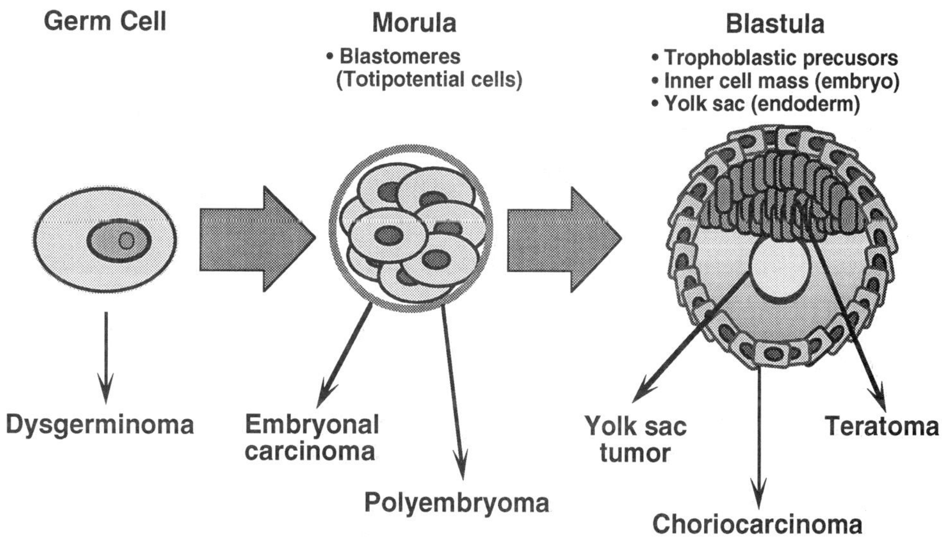

TABLE 10–1.
Classification of Germ Cell Tumors*

Dysgerminoma
Yolk sac tumor
Endodermal sinus tumor
Other
Teratoma
Immature
Low-grade
High-grade
Mature
Solid
Cystic
Mature cystic teratoma with malignant transformation
Monodermal or specialized
Struma ovarii
Carcinoid
Other
Choriocarcinoma
Embryonal carcinoma
Polyembryoma
Mixed germ cell tumor
Combination germ cell and sex-cord stromal tumor
Gonadoblastoma
Other

* Modified from the WHO Classification.

Germ cell tumors are currently staged on the basis of the most recent International Federation of Gynecology and Obstetrics (FIGO) Classification for Ovarian Cancer (see Chapter 9).[11] It must be remembered, however, that the earlier treatment and outcome data used previous FIGO staging systems.

TUMOR MARKERS

Germ cell tumors have various biologic markers that are useful in characterizing specific histopathologic types and in documenting the effective ness of adjunctive therapy against malignant types. These markers are often normally produced by the embryo or placenta during early gestation. The most useful markers have been α-fetoprotein (AFP) and human chorionic gonadotropin (hCG). More recently lactic dehydrogenase (LDH), placental alkaline phosphatase (PLAP), CA-125, CA 19-9, glial fibrillary acidic protein (GFAP), and the polysialic acid moiety of the neural cell adhesion molecule (NCAM) have been determined to be potentially useful. These markers can be identified and localized within tumor cells using a variety of histochemical stains and immunocytochemical techniques. Some of them are secreted and can be measured in the patient's serum.

AFP is a glycoprotein produced by endodermal cells in the yolk sac.[12, 13] AFP has been shown to be specifically present in cells of yolk sac tumors, particularly the endodermal sinus tumor (Fig. 10–3); it is secreted into the patient's serum.[14–16] Any tumor that has yolk sac elements will express AFP.[16, 17] Serial measurement of serum AFP

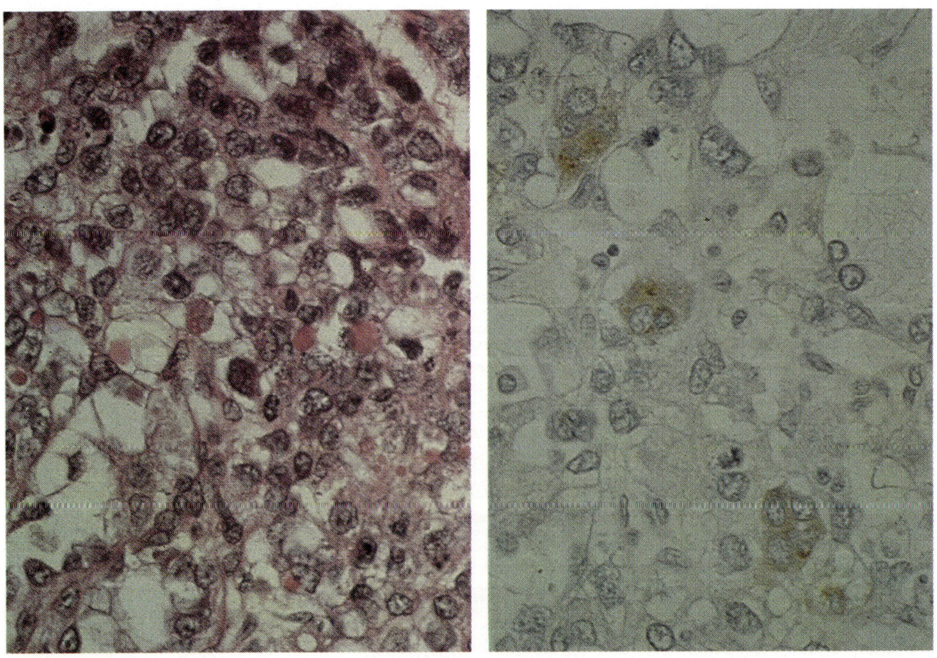

FIGURE 10–3
This is a microphotograph of a yolk sac tumor that demonstrates positive staining for α-fetoprotein. *Left,* A hematoxylin-eosin stained endodermal sinus tumor. *Right,* Individual endodermal cells that contain α-fetoprotein as demonstrated by the brown staining reaction (immunoperoxidase reaction using antibody to α-fetoprotein). (Courtesy of Dr. Richard Lieberman, Armed Forces Institute of Pathology, Washington, DC.)

can be used to monitor the efficacy of adjunctive chemotherapy in patients with these tumors. AFP levels drop to normal within 4 to 6 weeks after the yolk sac elements are completely removed. Persistent elevation may suggest metastatic disease, and a raise can identify disease progression.

HCG, the glycoprotein responsible for maintenance of the corpus luteum in early pregnancy, is produced primarily by the placental syncytiotrophoblast and to a lesser degree by the intermediate trophoblast.[18, 19] It is produced by tumors with trophoblastic cells, such as gestational trophoblastic neoplasia.[20, 21] Germ cell tumors with trophoblast (e.g., choriocarcinoma) also express hCG.[14] As with AFP, hCG is secreted into the serum and can be highly useful in identifying patients with metastatic or recurrent disease.

Alkaline phosphatase is an enzyme found in both the placenta[20, 27] and the plasma membrane of germ cells.[23] This marker has potential usefulness in identifying seminoma, the homolog of dysgerminoma in males.[24] LDH isoenzymes, which are normally produced by the liver and central nervous system, have been found in dysgerminoma and yolk sac tumor.[25–27] Tumor volume, however, must be large to produce a significant elevation in circulating LDH. Serum CA-125, of established value in monitoring the clinical course of patients with ovarian carcinoma, has also been identified in patients with yolk sac tumor, immature teratoma, and, less frequently, dysgerminoma.[26] Nevertheless, these markers have not demonstrated any advantage over AFP or hCG in monitoring the therapy of patients with those tumors. CA 19-9 has been identified in mature and immature teratoma.[26] GFAP and NCAM have demonstrated value in identifying neural tissue within teratoma.[28, 29] Table 10–2 summarizes the more important markers and the germ cell tumors in which they are found.

TABLE 10–2.
Tumor Markers in Malignant Germ Cell Tumors

Histologic Type	*AFP*	*hCG*	*LDH*	*PLAP*	*CA-125*
Dysgerminoma	–	+*	+	+	+
Yolk sac tumor	+*	–	+	–	+
Immature teratoma	+	–	–	–	+
Embryonal carcinoma	+*	+*	–	+	–
Choriocarcinoma	–	+*	–	+	–

Key: +, has been identified in at least some tumors; *, useful in monitoring treatment effectiveness; –, not identified in these tumors.

TUMOR TYPES

Dysgerminoma

Dysgerminoma is the most common malignant germ cell tumor of the ovary, representing approximately 1 to 3 percent of all ovarian malignancies. Although they can occur at any age, 5 percent of dysgerminomas occur in girls aged less than 10 years and 75 percent of patients are between 10 and 30 years of age. The median age at diagnosis is 20 years.[30, 31] Dysgerminoma is the most common ovarian malignancy of children and adolescents. In one study, 17 percent of the patients with dysgerminoma were pregnant at the time of diagnosis,[32] reflecting the fact that the majority of patients are of reproductive age. Paradoxically, exposure to large amounts of estrogen and progesterone (as seen during pregnancy) inhibits the growth of human dysgerminoma transplanted into thymic nude mice.[33]

Dysgerminoma is a frequent component of mixed germ cell tumors[31, 34, 35] and is a component of 50 percent of gonadoblastomas.[36] There is a tendency for dysgerminoma to arise in individuals who have dysgenetic gonads.[37, 38]

Clinical Presentation

Patients with dysgerminoma usually present with abdominal enlargement or a palpable abdominal mass. Necrosis, hemorrhage, and torsion can occur in cases in which the tumor exhibits rapid growth. These patients present with acute abdominal pain. In infants or young girls who have tumors that produce a considerable amount of hCG, precocious puberty or amenorrhea may be seen. In these cases a mixed germ cell tumor must be considered, since pure dysgerminomas do not produce such levels of hCG. However, the amount of hCG produced by a dysgerminoma can be enough to yield a positive pregnancy test. Hypercalcemia has also been reported in association with dysgerminoma.[39–41]

In the vast majority of patients, dysgerminoma is confined to the ovary (stage I). It is the only malignant germ cell tumor that may be bilateral (stage IB); the incidence of this is between 10 and 20 percent (Table 10–3).[30, 42]

Morphology

Dysgerminoma generally is a solid tumor, ranging in size from microscopic foci to 50 cm.[30] The surface is lobulated but smooth. The cut surface is typically cream to tan, but occasionally these

TABLE 10–3.
Incidence of Bilaterality of Germ Cell Tumors

Histologic Type	Bilaterality
Dysgerminoma	10–20%
Yolk sac tumor	None
Mature teratoma	10–20%
Immature teratoma	None*
Choriocarcinoma	None
Embryonal carcinoma	None
Gonadoblastoma	30–50%

* Five to ten percent of contralateral ovaries contain mature teratomas.

tumors are pinkish red. In areas of rapid growth, necrosis and hemorrhage may be present. Rupture can occur, particularly in large tumors. Previous sites of necrosis undergo scar formation and retract (Fig. 10–4). Some tumors have foci of calcification and cystic degeneration. If these are present, the possibility of a gonadoblastoma or a mixed germ cell tumor must be considered, since calcification and cystic change are more common in other germ cell tumor types.

Dysgerminoma has a very distinctive microscopic appearance, which is identical with that of testicular seminoma. There are three unique histologic elements: nests of germ cells, intervening fibrous septate bands, and lymphocytic infiltrate (Fig. 10–5). The hallmark feature, however, is the germ cell. These cells are uniform in size, round or polygonal, and have a diameter of approximately 20 μm. The cell borders are distinct. The cytoplasm is clear to slightly granular and contains glycogen. The presence of glycogen can be confirmed by a positive periodic acid–Schiff (PAS) staining reaction. Lipid can also be identified using fat stains on unfixed tissue. The nuclei are large and have a vesicular chromatin pattern; nuclear membranes are distinct. One or two prominent nucleoli are usually present. Mitotic activity is invariably present.

Immunocytochemical staining shows that dysgerminoma cells are negative for cytokeratin, carcinoembryonic antigen (CEA), AFP, and hCG but positive for PLAP. Ploidy studies done by flow cytometry identify a consistent increase in nuclear DNA content with either an aneuploid or a polyploid pattern. Electron microscopy shows that the cells have few organelles, glycogen-rich cytoplasm, surface filopods, annulate lamellae, and convoluted nucleoli—all morphologic features seen in normal primordial germ cells and in seminoma.[45,46]

Fibrous stroma separates the germ cells into islands or nests, imposing a trabecular arrangement on the tumor. The fibrous bands may be thin or broad and invariably are infiltrated by lymphocytes, which vary in amount from a few mononuclear cells to large numbers that can obscure the fibrous bands. Lymphoid follicles can sometimes develop. Immunocytochemical evaluation of these cells demonstrates that there is a predominance of T cells and macrophages; B cells are only rarely found.[47, 48] About 20 percent of dysgerminomas contain foreign body–type giant cells (Fig. 10–6); these cells, along with histiocytes, plasma cells, and fibrosis, may produce a granulomatous appearance.[30]

In 2 to 8 percent of dysgerminomas, giant cells

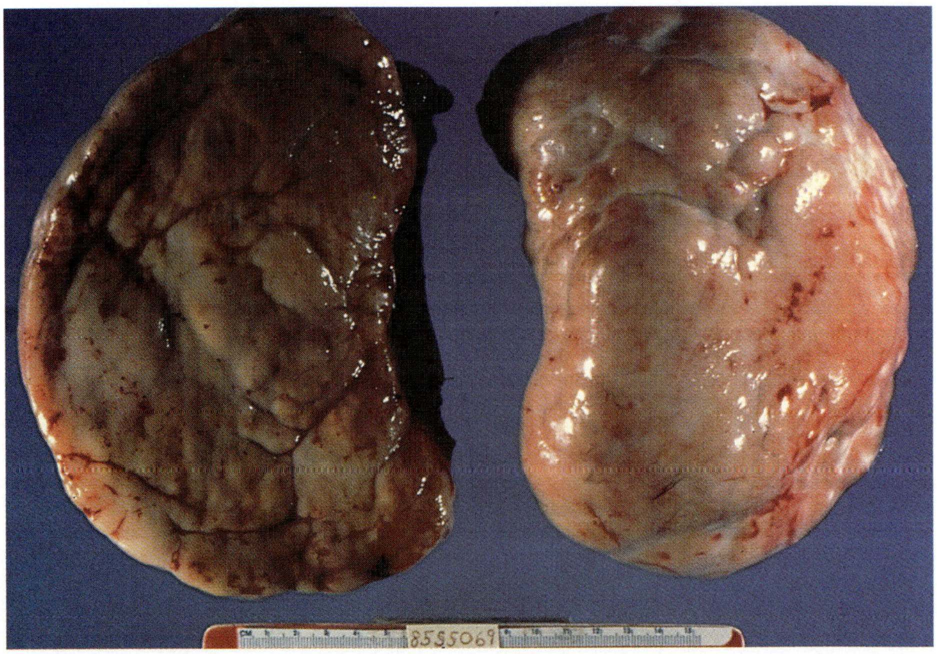

FIGURE 10–4
This large dysgerminoma is solid and pinkish yellow with focal areas of hemorrhage. The ovarian surface *(right)* is shiny and smooth. Indentations give it a lobulated appearance.

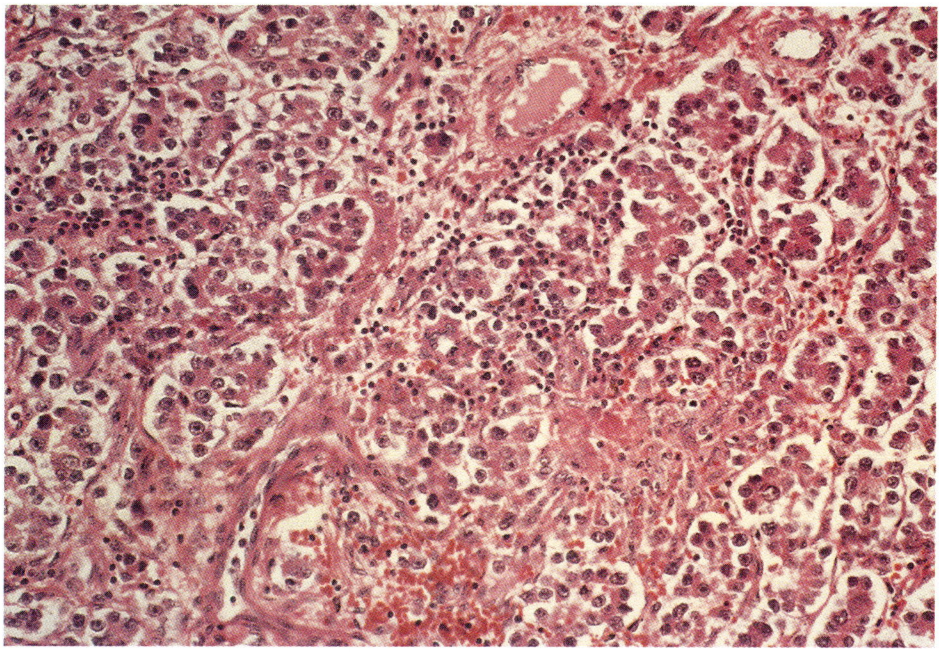

F I G U R E 1 0 – 5
The three characteristic histopathologic features of dysgerminoma (nests of primordial germ cells, fibrous septate bands, and lymphocytic infiltrate) are evident. The dysgerminoma cells are large compared with the lymphocytes. A fibrous septate band is seen diagonally crossing the center of the field.

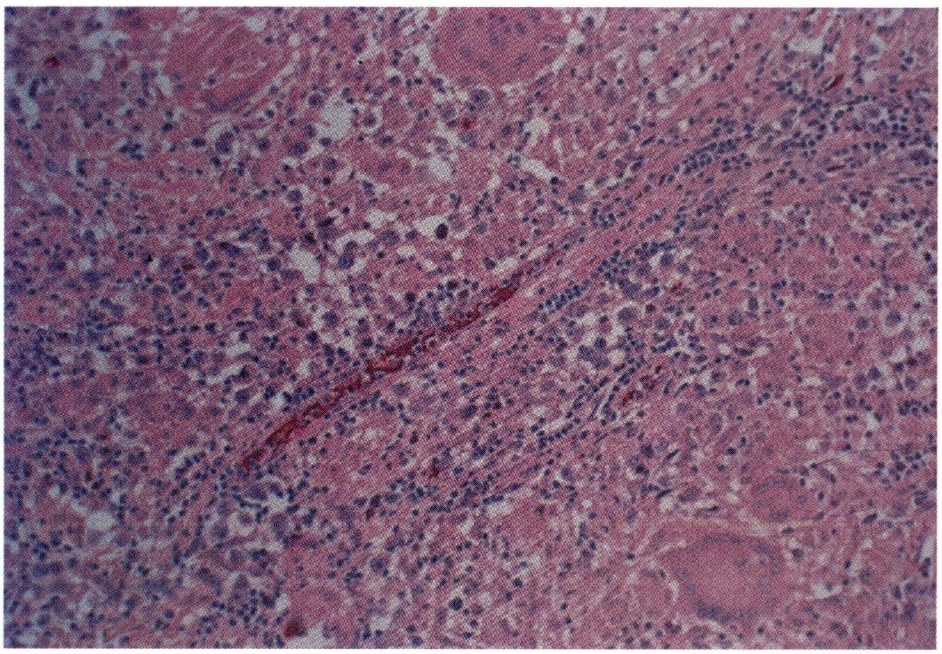

F I G U R E 1 0 – 6
The characteristic features of dysgerminoma are shown. There are numerous malignant germ cells. A prominent fibrous band is seen diagonally in the center. It is infiltrated by lymphocytes. Multinucleated giant cells are seen *(right bottom)*. These cells show the nuclei predominantly at the periphery of the cytoplasm consistent with foreign body type giant cells. A granulomatous appearance with multinucleate giant cells is seen *(top left)*. (Courtesy of Dr. Richard Lieberman, Armed Forces Institute of Pathology, Washington, DC.)

that resemble the syncytiotrophoblast can be detected (Fig. 10–7). HCG has been identified in these cells by immunocytochemistry.[49–51] The presence of syncytiotrophoblast does not warrant the diagnosis of a mixed germ cell tumor with choriocarcinoma if the histopathologic feature typical of choriocarcinoma (a diphasic trophoblastic population) is absent. However, a comment about the presence of syncytiotrophoblast should be made when rendering the diagnosis, as some clinicians would consider undertaking treatment for the possible choriocarcinoma component.

The differential diagnosis of dysgerminoma includes a high-grade lymphoma, clear cell carcinoma, and poorly differentiated adenocarcinoma. The unique histopathologic pattern of dysgerminoma and the absence of immunostaining of tumor cells for epithelial membrane antigen (EMA), cytokeratin (typical for carcinoma), or leukocyte common antigen (typical for lymphoma) usually leads to the correct diagnosis.

Clinical Management

Dysgerminoma is a malignant tumor. Tumor spread is by direct extension (Fig. 10–8), by lymphatics, or by blood vessels. The abdominal and pelvic lymph nodes, including high common iliac and periaortic nodes, are often involved (Fig. 10–9), and these areas must be sampled during exploratory laparotomy. Sites of distant metastasis include liver, bowel, and lungs.[35, 52] Metastatic spread to the breast has also been reported.[53] Adverse prognostic factors include metastatic disease, capsular rupture, surface adhesions to surrounding structures, and the presence of other germ cell elements. Abnormal DNA content does not appear to predict an adverse outcome.[43, 44] It has been suggested that the presence of an increased inflammatory or granulomatous infiltrate is associated with a good prognosis.[4]

Therapy for dysgerminoma is individualized according to the patient's age and childbearing wishes. The patient must be carefully staged at the time of exploratory laparotomy. Cell washings from the pelvis and both lateral gutters are obtained immediately after opening the abdomen. If ascites is present it is sent for cytopathologic evaluation. Scrapings of the right hemidiaphragm are taken for cytologic preparation. The omentum, pelvic, and paraaortic lymph nodes are sampled. The abdominal cavity is carefully evaluated, and suspicious areas and adhesions are submitted for biopsy. If the tumor is grossly confined to one ovary, a unilateral oophorectomy or salpingo-oophorectomy is recommended. Although a wedge biopsy of the contralateral ovary was recommended in the past, caution must be advised, as future childbearing potential in these young patients may be compromised by surgery and the resultant adhesive disease that may occur in the remaining adnexa. The contralateral ovary must be carefully inspected and any abnormalities sampled. Most patients (70 percent) with dysgerminoma have stage IA disease at diagnosis. Only 17 percent of these patients will experience a recurrence after conservative surgery only. Of those

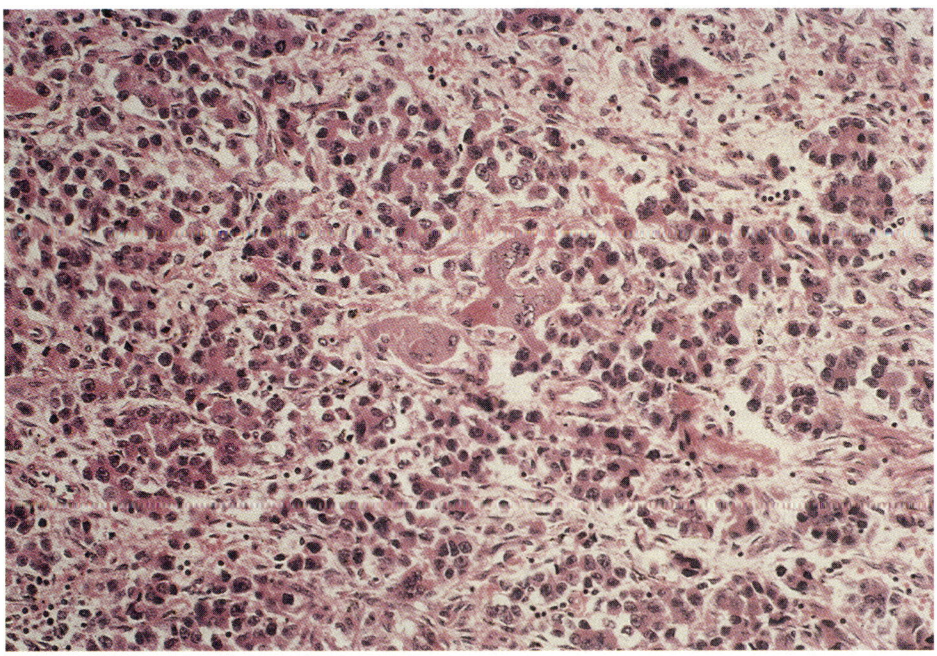

FIGURE 10–7
A dysgerminoma with two syncytiotrophoblastic cells in the center of the field is shown here. In contrast to the giant cells shown in Figure 10–6, the nuclei of the syncytiotrophoblasts are larger and pleomorphic. They show prominent nucleoli. The fibrous stroma divides the malignant germ cells into clusters or nests. (Courtesy of Dr. Richard Lieberman, Armed Forces Institute of Pathology, Washington, DC.)

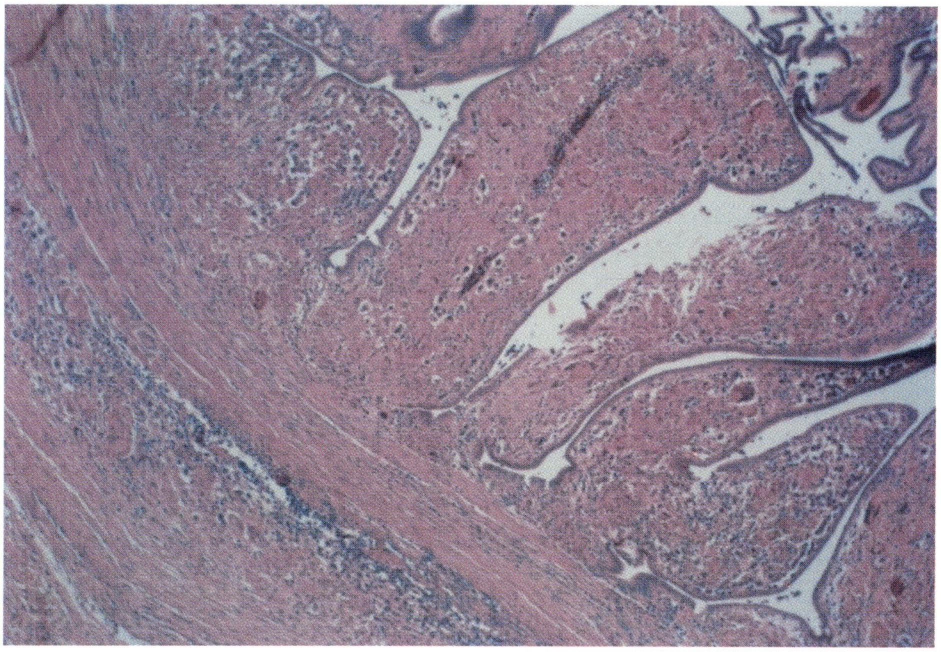

FIGURE 10-8
A section of fallopian tube with the lumen at the right upper corner is seen. The muscularis and tubal folds (i.e., plicae) are infiltrated by nests of dysgerminoma cells.

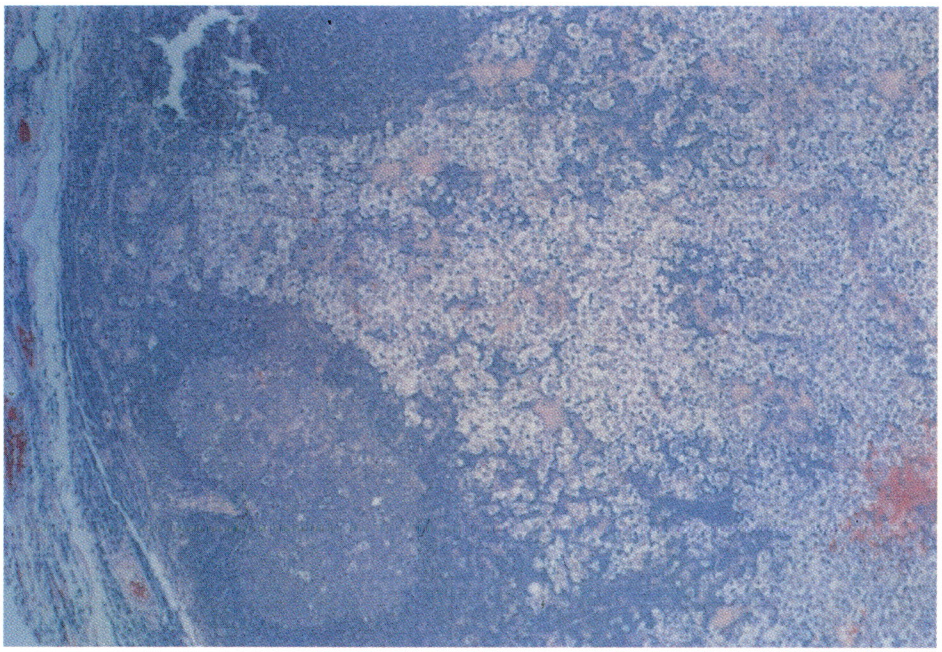

FIGURE 10-9
A mesenteric lymph node with metastatic dysgerminoma shows the normal lymphoid architecture at the *left*. A germinal center is seen *(left bottom)*. The dysgerminoma cells infiltrate the center of the lymph node. At low power the clear cytoplasm of these cells may be confused with a clear cell carcinoma. (Courtesy of Dr. Richard Lieberman, Armed Forces Institute of Pathology, Washington, DC.)

whose tumors recur, 92 percent can be salvaged with radiation or chemotherapy. Therefore, in adequately staged patients with dysgerminoma confined to one ovary, regardless of tumor size, conservative surgery alone is recommended. The 10-year survival of patients with stage IA dysgerminoma treated conservatively is better than 90 percent. If childbearing and ovarian and menstrual function are not considerations, a total abdominal hysterectomy and bilateral salpingo-oophorectomy could be performed. Bilateral salpingo-oophorectomy is also recommended for patients with dysgerminoma and dysgenetic gonads or those with abnormal karyotypes containing Y-chromosome. Patients with dysgerminoma have a good prognosis. However, if the dysgerminoma is one component of a mixed germ cell tumor, the prognosis and therapy are determined by the other elements. The uterus could be preserved.

Dysgerminomas are extremely radiosensitive; in the past, 10-year survival rates approaching 85 percent have been reported in patients treated with this modality.[30,54,55] Recently, use of megavoltage radiation has resulted in survival rates of 100 percent. Potential side effects related to radiation exposure of the bowel, bladder, uterus, and ovary are cause for concern. If a unilateral oophorectomy had been performed, radiation damage to the remaining ovary results in infertility. One review showed no significant adverse long-term effects in 43 patients who received radiation therapy for dysgerminoma, although none of the patients has conceived.[56] Combination chemotherapy has shown treatment efficacy comparable to that of radiation.[57] A Gynecologic Oncology Group study evaluating protocols known to be effective against other germ cell tumors (i.e., vincristine, actinomycin, and cyclophosphamide or cisplatin, bleomycin, and either vinblastine or etoposide) in women who had incompletely resected dysgerminoma has shown remission in 19 of 20 patients.[58] Patients with advanced dysgerminoma who wish to retain fertility could be cured by unilateral oophorectomy and combination chemotherapy and can preserve ovarian function. This treatment can have significant side effects,[59] but the substitution of etoposide for vinblastine lowers toxicity. As with other germ cell tumors, recurrence of dysgerminoma usually takes place within the first 2 years after diagnosis. Such patients are treated by tumor debulking followed by radiation or combination chemotherapy.[57,60,61]

Yolk Sac Tumor

Yolk sac tumor (endodermal sinus tumor) is the second most common ovarian malignant germ cell tumor.[62] Since most yolk sac tumors are of the endodermal sinus type, these two terms are frequently used synonymously. Yolk sac tumor represents about 1 percent of all ovarian malignancies and approximately 20 percent of malignant germ cell tumors.[63] In the past, confusion of endodermal sinus tumor with mesonephroid (clear cell) carcinoma and embryonal carcinoma has led to imprecise classification. New histopathologic variants are being described. Also, yolk sac elements may be found in many mixed germ cell tumors. Collected series of pure yolk sac tumor are few, and its true incidence is still not known.

Clinical Presentation

The age of patients with endodermal sinus tumor ranges from under 1 year to 50 years. Very few reported cases are of women over 40 years of age. The median age at the time of diagnosis is 19 years.[63] In contrast to patients who have dysgerminoma, those who have an endodermal sinus tumor frequently present with acute symptoms, since this tumor grows rapidly. Increase in abdominal girth or lower abdominal pain of no more than a week's duration secondary to tumor rupture or torsion occurs in approximately 50 percent of patients.[63] Rupture, hemorrhage, necrosis, and torsion can each result in acute abdominal pain. In contrast to dysgerminoma, endodermal sinus tumors do not lead to endocrine or menstrual abnormalities. Serum AFP levels are typically elevated, and this marker may be useful in the preoperative evaluation of young women with an adnexal mass. Pure endodermal sinus tumors do not produce hCG.

Owing to rapid growth, 25 percent of endodermal sinus tumors rupture before or during surgery. The majority of patients (70 percent) have stage I disease at diagnosis, 25 percent have stage III disease,[63] and the remainder have stage II or IV disease. Endodermal sinus tumors are unilateral. Involvement of the contralateral ovary indicates metastatic disease (see Table 10–3).

Morphology

Because of its rapid growth, yolk sac tumor is usually quite large at diagnosis. The majority are more than 10 cm in diameter. The surface is smooth unless rupture has occurred (Fig. 10–10). The cut surface reveals large and small cysts containing mucoid material. The coloration is pink to gray or yellow with gelatinous areas. Necrosis and hemorrhage are common.

As originally described by Teilum, numerous

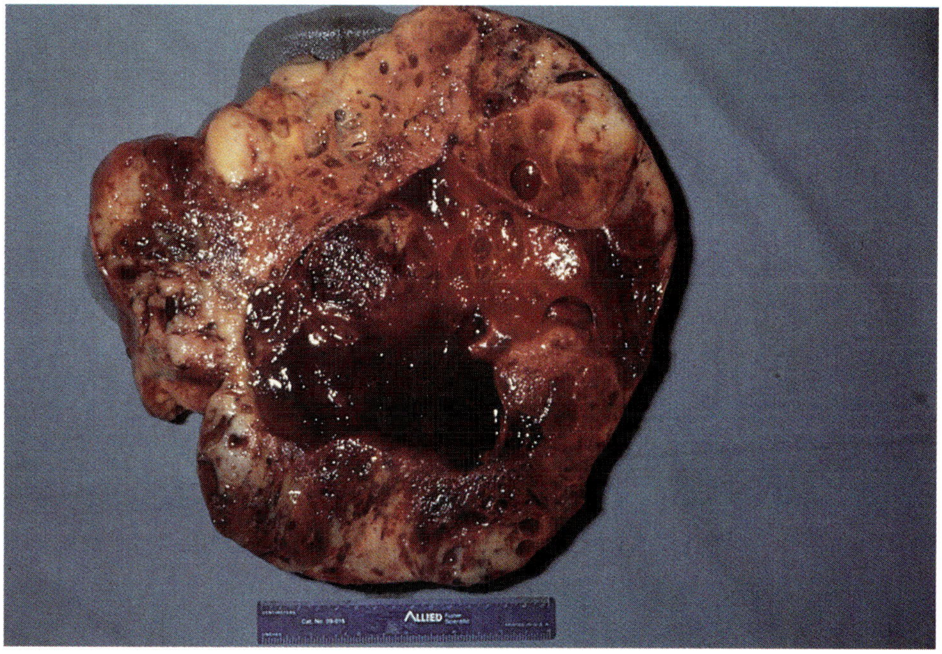

FIGURE 10–10
The gross appearance of an endodermal sinus tumor on cut section shows that the tumor is solid with cystic areas. A large area of hemorrhage is seen *(center)*. The outer tumor surface is smooth.

histopathologic patterns can be seen in yolk sac tumors.[64, 65] These include microcystic and macrocystic, solid, glandular-alveolar, endodermal sinus, polyvesicular-vitelline, and hepatoid. Recent studies of the secondary yolk sac demonstrate heterotopic endodermal structures that resemble many of these patterns (Fig. 10–11).[66,67]

Certain histopathologic features are very common, being present in almost all yolk sac tumors. There is a reticular meshwork composed of spaces and channels lined by flattened or cuboidal endodermal cells. These cells have scanty cytoplasm and indistinct borders (Fig. 10–12). Mitoses are frequent. DNA ploidy studies indicate that these cells usually are aneuploid.[68] Hyaline bodies, which are eosinophilic globules that stain positive with PAS, are common (Fig. 10–13).[63] Immunocytochemical studies have shown that these globules contain AFP and α-antitrypsin.[49,63,69]

Schiller-Duval bodies are rounded or elongated papillary structures that have a central vessel. This vessel is surrounded by primitive mesen-

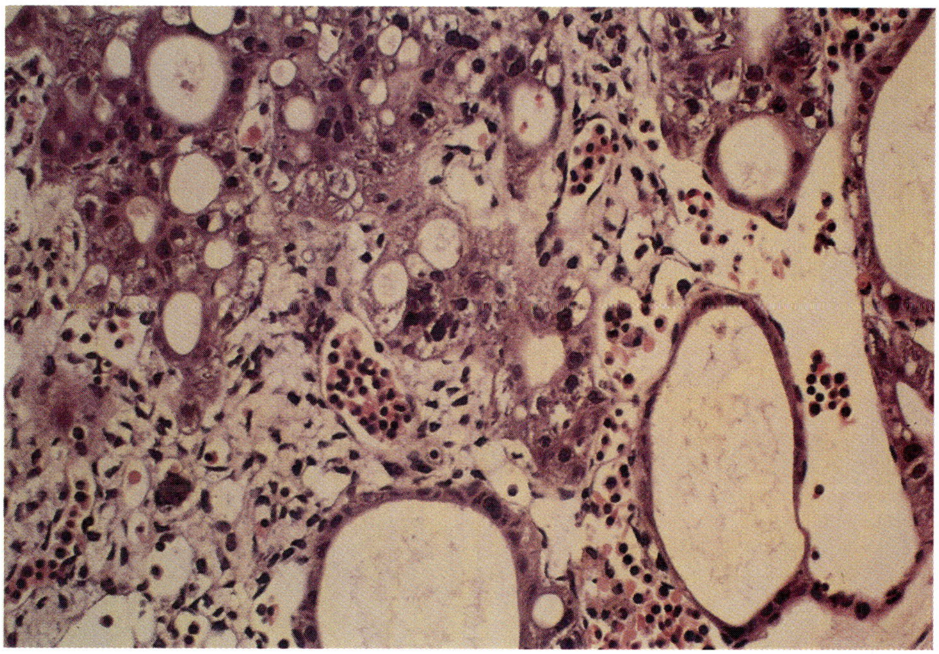

FIGURE 10–11
This is an embryonic secondary yolk sac. The endodermal cells are arranged in nests and lining cystlike spaces. Vascular spaces with nucleated blood cells are also seen. (Courtesy of Dr. Richard Lieberman, Armed Forces Institute of Pathology, Washington, DC.)

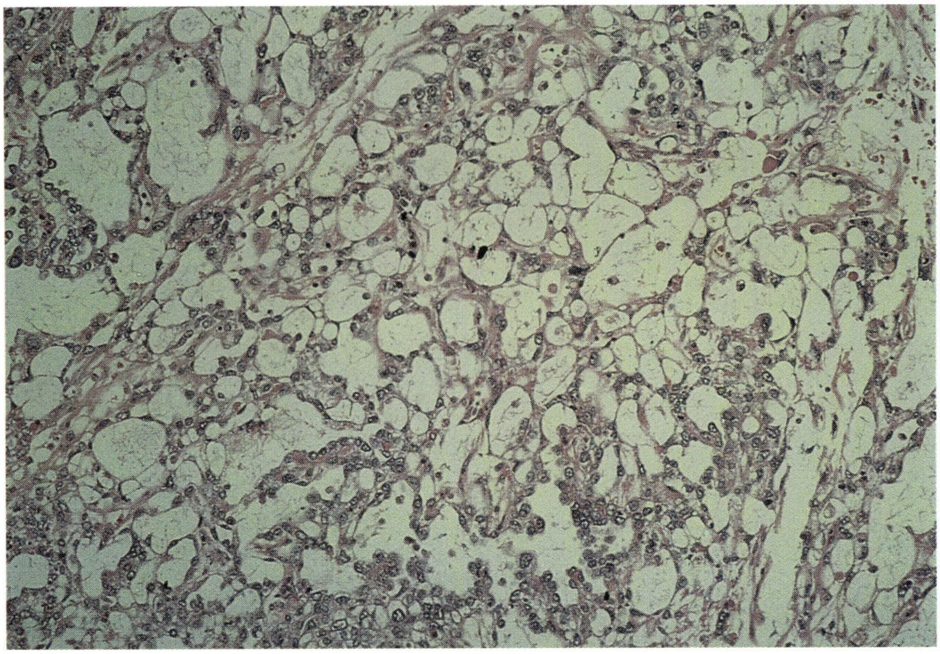

F I G U R E 1 0 - 1 2
This yolk sac tumor (endodermal sinus tumor) has large, pleomorphic endodermal cells that are admixed with flattened cells and line a meshwork of cystic spaces.

chyme covered by malignant endodermal cells. The nuclei are large and pleomorphic, and some have prominent nucleoli (Fig. 10–14). The Schiller-Duval bodies are characteristic of the endodermal sinus tumor but are not identified in every case. As originally described by Schiller, the resemblance of these structures to immature glomeruli led to the original misclassification of the tumor as a variant of ovarian mesonephroma.[70] Subsequent studies using three-dimensional models of these structures have demonstrated a lack of glomerular architecture.[71] The true origins of these structures were a puzzle until Teilum[64] associated their features to the endodermal sinuses of Duval,[72] which are found in the rat placenta. These structures have since been known as Schiller-Duval bodies.

Other patterns of yolk sac tumor are less common. The polyvesicular-vitelline pattern is characterized by cysts lined by flat or columnar epithelial cells that have clear cytoplasm. These cells lie within a dense fibroblastic stroma (Fig. 10–15). Central indentation gives an hourglass shape to the cysts. This pattern seldom is encountered in pure form. The solid pattern is composed of sheets

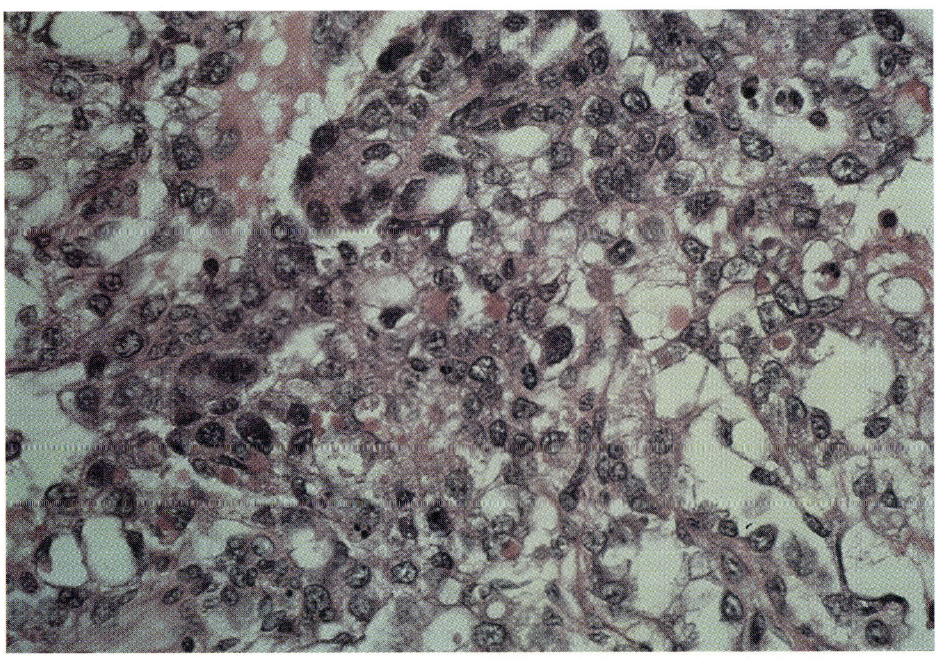

F I G U R E 1 0 - 1 3
This is a higher power view of a yolk sac tumor. The microcystic spaces are lined by large, pleomorphic endodermal cells or flat mesothelium-like cells. The cell borders are not clear. Some of the nuclei are larger and hyperchromatic. Several hyaline bodies are prominently seen as bright pink globules. (Courtesy of Dr. Richard Lieberman, Armed Forces Institute of Pathology, Washington, DC.)

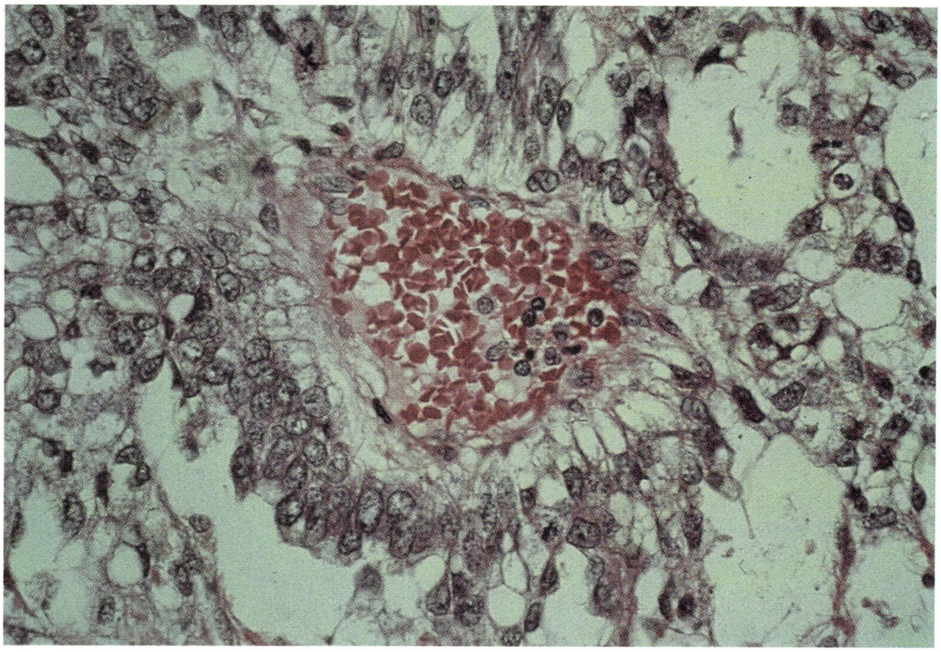

FIGURE 10-14
A Schiller-Duval body characteristic of endodermal sinus tumor is seen. A central vessel with red blood cells is surrounded by tumor mesenchyme, which is covered by malignant endodermal cells in a radiating pattern. Cystic spaces surround this structure. An abnormal mitosis is seen at the top of the field. (Courtesy of Dr. Richard Lieberman, Armed Forces Institute of Pathology, Washington, DC.)

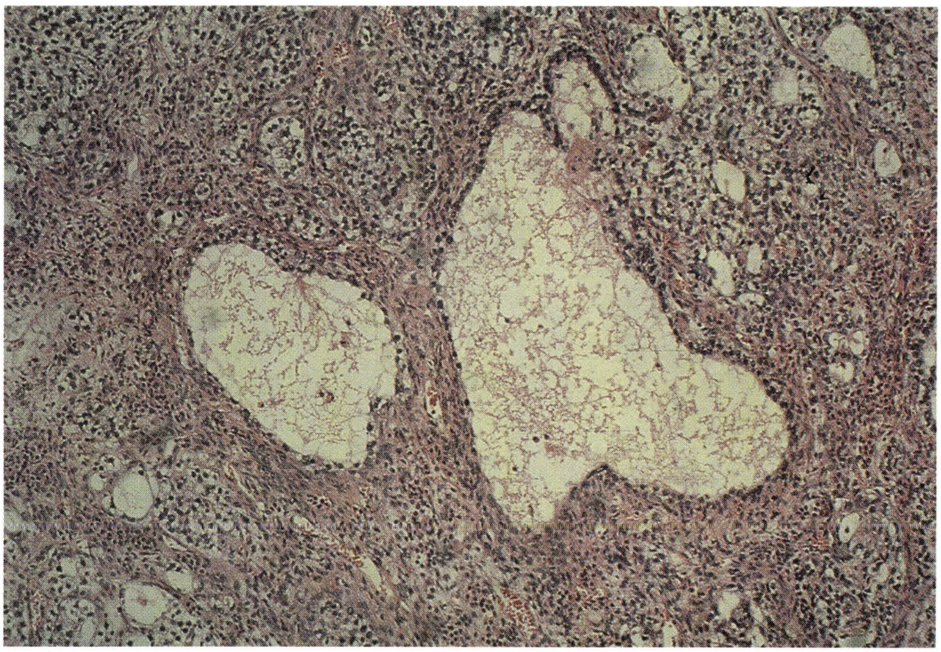

FIGURE 10-15
Two irregularly shaped large cystic spaces are lined by flattened to cuboidal cells. A cellular mesenchyme surrounds them. This constitutes the polyvesicular vitelline pattern. Smaller cysts and nests of malignant cells form the tumor background. (Courtesy of Dr. Richard Lieberman, Armed Forces Institute of Pathology, Washington, DC.)

of large, rounded, or polygonal cells that may have a similarity to embryonal carcinoma. In some instances, the cells have an eosinophilic granular cytoplasm that resembles hepatocytes (hepatoid pattern) (Fig. 10–16).[73] More recently, an intestinal pattern characterized by immature endodermal glands with goblet cells has been described.[74, 75] The lumen-like spaces in this variant may contain mucin-like secretions, leading to an overall resemblance to mucinous adenocarcinoma.

The differential diagnosis of yolk sac tumor includes dysgerminoma, embryonal carcinoma, clear cell carcinoma, and poorly differentiated adenocarcinoma. The presence of cystlike spaces and Schiller-Duval bodies helps in the diagnosis of yolk sac tumor. Immunocytochemistry may prove of value. Endodermal cells are positive for both cytokeratin and AFP, whereas the primordial germ cells of dysgerminoma are not.

Clinical Management

The metastatic spread of yolk sac tumors is similar to that of dysgerminoma. Tumor spread occurs by direct extension, by lymphatics, or by blood vessels. The prognostic variables that best predict outcome are extent of disease at the time of laparotomy and the presence of residual disease after surgery. The patient's age, preoperative AFP level, or tumor size does not affect the prognosis.[76] The microcytic and intestinal histopathologic patterns may be associated with a more favorable prognosis, possibly because of their having a diploid DNA content by flow cytometry.[68]

Before modern adjunctive therapy, the outlook for patients with a yolk sac tumor was dismal. Over three fourths of those with stage I disease experienced recurrence, and the mortality rate for all stages was 93 percent.[63] Ninety percent of recurrences were within 1 year of diagnosis, and nearly all those patients were dead within 2 years. More recently, chemotherapeutic regimens such as vincristine, actinomycin, and cyclophosphamide; vinblastine, bleomycin, and cisplatin; and bleomycin, etoposide, and cisplatin have shown cure rates of 50 to 70 percent.[77] Serum AFP measurements can be used to monitor therapeutic efficacy and detect subclinical recurrences. Fertility can be preserved in these patients if conservative surgery is followed by chemotherapy.[78]

Teratoma

The first detailed description of an ovarian teratoma was published in 1658 by Johann Sculteus. The monograph summarized the case of a German woman who experienced lower abdominal pain prior to death. The autopsy demonstrated an ovarian mass containing hair and "putrid" material.[5]

The term "dermoid cyst" was first coined by Lebert in 1857 to describe "cysts that show an organization similar to that of skin."[79] Virchow was the first to use the term "teratoma" to describe the finding of different tissue types in these tumors.[80]

During earlier times, teratomas were thought to originate from improper nutrition, demons, or unnatural sexual practices. By the nineteenth century, the majority of reports proposed abnormal

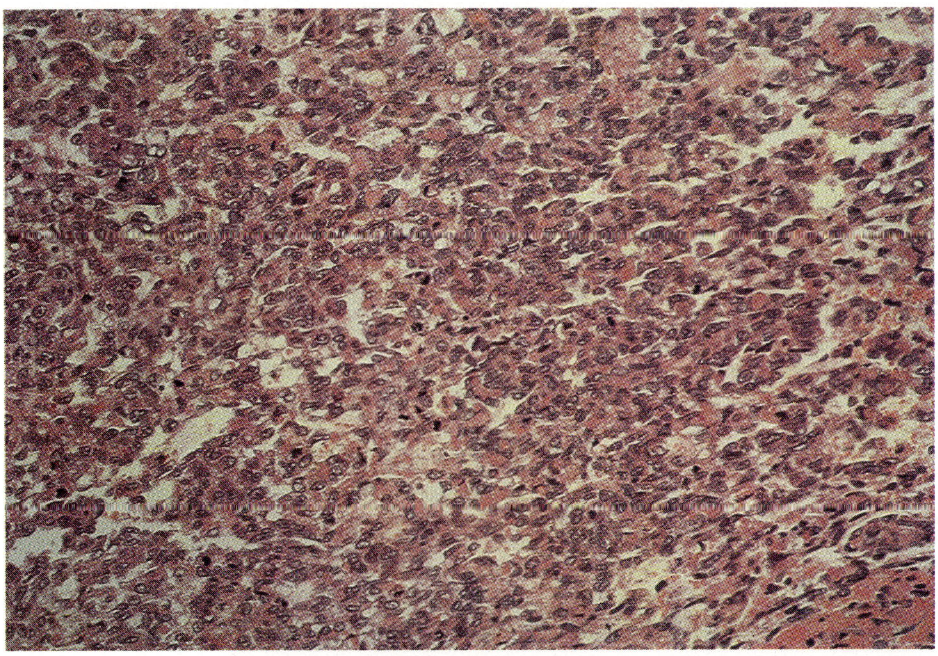

FIGURE 10–16
This yolk sac tumor shows sheets of cells with eosinophilic cytoplasm organized in a hepatoid pattern. (Courtesy of Dr. Richard Lieberman, Armed Forces Institute of Pathology, Washington, DC.)

fertilization as the most likely origin for these tumors; the idea of a "fetus in fetu" became popular. A teratoma found in a prepubertal infant with "an intact hymen" disputed this theory.[81] The usual lack of humanoid organization in mature teratomas was used to support the idea that these tumors arise de novo in the ovary.[82]

It is now believed that two thirds of mature teratomas are derived either from a single germ cell that fails to undergo the second meiotic division or from an endoreduplication of a mature ovum. The remainder, as well as the majority of immature teratomas, arise from either abnormal mitotic division of premeiotic germ cells or failure of the first meiotic division.[83–85] Some immature teratomas may also arise from fusion of two ova.[86] While the majority of teratomas have a 46,XX karyotype, a small number of tumors demonstrate deviations from the normal karyotype.[86] These abnormal karyotypes are found most frequently in immature teratomas of higher grade.[84]

Mature Cystic Teratoma

Mature teratomas are most commonly cystic. Mature solid teratomas do occur but are unusual. Although mesodermal and endodermal components can be present, the most common elements are ectodermally derived tissues. Mature teratomas account for approximately one quarter of all ovarian neoplasms and one half of all benign ovarian tumors. In patients under 30 years of age, they account for 70 percent of benign ovarian tumors.[3]

Clinical Presentation

Although most commonly encountered in young women, mature teratomas have been identified in postmenopausal women. A patient who has a mature teratoma is usually asymptomatic. The tumor is typically an incidental finding during a physical examination. It is uncommon for these tumors to demonstrate rapid growth. Nevertheless, when this does happen, the patient may complain of abdominal pain or increase in abdominal girth. Acute abdominal pain may indicate torsion, which is more common with teratoma than with other ovarian tumors. This occurs in 16 percent of cases.[2] Acute rupture with spillage of the cyst contents can cause an irritative peritonitis and shock. In rare instances, slow leakage of the cyst material can result in fistula formation into the bladder, vagina, or bowel.[86a]

Radiologic examination of the abdomen may show evidence of calcification, and, in rare instances, formed teeth (Fig. 10–17). Recently, the demonstration of hair in cystic teratomas by ultrasonography has proved useful in identifying these tumors preoperatively.[87]

Mature teratomas are bilateral in 10 to 20 percent of cases (see Table 10–3). Previous rupture and leakage of tumor contents into the abdomen can result in a granulomatous peritonitis that can resemble tuberculosis. Torsion of a teratoma may lead to infarction of the adnexa. Thrombosis of the utero-ovarian and infundibulopelvic vessels may also occur. Teratomas at other nonovarian abdominal sites are rare.[88]

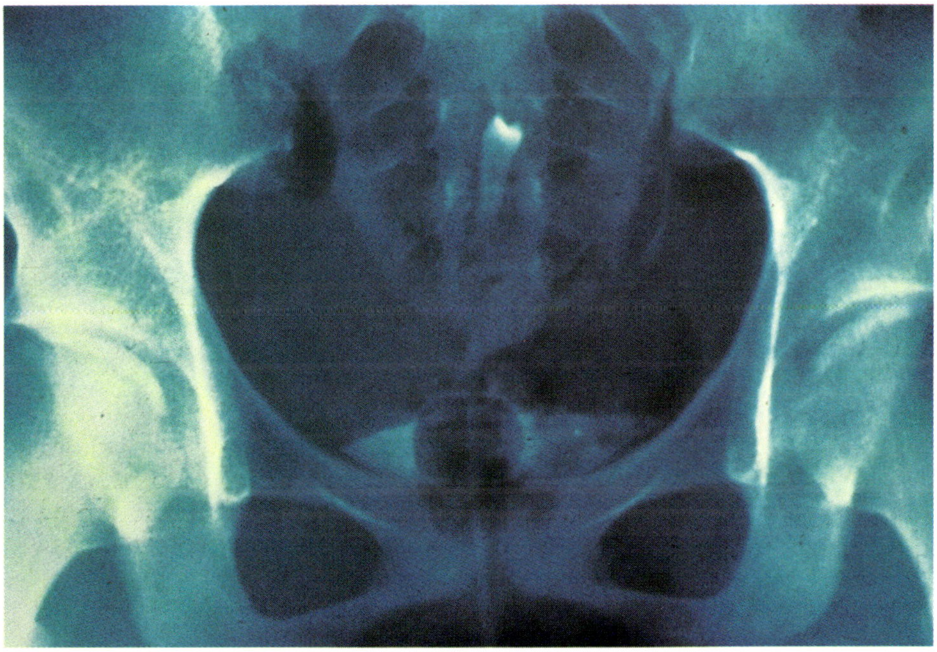

FIGURE 10-17
This pelvic radiograph shows a pelvic calcification, with the appearance of a tooth, that overlies the sacrum. This patient proved to have an ovarian mature cystic teratoma.

Morphology

Mature teratomas range in size from microscopic to very large neoplasms that extend to the upper abdomen. The usual size is between 5 and 10 cm. When the teratoma is large, a rim of normal ovary may be found around the tumor. The surface of a teratoma is smooth, pearl gray, and without adhesions. The tumor is generally cystic and most often unilocular. When opened, the cyst usually contains a semisolid, oily material that resembles sebum. Tufts of hair are also usually present. Some tumors with large cyst cavities contain clear cerebrospinal fluid. The inner cyst wall is yellow-pink, usually thickened, and generally smooth. At one pole, a raised nodule (Rokitansky's protuberance or the mamilla) can be identified; it is usually 0.5 to 2 cm in size (Fig. 10–18). When the tumor is cut, adipose tissue, calcified areas, and formed teeth may be seen. Rare cases of formation of fetus-like structures (homunculi) have been described.[89]

The inner wall of a mature cystic teratoma is usually lined by squamous epithelium. Often, owing to compression by the fluid in a large cyst, the epithelial surface is thinned. Hair shafts can be seen. The outer cyst wall is composed of a compressed rim of normal ovarian stroma that has become thinned and fibrotic. Chronic inflammation and foreign body giant cell reaction may be seen if microscopic rupture with exposure of the surrounding ovary to hair and sebaceous material has occurred.

The raised nodule (Rokitansky's protuberance) or other solid sites contain a variety of mature tissues from all three germ cell lines (Fig. 10–19). Although they are haphazardly arranged, the tissues are typically grouped in an organoid fashion. As an example, respiratory epithelium may be associated with mucous glands, cartilage, and smooth muscle, just as in a normal bronchus. Tissues that are commonly present include glia, retina, choroid, ameloblast (teeth anlage), thyroid, cartilage, bone, smooth muscle, fat, and intestine. It is important that any solid area be carefully sampled and evaluated, since immature or malignant mature elements, if present, will be found at these sites.

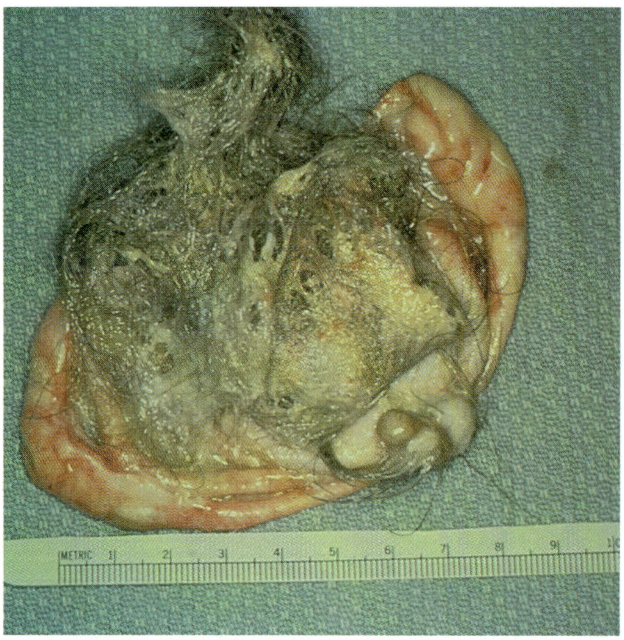

FIGURE 10–18
Cut surface of a mature cystic teratoma showing large amounts of hair and sebaceous material. The inner wall of the cyst is yellow-pink and smooth. Rokitansky's tubercle is seen *(lower right)*.

Clinical Management

A mature cystic teratoma can usually be removed by cystectomy. Since the capsule is thick, even large tumors can be enucleated from the surrounding ovary. The opposite ovary should be inspected but, if normal, not incised owing to the risk of subsequent ovarian scarring and adhesion formation. The likelihood that a normal-appearing ovary will contain a microscopic mature teratoma identified by random sampling is extremely small.[90]

Malignant Transformation of Mature Elements of Teratoma

Between 1 and 2 percent of mature cystic teratomas undergo malignant transformation of the mature tissues.[91–94] This occurs most frequently in postmenopausal women, who account for only 10 percent of patients. Of the malignancies arising in mature teratoma, squamous carcinoma is the most common (75 percent),[94] with adenocarcinoma, sarcoma, and carcinoid tumors making up most of the remainder.

Clinical Presentation

The clinical presentation of a patient with one of these tumors is no different from that of a patient with a mature teratoma without malignant transformation. However, if the malignant component demonstrates rapid growth, the symptoms are similar to those of a patient with immature teratoma. Ascites can occasionally be present. Eleva-

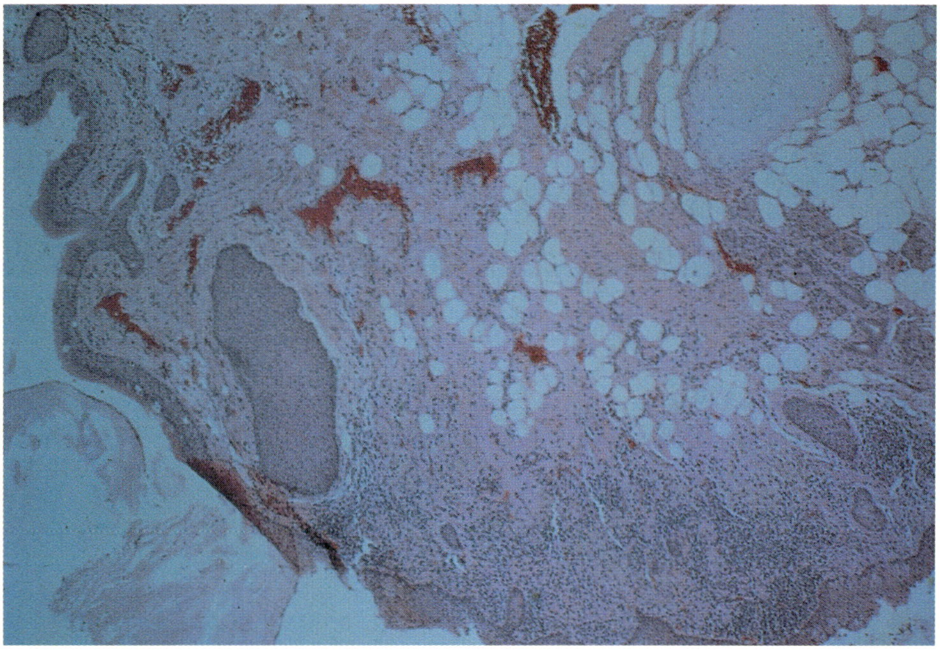

FIGURE 10-19
This mature cystic teratoma shows epidermis *(bottom right)* and adipose tissue and cartilage *(top right)*.

tion of serum squamous cell tumor antigen was found in three women who had squamous carcinoma arising in a mature cystic teratoma.[95]

Morphology

If the malignant element has not eroded through the ovarian capsule, the specimen externally will resemble a mature cystic teratoma as described above. When opened, a large solid area with evidence of hemorrhage and/or necrosis may be seen. Tumors that harbor squamous cell carcinoma may have a cauliflower-shaped mass. The carcinoma tends to grow through the teratoma wall and invade neighboring tissue.[91, 92] In 50 to 66 percent of cases, invasion of adjacent structures or metastasis is present at the time of diagnosis.[92,94]

Almost any component of a teratoma may undergo malignant change. In up to 80 percent of cases it is the epidermis that develops a squamous cell carcinoma.[91] Squamous intraepithelial lesions have also been reported.[96] Other tumor types are rare and usually described as case reports. These include leiomyosarcoma,[93] osteosarcoma, chondrosarcoma, basal cell carcinoma, Paget adenocarcinoma,[97] melanoma,[98] and thyroid carcinoma. Benign lesions include nevi[99] and sebaceous tumors. Sarcomatous or pseudosarcomatous changes of the stroma surrounding the carcinoma also occur. A fully developed gastric wall with a peptic ulcer and a spindle cell tumor arising in a mature cystic teratoma has been described.[100] Malignant degeneration of neural tissue, such as a high-grade glioma (glioblastoma), is best classified as a high-grade immature teratoma.

Clinical Management

Surgical treatment is total abdominal hysterectomy with bilateral salpingo-oophorectomy, with tumor debulking of any metastatic disease. The overall prognosis for a patient who has a mature cystic teratoma with malignant transformation has been described as poor. This is true only for patients who have tumors that extend beyond the ovary. In these cases, adjunctive therapy (radiation or chemotherapy) has not been shown to be of benefit. The 5-year survival rate of these patients approaches 30 percent.[92, 94] Patients with tumors that are confined to the ovary without spillage have a much better outlook, with reported survival rates as high as 85 percent.[94]

Tumor histopathology is also a prognostic indicator. The more unusual malignant cell types (e.g., adenocarcinoma, sarcoma) have worse 5-year survival rates than does squamous carcinoma.

Immature Teratoma

An immature teratoma as defined by WHO is one that contains variable amounts of immature tissue derived from any one of the three germ cell layers.[10] An immature teratoma with primitive cells has the potential for recurrence and metastasis. The risk for malignant behavior increases as the amount of immature tissue increases.[101–103] In describing a teratoma, the term malignant refers to the transformation of one of the mature tissue types into a carcinoma.[10]

Pure immature teratoma is the third most common malignant germ cell tumor of the ovary after dysgerminoma and endodermal sinus tumor.[62] However, immature teratomas represent only about 1 percent of all ovarian teratomas.[104]

Clinical Presentation

The immature teratoma usually occurs in children and young women. The reported mean age is between 17 and 20 years. Very few patients are over the age of 40 years.[101, 105, 106] Immature teratomas are slow-growing tumors, and symptoms (e.g., abdominal discomfort) may be present for a few weeks to months; occasionally symptoms are acute. A minority of patients have menstrual irregularities that are probably related to a reduction in amount of functioning ovarian tissue. Serum AFP and hCG levels are not elevated.

Patients who have either a history of a ruptured mature teratoma or multiple mature teratomas are at a slight increased risk for development of an immature teratoma.[107]

Approximately 80 percent of patients have stage IA disease at diagnosis. Although immature teratomas are unilateral tumors, a small percentage of patients will have a mature teratoma in the contralateral ovary (see Table 10–3).[102, 105, 106] Rupture or ascites is uncommon.

Morphology

Immature teratomas are usually large tumors. The median size is 16 cm, and the mean tumor weight is 1850 gm. Twenty-five percent of tumors weigh over 2000 gm.[106] The external surface is smooth and lobulated, although surface adhesions are sometimes present. On cut surface, the tumor is soft, fleshy, and variegated. It is gray and yellow to pink, and usually hemorrhage and necrosis are visible (Fig. 10–20). Hair, fat, teeth, and calcifications, all characteristic of teratomas, are commonly seen. A "cerebroid pattern," or areas of glial organization resembling brain, can be present. Although immature teratomas are predominantly solid, most have a cystic component. These cysts can be large and may contain a clear fluid.

A variety of mature and immature tissues may be present (Fig. 10–21). Glia constitutes most of the ectodermal tissue, but retinal components, nerve bundles, and skin structures are also prominent. Mesodermal elements such as connective tissue, cartilage, and smooth muscle can be present, but immaturity of these tissues has little or no influence on prognosis. Only a few teratomas composed only of endodermal tissue have been reported. These tumors stain positive for AFP.[108]

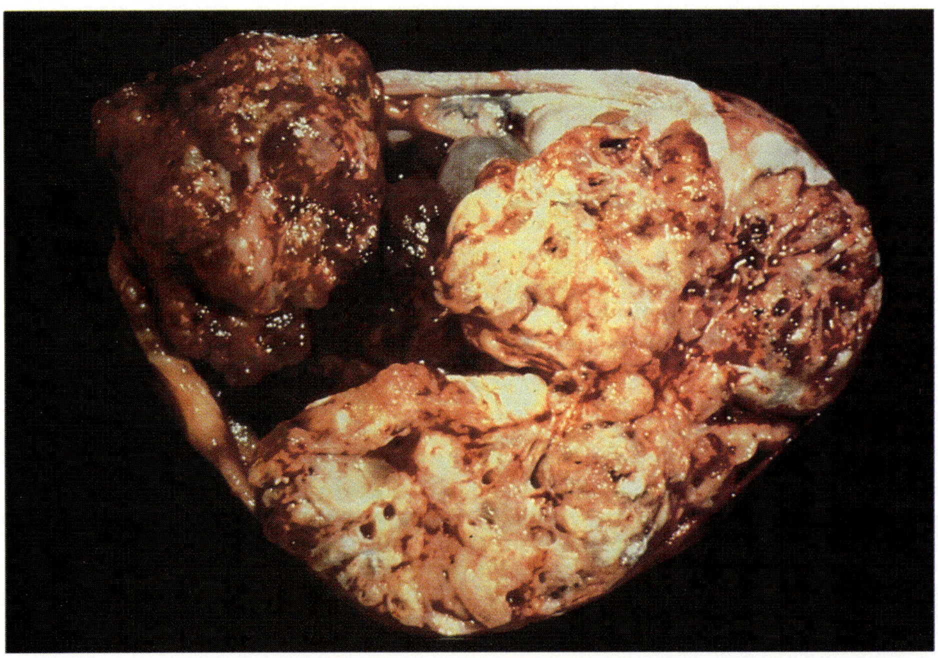

FIGURE 10–20
The gross appearance of an immature teratoma on cut section is shown. It is solid, fleshy, and yellow with multiple areas of hemorrhage. A large hemorrhagic and necrotic area is seen *(upper left)*. The tumor capsule is smooth.

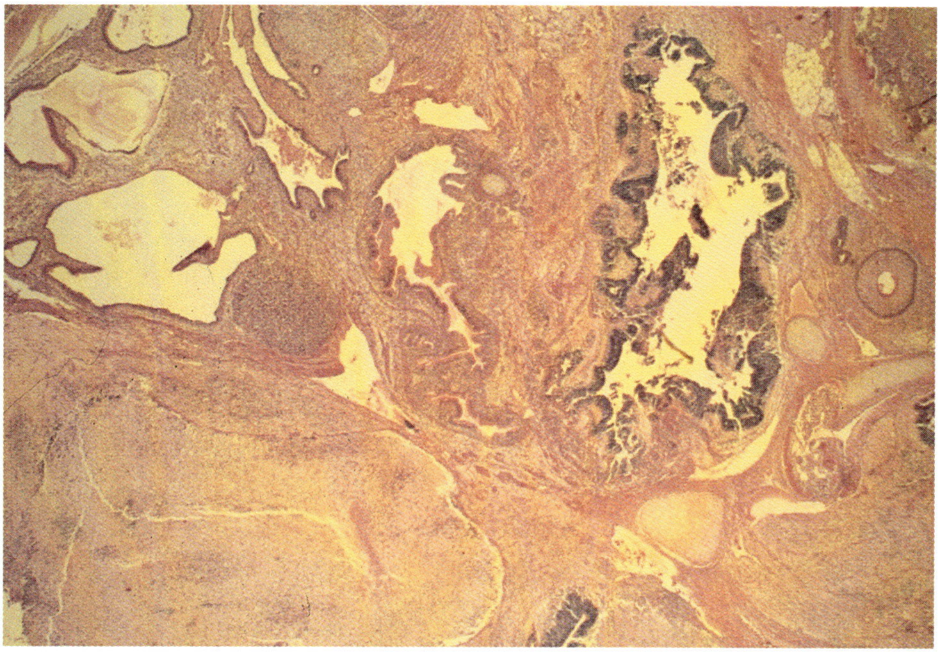

FIGURE 10-21
This immature teratoma has several types of tissue. Neuroectoderm (dark blue cells) lines a cystic area. Mature glia is present *(lower left)*. A hair follicle is seen to the right of the area of immature neuroectoderm. A structure recapitulating a bronchus is seen in the center.

The grade of immature teratoma is predictive of outcome. The immature element that is graded is the neuroepithelium. These cells are usually arranged in clusters or rosettes and may form glandlike spaces (Fig. 10–22); these often merge with sarcomatous areas. The latter can be confused with inflammatory or microglial cells (Fig. 10–23). Immature neuroepithelial cells are small cells with scant cytoplasm. The nuclei are hyperchromatic, of variable size and shape, and with brisk mitotic activity. Necrosis may be present (Fig. 10–24).

Early grading systems used a semiquantitative approach to assess the amount of immature tissue.[102, 109] In 1976, a system of quantifying the amount of immature neuroepithelium per low-power microscopic field was proposed (Table 10–4) and is used by many clinicians to determine the need for adjunctive therapy.[102] To evaluate the clinical usefulness and reproducibility of this grading system, an analysis of 244 immature teratomas accessioned at the Armed Forces Institute of Pathology (AFIP) was undertaken. The degree of agreement between two pathologists was at best

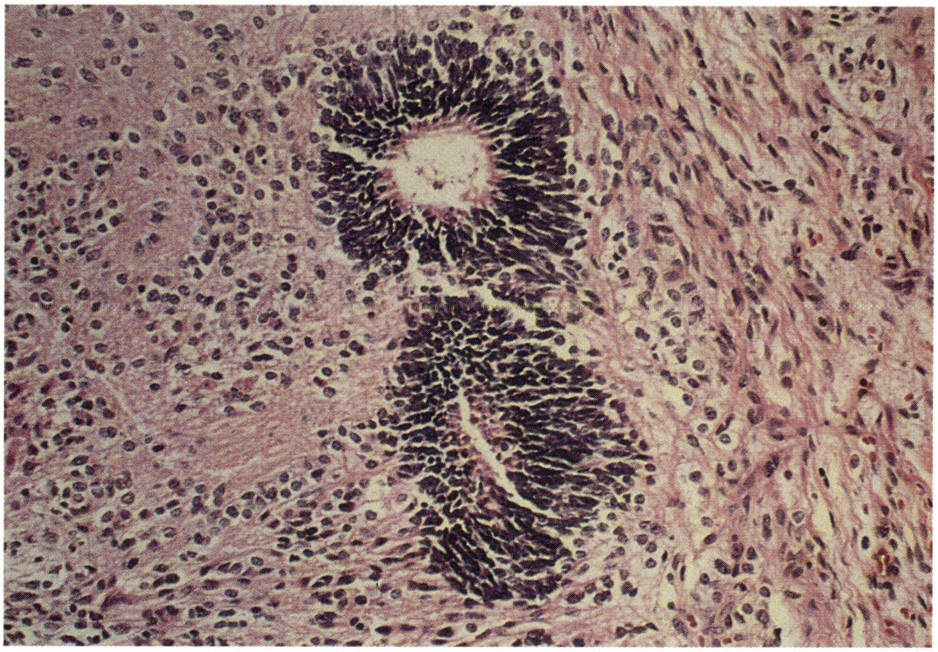

FIGURE 10-22
Neuroectoderm forming a rosette is shown in this high-power view of an immature teratoma.

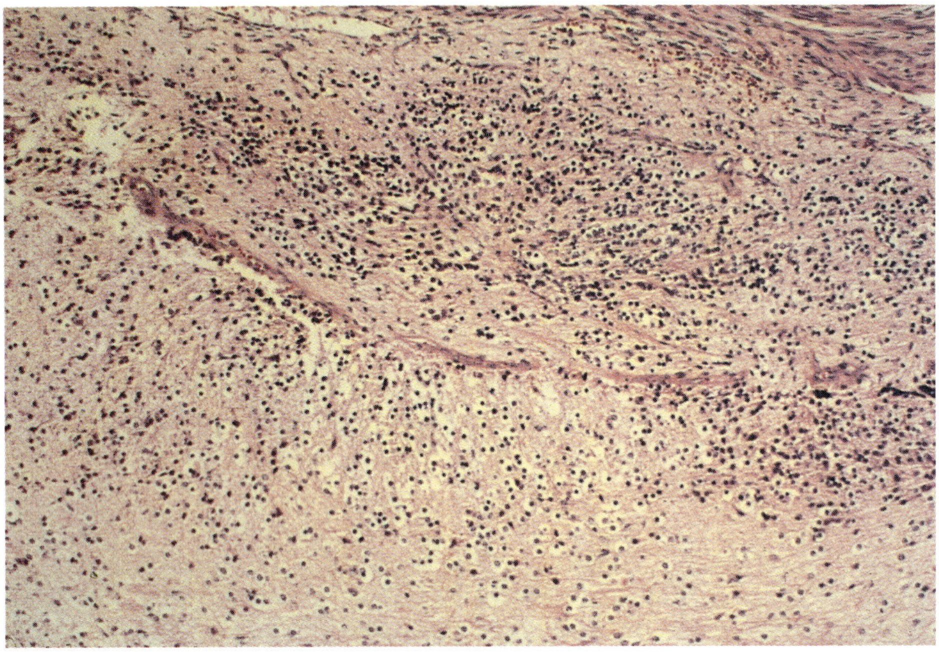

FIGURE 10-23
Glia is seen in an immature teratoma. The microglial cells have uniformly small, round, basophilic nuclei. Mitoses are absent. At low power these cells could be confused with an inflammatory infiltrate.

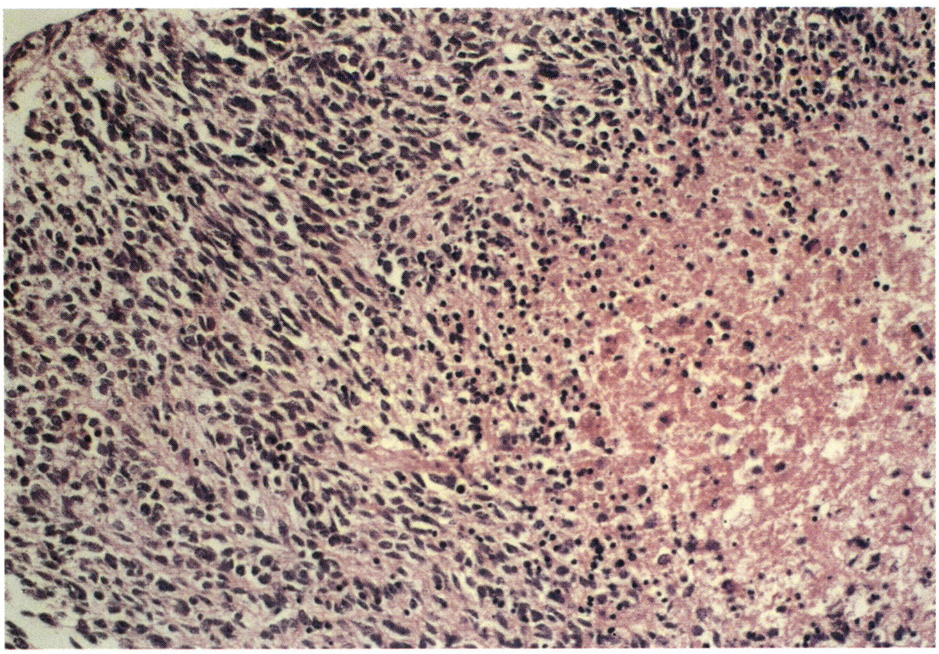

FIGURE 10-24
This section of an immature teratoma shows neuroectoderm arranged in a sarcomatoid pattern. The nuclei are irregular in size and shape (spindle-shaped to round). Necrosis is present on the right.

TABLE 10–4.
Grading of Immature Teratomas

Traditional Grading System	
Grade 0	All mature elements
Grade 1	Immature neuroepithelium occupying up to 1 low-power microscope field on any one slide
Grade 2	Immature neuroepithelium occupying between 1 and 4 low-power fields on any one slide
Grade 3	Immature neuroepithelium occupying more than 4 low-power fields on any one slide
Proposed Grading System	
Grade 0	All mature elements
Low grade	Immature neuroepithelium occupying up to 1 low-power field on any one slide
High grade	Immature neuroepithelium occupying greater than 1 low-power field on any one slide

moderate when this traditional grading system was used. Agreement improved substantially if the tumors were classified as low or high grade (see Table 10–4).[106] Since adjuvant therapy for patients with stage I immature teratoma is used only in instances of grade 2 or 3 tumor, dividing these tumors into low-grade (grade 1) and high-grade (grade 2 or 3) seems justified. Steeper and Mukai recommended using the proportion of tumor represented by neuroepithelium to indicate the tumor grade: <10 percent of immature neuroepithelium is grade 1; 10 to 50 percent is grade 2; and >50 percent is grade 3.[110] Estimating the percentage of a microscopic feature in a large teratoma is largely a guess and not quantitative. Other suggested methods to improve the ability to identify immature tissue have involved the use of immunocytochemistry with antibodies to GFAP[28] and NCAM.[29] However, GFAP and NCAM antibodies react with neuroectoderm without regard to immaturity or malignant potential and have not been tested statistically. The combination of image analysis systems (morphometry) and immunocytochemistry may allow for more accurate quantification of the immature elements.

Accurate grading requires adequate sampling. At least one block of tissue should be submitted for every 1 cm of maximum tumor diameter. Attention should be directed toward areas of necrosis and hemorrhage, as these areas are more likely to show immature tissue. Areas that appear solid and shiny also should be sampled.

Some immature teratomas have microscopic areas of other germ cell elements, particularly foci resembling yolk sac tumors. Such tumors are still classified as teratomas and are not considered to be combination germ cell tumors since the amount of nonteratomatous elements is small.

Clinical Management

Immature teratomas spread by direct extension and by abdominal seeding. The three cases of stage IV disease in the AFIP series had liver parenchymal metastasis; no extension beyond the abdomen was documented.[106] Prognosis is related to the stage of disease, the presence of postsurgical residual tumor, and the tumor grade. Since this tumor is never bilateral and patients are young at diagnosis, peritoneal washings, unilateral salpingo-oophorectomy, omentectomy, pelvic and periaortic node sampling, and wide sampling of peritoneal surfaces or implants constitute adequate surgical therapy.

Most patients (80 percent) have stage IA disease. Recurrences in patients with low-grade (i.e., grade 1), stage I tumors are so infrequent that additional therapy is not needed. Patients with stage I, grade 2 or 3 tumors experience recurrences with sufficient frequency that adjuvant therapy is recommended. Since therapy is the same for grades 2 and 3 tumors, these can be combined into a single group (high-grade).[106] Patients with disease other than stage I should also receive chemotherapy if the extraovarian lesions are not grade 0 (see below). Combination chemotherapy with vincristine, actinomycin, and cyclophosphamide produces an 85 percent cure rate.[105] Other regimens (i.e., cisplatin, bleomycin, and vinblastine; and cisplatin, bleomycin, and etoposide) have also been employed successfully.[105a] Figure 10–25 demonstrates the survival for patients with stage I teratoma diagnosed since 1977. The use of modern combination chemotherapy has led to excellent outcomes, as only 2 of 62 patients died of their disease.[106]

If metastases are present, the grade of the metastasis is a major prognostic indicator. Of patients who have a grade 1 primary tumor and grade 0 metastasis (gliomatosis peritonei) (Fig. 10–26), all survive when treated by surgery alone; therefore, they need only excision of the ovarian primary lesion and debulking of the implants. Patients who have high-grade primary tumors should receive chemotherapy regardless of the grade of metastasis. The presence of metastases other than grade 0 can adversely affect survival. These patients should also be treated with combination chemotherapy. In many cases, persistent tumor found at the time of re-exploration will show transformation into mature elements, usually glia (grade 0). This may occur either after treatment or spontaneously.[111] Although transformation from mature to immature tissue does not occur, cancerous transformation of a mature tissue element has been reported.[112]

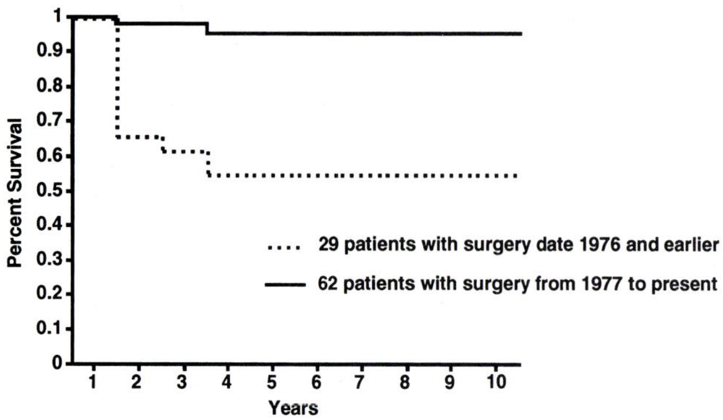

FIGURE 10-25
This graph shows the survival of patients with immature teratomas (all grades) diagnosed and managed before and after 1977. (From O'Connor DM, Norris HJ: The influence of grade on the outcome of stage I ovarian immature (malignant) teratomas and the reproducibility of grading. Int J Gynecol Pathol 1994;13:283–289.)

Monodermal and Highly Specialized Teratomas

These are teratomas with predominance of one particular tissue type. Although a variety of tissues are recognized, such as sebaceous melanotic, and pituitary, the two most common are thyroid and carcinoid. Some pure mucinous tumors that have intestinal differentiation may represent a monodermal teratoma. While mature neural teratomas are known to exist,[113] pure neuroectodermal tumors are best considered in the category of high-grade immature teratomas, since their clinical behavior is similar.

Struma Ovarii

Struma ovarii is a teratoma composed exclusively of thyroid tissue. While various definitions have been used in the past to signify struma ovarii (clinically functional thyroid tissue or malignant thyroid tissue), it is most appropriately defined by either of the following pathologic features: (1) a teratoma composed solely of thyroid tissue or one in which the thyroid tissue represents greater than one half of the tumor (this is the most commonly accepted definition); or (2) a teratoma in which the thyroid tissue is grossly recognizable.

Although thyroid tissue is found in approximately one fifth of mature teratomas, a diagnosis of struma ovarii is made in only 2 to 3 percent of mature teratomas.[1]

The age range of patients with struma ovarii is comparable to that of patients with mature cystic teratomas; the majority of patients are in the reproductive age group. The symptoms are likewise similar to those of mature teratomas, although a small number of patients have clinical evidence of thyrotoxicosis. In approximately 15 percent of cases, enlargement of the thyroid gland accompanies struma ovarii, and in affected patients it may be difficult to determine whether the excess thyroid hormones are from the thyroid gland or the ectopic thyroid tissue. The tumor is removed by cystectomy, if possible, or by oophorectomy. Even patients who were not thyrotoxic could exhibit postoperative symptoms of hyperthyroidism owing to manipulation of the thyroid tissue.[114] Ascites and hydrothorax have been reported with struma ovarii[115]; the cause for this is unknown.

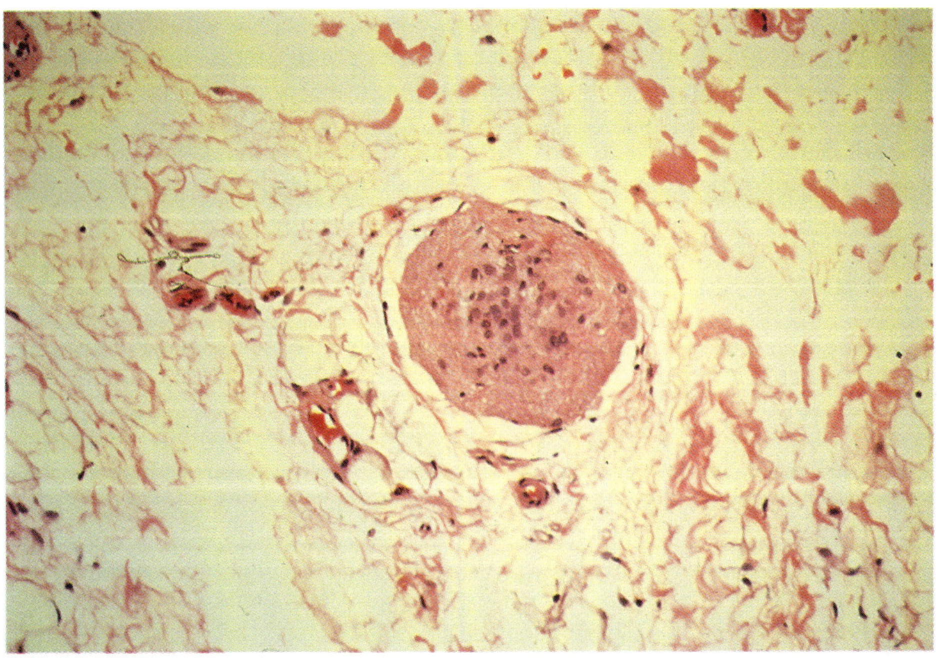

FIGURE 10-26
An extraovarian glial implant in a patient with an immature teratoma is seen. Peritoneal glial implants are considered grade 0. If the patient has a grade 1 immature teratoma with grade 0 peritoneal implants, her prognosis is excellent and conservative surgery is sufficient therapy.

On gross examination, the thyroid tissue has an appearance similar to that of normal thyroid gland. It is fleshy and gray-green to pinkish brown. Occasionally, the tumor is predominantly cystic; the larger spaces are often filled with a gelatinous, colloid-like fluid (Fig. 10–27). Thyroid tissue resembling normal thyroid gland is seen on microscopic examination (Fig. 10–28). The tissue is typically unencapsulated. The follicular structure and organization resemble normal thyroid, nodular goiter, or adenoma. Iodine, thyroglobulin, and triiodothyronine all have been demonstrated within the follicles. There have been reports of cases of struma ovarii resembling Graves' disease or Hashimoto's thyroiditis by histopathology.[114, 116]

Malignant struma ovarii is exceedingly rare. In the past the incidence was reported to be approximately 20 percent of all struma ovarii.[117] However, this number is probably an exaggeration, since metastasis occurred in only a minority of these cases.[116, 118] The criteria for malignancy are not well defined. Thyroid tissue within a teratoma is not encapsulated, and it gives the false impression of invasion. Papillary "hyperplasia" has also been reported to occur in struma ovarii, but it has no malignant potential.[119] The diagnosis of malignant struma ovarii should be made only when cytologic features of malignancy are present (Fig. 10–29). Very infrequently, peritoneal implants of benign thyroid tissue, termed strumosis, occur with struma ovarii; however, this condition behaves in a benign fashion.[4] The outlook for a patient with malignant struma ovarii depends on the presence of extraovarian tumor. Patients who have tumors confined to the ovary have an excellent prognosis and could be treated by unilateral oophorectomy and careful surgical exploration. However, patients who have metastatic disease have a worse prognosis. Treatment is hysterectomy and bilateral salpingo-oophorectomy to remove the diseased adnexa and surrounding structures. Debulking of metastases, if possible, is also recommended. Radioactive ^{131}I has been used as adjunctive therapy.[117] If conservation of ovarian and childbearing function is a concern and the uterus and contralateral ovary are not involved, conservation of these structures should be considered.

Carcinoid

Primary ovarian carcinoid tumors are unusual, and only a handful of cases have been reported.[120] This lesion accounts for less than 1 percent of ovarian teratomas.[121] The age of patients ranges from the third to the eighth decade. The tumor is a solid yellow or tan nodule within a cystic teratoma. In about one quarter of cases the carcinoid tumor is the only element. Primary ovarian carcinoid tumor must be differentiated from a gastrointestinal carcinoid tumor metastatic to the ovary. If there are other teratomatous elements, this suggests an ovarian primary tumor.

The most common histopathologic pattern is the insular, which resembles the midgut carcinoid tumor (Fig. 10–30). Islands of uniform small cells are surrounded by thick fibrous bands. The cells have small round nuclei and abundant cytoplasm. Mitotic activity is rare. Neurosecretory granules are present in 80 percent of cells. These have an affinity for silver salts and are argentaffin reaction positive. However, these granules are best demon-

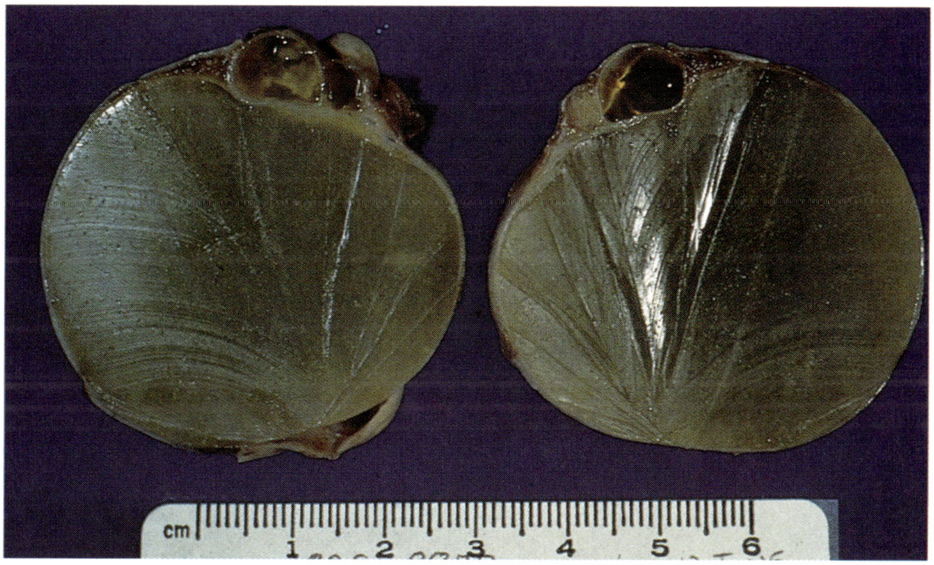

FIGURE 10–27
This struma ovarii has a large cavity filled with gelatinous, colloid-like fluid. The surrounding capsule is thin and smooth.

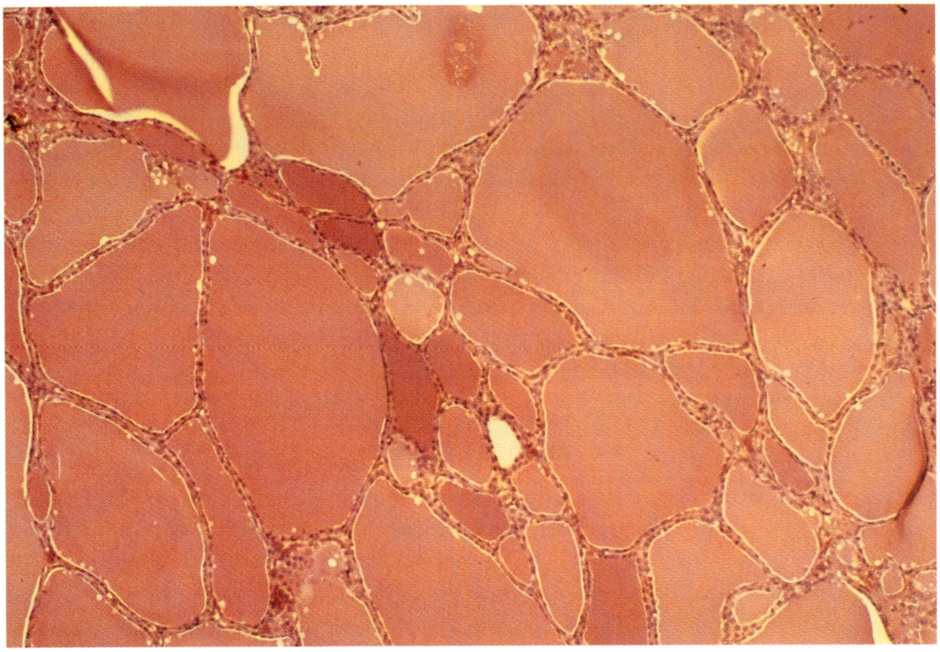

FIGURE 10-28
Colloid-filled follicles of various sizes lined by a single layer of cuboidal cells are characteristic of struma ovarii. This resembles a normal thyroid gland or nodular goiter.

strated by immunocytochemistry using antibodies to chromogranin, S100, and neuron-specific enolase. On electron microscopy, the granules show marked variation in size and a dumbbell shape.[122]

Acini with intraluminal eosinophilic secretions can be seen near the periphery of the islands, resembling a microfollicular granulosa cell tumor. The difference is that the nuclei of granulosa tumors cells are irregular and grooved. The immunocytochemistry findings described above are not present in granulosa cell tumor.

The carcinoid syndrome, which is characterized by diarrhea, abdominal pain, wheezing, flushing, and right heart murmurs, is present in approximately one third of patients with ovarian carcinoid tumor.[121] These symptoms are due to serotonin (5-hydroxytryptamine) production by the tumor cells. Intestinal carcinoid tumors produce the carcinoid syndrome only after metastasis to the liver has occurred. Ovarian carcinoid tumors, on the other hand, can produce the carcinoid syndrome without metastasis. The venous blood from the ovary

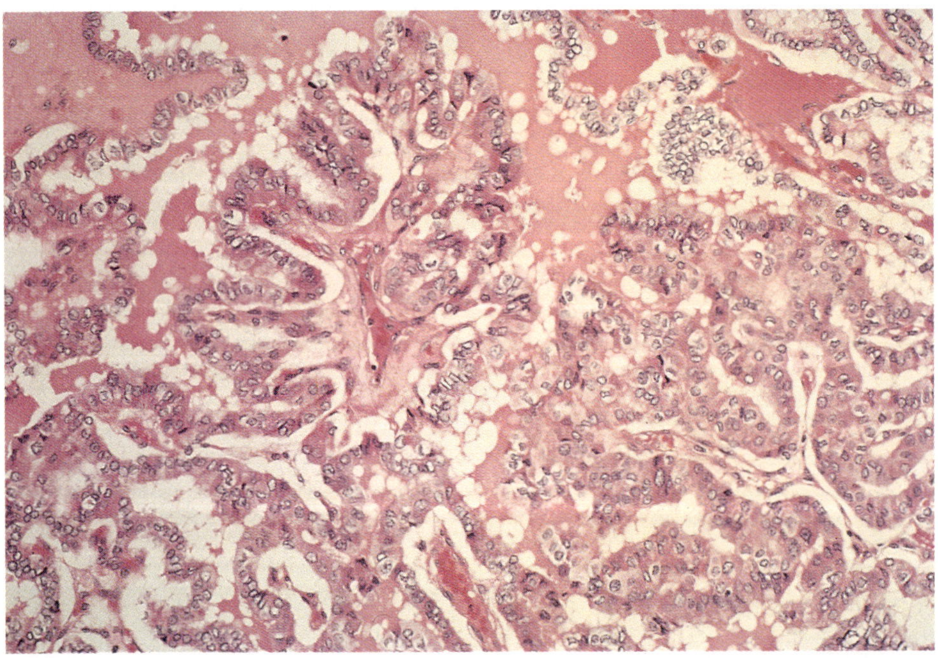

FIGURE 10-29
This malignant struma ovarii shows proliferation of the epithelium with cellular stratification and complex papillary structure. The nuclei show the chromatin clearing typical of papillary cancer of the thyroid. Colloid is seen. (Courtesy of Dr. Richard Lieberman, Armed Forces Institute of Pathology, Washington, DC.)

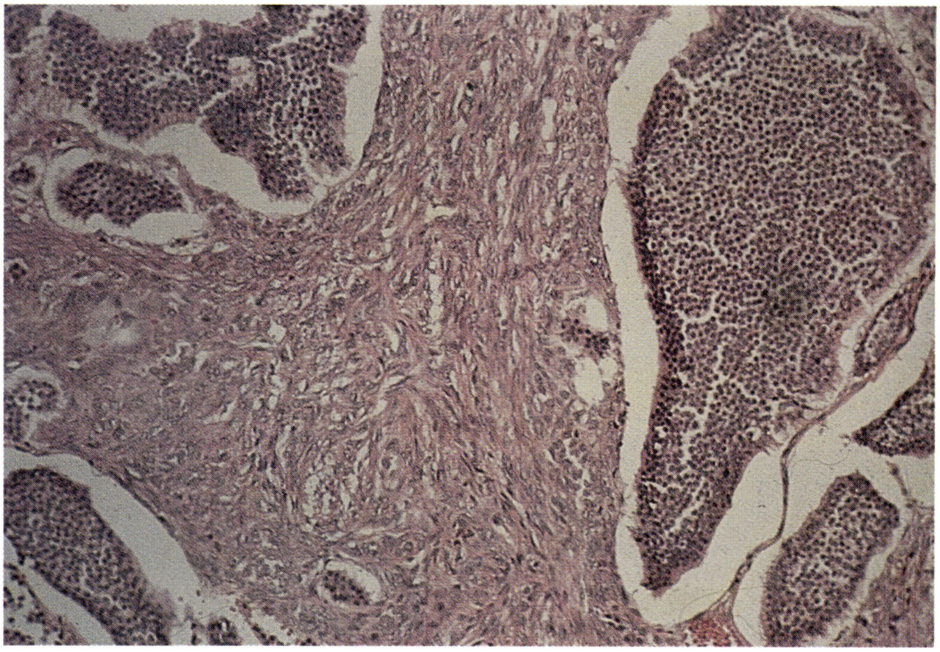

FIGURE 10–30
The insular pattern of carcinoid shows islands of round, uniform cells that are surrounded by fibroconnective tissue.

drains to the inferior vena cava and bypasses the portal circulation. Patients with primary ovarian carcinoid have early symptoms, and the symptoms abate after total excision. Abnormal 5-hydroxyindoleacetic acid (HIAA) levels measured in a 24-hour urine collection are present only in tumors that are at least 3 to 4 cm in diameter. Tricuspid valve involvement secondary to a carcinoid syndrome from an ovarian carcinoid has been reported.[123] Other substances produced by ovarian carcinoid tumors include insulin,[124] substance P,[125] and peptide tyrosine, which causes constipation.[126] Treatment of ovarian carcinoid tumor is surgical. Since these tumors have a limited capacity for metastatic spread, unilateral adnexectomy should be considered in the young patient without uterine or contralateral adnexal involvement.

The trabecular (foregut or hindgut) carcinoid is a much less common pattern.[127] The tumor is characterized by elongated narrow ribbons of carcinoid cells separated by fibrous trabeculae. Acini are usually absent. Neurosecretory granules are present in about one half of these cases and are positive for the same immunocytochemistry stains described above. On electron microscopy, the granules are round and of uniform size.[122] The carcinoid syndrome does not occur with trabecular carcinoid of the ovary. Except for one case,[120] metastases have not been reported. Unilateral adnexectomy and close follow-up should be adequate therapy.

Strumal carcinoid, originally described by Scully,[128] is a combination tumor with elements of both struma ovarii and carcinoid tumor. The origin of strumal carcinoid has been the subject of some debate.[129, 130] The tumor may represent differentiation of a primitive type of parafollicular C cell (the cell that leads to medullary carcinoma in the thyroid) or may result from thyroid differentiation in a carcinoid tumor. The tumor has been described as one of the components of type IIA multiple endocrine neoplasia syndrome.[131] Thyroid follicles are admixed with carcinoid tumor (Fig. 10–31). Myoglobin and secretory granules can occur in the same cell, as demonstrated by immunocytochemistry.[132] Calcitonin has also been identified in the carcinoid cells; this is the substance typically secreted by parafollicular cells and medullary thyroid carcinoma.[133] Only one malignant case has been documented.[120]

Choriocarcinoma

The finding of a choriocarcinoma in the ovary can be explained by a primary germ cell tumor, metastasis from gestational trophoblastic neoplasia arising in the uterus or tube, or degeneration of an ovarian pregnancy into gestational choriocarcinoma.

Primary ovarian choriocarcinoma may be pure choriocarcinoma or, more commonly, a component of a mixed germ cell tumor. It is unequivocally considered to be a primary germ cell tumor if diagnosed in a prepubertal child or in a reproductive age woman in association with other germ cell elements. Pure choriocarcinoma is more likely to be of gestational origin than of germ cell deriva-

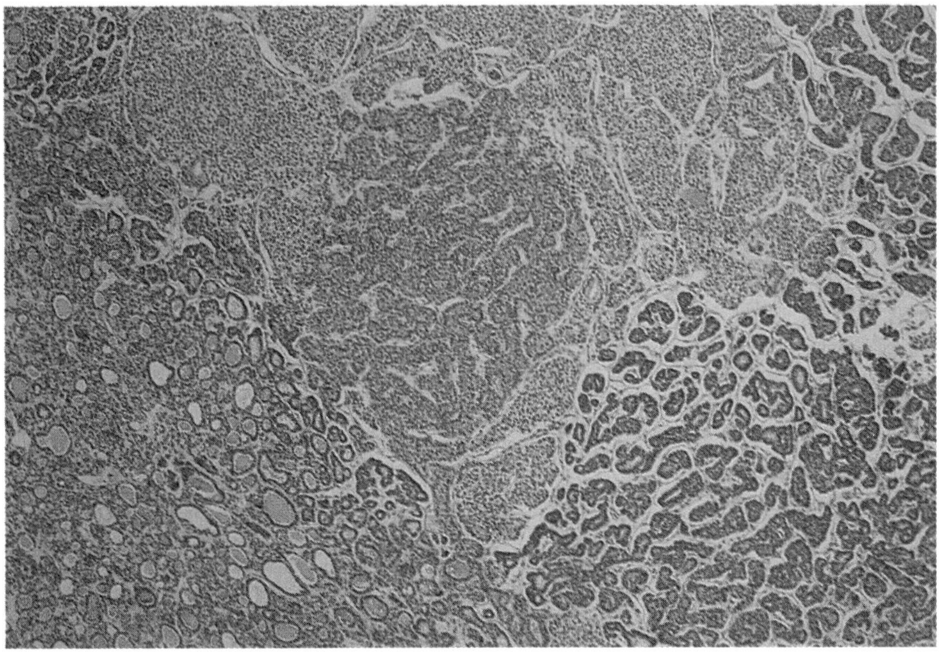

FIGURE 10–31
This is a strumal carcinoid. Normal thyroid-like tissue can be recognized *(lower left)*. The carcinoid is arranged in an insular pattern *(center)* and in a trabecular pattern *(lower right)*. (Courtesy of Dr. Richard Lieberman, Armed Forces Institute of Pathology, Washington, DC.)

tion. Metastatic gestational choriocarcinoma to the ovary is more common than a choriocarcinoma developing from an ovarian pregnancy.

Primary nongestational ovarian choriocarcinoma is extremely rare.[134–136] Two probable cases were encountered in the first 5000 ovarian tumors accessioned at the AFIP. Most nongestational choriocarcinoma of the ovary occurs in combination with teratoma, endodermal sinus tumor, dysgerminoma, or embryonal carcinoma. Of the first 40 examples of ovarian choriocarcinoma cited in the literature, only one half were pure.[134]

Clinical Presentation

In a review of published cases of both pure and mixed germ cell tumors with choriocarcinoma, the patients' ages ranged from 7 months to 35 years, with an average of 13 years.[134] Approximately one half of patients who have primary ovarian choriocarcinoma have abdominal enlargement and pain; hemoperitoneum is common. One half of premenarchal patients with choriocarcinoma have signs of precocious puberty. Theca lutein cysts have been reported in association with ovarian choriocarcinoma. This is due to high production of hCG by the tumor.[137] The hCG stimulates the ovary owing to its similarity to luteinizing hormone.

Morphology

Choriocarcinoma is typically a solid yellow or tan to brown mass of soft consistency. As with gestational choriocarcinoma, the center has abundant hemorrhage and necrosis, and there is a small rim of viable tumor at the periphery of the mass. Like most other malignant germ cell tumors, it is unilateral (see Table 10–3). If other germ cell elements are present, the appearance of the tumor may be similar to that described for the particular tumor whose element predominates.

Ovarian choriocarcinoma is composed of two populations of cells, cytotrophoblast and syncytiotrophoblast, which are arranged in a characteristic diphasic plexiform pattern (Fig. 10–32). Intermediate trophoblasts are not seen as with gestational choriocarcinoma (see Chapter 12). The multinucleate, eosinophilic to amphophilic syncytiotrophoblasts usually surround clusters of smaller mononuclear cytotrophoblasts. The cytotrophoblast has clear cytoplasm and an irregular nucleus. Both elements must be present to identify a case as choriocarcinoma and to avoid confusion with a germ cell tumor, such as dysgerminoma or embryonal carcinoma, which may contain trophoblastic cells. Extensive hemorrhage and necrosis may result in the recognition of only a small amount of viable trophoblastic tissue.

Clinical Management

Nongestational choriocarcinoma of the ovary has not been as responsive to chemotherapy as gestational choriocarcinoma. Treatment consists of surgical excision and combination chemotherapy.[134–136, 138] The surgery is tailored to the extent of tumor involvement found at exploration. The combination of vincristine, bleomycin, and cis-

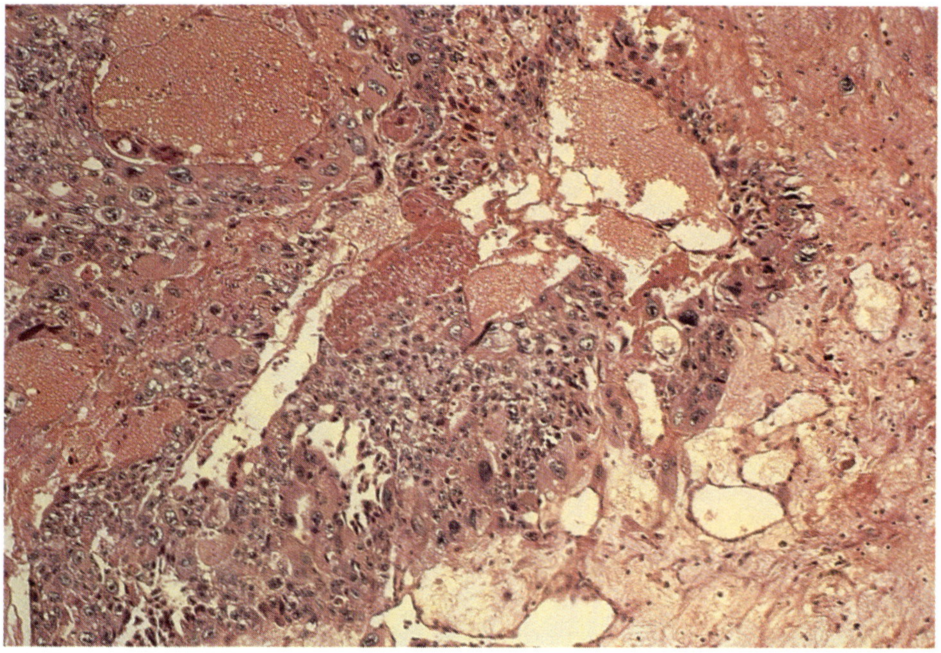

FIGURE 10-32
A primary ovarian choriocarcinoma composed of cyto- and syncytiotrophoblast accompanied by hemorrhage. The syncytiotrophoblasts are the larger cells with abundant cytoplasm and bizarre nuclei. Their cell borders are generally not well defined. The cytotrophoblasts are seen best in the center of the field. The cells and nuclei are smaller. Lakes of red cells are seen throughout the tumor.

platin has shown some success in the treatment of these tumors.[138] The combination of methotrexate, actinomycin, and cyclophosphamide has also been used.[77] Serial hCG determinations are used to monitor disease status and tumor response to therapy.

Embryonal Carcinoma

Although commonly seen in testicular germ cell tumors, ovarian embryonal carcinoma has only recently been characterized as a separate clinicopathologic entity.[139] In the past this tumor has been included in the category of endodermal sinus tumor. Review of the AFIP files identified 11 pure embryonal carcinomas and 4 mixed germ cell tumors with a predominantly embryonal carcinoma component.[139] Some of these tumors previously had been diagnosed as endodermal sinus tumors. Pure embryonal carcinoma is rare, accounting for less than 5 percent of malignant ovarian germ cell tumors. In common with other more differentiated germ cell tumors, it can express tumor markers (i.e., AFP, hCG).[140]

Clinical Presentation

The age of patients with embryonal carcinoma is between 4 and 28 years (median of 15 years). Nearly 50 percent are prepubertal.[139] The majority present with an abdominal or pelvic mass and 50 percent with abdominal pain. The duration of symptoms tends to be short (mean of 3 weeks). The symptoms can mimic those of appendicitis or ruptured ectopic pregnancy, and there can be confusion with ectopic pregnancy if the patient is of reproductive age and has a positive pregnancy test. Unlike patients who have endodermal sinus tumor, most of those with embryonal carcinoma have signs and symptoms secondary to abnormal hormone production. Signs of precocious puberty are present in almost one half of prepubertal girls.[139] Amenorrhea or abnormal vaginal bleeding is found in women of reproductive age. Mild hirsutism and virilization may also occur. Pregnancy tests are often positive.

Sixty percent of embryonal carcinomas are confined to one ovary (i.e., stage IA). The remainder divide equally between stage II and stage III. Stage IV disease is rarely encountered. Bilateral tumors (i.e., stage IB) do not occur.

Morphology

Embryonal carcinomas are typically large (median size, 17 cm), encapsulated, soft, and round. Focal hemorrhage and infarcts are common. The cut surface is gray-yellow, solid, and cystic.

Embryonal carcinoma is composed of solid sheets of large, primitive, pleomorphic cells that have amphophilic vacuolated cytoplasm. The nucleus has a vesicular chromatin pattern and one or more nucleoli (Fig. 10–33). These cells may form glandlike spaces and clusters suggesting an endodermal sinus tumor, but they lack the reticular background and Schiller-Duval bodies typical of that lesion. The relationship of embryonal carcinoma to endodermal sinus tumor is also demon-

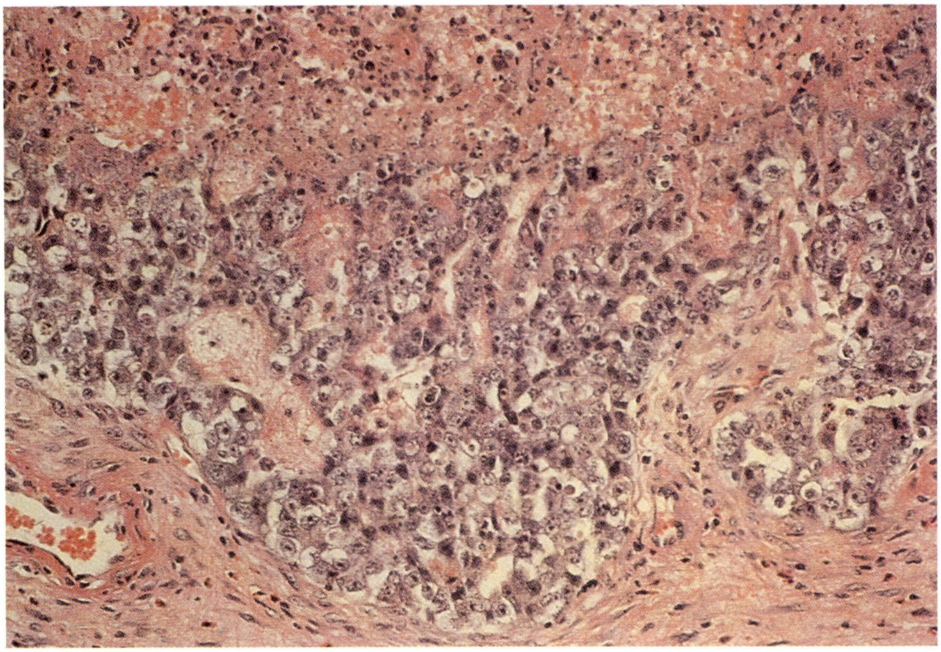

FIGURE 10-33
The primitive embryonal cells of embryonal carcinoma are arranged in sheets and ribbons. The cells are large with pleomorphic nuclei that have prominent nucleoli. These cells resemble cytotrophoblasts, but their cytoplasm is amphophilic, while that of the cytotrophoblast is often clear. (Courtesy of Dr. Richard Lieberman, Armed Forces Institute of Pathology, Washington, DC.)

strated by the presence of AFP (Fig. 10–34) and mucinous glands in both tumors. The stroma is variable; it can be either loose and myxoid or cellular with primitive fibroblastic mesenchymal cells.

All embryonal carcinomas contain isolated clusters of syncytiotrophoblasts (Fig. 10–35) and mononuclear cells that contain hyaline droplets. These droplets have been shown to contain hCG, AFP, and keratin by immunoperoxidase stains.[15, 139] The first two serve as tumor markers in tissue and serum (see Table 10–2). The close relationship of embryonal carcinoma to choriocarcinoma is illustrated by the presence of hCG and syncytiotrophoblastic cells and the occasional coexistence of both tumors. Embryonal carcinoma can also differentiate toward teratoma, as suggested by the presence of mature cartilage and squamous

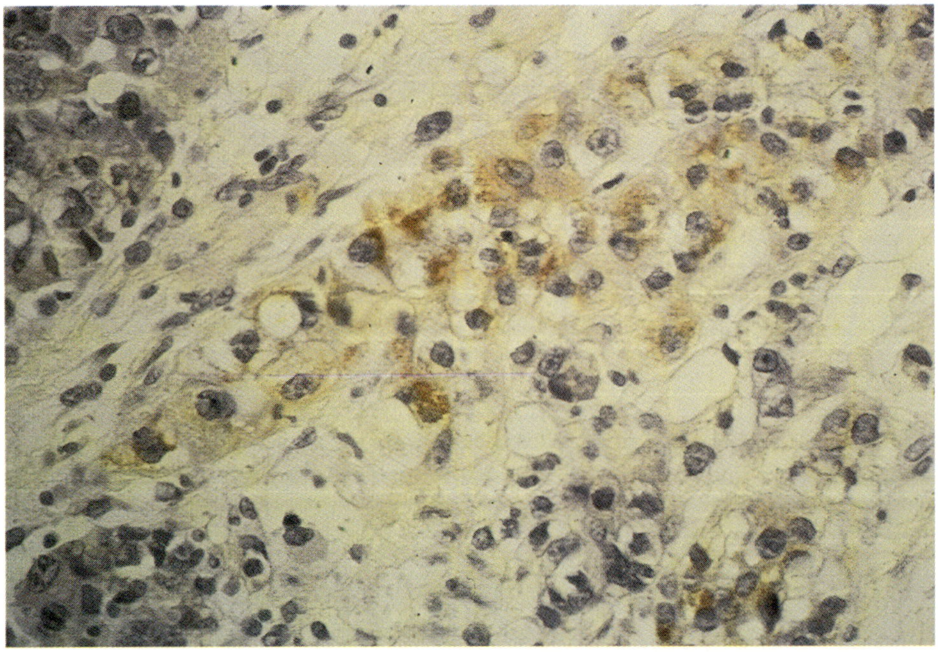

FIGURE 10-34
Embryonal cells with focal immunopositivity (brown stain) for α-fetoprotein are seen here.

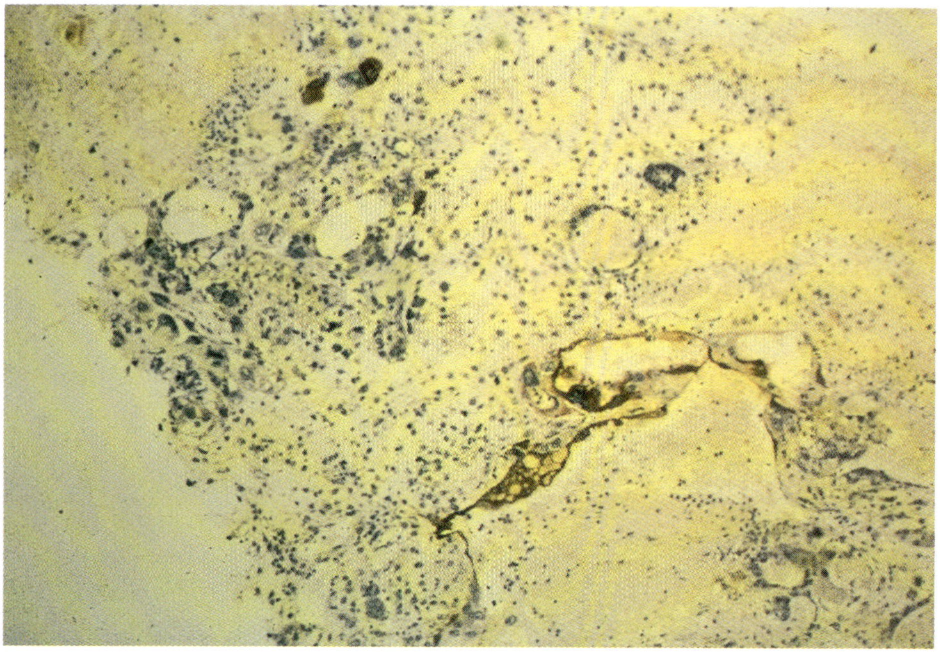

FIGURE 10–35
Focal trophoblastic cells of an embryonal carcinoma with immunopositivity (brown stain) for hCG are present.

epithelium in some cases. This is consistent with the ability of the totipotential embryonal cells to differentiate into mature tissue elements.

Clinical Management

Before combination chemotherapy, the 5-year actuarial survival for patients with embryonal carcinoma was 50 percent in stage I disease and 39 percent in all other stages combined. Patients who develop recurrences following treatment die within 2 years from widespread intraabdominal metastases.

The therapeutic approach to embryonal carcinoma is the same as for other malignant germ cell tumors and includes removal of the affected ovary, tumor debulking, and staging laparotomy. Because involvement of the contralateral ovary in the absence of visible metastases elsewhere is rare or nonexistent, unilateral salpingo-oophorectomy for stage I disease can be performed in the young patient. The opposite ovary, however, should be evaluated by wedge biopsy and frozen-section analysis. In two of six patients undergoing biopsy of the contralateral ovary, microscopic foci of pure dysgerminoma were found. In these cases the primary neoplasm also contained occult areas of dysgerminoma admixed with embryonal carcinoma.[139]

Since 50 percent of stage I patients die if treated by surgery alone, adjunctive chemotherapy must be given postoperatively. It is difficult to assess the value of adjunctive therapy in patients with embryonal carcinoma, since the number of cases is too small to draw meaningful conclusions. Nevertheless, the chemotherapeutic regimens that are effective in endodermal sinus tumors (e.g., bleomycin, etoposide, and cisplatin) should be as effective in patients with embryonal carcinomas. Monitoring of disease recurrence by serum AFP and hCG levels gives important information about disease status and the efficacy of chemotherapy.

Polyembryoma

This is a rare tumor pattern that occurs together with other malignant germ cell elements. Because it is never found in a pure form, it is best classified as a mixed germ cell tumor with embryoid formation rather than as a separate entity. Since its original description by Peyron[141] in a testicular teratoma, fewer than 50 cases have been reported in the ovaries; all tumors have arisen in individuals under the age of 40 years. Polyembryoma resembles embryonal carcinoma in appearance. The characteristic microscopic feature is the embryoid body, a microscopic structure that recapitulates the features of a presomite embryo of 13- to 15-day gestational age (Fig. 10–36).[142] Structures resembling the embryonic disk, yolk sac, and amniotic cavity can usually be identified. Embryoid types are described as complete, imperfect, or amorphous, depending on the degree of organization.[143] Laboratory studies have shown that embryoids are observed in transplanted embryonal carcinoma after germ cells are no longer identifiable. This suggests that they are a stage in the differentiation of embryonal carcinoma or primitive totipotential cells.[144] Other tumors that may

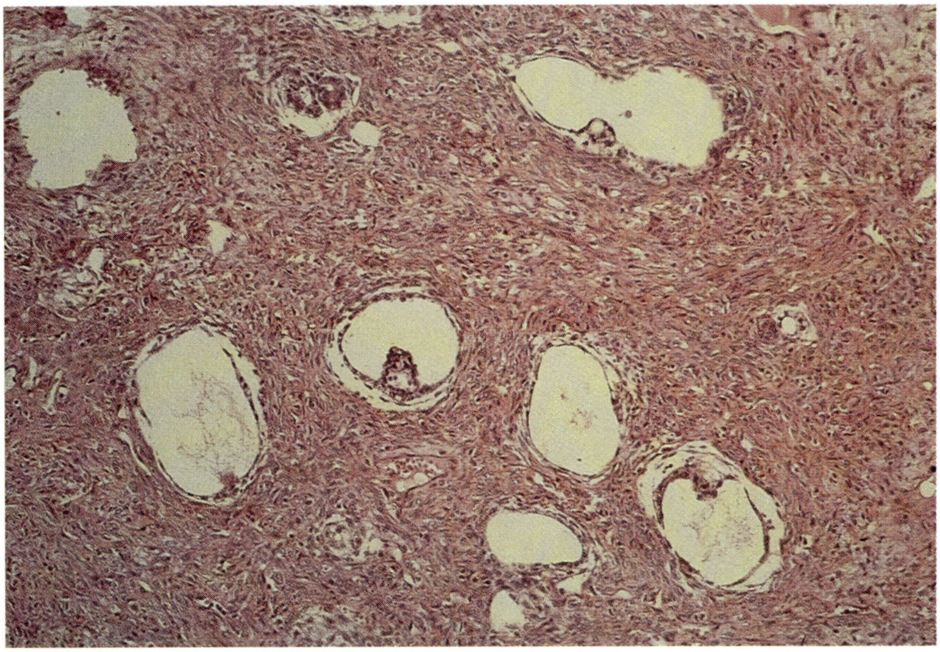

FIGURE 10–36
In this polyembryoma numerous embryoid bodies in various stages of development are seen. They resemble a 13- to 15-day embryo. (Courtesy of Dr. Richard Lieberman, Armed Forces Institute of Pathology, Washington, DC.)

be present in combination with polyembryoma include dysgerminoma, endodermal sinus tumor, embryonal carcinoma, and teratoma. The clinical behavior of this neoplasm is consistent with that of the other malignant germ cell tumors that it accompanies. Its treatment is similar to that to be described for mixed germ cell tumors.

Mixed Germ Cell Tumor

Mixed germ cell tumors are defined as tumors that contain two or more malignant germ cell elements. Dysgerminoma with endodermal sinus tumor is the most common combination; however, all types of ovarian malignant germ cell tumors have been identified in some combination or various combinations.

These tumor are not as common in women as in the male testis. They account for about 8 percent of malignant germ cell tumors of the ovary, compared with 60 percent in the testis. Their true incidence is difficult to ascertain. Extensive sampling of large germ cell tumors may result in the more frequent finding of additional germ cell elements.

Clinical Presentation

Patients are between 5 and 33 years of age, with a median of 16 years. Forty percent are prepubertal, and one third of these are children with signs of precocious puberty.[145] Pregnancy tests are positive in 38 percent of nonpregnant patients, reflecting the presence of syncytiotrophoblasts in the tumor. Although the majority of patients present with a relatively asymptomatic abdominal or pelvic mass, 20 percent will have acute abdominal pain and 20 percent will have a fever. The mean interval between onset of symptoms and diagnosis is 4 weeks.

Two thirds of patients have stage I disease at laparotomy, with no macroscopic involvement of the opposite ovary. Most of the remainder have either stage II or stage III disease in equal numbers. In advanced disease, the abdominal and pelvic peritoneum and organs are the principal sites of metastasis.

Morphology

Like other germ cell tumors, these neoplasms tend to be large with a mean diameter of 15 cm. The outer surface is smooth, but the appearance of the cut surface depends on the type and quantity of its components. Solid fleshy areas correspond with dysgerminoma, and mucoid cystic areas with teratoma; hemorrhage and necrosis correlate most frequently with endodermal sinus tumor or choriocarcinoma. Careful examination of the gross specimen and selective sampling are essential for accurate histopathologic diagnosis.

By definition, at least two malignant elements must be present for a lesion to be called a mixed germ cell tumor (Fig. 10–37). The most common element is dysgerminoma, which is found in 80 percent of tumors, followed by endodermal sinus tumor in 70 percent, immature teratoma in 53

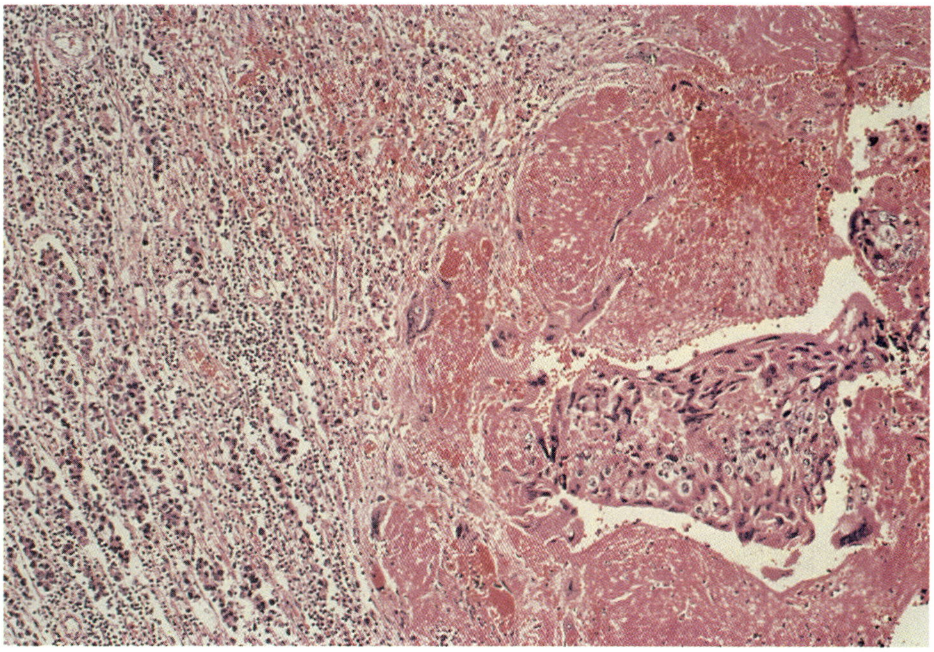

FIGURE 10-37
A choriocarcinoma with the characteristic diphasic pattern is seen on the right. There are cytotrophoblasts, syncytiotrophoblasts, and hemorrhage. A dysgerminoma is seen on the left. There are cords of germ cells separated by a stroma that is infiltrated by lymphocytes. (Courtesy of Dr. Richard Lieberman, Armed Forces Institute of Pathology, Washington, DC.)

percent, choriocarcinoma in 20 percent, and embryonal carcinoma in 13 percent.[145]

In two thirds of tumors, only two malignant components are present. The most common combination is dysgerminoma and endodermal sinus tumor. The combination represents a third of all mixed germ cell tumors. When immature teratoma is present, it is grade 1 in half the cases. When the opposite ovary is evaluated microscopically and found to contain malignancy, it is dysgerminoma. The other components are not found bilaterally.

Clinical Management

Before modern combination therapy, the actuarial 5-year survival of patients with stage I disease was 50 percent.[145] The introduction of chemotherapeutic regimens has improved the survival of patients with stage I disease to 79 percent.[146] The factors that are predictive of survival in stage I disease are the size and composition of the neoplasm.[145] If more than one third of a stage I tumor is composed of endodermal sinus tumor, choriocarcinoma, or grade 3 teratoma, the tumor behaves very aggressively; however, if it contains less than one third of these elements or contains combinations of dysgerminoma, embryonal carcinoma, and low-grade immature teratoma, it behaves slightly less aggressively. Patients who have tumors that are less than 10 cm in diameter are likely to survive regardless of the composition of the tumor.

The surgical treatment of patients with mixed germ cell tumors is similar to that utilized for malignant pure germ cell tumors and is dependent on the patient's desire to maintain childbearing potential and on the extent of disease. It is appropriate to perform an initial conservative procedure and wait for the complete pathologic evaluation. A second operation can be performed if indicated. If a unilateral adnexectomy is performed, the opposite ovary should be carefully inspected, at least, since mixed tumors with dysgerminoma elements can have contralateral ovarian involvement.

Combined Germ Cell and Sex Cord Stromal Tumor

This category includes tumors that contain germ cells admixed with ovarian stromal cells. The only tumor of numerical significance is the gonadoblastoma. A very small number of other types have been described.[147, 148] Their clinical and pathologic features justify distinguishing them from gonadoblastoma, but they are very rare.[149]

Gonadoblastoma

This neoplasm arises almost exclusively in dysgenetic gonads.[36] The true incidence may be difficult to determine, since many gonadoblastomas hyalinize and calcify with time or become overgrown by dysgerminoma. Nevertheless, over 150 cases have been reported.[148] Twenty-two percent arise in a streak gonad, 18 percent in an undescended dysgenetic testis, and the majority in an abnormal gonad of indeterminate type. Over 80 percent of patients are phenotypic females who are usually virilized. Ninety percent of all patients have a Y chromosome,[36] although this is not essential for the diagnosis.[15] An abnormal ring type of Y chromosome has been reported.[151] Gonadoblastoma has been very rarely reported in women who have a normal 46,XX karyotype[152, 153] or in fertile women.[36, 152, 154] It is very rare in true hermaphrodites.[155, 156] These patients may actually be mosaics, since gonadal mosaicism can be difficult to establish reliably. Y chromosome material may be present in a somatic chromosome.[153] The presence of gonadoblastoma in patients who have a male karyotype and abnormal gonads as well as its unique histopathology suggests that this tumor represents an abortive attempt at testes development.

Clinical Presentation

The age of the patients is between 1 and 38 years. The clinical presentation depends upon the nature of the underlying gonadal abnormality. Primary amenorrhea with or without signs of virilization is common in phenotypic females, while abnormal genitalia is frequent in phenotypic males. Owing to gonadal failure, most patients have high serum and urinary gonadotropin levels.[157]

Morphology

Gonadoblastomas vary in size from a few millimeters to a large, solid, soft, or firm and gritty mass. These characteristics depend on the degree of calcification and the contribution of different germ cell elements. Most gonadoblastomas are only a few centimeters in diameter. Calcifications can be found in 50 percent of cases and may be recognized by plain abdominal radiographs. Bilaterality is common, occurring in one third to one half of patients (see Table 10–3).

The essential histopathologic feature is the presence of circumscribed nests of primordial germ cells surrounded by ovarian specialized stromal cells. Although the nature of the stromal cells is not clear, immunocytochemical positivity for keratin and vimentin and the presence of Charcot-Böttcher crystals on electron microscopy favor a Sertoli type of cell differentiation.[158] The sex cord stromal cells typically form three distinctive patterns: (1) a circumferential arrangement of cells around a central nest of germ cells, (2) cells surrounding an individual germ cell, or (3) clusters of germ cells or cells surrounding spaces resembling Call-Exner bodies (Fig. 10–38). PAS-positive hyaline material can be found in the rosette-lined spaces, a pattern resembling the one that is typical of sex cord tumors with annular tubules (Fig. 10–39). In two thirds of gonadoblastomas, cells that look like Leydig cells and luteinized stromal cells are present.[36] This may, however, reflect stimulation of stromal cells by trophic hormones. Calcification and overgrowth by malignant germ cells occur to varying degrees.

Approximately 50 percent of gonadoblastomas have a significant component of dysgerminoma.[153] Ten percent are associated with endodermal sinus tumor, embryonal carcinoma, or choriocarcinoma.[159] Comprehensive sampling of these tumors

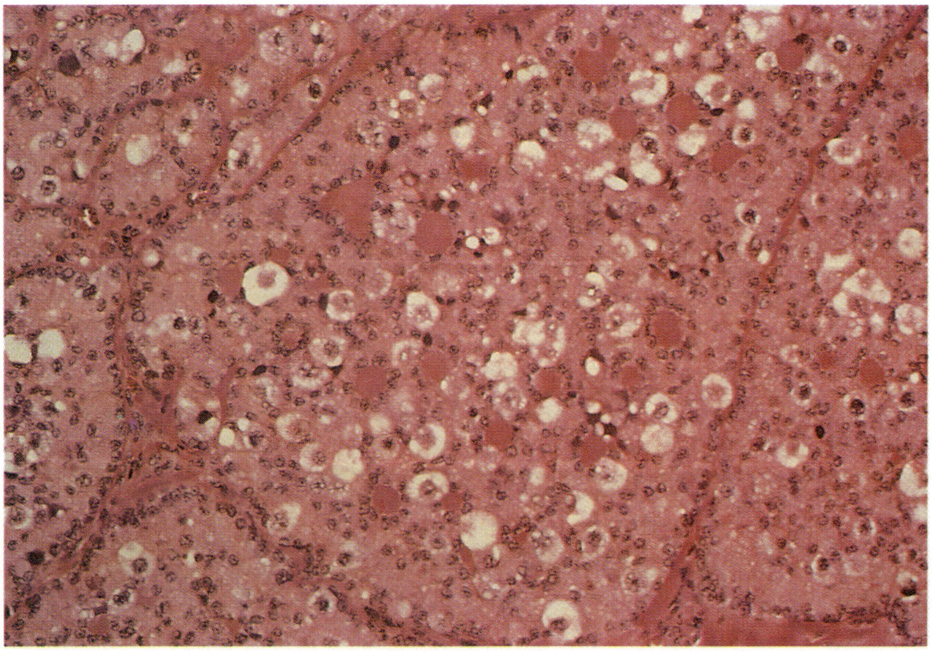

FIGURE 10–38
A gonadoblastoma is shown. The large germ cells with clear cytoplasm are surrounded by the smaller stromal cells. Some of the stromal cells surround brightly eosinophilic globules of acellular material (i.e., hyaline globules that stain positive with PAS). (Courtesy of Dr. Richard Lieberman, Armed Forces Institute of Pathology, Washington, DC.)

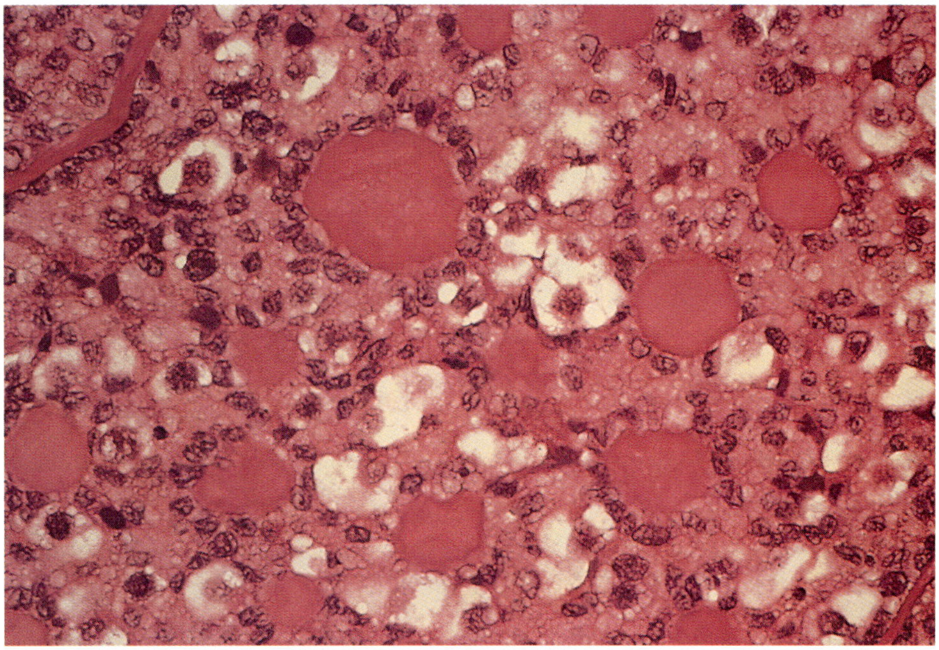

FIGURE 10–39
A high-power view of Figure 10–38. The round eosinophilic material is surrounded by a single layer of stromal cells in a rosette pattern. This is reminiscent of the sex cord tumor with annular tubules (see Chapter 11). (Courtesy of Dr. Richard Lieberman, Armed Forces Institute of Pathology, Washington, DC.)

is important, since the clinical behavior of gonadoblastoma depends on the presence of the other malignant elements. Metastasis of a dysgerminoma component in gonadoblastoma is uncommon even if the tumor is bilateral and large. In contrast, other malignant combinations have been fatal within 18 months.[154]

Clinical Management

Pure gonadoblastomas behave in a benign fashion. However, because of their potential to contain malignant germ cell elements and the high probability of an abnormal contralateral ovary as well as their origin in dysgenetic gonads, bilateral gonadectomy is indicated. If the tumor is small, laparoscopic gonadectomy can be considered.[160] Further treatment is determined by the presence of other malignant elements and the stage of disease.[153,161]

Combined Germ Cell and Sex Cord Stromal Tumors Other Than Gonadoblastoma

These tumors occur in males and females of all ages and are not associated with a chromosomal abnormality. These neoplasms are composed of two intimately admixed cellular elements and must be differentiated from gonadoblastoma. There is a lack of bilaterality and absence of calcification or nestlike pattern as well as a paucity of germ cells. The two cell types are arranged in either a diffuse or a tubular pattern, the latter resembling Pflüger's tubules of the embryonic gonad. The sex cord stromal type cells resemble Sertoli cells more than granulosa cells. Heterologous elements similar to those occasionally seen in Sertoli tumors have been identified in one case.[162] An association with a significant dysgerminoma component has not been described. The neoplasm is dominated by stromal proliferation.

With rare exception, these tumors are benign.[148] The metastasis in one case contained both tumor components.[147] In a second case the metastasis was of the dysgerminoma component and, in a third case, of the gonadoblastoma.[148] Conservative therapy (i.e., unilateral adnexectomy and staging laparotomy) is the treatment of choice. Karyotyping is recommended. If the patient is 46,XX, removal of the contralateral gonad may not be necessary.

MALIGNANT GERM CELL TUMORS AND GONADAL DYSGENESIS

Any patient who has gonadal dysgenesis and a Y chromosome is at high risk for developing a germ cell tumor, particularly gonadoblastoma. In one review at least nine tenths of gonadoblastomas arose in these patients.[36] Dysgerminoma may also occur in a dysgenetic gonad[153]; however, this may be a gonadoblastoma that has been overgrown by a dysgerminoma component.

A review of several studies determined that 25 percent of germ cell tumors in patients with gonadal dysgenesis and a Y chromosome are malignant.[163] Others have reported that approximately 40 percent are malignant.[153, 164, 165] The karyotype rather than the type of gonadal dysgenesis is decisive in assessing the risk of malignancy in an individual. The risk is increased by the presence of a Y chromosome.[153] Despite clarification of the histopathologic sequence in gonadal differentiation, the study of gonadal dysgenesis is still hampered by imprecise nomenclature and criteria. Individual cases may not fit a particular category,[166] or precise classification may be impossible because the tumor has destroyed the original gonadal tissue. In addition, mosaicism may be difficult to exclude because it can be incomplete or limited to the gonads.

Pure Gonadal Dysgenesis

Pure gonadal dysgenesis is the result of early embryonic testicular regression. These patients have bilateral streak gonads as well as a female phenotype and normal height. They lack the stigmata of Turner syndrome. The majority have either a 46,XY (male) karyotype or XY mosaicism. Less commonly, a 46,XX karyotype is found.

Gonadal tumors are very rare in patients with pure gonadal dysgenesis and 46,XX karyotype, however, among 15 patients with 46,XY karyotype, Teter found 3 with gonadoblastoma and 4 with dysgerminoma.[165] The calculated risk for gonadal neoplasia in patients with pure gonadal dysgenesis and a Y chromosome is about 30 percent.[167] Because of this, prophylactic gonadectomy is recommended for these individuals.

Mixed Gonadal Dysgenesis

These phenotypic females usually have a streak ovary on one side and a dysgenetic testis on the other. This condition may be regarded as intermediate between pure gonadal dysgenesis and Turner syndrome. In most cases affected patients are 45,XO/46,XY mosaics. Depending on the criteria selected, stigmata suggesting Turner syndrome are present in approximately 50 percent of patients. In 51 cases of 45,XO/46,XY mosaicism, of which two fifths were classified as mixed gonadal dysgenesis, 9 patients (18 percent) had a neoplasm.[168] The incidence was 23 percent among individuals who had abnormal external genitalia. Prophylactic gonadectomy is recommended in these instances.

Turner Syndrome

Patients with Turner syndrome have the typical 45,XO karyotype (or less frequently 45,XO/46,XX) and no signs of virilization. This chromosomal abnormality results in gonadal dysgenesis (i.e., streak gonads). Gonadal neoplasms are rare in these individuals.[165, 168] Although germ cells are rarely identified in the gonads of 45,XO patients, they occur occasionally, and there are reports of such women having a full-term pregnancy.[169] In contrast, among four women who had a Turner syndrome phenotype with virilization (which is usually associated with a Y chromosome), Teter reported one gonadoblastoma and one interstitial hilar cell tumor.[165, 170] Patients with Turner syndrome who developed germ cell tumors have all been found by sensitive hybridization techniques to harbor Y chromosome fragments. Thus, in these individuals, a complete and thorough chromosome analysis should be performed to exclude the presence of Y chromosome material. If the complete absence of Y chromosome material cannot be excluded, a bilateral gonadectomy should be performed.[171]

Testicular Feminization

Individuals with testicular feminization have a 46,XY karyotype and target organ androgen insensitivity. Because of this they are phenotypic females. They commonly present with primary amenorrhea or inguinal hernias. They have abdominal or labial testes, and some have gonadal tumors within the small abnormal testes. Most of these tumors are either hamartomas or Sertoli cell adenomas. The incidence of malignant germ cell tumor is difficult to ascertain, since most reported cases of testicular feminization are of young patients whose gonads have already been removed. It is estimated that about one third will develop a gonadal tumor with malignant potential (most commonly gonadoblastoma or dysgerminoma) by the age of 50 years; yet the calculated risk is only 2 percent before puberty.[167] Prophylactic gonadectomy is recommended for these patients; however, the procedure can be delayed until puberty.

Hermaphroditism

Hermaphrodites either have ovarian and testicular tissue in the same gonad or have a unilateral ovary and a contralateral testis. Most true hermaphrodites (60 percent) have a 46,XX karyotype.[172] Dysgerminoma has been reported in true hermaphrodites. Gonadoblastoma has also been reported in hermaphrodites who have either 46,XY or 46,XX karyotype.[155] However, modern, more sensitive techniques may be able to detect Y chromosome material in the 46,XX individual.[153] The factors predisposing to malignancy are the Y chro-

TABLE 10–5.
Proportion of Patients with Gonadal Dysgenesis Who Develop Germ Cell Neoplasms

Type of Gonadal Dysgenesis	*Karyotype*	*Proportion with Neoplasia*
Pure gonadal dysgenesis	46,XY	30%
	46,XX	Rare
Mixed gonadal dysgenesis	45,XO/46,XY	18–23%
Turner syndrome	45,XO	Rare
Testicular feminization	46,XY	30%
Hermaphroditism	46,XX	<5%
	46,XY	<5%

mosome and the abdominal, inguinal, or labial position of the gonad.

Table 10–5 summarizes the proportion of patients with dysgenetic gonads who develop germ cell neoplasms. It can be seen that the likelihood of an individual who has abnormal gonads developing a germ cell tumor depends on the karyotype rather than on classification of the dysgenesis. Those with undescended gonads and XY karyotypes or XY mosaicism have a high incidence of malignancy regardless of the clinical features. Individuals who have a normal 46,XX karyotype, 45,XO karyotype, or mosaic karyotype without Y chromosome material are at low risk for malignancy. Therefore, a careful search for Y chromosome material is of utmost importance.

REFERENCES

1. Talerman A: Germ cell tumors of the ovary. *In* Kurman RJ (ed): Blaustein's Pathology of the Female Genital Tract, 3rd ed. New York, Springer-Verlag, 1987, pp 559–560.
2. Scully RE: Germ cell tumors. *In* Tumors of the Ovary and Maldeveloped Gonads (Second Series, Fascicle 16). Washington, DC, Armed Forces Institute of Pathology, 1978, pp 226–310.
3. Koonings PP, Campbell K, Mishell DR, et al: Relative frequency of primary ovarian neoplasms. Obstet Gynecol 1989;74:921.
4. Norris HJ, O'Connor DM: Pathology of malignant germ cell tumors. *In* Coppleson M (ed): Gynecologic Oncology, 2nd ed. London, Churchill Livingstone, 1992, pp 917–934.
5. Wheeler JE: History of teratomas. *In* Damjanov I, Knowles BB, Stolter D (eds): The Human Teratomas (Experimental and Clinical Biology). Clifton, NJ, Humana Press, 1983, pp 1–15.
6. Teilum G: Homologous tumors of the ovary and testis: contribution to classification of gonadal tumors. Acta Obstet Gynecol Scand 1944;24:480.
7. Teilum G: Classification of endodermal sinus tumor (mesoblastoma vitellinum) and so-called embryonal carcinoma of the ovary. Acta Pathol Microbiol Scand 1965;64:407.
8. Iyengar B: The germ cell—oncogenic and embryogenic correlates. Experientia 1982;38:1239.
9. Steinhauer WR, Kalfayan LJ: A specific ovarian tumor protein isoform is required for efficient differentiation of germ cell Drosophila oogenesis. Genes Dev 1992;6:233.
10. Serov SF, Scully RE, Sobin LH: Histological typing of ovarian tumors. *In* International Histologic Classification of Tumors (No. 9). Geneva, World Health Organization, 1973.
11. FIGO Cancer Committee: Staging-grouping for primary carcinoma of the ovary. Gynecol Oncol 1986;25:383.
12. Gitlin D, Perricelli A: Synthesis of serum albumin, prealbumin, alpha-fetoprotein, alpha-1-antitrypsin and transferrin by the human yolk sac. Nature 1970;228:995.
13. Gitlin D, Perricelli A, Gitlin GM: Synthesis of alpha-fetoprotein by liver, yolk sac and gastrointestinal tract of the human conceptus. Cancer Res 1972;32:979.
14. Jacobsen GK: Alpha-fetoprotein (AFP) and human chorionic gonadotropin (HCG) in testicular germ cell tumors: A comparison of histologic and serologic occurrence of tumor markers. Acta Pathol Microbiol Scand 1983;91:183.
15. Kurman RJ, Scardino PT, McIntire KR, et al: Malignant germ cell tumors of the ovary and testis: An immunologic study of 69 cases. Ann Clin Lab Sci 1979;9:462.
16. Talerman A, Haije WG, Baggerman L: Serum alpha-fetoprotein in patients with germ cell tumors of the gonads and extragonadal sites: correlation between endodermal sinus (yolk sac) tumor and raised serum AFP. Cancer 1980;46:380.
17. Norgaard-Pedersen B, Schultz HP, Arends J, et al: Tumour markers in testicular germ cell tumours: Five-year experience from the DATECA Study, 1976–1980. Acta Radiol 1984;23:287.
18. Kurman RJ, Main CS, Chen H: Intermediate trophoblast: A distinctive form of trophoblast with specific morphological, biochemical and functional features. Placenta 1984; 5:349.
19. Yeh I, O'Connor DM, Kurman RJ: Intermediate trophoblast: Further immunocytochemical characteristics. Mod Pathol 1990;3:382.
20. Brescia RJ, Kurman RJ, Main CS, et al: Immunocytochemical localization of chorionic gonadotrophin, placental lactogen, and placental alkaline phosphatase in the diagnosis of complete and partial moles. Int J Gynecol Pathol 1987;6:213.
21. Kurman RJ, Young RH, Norris HJ, et al: Immunocytochemical localization of placental lactogen and chorionic gonadotropin in the normal placenta and trophoblastic tumors, with emphasis on intermediate trophoblast and the placental site trophoblastic tumor. Int J Gynecol Pathol 1984;3:101.
22. Yeh I, O'Connor DM, Kurman, RJ: Vacuolated trophoblast: A subpopulation of trophoblast in the chorion laeve. Placenta 1989;10:429.
23. Larson WJ: Human Embryology. New York, Churchill Livingstone, 1993, pp 3–4.
24. Jacobsen GK, Norgaard-Pedersen B: Placental alkaline phosphatase in testicular germ cell tumors and in carcinoma in situ of the testis. Acta Pathol Microbiol Scand 1984;92:323.
25. Fujii S, Konishi A, Suzuki A, et al: Analysis of lactic

dehydrogenase levels and its isoenzymes in ovarian dysgerminoma. Gynecol Oncol 1985;22:65.

26. Kawai M, Kano T, Kikkawa F, et al: Seven tumor markers in benign and malignant germ cell tumors of the ovary. Gynecol Oncol 1992;45:248.
27. Schwartz PF, Morris JM: Serum lactic dehydrogenase: A tumor marker for dysgerminoma. Obstet Gynecol 1988; 72:511.
28. Steeper TA, Mukai K: Solid ovarian teratomas: An immunocytochemical study of thirteen cases with clinicopathologic correlation. Pathol Annu 1984;19:81.
29. Notohara K, Hseuh CL, Awai M: Glial fibrillary acidic protein immunoreactivity of chondrocytes in immature and mature teratomas. Acta Pathol Jpn 1990;40:335.
30. Asadourian, LA, Taylor HB: Dysgerminoma: an analysis of 105 cases. Obstet Gynecol 1969;33:370.
31. Higuchi K, Kato T: Dysgerminoma of the ovary. J Jpn Obstet Gynecol Soc 1958;5:206.
32. Krepart G, Smith JP, Rutledge F, Delclos L: The treatment for dysgerminoma of the ovary. Cancer 1978;41:897.
33. Ochiai D, Isonishi S, Hirama Y: Effect of estrogen and progesterone on the growth of human ovarian dysgerminoma heterotransplanted to athymic nude mice. Asia Oceania J Obstet Gynaecol 1991;17:147.
34. Jackson SM: Ovarian dysgerminoma. Br J Radiol 1967; 40:459.
35. Talerman A, Huyzinga WT, Kuipers T: Dysgerminoma: Clinicopathologic study of 22 cases. Obstet Gynecol 1973;41:137.
36. Scully RE: Gonadoblastoma: A review of 74 cases. Cancer 1970;25:1340.
37. Manuel M, Katayama KP, Jones HW Jr: The age of occurrence of gonadal tumors in intersex patients with a Y-chromosome. Am J Obstet Gynecol 1976;124:293.
38. Talerman A, Jarabak J, Amarose A: Gonadoblastoma and dysgerminoma in a true hermaphrodite with 46,XX karyotype. Am J Obstet Gynecol 1981;140:175.
39. Bakri YN, Akhtar M: Gonadal dysgerminoma—seminoma associated with severe hypercalcemia. Acta Obstet Gynecol Scand 1993;72:57.
40. Giebel SC, Stanhope CR, Malkasian GD Jr, et al: Humoral hypercalcemia associated with a dysgerminoma. Mayo Clin Proc 1992;67:966.
41. Anstey A, Gowers L, Vass A: Ovarian dysgerminoma presenting with hypercalcemia: Case report and review of the literature. Gynaecology 1990;97:641.
42. Mueller CW, Topkins P, Lapp WA: Dysgerminoma of the ovary: An analysis of 427 cases. Am J Obstet Gynecol 1950;60:153.
43. Palmquist MB, Webb MJ, Lieber MM, et al: DNA ploidy of ovarian dysgerminomas: Correlation with clinical outcome. Gynecol Oncol 1992;44:13.
44. Oud PS, Soeters RP, Pahlplatz MM, et al: DNA cytometry of pure dysgerminoma of the ovary. Int J Gynecol Pathol 1988;7:258.
45. Hou-Jensen K, Kempson RL: The ultrastructure of gonadoblastoma and dysgerminoma. Hum Pathol 1974;5:79.
46. Hees K, de Jonge JP, von Kortzfleisch DH: Dysgerminoma of the ovary: cytologic and electron microscopic study of a case. Acta Cytol 1991;3:341.
47. Stewart CJ, Farquharson MA, Foulis K: Characterization of the inflammatory infiltrate in ovarian dysgerminoma: An immunocytochemical study. Histopathology 1992; 20:491.
48. Dietl J, Horny HP, Ruck P: Dysgerminoma of the ovary: An immunohistochemical study of tumor infiltrating lymphoreticular cells and tumor cells. Cancer 1993;15:2562.
49. Kurman RJ, Scardino PT, McIntire KR, et al: Cellular localization of AFP and hCG in germ cell tumors of the testis and ovary. Scand J Immunol 1978;8(Suppl 8):127.
50. Ueda G, Hamanaka N, Hayakawa K, et al: Clinical, histochemical and biochemical studies of an ovarian dysgerminoma with trophoblasts and Leydig cells. Am J Obstet Gynecol 1972;114:748.
51. Zaloudek CS, Tavassoli FA, Norris HJ: Dysgerminoma with syncytiotrophoblastic giant cells: A histologically distinct subtype of dysgerminoma. Am J Surg Pathol 1981;5:361.
52. Freel JH, Cassir JF, Pierce VK, et al: Dysgerminoma of the ovary. Cancer 1979;42:798.
53. Kattan J, Droz JP, Charpentire P, et al: Ovarian dysgerminoma metastatic to the breast. Gynecol Oncol 1992; 46:104.
54. Afridi MA, Vongtama V, Tsukada Y, et al: Dysgerminoma of the ovary: Radiation therapy for recurrence and metastases. Am J Obstet Gynecol 1976;126:190.
55. Bjorkholm E, Lundell M, Gyftodimos A, et al: Dysgerminoma: The Radiumhemmet series 1927–1984. Cancer 1990;1:38.
56. Mitchell MF, Gershensn DM, Soeters RP, et al: The long-term effects of radiation therapy on patients with ovarian dysgerminoma. Cancer 1991;67:1084.
57. Thomas GM, Dembo AJ, Hacher NF, Depetrillo AD: Current therapy for dysgerminoma of the ovary. Obstet Gynecol 1987;70:268.
58. Williams SD, Blessing JA, Hatch KD, et al: Chemotherapy of advanced dysgerminoma: Trials of the Gynecology Oncology Group. J Clin Oncol 1991;9:1950.
59. Young DC, Mitchell A, Kessler J, et al: Cortical blindness and seizures possibly related to cisplatin, vinblastine, and bleomycin treatment of ovarian dysgerminoma. J Am Osteopath Assoc 1993;93:502.
60. Boyes DA, Pankratz E, Galliford BW, et al: Experience with dysgerminomas at the Cancer Control Agency of British Columbia. Gynecol Oncol 1978;6:123.
61. Burkons DM, Hart WR: Ovarian germinomas (dysgerminomas). Obstet Gynecol 1978;51:221.
62. Norris HJ, Jensen RD: Relative frequency of ovarian neoplasms in children and adolescents. Cancer 1972;30:713.
63. Kurman RJ, Norris HJ: Endodermal sinus tumor of the ovary: A clinical and pathologic analysis of 71 cases. Cancer 1976;38:2404.
64. Teilum G: Endodermal sinus tumors of the ovary and testis: comparative morphogenesis of the so-called mesonephroma ovarii (Schiller) and extraembryonic (yolk sac–allantoic) structures of the rat's placenta. Cancer 1959; 12:1092.
65. Teilum G: The concept of endodermal sinus (yolk sac) tumor. Scand J Immunol 1978;8(Suppl 8):75.
66. Nogales FF, Beltran E, Pavcovich M, Bustos M: Ectopic somatic endodermal in secondary yolk sac. Hum Pathol 1992;23:921.
67. Nogales FF: Embryologic clues to human yolk sac tumors: A review. Int J Gynecol Pathol 1993;12:101.
68. Kommoss F, Bibbo M, Talerman A: Nuclear deoxyribonucleic acid content (ploidy) of endodermal sinus (yolk sac) tumor. Lab Invest 1990;62:223.
69. Palmer PE, Safaii H, Wolfe HJ: Alpha-antitrypsin and alpha-fetoprotein: Protein markers in endodermal sinus (yolk sac) tumors. Am J Clin Pathol 1976;65:575.
70. Schiller W: Mesonephromal ovarii. Am J Cancer 1939; 35:1.
71. Kazancigil TR, Laqueur W, Ladewig P: Papillo-endothelioma ovarii: Report of 3 cases and a discussion of Schiller's "mesonephroma ovarii." Am J Cancer 1940; 40:199.
72. Duval M: Le placenta de rongeurs. J Anat Physiol (Paris) 1891;27:515.
73. Prat J, Bhah AK, Dickersin GR, et al: Hepatoid yolk sac tumor of the ovary (endodermal sinus tumor with hepatoid differentiation). Cancer 1982;50:2355.
74. Cohen MB, Mulchahey KM, Molnar JJ: Ovarian endodermal sinus tumor with intestinal differentiation. Cancer 1986;57:1580.
75. Cogen MB, Friend DS, Molnar JJ, et al: Endodermal sinus tumor with intestinal differentiation: a new histologic type. Pathol Res Pract 1987;182:609.
76. Kawai M, Kano T, Furuhashi Y, et al: Prognostic factors

in yolk sac tumors of the ovary: A clinical pathologic analysis of 29 cases. Cancer 1991;1:184.
77. DiSaia PJ, Creasman WT: Germ cell, stromal and other ovarian tumors. *In* DiSaia PJ, Creasman WT (eds): Clinical Gynecologic Oncology, 4th ed. St. Louis, Mosby Year Book, 1993, pp 426–445.
78. Wu PC, Huang RL, Lang JG, et al: Treatment of malignant germ cell tumors with preservation of fertility: A report of 28 cases. Gynecol Oncol 1991;40:2.
79. Lebert H: Anatomie Pathologique Générale et Spéciale. Paris, Bailliere, 1857.
80. Virchow R: Vorlesungun über Pathologie. Berlin, Hirschwald, 1863, p 96.
81. Pauley J: On dermoid cysts of the ovary. Am J Obstet 1875;8:404.
82. Willis RA: The structure of teratomata. J Pathol Bacteriol 1935;40:1.
83. Surti U, Hoffner L, Chakravarti A, et al: Genetics and biology of human ovarian teratomas: I. Cytogenetic analysis and mechanism of origin. Am J Hum Genet 1990;47:635.
84. Ihara T, Ohama K, Saton N, et al: Histologic grade and karyotype of immature teratoma of the ovary. Cancer 1984;54:2988.
85. Ohama K, Nomura F, Okamoto E, et al: Origin of immature teratoma. Am J Obstet Gynecol 1985;152:896.
86. Hoffner L, Shen-Schwarz S, Deka R, et al: Genetics and biology of human ovarian teratomas: III. Cytogenetics and origins of malignant ovarian germ cell tumors. Cancer Genet Cytogenet 1992;62:58.
86a. Shiel WE, Dueno F, Hernandez E: Ovarian dermoid cyst complicated by an entero-vaginal fistula. Radiology 1986;160:443.
87. Bronstein M, Yoffe N, Brandes JM, et al: Hair as a sonographic marker of ovarian teratomas: Improved identification using transvaginal sonography and simulation model. J Clin Ultrasound 1991;19:351.
88. Smith R, Deppe G, Selvaggi S: Benign teratoma of the omentum and ovary coexisting with an ovarian neoplasm. Gynecol Oncol 1990;39:204.
89. Weldon-Linne CM, Rushovich AM: Benign ovarian cystic teratomas with homunculi. Obstet Gynecol 1983; 61(Suppl):88.
90. Doss N Jr, Forney P, Vellios F: Covert bilaterality of mature ovarian teratomas. Obstet Gynecol 1977;50:651.
91. Kelly RR, Scully RE: Cancer developing in dermoid cysts of the ovary. Cancer 1961;14:989.
92. Peterson WF: Malignant degeneration of benign cystic teratomas of the ovary: A collective review of the literature. Obstet Gynecol Surv 1957;12:793.
93. Climie ARW, Heath LP: Malignant degeneration of benign cystic teratomas of the ovary. Cancer 1968;22:824.
94. Chadha S, Schaberg A: Malignant transformation in benign cystic teratomas: Dermoids of the ovary. Eur J Obstet Gynecol 1988;29:329.
95. Miyazaki K, Tokunage T, Katabuchi H, et al: Clinical usefulness of serum sqauamous cell carcinoma antigen for early detection of squamous cell carcinoma arising in mature cystic teratoma of the ovary. Obstet Gynecol 1991;78:562.
96. Tobon H, Surti U, Naus GJ, et al: Squamous cell carcinoma in situ arising in an ovarian mature cystic teratoma: Report of one case with histopathologic, cytogenetic, and flow cytometric DNA content analysis. Arch Pathol Lab Med 1991;115:172.
97. Randall BJ, Ritchie C, Hutchison RS: Paget's disease and invasive undifferentiated adenocarcinoma occurring in a mature cystic teratoma of the ovary. Histopathology 1991;18:469.
98. Leo S, Rorat E, Parekh M: Primary malignant melanoma in a dermoid cyst of the ovary. Obstet Gynecol 1973;41:205.
99. Hermann WJ Jr, Humes JJ: A compound nevus in a benign cystic teratoma of the ovary. Am J Clin Pathol 1976;66:54.
100. Sahin AA, Ro JY, Chen J, et al: Spindle cell nodule and peptic ulcer arising in a fully developed gastric wall in a mature cystic teratoma. Arch Pathol Lab Med 1990; 114:529.
101. Nogales FF, Favara BE, Major FJ, et al: Immature teratoma of the ovary with a neural component ("solid teratoma"). Hum Pathol 1976;7:625.
102. Norris JH, Zirkin HJ, Benson WL: Immature (malignant) teratoma of the ovary: A clinical and pathologic study of 58 cases. Cancer 1976;37:2359.
103. Robboy SJ, Scully RE: Ovarian teratoma with glial implants on the peritoneum: an analysis of 12 cases. Hum Pathol 1970;1:643.
104. Caruso PA, Marsh MR, Minkowitz S, et al: An intense clinicopathologic study of 305 teratomas of the ovary. Cancer 1971;27:343.
105. Gershenson DM, Del Junco G, Silva E, et al: Immature teratoma of the ovary. Obstet Gynecol 1986;68:624.
106. O'Connor DM, Norris HJ: The influence of grade on the outcome of stage I ovarian immature teratomas and the reproducibility of grading these neoplasms. Int J Gynecol Pathol, 1994;13:283.
106a. Coussens PD, Hernandez E, Miyazawa K: Pregnancy after intensive chemotherapy for an immature teratoma. Mil Med 1985;150:559.
107. Yanai-Inbar I, Scully RE: Relation of ovarian dermoid cysts and immature teratomas: An analysis of 350 cases of immature teratoma and 10 cases of dermoid cyst with microscopic foci of immature tissue. Int J Gynecol Pathol 1987;6:203.
108. Nogales FF, Ruiz Avila I, Concha A: Immature endodermal teratomas of the ovary: Embryologic correlations and immunohistochemistry. Hum Pathol 1993;24:364.
109. Thurlbeck WM, Scully RE: Solid teratoma of the ovary. Cancer 1960;13:801.
110. Steeper TA, Mukai K: Solid ovarian teratomas: an immunocytochemical study of thirteen cases with clinicopathologic correlation. Pathol Annu 1984;19:81.
111. Benjamin F, Rorat E: Solid ovarian teratoma with peritoneal and abdominal wall implants, progressive in vivo maturation, and probable cure. Gynecol Oncol 1975;3:308.
112. Jumean HG, Komorowski R, Mahvi D: Immature teratoma of the ovary: an unusual case. Gynecol Oncol 1992;46:111.
113. Spaun E, Rix P: Benign cystic monodermal teratoma of neurogenic type. Int J Gynecol Pathol 1990;9:283.
114. Kung AW, Ma JT, Wang C: Hyperthyroidism during pregnancy due to coexistence of struma ovarii and Graves' disease. Postgrad Med J 1990;66:132.
115. Kawahara H: Struma ovarii with ascites and hydrothorax. Am J Obstet Gynecol 1963;85:85.
116. Farrell DJ, Bioxham CA, Scott DJ: Hashimoto's disease in a benign cystic teratoma of the ovary. Histopathology 1991;19:283.
117. Yannopoulos D, Yannopolulos K, Ossowski R: Malignant struma ovarii. Pathol Annu 1976;11:403.
118. Williamse PH, Oosterhuis JW, Aaldus JG: Malignant struma ovarii treated by ovariectomy, hysterectomy, and ^{131}I administration. Cancer 1987;60:178.
119. Devaney K, Snyder R, Norris JH, et al: Proliferative and histologically malignant struma ovarii: A clinicopathologic study of 54 cases. Int J Gynecol Pathol 1993;12:333.
120. Talerman A: Carcinoid tumors of the ovary. J Cancer Res Clin Oncol 1984;107:125.
121. Robboy SJ, Norris JH, Scully RE: Insular carcinoid primary in the ovary: A clinicopathologic analysis of 48 cases. Cancer 1975;36:404.
122. Serratini FT, Robboy SJ: Ultrastructure of primary and metastatic carcinoids: Analysis of 11 cases. Cancer 1975;36:157.
123. Artaze A, Beiner JT, Gonzales H, et al: Carcinoid heart disease: Report of a case secondary to pure carcinoid tumor of the ovary. Eur Heart J 1985;6:800.
124. Morgello S, Schwartz I, Horwith M, et al: Ectopic insulin

production by primary ovarian carcinoid. Cancer 1988;61:800.
125. Strodel WE, Vinik AI, Jaffe BM, et al: Substance P in the localization of carcinoid tumor. J Surg Oncol 1984;27:106.
126. Motoyama T, Katayama Y, Watanabe H, et al: Functioning ovarian carcinoids induce severe constipation. Cancer 1992;70:513.
127. Robboy SJ, Scully RE, Norris JH: Primary trabecular carcinoid of the ovary. Obstet Gynecol 1977;49:202.
128. Scully RE: Recent progress in ovarian cancer. Hum Pathol 1970;1:73.
129. Ranchod M, Kempson RL, Dorgeloh JR: Strumal carcinoid of the ovary. Cancer 1976;37:1913.
130. Robboy SJ, Scully RE: Strumal carcinoid of the ovary: An analysis of 50 cases of a distinctive tumor composed of thyroid tissue and carcinoid. Cancer 1980;46:2019.
131. Tamsen A, Mazur MT: Ovarian strumal carcinoid in association with multiple endocrine neoplasia, type IIA. Arch Pathol Lab Med 1992;116:200.
132. Snyder RR, Tavassoli FA: Ovarian strumal carcinoid: immunohistochemical, ultrastructural and clinicopathologic observations. Int J Gynecol Pathol 1986;5:187.
133. Greco MA, LiVolsi VA, Pertschuk LP, et al: Strumal carcinoid of the ovary: analysis of its components. Cancer 1979;43:1389.
134. Axe SR, Klein VR, Woodruff JD: Choriocarcinoma of the ovary. Obstet Gynecol 1985;66:111.
135. Gerbie MV, Brewer JI, Tamimi H: Primary choriocarcinoma of the ovary. Obstet Gynecol 1975;46:720.
136. Vance RP, Geisenger KR: Pure nongestational choriocarcinoma of the ovary: report of a case. Cancer 1985;56:2321.
137. Wheeler CA, Davis S, Degefu S: Ovarian choriocarcinoma: a difficult diagnosis of an unusual tumor and a review of the hook effect. Obstet Gynecol 1990;75:547.
138. Grover V, Grover RK, Usha R, et al: Primary pure choriocarcinoma of the ovary. Gynecol Obstet Invest 1990;30:61.
139. Kurman RJ, Norris HJ: Embryonal carcinoma of the ovary: A clinicopathologic entity distinct from endodermal sinus tumor resembling embryonal carcinoma of the adult testis. Cancer 1976;38:2420.
140. Sediya S, Ishige K, Yamazawa M: The capacity for differentiation and production of human chorionic gonadotropin and alfa-fetoprotein in human embryonal carcinoma cell lines. Int J Gynecol Pathol 1988;7:373.
141. Peyron A: Faits nouveaux relatifs à l'origine et à l'histogenèse des embryones. Bull Cancer (Paris) 1939;28:658.
142. Takeda A, Ishizuku T, Goto S: Polyembryoma of ovary producing alpha-fetoprotein and hCG. Cancer 1982; 49:1878.
143. Marin-Padilla M: Origin, nature and significance of the "embryoids" of human teratomas. Virchows Arch Pathol Anat 1965;340:105.
144. Stevens LC Jr: Embryonic potency of embryoid bodies derived from a transplantable testicular teratoma of the mouse. Dev Biol 1960;2:285.
145. Kurman RJ, Norris HJ: Malignant mixed germ cell tumors of the ovary: a clinical and pathologic analysis of 30 cases. Obstet Gynecol 1976;48:579.
146. Gershenson DM, Del Junco G, Copeland LJ, et al: Mixed germ cell tumors of the ovary. Obstet Gynecol 1984; 64:200.
147. Lacson AG, Gillis DA, Shawwa A: Malignant mixed germ cell—sex cord stromal tumor of the ovary associated with isosexual precocious puberty. Cancer 1988;61:2122.
148. Talerman A: The pathology of gonadal neoplasms composed of germ cells and sex cord stromal derivatives. Pathol Res Pract 1980;170:21.
149. Hughesdon PE, Kumarasamy T: Mixed germ cell tumors (gonadoblastomas) in normal and dysgenetic gonads. Virchows Arch Pathol Anat 1970;349:258.
150. Williamson HO: Gonadoblastoma: Histologic, ultrastructural and histochemical observations in five cases. Am J Obstet Gynecol 1976;125:459.
151. Khudr G, Bernirschke K: Y ring chromosome associated with gonadoblastoma in situ. Obstet Gynecol 1973;41:897.
152. de Bacalao EB, Dominguez I: Unilateral gonadoblastoma in a pregnant woman. Am J Obstet Gynecol 1969; 105:1279.
153. Troche V, Hernandez E: Neoplasia arising in dysgenetic gonads. Obstet Gynecol Surv 1986;41:74.
154. Erhan Y, Toprak AS, Ozdemir N: Gonadoblastoma and fertility. J Clin Pathol 1992;45:828.
155. McDonough PG, Rogers-Byrd J, Tho PT: Gonadoblastoma in a true hermaphrodite with a 46,XX karyotype. Obstet Gynecol 1976;47:355.
156. Szokol M, Kondrai G, Papp Z: Gonadal malignancy and 46,XY karyotype in a true hermaphrodite. Obstet Gynecol 1977;49:358.
157. Winter JSD, Faiman C: Serum gonadotrophin concentrations in agonadal children and adults. J Clin Endocrinol Metab 1972;35:561.
158. Roth LM, Eglen DE: Gonadoblastoma: immunohistochemical and ultrastructural observations. Int J Gynecol Pathol 1988;8:72.
159. Talerman A: Gonadoblastoma associated with embryonal carcinoma. Obstet Gynecol 1974;43:138.
160. Wilson EE, Vuitch F, Carr BR: Laparoscopic removal of dysgenetic gonads containing a gonadoblastoma in a patient with Swyer syndrome. Obstet Gynecol 1992;79:842.
161. Parker M, Teneriello M, Barnhill D: Metastatic dysgerminoma in a patient with Swyer's syndrome. Obstet Gynecol 1992;80:697.
162. Zuntova A, Motlik K, Horejsi J, Eckschlager T: Mixed germ cell—sex cord stromal tumor with heterologous elements. Int J Gynecol Pathol 1991;35:83.
163. Schellhas HF: Malignant potential of the dysgenetic gonad. Obstet Gynecol 1974;44:302.
164. Andrews J: Streak gonads and the Y-chromosome. J Obstet Gynaecol Brit Commonw 1971;78:448.
165. Teter J: Rare gonadal tumors occurring in intersexes and their classification. Int J Gynaecol Obstet 1969;7:183.
166. Adshi E, Farrber M, Safaii HS, et al: Mixed gonadal dysgenesis without virilization. Obstet Gynecol 1977;50:397.
167. Manuel M, Katayama KP, Jones HW Jr: The age of occurrence of gonadal tumors in intersex patients with a Y-chromosome. Am J Obstet Gynecol 1976;124:293.
168. von Camperhout J, Lord J, Lanthier A, et al: The phenotype and gonadal history in XO/XY mosaic individuals: Report of two personal cases. J Obstet Gynaecol Brit Commonw 1969;76:631.
169. Nakashima I, Robinson A: Fertility in a 45,X female. Pediatrics 1971;47:770.
170. Teeter J, Bozkowski K: Occurrence of tumors in dysgenetic gonads. Cancer 1967;20:1301.
171. Krasna IH, Lee ML, Smilow P, et al: Risk of malignancy in bilateral streak gonads: The role of the Y-chromosome. J Pediatr Surg 1992;27:1376.
172. Simpson JL: Genetics of sexual differentiation. *In* Carpenter SEK, Rock JA (eds): Pediatric and Adolescent Gynecology. New York, Raven Press, 1992, pp 1–37.

11

Tumors of the Ovarian Stroma

Cornelia Liu Trimble / Edward L. Trimble / Enrique Hernandez

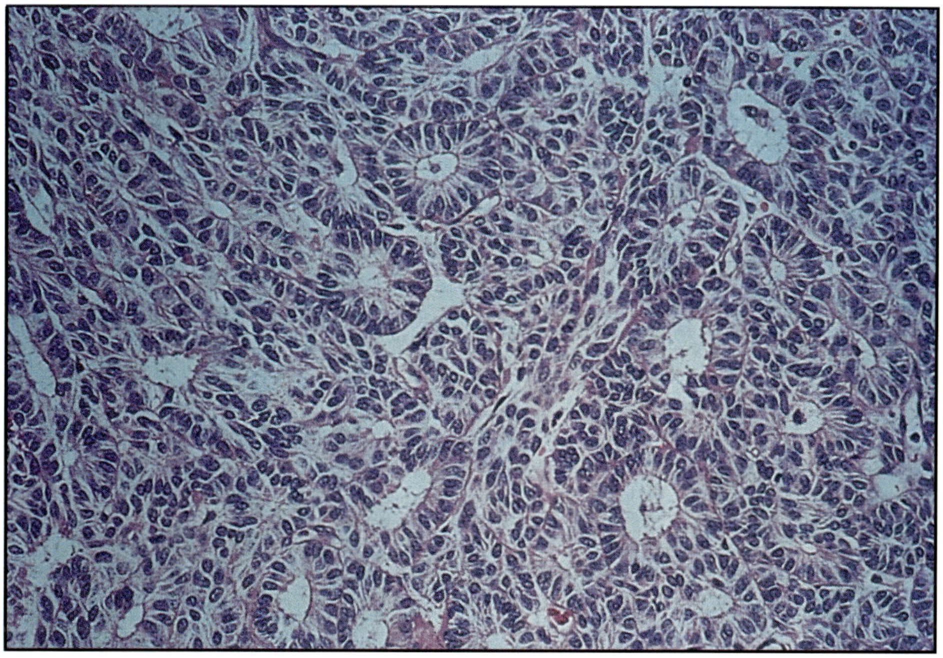

EMBRYOLOGY

By the third week post conception the embryo develops three different germ layers: ectoderm, mesoderm, and endoderm. By the fourth week post conception the embryo folds and forms a tubular structure. The ectoderm covers the external surface, while the endoderm is inside the tube and the mesoderm lies between the ectoderm and the mesoderm. The mesoderm organizes into paraaxial, intermediate, and lateral plate areas. The paraaxial mesoderm lies immediately lateral to the neural tube. It gives rise to musculoskeletal structures. The intermediate mesoderm gives rise to the embryonic kidney (mesonephros), the adult kidney (nephros), and the wolffian (mesonephric) ducts. The lateral plate mesoderm splits into the somatic and splanchnic mesoderm. The splanchnic mesoderm covers the peritoneal surfaces. By now the lateral plate mesoderm is in a ventral location, while the intermediate mesoderm is dorsal (Fig. 11–1). Besides giving rise to the peritoneal cavity and peritoneum, the lateral plate mesoderm gives rise to the müllerian (paramesonephric) structures and the ovaries.[1]

The predecessor of the ovaries is the gonadal ridge, which develops by the fourth week of embryonic life. This longitudinal ridge lies on either side of the midline between the dorsal mesentery and the mesonephric ridge. The germ cells are initially found in the wall of the yolk sac. They then migrate along the dorsal mesentery and reach the gonadal ridge during the sixth week of embryonic life. If germ cells do not reach the gonadal ridge, the ovary does not develop. The arrival of the germ cells at the gonadal ridge causes its surface mesoderm, which is now the coelomic epithelium, to proliferate and penetrate the underlying mesenchyme. This coelomic epithelium, which proliferates to cover the gonadal ridge, becomes the specialized stroma of the gonads. In the male this proliferation takes the form of cords that lead to the seminiferous tubules of the adult male. In females, the proliferating epithelium does not arrange itself into cords but rather stays close to the surface and surrounds individual germ cells. The germ cells eventually develop into the oogonia. The envelope of coelomic epithelium, which is of mesodermal origin, forms the follicular cells (Fig. 11–2).[1, 2]

Tumors of the specialized ovarian stroma account for approximately 5 percent of all ovarian tumors.[3] The great majority of these tumors are benign. The term sex cord–stromal tumors was adopted by the World Health Organization (WHO) in 1973 to describe these lesions. The WHO classification was subsequently modified by Young and Scully to include several types of tumors that have been recognized since that time.[4] However, as described above, the sex cords are never well defined in the female gonad.[1] Tumors that arise from the nonspecific ovarian mesenchyme are similar to those that arise at other soft tissue sites.

TUMORS OF THE SPECIALIZED OVARIAN STROMA

Tumors of the specialized ovarian stroma are characterized by their production of hormones. However, hormone production is not universally present. A patient with a tumor of the specialized ovarian stroma may present with signs and symptoms of estrogen, androgen, and/or progesterone excess, or the tumor may not be hormonally active at all. Also, hormonal production is not a characteristic limited to this group of neoplasms. Other tumors, including metastatic tumors that stimulate the ovarian stroma, may lead to hormone production. We have found a patient (E. Hernandez,

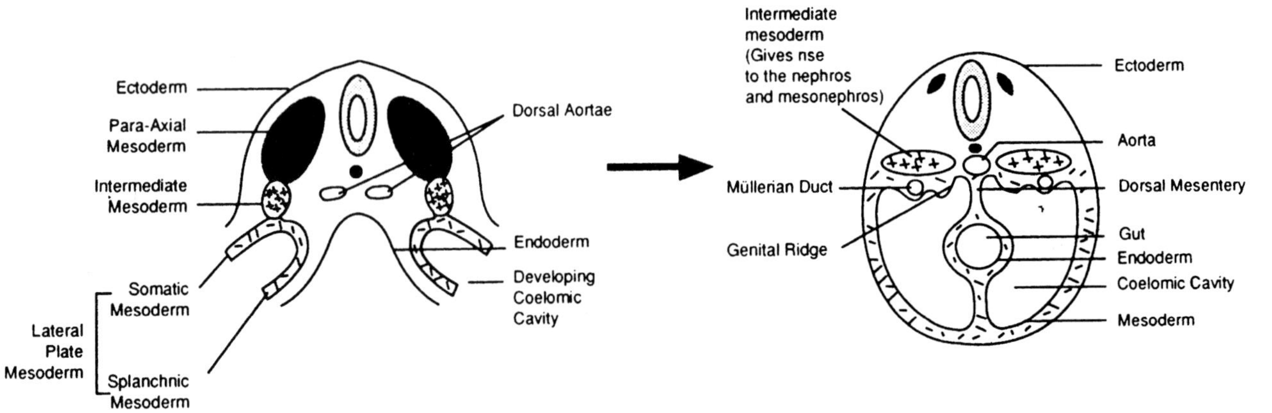

FIGURE 11–1
This is a diagrammatic representation of early (3 to 4 weeks post conception) embryonic development.

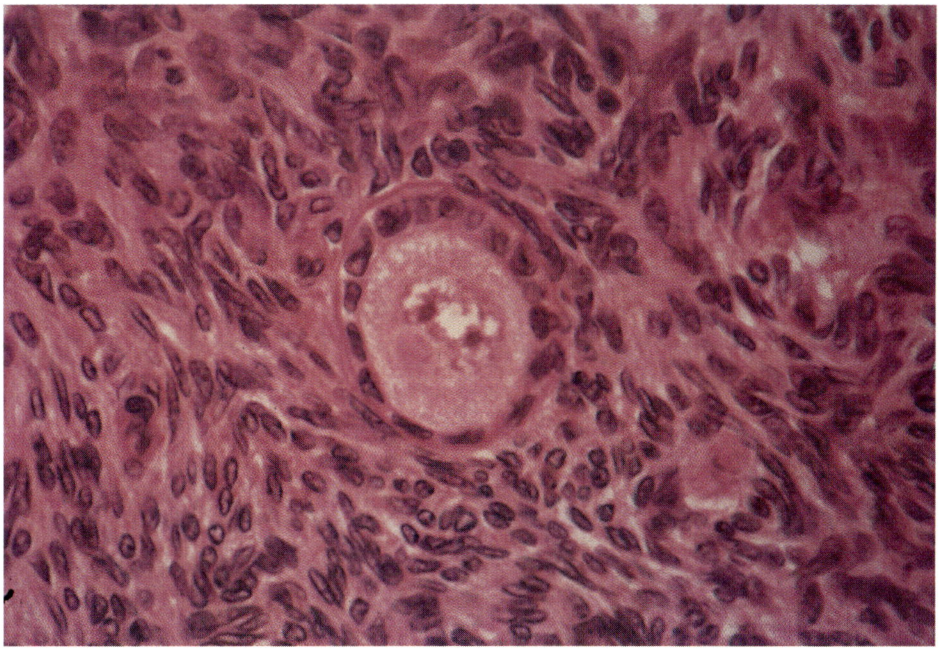

FIGURE 11-2
This microphotograph of a primary follicle shows a large oocyte surrounded by a single layer of granulosa cells that are of mesodermal origin. This primary follicle is in a background of nonspecific ovarian stroma.

unpublished case) who had an ovarian mucinous cystadenoma with mucin infiltrating the ovarian stroma, the endometrium showed decidualization and an Arias-Stella reaction, both the result of a progesterone excess. This and other reported cases seem to exemplify the ability of the normal ovarian stroma to produce and secrete hormones when stimulated.

Granulosa Cell Tumors

Adult Granulosa Cell Tumor

Adult granulosa cell tumor constitutes 1 to 2 percent of all ovarian tumors and 95 percent of all granulosa cell tumors. The reported mean and median age of patients is between 42 and 54 years. However, the age range is wide. This tumor has been found in newborns and in elderly women. Over one half of patients are postmenopausal. Two to four percent of patients are prepubertal. In about 85 percent of prepubertal patients the tumor has distinctive features and are designated as juvenile granulosa cell tumors (see below). About 50 percent of patients report symptoms suggestive of endocrinologic disturbance (e.g., abnormal uterine bleeding, breast tenderness, changes in libido). Other symptoms, including abdominal pain, backache, abdominal swelling, dysuria, and dyspareunia, occur in 20 to 30 percent of patients. Both endometrial hyperplasia and endometrial carcinoma have been reported in patients who have estrogen-producing granulosa cell tumors.[5,6] In one large series, 6 percent of patients with a granulosa cell tumor had an endometrial adenocarcinoma.[6] Three percent of patients who have a granulosa cell tumor have no symptoms, and the tumor is discovered only by chance. Virilizing granulosa cell tumors are rare.

Less than 10 percent of granulosa cell tumors are bilateral. Their size may range from a microscopic focus found incidentally in an ovary removed for an unrelated indication to a large mass that fills the abdomen. In a review of 198 cases of granulosa cell tumor, 123 (64 percent) were larger than 5 cm in diameter.[6] These have a soft consistency and are usually solid, although they frequently contain cystic areas (Fig. 11–3). An occasional tumor is entirely cystic.[7] The cut surface is yellowish white, the color depending on the amount of intervening fibrous stroma, which makes the tumor white, and the lipid content of the granulosa cells, which is responsible for the yellow hue (Fig. 11–4). Areas of hemorrhagic degeneration are frequently present. Perforation of the tumor capsule can result in hemoperitoneum and an acute abdomen.

The well-differentiated adult granulosa cell tumor can exhibit several histopathologic patterns including microfollicular, macrofollicular, trabecular, and insular. The less differentiated tumors display more solid growth or undulating cords forming a gyriform (wavelike) or watered-silk pattern. The granulosa cell itself has a bland appearance, with scanty and delicate cytoplasm and a pale nucleus that often displays a prominent longitudinal groove. These cellular features are different from those typical of a juvenile granulosa cell tumor, which has cells with a rounded nucleus and abundant cytoplasm.

The microfollicular pattern is characterized by

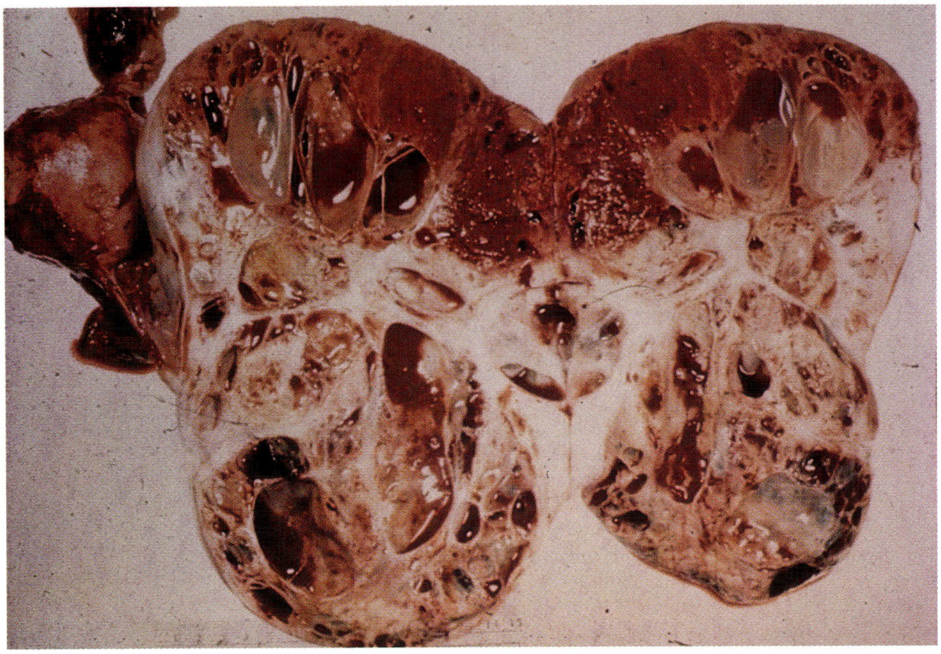

FIGURE 11-3
The cut surface of this granulosa cell tumor shows multiple cystic spaces. The tumor is tan with white fibrous septa and hemorrhage at its superior pole. (Courtesy of Dr. J. Donald Woodruff, The Johns Hopkins Hospital, Baltimore, MD.)

granulosa cells that surround small round spaces (Fig. 11–5). The spaces contain eosinophilic material that stains positive with periodic acid–Schiff (PAS). These structures recapitulate the Call-Exner body seen in the developing graafian follicle (Fig. 11–6). The nuclei in the cells, in both the Call-Exner bodies and the cells between them, are haphazardly placed.

It is important to distinguish adult granulosa cell tumor from well-differentiated adenocarcinoma and from carcinoid tumor, since the clinical implications differ considerably. Acinar structures in well-differentiated adenocarcinoma display a more regular basally oriented arrangement of nuclei than that observed in granulosa cell tumors with a microfollicular pattern. The typical granulosa cell, which was described above, differs from the cells of ovarian adenocarcinoma and carcinoid tumor. The cells of adenocarcinoma are often larger and have more distinct cell borders and a more prominent nucleolus. The cells of a carcinoid tumor often have granular, eosinophilic cytoplasm, but

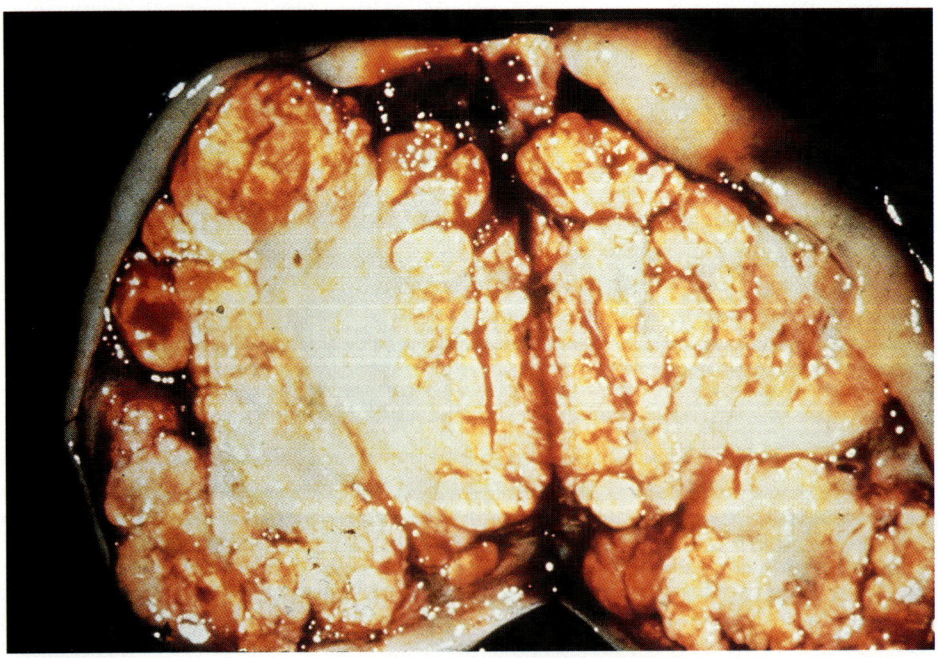

FIGURE 11-4
This granulosa cell tumor is solid. The cut surface is yellow. Areas of hemorrhage are seen. (Courtesy of Dr. J. Donald Woodruff, The Johns Hopkins Hospital, Baltimore, MD.)

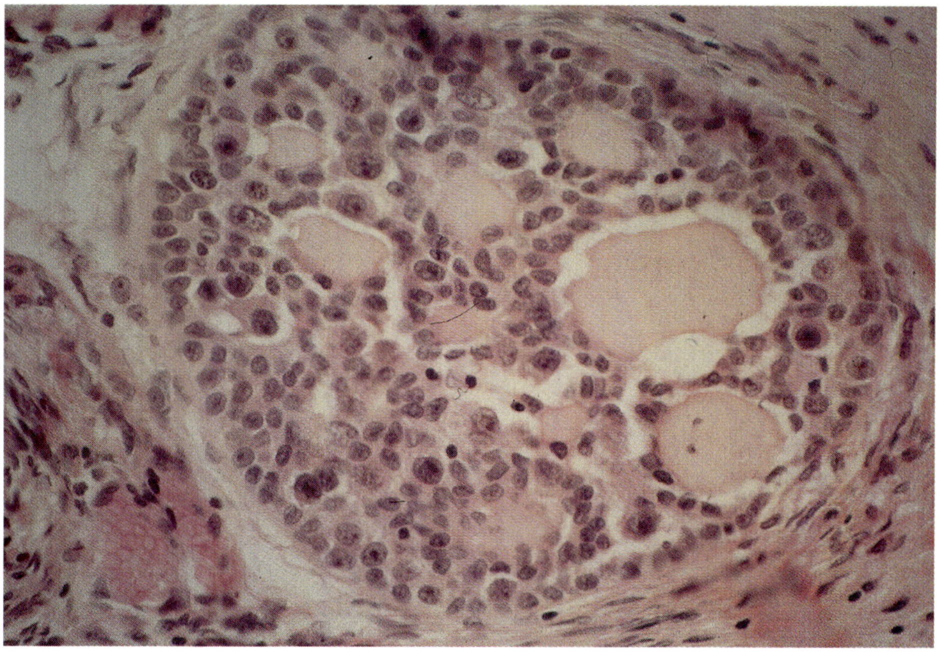

FIGURE 11–5
This microphotograph shows the microfollicular pattern of a granulosa cell tumor. The granulosa cells haphazardly surround eosinophilic material. Close inspection reveals that a few nuclei have longitudinal grooves (i.e., coffee bean nucleus). A few nuclei are larger and have variable chromatin patterns.

the nucleus may resemble that of a granulosa cell. A Grimelius stain can demonstrate argyrophil cells in carcinoid tumors. Immunocytochemical techniques reveal that the carcinoid cells have neurosecretory granules that stain positive for neuron-specific enolase, S100, and chromogranin (Fig. 11–7).

The macrofollicular pattern of adult granulosa cell tumor is much less common than the microfollicular pattern. This macrofollicular pattern consists of large, irregular cystic structures lined by granulosa cells that are often surrounded by theca cells (Fig. 11–8). A granulosa cell tumor composed entirely of this pattern is rare. When it occurs it must be distinguished from a cystic benign tumor such as serous cystadenoma and from normal cystic ovarian follicles.

The trabecular pattern of granulosa cell tumor displays ribbons and cords of granulosa cells, often interspersed with fibrous stroma (Fig. 11–9). The insular pattern is the variant that most closely resembles the carcinoid tumor. This pattern is

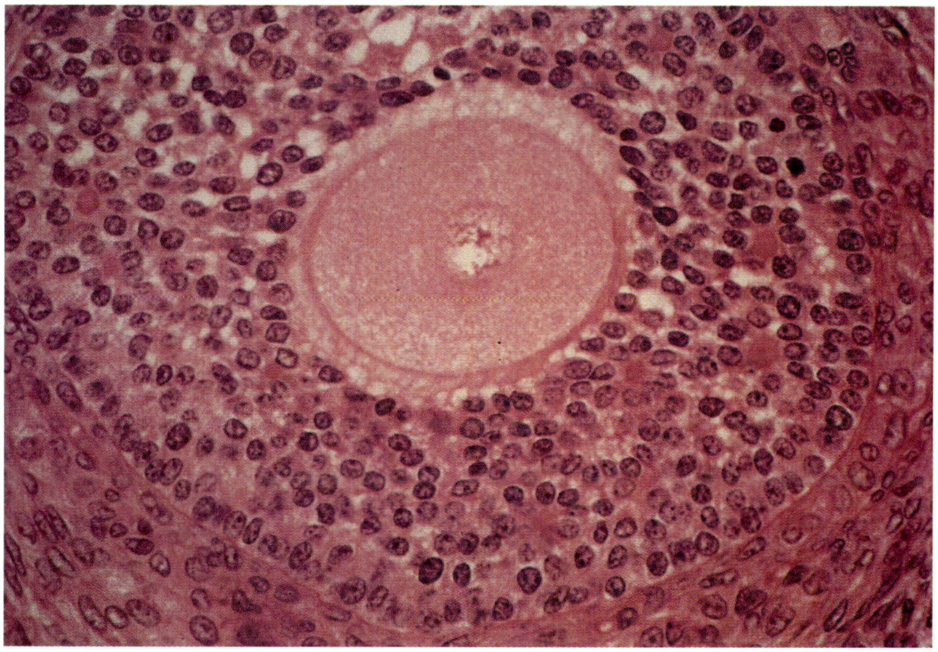

FIGURE 11–6
A developing graafian follicle is shown. The central oocyte is surrounded by multiple layers of granulosa cells. Eosinophilic material surrounded by granulosa cells is also seen.

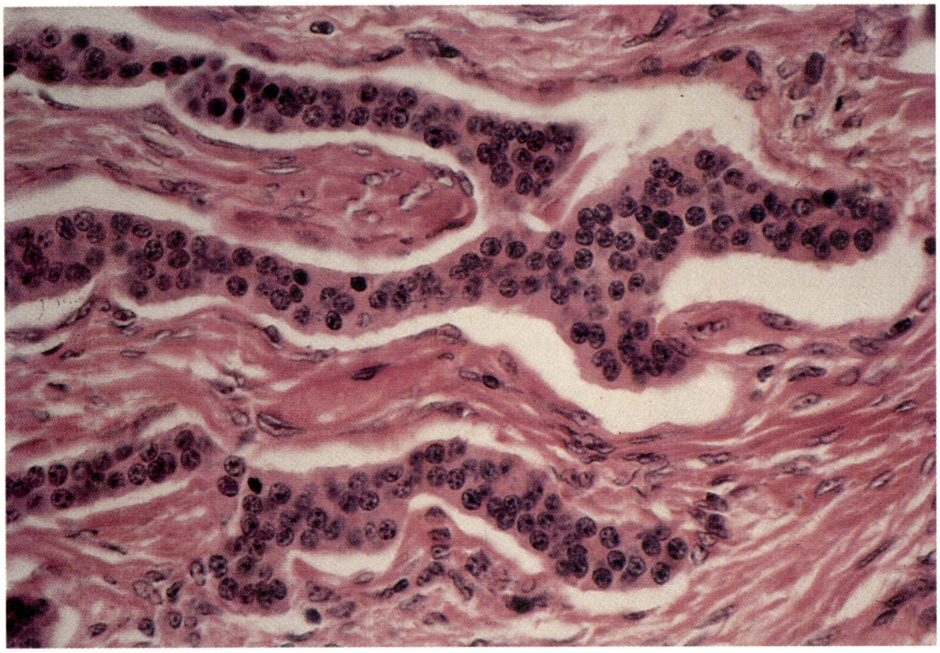

FIGURE 11–7
A trabecular pattern of a carcinoid tumor of the ovary is seen. The cells are similar to those of the granulosa cell tumor, but the nuclei are more round and uniform. The presence of other architectural patterns typical of granulosa cell tumor may aid in the differential diagnosis. Special stains reveal the neurosecretory granules of the carcinoid tumor.

characterized by tumor cells that are arranged in nests or islands, separated by fibrous stroma. The cells on the periphery of the nests are often arranged in a palisade-like pattern. The tubular pattern of granulosa cell tumor cannot be differentiated from Sertoli cell tumor if it is present in a pure form. It is unusual to find a granulosa cell tumor consisting solely of one of these patterns.

A moderately differentiated granulosa cell tumor typically contains less intervening fibrous stroma than the well-differentiated tumor and may display a watered-silk pattern (Fig. 11–10). The poorly differentiated granulosa cell tumor may appear as sheets of spindle-shaped cells, which give it a sarcomatoid appearance. The differential diagnosis of poorly differentiated granulosa cell tumor includes metastatic endometrial stromal sarcoma and primary or metastatic small cell carcinoma. In all the histopathologic grades and patterns of a granulosa cell tumor, the granulosa cells may con-

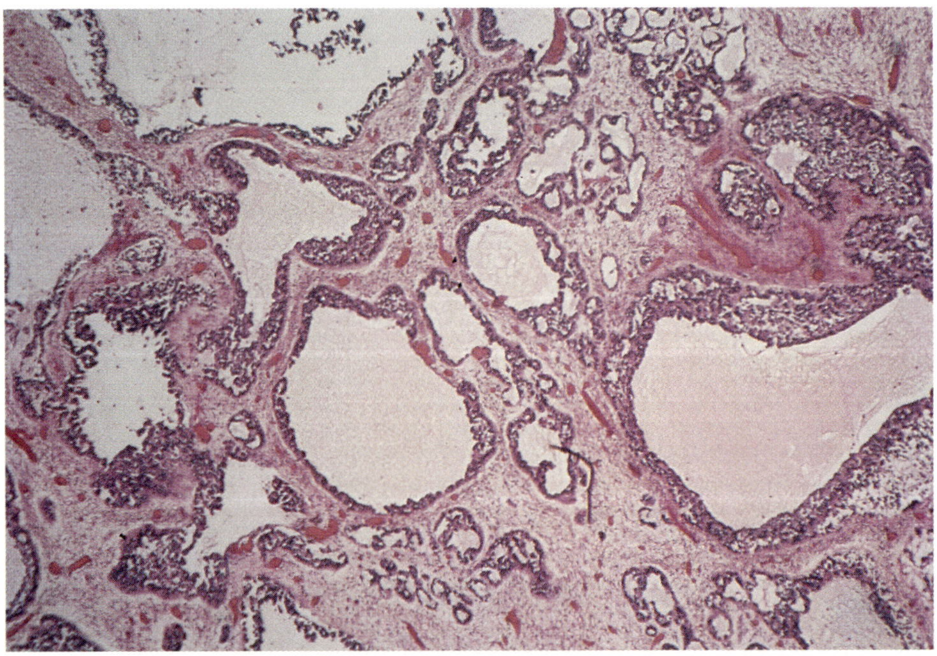

FIGURE 11–8
Large, irregular cystic structures lined by granulosa cells represent the macrofollicular pattern of granulosa cell tumor.

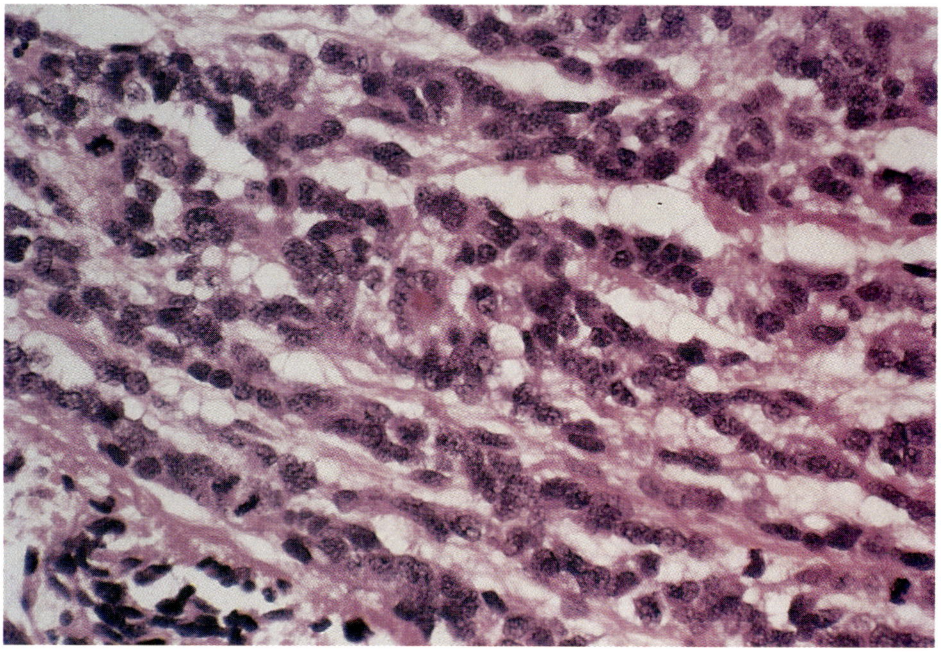

FIGURE 11–9
This is a juvenile granulosa cell tumor showing a trabecular pattern. The tumor cells are arranged in cords with intervening connective tissue. Mitotic figures are seen.

tain abundant pale cytoplasm, resembling the luteinized granulosa cells of the corpus luteum (Fig. 11–11).

The cornerstone of therapy for a patient who has a granulosa cell tumor is excision and surgical staging. Total abdominal hysterectomy and bilateral salpingo-oophorectomy is performed in a postmenopausal patient. Since granulosa cell tumor is rarely bilateral, unilateral salpingo-oophorectomy can be done in the younger woman who has apparent stage IA disease (confined to the ovary) and who wishes to preserve fertility. A complete surgical staging procedure is recommended, however, including a thorough inspection of pelvic and abdominal organs and all peritoneal surfaces. Peritoneal washings for cytologic evaluation are obtained prior to any manipulation. Selective biopsies of pelvic and paraaortic nodes as well as biopsy of the omentum, peritoneal adhesions, and any peritoneal lesions are performed. Scrapings of the diaphragm for cytologic evaluation are obtained.

Granulosa cell tumors tend to be indolent, but

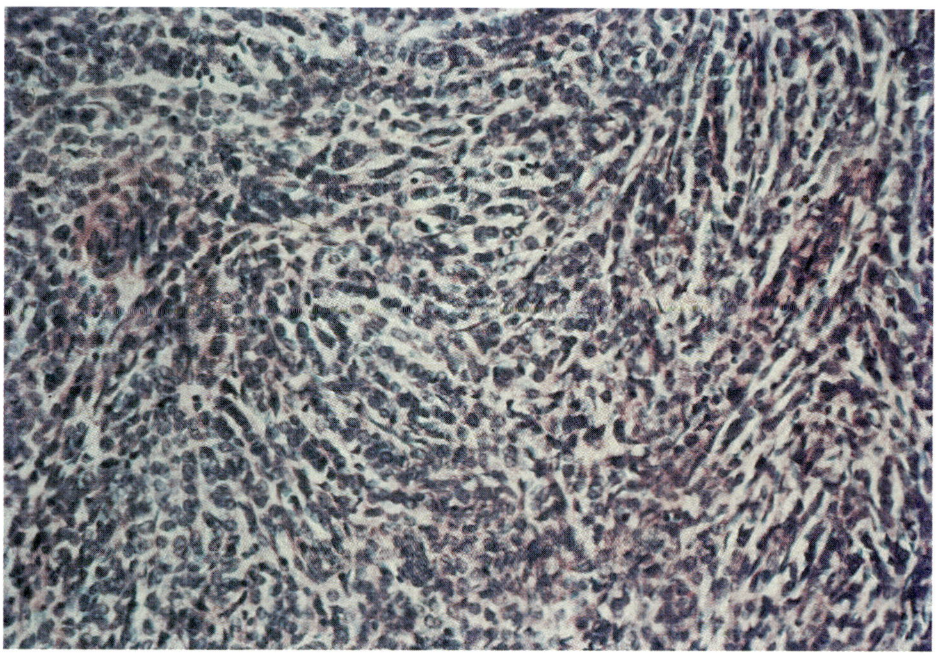

FIGURE 11–10
The watered-silk pattern of the granulosa cell tumor shows tumor cells arranged in cords and forming a wavelike (gyriform) pattern. There is little intervening stroma. (Courtesy of Dr. J. Donald Woodruff, The Johns Hopkins Hospital, Baltimore, MD.)

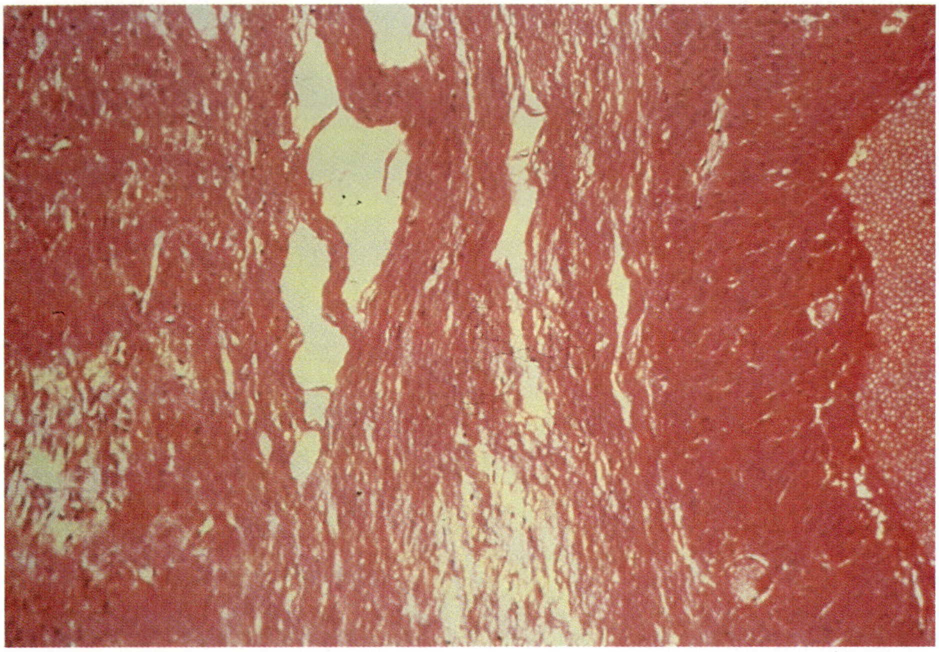

FIGURE 11-11
A luteinized granulosa cell tumor is seen. The luteinized granulosa cells are seen as shadowy outlines on the right and are also present on the left. There is intervening stroma. The cytoplasm of the luteinized cells is abundant and eosinophilic. (Courtesy of Dr. J. Donald Woodruff, The Johns Hopkins Hospital, Baltimore, MD.)

late recurrences are common. Reported 20-year survival rates suggest that up to 50 percent of patients may die from this tumor. Over 80 percent of patients have stage IA disease at presentation. The 10-year survival rate for patients who have stage I disease is approximately 90 percent, compared with 30 to 40 percent for those who have stage III or IV disease.[6–10] Tumor rupture is associated with a poorer prognosis. Even though the 5- and 10-year survival for patients with stage I disease is the same whether or not there was tumor rupture, the 20-year survival is 85 percent if the tumor has not ruptured and 65 percent if it has.[6] Clinicopathologic factors other than stage that adversely affect prognosis include large tumor size and high mitotic rate.[6, 10a] Histopathologic grading is of little prognostic value.[5, 8] Although responses to radiotherapy and chemotherapy have been documented in patients who had measurable disease, neither has shown an impact on survival when given in the adjuvant setting (i.e., after complete tumor excision). Radiotherapy has included radiation to the pelvis only or to the whole abdomen and pelvis. Chemotherapy regimens have included melphalan alone, cisplatin/vinblastine/bleomycin, cisplatin/etoposide/bleomycin, and cisplatin/doxorubicin/cyclophosphamide.[11–13] Since granulosa cell tumor arises from hormonally sensitive mesoderm, at the Medical College of Pennsylvania two recent patients who had stage I tumors that ruptured are being indefinitely treated with megestrol acetate. They have been followed for over 5 years, and there is no evidence of recurrence (E. Hernandez, unpublished report). A patient who had stage IIIA completely excised disease was treated with six courses of megestrol acetate, cyclophosphamide, and cisplatin. Megestrol acetate was continued after completion of the chemotherapy. She also has been free of disease for more than 5 years. Since this is such an indolent tumor, longer follow-up is required before firm conclusions can be made.

After completion of therapy we follow patients every 3 months for 2 years and then every 6 months indefinitely. A thorough physical examination is done at each visit. Liver enzymes are evaluated every 6 to 12 months. Although liver metastasis is rare, if it occurs it can be easily detected by this study. Radiation therapy has been used successfully in controlling metastatic disease.[14] The measurement of serum estradiol and serum inhibin levels has been proposed as valuable for the early detection of recurrence at a time when multiagent chemotherapy may be more effective.[15] Measurement of serum inhibin levels is not readily available in most clinical laboratories. Serum estradiol level determinations are relatively easy to obtain, but not all granulosa cell tumors produce this hormone, and when they do, the detection of elevated levels in serum may lag behind that of serum inhibin.[15] Granulosa cell tumor that is metastatic to peritoneal surfaces may cause the secretion of the antigen CA 125, which can be detected in the serum as occurs with a number of other conditions.[16] At the present time we follow patients who have had a granulosa cell tumor with serial determinations of serum estradiol level if it was elevated at the time of diagnosis. We also obtain serial determinations of CA 125, although the value of this approach has yet to be proved.

Juvenile Granulosa Cell Tumor

Ovarian neoplasms are rare in children and adolescents. They account for less than 1 percent of all cancers diagnosed in women during their first two decades of life.[17] Most malignant ovarian neoplasms in this age group are germ cell tumors,[18] and only 5 percent arise from the specialized ovarian stroma. Most of these are granulosa cell tumors. Two to four percent of granulosa cell tumors occur in girls before the normal age of puberty. Approximately 85 percent of granulosa cell tumors occurring before the age of normal puberty have clinical and pathologic features that differ from the adult granulosa cell tumor described above. These cases are designated juvenile granulosa cell tumors.[19, 20] The juvenile variant of granulosa cell tumor is not limited to prepubertal girls. Fifty-three percent of juvenile granulosa cell tumors occur in women in the second and third decades of life.[21] Three percent are found in women older than 30 years. The juvenile granulosa cell tumor may be associated with isosexual pseudoprecocious puberty, Ollier disease (enchondromatosis), Maffucci syndrome (enchondromatosis and hemangiomas), and abnormal karyotypes with ambiguous genitalia.[21] In girls who are 8 years of age or younger, isosexual pseudoprecocious puberty develops in 75 percent of cases.[17] Signs and symptoms due to hyperestrogenemia are frequent in all age groups. These disappear after removal of the tumor. Juvenile granulosa cell tumors are almost always unilateral (98 percent) and are confined to the ovary.[17, 19, 20]

As with the adult granulosa cell tumor, the juvenile variant is commonly described as being solid and cystic. The solid component is often yellow-tan or gray (Fig. 11–12). On microscopic examination it generally contains granulosa cells arranged in sheets or nodules. It may be completely solid or include irregular, cystic follicular spaces of various size (Fig. 11–13). The granulosa cells exhibit pleomorphism and mitotic activity (Fig. 11–14). They have round nuclei and abundant pale cytoplasm (Fig. 11–15). Most juvenile granulosa cells lack the nuclear grooving seen in adult granulosa cell tumors. A thecomatous component is common. The differential diagnosis includes embryonal carcinoma, choriocarcinoma, endodermal sinus tumor, small cell carcinoma, Sertoli cell tumor, and clear cell carcinoma.

The recommended treatment for patients who have a juvenile granulosa cell tumor confined to one ovary is either unilateral oophorectomy or salpingo-oophorectomy. The cure rate by surgery alone approaches 95 percent. Unlike an adult granulosa cell tumor, which, if it recurs, tends to do so more than 5 years after diagnosis, a juvenile granulosa cell tumor tends to recur within months to 3 years after surgery.[17] Moderate responses to cisplatin/vincristine/bleomycin, cisplatin/etoposide/bleomycin, and cisplatin/doxorubicin/cyclophosphamide have been reported.[17, 21, 22] Although juvenile

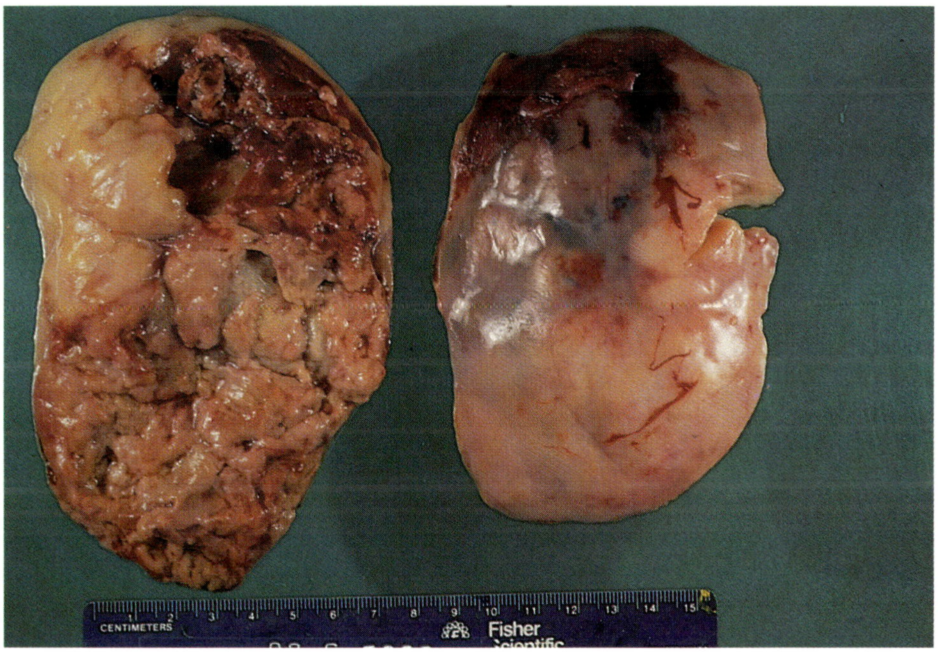

FIGURE 11-12
This juvenile granulosa cell tumor has an outer surface that is smooth and shiny. The cut surface is fleshy and yellow and pinkish-tan. There is a cystic area and hemorrhage.

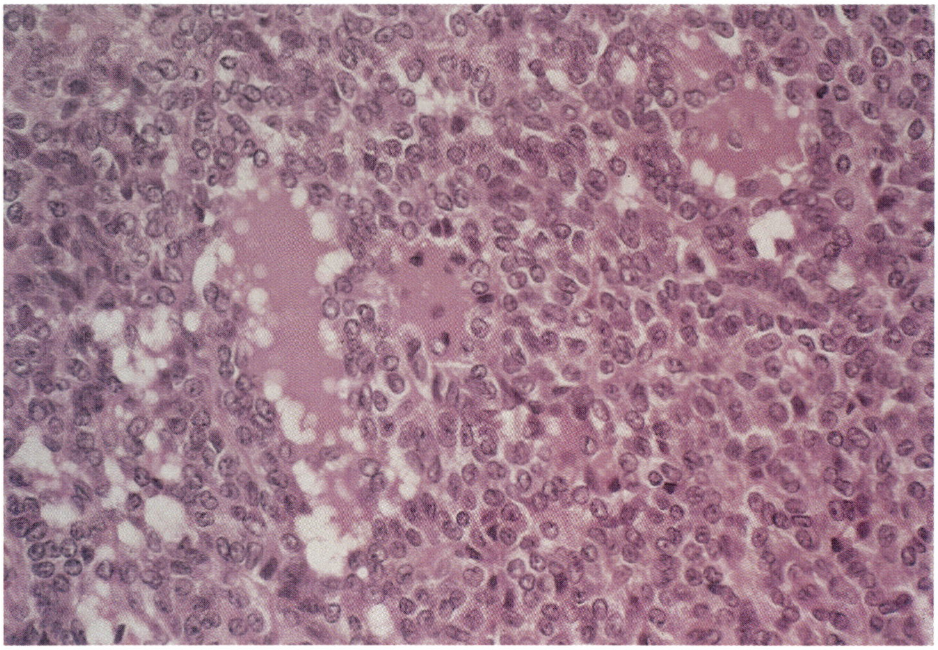

FIGURE 11-13
A juvenile granulosa cell tumor is shown. Small irregular spaces filled with eosinophilic material are seen. The cellular lining is scalloped in these spaces. There is pleomorphism of nuclear shape. Nucleoli are present.

granulosa cell tumor recurrences or residual postsurgical disease can be controlled locally with radiation, metastases tend to be widely disseminated and may involve extrapelvic and extraabdominal sites including lungs, bone, bone marrow, inguinal nodes, and mediastinum.

Histopathologic findings do not predict the biologic behavior of a juvenile granulosa cell tumor. The stage of disease is the most significant prognostic indicator. No association was found between prognosis and an aneuploid DNA content in stage IA tumors.[23] However, analysis of tumor DNA content may predict clinical outcome in patients who have stage III disease. In one study of four patients who had stage III disease, the two who had aneuploid tumors with a high S-phase fraction

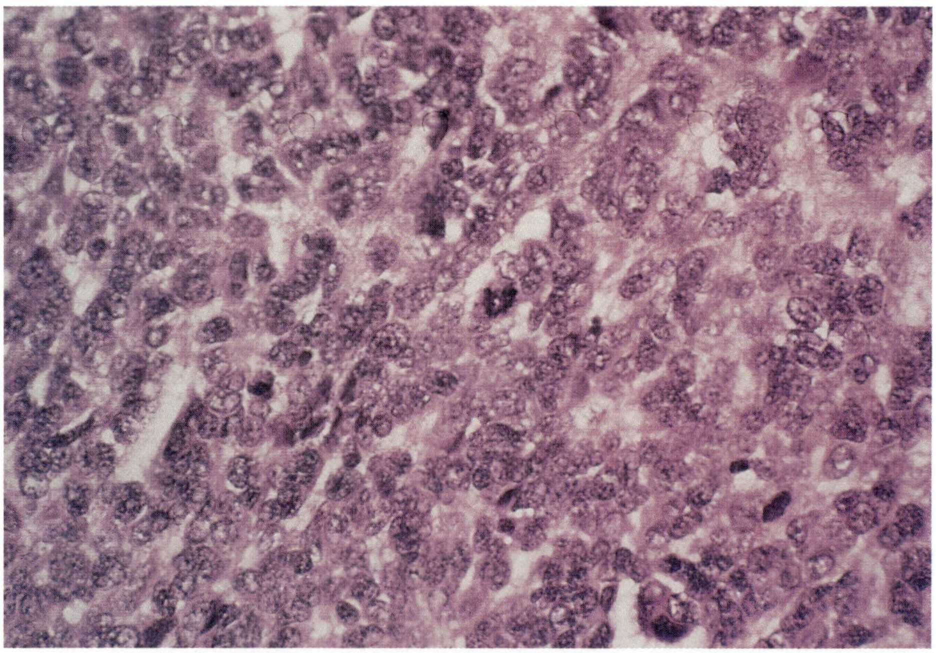

FIGURE 11-14
Juvenile granulosa cells show marked pleomorphism and mitotic activity. These nuclei are hyperchromatic and more pleomorphic than those shown in Figure 11-13.

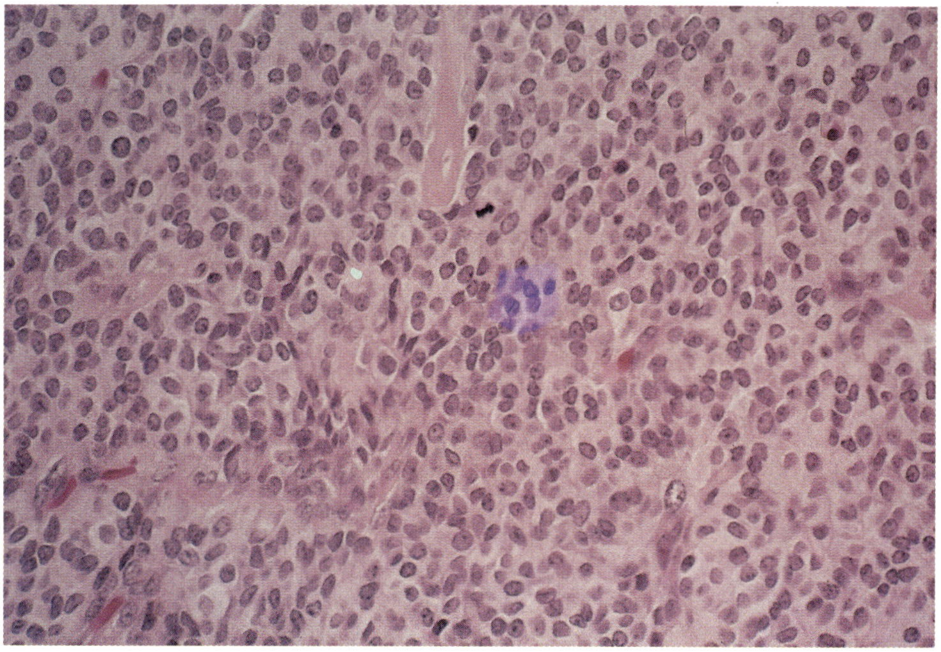

FIGURE 11-15
The juvenile granulosa cell tumor may have sheets of granulosa cells with abundant cytoplasm. A mitotic figure is seen near the center.

experienced recurrences. The two who had diploid tumors with low S-phase fraction are free of recurrence 1 year and 8 years after diagnosis.[23]

Fibrothecoma

As described above, granulosa cell tumors frequently have a theca cell component. Likewise, granulosa cells are often found in tumors that are predominantly of theca cell origin.[17, 24] In these cases the term granulosa-theca cell tumor is used. In some cases it may be difficult to distinguish a fibroma from a thecoma, and so the term fibrothecoma is used. Cell characteristics, the presence of granulosa cells that are found in thecomas, and positive staining of theca cells with fat-specific stains (e.g., Sudan red) help in making the differentiation.[25] Evidence of hormonal production by the theca cells is commonly seen in patients who have a thecoma. Fibrothecomas are benign neoplasms. Those cases reported in the literature as malignant thecomas are most likely fibrosarcomas or poorly differentiated granulosa cell tumors.[3]

Thecoma

Thecomas account for 1 percent of all ovarian tumors. They are rarely bilateral. If malignant behavior is encountered a misdiagnosis must be suspected.[26] The mean age at diagnosis is 55 years, most patients being postmenopausal. Thecomas are rare in children and are uncommon before the age of 30 years.[27] The most common presenting symptoms are the sensation of a pelvic or abdominal mass and abnormal uterine bleeding. The latter is due to production of estrogen by the tumor. As with patients who have a granulosa cell tumor, endometrial hyperplasia and endometrial carcinoma are also found in association with thecomas.[24, 28, 29]

Thecomas may range in size from small nodules to large, firm, solid tumors. Cystic areas are present in some cases. The cut surface is typically bright yellow to orange (Fig. 11–16). Two patterns are seen on microscopic examination. The more common pattern is composed of large, ill-defined sheets of spindle-shaped to rounded cells that contain abundant pale cytoplasm (Fig. 11–17). The cytoplasm stains with fat-specific stains that identify the presence of lipid. The nuclei of these cells are round to oval without atypia. Longitudinal grooves, which are seen in the cells of adult granulosa cell tumor, are not present. Mitoses are rare. The theca cells may be separated into nests or sheets by bands of fibroconnective tissue, which in some cases may be hyalinized or even calcified. If the fibroconnective tissue component is significant, the cut surface on gross examination is white with focal yellow areas. Over 50 percent of thecomas are associated with stromal hyperplasia (i.e., hyperthecosis) in the same or contralateral ovary. This stromal hyperplasia may be nodular or diffuse.

The second pattern is characterized by both theca cells and fibroconnective tissue but also contains clusters or masses of large, eosinophilic,

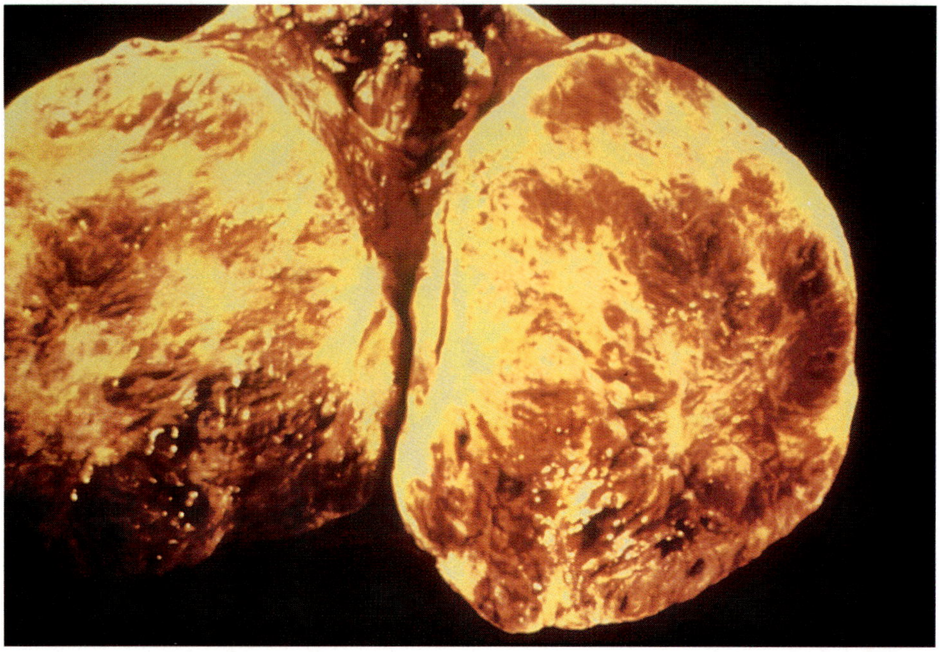

FIGURE 11–16
The cut surface of a thecoma is shown. The tumor is solid and colored yellow and orange. (Courtesy of Dr. J. Donald Woodruff, The Johns Hopkins Hospital, Baltimore, MD.)

lipid-containing, luteinized cells. These are known as luteinized thecomas. They should not be confused with luteoma of pregnancy (see Chapter 8) or with the hilar or Leydig cell tumor, which has cells that contain Reinke crystalloids. If the luteinized cells are so extensive that the other elements are not recognized, a diagnosis of steroid cell tumor is made (Fig. 11–18). These are also known as lipoid or lipid cell tumor, but since approximately 40 percent do not stain for lipid, the term steroid cell tumor is preferred.[30] They can produce androgens, estrogens, or corticosteroids. The steroid cell tumor, in contrast to thecoma, frequently exhibits malignant behavior.[30a] A tumor size greater than 8 cm, the presence of extraovarian tumor, necrosis, hemorrhage, nuclear atypia, and increased mitotic activity are associated with malignancy.

Patients who have luteinized thecomas tend to be younger than those whose tumors are not luteinized. Although luteinized thecomas usually produce estrogen, defeminization or virilization is

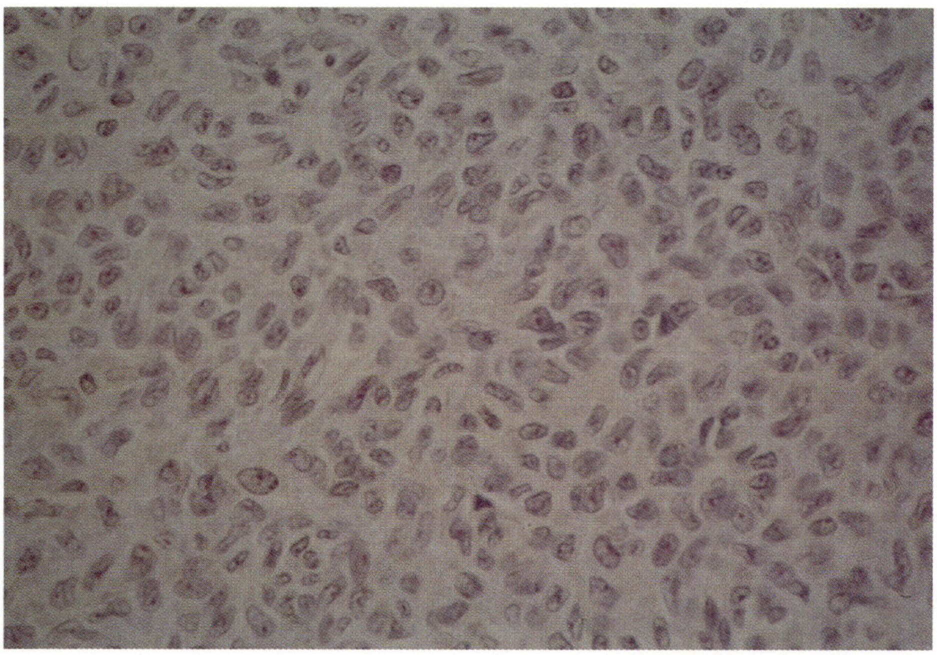

FIGURE 11–17
This thecoma is composed of sheets of spindle-shaped cells without distinct cell borders. The nuclei are vesicular, and nucleoli are present.

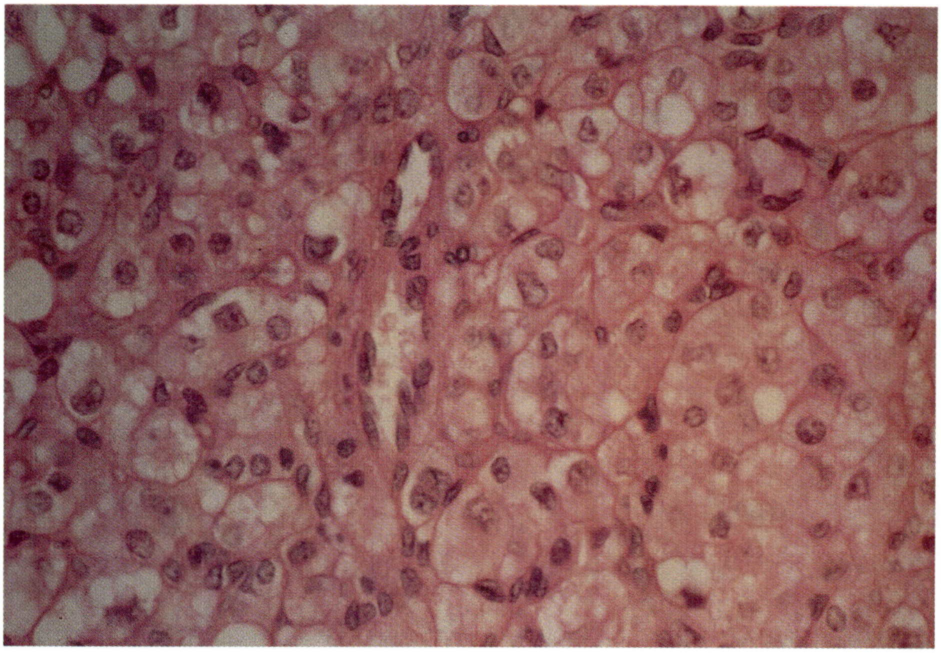

FIGURE 11–18
Sheets of cells containing a large amount of eosinophilic, vacuolated cytoplasm are characteristic of the steroid cell tumor.

sometimes observed. Androgen production is identified in 10 percent of cases.[30] As with the nonluteinized thecomas, luteinized thecomas are almost always unilateral and exhibit benign behavior.

If a solid adnexal mass is present and the diagnosis of thecoma is clinically suspected, evaluation of the endometrium prior to surgery should be considered in view of the frequent association of thecoma with endometrial hyperplasia or adenocarcinoma. In patients who wish to preserve fertility and have no evidence of endometrial carcinoma, a unilateral oophorectomy is performed. In patients in whom preservation of the uterus is not an issue, total abdominal hysterectomy with bilateral salpingo-oophorectomy is standard treatment. Since thecomas are benign, no other therapy is indicated.

Sclerosing Stromal Tumor

This is a rare tumor of the specialized ovarian stroma. Some believe it to be a variant of luteinized thecoma.[25] It tends to occur in younger women (mean age, 27 years). Sclerosing stromal tumors are unilateral. Hormone production by the tumor is rare, although on occasion it can secrete estrogen, progesterone, or testosterone.[31–33]

On gross examination sclerosing stromal tumors are sharply circumscribed from the adjacent ovarian tissue. The cut surface is off-white, and there are yellow areas. Focal edema and cyst formation may be present. Microscopic examination shows a pseudolobular pattern of cellular zones separated by acellular sclerotic or edematous areas (Fig. 11–19). Two cell types are seen: spindle-shaped cells, which produce collagen; and round to oval cells, which have vacuolated cytoplasm. The nuclei of the latter cells are small, dark, and nongrooved (Fig. 11–20). Mitoses are rare or absent. In an occasional tumor these cells are similar to those of the luteinized thecoma. They have dense eosinophilic cytoplasm and large nuclei with prominent nucleoli. The theca cells of sclerosing stromal tumor on rare occasions have eccentric, compressed nuclei and resemble the signet ring cells of Krukenberg tumor (i.e., gastric carcinoma metastatic to the ovary). However, the vacuoles in the cytoplasm of the theca cells of sclerosing stromal tumor contain lipid, in contrast to tumors of gastrointestinal origin, which often contain mucin. The sclerosing stromal tumor also has a network of thin-walled blood vessels, which may suggest a hemangiopericytoma.

This tumor is benign, and no further therapy is indicated after its removal.

Sertoli and Leydig Cell Tumors

Several terms have been used to identify this class of tumors, including androblastoma, arrhenoblastoma, and Sertoli-Leydig cell tumors.[34] This category encompasses tumors composed of cells of the specialized gonadal stroma that recapitulate the Sertoli cells or Leydig cells of the testis. These tumors may be formed by Sertoli cells only, Leydig cells only, or both. Sertoli and Leydig cell tumors are rare and account for less than 0.2 percent of all ovarian neoplasms. Tumors with both Sertoli-

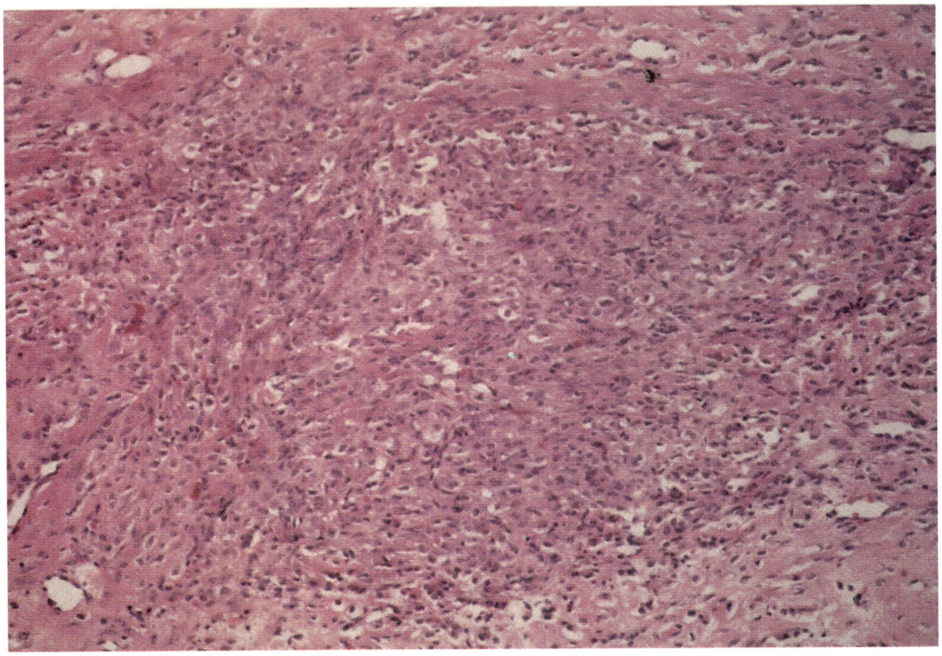

FIGURE 11-19
A cellular pseudolobule is circumscribed by a sclerotic, less cellular area. Small capillaries are seen in the cellular area and ectatic vessels in the surrounding collagenous area. These are characteristics of the ovarian sclerosing stromal tumor.

Leydig and granulosa-theca cell elements are called gynandroblastomas (see below). Sertoli and Leydig cell tumors may produce androgens, estrogens, both, or neither.

Sertoli Cell Tumor

Pure Sertoli cell tumors are extremely rare, constituting only 4 percent of all Sertoli and Leydig cell tumors. They may occur at any age. Seventy percent of patients who have a pure Sertoli cell tumor report symptoms caused by an excess of circulating estrogens produced by the tumor. In 20 percent of patients, androgen production by the tumor is responsible for the signs and symptoms. Isosexual precocity and increased libido can be seen in association with Sertoli cell tumors.[35–37]

A Sertoli cell tumor is almost always unilateral. It appears as a well-encapsulated, lobulated, solid mass, which typically is yellow or brown. The ma-

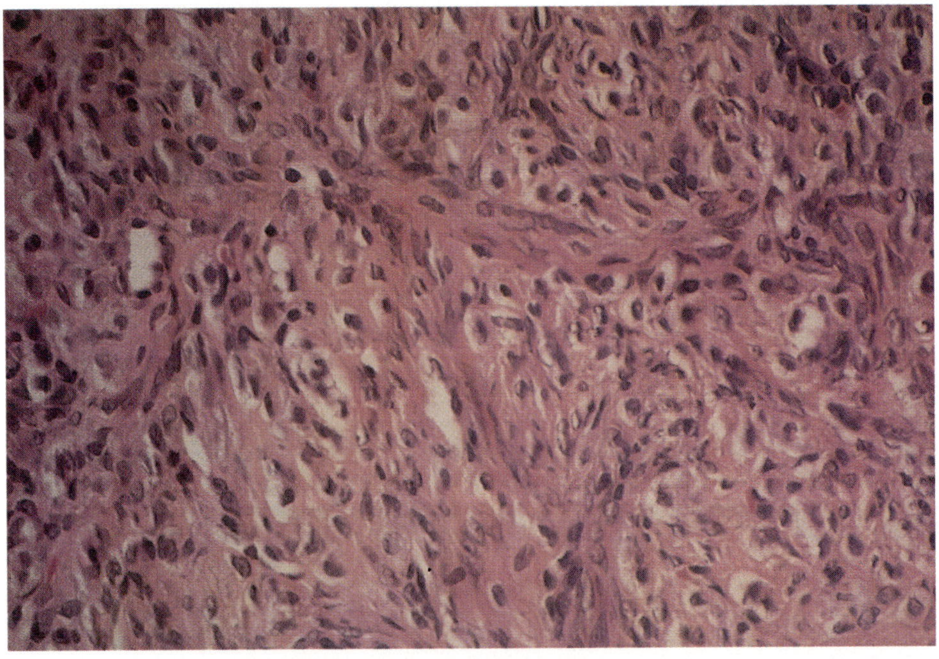

FIGURE 11-20
Bands of spindle-shaped cells separate clusters of round cells with clear cytoplasm. Small, dark nuclei are seen in the round cells. This is a high-power view of an ovarian sclerosing stromal tumor.

jority of Sertoli cell tumors are less than 5 cm in diameter. Microscopically they are composed of lobules of uniform, tortuous tubules, lined by one or more layers of cuboidal to columnar cells. These cells have slightly eosinophilic or pale vacuolated cytoplasm (Fig. 11–21). The nucleus is round to oval, basally oriented, and chromatin that is often dark. Mitoses are rare. A variant pattern is composed of tubules with cells that contain generous amounts of intracytoplasmic lipid. This has been called lipid-rich Sertoli cell tumor or "folliculome lipidique." In the past some have included this tumor in the granulosa cell group.[25]

Simple oophorectomy is sufficient treatment and is the choice if a woman wishes to conserve her uterus. Total abdominal hysterectomy with bilateral salpingo-oophorectomy is appropriate in a postmenopausal or perimenopausal woman. In general, these tumors are benign; only one death from metastatic disease has been reported.[10]

Leydig Cell Tumor

The majority (80 percent) of Leydig cell tumors are androgenic, 10 percent are estrogenic, and the rest do not produce hormones. Premenarchal girls who have a Leydig cell tumor may experience growth of pubic and axillary hair as well as clitoral hypertrophy. Women in the reproductive years may report breast atrophy, temporal balding, acne, deepening of the voice, and clitoral hypertrophy. In postmenopausal women, alopcia, hirsutism, and clitorimegaly are seen. Despite these manifestations of obvious androgen excess, the endometrium may show hyperplasia or adenocarcinoma.[25] This phenomenom may be the result of peripheral conversion of androgens to estrogens. This tumor is found most often in women between the ages of 50 and 70 years and is generally unilateral. Since these lesions rarely exceed 5 cm in diameter, they are usually brought to medical attention when the patient complains of symptoms attributable to the hormones produced by the tumor.[38, 39]

Leydig cell tumor is well-circumscribed, soft, and fleshy; (Fig. 11–22) reddish brown, yellow, or olive; and composed of hilar cells (Fig. 11–23). These cells are found in the stroma of the hilum of over 80 percent of ovaries removed from postmenopausal women. The cells are polygonal, sometimes oval, and contain eosinophilic, finely granular cytoplasm. The nucleus is round and central and may contain one to three basophilic nucleoli. Mitoses are rare. Reinke crystalloids may be seen when the tissue sections are stained with Mallory trichrome stain. The Reinke crystalloids are rodlike, intracytoplasmic, eosinophilic structures that measure 10 to 30 μm (Fig. 11–24). Their ends are rounded, tapered, or blunt. A straight clear line bisects the crystalloid longitudinally. The exact nature and function of the Reinke crystalloid remain obscure.

The hilar cell is identical to the Leydig cell of the testis. Thus the term Leydig cell tumor is used to describe a uniform mass of these cells that measures more than 1 cm.[40] A smaller proliferation is referred to as hilar cell hyperplasia. Some

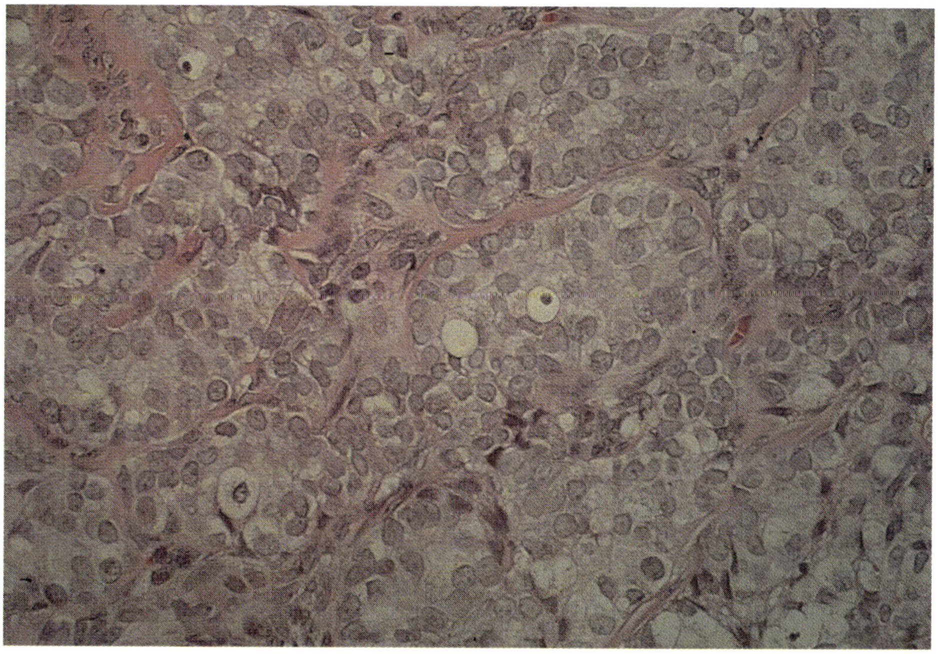

FIGURE 11–21
Sertoli cells fill poorly formed tubules. The cells are cuboidal and have abundant pale or vacuolated cytoplasm. The nuclei are round to oval. Some nucleoli are seen. This is a poorly differentiated Sertoli cell tumor. (Courtesy of Dr. Dennis O'Connor, University of Louisville, Louisville, KY.)

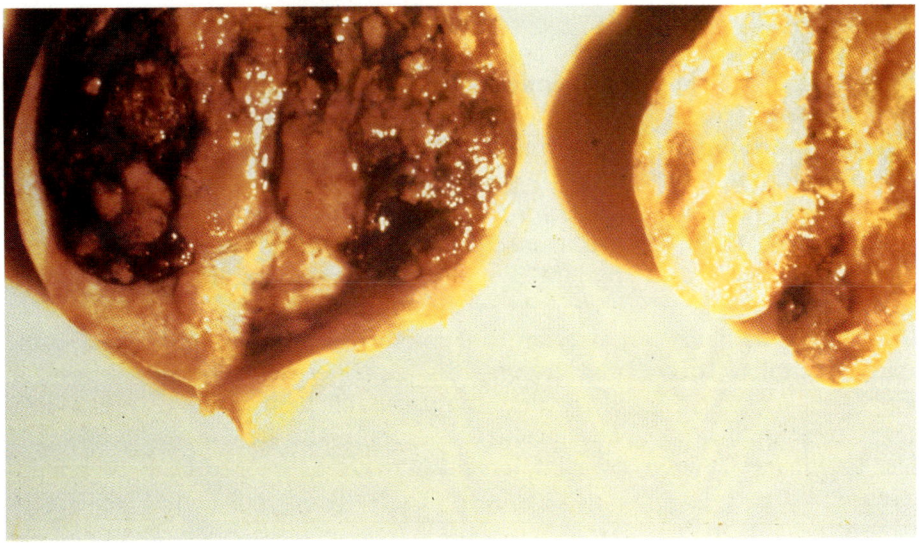

FIGURE 11-22
The cut surface of a normal ovary is shown on the right. The ovary on the left contains a Leydig cell tumor. The tumor is fleshy and orange. (Courtesy of Dr. J. Donald Woodruff, The Johns Hopkins Hospital, Baltimore, MD.)

argue that the term Leydig cell tumor should be used only when Reinke crystalloids are identified; otherwise, the term hilar cell tumor should be used.[30] Since the Leydig cell tumor and the hilar cell tumor are pathologically identical, except for the presence or absence of Reinke crystalloids and location (Leydig cell tumors may be found in the ovarian hilum or within the ovarian stroma), the term Leydig cell tumor can be applied to both.

Leydig cell tumors of the ovary are benign neoplasms; malignant Leydig cell tumors have been described in the testis.[41] In one well-documented testicular Leydig cell tumor there was a high mitotic count (15 mitoses per 10 high-power fields [HPFs]). This finding has been rare or absent in the ovarian Leydig cell tumors described so far.[41] Unilateral oophorectomy or salpingo-oophorectomy is sufficient therapy for ovarian Leydig cell tumor. The patient's endometrium needs to be evaluated, particularly if there has been abnormal uterine bleeding. Total abdominal hysterectomy and bilateral salpingo-oophorectomy may be performed in the postmenopausal woman.

Sertoli-Leydig Cell Tumor

In two thirds of cases of Sertoli and Leydig cell tumors, both Sertoli and Leydig cells are present.

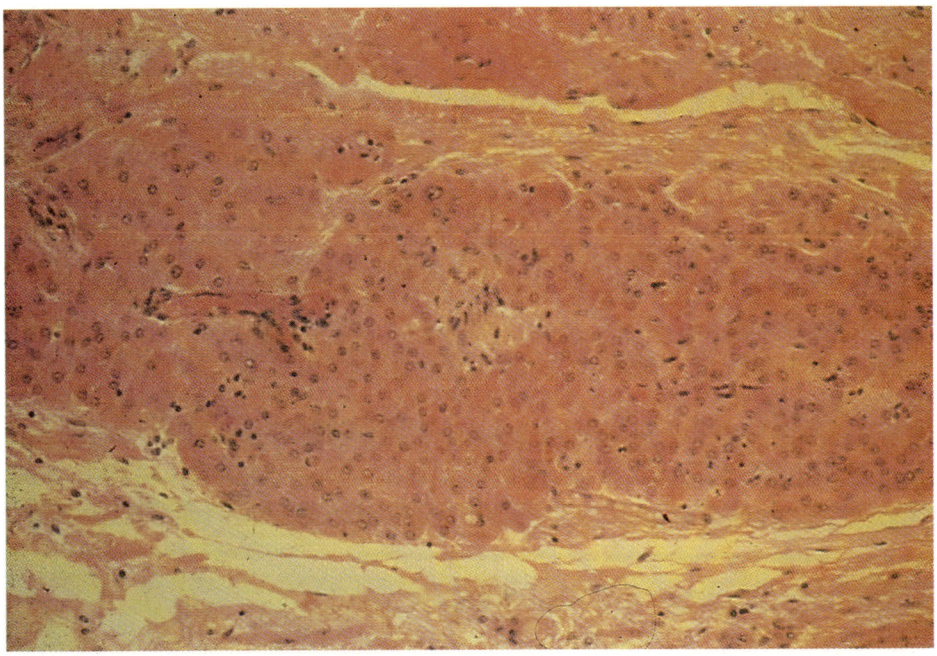

FIGURE 11-23
Hilar cell hyperplasia is shown. The hilar cells have round, uniform nuclei and abundant eosinophilic cytoplasm. (Courtesy of Dr. J. Donald Woodruff, The Johns Hopkins Hospital, Baltimore, MD.)

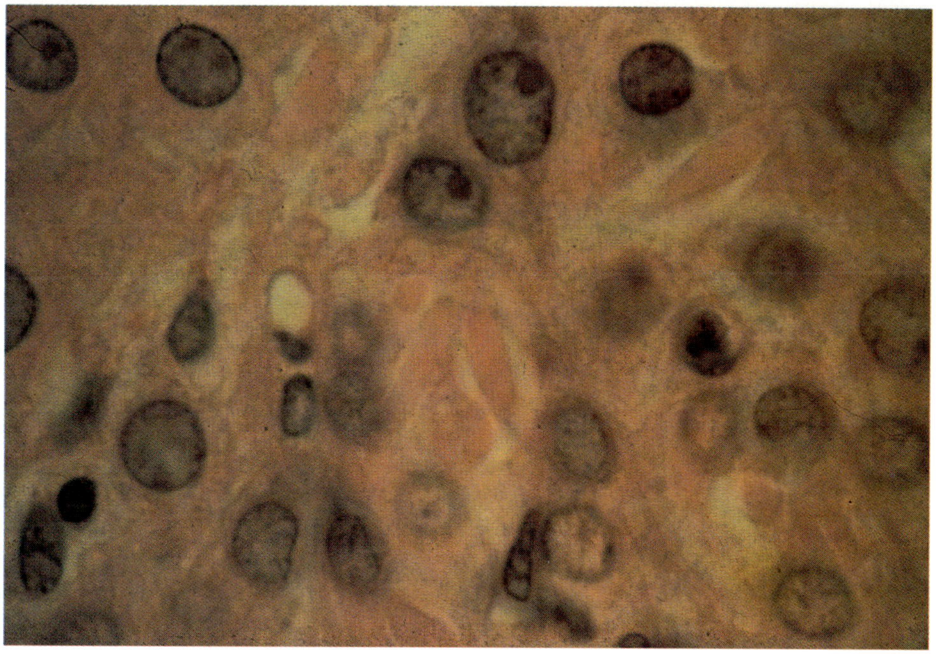

FIGURE 11-24
Under oil immersion the Reinke crystalloids are seen within the area of hilar cell hyperplasia. The etiology of these eosinophilic, rodlike structures is not known. Prominent nucleoli are seen in some of the cells.

It has been suggested that these tumors be classified in one of five categories: well-differentiated tumors, moderately differentiated tumors, poorly differentiated tumors, tumors with heterologous elements, and tumors with a retiform pattern.[30] Up to 30 percent of Sertoli-Leydig cell tumors are malignant. Evidence of extraovarian disease at the time of staging laparotomy is associated with a two-thirds recurrence rate within 1 year. However, the vast majority of these lesions are unilateral and confined to the ovary (80 percent stage IA). Only 2.5 percent have spread beyond the ovary at the time of diagnosis. Sertoli-Leydig cell tumors may occur in all age groups but are most often seen in young women. Tumors with a retiform pattern occur in younger women (mean age, 17 years) and are more common in the first decade of life than any of the other four types.[42] They are less likely to cause virilization than are the Sertoli-Leydig cell tumors in the other categories. Moderately and poorly differentiated tumors occur in slightly older patients (mean age, 25 years), while well-differentiated tumors occur at a mean age of 35 years. Sixty percent of patients who have a Sertoli-Leydig cell tumor have no endocrine abnormalities. The patients present with abdominal swelling or pain. One third present with signs and symptoms of androgen excess, which include breast atrophy, acne, hirsutism, temporal balding, deepening of the voice, and clitoral hypertrophy. Plasma levels of testosterone, androstenedione, and other androgens may be elevated.[43–45]

Sertoli-Leydig cell tumors tend to be large; the average diameter is 13 cm. Clinically malignant tumors tend to be larger than nonmalignant ones, having a mean diameter of 17.8 cm.[46] Only 2 percent are bilateral. Typically they are firm with a smooth or bosselated outer surface; the cut surface is tan or yellow (Fig. 11–25). The tumor is usually solid or may have cysts, particularly if heterologous elements (e.g., gastrointestinal mucinous epithelium) are present. The solid portion of the tumor is lobulated. Poorly differentiated tumors and those with heterologous elements in the form of skeletal muscle and cartilage tend to be fleshy and exhibit areas of necrosis and hemorrhage.[47]

Well-differentiated Sertoli-Leydig cell tumors have a predominantly tubular pattern (Fig. 11–26). The tubules are divided into lobules by intersecting fibrous bands, a prominent feature that can be easily observed on low-power microscopic examination. The tubules can be solid or hollow. The hollow tubules are typically round and small and contain no luminal secretions; occasionally, they have an irregular shape and contain eosinophilic acellular material in the lumen. Some of the tubules may be large. The tubules are lined by cuboidal to columnar epithelial cells with round to oblong nuclei. Nucleoli are not prominent; nuclear grooves are absent; and nuclear atypia and mitoses are rare. Leydig cells may be seen in the bands of fibrous tissue. Reinke crystalloids are occasionally identified in the Leydig cells.[48]

A variety of patterns and combinations of cell types are seen in moderately and poorly differentiated Sertoli-Leydig cell tumors. Both Sertoli and Leydig cells may display varying degrees of immaturity. The immature Sertoli cell has a small,

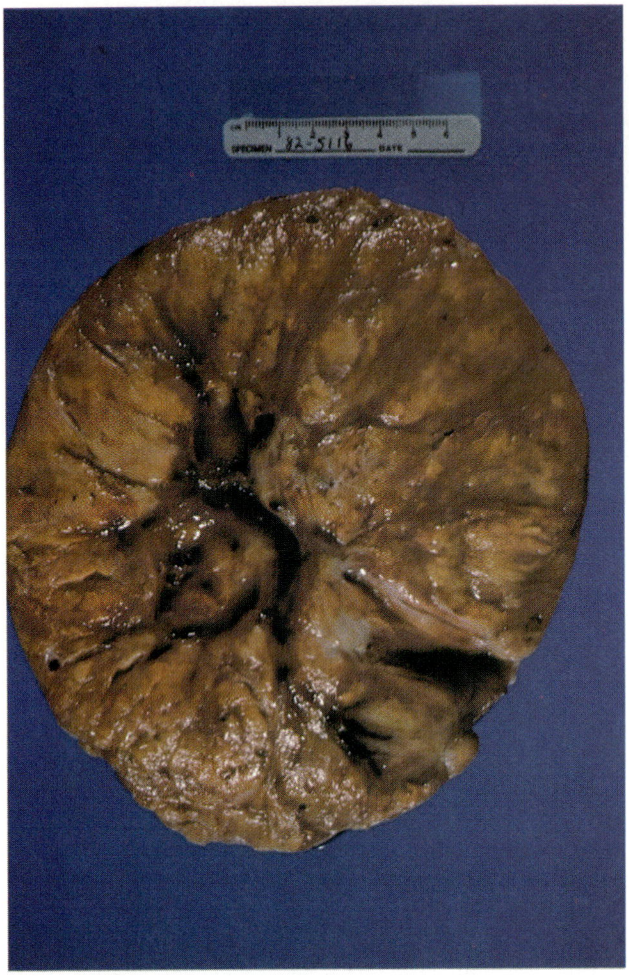

FIGURE 11–25
This is a large, solid Sertoli-Leydig cell tumor, which on cut section appears tan-yellow. Areas of hemorrhage are seen. (Courtesy of Dr. Fred B. Askin, The Johns Hopkins Hospital, Baltimore, MD.)

dark-staining, round to oval nucleus and scant cytoplasm. In some cases, the immature Sertoli cell contains abundant pale, vacuolated, or eosinophilic cytoplasm. In moderately differentiated tumors the Sertoli cells may be arranged in poorly defined masses, which have a lobulated appearance on low-power microscopic examination. Leydig cells are commonly found admixed with the Sertoli cells. The Sertoli cells may also form short thin cords or true hollow tubules. Poorly differentiated Sertoli-Leydig cell tumors consist of sheets of spindle-shaped cells and occasional cordlike structures or tubules (Fig. 11–27). The stroma may be fibromatous, cellular, or edematous. On occasion the stroma may be composed of immature cellular mesenchymal tissue. The poorly differentiated Sertoli-Leydig cell tumor is distinguished from a sarcoma by the presence of Leydig cells, Sertoli cell cords or tubules, or other Sertoli-Leydig cell patterns. In moderately differentiated Sertoli-Leydig cell tumors, mitoses are infrequent; in contrast, the sarcoma-like areas of poorly differentiated tumors may contain numerous mitoses, more than 1 per HPF.[46]

Fifteen percent of Sertoli-Leydig cell tumors may have tubular structures arranged in a pattern recapitulating that of the rete testis. When 5 percent or more of the mass consists of this pattern, the tumor is classified as a Sertoli-Leydig cell tumor with retiform differentiation.[44] This pattern is seen only in moderately differentiated and poorly differentiated tumors and those that contain heterologous elements. It is characterized by a network of long, narrow tubules and cysts, into

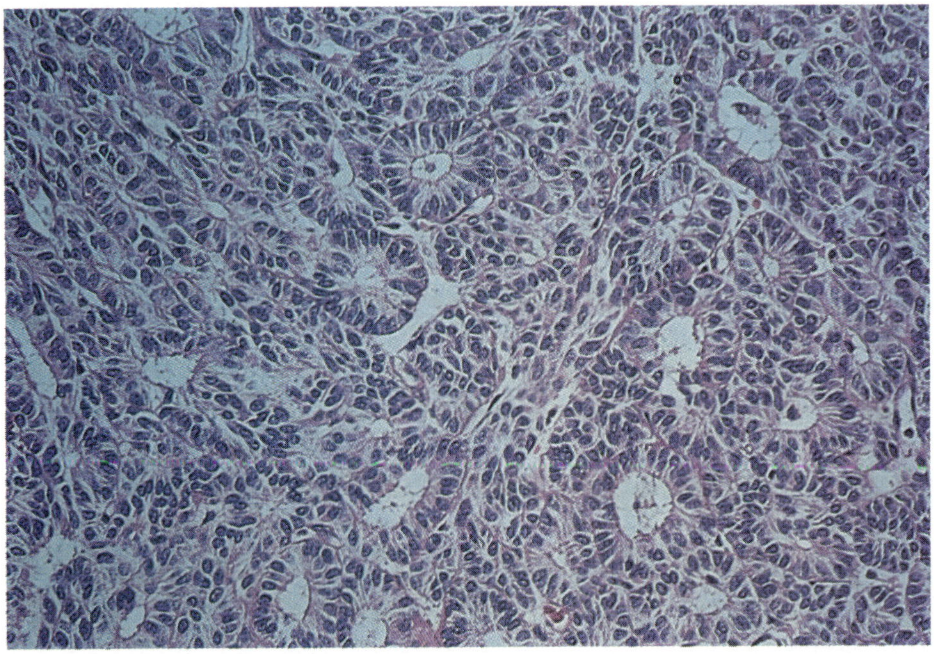

FIGURE 11–26
Small, round tubules are seen in this well-differentiated Sertoli-Leydig cell tumor. Many of the cells that line the tubules are columnar and have a basally oriented nucleus. The tubules are separated by thin fibrous bands. A cluster of Leydig cells with abundant eosinophilic cytoplasm is seen at the bottom center. (Courtesy of Dr. Fred B. Askin, The Johns Hopkins Hospital, Baltimore, MD.)

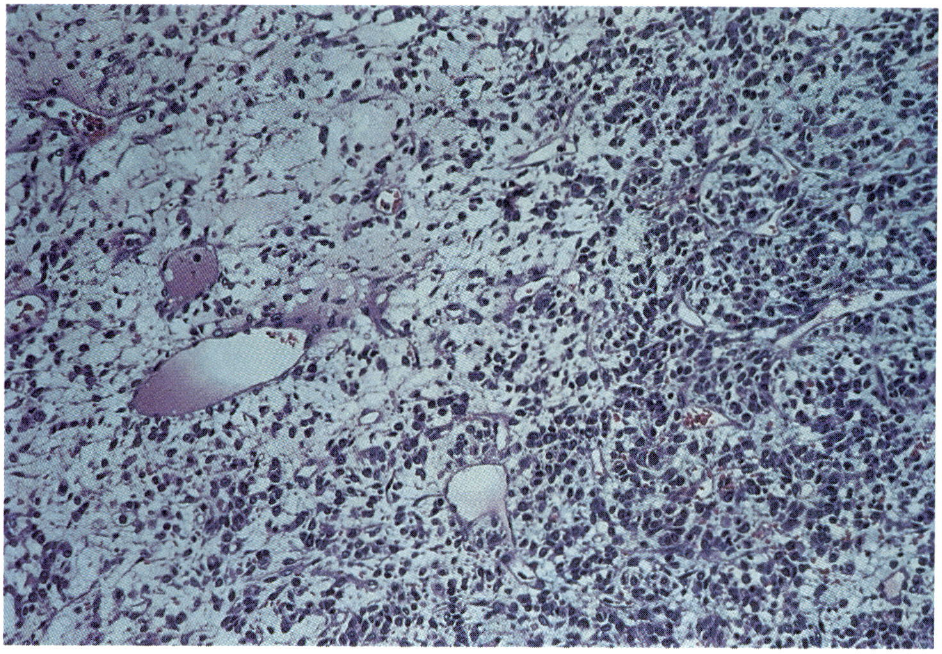

FIGURE 11-27
This poorly differentiated Sertoli-Leydig cell tumor shows an edematous stroma *(left)*. Atypical Sertoli cells are dispersed within the stroma. The cells on the right are attempting to form tubules. (Courtesy of Dr. Fred B. Askin, The Johns Hopkins Hospital, Baltimore, MD.)

which papillae may project (Fig. 11–28). These papillae may be small and rounded, large and bulbous, or delicate with extensive branches.[49] The tubules, cysts, and papillae are lined by one or several layers of cuboidal cells that contain a scant amount of cytoplasm. The nucleus of these cells is regular and has a small nucleolus. Mitotic figures are uncommon. Psammoma bodies are occasionally seen. This, together with the papillary features, may cause an erroneous diagnosis of ovarian papillary serous adenocarcinoma. However, patients who are diagnosed with Sertoli-Leydig cell tumor are young, whereas those who have ovarian epithelial tumors tend to be postmenopausal. In addition, areas more typical of Sertoli-Leydig cell tumor are usually present in conjunction with the retiform differentiation. The Sertoli-Leydig cell tumor may be confused with a yolk sac tumor because of the patient's young age. However, the histopathologic features of these two tumors are quite different (see Chapter 10).

Up to 20 percent of Sertoli-Leydig cell tumors

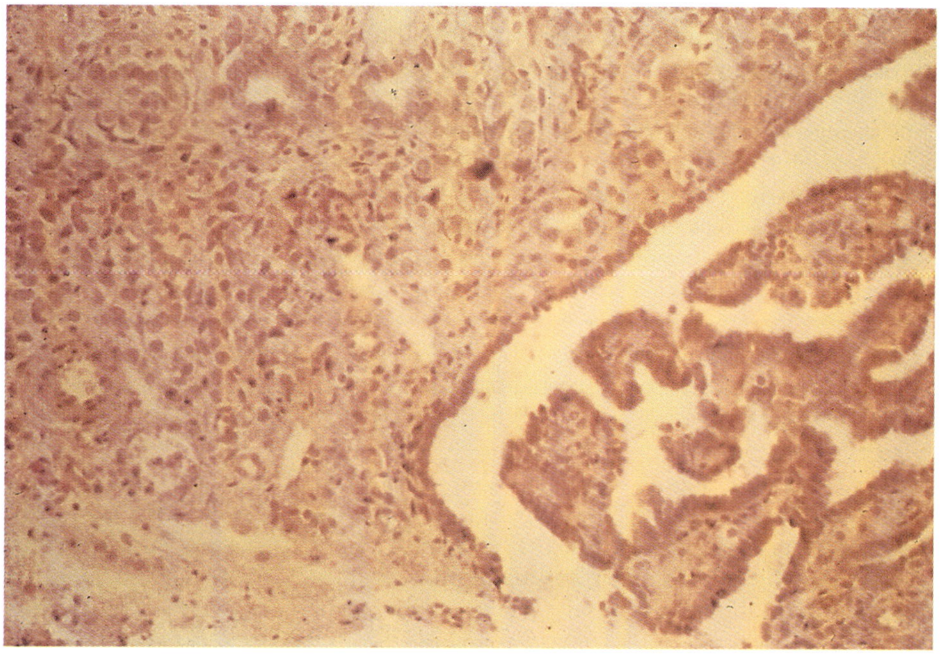

FIGURE 11-28
Tubules lined by Sertoli cells and separated by Leydig cells are seen on the left. A papillary structure projects into a space lined by cuboidal cells. This is a Sertoli-Leydig cell tumor with retiform differentiation. (Courtesy of Dr. J. Donald Woodruff, The Johns Hopkins Hospital, Baltimore, MD.)

contain heterologous elements. These include intestinal type epithelium, carcinoid tumor, cartilage, rhabdomyosarcoma, and neuroblastoma.[46, 47] The most common of these is the gastrointestinal type mucinous epithelium. This entity is usually benign but occasionally may be a low-grade carcinoma.[50] The Sertoli-Leydig cell tumor with heterologous elements must not be confused with a teratoma (see Chapter 10). The presence of areas of typical Sertoli-Leydig cell tumor and the absence of squamous epithelium with skin appendages should clarify the diagnosis.

Stage of disease, degree of tumor differentiation, the presence of heterologous elements other than gastrointestinal, and tumor rupture at the time of surgery all affect the prognosis. Well-differentiated Sertoli-Leydig cell tumors are stage IA and do not recur.[46] Eleven percent of moderately differentiated Sertoli-Leydig cell tumors exhibit malignant behavior; this increases to 60 percent if the tumor is poorly differentiated.[4] In one series of six cases of Sertoli-Leydig cell tumor with retiform differentiation, all tumors had areas typical of the moderately or poorly differentiated type.[42] Only one of these six patients (17 percent) had a recurrence and died 3 1/2 years after diagnosis. The presence of heterologous elements other than gastrointestinal type epithelium is associated with an extremely poor prognosis.[47] These elements are usually found in a background of poorly differentiated Sertoli-Leydig cell tumor. Of 12 patients whose tumors contained chondrosarcoma, rhabdomyosarcoma, or neuroblastoma components, follow-up was available on ten. Eight (80 percent) had died of tumor. Of tumors that rupture, 30 percent are malignant compared with only 7 percent malignancy in those that are intact.[46] Tumor rupture seems to be associated with poor tumor differentiation and the presence of nongastrointestinal heterologous elements.[47]

Although both chemotherapy and radiation therapy have produced responses in patients who have advanced or metastatic disease, there is little evidence that either is useful in the adjuvant setting (i.e., in the patient whose tumor was completely excised). The combination of vincristine, actinomycin D, and cyclophosphamide has been the chemotherapeutic regimen most often utilized.[44, 45]

Unilateral oophorectomy appears to be reasonable treatment for the patient with stage IA disease who wishes to retain her fertility. Complete surgical staging should be performed, including pelvic and paraaortic node sampling. In patients who have more advanced disease, resection of all gross tumor in addition to total abdominal hysterectomy and bilateral salpingo-oophorectomy is performed. In the absence of prospective data to support it, adjuvant chemotherapy or radiation therapy is not appropriate. These modalities should be reserved for patients who have persistent, metastatic, or recurrent disease.

Gynandroblastoma

Gynandroblastomas are exceedingly rare. To make this diagnosis the presence of both granulosa-theca and Sertoli-Leydig cell types is required. The minor component must constitute at least 10 percent of the tumor. As with other tumors of the specialized ovarian stroma, these may be associated with signs and symptoms of androgen excess, estrogen excess, or normal endocrine function. The mean age at presentation is 27 years. All reported cases have been unilateral, and to date, none has had a malignant course.[51]

These are small (2 to 6 cm), solid, pale tumors. The cut surface may show pink to yellow fleshy nodules. Microscopic examination reveals varying numbers of mature granulosa cells and Call-Exner bodies as well as tubules lined with typical Sertoli cells and the presence of Leydig cells in which Reinke crystalloids are sometimes identified.

Sex Cord Tumor with Annular Tubules

The sex cord tumor with annular tubules (SCTAT) was first described by Scully in 1970.[52] One third of SCTATs are found in conjunction with the Peutz-Jeghers syndrome, an autosomal dominant disorder consisting of gastrointestinal polyposis and oral and cutaneous melanin pigmentation. Ovarian tumors are found in 15 percent of women who have Peutz-Jeghers syndrome, many of which are SCTAT, although other types are found as well. The lesions of SCTAT in patients with Peutz-Jeghers syndrome are typically very small, bilateral, multifocal, and an incidental finding. Those SCTAT tumors not associated with Peutz-Jeghers syndrome are unilateral and usually large.[53] Adenoma malignum of the cervix has been reported in a few patients with Peutz-Jeghers syndrome and SCTAT.[53] Approximately 40 percent of patients who have SCTAT with or without Peutz-Jeghers syndrome show signs and symptoms of estrogen excess.[53, 54] An occasional SCTAT produces progesterone.[55]

The SCTAT has histopathologic features intermediate between those of the granulosa cell tumor and a Sertoli-Leydig cell tumor. It is composed of sharply circumscribed nests of ring-shaped tubules that encircle hyalinized basement membrane–like material. The tubules may be single or may communicate and encircle multiple hyaline masses. The cells lining the tubules are tall columnar and have basally located nuclei. The nuclei of opposed columnar cells are found at opposite poles. The cytoplasm is abundant, pale, and rich in lipids. Calcifications are common when SCTAT is associated with Peutz-Jeghers syndrome. Areas of granulosa cell and/or Sertoli cell tumor are frequently seen in SCTAT not associated with Peutz-Jeghers syndrome (Fig. 11–29).

The SCTAT tumors associated with Peutz-Jeghers syndrome are benign. However, 20 percent of SCTATs not so associated behave in a malignant fashion. Primary treatment consists of surgical excision. Radiotherapy appears to be of benefit in patients who have metastatic disease; chemotherapy does not.[53, 55, 56]

TUMORS OF NONSPECIFIC OVARIAN STROMA

Fibromas and Fibrosarcomas

Fibroma is the most common tumor of the ovarian stroma. It accounts for 4 percent of all ovarian neoplasms and constitutes two thirds of the ovarian stromal tumors. Ninety percent occur in women who are over the age of 30 years. The mean age at tumor removal is 48 years. Ovarian fibromas are bilateral in 15 percent of cases.[57] Ascites occurs in 10 to 15 percent of women in whom the lesion is greater than 10 cm. Meigs syndrome (ascites and pleural effusions) has been reported in 1 percent of patients who have an ovarian fibroma. This is probably due to partial torsion of the ovarian vascular pedicle, which results in venous engorgement and transudation into the peritoneal cavity. The accumulated peritoneal fluid eventually finds its way to the pleural space through the diaphragmatic lymphatics.

Fibromas have a smooth or slightly bosselated serosal surface (Fig. 11–30). They are rubbery to hard, with a white cut surface (Fig. 11–31). Bundles of spindle-shaped cells with elongated nuclei are seen; these bundles are intersected by bands of collagenous fibrous tissue. Nuclear atypia and mitoses are rarely seen. As with a thecoma (see above), the uninvolved portion of the ovary or the contralateral ovary may show nodular or diffuse stromal hyperplasia (i.e., hyperthecosis). Degenerative changes similar to those seen in uterine leiomyoma (e.g., hyalinization, calcification, cystic degeneration) are frequent, particularly in a large fibroma.

Fibromas are occasionally hypercellular. Those containing one to three mitoses per ten microscopic HPF have been called cellular fibromas. They are usually benign, although local recurrences have been reported. Those containing four or more mitoses per ten HPF are considered to be malignant and are diagnosed as fibrosarcoma.[58]

Other Tumors of the Nonspecific Ovarian Stroma

Soft tissue tumors, similar to those of other connective tissue sites, occasionally arise in the ovary.

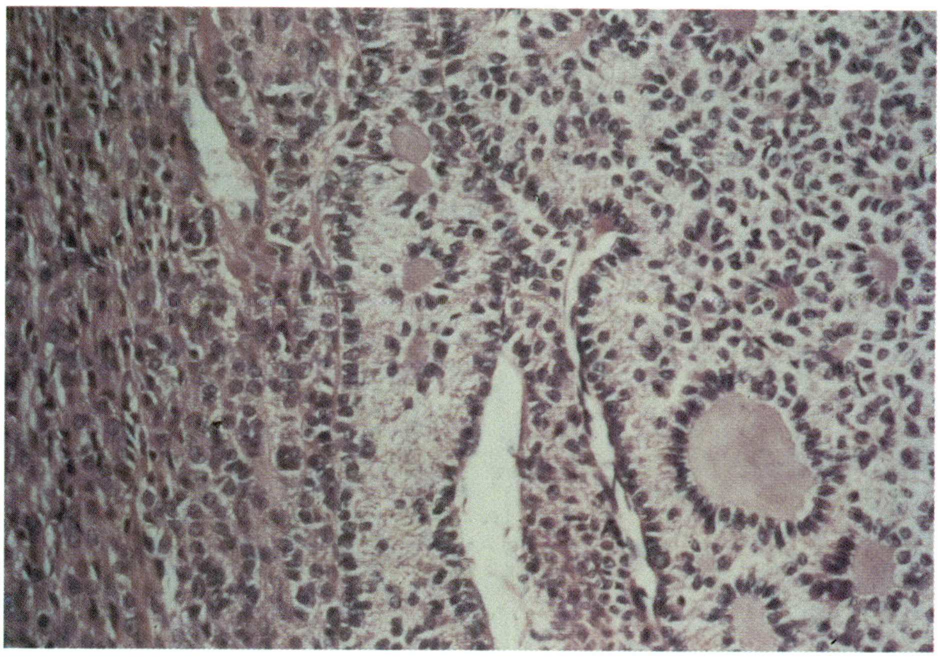

FIGURE 11-29
Tubules of various sizes surround hyaline masses. Leydig cells are seen on the left. This is a Sertoli-Leydig cell tumor with annular tubules also known as a sex cord–stromal tumor with annular tubules. (Courtesy of Dr. J. Donald Woodruff, The Johns Hopkins Hospital, Baltimore, MD.)

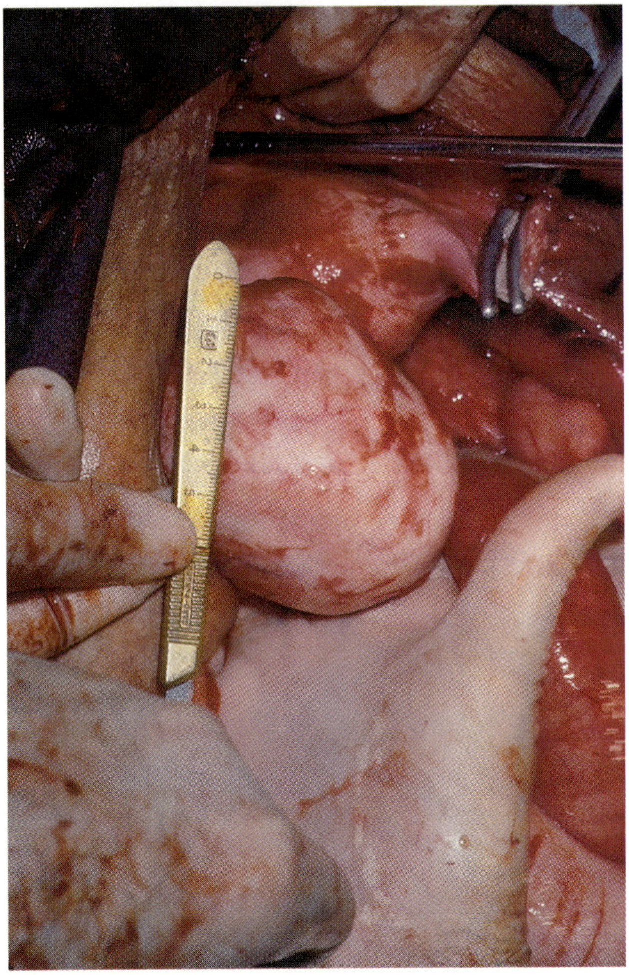

FIGURE 11-30
A fibroma that replaces the left ovary is shown. The surface is off-white and smooth. This tumor was firm.

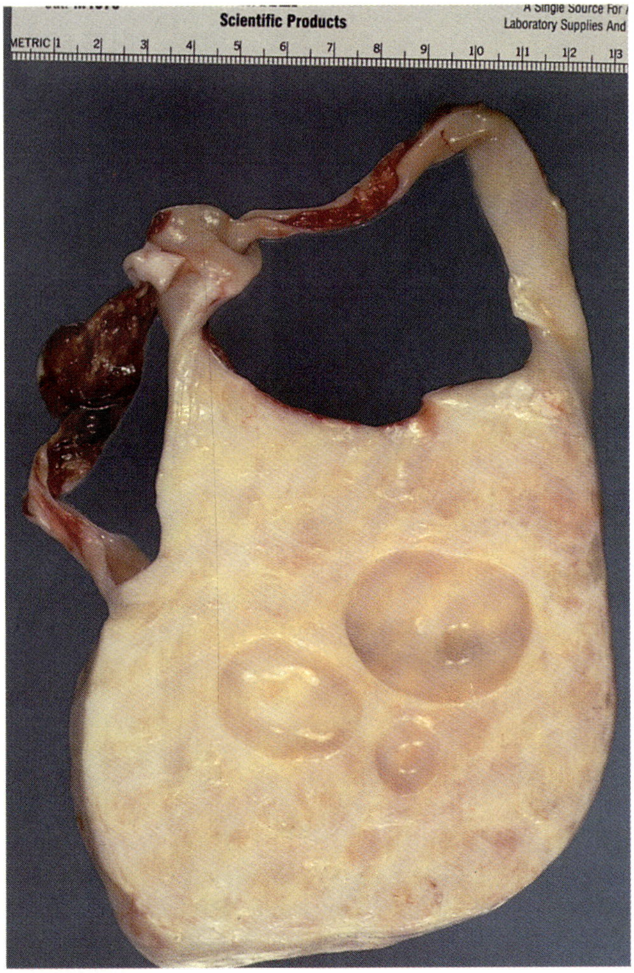

FIGURE 11-31
This solid tumor with cystic areas is a cystadenofibroma. The fibromatous areas are composed of white, shiny, interlacing bundles of fibrous tissue.

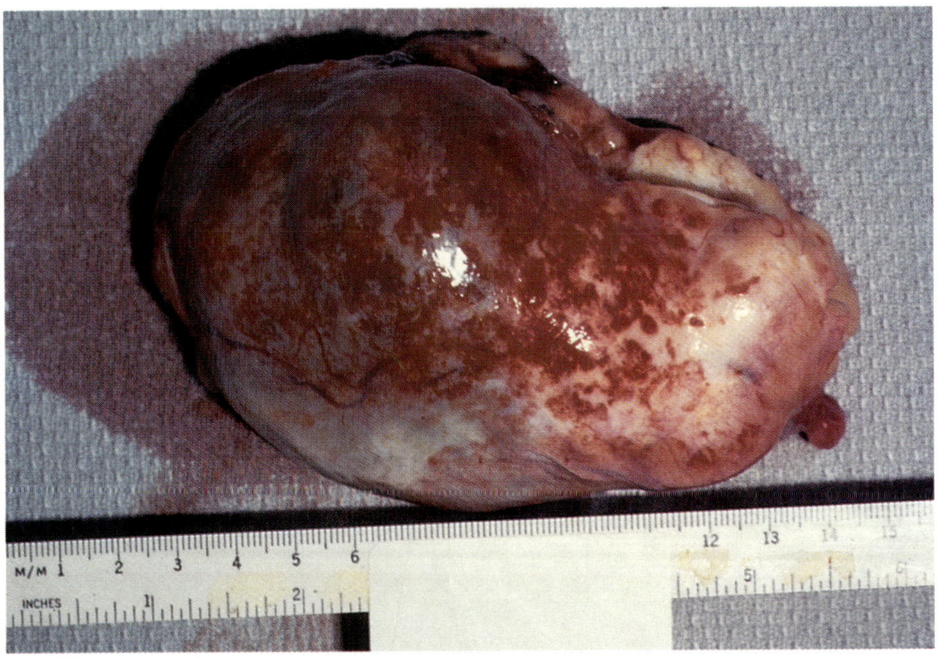

FIGURE 11-32
This large ovarian carcinosarcoma has an irregular surface and extensive hemorrhage.

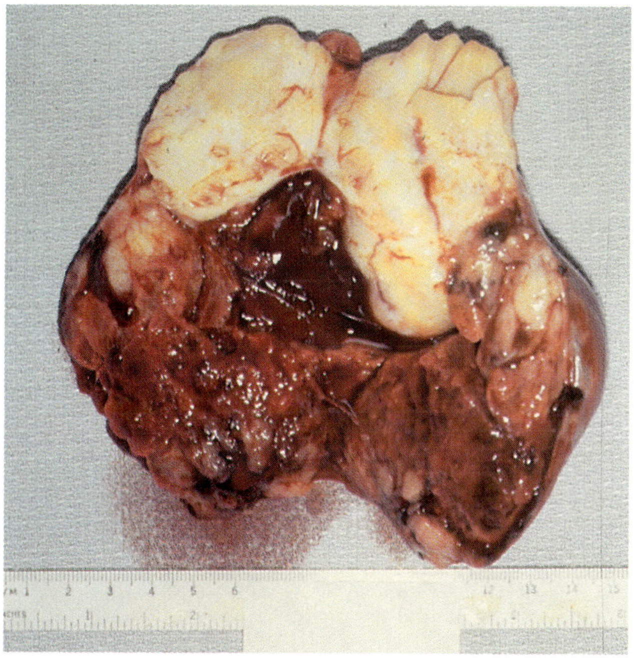

FIGURE 11-33
The cut surface of the carcinosarcoma shown in Figure 11-32 demonstrates a solid, white-yellow area as well as extensive hemorrhage and necrosis.

These tumors include leiomyoma, hemangioma, leiomyosarcoma, lymphoma, carcinosarcoma, and other rare mesenchymal neoplasms.[3, 25] Of these, the most common and important are carcinosarcoma (malignant mixed mesodermal tumor) and lymphoma.

Carcinosarcoma of the ovary is a highly malignant tumor; it is identical to that found in the uterus (see Chapter 6).[59] Most patients are in the sixth decade of life. These tumors present as a large solid and cystic mass having a gray irregular surface and hemorrhagic areas (Fig. 11-32). The cut surface is fleshy and has extensive hemorrhage and necrosis (Fig. 11-33). Widespread involvement of other pelvic and abdominal strucures is almost invariably found. Hemoperitoneum may be present. The tumor is composed of a malignant epithelial component (i.e., adenocarcinoma) and a sarcomatous component that may contain heterologous elements (Fig. 11-34). Seventy-five percent of patients with stage III ovarian carcinosarcoma are dead of tumor within 6 months of the diagnosis. One case of a patient who had metastatic disease and who responded to multiagent chemotherapy consisting of doxorubicin, ifosfamide, dacarbazine, and mesna has been documented.[60] As in cases of uterine carcinosarcoma, the combination of cisplatin and ifosfamide may have some effect.

Most lymphomas found in the ovary have spread from other sites. A few cases of primary ovarian lymphoma have been documented.[61, 62] Metastatic ovarian lymphoma does not require removal of the ovaries if the diagnosis has already been established by examination of other involved sites. Lymphoma involving the ovary may be misdiagnosed as either a granulosa cell tumor or dysgerminoma and vice versa.[63] Identification of architecture and growth patterns is the key to recognizing that the tumor is not a lymphoma.

FIGURE 11-34
This ovarian carcinosarcoma shows immature cartilage *(left)*. Several malignant glands are seen in a background of malignant stroma.

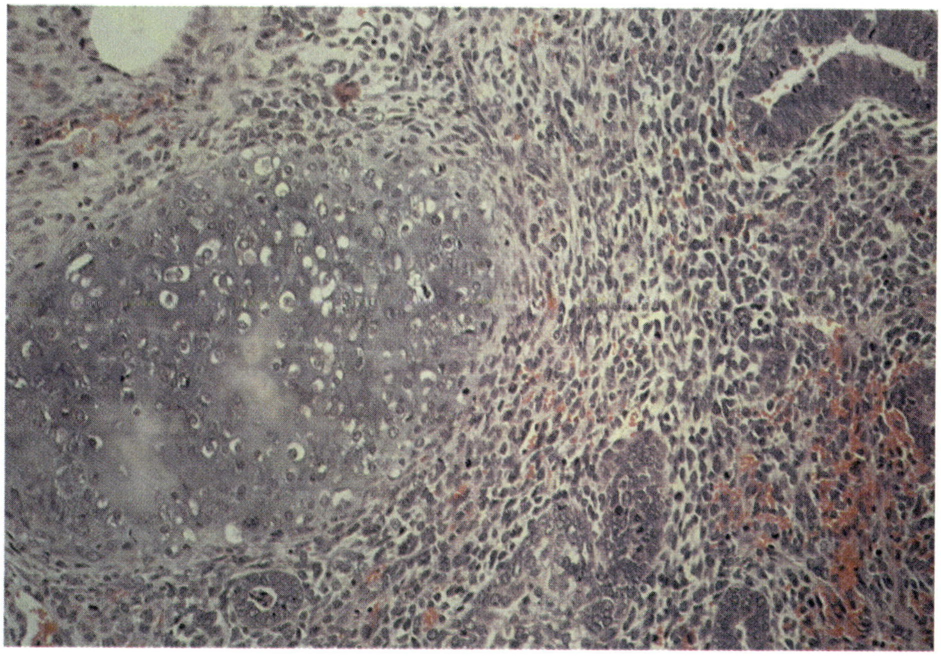

Lymphoma usually has a rapid response to chemotherapy, but recurrence is frequent. Primary ovarian lymphoma is usually not diagnosed until the ovarian mass is removed. The staging of this disease is clinical and includes computed tomography and bone marrow biopsy. Therapy is dictated by the histopathologic type.

REFERENCES

1. Parmley TH: Clinical Review of the Embriology of the Female Genital Canal. Wichita, KS, Eagle Press, 1988, pp 3–5.
2. Langman J: Medical Embriology, 2nd ed. Baltimore, Williams & Wilkins, 1969, pp 148–167.
3. DiSaia PJ, Creasman WT: Clinical Gynecologic Oncology, 2nd ed. St. Louis, Mosby-Year Book, 1993, pp 445–451.
4. Young RH, Scully RE: Sex cord–stromal, steroid cell, and other ovarian tumors with endocrine, paraendocrine, and paraneoplastic manifestations. *In* Kurman RJ (ed): Blaustein's Pathology of the Female Genital Tract, 3rd ed. New York: Springer-Verlag, 1987, pp 607–658.
5. Evans AT, Gaffey TA, Malkasian GD, Annegers JF: Clinicopathologic review of 118 granulosa cell and 82 theca cell tumors. Obstet Gynecol 1980;55:231–238.
6. Björkholm E, Silverswärd C: Prognostic factors in granulosa-cell tumors. Gynecol Oncol 1981;11:261–274.
7. Novak ER, Kutchmeshgi J, Mupas RS, Woodruff JD: Feminizing gonadal stromal tumors: analysis of the granulosa-theca cell tumors of the Ovarian Tumor Registry. Obstet Gynecol 1971;38:701–713.
8. Norris HJ, Taylor HB: Prognosis of granulosa-theca tumors of the ovary. Cancer 1968;21:255–263.
9. Fox H, Agrawal K, Langley FA: A clinicopathologic study of 92 cases of granulosa cell tumors of the ovary with special reference to the factors influencing prognosis. Cancer 1975;35:231–241.
10. Stenwig JT, Hazekamp JT, Beechamp JB: Granulosa cell tumors of the ovary: a clinicopathologic study of 118 cases with long-term follow-up. Gynecol Oncol 1979;7:136–152.

10a. Malmström H, Högberg T, Risberg B, Simonsen E: Granulosa cell tumors of the ovary: prognostic factors and outcome. Gynecol Oncol 1994;52:50–55.

11. Schwartz PE, Smith JP: Treatment of ovarian stromal tumors. Am J Obstet Gynecol 1976;125:402–411.
12. Zambeti M, Escobedo A, Pilotti S, De Paolo G: cis-Platinum/vinblastine/bleomycin combination chemotherapy in advanced or recurrent granulosa cell tumors of the ovary. Gynecol Oncol 1990;36:317–320.
13. Gershenson DM, Copeland LJ, Kavanagh JJ, et al: Treatment of metastatic stromal tumors of the ovary with cisplatin, doxorubicin, and cyclophosphamide. Obstet Gynecol 1987;70:765–769.
14. Kumar PP, Good RR, Linder J: Complete response of granulosa cell tumor metastatic to liver after hepatic irradiation: a case report. Obstet Gynecol 1986;67(Suppl):95S–98S.
15. Lappöhn RE, Burger HG, Bouma J, et al: Inhibin as a marker for granulosa-cell tumors. N Engl J Med 1989;321:790–793.
16. Bast RC, Hunter V, Knapp RC: Pros and cons of gynecologic tumor markers. Cancer 1987;60:1984–1992.
17. Vassal G, Flamant F, Caillaud JM, et al: Juvenile granulosa cell tumor of the ovary in children: a clinical study of 15 cases. J Clin Oncol 1988;6:990–995.
18. La Vecchia C, Morris HB, Draper GJ: Malignant ovarian tumors in childhood. Br J Cancer 1983;48:363–374.
19. Scully RE: Ovarian tumors: a review. Am J Pathol 1977;87:686–720.
20. Young RH, Dickersin GR, Scully RE: Juvenile granulosa cell tumor of the ovary. Am J Surg Pathol 1984;8:575–596.
21. Powell JL, Johnson NA, Bailey CL, Otis CN: Management of advanced granulosa cell tumor of the ovary. Gynecol Oncol 1993;48:119–123.
22. Takeuchi H, Hamada H, Sodemoto Y, Ushigome S: Juvenile granulosa cell tumor with rapid distant metastases. Acta Pathol Jpn 1983;33:537–546.
23. Jacoby AF, Young RH, Colvin RB, et al: DNA content in juvenile granulosa cell tumors of the ovary: a study of early- and advanced-stage disease. Gynecol Oncol 1992; 46:97–103.
24. Anikwue C, Dawood MY, Kramer E: Granulosa and theca cell tumors. Obstet Gynecol 1978;51:214–220.
25. Novak ER, Woodruff JD: Novak's Gynecologic Pathology, 8th ed. Philadelphia, WB Saunders, 1979, pp 451–460, 511–512.
26. Waxman M, Vuletin JC, Urcyo R, Belling CG: Ovarian low grade stromal sarcoma with thecomatous features: a critical reappraisal of the so-called "malignant thecoma." Cancer 1979;44:2206–2217.
27. Björkholm E, Silverswärd C: Theca-cell tumors: clinical features and prognosis. Acta Radiol Oncol Radiat Phys Biol 1980;19:241–244.
28. Norris HJ, Taylor HB: Prognosis of granulosa-theca tumors of the ovary. Cancer 1968;21:255–263.
29. Björkholm E, Petterson F: Granulosa-cell and theca-cell tumors: the clinical picture and long-term outcome for the Radiumhemmet series. Acta Obstet Gynaecol Scand 1980;59:361–365.
30. Young RH, Clement PB, Scully RE: The ovary. *In* Sternberg SS, Mills SE (eds): Surgical Pathology of the Female Reproductive System and Peritoneum. New York; Raven Press, 1991, pp 169–248.

30a. Hayes MC, Scully RE: Ovarian steroid cell tumors (not otherwise specified): a clinicopathological analysis of 63 cases. Am J Surg Pathol 1987;11:835–845.

31. Chalvardjian A, Scully RE: Sclerosing stromal tumors of the ovary. Cancer 1973;31:664–670.
32. Quinn MA, Oster AO, Fortune D, Hudson B: Sclerosing tumor of the ovary: case report with endocrine studies. Br J Obstet Gynaecol 1981;88:555–558.
33. Tang M, Liu T: Ovarian sclerosing stromal tumors: clinicopathologic study of 10 cases. Chin Med J 1982;95:186–190.
34. Ireland K, Woodruff JD: Masculinizing ovarian tumors. Obstet Gynecol Surv 1917;31:83–111.
35. Tavassoli FA, Norris HJ: Sertoli tumors of the ovary: a clinicopathologic study of 28 cases with ultrastructural considerations. Cancer 1980;46:2282–2297.
36. Young RH, Scully RE: Ovarian Sertoli cell tumors: a report of 10 cases. Int J Gynaecol Pathol 1984;2:349.
37. Young RH, Scully RE: Ovarian sex cord-stromal tumors: recent advances and current status. Clin Obstet Gynecol 1984;11:93–134.
38. Dunnihoo DR, Grieme DL, Woolf RB: Hillar-cell tumors of the ovary: report of 2 new cases and a review of the world literature. Obstet Gynecol 1966;27:703–712.
39. Sternberg WH, Dhuranandhar HN: Functional ovarian tumors of stromal and sex cord origin. Hum Pathol 1977;8:565–582.
40. Novak ER, Mattingly RF: Hilus cell tumor of the ovary. Obstet Gynecol 1960;15:425–432.
41. Bertram KA, Bratloff B, Hodges GF, Davidson H: Treatment of malignant Leydig cell tumor. Cancer 1991; 68:2324–2329.
42. Roth LM, Slayton RE, Brady LW, et al: Retiform differentiation in ovarian Sertoli-Leydig cell tumors: a clinicopathologic study of six cases from a Gynecologic Oncology Group study. Cancer 1985;55:1093–1098.
43. Genton CY: Ovarian Sertoli-Leydig cell tumors: a clinical, pathological, and ultrastructural study with particular reference to the histogenesis of these tumors. Arch Gynecol 1980;230:49–75.
44. Roth LM, Anderson MC, Govan ADT, et al: Sertoli-Leydig cell tumors: a clinocopathologic study of 34 cases. Cancer 1981;48:187–197.

45. Zaloudek C, Norris HJ: Sertoli-Leydig cell tumors of the ovary: a clinicopathologic study of 64 intermediate and poorly differentiated neoplasms. Am J Surg Pathol 1984;8:405–418.
46. Young RH, Scully RE: Ovarian Sertoli-Leydig cell tumors: a clinicopathologic analysis of 207 cases. Am J Surg Pathol 1985;9:543–569.
47. Prat J, Young RH, Scully RE: Ovarian Sertoli-Leydig cell tumors with heterologous elements: II. Cartilage and skeletalmuscle; clinicopathologic analysis of twelve cases. Cancer 1982;50:2465–2475.
48. Young RH, Scully RE: Well-differentiated ovarian Sertoli-Leydig cell tumors: a clinicopathologic analysis of 23 cases. Int J Gynecol Pathol 1984;3:277–290.
49. Young RH, Scully RE: Ovarian Sertoli-Leydig cell tumors with a retiform pattern: a problem in histopathologic diagnosis: a report of 25 cases. Am J Surg Pathol 1983;7:755–771.
50. Young RH, Prat J, Scully RE: Ovarian Sertoli-Leydig cell tumors with heterologous elements: I. Gastrointestinal epithelium and carcinoid: a clinicopathologic analysis of thirty-six cases. Cancer 1982;50:2448–2456.
51. Chalvardjian A, Derzko C: Gynandroblastoma: its ultrastructure. Cancer 1982;50:710–721.
52. Scully RE: Sex cord tumors with annular tubules: a distinctive ovarian tumor of the Peutz-Jeghers syndrome. Cancer 1970;25:1107–1121.
53. Young RH, Welch WR, Dickersin R, Scully RE: Ovarian sex cord tumor with annular tubules: review of 74 cases including 27 with Peutz-Jeghers syndrome and four with adenoma malignum of the cervix. Cancer 1982;50:1384–1402.
54. Young RH, Dickersin R, Scully RE: A distinctive ovarian sex cord–stromal tumor causing sexual precocity in the Peutz-Jeghers syndrome. Am J Surg Pathol 1983;7:233.
55. Shen K, Wu P-C, Lang J-H, et al: Ovarian sex cord tumor with annular tubules: a report of six cases. Gynecol Oncol 1993;48:180–184.
56. Young RH, Scully RE: Ovarian sex cord–stromal tumors: recent progress. Int. J Gynecol Pathol 1982;1:101–123.
57. Dockerty MB, Mason JC: Ovarian fibromas: a clinical and pathologic study of 283 cases. Am J Obstet Gynecol 1944;47:741–752.
58. Prat J, Scully RE: Cellular fibromas and fibrosarcomas of the ovary: a comparative clinicopathologic analysis of 17 cases. Cancer 1981;47:2663–2670.
59. Hernandez W, DiSaia PJ, Morrow CP, Townsend DE: Mixed mesodermal sarcoma of the ovary. Obstet Gynecol 1977;49(Suppl):59S–63S.
60. Simon SR, Wang SE, Uhl M, Schakney S: Complete response of carcinosarcoma of the ovary to therapy with doxorubicin, ifosfamide, and dacarbazine. Gynecol Oncol 1991; 41:161–166.
61. Freeman C, Berg JW, Cutler S: Occurrence and prognosis of extranodal lymphomas. Cancer 1972;29:252–260.
62. Rotmensch J, Woodruff JD: Lymphoma of the ovary: report of twenty new cases and update of previous series. Am J Obstet Gynecol 1982;143:870–875.
63. Osborne BM, Roboy SJ: Lymphomas or leukemia presenting as ovarian tumors: an analysis of 42 cases. Cancer 1983;52:1933–1943.

12

Gestational Trophoblastic Disease

Enrique Hernandez / Gulnar Balsara

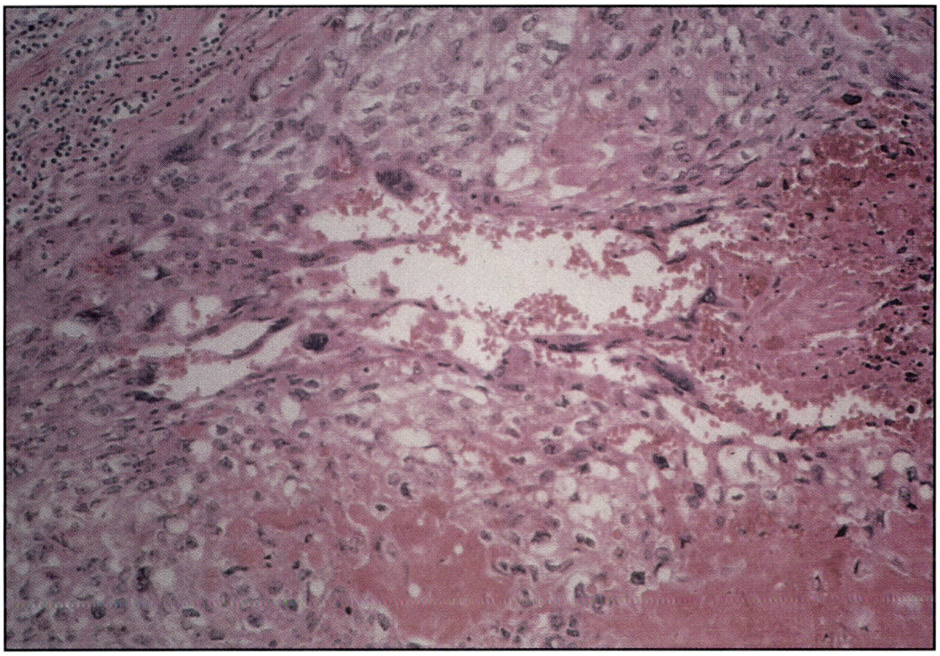

Gestational trophoblastic disease (GTD) encompasses a diverse group of lesions, all characterized by abnormalities of the trophoblast. They include hydatidiform mole, choriocarcinoma, and placental site trophoblastic tumor (PSTT). Cytogenetic and immunocytochemical studies suggest that the various forms of GTD are related to specific pathologic deviations from the normal development of the zygote and formation of the placenta.

All forms of hydatidiform mole are the result of genetic aberrations related to the villous trophoblast. They are generally benign. In 15 to 20 percent of cases they persist or metastasize, and the patient requires chemotherapy.[1, 2] Persistence of a hydatidiform mole after uterine evacuation is determined by a plateau or rise in the patient's serum beta-human chorionic gonadotropin (β-hCG) produced by the molar trophoblast. Choriocarcinomas arise from the previllous trophoblast and are by definition malignant. When this pathologic diagnosis is rendered, the clinician should initiate a thorough search for metastases, since their presence or absence may dictate the type of adjunctive therapy. PSTT arises from the extravillous trophoblast. The clinical behavior of PSTT is inconsistent, and the current treatment recommendation is hysterectomy.[3]

Historically, these heterogeneous lesions have been grouped under the heading of GTD because clinical management is dictated by clinical behavior rather than by histologic type. Histopathologically, these lesions are classified according to the system developed by the International Society of Gynecologic Pathologists, which was adopted by the World Health Organization (WHO).[4] The diagnoses in the WHO classification include hydatidiform mole (complete or partial), invasive hydatidiform mole, choriocarcinoma, PSTT, and unclassified trophoblast lesions. These will be discussed in detail in the following sections. To better understand the spectrum of abnormalities seen with GTD, a basic understanding of the development, morphology, and function of the normal placenta is essential.

NORMAL PLACENTA

Embryology

The morphology of the mature placenta is the end result of a series of developmental changes that starts with the implantation of the blastocyst in the endometrial stroma. The function of the placental trophoblast is to maintain this implantation and to establish the maternal-fetal circulation. uring the first 2 weeks after implantation, the trophoblastic cell mass of the outer cell layer of the blastocyst proliferates rapidly and differentiates into the inner cytotrophoblast and the outer syncytiotrophoblast. Between these two layers lies the intermediate trophoblast. This early proliferation, prior to the development of the chorionic villi, is the previllous trophoblast. As the trophoblast proliferates and further invades the endometrium, it erodes and destroys the capillaries to produce blood-filled lacunae separated by trophoblastic trabeculae. Choriocarcinoma recapitulates this previllous trophoblastic proliferation and vascular invasion.

After the second week of development, the invasive trophoblastic columns, composed of peripherally oriented syncytiotrophoblasts, are penetrated by mesoderm. This represents the earliest stem villi. The mesodermal cores of these villi contain small vessels and motile macrophages, the Hofbauer cells. New villi form through proliferation and branching of the trophoblastic columns, and then the column is invaded by vascularized mesenchyme. Hydatidiform moles are an abnormal development of the villous trophoblast. Concurrent with this growth is the coalescence of the lacunae to form the intervillous spaces that contain maternal blood. The terminal villi with their fetal capillaries protrude into these spaces, which form the region of maternal-fetal metabolic interactions.

The growth of the trophoblast is asymmetrical. It is greatest at the base of the implantation site and is responsible for the discoid configuration of the term placenta. The intermediate trophoblast is the cell that is predominantly involved in the invasion of the endomyometrium at the base of the implantation site. These cells infiltrate between the decidual cells of the endometrial stroma, leaving the endometrial glands intact. They also invade the spiral arterioles in a characteristic pattern. The smooth muscle of the arterial wall is invaded by the intermediate trophoblast, which ultimately disintegrates to form a fibrinoid matrix. The vessels remain intact but lose their ability to constrict, thus providing a physiologic low-pressure uteroplacental circulation. The intermediate trophoblast is particularly able to effect this invasion of the uterine wall because of the action of plasminogen activators, which play a major role in the destruction of extracellular matrix.[5, 6] The intermediate trophoblast in this location is referred to as the extravillous trophoblast; this is the cell of origin of PSTT.

By the twentieth week of gestation, as growth and enlargement of the chorion occurs, the decidua

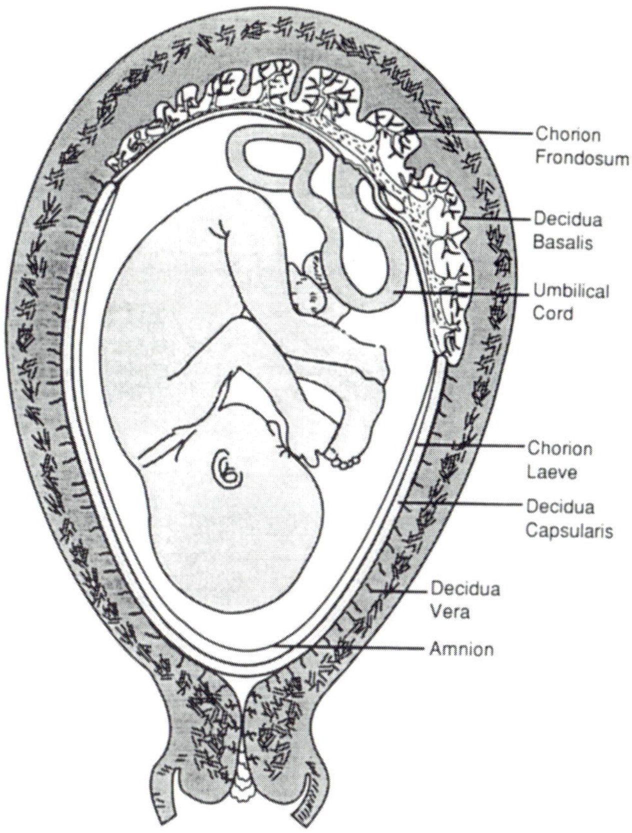

FIGURE 12-1
A normal pregnancy at 20 weeks of gestation is shown.

capsularis fuses to the decidua vera and then the uterine cavity is obliterated. This is accompanied by growth and enlargement of the amnion. The embryo, which is derived from the inner cell mass of the blastocyst, and the umbilical cord, which originates from extraembryonic mesenchyme, ultimately occupy most of the amniotic cavity (Fig. 12–1).

Septa, composed of folds of the basal plate, then divide the maternal surface of the placenta into 15 to 20 cotyledons. These divisions do not have any physiologic significance. It is the terminal villus that forms the functional unit of the placenta. To facilitate the exchange of nutrients and gases, the terminal villi undergo a series of changes during the gestational period. The terminal villi seen during the first trimester are large, approximately 170 μm in diameter, and have a loose edematous stroma containing small, centrally placed fetal capillaries, stellate mesenchymal cells, and Hofbauer cells. These villi have a double layer of trophoblasts, including an inner layer of cytotrophoblasts and an outer layer of syncytiotrophoblasts (Fig. 12–2). As placental growth proceeds through pregnancy, the villi become smaller. Second trimester villi average approximately 70 μm in diameter. They have a more condensed stromal core containing dilated fetal capillaries that come to occupy an increasingly large proportion of the villous cross-sectional area. The cytotrophoblastic layer becomes a thin discontinuous layer, and the syncytiotrophoblastic nuclei are gathered focally into "syncytial knots." These knots are better defined in the third trimester villi, which are approximately 50 μm in diameter, and the cores are completely overrun by dilated capillaries. Between the syncytial knots, the trophoblastic layer overlying the fetal capillaries

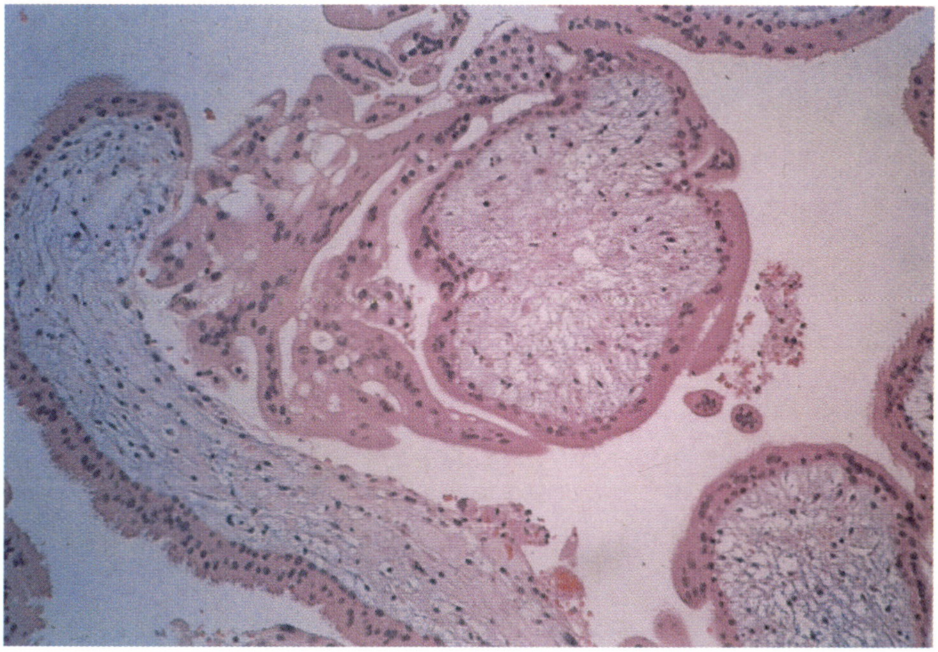

FIGURE 12-2
First trimester chorionic villi with a loose edematous stroma and stellate mesenchymal cells. The villi are surrounded by a double layer of trophoblasts seen best in the lower left corner. There is polar proliferation of the trophoblasts as seen to the left of the villus in the center.

becomes attenuated and anuclear. These are the "vasculosyncytial membranes," which are believed to be important areas for gas transfer.

Morphology

The normal term placenta is an oval or circular disk measuring 15 to 20 cm in diameter and 1.5 to 3 cm in thickness. The placenta with its attached umbilical cord and membranes weighs approximately 450 to 600 gm. The fetal surface is covered by amnion overlying the chorionic plate. The major fetal vessels course over the surface of the chorionic plate with the thick-walled arteries lying superficial to the thin-walled wider veins (Fig. 12–3*A*). The maternal surface is partly subdivided

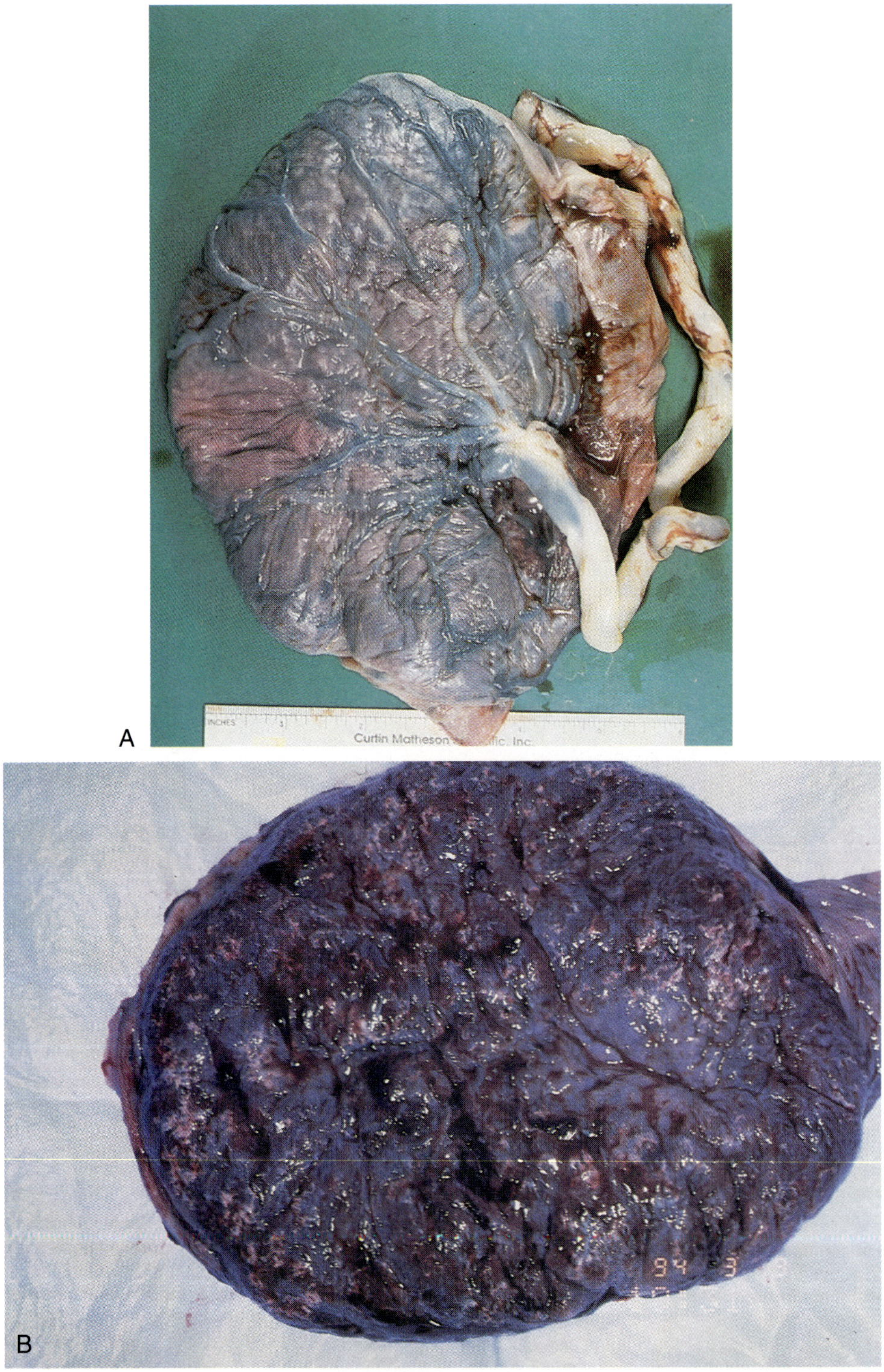

FIGURE 12–3
A, The fetal surface of normal-term placenta is seen. The umbilical cord is attached off center. The shiny amnion covers the placental vessels. *B,* Maternal surface of 32-week placenta is shown.

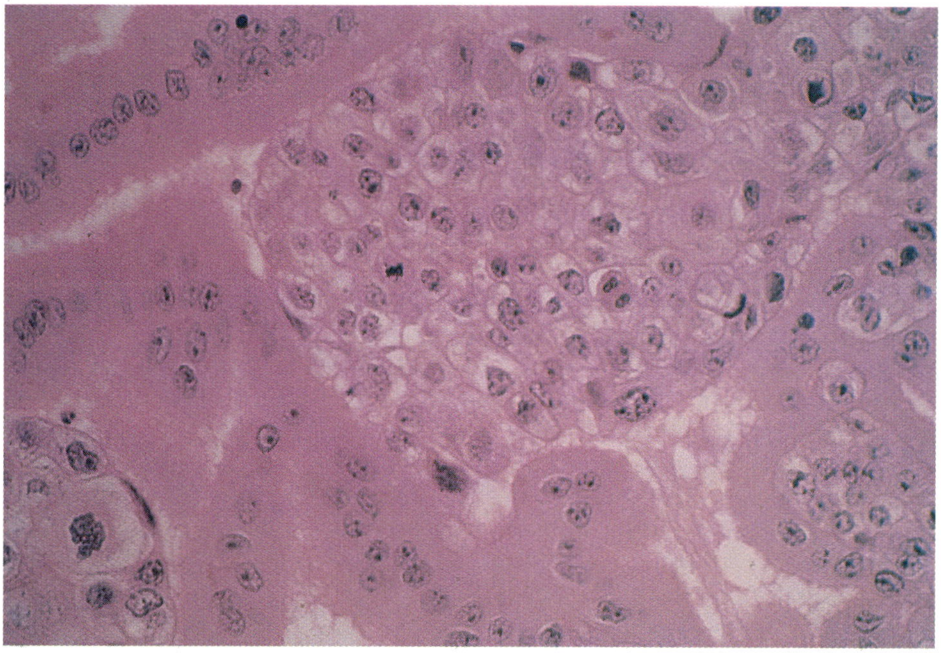

FIGURE 12-4
Cytotrophoblasts are seen in the center of this field. They are polygonal cells with distinct cell borders, clear cytoplasm, and round, large, vesicular nuclei with prominent nucleoli. A mitosis is seen in the central mass of cytotrophoblasts. The syncytiotrophoblasts are seen at the periphery. They are multinucleated cells with glassy, eosinophilic cytoplasm and prominent nucleoli.

into fleshy, maroon cotyledons to which are attached small fragments of maternal decidua (Fig. 12–3*B*).

Cytotrophoblasts are polygonal cells with distinct cell borders, clear cytoplasm, and large round vesicular nuclei. Nucleoli and mitotic activity are prominent, reflecting the undifferentiated germinative nature of the cytotrophoblast (Fig. 12–4). These are functionally inactive cells and do not synthesize any hormones. With immunocytochemical techniques they stain for cytokeratin, which reflects their epithelial nature. The syncytiotrophoblasts are multinucleated and have pyknotic chromatin. There is abundant eosinophilic or amphophilic cytoplasm that contains vacuoles of various sizes caused by infoldings of the surface membrane (see Fig. 12–4). These cells are differentiated and therefore lack mitotic activity. Syncytiotrophoblasts are responsible for most of the hormonal production of the placenta. The intermediate trophoblast, as the name suggests, shows morphologic features of both the cytotrophoblast and the syncytiotrophoblast. They generally are large mononucleate cells that have a spindle to

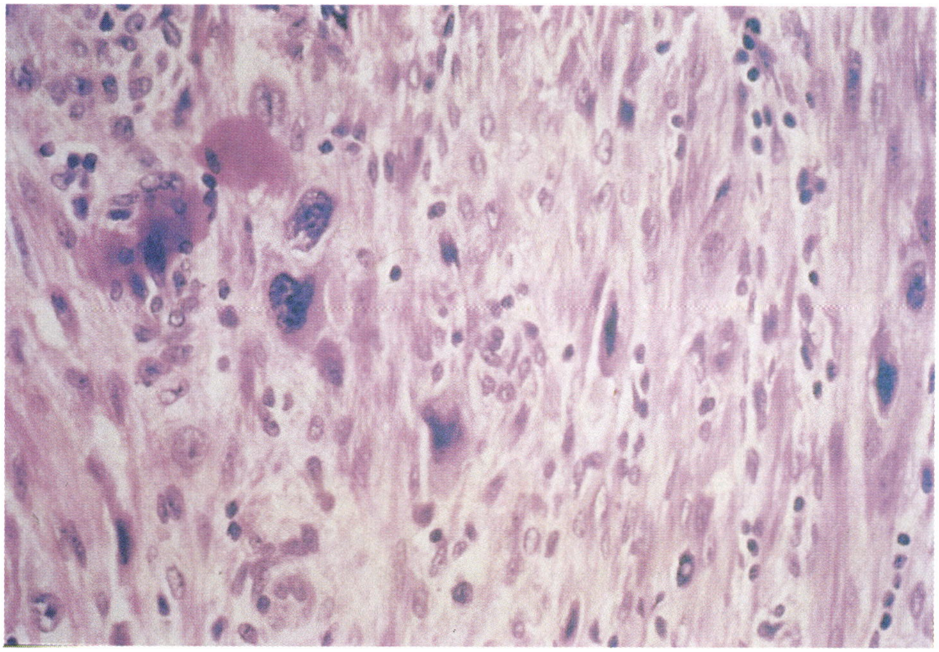

FIGURE 12-5
This is a histologic section of placental site trophoblastic tumor showing a scattering of intermediate trophoblasts between myometrial fibers. The cells are large and polyhedral with opaque eosinophilic cytoplasm and a single hyperchromatic nucleus. Two spindle-cell variants are seen to the right of center.

polyhedral shape. They have abundant eosinophilic to amphophilic cytoplasm without vacuoles. The nuclei of the intermediate trophoblasts are large and more hyperchromatic than those of either the cytotrophoblast or the syncytiotrophoblast (Fig. 12–5).

Both the syncytiotrophoblast and the intermediate trophoblast secrete a variety of enzymes and also steroid and protein hormones, of which hCG and human placental lactogen (hPL) are the most significant. The localization of these hormones in the normal placenta varies with gestational age. Syncytiotrophoblasts contain abundant hCG during the first trimester. By the third trimester hCG is present only focally in these cells. Human placental lactogen is present in small amounts in syncytiotrophoblasts in the first trimester. It steadily increases through gestation so that by term all syncytiotrophoblasts stain for hPL. Intermediate trophoblasts contain small amounts of poorly distributed hCG in the first trimester, which disappears totally as pregnancy advances. These cells also contain hPL, which increases with gestation to reach abundant proportions in the third trimester. The changing pattern of distribution of these hormones during the different stages of placental development suggests that hormone synthesis is linked to trophoblast maturation and may be related to tumorigenesis.[7]

HYDATIDIFORM MOLE

Epidemiology

The incidence of hydatidiform mole in the United States, as estimated by hospital-based studies, is between 1 in 1250 and 1 in 1500 pregnancies, in contrast to a reported incidence of 1 in 200 pregnancies in Mexico and 1 in 100 pregnancies in Indonesia.[8] However, it is believed that in countries where a large proportion of deliveries occur at home or in hospitals that attract GTD referrals from a wide area, there may be an overestimate of the incidence of hydatidiform mole.[9] Population-based studies estimate the incidence of hydatidiform mole as 1 in 900 pregnancies in the United States, 1 in 1666 pregnancies in Sweden, and 1 in 5000 pregnancies in Paraguay.[8] These differences are believed to be due in part to the difference in denominator employed to determine incidence rates in different studies. Compounding the problem is the lack of accurate statistics on the total number of pregnancies during the study period (live births, stillbirths, ectopic pregnancies, induced and spontaneous abortions). Another difficulty is the problem of determining the total number of cases of hydatidiform mole because some cases are terminated by either spontaneous or induced abortion. In a study designed to address these issues, 84,318 cases of elective first- and second-trimester pregnancy terminations were studied.[9] The incidence of hydatidiform mole in the United States was estimated as 1 in 1333 pregnancies. Among many possible risk factors for developing hydatidiform mole, the only one that has been consistently reported is maternal age.[9–11] The risk of a molar pregnancy increases after the age of 39 years.[12] Atrash et al reported an incidence of hydatidiform mole of 1 in 63 pregnancies in women 45 years of age or older.[9] In contrast, the incidence was 1 in 6666 pregnancies in women aged 30 to 34 years. An increased risk of molar gestation is also seen among teenagers.[9–11]

Hydatidiform moles are classified as either complete or partial. The presence of a fetus coexisting with a hydatidiform mole is identified as a partial mole. This is a rare occurrence that has a reported incidence of between 1 in 10,000 and 1 in 100,000 pregnancies.[13] In addition to differences in incidence and morphology between complete moles and partial moles, there are also differences in clinical behavior and pathogenesis. These will be discussed next.

Pathogenesis

Complete Mole

Cytogenetic studies have shown that chromosomal abnormalities play a major role in the development of both complete and partial moles.[14] Most complete moles have a 46,XX androgenic chromosomal complement.[15] This is believed to be the result of a single sperm fertilizing an ovum that is devoid of chromosomal material, the so-called empty egg.[16] After fertilization the paternal chromosomal component duplicates, resulting in a double male haploid set without a maternal chromosomal component (Fig. 12–6). However, gene amplification by polymerase chain reaction has shown that the mitochondrial DNA of complete moles coincides with the maternal mitochondrial DNA.[17] This suggests that the mitochondrial DNA of complete moles is inherited from the ovum.

Approximately 4 percent of complete moles have a 46,XY chromosomal component.[18, 19] By studying Q- and R-banding heteromorphism, HLA polymorphism, and chromosomal markers such as esterase D as well as phosphoglucomutase of the molar stromal cells and the parental peripheral blood lymphocytes, it was determined that these 46,XY

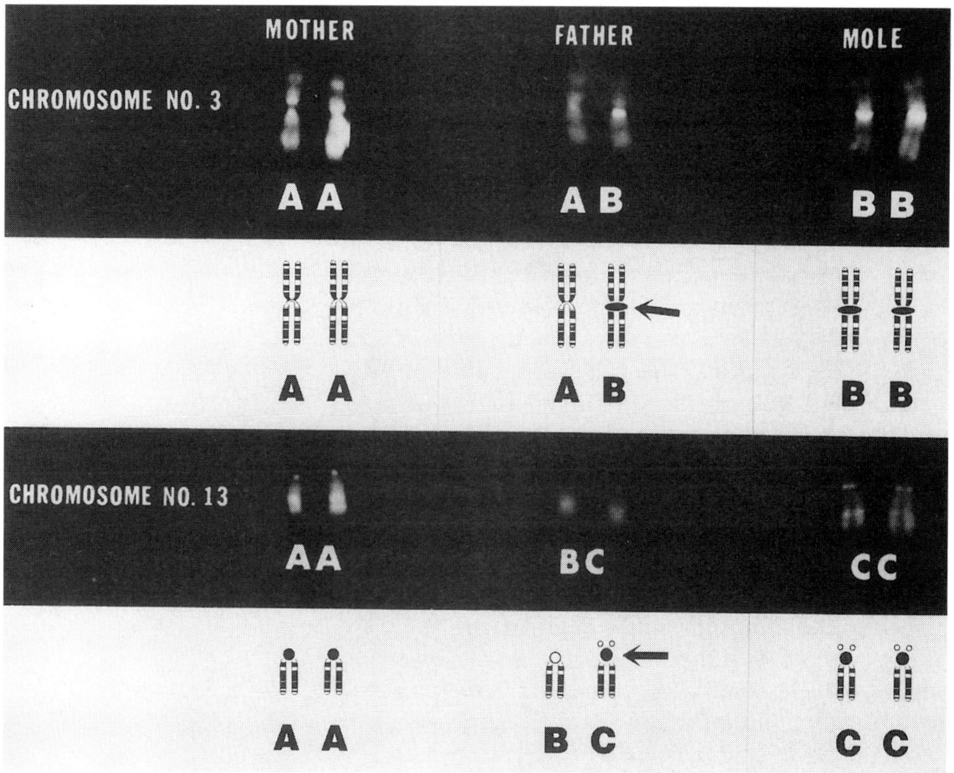

FIGURE 12–6 Chromosomal polymorphism is demonstrated: Banding pattern of chromosome 3 shows that the band *(arrow)* seen on the paternal chromosome and not seen on the maternal chromosome is present in both molar chromosomes. This is the result of one sperm fertilizing an "empty egg" and subsequently duplicating its chromosomal complement. All chromosomes of a complete hydatidiform mole are of paternal (androgenic) origin. The same applies to chromosome 13. (Courtesy of Dr. Urvashi Surti, Magee-Women's Hospital, Pittsburgh, PA.)

moles are usually the result of dispermy, two haploid sperm fertilizing an empty egg. A few dispermic 46,XX complete moles have also been reported.[18, 19] In addition, a few cases of triploid and tetraploid complete mole have been described.[20] The mechanism that appears to be involved in the origin of these moles is fertilization of a normal haploid ovum by three sperm or by two sperm, one of which is diploid. The reported proportion of complete moles that show paternal heterozygosity (fertilization by more than one sperm) ranges from 3 to 13 percent.[20] Moles that have a 46,YY karyotype are never found because at least one X chromosome is essential for cell survival.

Partial Mole

Partial moles are generally triploid and have 69 chromosomes, the extra haploid set being paternal in origin.[21] This may result from dispermy (fertilization of a normal egg by two independent sperm) or fertilization of a normal egg by a sperm with failure of the first meiosis. In the latter case, the paternal chromosomes fail to undergo a reduction division during gametogenesis, and this results in a 46,XY sperm. Fertilization of a 46,XX egg with a normal sperm does not produce a mole.[21]

The hypothesis that diploid partial moles exist has been challenged.[20] Karyotyping of a morphologically typical partial mole as 46,XX may result if the cell culture is overgrown by maternal cells. The presence of a normal fetus with a hydatidiform mole that has a normal karyotype is the result of a twin gestation.[20] The fetus is a product of a normal conception, and there should be an equal number of paternally and maternally derived chromosomes. The mole is a complete one with an androgenic chromosomal complement as described previously. Analysis of cytogenetic markers may clarify these situations.[22]

A case of a triploid molar pregnancy and a diploid normal fetus has been described.[23] This can be explained by the presence of mosaicism confined to the placenta that is the result of a postzygotic mitotic error occurring in the placenta.

DNA fingerprinting has been advanced as a technique that could be used to evaluate the genetic origin of the hydatidiform mole. It would avoid the need to culture fresh tissue for karyotyping.[23a]

Clinical Presentation and Diagnosis

Complete Mole

Vaginal bleeding in the first or early second trimester of gestation is the most frequent symptom in patients who have a hydatidiform mole. Bleeding occurs in almost every case.[24] Preeclampsia and prolonged hyperemesis gravidarum are also common presentations (30 percent of cases).[1, 24] Although pregnancy-induced hypertension typically occurs in the last trimester of a normal gestation, it may occur in the late first or early second trimester in a molar pregnancy. Thyrotoxicosis occurs in a few cases (3 percent).[1] The cause of the thyrotoxicosis is controversial,[25] but some investigators believe that the observed elevation of circulating thyroid hormones is due to the production by the molar tissue of a yet to be isolated thyrotropin.[26] Others believe it to be the result of very high levels of hCG.[25] Similarities between hCG and thyroid-stimulating hormone (TSH) may lead to binding of hCG to the TSH receptors on the thyroid cells. When the hCG level is sufficiently high, significant stimulation of the thyroid could occur, resulting in production of an excessive amount of circulating thyroid hormone. Whatever the explanation, thyrotoxicosis and thyroid storm, although rare, are possible complications of GTD.

The uterus is larger than expected for gestational age, as calculated from the last menstrual period, in approximately half of patients with complete hydatidiform mole.[1, 24, 27] However, the uterus is smaller than expected in one fourth of cases and is consistent with dates in the remaining patients. Spontaneous abortion of complete moles usually occurs at between 16 and 18 weeks of gestation, in contrast to nonmolar spontaneous abortions, which occur between 10 and 12 weeks.[1] In approximately half of the patients the diagnosis of hydatidiform mole is made when the characteristic hydatidiform vesicles (Fig. 12–7) are seen as they are expelled from the uterine cavity.[1, 24] In the absence of this pathognomonic sign, the clinical diagnosis is based on an elevated serum β-hCG level and the typical ultrasonographic findings (Fig. 12–8).

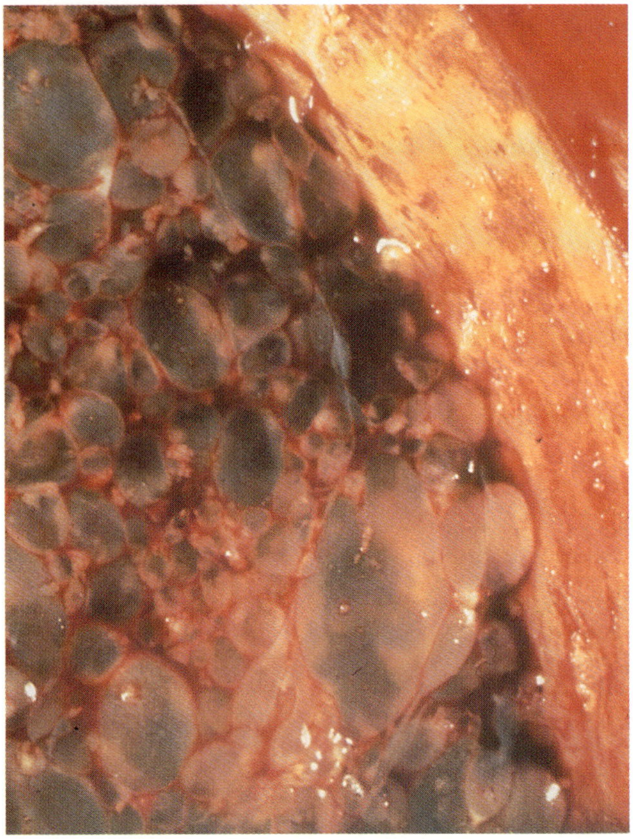

FIGURE 12–7
Complete hydatidiform mole is seen within uterine cavity. Edematous villi are grossly seen as fluid-filled vesicles of varying size (0.5 to 1.5 cm). The mole does not invade the myometrium *(right)*. (From Hernandez E, Rosenshein NB: Manual of Gynecologic Oncology. New York, Churchill Livingstone, 1989.)

Serum β-hCG levels greater than 100,000 mIu/ml are frequently seen in women with complete hydatidiform mole.[28] However, a lower titer does not exclude the diagnosis of a hydatidiform mole, and high levels may occur early in pregnancy in normal twin gestations. The typical sonographic appearance is that of a "snowstorm pattern" as seen with gray scale ultrasound.[29] On real-time ultrasonography the actual hydatidiform vesicles can be seen (see Fig. 12–8). In patients who have a complete mole no fetal parts and no fetal heart can be identified. In 30 to 40 percent of cases theca lutein cysts are present (Fig. 12–9).[28, 29] These are caused by high levels of circulating hCG, which may act like luteinizing hormones (LH), producing ovarian hyperstimulation.[30] Once the clinical diagnosis of hydatidiform mole is made, evacuation of the uterus by suction curettage should be done without delay. Involution of the theca lutein cysts, if present, may take up to 12 weeks after evacuation.[28]

The rare occurrence of a complete mole in an ectopic tubal pregnancy has been reported.[31] A review of the files of the New England Trophoblastic Center identified 2100 patients with GTD, of whom 16 (0.8 percent) had GTD in the fallopian tubes. A complete mole was identified in 5 of the 16 patients who had tubal GTD. Of the other 11, five had a partial mole and six a choriocarcinoma. The five patients with tubal complete mole presented with the classic signs and symptoms of ectopic pregnancy: amenorrhea or irregular vaginal bleeding, abdominal pain, and a positive pregnancy test. None of the patients with tubal GTD had toxemia, hyperemesis, or hyperthyroidism. None had ovarian theca lutein cysts or markedly elevated serum β-hCG titers. One patient with a tubal complete mole developed metastasis. However, all achieved long-term normalization of the serum β-hCG titers.

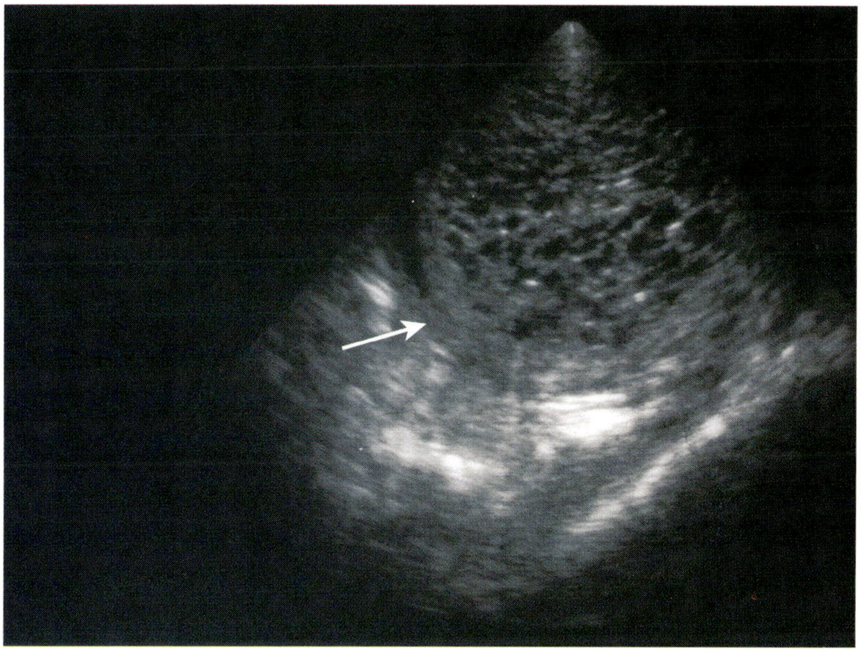

FIGURE 12-8
Real-time ultrasound study of hydatidiform mole shows the edematous villi as multiple hypoechoic (dark) areas within the uterus. An arrow identifies the uterine wall. (Courtesy of Dr. Arnold Friedman, Medical College of Pennsylvania, Philadelphia, PA.)

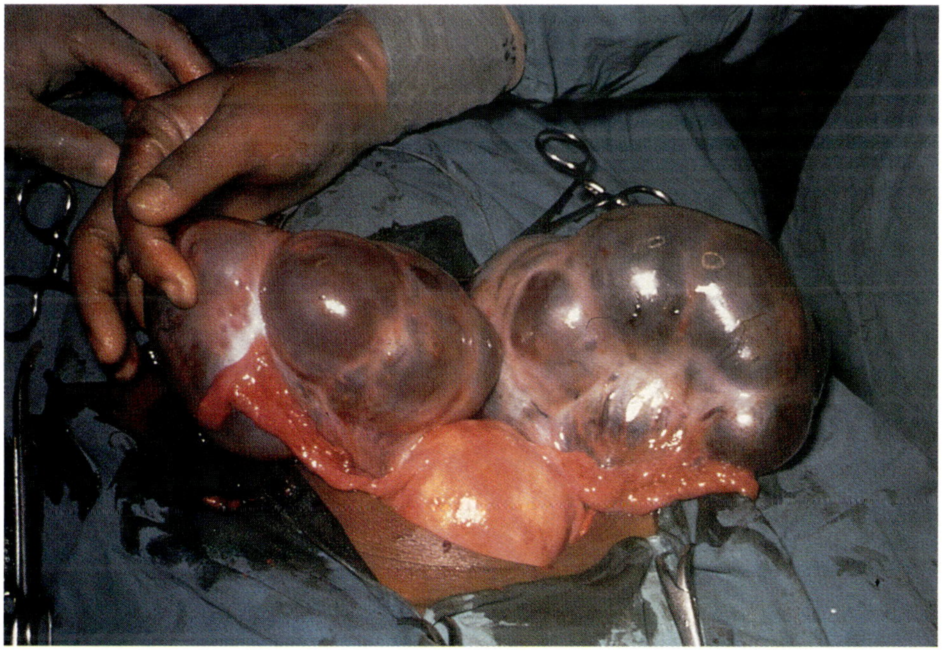

FIGURE 12-9
Intraoperative photograph showing bilateral theca lutein cysts flanking the uterine fundus. Normal fallopian tubes are seen. (Courtesy of Dr. J. Donald Woodruff, The Johns Hopkins Hospital, Baltimore, MD.)

Partial Mole

Partial moles are a rare clinical occurrence.[32] Most patients with partial moles present with vaginal bleeding. Berkowitz et al reported on 81 patients with partial molar pregnancy observed at the New England Trophoblastic Center.[33] Vaginal bleeding was the presenting symptom in 72.8 percent. Pregnancy-induced hypertension occurred in only 2.5 percent. In contrast, at the Magee Womens Hospital 8 percent of patients with partial molar pregnancy and 6 percent with complete mole presented with preeclampsia.[21] Preeclampsia tended to become manifest a month later in patients with partial mole. Berkowitz et al reported no cases of hyperemesis gravidarum and no cases of thyrotoxicosis.[33] Of 55 patients with partial mole reported by Watson et al, one patient was clinically and chemically hyperthyroid.[13] In contrast to complete mole, with partial mole the uterus is larger than expected for gestational age in only 4 to 11 percent of patients (Table 12–1).[21, 33] The uterus is small for gestational age in 65 to 67 percent.[32, 33]

The diagnosis of partial mole is seldom made prior to evacuation of the uterus. The preevacuation clinical diagnosis in most cases is incomplete or missed abortion.[33] The ultrasonographic findings are interpreted as consistent with incomplete or missed abortion in 74 percent of cases. Theca lutein cysts were not identified in 61 patients who had partial mole and who underwent preevacuation ultrasonography.[33] The serum β-hCG levels tend to be lower in women with a partial molar pregnancy than in those with a complete mole.[21] A serum β-hCG titer of greater than 100,000 mIu/ml is seen in only 7 percent of patients with partial mole; in 63 percent the titers are less than 10,000 mIu/ml.[33]

The average gestational age at the time of evacuation of a partial mole is 24 weeks (range, 9 to 40 weeks).[13] The two most common methods of evacuation are induction of uterine contractions with oxytocin or prostaglandins and cervical dilation and uterine curettage. Following evacuation, serial serum β-hCG titers should be obtained because malignant sequelae have been reported in 4 to 14 percent of patients.

Rare cases of a partial mole occurring in an ectopic tubal pregnancy have been reported.[31] Five cases of tubal partial mole were identified in the files of the New England Trophoblastic Center. All patients presented with the classic signs and symptoms of an ectopic pregnancy: amenorrhea or irregular vaginal bleeding, abdominal pain, and a positive pregnancy test. None of the five patients had toxemia, hyperemesis, hyperthyroidism, theca lutein cysts, or markedly elevated serum β-hCG titers. None developed malignant sequelae.

Morphology

A *complete mole* is composed of large amounts of bloody, purple-brown, placental-like tissue (Fig. 12–10). Multiple thin-walled vesicles of varying sizes containing clear fluid are identified, imparting the classic grapelike appearance to the lesion (see Fig. 12–7). The fluid-filled vesicles represent edematous placental villi. The size of the hydropic villi varies with the degree of edema and degenerative changes. Most vesicles measure 1 to 2 cm.[15, 18] The procedure of suction curettage sometimes leads

TABLE 12–1.

General Characteristics of Complete and Partial Hydatidiform Moles

	Complete	*Partial*
Vaginal bleeding	++++	++++
Toxemia	++	++
Hyperthyroidism	+	Rare
β-hCG > 100,000 mIu/ml	+++	+
Large uterus	++	+
Theca lutein cyst	++	−
Vesicles	Generalized	Focal
Fetal parts or membranes	No	Yes
Microscopic	Universal hydropic swelling of villi, trophoblastic hyperplasia and anaplasia, no fetal blood vessels	Focal hydropic swelling of villi and focal trophoblastic hyperplasia, presence of fetal blood vessels, scalloping of villi and trophoblastic inclusions
Karyotype	46,XX/46,XY	69,XXY/69,XXX/69,XYY
Malignant potential	Yes	Yes

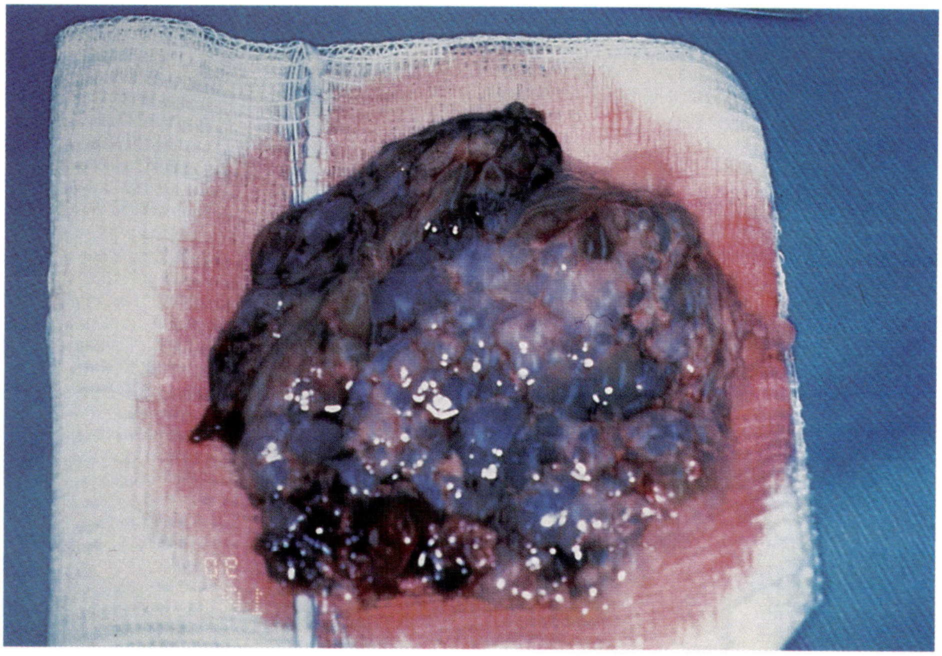

FIGURE 12-10
A suction curettage specimen of a complete hydatidiform mole is seen. Purple-brown, placenta-like tissue with fluid-filled vesicles of varying size. No fetal parts could be identified.

to collapse and distortion of the molar villi. In such situations, the diagnosis is established by histopathologic evaluation of the specimen. No embryo or fetus is present in a complete mole. In rare instances of twin gestation (as described previously), a complete hydatidiform mole and a fetus may coexist.

In cases of *partial mole,* the tissue obtained is less voluminous. The fluid-filled vesicles do not involve the entire placenta. Fetal parts or membranes are frequently present. Their absence does not rule out a partial mole; however, the definitive diagnosis of a partial mole is made by histologic and cytogenetic examination of the tissue.

Complete moles are characterized by (1) varying degrees of hydropic swelling of all the villi and (2) trophoblastic proliferation. The rapid accumulation of fluid in the center of the villi surrounded by maturing mesenchyme leaves hollow spaces known as cisternae. The villi are generally avascular. Small attenuated stromal capillaries lacking nucleated red cells are found in approximately 80 percent of complete moles.[18] Trophoblastic proliferation is variable in degree and may be focal and minimal or marked. On occasion, large sheets of trophoblasts, seemingly unattached to villi, are present. Typically, the trophoblastic proliferation is circumferential with an admixture of cytotrophoblasts, syncytiotrophoblasts, and intermediate trophoblasts haphazardly projecting from the villous surface (Fig. 12–11). The trophoblasts of a hydatidiform mole exhibit varying degrees of cellular anaplasia. An attempt to correlate malignant potential with the degree of trophoblastic hyperplasia and anaplasia has been made.[34, 35] However, at present such an approach is considered unreliable; malignant potential is currently evaluated by carefully monitoring the serum β-hCG regression curve.[36]

The pleomorphism and giant nuclei seen in hydatidiform moles appear to be caused by the process of endomitosis. In this process DNA is duplicated without accompanying nuclear division. Sarto et al identified three types of cells in hydatidiform moles.[37] The smaller cells range in size from 10 to 15 μm. Some of these small cells demonstrate no DNA synthesis, whereas other cells are dividing actively. The intermediate cells measure 15 to 50 μm. These cells are the ones that show active endomitosis by autoradiography. The giant cells have nuclei that exceed 50 μm in diameter. These large nuclei do not undergo mitosis.

No differences have been found between XY and XX complete moles, but differences between younger moles (12 weeks or less of gestational age) and older moles have been described.[18] The younger moles have smaller elliptic or club-shaped villi with numerous secondary villous sprouts. Remnants of mesenchymal capillaries are more frequently found in the younger moles. Also in the younger moles the central cisternae are poorly developed.

Partial moles are generally associated with the presence of a fetus. When fetal demise and degeneration have occurred, identification of fetal structures may be difficult. In these situations the

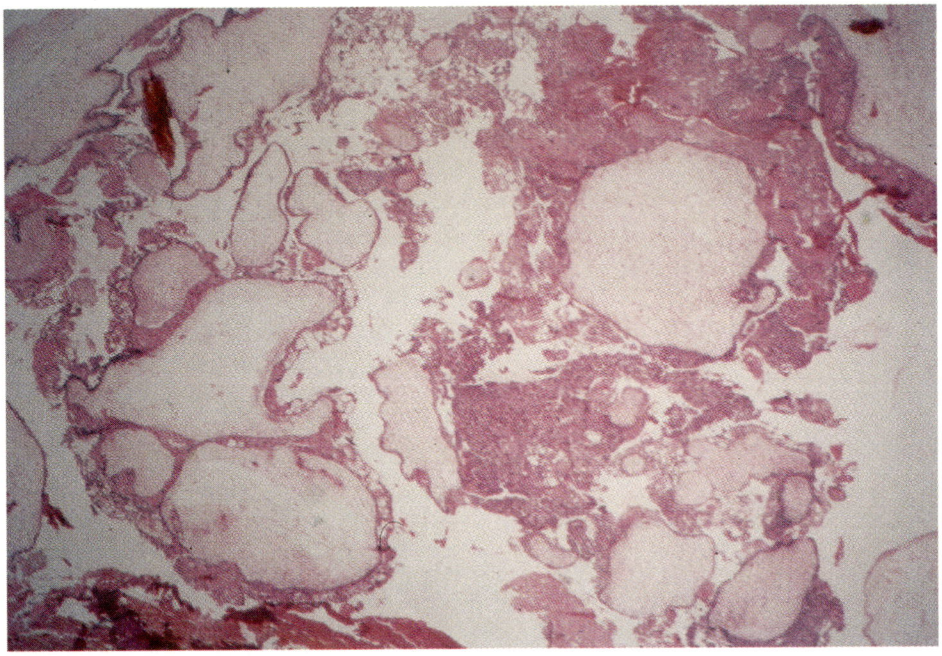

FIGURE 12–11
This is a complete hydatidiform mole showing hydropic villi of varying size with central cisternae. Many of the villi show circumferential trophoblastic proliferation.

presence of villous capillaries containing nucleated red blood cells is indicative of fetal development.[38] Partial moles are characterized by a variable villous morphology.[38] Some of the villi are similar to the large edematous villi encountered in complete moles. The changes are not as pronounced as those seen in complete moles. The central cisternae are less conspicuous, and trophoblastic hyperplasia is focal, with no atypia.[21] Many of these villi have a scalloped border with mesenchymal trophoblastic inclusions (Fig. 12–12). Small and normal sized villi are also present, and there is stromal fibrosis similar to that encountered in missed abortions.[39]

Differential Diagnosis

Both complete and partial moles must be distinguished from hydropic degeneration in an abortus. Spontaneous abortions, particularly those associated with a blighted ovum, have edematous villi lacking blood vessels, and trophoblastic proliferation is present. The villi in nonmolar abortions have less pronounced edema, lack cisternae, and

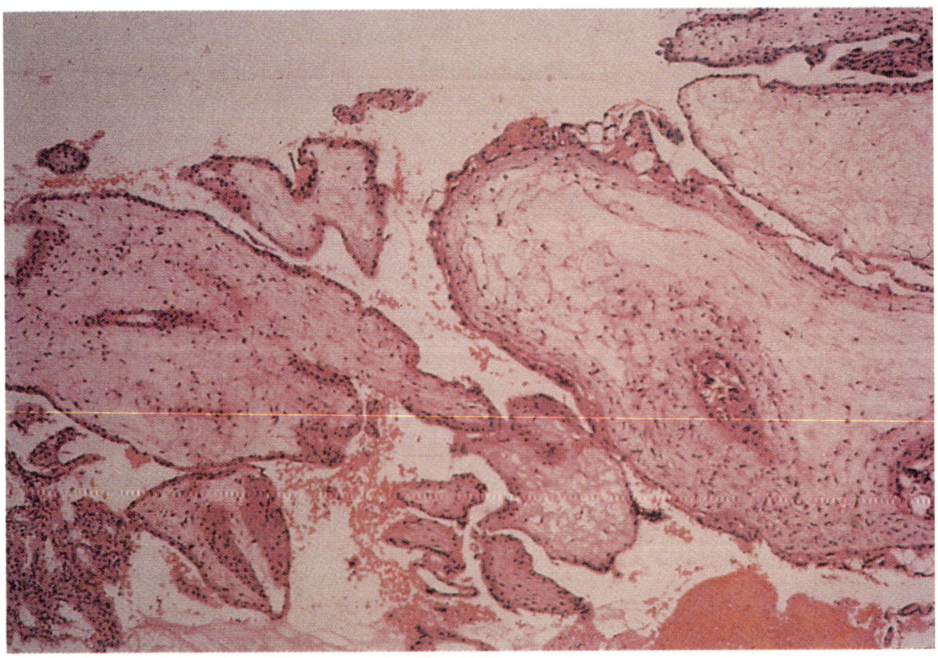

FIGURE 12–12
A histopathologic section of a partial hydatidiform mole is seen. Dilated villi with trophoblasts that appear to be within the mesenchyme are seen (trophoblastic inclusions). This is the result of infoldings (scalloping) of the villous surface as seen in the hydropic villus on the left. Small fibrotic villi are seen *(bottom center)*. (Courtesy of Dr. Ross Berkowitz, Brigham and Women's Hospital, Boston, MA.)

are not macroscopically visible. The trophoblastic proliferation is generally mild and lacks cellular atypia. Nonmolar hydropic villi also lack the scalloping and trophoblastic inclusions of a partial mole. Immunocytochemistry may be helpful in some cases. Placental alkaline phosphatase is focally present in hydropic villi of abortions, but it is present in a diffuse pattern in partial moles.[40]

The trophoblastic hyperplasia of hydatidiform mole must also be distinguished from the proliferative trophoblast of very early pregnancy. In the latter situation the trophoblast proliferates in a polar fashion, growing in the direction of implantation, in contrast to the disorderly circumferential proliferation seen in a hydatidiform mole.

When distinction between complete and partial moles is problematic, cytogenetic studies, flow cytometry, and immunocytochemical techniques may be helpful.[41] In complete moles, hCG staining is uniform and strongly positive whereas placental alkaline phosphatase staining is only focally positive. Partial moles show the reverse staining pattern.[40]

Clinical Management

Following the diagnosis of hydatidiform mole a quantitative serum β-hCG titer and chest radiograph are obtained. The latter is obtained to rule out metastasis and to establish a baseline for future follow-up. If metastasis is found on chest radiography, a diagnosis of metastatic GTD is made and the patient is managed as outlined later. Evacuation of the mole should be performed without undue delay. Evacuation of the complete mole is usually accomplished by dilatation of the cervix and uterine suction curettage. Most partial moles can also be evacuated by suction curettage. However, partial moles are frequently diagnosed late in the second trimester or in the third trimester.[13] These advanced gestations may require induction with prostaglandin or oxytocin to achieve evacuation of the molar gestation safely from the uterus. Although there is a risk of trophoblastic embolization during evacuation by induction of a partial mole, metastatic disease is rarely seen in these patients.[13] If no future childbearing is desired, hysterectomy with the mole in situ could be performed.[1] Trophoblastic cells express Rh-D blood group antigens on their surface membranes. Therefore, previously unsensitized Rh-negative women should receive Rho(D) immune globulin following molar evacuation.[1]

Amniocentesis should be performed if ultrasonography identifies placental changes consistent with a hydatidiform mole and a normal fetus. This may represent a twin gestation. In the presence of a normal fetal karyotype, no evidence of fetal anomalies on ultrasound, and no maternal complications, the pregnancy may be continued until fetal maturity is reached.[13]

After evacuation of the mole, there is a logarithmic drop in serum β-hCG titers, which then become normal by 12 to 15 weeks.[28, 42] Patients should have weekly quantitative serum β-hCG determinations until three to four normal titers are obtained. In most clinical laboratories the normal serum β-hCG titer is reported as less than 3 to 5 mIu/ml. However, it has been demonstrated in vitro that 100,000 trophoblasts produce 1 mIu/ml of β-hCG.[1] Therefore, a significant number of residual trophoblastic cells may still be present when the first normal serum β-hCG titer is obtained. After at least three normal values have been obtained, monthly serum β-hCG titers are obtained for at least 6 months. During the follow-up period the patient should be using reliable contraception, preferably oral contraceptives. Oral contraceptives have not been found to affect the serum β-hCG regression curve.[43, 44] If an elevation in serum β-hCG titer occurs after it has been persistently normal, a pelvic ultrasound should be obtained to rule out a possible normal pregnancy. Repeat molar gestations occur in 0.6 to 2.0 percent of cases.[45] However, patients who have had two molar gestations have a 28 percent chance of having a third.[46]

In 15 to 20 percent of patients with complete mole and in 3 to 11 percent of those with partial mole the serum β-hCG titers reach a plateau or rise.[13, 47, 48, 49] These patients should undergo a thorough search for metastases. Such a search includes a chest radiograph and a computed tomogram of the head, abdomen, and pelvis. If no metastases are found, a diagnosis of nonmetastatic GTD is made. Treatment consists of single-agent chemotherapy with methotrexate or actinomycin D.[50] If the patient is not interested in future childbearing and other indications exist, hysterectomy during the first course of chemotherapy will decrease the number of courses of chemotherapy necessary to achieve remission.[1] Weekly serum β-hCG titers are obtained while the patient is receiving therapy. Chemotherapy is continued for one cycle after a normal serum β-hCG level has been achieved. If the serum β-hCG titers plateau or rise during chemotherapy, the treatment is changed to the alternate drug (i.e., methotrexate or actinomycin D). After three to four normal serum β-hCG titers have been obtained, the patient is followed with monthly serum β-hCG determinations for 1 year. Reliable contraception during treatment and follow-up is mandatory. This therapeutic approach results in a sustained remission or "cure" rate of almost 100 percent.[1] Late recurrences are rare and will occur within 36 months of primary remission.[51] Patients with sustained remission lasting 18 months after primary therapy have a 1 percent risk of subsequent recurrence.[51] Subsequent pregnancies should be evaluated early with ultrasonography to exclude the presence of a recurrent molar gestation. However, those patients who are treated successfully for nonmetastatic malignant GTD can be reassured of a normal reproductive outcome in subsequent conceptions.[52]

If metastases are demonstrated, a diagnosis of metastatic GTD is made. Such a patient is classified as having a good or poor prognosis according to the National Institutes of Health classification (Table 12–2) or as having low-, medium-, or high-risk disease according to the Bagshawe classification as adopted and modified by WHO (Table 12–3).[53] Patients with low-risk or good-prognosis metastatic GTD are treated with single-agent chemotherapy as described for nonmetastatic malignant GTD.

Patients with poor-prognosis metastatic GTD are treated with multiagent chemotherapy. One of the most popular regimens consists of a combination of methotrexate, actinomycin D, and cyclophosphamide (MAC).[50] Patients with high-risk disease according to the WHO classification should be considered for a more intensive regimen.[53] The combination of etoposide, methotrexate, and actinomycin D given in week 1, followed by vincristine (Oncovin) and cyclophosphamide given in week 2, (EMA/CO regimen) has been shown to be highly effective. Cisplatin-based regimens have been successfully used for salvage therapy.[54] Chemotherapy is continued for two courses past achievement of a normal serum β-hCG titer. Patients with brain metastasis receive whole brain irradiation and high-dose corticosteroids in conjunction with chemotherapy.[55] Patients with liver metastasis are considered for whole liver irradiation.[56] Follow-up consists of periodic physical examinations and monthly serum β-hCG determinations for 1 year, one every 3 months during the second year after remission, and one every 6 months thereafter.[50] Subsequent pregnancies should be evaluated by early ultrasound examination.

The cure rate for patients with good-prognosis metastatic GTD approaches 100 percent and is 70 percent for patients in the poor-prognosis category.[1, 57, 58] However, the survival of patients with liver metastasis is only 13 to 33 percent, and only 25 to 50 percent of patients with brain metastases survive.[55, 56, 59, 60] Modern aggressive combination chemotherapy may now result in achievement of sustained remissions in almost all patients in the poor-prognosis category.[54] Patients with poor-prognosis metastatic GTD who do not respond to initial single-agent chemotherapy have a 14 percent chance of sustained remission with subsequent multiagent chemotherapy.[58, 61] This underscores

TABLE 12–2.

National Institute of Health Classification of Gestational Trophoblastic Disease

I. Nonmetastatic disease: no evidence of disease outside of uterus

II. Metastatic disease: any disease outside of uterus
   - A. Good prognosis
     1. Short duration (last pregnancy < 4 months)
     2. Low pretreatment serum β-hCG liter titer (< 40,000 mIu/ml)
     3. No metastasis to brain or liver
     4. No significant prior chemotherapy
   - B. Poor prognosis*
     1. Long duration (last pregnancy > 4 months)
     2. High pretreatment serum β-hCG titer (> 40,000 mIu/ml)
     3. Brain or liver metastasis
     4. Significant prior chemotherapy
     5. Disease following term pregnancy

* The presence of any one of these classifies the patient in the poor-prognosis category.

TABLE 12–3.

World Health Organization Classification of Gestational Trophoblastic Disease

	Score			
Prognostic Factor	*0*	*1*	*2*	*4*
Age (years)	< 39	> 39	—	—
Antecedent pregnancy	Mole	Abortion	Term	—
Interval (months) between end of antecedent pregnancy and start of chemotherapy	< 4	4–6	7–12	—
β-hCG (mIU/ml)	$< 10^3$	$10^3–10^4$	$10^4–10^5$	$> 10^5$
ABO groups (female × male)	—	O × A A × O	B AB	—
Largest tumor, including uterine	—	3–5 cm	> 5 cm	—
Site of metastases	—	Spleen Kidney	GI tract Liver	Brain
No. metastases	—	1–4	4–8	> 8
Prior chemotherapy	—	—	Single drug	≥ 2 more drugs

Total score: Low risk = 0–4; Medium risk = 5–7; High risk = 8 or higher. Modified from Bagshawe KD: Treatment of high-risk choriocarcinoma. J Reprod Med 1984; 29: 813–820.

TABLE 12–4.
FIGO Staging of Gestational Trophoblastic Disease

Stage I	Confined to the uterus
Stage II	Limited to the genital structures
Stage III	Lung metastases
Stage IV	Other metastases
	A. No risk factors
	B. One risk factor
	C. Two risk factors

Risk Factors:
1. Serum β-hCG greater than 100,000 mIu/ml
2. Duration of disease greater than 6 months

the need for immediate, adequate, and aggressive chemotherapy in patients who have high-risk disease.

The official staging of malignant GTD as approved by the International Federation of Gynecology and Obstetrics (FIGO) is presented in Table 12–4.[53] Although this classification is used to report and compare international survival data, it is not routinely used in the United States to guide therapy.[53]

INVASIVE MOLE

Clinical Presentation and Diagnosis

This lesion, at one time called chorioadenoma destruens, can complicate a partial or complete hydatidiform mole. Confirmation of the clinical diagnosis of invasive mole requires the identification of molar villi invading the myometrium or vascular spaces or the identification of metastasis in a patient with histologically confirmed hydatidiform mole. The first situation requires a hysterectomy in order to make this diagnosis and this procedure is seldom necessary for the treatment of GTD. Therefore, the diagnosis of invasive mole is seldom histopathologically confirmed, and the true incidence of this condition is not known. Some authors suggest that invasive mole constitutes 15 percent of GTD.[1] However, this figure includes patients with hydatidiform mole who have persistent elevation of β-hCG titers and in whom choriocarcinoma is not diagnosed. This is probably a good estimate of the incidence because Hammond et al[57] found disease in the myometrium in over 90 percent of women undergoing a hysterectomy for nonmetastatic malignant GTD. This report included 17 women with nonmetastatic malignant GTD who underwent elective hysterectomy as well as 13 women who had failed chemotherapy and underwent "secondary" hysterectomy. This second group was at higher risk of having intramyometrial disease that was inaccessible to systemic chemotherapy.

In patients with nonmetastatic malignant GTD who are unresponsive to systemic chemotherapy and in whom uterine preservation is desired, the identification of GTD in the myometrium can be made by angiography or by duplex ultrasonography.[57,62,63]

Occasionally, an invasive mole invades as far as the serosa of the uterus, and the patient presents with signs and symptoms of hemoperitoneum. These patients require immediate abdominal exploration and hysterectomy. Even if a patient wishes a future pregnancy, hysterectomy is necessary if other techniques (e.g., uterine artery ligation) fail to control the bleeding.

Morphology

The gross appearance of the invasive mole is similar to that described for noninvasive hydatidiform mole except that hemorrhagic invasion of villi into the myometrium has occurred (Fig. 12–13). This invasion of the myometrium by the molar tissue may be very superficial or may extend deep into the uterine wall, leading to perforation and involvement of the broad ligament and adnexa. Due to the destructive nature of this lesion and the smaller size of the villi, the molar vesicles may not always be grossly apparent.

The histopathologic diagnosis of invasive mole is made when there is destructive invasion of the myometrium or extrauterine sites by villi and trophoblasts. The hydropic villi of the invasive mole are smaller than those of its noninvasive counterpart. They measure 2 to 4 mm in diameter on average. The trophoblastic hyperplasia and cellular anaplasia range from mild to marked. Invasive mole can involve extrauterine sites, most notably the vagina, vulva, and lungs.[1] In both uterine and extrauterine sites the molar villi may not be identified if they are overshadowed by marked trophoblastic hyperplasia. If no villi are identified at any of the examined sites (uterine or extrauterine) a diagnosis of choriocarcinoma is appropriate, but to avoid misclassifying the lesion it is essential to sample all tissue extensively using serial sectioning in an effort to identify the villi. Currently, there is no difference in the clinical management of patients with invasive mole and those with choriocarcinoma. In extrauterine sites the lesion characteristically demonstrates molar villi within the lumens of blood vessels, and invasion into the adjoining parenchyma is absent. Be-

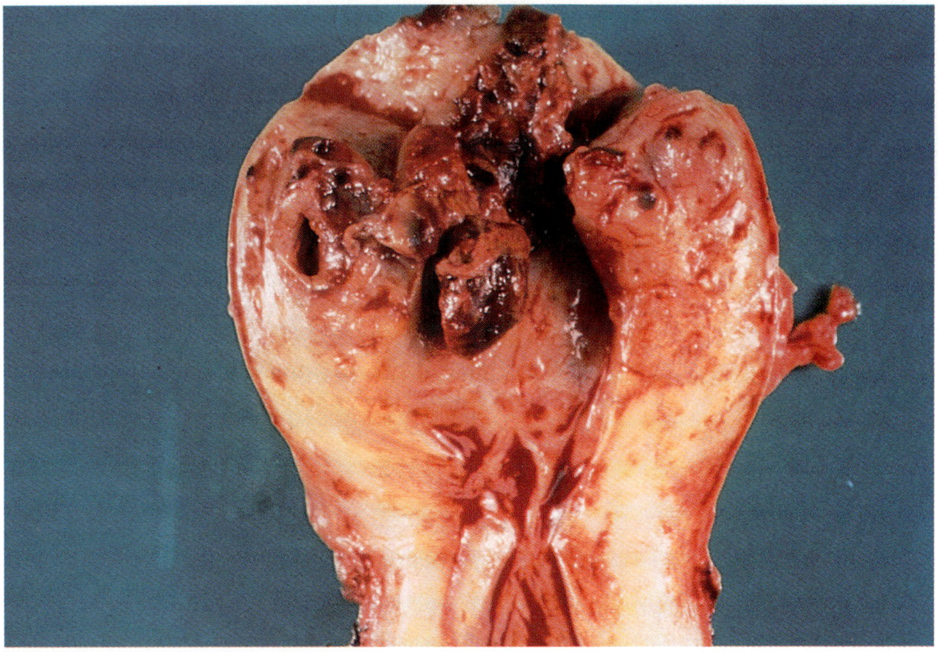

FIGURE 12-13
This hysterectomy specimen has a partial hydatidiform mole invading the myometrium of the fundus on both sides. The invasive process is poorly circumscribed and hemorrhagic. No fetal parts are seen.

cause of this property the extrauterine lesions are considered "deportation lesions" rather than metastases.

Differential Diagnosis

Invasive moles should be distinguished from abnormalities in placental implantation such as placenta increta or percreta, exaggerated placental site reaction, noninvasive hydatidiform moles, and choriocarcinoma. In placenta increta or percreta the cardinal feature is absence of the decidua basalis and adherence of the villi directly to the myometrium. The chorionic villi lack the hydropic change characteristic of an invasive mole. An exaggerated placental site reaction can be difficult to distinguish from invasive mole, particularly if the invasive mole has scant villi that are difficult to identify. Exaggerated placental site reaction is characterized by extensive trophoblastic invasion of both the endometrium and the myometrium by intermediate and syncytiotrophoblastic cells. Molar villi generally do not invade the myometrium as invasive moles do. In noninvasive hydatidiform moles sections of the myometrium lack the presence of molar villi within the muscle or blood vessels. As mentioned previously, if the tissue is sampled extensively and villi are identified, invasive moles will not be misdiagnosed as choriocarcinoma.

Clinical Management

When a pathologic diagnosis of invasive mole is rendered, the patient should undergo a careful search for metastasis. This includes a complete and thorough medical history and physical examination, chest radiograph, and computed tomography of the head, abdomen, and pelvis. Laboratory studies include a hemogram, liver profile, serum chemistries, and a quantitative serum β-hCG. If no metastases are identified, nonmetastatic GTD is diagnosed and the patient is treated with single-agent chemotherapy (e.g., methotrexate, actinomycin D) as described earlier for patients with persistent hydatidiform mole (i.e., plateauing or rising β-hCG titers).

The presence of invasive mole deep in the myometrium may serve as a sanctuary site that is protected from the chemotherapy. Frequently, after the initial drop in serum β-hCG titers the titers plateau or begin to rise. Angiography or duplex ultrasonography can be used to identify persistent disease in the myometrium.[57, 62, 63] When systemic chemotherapy fails, intraarterial chemotherapy instilled directly into the uterine arteries has been used with limited success.[57] Hysterectomy is usually necessary to achieve a cure in these situations.[57]

If a patient with invasive mole has extrauterine metastasis, a diagnosis of metastatic GTD is made. The disease is classified and treated as described earlier in this chapter.

CHORIOCARCINOMA

Epidemiology

The true incidence of choriocarcinoma is difficult to ascertain. Population studies are fraught with the same methodologic problems as those described for hydatidiform mole. The reported incidence of gestational choriocarcinoma throughout the world varies from 1 in 50,000 pregnancies in some countries in Latin America and Europe to 1 in 5000 in South Asia.[8] In the United States an incidence of 1 in 20,000 to 1 in 33,000 pregnancies has been reported.[8] The histologic confirmation of choriocarcinoma is not considered clinically necessary in cases of metastatic GTD, and when metastases are identified during follow-up of a patient with hydatidiform mole it is assumed that it represents a choriocarcinoma.[34, 64] It is accepted that approximately 3 percent of patients with hydatidiform mole develop choriocarcinoma.[1, 10] In most cases this assumption is probably true because histologic evaluation of the metastatic sites in patients being followed for hydatidiform mole has shown choriocarcinoma.[65, 66]

Most cases of gestational choriocarcinoma occur after a hydatidiform mole. As in patients with hydatidiform mole, advanced maternal age is associated with an increased incidence of choriocarcinoma.[10] A weaker association has been cited with particular ABO blood groups and with some dietary factors.[12, 67–69] Buckley pooled the data from nine studies from the international literature that had a total of 588 patients with choriocarcinoma.[10] Hydatidiform mole was the antecedent pregnancy in 57 percent, an abortion in 17 percent, and a normal pregnancy in 26 percent. Occasionally a choriocarcinoma is associated with an ectopic pregnancy.[31, 70] The John I. Brewer Trophoblastic Disease Center reported that choriocarcinoma associated with ectopic pregnancy constituted 4 percent of their patients receiving chemotherapy for choriocarcinoma.[70] In the United States approximately 50 percent of gestational choriocarcinomas are preceded by a molar pregnancy, 25 percent by a spontaneous abortion, 22 percent by a pregnancy delivered at term, and 3 percent by an ectopic pregnancy.[1] About 1 of every 40 hydatidiform moles is followed by choriocarcinoma, and approximately 1 of every 160,000 term deliveries is followed by choriocarcinoma. The incidence of choriocarcinoma associated with an ectopic pregnancy is 1 in 5333, but it is 1 in 15,386 following a spontaneous abortion.[70, 71] The time interval between the antecedent pregnancy and metastatic GTD (i.e., choriocarcinoma) is usually a few months to 2 years; however, longer intervals have been reported.[53]

A very early unrecognized spontaneous abortion may explain cases of choriocarcinoma with no history of a previous gestation. Additional cases of choriocarcinoma unrelated to pregnancy, germ cell tumors, or teratomas have been described. These are believed to arise from a poorly differentiated carcinoma or to develop as carcinoma with trophoblastic differentiation.[72]

Pathogenesis

The pathogenesis of choriocarcinoma is not as well understood as that of hydatidiform mole. Karyotype analysis of choriocarcinoma is variable because there are frequent chromosomal changes in malignant cells. A change in chromosome number, gain or loss of parts of chromosomes, or chromosome rearrangements can occur.[73, 74] DNA analysis by restriction fragment length polymorphisms (RFLP) has helped to elucidate the pathogenesis of choriocarcinoma and has been useful in differentiating gestational from nongestational choriocarcinoma.[74] By using RFLP techniques the genome of choriocarcinoma has been shown to reflect that of the pregnancy of origin.[74, 75] Choriocarcinoma that arises from a hydatidiform mole contains DNA of paternal origin only, whereas choriocarcinoma that arises from a normal pregnancy contains both paternal and maternal DNA.[74, 75] When only maternal DNA is identified, it is believed to represent a nongestational choriocarcinoma.[74]

Clinical Presentation and Diagnosis

A frequent clinical presentation of choriocarcinoma is abnormal uterine bleeding.[76] If the lesion is confined to the myometrium or if the primary tumor in the uterus undergoes regression, the patient may be asymptomatic and the first indication of choriocarcinoma may be symptoms related to the blood-borne metastases.[77] The most frequent metastatic sites identified clinically are the lungs, vagina, brain, liver, gastrointestinal tract, and spleen.[78–81] A few cases of maternal choriocarcinoma with metastases to the fetus have been reported.[82] Patients with pulmonary metastases may present with hemoptysis or respiratory distress.[83] Computed tomography was able to identify micrometastases in 41 percent of patients in whom no metastasis was identified by routine chest radiograph.[84] Jaundice and right upper quadrant pain are often the presenting symptoms in the presence of liver metastases. Headaches, focal neurologic deficits or dysfunction, decreased sensorium, seizures, or even coma may occur in patients with brain metastases.[55, 65] Gastrointestinal or genitourinary bleeding are the presenting complaints with intestinal or renal metastases. The clinician caring for women in the reproductive age group must consider choriocarcinoma in the differential diagnosis of a woman with any of these symptoms

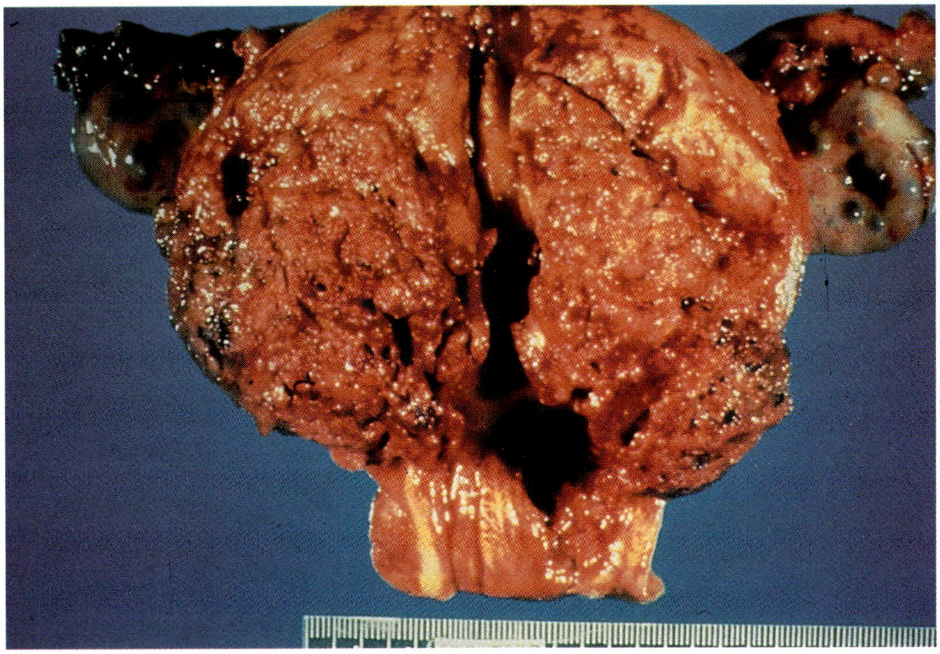

FIGURE 12–14
This hysterectomy specimen shows a large, fleshy, shaggy mass deeply invading the myometrium through to the serosa. This is the gross appearance of a gestational choriocarcinoma.

and a positive pregnancy test. Extrapulmonary metastases rarely occur in the absence of lung metastases.[53]

If a patient with hydatidiform mole is followed closely, the diagnosis of choriocarcinoma can be made before the patient becomes symptomatic. A rise or plateau in serum β-hCG titers should trigger a search for metastases. If metastases are found, a diagnosis of metastatic GTD (i.e., choriocarcinoma) is made, and appropriate therapy is then instituted. Histologic confirmation in this situation is not deemed necessary.

Morphology

Uterine choriocarcinoma is a hemorrhagic, dark red, irregular fleshy, shaggy mass that infiltrates and destroys the myometrium (Fig. 12–14). The size of the lesion can vary and ranges from a microscopic tumor to a very large mass. Extrauterine

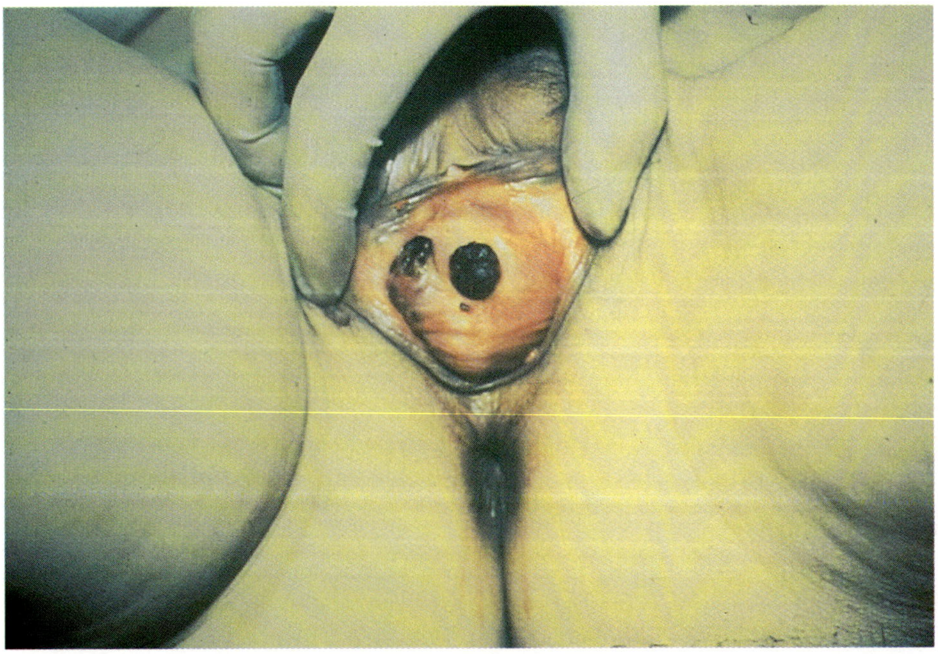

FIGURE 12–15
Choriocarcinoma metastatic to lower genital tract. Well-defined blue-black nodules with smaller satellite lesions are seen. (From Hernandez E, Rosenshein NB: Manual of Gynecologic Oncology. New York, Churchill Livingstone, 1989.)

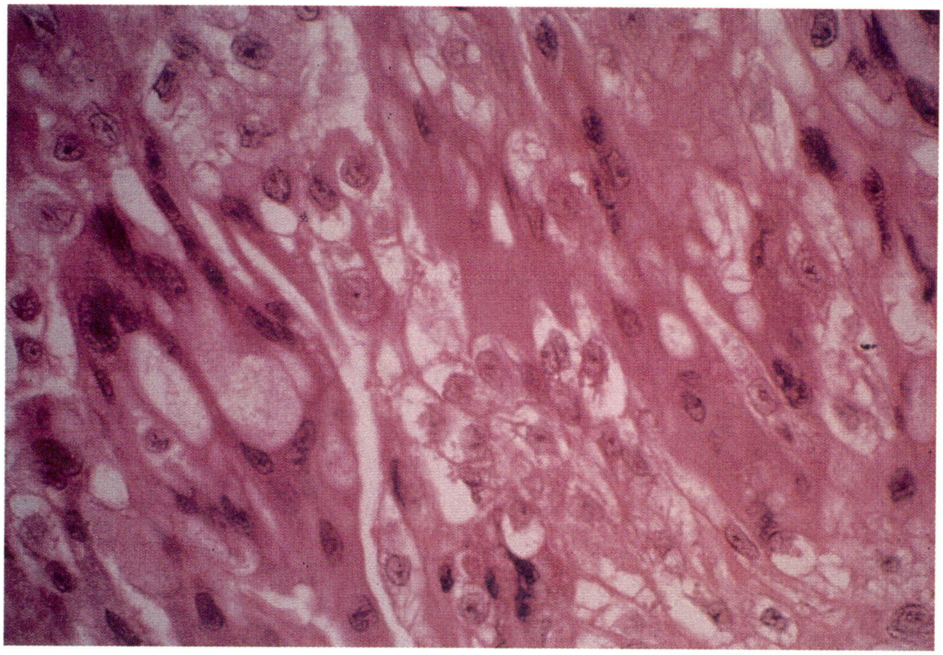

FIGURE 12–16
This illustrates a diphasic pattern of choriocarcinoma. There is a mix of cyto- and syncytiotrophoblasts. The cytotrophoblasts have clear cytoplasm and distinct cytoplasmic outlines. The cytoplasm of the syncytiotrophoblasts stains eosinophilic. The syncytiotrophoblasts on the left are forming lacunae where red blood cells are found.

metastases are generally well circumscribed and hemorrhagic. In the vagina, blue-black irregular nodules with well-defined borders and satellite lesions are seen (Fig. 12–15). They tend to bleed profusely if biopsy is performed. On chest radiograph pulmonary metastases most often appear as multiple discrete nodules, although fluffy alveolar opacities have also been described.[85]

The pattern of trophoblastic growth in choriocarcinoma recapitulates the primitive trophoblast (previllous) of the implanting blastocyst. The classic histologic pattern is described as "diphasic" with islands and sheets of cytotrophoblasts interspersed with syncytiotrophoblasts and scattered intermediate trophoblasts (Fig. 12–16). Variant patterns of growth have also been described, e.g., a focal overgrowth of one of the cell types.[66] Choriocarcinoma generally does not have an intrinsic vascular stroma. The tumor grows rapidly and invades the surrounding tissue, thereby gaining access to the host's blood supply. The syncytiotrophoblast does this by permeating and replacing the uterine vessels. The lesion is therefore characterized by sheets of alternating trophoblasts on a background of hemorrhage (Fig. 12–17). Chorionic villi are not a component of choriocarcinoma, and

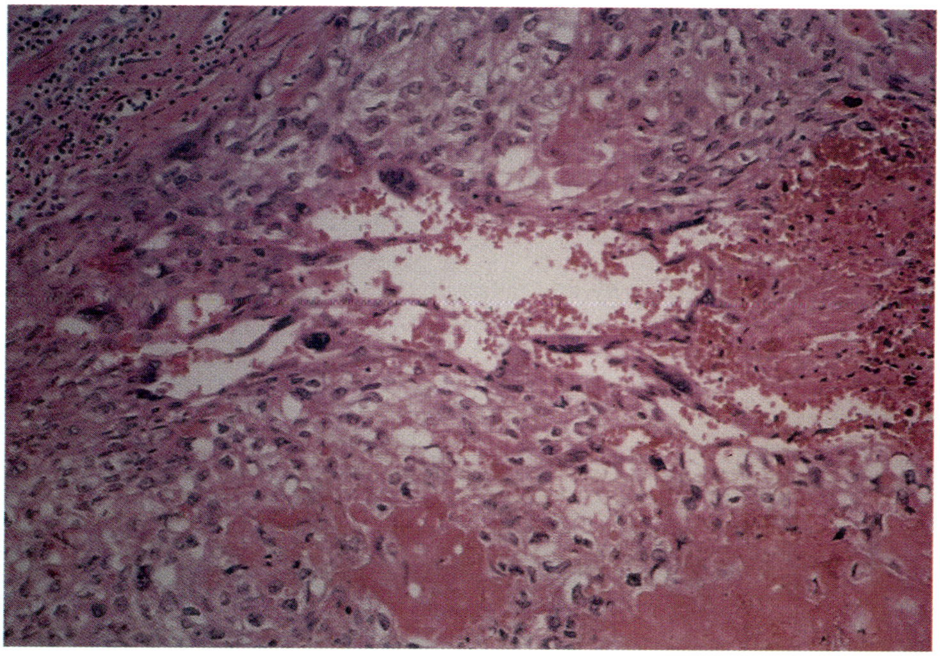

FIGURE 12–17
A photomicrograph of gestational choriocarcinoma shows sheets of cytotrophoblasts interspersed with syncytiotrophoblasts. Hemorrhage and red blood cells filled spaces lined by trophoblasts *(center)*. Myometrial fibers with an inflammatory infiltrate are seen *(upper left)*.

their presence negates this diagnosis. In rare cases in which the choriocarcinoma develops during a normal gestation, it arises from the trophoblasts covering the normal placental villi.[86]

All three trophoblastic cell types encountered in choriocarcinoma may show varying degrees of cytologic atypia. Nuclear pleomorphism and hyperchromasia vary from mild to marked. Nucleoli vary from insignificant to prominent. The typical appearance of the trophoblasts is also altered by cytotoxic therapy.[66] The syncytiotrophoblast often becomes small and dark, and the nucleus becomes pyknotic. The treated cytotrophoblast may have indistinct cell borders and irregular nuclei.

Immunocytochemical studies for hCG and hPL may be helpful in recognizing the characteristic diphasic pattern.[87] The syncytiotrophoblasts are strongly positive for hCG and weakly positive for hPL, whereas the intermediate trophoblasts are variably positive for hCG and hPL. Cytotrophoblasts do not stain for hCG or hPL. Because of the propensity of this tumor to undergo extensive hemorrhage and necrosis, only scant amounts of viable tumor may be present at the periphery, and multiple sections may be necessary to find the diagnostic trophoblastic cells.

Differential Diagnosis

Although the majority of choriocarcinomas have the typical diphasic pattern, variations exist. Occasionally there is focal overgrowth of one of the cell types.[66] When this involves cytotrophoblasts or intermediate trophoblasts, the lesion may mimic a poorly differentiated carcinoma. Spindle cell variants of intermediate trophoblasts can resemble sarcomas. In such situations, extensive sampling usually reveals the characteristic diphasic nature of the lesion. In addition, immunocytochemical localization, particularly of syncytiotrophoblasts, will confirm the correct diagnosis.

Trophoblastic proliferation of choriocarcinoma must also be distinguished from that seen in molar and early normal gestations. The presence of villi in these latter two situations makes it relatively easy to distinguish them from choriocarcinoma. On the other hand, when uterine curettings show no chorionic villi and only trophoblastic tissue, the differential diagnosis must include both choriocarcinoma and an incomplete abortion in which the villi had been passed prior to the curettage. Histologic features that favor choriocarcinoma in such situations include extensive trophoblastic proliferation with the typical diphasic pattern, significant cytologic atypia, and tumor necrosis with hemorrhage. Serum β-hCG levels, the previous obstetric history, and the presence of extrauterine lesions also aid in establishing the correct diagnosis.

Metastatic choriocarcinoma must be distinguished from invasive moles with deportation of trophoblasts to extrauterine sites. If the metastatic lesion contains chorionic villi or if the trophoblasts lack the diphasic pattern or consist almost entirely of intermediate trophoblasts, a diagnosis of invasive mole is supported. Choriocarcinoma must also be differentiated from the nongestational choriocarcinoma of germ cell origin. Fortunately, in its pure form the latter is very rare. More often, it is one component of a mixed germ cell tumor, and identification of the other germ cell elements resolves the problem. The differentiation of choriocarcinoma from placental site trophoblastic tumor will be discussed in the next section. The differential diagnosis at metastatic sites also includes primary carcinomas of organs such as the bladder, breast, liver, and gastrointestinal tract with choriocarcinomatous differentiation. Generally, multiple sections will reveal the histology of the primary tumor. In poorly differentiated carcinomas with tumor giant cells that mimic syncytiotrophoblast, immunoreactivity for hCG can be used to establish the diagnosis of choriocarcinoma.[88]

Clinical Management

The therapy of the patient with gestational choriocarcinoma is dictated by the presence or absence of metastases and whether the metastatic disease is considered low or high risk. Therefore, when a histologic diagnosis of choriocarcinoma is made, a thorough search for metastases is undertaken, and the disease is classified as previously described for patients with persistent hydatidiform mole (i.e., plateauing or rising β-hCG titers). However, it should be clear that the therapy is not dictated by the histologic type of GTD but by the clinical classification. There have been some reports that correlate morphology with therapeutic response.[89] Choriocarcinoma with little syncytiotrophoblastic differentiation appears to have a worse prognosis. The therapy for good-prognosis metastatic GTD is the same whether the pathologic diagnosis is invasive mole or choriocarcinoma. The treatment of malignant GTD was discussed in some detail in the previous section on the clinical management of hydatidiform mole. In the treatment of malignant GTD, resistant focal disease may be curable by surgical excision and further chemotherapy.[90, 91] With the advent of chemotherapy, the prognosis of choriocarcinoma has improved dramatically, and survival rates are now over 90 percent.[92] Mortality from choriocarcinoma is related to hemorrhage at metastatic sites (e.g., lung, liver, brain) and the adverse effects of chemotherapy.

PLACENTAL SITE TROPHOBLASTIC TUMOR

Clinical Profile

PSTT is a rare form of GTD that can follow or complicate any type of pregnancy.[93–97] The relationship to the previous gestation is uncertain because the interval between the last documented pregnancy and the diagnosis of PSTT ranges from weeks to years, with one reported case occurring 18 years after the last known pregnancy.[94, 97] This is a disease of the reproductive years. Most patients are in their twenties or thirties at the time of diagnosis.[93, 94, 96, 97] Two cases that occurred in postmenopausal women have been reported.[97] Patients with PSTT usually present with amenorrhea accompanied by uterine enlargement. Normal pregnancy is simulated, and if a sensitive immunologic assay is employed, the pregnancy test may be positive.[98] Abnormal vaginal bleeding is the most frequent presenting symptom.[94, 97] Virilization, polycythemia, and nephrotic syndrome are other presenting symptoms reported with PSTT.[94, 97]

The pathogenesis of this rare but interesting form of GTD is not clearly understood. It is a neoplasm composed predominantly of intermediate trophoblasts and generally follows a benign course but has the potential to be highly malignant. The morphology of this neoplasm recapitulates the normal infiltration of the intermediate trophoblast at the implantation site as discussed in the section on embryology.[100] The intermediate trophoblast is also known as the extravillous trophoblast—hence the earlier name of trophoblastic "pseudotumor" to describe the entity.[100] The immunocytochemical distribution of hCG and hPL is similar in both the normal implantation site and PSTT. The increased staining for hPL relative to hCG in PSTT is the opposite of the situation encountered in choriocarcinoma and suggests that PSTT does not arise from as primitive a cell as choriocarcinoma. This probably accounts for its more benign behavior. The serum β-hCG titers are elevated but are usually less than 1000 mIu/ml.[94, 97] Although some authors have advocated the measurement of serum hPL titers for the diagnosis and follow-up of this disease, serum hPL is frequently undetectable in these patients.[93,97]

Morphology

The gross appearance of PSTT is variable. The tumors range from microscopic lesions to large masses that expand and distort the uterus. They may protrude into the endometrial cavity as yellow-tan, soft, polypoid masses (Fig. 12–18). In this setting endometrial curettage produces abundant diagnostic tissue.[93, 96, 97] When the tumors are confined to the myometrium, endometrial curettage is nondiagnostic. The neoplasm may be circumscribed or poorly defined, and there are usually areas of hemorrhage and necrosis. Many of these tumors have invaded through the entire thickness

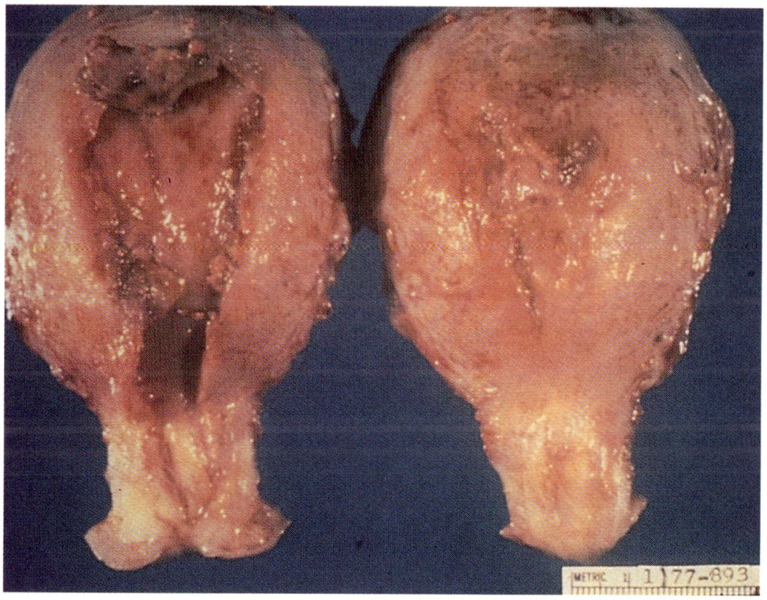

FIGURE 12-18
This is a hysterectomy specimen from a patient with placental site trophoblastic tumor. A shaggy yellow-tan, irregular mass protrudes from the uterine fundus. Lesions are also seen on the lateral walls. (Courtesy of Dr. Neil B. Rosenshein, The Johns Hopkins Hospital, Baltimore, MD.)

of the myometrium and involve the serosa. In cases of deep penetration by the tumor, curettage may result in perforation.[101] Involvement of the adnexal structures is rare.[93]

The tumor is characterized by anastomosing cords and sheets as well as by single mononuclear cells infiltrating the myometrium and its blood vessels. The predominant cell of the PSTT is the intermediate trophoblast. These cells are generally mononuclear and polyhedral to spindled in shape. There is a centrally placed, medium-size, round to oval nucleus that has an irregular membrane. The cytoplasm is eosinophilic to amphophilic and finely granular. Cytotrophoblasts and syncytiotrophoblasts form a lesser component of this neoplasm. The neoplastic cells infiltrate between the smooth muscle fibers of the myometrium, splitting the muscle bundles and producing very little necrosis (Figs. 12–5 and 12–19). In contrast to the very hemorrhagic appearance of choriocarcinoma, PSTT shows only focal hemorrhage, and this is usually at the site of vascular invasion. PSTT characteristically involves the walls of the uterine blood vessels, replacing them entirely in a manner similar to that associated with extravillous trophoblasts. Deposition of fibrinoid material both in the vessel walls and in the myometrium is another hallmark of this lesion. Erythrocytes within a space surrounded by fibrinoid material may be the only indication of the prior presence of a blood vessel. Chorionic villi are not present in PSTT.

A number of histologic features have been assoaciated with an aggressive clinical behavior, including large sheets of cells diffusely invading the myometrium. These are often associated with necrosis. Many of these cells have clear cytoplasm and evidence of increased mitotic activity. In benign PSTT the average mitotic rate is only two per 10 high-power fields (HPF). In general, PSTT that has a mitotic count of more than five per 10 HPF is associated with a fatal outcome.[102]

On immunocytochemistry the cells of the intermediate trophoblast of PSTT are strongly positive for hPL, and occasional cells show weak to moderate positivity for hCG. The malignant variants of PSTT show more diffuse staining for hCG than for hPL; thus, the hormonal distribution resembles that of choriocarcinoma.

Differential Diagnosis

PSTT is generally easily distinguished from choriocarcinoma. PSTT is composed predominantly of intermediate trophoblasts with only rare interspersed syncytiotrophoblasts.[103] It lacks the characteristic diphasic architecture of choriocarcinoma and also has a characteristic pattern of vascular invasion with replacement of vessel walls by a fi-

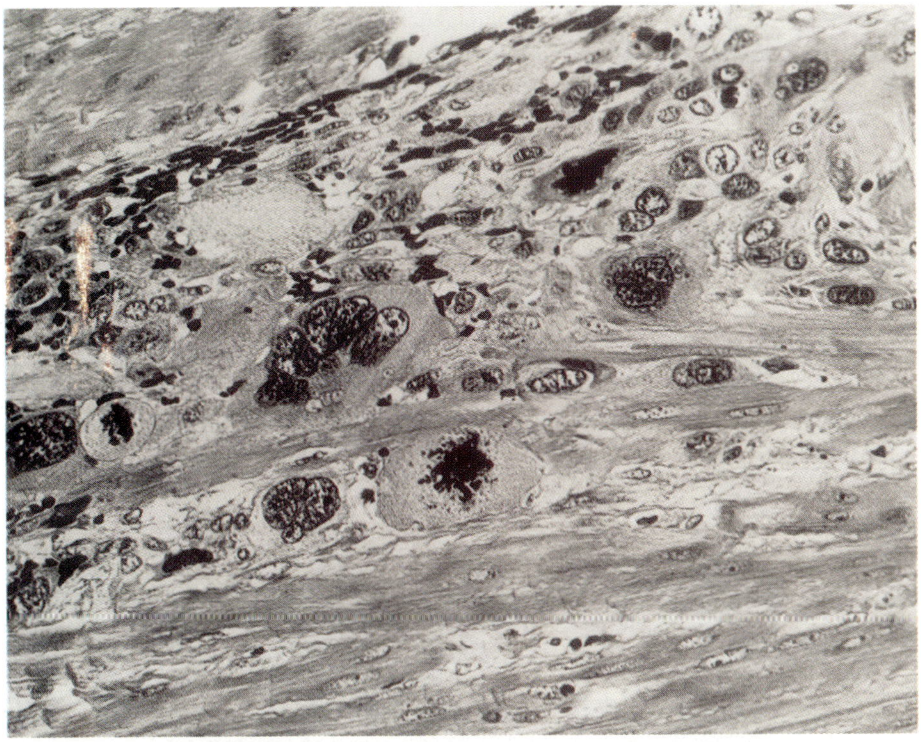

FIGURE 12–19
This photomicrograph shows a placental site trophoblastic tumor. The malignant intermediate trophoblasts are seen splitting the myometrial bundles, and there is no necrosis. A rare, multinuclear form of intermediate trophoblast is seen in the center. (From McLellan R et al: Placental site trophoblastic tumor in a postmenopausal woman. Am J Clin Pathol 1991;95:670–675.)

brinoid matrix. This fibrinoid material is not a component of choriocarcinoma. PSTT has an infiltrating peripheral border in contrast to the pushing expansile margin of choriocarcinoma. Finally, in cases in which difficulty arises, the distribution of hPL and hCG by immunocytochemical techniques may be helpful.

More difficult to separate from PSTT is the implantation site reaction, particularly when it is a florid "exaggerated placental site." This is especially true in curettings that do not contain chorionic villi or villous trophoblast (i.e., cytotrophoblast and syncytiotrophoblast). The placental site reaction, however, is a purely physiologic phenomenon and does not produce a mass that distorts the endomyometrial architecture. Monitoring of serum hCG levels may also be helpful in excluding PSTT. If, after curettage, hCG levels return to normal and menstruation commences, PSTT can be ruled out. If, on the other hand, moderately elevated hCG levels persist after curettage, the possibility of PSTT must be entertained, and close clinical evaluation is critical.

Rarely, PSTT can mimic epithelioid leiomyosarcomas or clear cell carcinomas of the cervix or endometrium on histopathologic evaluation. In these situations, use of immunocytochemical techniques can lead to the correct diagnosis.

Clinical Management

A review of 52 reported cases of PSTT revealed 12 deaths despite aggressive therapy.[97] The lung is the most frequent site of metastasis. Other sites include the brain, liver, kidney, vagina, stomach, spleen, and lymph nodes.[94, 96] When a diagnosis of PSTT is rendered, the patient should undergo a thorough search for metastases. This includes a complete physical examination, hemogram, hepatorenal profile, serum β-hCG determination, chest radiograph, and computed tomography of the head, abdomen, and pelvis. Magnetic resonance imaging and color flow Doppler ultrasonography may help to evaluate the extent of uterine involvement.[96]

Because there is no reliable way to predict the possible malignant behavior of PSTT, following uterine evacuation and diagnosis the patient should undergo abdominal exploration and excision of the tumor.[94, 96] In most instances this is accomplished by a simple total abdominal hysterectomy.[94] In a young woman, the ovaries can be preserved if they appear grossly normal.[93] Some investigators have suggested obtaining peritoneal washings and pelvic and paraaortic node sampling in an effort to better understand the behavior of this disease.[93, 96] The majority of patients do not have metastasis. If metastatic disease is not present, the patient is closely followed with physical examinations, chest radiographs, and serial serum β-hCG titers over a long period of time. Metastases have occurred as late as 10 years after the initial diagnosis.[94] Because the tumor secretes little hCG, a large tumor burden may be present when the first elevation in serum β-hCG is noted. Metastatic disease is uniformly resistant to chemotherapy.[97] Radiation therapy can be used for local control and palliation of symptoms. Surgical excision of localized metastases followed by aggressive chemotherapy may offer some hope.[96]

REFERENCES

1. McDonald TW, Ruffolo EH: Modern management of gestational trophoblastic disease. Obstet Gynecol Surv 1983; 38:67–83.
2. Lurain JR, Brewer JI, Torok EE, Halpern B: Natural history of hydatidiform mole after primary evacuation. Am J Obstet Gynecol 1983;145:591–595.
3. McLellan R, Buscema J, Currie JL, Woodruff JD: Placental site trophoblastic tumor in a postmenopausal woman. Am J Clin Pathol 1991;95:670–675.
4. Silverberg SG, Kurman RJ: Tumors of the uterine corpus and gestational trophoblastic disease. *In* Armed Forces Institute of Pathology: Atlas of Tumor Pathology. Third Series, Fascicle 3. 1991;3:233–282.
5. Blasi F, Vassali JD, Dano K: Urokinase-type plasminogen activator: proenzyme receptor and inhibitors. J Cell Biol 1987;104:801–804.
6. Mignatti P, Robbins E, Rifkin DB: Tumor invasion through the human amniotic membrane: Requirement for a proteinase cascade. Cell 1986;47:487–498.
7. Hoshima M, Boothby M, Hussa R, Patillo R, Camel HM, Boime I: Linkage of HCG and placental lactogen biosynthesis to trophoblast differentiation and tumorigenesis. Placenta 1985;6:163–172.
8. Grimes DA: Epidemiology of gestational trophoblastic disease. Am J Obstet Gynecol 1984;150:309–318.
9. Atrash HK, Hogue CJR, Grimes DA: Epidemiology of hydatidiform mole during early gestation. Am J Obstet Gynecol 1986;154:906–909.
10. Buckley JD: The epidemiology of molar pregnancy and choriocarcinoma. Clin Obstet Gynecol 1984;27:153–159.
11. Bandy LC, Clarke-Pearson DL, Hammond CB: Malignant potential of gestational trophoblastic disease at the extreme ages of reproductive life. Obstet Gynecol 1984; 64:395–399.
12. Berkowitz RS, Cramer DW, Bernstein MR, Cassells S, Driscoll SG, Goldstein DP: Risk factors for complete molar pregnancy from a case-control study. Am J Obstet Gynecol 1985;152:1016–1020.
13. Watson EJ, Hernandez E, Miyazawa K: Partial hydatidiform moles: A review. Obstet Gynecol Surv 1987;42:540–544.
14. Dodson MG: New concepts and questions in gestational trophoblastic disease. J Reprod Med 1983;28:741–749.
15. Vassilakos P, Riotton G, Kajii T: Hydatidiform mole: Two entities. Am J Obstet Gynecol 1977;127:167–170.
16. Kajii T, Ohama K: Androgenetic origin of hydatidiform mole. Nature 1977;268:633–634.
17. Azuma C, Saji F, Tokugawa Y, Kimura T, Nobunaga T,

Takemura M, Kameda T, Tanizawa O: Application of gene amplification by polymerase chain reaction to genetic analysis of molar mitochondrial DNA: The detection of anuclear empty ovum as the cause of complete mole. Gynecol Oncol 1991;40:29–33.
18. Kajii T, Kurashige H, Ohama K, Uchino F: XY and XX complete moles: Clinical and morphologic correlations. Am J Obstet Gynecol 1984;150:57–64.
19. Surti U, Szulman AE, O'Brien S: Dispermic origin and clinical outcome of three complete hydatidiform moles with 46,XY karyotype. Am J Obstet Gynecol 1982;144:84–87.
20. Vejerslev LO, Fisher RA, Surti U, Walke N: Hydatidiform mole: Cytogenetically unusual cases and their implications for the present classification. Am J Obstet Gynecol 1987;157:180–184.
21. Szulman AE, Surti U: The syndromes of partial and complete molar gestations. Clin Obstet Gynecol 1984;27:172–180.
22. Vejerslev LO, Dueholm M, Nielsen FH: Hydatidiform mole: Cytogenetic marker analysis in twin gestation: Report of two cases. Am J Obstet Gynecol 1986;155:614–617.
23. Sarno AP Jr, Moorman AJ, Kalousek DK: Partial molar pregnancy with fetal survival: An unusual example of confined placental mosaicism. Obstet Gynecol 1993;82:716–719.
23a. Takahashi H, Kanazawa K, Ikarashi T, Sudo N, Tanaka K: Discrepancy in the diagnosis of hydatidiform mole by macroscopic and microscopic findings and the deoxyribonucleic acid fingerprint method. Am J Obstet Gynecol 1990;163:112–113.
24. DiSaia PJ, Creassman WT: Clinical Gynecologic Oncology, 4th ed. St. Louis, Mosby–Year Book, 1993, pp 212–213.
25. Amir SM, Osathanondh R, Berkowitz RS, Goldstein DP: Human chorionic gonadotropin and thyroid function in patients with hydatidiform mole. Am J Obstet Gynecol 1984;150:723–728.
26. Galton VA, Ingbar SH, Jimenez-Fonseca J, Hershman JM: Alterations in thyroid hormone economy in patients with hydatidiform mole. J Clin Invest 1971;50:1345–1354.
27. Goldstein DP, Berkowitz RS: Gestational Trophoblastic Neoplasms. Clinical Principles of Diagnosis and Management. Philadelphia, WB Saunders, 1982.
28. Morrow CP, Kletzky OA, DiSaia PJ, Townsend DE, Mishell DR, Nakamura RM: Clinical and laboratory correlates of molar pregnancy and trophoblastic disease. Am J Obstet Gynecol 1977;128:424–429.
29. Rinehart JS, Hernandez E, Rosenshein NB, Sanders RC: Degenerating leiomyomata uteri: An ultrasonic mimic of hydatidiform mole. J Reprod Med 1981;26:142–144.
30. Morrow CP, Townsend DE: Synopsis of Gynecologic Oncology, 3rd ed. New York, Churchill Livingstone, 1987, pp 355–356.
31. Muto M, Lage JM, Berkowitz RS, Goldstein DP, Bernstein MR: Gestational trophoblastic disease of the fallopian tube. J Reprod Med 1991;164:611–616.
32. Szulman AE, Surti U: The clinicopathologic profile of the partial hydatidiform mole. Obstet Gynecol 1982;59:597–602.
33. Berkowitz RS, Goldstein DP, Bernstein MR: Natural history of partial molar pregnancy. Obstet Gynecol 1983; 66:677–681.
34. Goldstein DP: Worldwide controversies in gestational trophoblastic neoplasms. Int J Gynaecol Obstet 1977;15:207–215.
35. Hertig AT, Sheldon WH: Hydatidiform mole: A pathologic-clinical correlation of 200 cases. Am J Obstet Gynecol 1947;53:1–36.
36. Genest DR, Laborde O, Berkowitz RS, Goldstein DP, Bernstein MR, Lage J: A clinicopathologic study of 153 cases of complete hydatidiform mole (1980–1990): Histologic grade lacks prognostic significance. Obstet Gynecol 1991;78:402–409.
37. Sarto GE, Stubblefield PA, Lurrain J, Therman E: Mechanisms of growth in hydatidiform moles. Am J Obstet Gynecol 1984;148:1014–1023.
38. Szulman AE, Surti U: The syndromes of hydatidiform mole. II. Morphologic evolution of the complete and partial mole. Am J Obstet Gynecol 1978;132:20–27.
39. Czernobilsky B, Barash A, Lancet M: Partial moles: a clinicopathologic study of 25 cases. Obstet Gynecol 1982;59:75–77.
40. Brescia RJ, Kurman RJ, Main C, Surti U, Szulman AE: Immunocytochemical localization of chorionic gonadotropin, placental lactogen, and placental alkaline phosphatase in the diagnosis of complete and partial hydatidiform moles. Int J Gynecol Pathol 1987;6:213–219.
41. Lage JM, Driscoll SG, Yaven DL, Oliver AP, Mark SD, Weinberg DS: Hydatidiform moles. Am J Clin Pathol 1988;89:596–600.
42. Rotmensch J, Rosenshein NB, Block BS: Comparison of human chorionic gonadotropin regression in molar pregnancies and postmolar nonmetastatic gestational trophoblastic neoplasia. Gynecol Oncol 1988;29:82–86.
43. Morrow P, Nakamura R, Schlaerth J, Gaddis O Jr, Eddy G: The influence of oral contraceptives on the postmolar human chorionic gonadotropin regression curve. Am J Obstet Gynecol 1985;151:906–914.
44. Curry SL, Schlaerth JB, Kohorn EI, Boyce JB, Gore H, Twiggs LB, Blessing JA: Hormonal contraception and trophoblastic sequelae after hydatidiform mole (A Gynecologic Oncology Group study). Am J Obstet Gynecol 1989;150:805–811.
45. Rice LW, Lage JM, Berkowitz RS, Goldstein DP, Bernstein MR: Repetitive complete and partial hydatidiform mole. Obstet Gynecol 1989;74:217–219.
46. Sand PK, Lurain JR, Brewer JI: Repeat gestational trophoblastic disease. Obstet Gynecol 1984;63:140–144.
47. Berkowitz RS: Gestational trophoblastic disease: Recent advances in the understanding of cytogenetics, histopathology, and natural history. Curr Opin Obstet Gynecol 1992;4:616–620.
48. Lurain JR, Brewer JI, Torok EE, Halpern B: Natural history of hydatidiform mole after primary evacuation. Am J Obstet Gynecol 1983;145:591–595.
49. Goto S, Yamada A, Ishizuka T, Tomoda Y: Development of postmolar trophoblastic disease after partial molar pregnancy. Gynecol Oncol 1993;48:165–170.
50. Hernandez E, Rosenshein NB: Manual of Gynecologic Oncology. New York, Churchill Livingstone, 1989, pp 75–85.
51. Mutch DG, Soper JT, Babcock CJ, Clarke-Pearson DL, Hammond CB: Recurrent gestational trophoblastic disease: Experience of the Southeastern Regional Trophoblastic Disease Center. Cancer 1990;66:978–982.
52. Berkowitz RS, Goldstein DP, Bernstein MR: Reproductive experience after complete and partial mole pregnancy and gestational trophoblastic tumors. J Reprod Med 1991;36:3–8.
53. Duduc-Lissoir J, Sweizig S, Schlaerth JB, Morrow CP: Metastatic gestational trophoblastic disease: A comparison of prognostic classification systems. Gynecol Oncol 1992;45:40–45.
54. Schink JC, Singh DK, Rademaker AW, Miller DS, Lurain JR: Etoposide, methotrexate, actinomycin D, cyclophosphamide, and vincristine for the treatment of metastatic, high-risk gestational trophoblastic disease. Obstet Gynecol 1992;80:817–820.
55. Yordan EL Jr, Schlaerth J, Gaddis O, Morrow CP: Radiation therapy in the management of gestational choriocarcinoma metastatic to the central nervous system. Obstet Gynecol 1987;69:627–630.
56. Barnard DE, Woodward KT, Yancy SG, Weed JC Jr, Hammond CB: Hepatic metastases of choriocarcinoma: A report of 15 patients. Gynecol Oncol 1986;25:73–83.
57. Hammond CB, Weed JC Jr, Currie JL: The role of operation in the current therapy of gestational trophoblastic disease. Am J Obstet Gynecol 1980;136:844–858.

58. DuBeshter B, Berkowitz RS, Goldstein DP, Cramer DW, Bernstein MR: Metastatic gestational trophoblastic disease: Experience at the New England Trophoblastic Disease Center, 1965 to 1985. Obstet Gynecol 1987;69:390–395.
59. Jones WB, Wagner-Reiss K, Lewis JL Jr: Intracerebral choriocarcinoma. Gynecol Oncol 1990;38:234–243.
60. Weed JC Jr, Hammond CB: Cerebral metastatic choriocarcinoma: Intensive therapy and prognosis. Obstet Gynecol 1980;55:89–94.
61. Hammond CB, Borchert LG, Tyrey L, Creasman WT, Parker R: Treatment of metastatic trophoblastic disease: Good and poor prognosis. Am J Obstet Gynecol 1973;115:451–457.
62. Dobkin GR, Berkowitz RS, Goldstein DO, Bernstein MR, Doubilet PM: Duplex ultrasonography for persistent gestational trophoblastic tumor. J Reprod Med 1991;36:14–16.
63. Oka M, Fukuda O, Katabuchi H, Maeyama M, Takahashi M: Digital subtraction angiography for the evaluation of persistent uterine trophoblastic disease. Obstet Gynecol 1984;63S:66–71.
64. Nishikawa Y, Kaseki S, Tomoda Y, Ishizuka T, Asai Y, Suzuki T, Ushijima H: Histopathologic classification of uterine choriocarcinoma. Cancer 1985;55:1044–1051.
65. Ilancheran A, Ratnam SS, Baratham G: Metastatic cerebral choriocarcinoma with primary neurological presentation. Gynecol Oncol 1988;29:361–364.
66. Mazur MT: Metastatic gestational choriocarcinoma: Unusual pathologic variant following therapy. Cancer 1989;63:1370–1377.
67. Bagshawe KD: Risk and prognostic factors in trophoblastic neoplasia. Cancer 1976;38:1373–1385.
68. Mittal KK, Kachrn RB, Brewer JI: The HLA and ABO antigens in trophoblastic disease. Tissue Antigens 1975;6:57–69.
69. Sasaki K, Hata H, Nakano R: ABO blood group in patients with malignant trophoblastic disease. Gynecol Obstet Invest 1985;20:23–26.
70. Lurain JR, Sand PK, Brewer JI: Choriocarcinoma associated with ectopic pregnancy. Obstet Gynecol 1986; 68:286–287.
71. Hertig AT, Mansell H: Tumors of the female sex organs: Part I. Hydatidiform mole and choriocarcinoma. *In* Armed Forces Institute of Pathology: Atlas of Tumor Pathology, Section 9, Fascicle 33. Washington, DC, Armed Forces Institute of Pathology, 1956.
72. Savage J, Subby W, Okagaki T: Adenocarcinoma of the endometrium with trophoblastic differentiation and metastases as choriocarcinoma: A case report. Gynecol Oncol 1987;26:257–262.
73. Azuma C, Saji F, Nobunaga S, Kamiura S, Kimura T, Tokugawa Y, Koyama M, Tanizawa O: Studies on the pathogenesis of choriocarcinoma by analysis of restriction fragment length polymorphisms. Cancer Res 1990;50:488–491.
74. Fisher RA, Newlands ES, Jeffreys AJ, Boxer GM, Begent RHJ, Rustin GJS, Bagshawe KD: Gestational and nongestational trophoblastic tumors distinguished by DNA analysis. Cancer 1992;69:839–845.
75. Chaganti RSK, Koduru PRK, Chakraborty R, Jones WB: Genetic origin of a trophoblastic choriocarcinoma. Cancer Res 1990;50:6330–6333.
76. Olive DL, Lurain JR, Brewer JI: Choriocarcinoma associated with term gestation. Am J Obstet Gynecol 1984;148:711–716.
77. Hou PC, Pang SC: Chorioepithelioma: An analytical study of 28 necropsied cases with special references to the possibility of spontaneous retrogression. J Pathol Bacteriol 1956;72:95–104.
78. Azab MB, Pejovic M-H, Theodore C, George M, Droz J-P, Bellet D, Michel G, Amiel J-L: Prognostic factors in gestational trophoblastic tumors: A multivariate analysis. Cancer 1988;62:585–592.
79. Gordon AN, Gershenson DM, Copeland LJ, Saul PB, Kavanagh JJ, Edwards CL: High-risk metastatic gestational trophoblastic disease. Obstet Gynecol 1985;65:550–556.
80. Soper JT, Clarke-Pearson D, Hammond CB: Metastatic gestational trophoblastic disease: Prognostic factors in previously untreated patients. Obstet Gynecol 1988;71:338–343.
81. Soper JT, Mutch DG, Chin N, Clarke-Pearson DL, Hammond CB: Renal metastases of gestational trophoblastic disease: A report of eight cases. Obstet Gynecol 1988;72:796–798.
82. Tsukamoto N, Matsumura M, Matsukuma K, Kamura T, Baba K: Choriocarcinoma in mother and fetus. Gynecol Oncol 1986;24:113–119.
83. Kelly MP, Rustin JS, Ivory C, Phillips P, Bagshawe KD: Respiratory failure due to choriocarcinoma: A study of 103 dyspneic patients. Gynecol Oncol 1990;38:149–154.
84. Mutch DG, Soper JT, Baker ME, Bandy LC, Cox EB, Clarke-Pearson DL, Hammond CB: Role of computer axial tomography of the chest in staging patients with nonmetastatic gestational trophoblastic disease. Obstet Gynecol 1986;68:348–352.
85. Hendin AS: Gestational trophoblastic tumors metastatic to the lung: Radiologic-clinical correlations. Cancer 1984;53:58–61.
86. Brewer JI, Mazur MT: Gestational choriocarcinoma: Its origin in the placenta during seemingly normal pregnancy. Am J Surg Pathol 1981;5:267–277.
87. Kurman RJ, Young RH, Norris HJ, Main CS, Lawrence WD, Scully RE: Immunocytochemical localization of placental lactogen and chorionic gonadotropin in the normal placenta and trophoblastic tumors, with emphasis on intermediate trophoblast and the placental site trophoblastic tumor. Int J Gynecol Pathol 1984;3:101–121.
88. Civantos F, Rywlin AM: Carcinoma with trophoblastic differentiation and secretion of chorionic gonadotrophins. Cancer 1972;29:789–798.
89. Deligdisch L, Driscoll SG, Goldstein DP: Gestational trophoblastic neoplasms: Morphologic correlates of therapeutic response. Am J Obstet Gynecol 1978;130:801–806.
90. Bagshawe KD: Treatment of high-risk choriocarcinoma. J Reprod Med 1984;29:813–820.
91. Surwit EA, Alberts DS, Christian CD, Graham VE: Poor-prognosis gestational trophoblastic disease: An update. Obstet Gynecol 1984;64:21–26.
92. Lurain JR, Brewer JI, Torok EE, Halpern B: Gestational trophoblastic disease: Treatment results at the Brewer Trophoblastic Disease Center. Obstet Gynecol 1982; 60:354–360.
93. Berkowitz BJ, Jones JG, Merkatz IR, Runowicz CD: Ovarian conservation in placental site trophoblastic tumor. Gynecol Oncol 1990;37:239–243.
94. Finkler NJ: Placental site trophoblastic tumor: Diagnosis, clinical behavior and treatment. J Reprod Med 1991;36:27–30.
95. Fisher RA, Paradinas FJ, Newlands ES, Boxer GM: Genetic evidence that placental site trophoblastic tumor can originate from a hydatidiform mole or a normal conceptus. Br J Cancer 1992;65:355–358.
96. Hoffman JS, Silverman AD, Gelber J, Cartun R: Placental site trophoblastic tumor: A report of radiologic, surgical, and pathologic methods of evaluating the extent of disease. Gynecol Oncol 1993;50:110–114.
97. McLellan R, Buscema J, Currie JL, Woodruff JD: Placental site trophoblastic tumor in a postmenopausal woman. Am J Clin Pathol 1991;95:670–675.
98. Finkler NJ, Berkowitz RS, Driscoll SG, Goldstein DP, Bernstein MR: Clinical experience with placental site trophoblastic tumors at the New England Trophoblastic Disease Center. Obstet Gynecol 1988;71:854–857.
99. Brewer CA, Adelson MD, Elder RC: Erythrocytosis associated with a placental-site trophoblastic tumor. Obstet Gynecol 1992;79:846–849.
100. Kurman RJ, Main CS, Chen HC: Intermediate tropho-

blast: A distinctive form of trophoblast with specific morphological, biochemical and functional features. Placenta 1984;5:349–369.

101. Kurman RJ, Scully RE, Norris HJ: Trophoblastic pseudotumor of the uterus: An exaggerated form of "syncytial endometritis" simulating a malignant tumor. Cancer 1976;38:1214–1226.

102. Silverberg SG, Kurman RJ: Atlas of Tumor Pathology: Tumors of the uterine corpus and gestational trophoblastic disease. AFIP 1991;3:233–282.

103. Patillo RA: Gestational and non-gestational trophoblastic neoplasms: New developments in DNA analysis, metabolic function, diagnosis and treatment. Curr Opin Obstet Gynecol 1993;5:486–489.

Index

Note: Page numbers in *italics* refer to illustrations; page numbers followed by t refer to tables.

D

E

H

M

R

S

W

X

Y

Z

ISBN 0-7216-5170-4

90071

9 780721 651705